# BREAKTHROUGHS IN MELANOMA RESEARCH

Edited by **Yohei Tanaka**

**Breakthroughs in Melanoma Research**
Edited by Yohei Tanaka

**Published by InTech**
Janeza Trdine 9, 51000 Rijeka, Croatia



**Publishing Process Manager** Sandra Bakic

**Technical Editor** Teodora Smiljanic

**Cover Designer** InTech Design Team

Additional hard copies can be obtained from orders@intechopen.com

Breakthroughs in Melanoma Research, Edited by Yohei Tanaka
p. cm.
ISBN 978-953-307-291-3

For EU product safety concerns:
IN TECH d.o.o., Prolaz Marije Krucifikse Kozulić 3, 51000 Rijeka, Croatia,
info@intechopen.com or visit our website at intechopen.com.

# Meet the editor

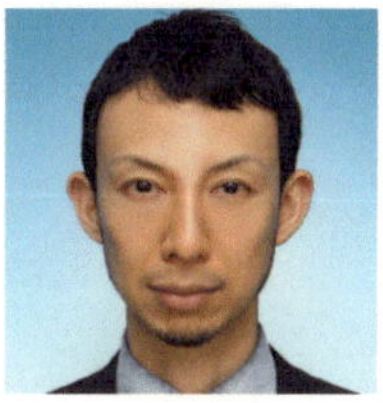

Dr. Yohei Tanaka is a board certified plastic surgeon who is dedicated to his patients as well as an enthusiastic researcher. He received his MD from Shinshu University School of Medicine in 2000., followed by a Ph.D. from Shinshu University Graduate School of Medicine in 2010. In addition to being a clinical assistant professor at the department of plastic and reconstructive surgery of Shinshu University School of Medicine, he is also the founder of the Clinica Tanaka Plastic and Reconstructive Surgery and Anti-aging Center, and the Society for Near-infrared rays Research. Dr. Yohei Tanaka enthusiastically performs various researches at Shinshu University, his own clinic, and his laboratory. He now specializes in blepharoplasty, filler injection, and the biological investigation of near-infrared radiation.

# Contents

# Preface

Melanoma is considered to be one of the most aggressive forms of skin neoplasms.

Over the past few decades, the incidence rate of melanoma has steadily risen throughout the world, and malignant melanoma is one of most resistant skin neoplasms to anti-cancer treatments. Despite aggressive research towards finding treatments, no effective therapy exists to inhibit the metastatic spread of malignant melanoma.

This book covers a wide range of aspects and issues related to melanoma, and brings together researchers from 19 different countries. The book consists of 29 chapters written by over 100 authors.

The first 9 chapters describe several aspects of the biology of melanoma. The subsequent sections, including 10 chapters, describe pigmentations, pathways, receptors and diagnosis. The last 10 chapters discuss treatments and therapies.

An understanding of how melanoma cells differ from normal tissues and how normal cells develop into malignant cells is essential for making potential new therapeutic discoveries.

The early detection and removal of melanoma at an early stage are particularly important, since it is one of the most fatal forms of skin neoplasms. Additionally, the 5-year survival rate of metastatic melanoma is still significantly low, and there is an earnest need to develop more effective therapies with greater anti-melanoma activity.

It is a distinct honor for me to edit this book. I believe I was appointed editor of this book to encourage melanoma investigations from another viewpoint, although I am neither an oncologist nor a researcher specializing in melanoma, but rather a plastic surgeon who enthusiastically uses near-infrared irradiation.

Here, I would like to suggest that near-infrared radiation may affect the etiology of melanoma, since I am now specializing in the biological investigation of this type of radiation.

I would like to express my sincere appreciation and gratitude to all authors who contributed to this book with their research and to the InTech team who accomplished their mission with professionalism and dedication.

I hope that this book will not only be beneficial for readers, but will also contribute to scientists making continued breakthroughs in melanoma research.

**Yohei Tanaka, MD, PhD.**
Department of Plastic and Reconstructive Surgery,
Shinshu University School of Medicine,
Japan

# Part 1

## Biology

# 1

# Reactive Oxygen Species in the Biology of Melanoma

Irene L. Ibañez[1,2], Cintia Notcovich[1],
Lucía L. Policastro[1,2] and Hebe Durán[1,2,3]
[1]*Comisión Nacional de Energía Atómica;*
[2]*Consejo Nacional de Investigaciones Científicas y Técnicas;*
[3]*Escuela de Ciencia y Tecnología, Universidad Nacional de San Martín;*
*Argentina*

## 1. Introduction

The incidence of melanoma has been increasing at an alarming rate worldwide. Although melanoma accounts for only 10% of skin cancer, it is responsible for at least 80% of skin cancer deaths. Malignant melanoma remains one of the cancers most resistant to treatment. Moreover, no effective therapy exists to inhibit the metastatic spread of this type of cancer. Research to further understanding of how melanoma cells differ from normal tissues is essential to make the discovery of potential new ways of attack. Increased reactive oxygen species (ROS) levels have been associated with numerous pathological conditions, including cancer. Particularly, melanoma cells constituvely produce high amounts of ROS as compared with their non-tumoural counterpart, melanocytes (Policastro et al, 2009). In relation to this, one promising strategy relates to the development of new therapies taking advantage of the excess of ROS produced by melanomas. In this chapter, we review: our current understanding of the involvement of ROS in cancer and particularly in the biology of melanocytes and melanoma, therapeutic approaches related to intracellular ROS modulation and emerging gene therapy strategies based on intracellular ROS levels of melanoma.

### 1.1 Role of reactive oxygen species in cancer

In order to further understand the involvement of ROS in the biology of melanoma, we will briefly introduce state-of–the-art advances regarding ROS and cancer. ROS are largely generated as oxidative by-products of normal cellular metabolism which include highly reactive radicals (e.g. superoxide anion, $O_2^{\bullet -}$ and hydroxil radical •OH) and milder oxidants such as hydrogen peroxide ($H_2O_2$). ROS were traditionally considered as toxic products leading to cellular damage. However, at physiological concentrations, some of these species are involved in the regulation of cellular processes and their levels are tightly controlled by specific antioxidant scavenging systems (Halliwell & Gutteridge, 2007). Antioxidants can be synthesized *in vivo* or taken from the diet. These antioxidant defences contribute to preserve the redox state of cell in homeostatic balance and they comprise enzymes, like superoxide dismutase (SOD), catalase, glutathione peroxidase (GPx), peroxiredoxins and non-enzymatic agents such as low molecular weight antioxidants (Fig. 1). Differences in level and composition of antioxidant defences can be found from tissue to tissue and cell type to cell type within a given tissue depending on which ROS are generated, the manner, the time and which of the targets is affected (Halliwell & Gutteridge, 2007).

An imbalance between ROS generation and their removal may induce an oxidative stress or a prooxidant state, which in turn may result in increased proliferation, adaptation, cell injury, apoptosis, senescence, cytotoxicity and cell death. On the other hand, physiological levels of ROS are necessary for proper functioning of cellular processes such as proliferation, whereas scavenging of $H_2O_2$ inhibits cell proliferation (Stone & Yang, 2006).

ROS have been reported to be involved in over 150 human disorders, e.g. atherosclerosis and cardiovascular diseases, autoimmune and neurodegenerative disorders and cancer (Halliwell & Gutteridge, 2007). ROS may play a role in tumour development, not only as DNA-damaging agents that increase the mutation rate and promote oncogenic transformation (Halliwell, 2007) but also as mediators of signal transduction pathways related to cell proliferation, angiogenesis and migration (Nishikawa, 2008).

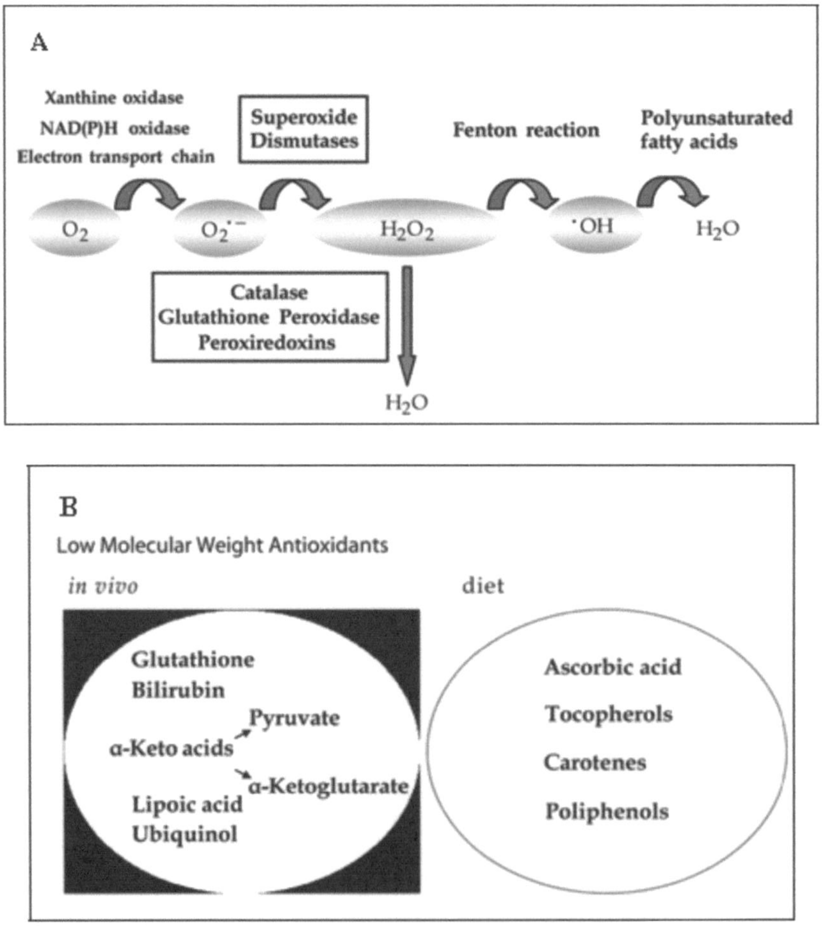


Fig. 1. Antioxidant defence systems. (A) Enzymatic and (B) Non-enzymatic antioxidant defences

One of the major endogenous sources of DNA damage is that produced by ROS (Jackson & Loeb, 2001). It has been estimated that approximately 20,000 bases in DNA are damaged in each human cell per day by ROS (Jackson & Loeb, 2001). Some of the oxidative modified bases constitute blocks to replication, while others are able to misrepair at high frequency, leading to base substitutions (Jackson & Loeb, 2001). Thus, DNA damage induced by ROS in cells exposed to a prooxidant state could result in an overwhelming mutational load that could contribute to carcinogenesis. Indeed, many chemical carcinogens act through free radical metabolites (Guyton & Kensler, 1993), some tumour promoters stimulate the production of free radicals in several cell types and tissues (Cerutti, 1985; Duran & de Rey, 1991), whereas free radical-scavengers protect against cancer development in animal models (Hyoudou et al, 2009) and may be chemoprotective in humans (Cerutti, 1985; Guyton & Kensler, 1993). In addition, $O_2^{\bullet-}$ and $H_2O_2$ can enhance cell survival and stimulate proliferation. The production of large amounts of $H_2O_2$ was reported in cancer cells and tissues (breast, colorectal and renal cell carcinoma and melanoma) as compared with its non-tumoural counterpart (Policastro et al, 2004; Policastro et al, 2009; Szatrowski & Nathan, 1991; Toyokuni et al, 1995). This could be attributed in part to deregulation of antioxidant enzymes, which could lead to an increased ROS accumulation. Particularly, an increase in superoxide dismutase and a decrease in catalase activities were found in epithelial tumour cells and in human melanoma cells. In this sense, a correlation between the endogenous levels of $H_2O_2$ and the degree of malignancy was demonstrated in epithelial tumour cell lines from skin, breast and bladder (Hempel et al, 2009; Policastro el al, 2004). These characteristics further perpetuate a state of oxidative stress in cancer cells. In agreement with this concept, the scavenging of ROS inhibits cell proliferation in tumour cells, as described in cells treated with catalase, glutathione (GSH) or N-acetylcysteine (NAC) (Laurent et al, 2005; Onumah et al, 2009; Policastro et al, 2004).

It is well documented that $H_2O_2$ is involved in signal transduction pathways (Fig. 2), e.g. increased levels of $H_2O_2$ induce mitogenic signals, such as those related to epidermal growth factor receptor (EGFR)/Ras/ extracellular signal-regulated kinases 1 and 2 (ERK1/2) pathway, and stress-responsive signals, such as those related to Jun N-terminal kinases (JNKs) and p38 mitogen-activated protein kinase (MAPK) pathways. Moreover, ROS and $H_2O_2$ were also implied in the modulation of receptor tyrosine kinases (RTK) and phosphatidylinositol 3-kinase (PI3K)/AKT pathways (Stone & Yang, 2006). These redox-dependent signalling cascades converge on core cell cycle regulators (Burhans & Heintz, 2009). The regulation of cell cycle is highly coordinated by sequential assembly and activation of phase-specific protein kinase complexes (Elledge, 1996; Sherr, 1996), formed by cyclins and cyclin dependent kinases (CDKs), which are also regulated by the INK4 proteins and the CDK inhibitors (CDKIs). D-type cyclins are expressed throughout the cycle in response to mitogen stimulation (Sherr, 1996). Fluctuations observed in the intracellular redox state during cell cycle progression could link oxidative metabolic processes to cell cycle regulation (Menon et al, 2003; Sarsour et al, 2009). The regulation of cyclin D1 expression was connected to $H_2O_2$ variations along the cell cycle (Burch & Heintz, 2005). Thus, the removal of endogenous $H_2O_2$ by overexpression of catalase and glutathione peroxidase induces G0/G1 arrest (Ibanez et al, 2011; Onumah et al, 2009) and decreases cell DNA synthesis (Felty et al, 2005). We demonstrated that the scavenging of $H_2O_2$ by catalase in tumour cells induced G1/S arrest by modulating the levels of specific regulatory proteins of early to mid G1 (cyclin D1) and G1/S transition ($p27^{KIP1}$). Moreover, we found a modification in the intracellular localization of the inhibitory protein $p27^{KIP1}$. This protein remained in the nucleus where it inhibits the cyclin E-CDK2 complex after catalase treatment, whereas it showed cytoplasmic localization in proliferating cells. In addition, we demonstrated an increase of $p27^{KIP1}$ in response to $H_2O_2$ scavenging *in vivo* related to the inhibition of tumour growth after catalase treatment in agreement with *in vitro* results (Ibanez et al, 2011). In view of the aforementioned, the prooxidant state of tumour cells may confer them a proliferative advantage and contribute to the acquisition of a malignant phenotype.

Furthermore, a role of oxidative stress in the regulation of metastasis and tumour progression has been reported. It is becoming clear that a number of steps in the metastatic cascade, such as invasion, intravasation and extravasation, as well as, the angiogenic response are regulated by redox signalling. Particularly, ROS increase the expression and/or activate matrix metalloproteinases (MMPs), adhesion molecules, EGFR, vascular endothelial growth factor (VEGF) and the hypoxia-inducible factor (HIF) transcription factor (Nishikawa, 2008; Toullec et al, 2010). In the process of cancer cells forming metastatic colonies, active MMPs are required to destroy the extracellular matrix and basement membranes for the migration of tumour cells. These cells and their surrounding cells secrete MMPs in latent forms which are activated by ROS (Nishikawa, 2008). The $H_2O_2$-dependent expression of both MMP-9 and VEGF was demonstrated as removal of $H_2O_2$ by overexpression of catalase attenuated their expression (Hempel et al, 2009).

In addition, it has been proposed that cancer cells could induce oxidative stress in the tumour microenvironment, resulting in the amplification of oxidative stress in a given tissue area. This would then provide a mutagenic/oxidative field resulting in widespread ROS production and DNA damage. This bystander oxidative stress could favour an increase in the mutation rate of adjacent normal epithelial cells or cancer cells, resulting in more aggressive cancer cells (Martinez-Outschoorn et al, 2010).

## 2. Reactive oxygen species in melanocytes and melanoma

### 2.1 ROS in the physiology of melanocytes. Involvement of reactive oxygen species in melanogenesis

The skin represents one of the largest organs of the human body and is a constant target of endogenous and exogenous ROS, counteracted by a powerful defence system, particularly, the biopolymer melanin functions as an intrinsic free radical trap. Also, the UV properties of melanin have a preventive action to protect epidermal proliferating cells (Schallreuter & Wood, 2001)

The pigmentation process takes place in melanocytes, which produce melanin through the process called melanogenesis. The specific organelle involved in this process is the melanosome, which has the full capacity for the biosynthesis and distribution of both eumelanin and pheomelanin.

Tyrosinase, the key enzyme in melanogenesis, contains two copper atoms in its active site, which are primarily coordinated to histidine residues. In its Cu(II) oxidation state, the enzyme is inactive representing met-tyrosinase. Consequently met-tyrosinase has to be activated by the reduction of the two Cu(II) centres to Cu(I) by single electron donors, such as L-DOPA, ascorbic acid or superoxide anion (Schallreuter et al, 2008). Tyrosinase catalyses the hydroxylation of L-tyrosine to L-DOPA and the oxidation of this to dopaquinone. These quinones evolve through a series of steps, both enzymatically and non-enzymatically, to generate several unstable intermediates, which polymerize to melanins (Munoz-Munoz et

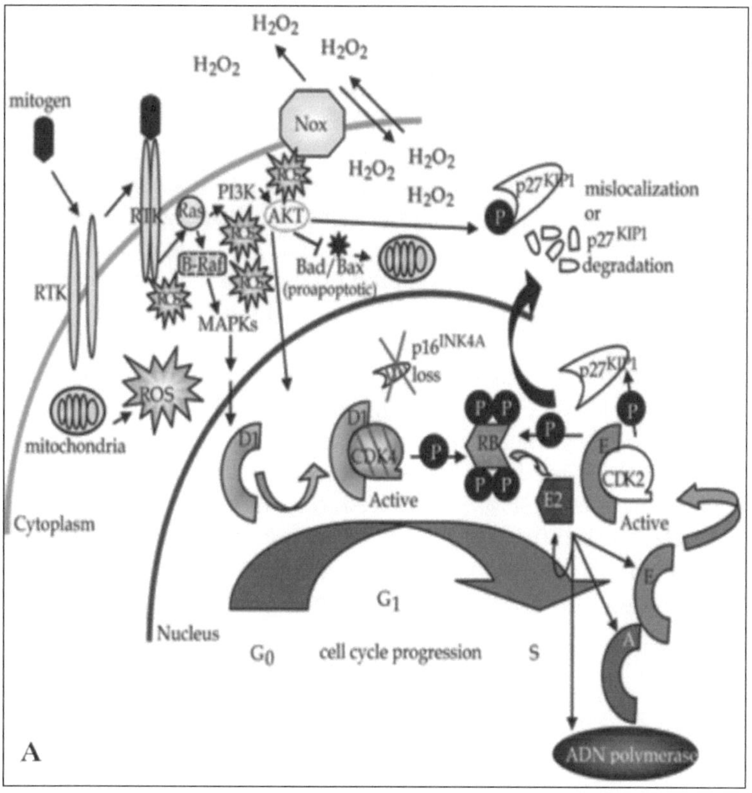


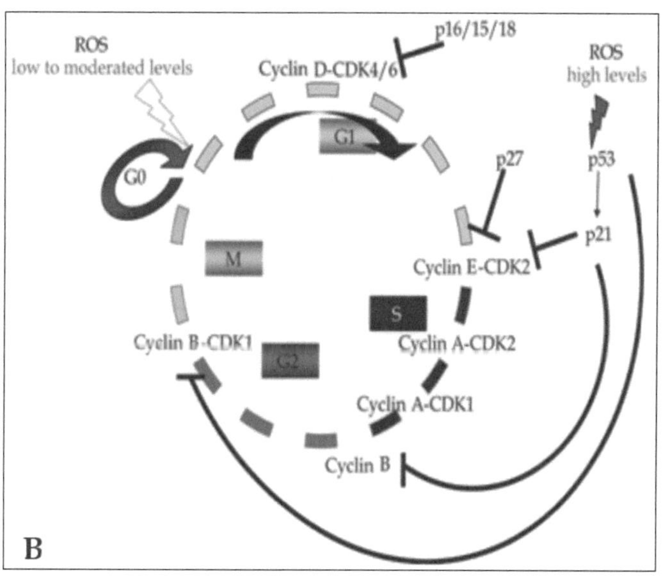


Fig. 2. ROS involvement in cell cycle regulation. (A) Redox-dependent signalling cascades involved in the regulation of G1/S transition in cancer and, in particular, in melanoma. (B) Low to moderate levels of ROS may initiate cell cycle division whereas high levels of ROS may induce cell cycle arrest, apoptosis, terminal differentiation or cytotoxicity

al, 2009). Moreover, L-DOPA is mainly formed from L-tyrosine by tyrosine hydroxylase isoform I (THI). Thus, the availability of L-tyrosine is essential for melanocytes. This aminoacid is provided by facilitated diffusion and by the intracellular enzymatic conversion of the essential aminoacid L-phenylalanine via phenylalanine hydroxylase (PAH) (Schallreuter et al, 2008). The activities of PAH, THI and tyrosinase are controlled by the cofactor 6-tetrahydrobiopterin (6BH4). High levels of ROS, such as $O_2^{\bullet-}$ and $H_2O_2$, can directly inhibit tyrosinase activity, by leading to structural changes of the enzyme due to the presence of cysteine residues susceptible to be oxidized or by deactivation of the enzyme by the oxidation of a methionine residue to methionine sulfoxide at the active site. Moreover, the oxidation of the cofactor 6BH4 to 6 biopterin may be generated by both $H_2O_2$ and also by UV-B exposure (Schallreuter et al, 2008; Schallreuter & Wood, 2001). However, low concentrations of $H_2O_2$, in the micromolar range, are needed to upregulate or activate tyrosinase and other proteins related to melanogenesis. In addition, both tyrosine-related proteins, TRP1 and TRP2, which are located close to tyrosinase in the melanosomal membrane, protect this enzyme from ROS attack. These proteins also contain cysteine rich domains, which are targets of $H_2O_2$ mediated oxidation. Thus, the levels of ROS and particularly of $H_2O_2$ are tightly controlled under physiological conditions, maintaining redox homeostasis in the melanosome and regulating the melanogenesis process. Particularly, catalase is an important antioxidant enzyme that regulates this process by $H_2O_2$ removal.

Regarding the alterations of melanogenesis in melanoma, the loss of pigmentation is very common in advanced and in metastatic lesions because of the dysfunction of melanocyte-specific proteins involved in melanogenesis (Watabe et al, 2004). The main regulator of melanogenesis at the transcriptional level is microphtalmia-associated transcription factor (MiTF). This factor controls the expression of all known melanosomal proteins (Levy & Fisher, 2011). However, post-transcriptional processes may also be involved in the pigmentation phenotype of melanoma, particularly the activation of tyrosinase as an important control point for melanin biosynthesis. In this sense, several events have been suggested to be involved in the hypopigmentation of amelanotic melanoma, such as disruption of melanosomal maturation and alterations on the glycosylation and stability of tyrosinase. Moreover, considering the ability of $H_2O_2$ to inhibit tyrosinase and other proteins involved in the melanogenesis process (Jimenez-Cervantes et al, 2001), the high levels of $H_2O_2$ associated to a decrease in catalase activity (Picardo et al, 1996; Policastro et al, 2009; Szatrowski & Nathan, 1991) would be relevant in the induction of the amelanotic phenotype. In addition, the down-regulation of melanocyte differentiation markers was preceded by a decrease in microphthalmia transcription factor gene (MITF) expression in $H_2O_2$-treated melanoma cells. Therefore, it was suggested that oxidative stress may lead to hypopigmentation by mechanisms that include a MiTF-dependent downregulation of the melanogenic enzymes (Jimenez-Cervantes et al, 2001).

### 2.2 Involvement of ROS in the development of melanoma

Many of the general risk factors for developing melanoma include sun exposure, previous melanoma or non-melanoma skin cancer, family history of melanoma and large numbers of moles (Satyamoorthy & Herlyn, 2002; Wang et al, 2010). The human melanocyte is continuously exposed to reactive biochemical species, but is finely tuned via the intrinsic antioxidant and radical properties of melanin to suppress the build-up of an altered redox phenotype. Meyskens *et al.* propose that this control is lost during the development of

melanoma (Meyskens et al, 2001), moreover they hypothesize that the disruption of melanosomal melanin might be an early event in the etiology of melanoma, leading to increased oxidative stress and mutation (Gidanian et al, 2008).
Sunlight exposure is the major cause of skin cancers, including melanoma. Epidemiological studies implicate ultraviolet radiation (UV) B (290-320 nm) and UVA (320-400 nm) in the development of nonmelanoma skin cancer and melanoma respectively. Although the action of UVB radiation is mediated by specific photoproducts, such as pyrimidine dimers, it is well known that UVA acts mainly through the induction of ROS. The most important source of $H_2O_2$ is represented by the free radicals generated after UV exposition, though $H_2O_2$, as a product of melanogenesis itself, also plays an important role since it is able to diffuse outside the melanosome to reach other cellular compartments. Moreover, structural alterations of melanosomal membrane in pigmented melanomas may lead to significant leakage of reactive melanin precursors including free radical species (Borovansky et al, 1991).
As described in the introduction tumour cells produce high amounts of ROS. Regarding melanoma, we demonstrated an increase in the levels of $H_2O_2$ in human melanoma cells as compared to melanocytes (Policastro, 2009). Figure 3 shows the differences in ROS levels between melanocytes and melanoma. Moreover, an imbalance in the antioxidant system has been described in human melanomas, which can lead to endogenous generation of ROS and to cellular incapability of coping with exogenous peroxidative attacks. In addition, it has been proposed that the functional effect of melanin dysregulation is its evolution to a prooxidant behaviour (Gidanian et al, 2008) and melanin is able to induce DNA damage. Thus, the oxidative stress characteristic of melanoma cells is associated with increased DNA damage and high rates of mutation. In relation to this, we demonstrated high levels of basal DNA damage in melanoma cells (Ibanez et al, 2009) in agreement with other authors (Warters et al, 2005).

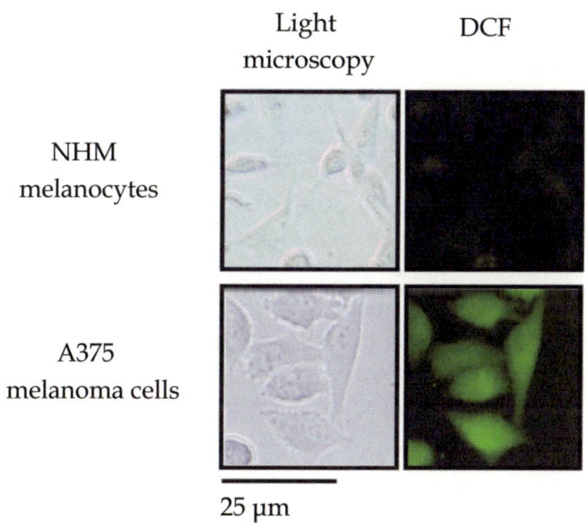


Fig. 3. ROS levels on normal human melanocytes (NHM) and A375 melanoma cells. Representative images of NHM and A375 cells, showing the intracellular ROS levels determined by 2′, 7′-dichlorodihydro-fluorescein diacetate (DCFH-DA) assay, as described by Tarpey *et al.*, 2004. DCF: oxidized 2′, 7′-dichloro-fluorescein

### 2.3 Redox regulation in melanocytes and melanoma

Redox regulation of protein activity is an important mechanism involved in the modulation of signalling and transcription, as part of the large array of posttranslational modifications, including, acetylation, carboxylation, glycosylation, hydroxylation or methylation. Different mechanisms for sensing have been observed in the various redox-regulated proteins. While in many of them, reactive cysteine(s) residues function as redox sensors, others use the metal iron, coordinated in Fe–S clusters as a sensor and, lastly, other use their thiol-coordinated zinc sites as redox switches stimuli (Shlomai, 2010).

#### 2.3.1 Redox regulation of transcription factors

Several master transcription regulators, which control cell growth, development and survival have redox control, many of which are involved in the regulation of signalling transduction pathways in melanocytes and melanoma.

##### 2.3.1.1 Hypoxia inducible factors (HIF)

HIF play a key role in the maintenance of oxygen homeostasis. They are involved in facilitating cell survival and energy supply in reduced oxygen condition. HIF activation affects principally the shift of energy production by increasing glycolysis and decreasing mitochondrial function under hypoxic condition (Denko, 2008). HIF-1, the most studied HIF factor, was initially identified by its response to low oxygen concentration, but it is now apparent that HIF-1 is also crucial in cancer development and progression including angiogenesis and tumour invasion (Harris, 2002). HIF-1 is a heterodimeric complex comprised of an unstable and oxygen regulated subunit (HIF-1$\alpha$) and a constitutively expressed subunit (HIF-1$\beta$), also referred to as the arylhydrocarbon receptor nuclear translocator (ARNT). HIF-1 is constitutively transcribed and translated, however under normoxia it is rapidly degraded by the ubiquitin-proteasome system. Under sustained hypoxia, degradation of the HIF-subunit is inhibited allowing the protein to accumulate, heterodimerize and translocate to the nucleus. Thus, in hypoxia conditions, the functional HIF-1 dimer, binds to a consensus core sequence namely hypoxia response elements (HREs) in the promoter or enhancer of its target genes (Harris, 2002).

A large body of evidence suggests that ROS modulate HIF-1 activity. $H_2O_2$ and nitric oxide (NO) donors were found to stabilize HIF-1, and genetic and pharmacological interventions modulating ROS generation have been shown to affect the accumulation of HIF-1$\alpha$ (Brune & Zhou, 2007; Kietzmann & Gorlach, 2005). It is well demonstrated that during hypoxia, ROS production is increased at complex III levels in mitochondria, and this condition is necessary for HIF-1$\alpha$ stabilization during hypoxia (Chandel et al, 1998).

A direct role of hypoxia in advanced melanoma is slowly starting to emerge (Bedogni & Powell, 2009). HIF-1 has been shown to play a critical role in uveal melanoma progression and is regarded as one of the critical biomarkers to predict uveal melanoma metastasis (Chang et al, 2008; Victor et al, 2006). The overexpression of HIF-1$\alpha$ and HIF-2$\alpha$ in human melanoma of the skin was reported, and HIF-2$\alpha$, along with VEGF and vascular density, was associated with poor overall disease survival (Giatromanolaki et al, 2003). Melanoma cells have also shown a marked HIF-1$\alpha$ activity under normoxic conditions. Immunohistochemistry of malignant melanoma showed the focal expression of HIF-1$\alpha$ in cancer tissue independent of regional hypoxia. In this work, it has been demonstrated that constitutive HIF-1$\alpha$ activity under normoxic conditions is associated with the ROS microenvironment around melanoma cells. The inhibition or induction of ROS decreased or activated, respectively, HIF-1 activity and HIF-1alpha protein expression. In addition, the involvement of nuclear factor kappa B (NF-κB) was demonstrated in the regulation of HIF expression by ROS in melanoma cells (Kuphal et al, 2010).

### 2.3.1.2 Nuclear factor kappa B (NF-κB)

NF-κB is a conserved inducible transcription factor that plays a key role in the control of a diverse range of genes involved in inmunological response, cell proliferation, apoptosis, tissue remodelling, cellular responses to stress and oncogenesis (Ghosh & Hayden, 2008). In mammalian cells, the NF-κB family comprises five related proteins: p50, p52, RelA (also known as p65), c-Rel, and RelB which can homo- and heterodimerize through the rel homology domain (RHD). Only RelA, c-Rel, and RelB contain a transcriptional activation domain, while p50 and p52 can only activate transcription through heterodimerization with RelA, c-Rel, or RelB. NF-κB dimers are generally found inactive in the cytoplasm bound to inhibitory proteins IκB (IκB-α and IκB-β). In response to a wide array of stimuli, IκB proteins are phosphorylated and NF-κB dimeric complex is released and its nuclear localization signal is unmasked. NF-κB translocates to the nucleus, where it can 'turn on' the expression of specific genes that have DNA-binding sites for NF-κB (Perkins, 2007). ROS have long been known to activate NF-κB; however, the role of redox in NF-κB regulation is apparently different in cytoplasm and in the nucleus (Kabe et al, 2005). Whereas in the cytoplasm ROS have been described in multiple reports to enhance signal transduction pathways, leading to NF-κB activation and translocation into the nucleus, it was shown to significantly inhibit the capacity of NF-κB to bind the DNA in the nucleus, a capacity that is consequently restored through the action of reducing enzymes (Kabe et al, 2005).

In melanoma, NF-κB is constitutively active unlike to normal melanocytes and is increased under conditions of oxidative stress (Meyskens et al, 1999). In this study, the basal DNA-binding activity of NF-κB in metastatic melanoma cells was found to increase 4-fold as compared with normal melanocytes. This level of binding was paralleled by a 1.5- to 4-fold increase in the expression of p50, p65 (RelA), and IκB-α. In contrast, the expression of c-Rel was markedly decreased (60%) in melanoma cells as compared with normal melanocytes. Following oxidative stress produced by enzyme-generated $H_2O_2$, free $H_2O_2$, or incubation with buthionine sulfoximine, NF-κB binding activity increased 1.5- to 2.5-fold in melanoma cells, but only slightly in normal melanocytes (Meyskens et al, 1999). Shattuck-Brandt and Richmond reported an endogenous activation of NF-κB in melanoma due to posttranslational modification of the inhibitory element IκB, as a result of oxidative processes, that enhances its degradation (Shattuck-Brandt & Richmond, 1997). In addition, melanoma cell lines that exhibit high or low activity of the membrane-bound gamma-glutamyl transpeptidase (GGT), a basal source of $H_2O_2$ in the extracellular space, were associated either with higher or lower levels of NF-κB respectively (Maellaro et al, 2000). Moreover, stimulation or inhibition of GGT activity in higher GGT activity cells resulted in progressive activation or inactivation of NF-κB, respectively. A role of NAD(P)H oxidase and NAD(P)H:quinone oxidoreductase in oxidant signalling of melanoma cell growth has also been demonstrated by activating the redox-regulated NF-κB transcription factor (Brar et al, 2003).

### 2.3.1.3 Activating protein 1 (AP-1)

AP-1 is a dimeric transcription factor comprising proteins from several families whose common denominator is the possession of basic leucine zipper (bZIP) domains that are essential for dimerization and DNA binding. The Jun (c-Jun, JunB and JunD) and Fos (c-Fos, FosB, Fra1 and Fra2) subfamilies are the major AP-1 proteins. Activating transcription factor (ATF) proteins ATF2, LRF1/ATF3, B-ATF, JDP1 and JDP2 are also components of AP-1. The last group of AP-1 proteins, and the least studied, is the Maf subfamily, which includes c-Maf, MafB, MafA, MafG/F/K and Nrl (Eychene et al, 2008). Different combinations of these proteins in the AP-1 complex bind to their specific DNA consensus sequences, determining which genes are regulated (Chinenov & Kerppola, 2001). AP-1 family is involved in the regulation of central cellular processes, including cell proliferation, survival, growth, differentiation, apoptosis, migration, and transformation. AP-1 proteins can function as anti-oncogenic factors, by inducing apoptosis, or as oncogenic factors, by signalling cell survival (Eferl & Wagner, 2003; Hess et al, 2004; Shaulian & Karin, 2002; Verde et al, 2007). Multiple different stimuli induce AP-1, including cytokine, growth factors, neurotransmitters, hormones, bacterial and viral infections, stress signals, and oncogenic stimuli. Its activity can be regulated at the levels of transcription of the genes encoding AP-1 subunits, mRNA stability and translation, protein turnover, and posttranslational modification (Vesely et al, 2009). AP-1 transcriptional activity is controlled by ROS and reactive nitrogen species (RNS) at several levels of its regulation. This includes the regulation of expression of the genes encoding AP-1 subunits, the interactions of the AP-1 proteins with their DNA-binding sites, their interactions with co-activators, as well as at the level of chromatin remodelling, through the modulation of histone acetyltransferase and histone deacetylase (Shlomai, 2010).

Abnormal redox regulation of AP-1 has been reported in melanoma (Yang & Meyskens, 2005). Treatment of human metastatic melanoma cells with resveratrol, a potent ROS scavenger, produces some morphological changes, such as reduced anchorage-independent growth and decreased AP-1 binding and transcriptional activities. These changes in AP-1 activities were related to different AP-1 composition, where c-Jun/JunD/Fra1 turned to JunD/Fra1/Fra2, with increased levels of JunD, Fra1, and Fra2 expression in the nucleus. Furthermore, the overexpression of Fra2 in human melanoma cells reduced significantly both AP-1 transcriptional activity and 12-*O*-tetradecanoylphorbol-induced transcriptional transactivation. Addition of $H_2O_2$ partially reversed the inhibition of colony proliferation. Although $H_2O_2$ restored participation of c-Jun in AP-1 complexes, $H_2O_2$ addition did not affect the induction of Fra1 and Fra2 by resveratrol nor the morphological changes. The authors hypothesized that alterations in AP-1 composition and reduction of intracellular oxidative status by resveratrol might contribute to the recruitment of normal AP-1 transcription signalling in melanoma and subsequently induce cellular biological features consistent with a more normal phenotype.

#### 2.3.1.4 Forkhead box O (FoxO) family of transcription factors

FoxO transcription factors regulate development, proliferation, survival and longevity. Members of the mammalian FoxO family, which include FoxO1, FoxO3, FoxO4 and FoxO6, are relatively expressed in an ubiquitous way. However, FoxO proteins are not equally expressed in all tissues, thus individual FoxO proteins may have specificity in regards to cellular function (Maiese et al, 2009). Moreover, target gene regulation appears to be controlled in a cell-type-specific manner due to association of FoxO isoforms with specific cofactors. Many of the cellular processes modulated by FoxO are themselves deregulated in tumorigenesis, and deletion of FOXO genes has demonstrated that these transcription factors function as tumour suppressors (van der Vos & Coffer, 2011). FOXOs were originally identified as downstream components of insulin/insulin-like growth factor signalling through phosphoinositide 3-kinase (PI3K) and AKT (Brunet et al, 1999; Kops et al, 1999). In mice, FoxOs act as functionally redundant tumour suppressors (Paik et al, 2009), and in cell systems, FoxOs can either mediate apoptosis or quiescence in response to growth factor deprivation (Medema et al, 2000). The DNA binding domain (DBD) is highly conserved between FoxO proteins. FoxOs can function both as transcriptional activators and repressors, depending on the associated cofactors that they recruit upon DNA binding. Growth factors, cytokines, and hormones negatively regulate FoxO transcriptional activity through inhibitory phosphorylation predominantly mediated by AKT.

Regulation of FoxOs by ROS occurs through numerous posttranslational modifications (van der Horst & Burgering, 2007). Besides, FoxO activation increases resistance to oxidative stress through transcription of antioxidant enzymes as MnSOD and catalase as a result of a negative feedback loop (Kops et al, 2002).

It has been described that FoxO4 is involved in oncogene-induced senescence (OIS) through redox mechanisms. Oncogenic BRAF signalling through mitogen-activated protein kinase/extracellular signal-regulated kinase kinase results in increased ROS levels and JNK-mediated activation of FoxO4 via its phosphorylation, which induces $p21^{CIP1}$-mediated cell senescence (de Keizer et al, 2010). In this sense, the ectopic introduction of FoxO4 in endogenous oncogenic BRAF-expressing melanoma cells induces a growth arrest through cellular senescence (de Keizer et al, 2010). OIS represents a barrier for tumour formation, and consequently, the melanoma cells have to bypass this barrier, suggesting that FoxO inactivation is one of the requirements for senescence bypass and melanoma growth (de Keizer et al, 2010).

**2.3.1.5 p53 tumour suppressor protein**

The tumour suppresor protein p53 (encoded by TP53 gene) is an important transcription factor that is induced in response to many forms of cellular stress. This protein has been named "the guardian of the genome" because it plays a central role in coordinating the cellular responses to a broad range and levels of cellular stress factors, leading to apoptosis, cell cycle arrest, senescence, DNA repair, changes in cell metabolism, or autophagy (Green & Kroemer, 2009; Helton & Chen, 2007). There are hundreds of p53 DNA-specific binding sequences located close to promoters of target genes in the human genome.

The role of redox signalling in the regulation of p53 has been well demonstrated. The p53 DNA-binding activity depends on redox regulation by the oxidation of several reactive cysteine residues located within its DNA binding domain (Hainaut & Mann, 2001). ROS can also regulate the function of p53 through indirect oxidative modifications of its interacting partners such as Mdm2 (Shlomai, 2010). Moreover, it was demonstrated that p53 regulates energy metabolism and its resulting ROS generation by modulating the transcription of p53 target genes that control mitochondrial respiration, glycolysis, and the pentose phosphate shunt (Bensaad & Vousden, 2007).

Approximately half of human cancers were found to have inactivating mutations of TP53. Although most melanomas have wild type TP53, loss of function of p53 is rather common. This protein is kept inactive and at low levels predominantly bound to Mdm2, targeting it for proteasomal degradation (Box & Terzian, 2008).

**2.3.1.6 Microphthalmia-associated transcription factor (MiTF)**

MITF is the master control gene for melanocyte lineage survival. The mutation of MITF gene causes a microphthalmia phenotype in mice, deafness and lack of pigmentation

(Steingrimsson et al, 2004). In humans, mutations of MITF gene cause Waardenburg syndrome type IIA in which patients exhibit deafness and pigment disturbances because of a lack of melanocytes (Tassabehji et al, 1994). The role of MiTF in differentiation and development is well established, but evidence of its role in tumorigenesis remains contradictory. In human melanocytes transfected with mutant BRAF, overexpression of MiTF leads to transformation (Garraway et al, 2005). As the MITF gene is amplified in some melanomas, it has been suggested that MITF can function as a melanoma oncogene (Levy et al, 2006). In another report, however, MiTF was downregulated in Braf-transformed murine melanocytes and BRAF-expressing human melanocytes; reexpression of MiTF in these cells inhibited cell proliferation (Wellbrock & Marais, 2005). These contradictions have been elegantly reconciled in a recent review that has pointed out that an optimal amount of MiTF is required for maintaining proliferation and differentiation, whereas MiTF levels that are too low or too high may cause cell-cycle arrest and apoptosis (Gray-Schopfer et al, 2007).

It has been demonstrated that MiTF regulates cellular response to ROS by upregulating APE-1 at the basal level as well as enhancing its stimulation by ROS (Liu et al, 2009). APE-1 has two essential well characterized functions: a DNA endonuclease activity, which has a key role in the base excision DNA repair pathway and a role as redox sensor that enhances the DNA binding activities of a large number of transcription factors, including p53, HIF-1α, AP-1, and NF-κB upon an increase of intracellular ROS. Depletion of APE-1 by siRNA leads to apoptosis in human cells due to accumulation of damaged DNA, especially when ROS increase (Fung & Demple, 2005).

### 2.3.2 Redox regulation in the melanoma signalling network

Melanocyte and melanoblast proliferation, survival, differentiation and migration are all critical elements of normal developmental physiology. The signalling circuitry that regulates these events is often indelibly altered at the genetic level by the potential melanoma cell (Fig. 4).

At least four major signalling abnormalities have been described in melanoma. They include the Ras signalling network, both through RAF/ERK MAPK and PI3K/AKT cascades; the $p16^{INK4A}$/CDK4 network; the Bcl-2/p53 network and the melanocyte developmental pathways that involve receptor tyrosine kinase (KIT), microphtalmia transcription factor (MITF) and β-Catenin. The abnormalities in these signalling cascades are involved in the different steps of promotion and progression of melanoma, from the radial growth, the resistance to apoptosis and radio- and chemotherapy up to the vertical growth and the invasion and metastasis processes (Hocker et al, 2008).

#### 2.3.2.1 The Ras signalling network

The Ras signalling network regulates cell growth, cell proliferation, survival and invasion through two distinct cascades, the Ras/MAPK and the Ras/PI3K signalling streams.

One of the first genes shown to be specifically mutated in melanoma was NRAS, a gene encoding a member of the Ras family of small GTP-binding proteins (Berger & Garraway, 2009). These proteins lie at the top of the Ras/Raf/MEK/ERK MAPK pathway. This activates a large number of growth-promoting genes in response to growth factors and cytokines. NRAS is mutated in 15-30% of melanomas (Demunter et al, 2001; van Elsas et al, 1996). These mutations impair GTPase catalytic activity of Ras, resulting in a constitutively GTP-bound and active state. It has been suggested that the spatial distribution of NRAS-mutated tumours on the skin and their proclivity for dipyrimidine mutations have a possible correlation with UV exposure (Berger & Garraway, 2009).

As noted above, Ras works in the MAPK pathway (Fig. 2A and 4). This pathway is hyperactivated in up to 90% of human melanomas (Cohen et al, 2002). This emphasizes the contribution of NRAS mutations to the development of melanoma but also indicates the involvement of other genes in the pathway. The BRAF gene was observed to be mutated in 80% of short-term melanoma cell cultures and 66% of uncultured melanomas thereby making BRAF the single most commonly mutated gene in melanoma (Hocker et al, 2008). The product of BRAF gene is a serine-threonine kinase that induces MEK to phosphorylate ERK, which enhances cell growth and proliferation (Berger & Garraway, 2009). Notably, up to 90% of the BRAF mutations in melanoma involved a single substitution of valine to glutamic acid in the kinase domain (V600E) (Berger & Garraway, 2009; Davies et al, 2002). The oncogenic potential lies in the ability of the V600E mutant to lead to a constitutively active BRAF product (Berger & Garraway, 2009; Davies et al, 2002; Shinozaki et al, 2004; Wan et al, 2004). Unlike the mutation patterns observed in NRAS, the T>A transversion at the 1799 position associated with the V600E mutation is not suggestive of UV-induced DNA damage, although there is an apparent association between this mutation and intermittent exposure to sun (Maldonado et al, 2003). Thus, mutations in both NRAS and BRAF occur in a mutually exclusive manner suggesting some degree of functional redundancy between these genetic events (Hocker et al, 2008).

Once activated, Ras induces the membrane translocation and activation of PI3K, which leads to activation of a prominent downstream oncogenic effector, AKT (Fig. 2A and 4). Downstream effectors of AKT promote proliferation, survival and invasion (Hocker et al, 2008). Downstream components of the PI3K pathway have been shown to be altered in up to 50-60% of melanomas (Stahl et al, 2004; Zhou et al, 2000) The expression of PI3K and AKT have shown to gradually increase during the progression from benign nevi to early melanoma, and finally, to metastasic disease (Hocker et al, 2008; Stahl et al, 2004). Interestingly, the AKT3 isoform is highly expressed in neural crest-derived cells such as melanocytes, and AKT3 has been found undergo chromosomal copy gains and/or overexpression in up to 60% of melanomas (Stahl et al, 2004). Moreover, activating point mutations in AKT3 have also been described in melanoma (Davies et al, 2008).

A key downstream component of the PI3K pathway, PTEN (also named PTEN/MMAC1), is frequently altered in melanoma and is thought to be one of the main mediators of PI3K pathway activation and melanoma tumorigenesis (Fig. 4). Deletions or loss-of-function mutations in PTEN were observed in 40% of melanoma cell lines (Guldberg et al, 1997; Wu et al, 2003). Inactivating mutations in PTEN and activating mutations in NRAS were proved to exist in reciprocal fashion. This suggests that the loss of PTEN and the activation of NRAS product may functionally overlap (Hocker et al, 2008). The protein PTEN is involved in the termination of PI3K signalling, upregulation of cell cycle arrest and proapoptotic proteins, and downregulation of antiapoptotic proteins of the Bcl-2 family. The expression of PTEN is lost or decreased in 15-50% of melanomas even in the absence of demonstrable mutations (Zhou et al, 2000). Remarkably, ROS participate as second messengers both in RAF/MAPK and PI3K/AKT cascades stimulating cell proliferation (Fig. 2A and 4). ROS often go along with aberrant Ras signalling, either caused by oncogenic forms of the protein or by strong upstream growth factor signalling through the Ras/Raf/MAPK pathway (Finkel, 2006; Kopnin et al, 2007). Moreover, Ras can be activated by UV radiation, ROS, metals and mitogenic stimuli (Valko et al, 2006). It has been reported that the serine/threonine kinases of the MAPK family can be regulated by oxidants. In this sense, $O_2^{\bullet -}$ and $H_2O_2$ can activate the MAPK cascade at the level of MEK and ERK1/2 (Valko et al, 2006). Disregulation of

MAPK function was found in human skin cancers (Valko et al, 2006) and this pathway is invariably activated in early-, intermediate-, and last-stage melanomas (Verhaegen et al, 2006). Moreover interplay among the MAPK pathway, ROS and antiapoptotic factors in the control of melanoma viability was demonstrated. Verhaegen *et al* reported a tumour cell-selective role of the MAPK pathway upstream of the mitochondria, controlling ROS production. This function was critical to prevent the activation of proapoptotic functions of p53 in melanoma cells, but it was dispensable for normal melanocytes (Verhaegen et al, 2006).
In addition to PTEN and BRAF mutations, proto-oncogene pathway activation can occur in melanoma as a result of ROS potentiating AKT signalling by inhibition of PTEN phosphatase activity (Fruehauf & Trapp, 2008). Moreover, as described in 2.3.1.2 section, the NF-κB transcription factor is constitutively active in melanoma (Meyskens et al, 1999). Furthermore, it is well known that this transcription factor is usually activated under prooxidant conditions (Stone & Yang, 2006). Govindarajan *et al.* found that $O_2^{\bullet -}$ can be induced by AKT in melanoma, and AKT can prevent cells from superoxide mediated cell death. Thus AKT may serve as a molecular switch that enhances aggressiveness through tumour angiogenesis and the generation of $O_2^{\bullet -}$. The payoff for the tumour is generating ROS-NF-κB signalling, which allows increased angiogenesis and resistance to chemotherapy (Govindarajan et al, 2007).

**2.3.2.2 The p16$^{INK4A}$/CDK4/Cyclin D1 network**

Although NRAS and BRAF play a key role in melanocytes proliferation, activating mutations in those genes are alone insufficient to lead to malignant transformation. Consequently the requirement for cooperation of other pathways is highlighted. In order for malignant transformation to occur, the mechanisms that mediate senescence must be overridden. Oncogene-induced senescence is thought to involve activation of tumour suppressors such as CDKN2A, RB and TP53 (Mooi & Peeper, 2006). Increased susceptibility to melanoma was observed in patients with germline mutations in these genes. The CDKN2A gene encodes two proteins: p16$^{INK4A}$ and p14$^{ARF}$, and both of them are involved in melanoma growth and survival (Sharpless et al, 2003). The p16$^{INK4A}$ protein inhibits the phosphorylation of the retinoblastoma protein by CDK4/6. On the other hand, p14$^{ARF}$ inhibits the p53 antagonist Mdm2 and it is suggested that p14$^{ARF}$ also possessed tumour-suppressive effects that are independent of p53 (Ha et al, 2007). Thus CDKN2A appears to play a major role in preventing cancer formation by mediating a senescence-like state upon oncogenic stress (Hocker et al, 2008; Serrano et al, 1997) Melanoma cell lines often exhibited loss of both CDKN2A copies (Fig. 4). Those that retain at least one copy of CDKN2A frequently carried nonsense, missense or frameshift mutations of the remaining allele (Hocker et al, 2008). This loss of CDKN2A is required in addition to NRAS mutations in order to progress to frank melanoma (Hocker et al, 2008).
Moreover, both somatic and germline mutations in CDK4 have been detected in melanoma (Hocker et al, 2008). The mutations in CDK4 fall in the p16$^{INK4A}$ binding region (Lys22 or Arg24) and prevent p16$^{INK4A}$ from binding to and inhibiting CDK4 protein (Hocker et al, 2008). Thus, these alterations in CDK4 mimic p16$^{INK4A}$ loss.
Cyclin D (encoded by CCND1) is another fundamental component of the CDK4/6 complex. Oncogenic Ras positively impacts the cell cycle by upregulating cyclin D1 through MAPK signalling, drawing another link between Ras network and p16$^{INK4A}$/CDK4 network (Fig. 4). A less common melanoma subtype, acral lentiginous melanoma, frequently exhibits amplification of the chromosomal region that encompasses the CCND1 locus (Bastian et al,

2000; Sauter et al, 2002). Additionally, CCDN1 amplifications were noted to occur more often on melanomas that take place on skin with chronic sun-induced damage (Curtin et al, 2005). The tumour-suppressor $p16^{INK4A}$ was recently suggested as an endogenous regulator of carcinogenic intracellular oxidative stress and the increased susceptibility of melanocytes to elevated ROS in the context of the characteristic oncogenic $p16^{INK4A}$ depletion was reported (Jenkins et al, 2010). Considering the importance of cell cycle regulation tightly bound to Ras/MAPK and PI3K/AKT signalling cascades and to the $p16^{INK4A}$/CDK4 network, we studied the effects of ROS modulation on cell cycle and we demonstrated that the high levels of intracellular ROS of melanoma cells are associated with increased levels of cyclin D1 and mislocalization of the negative regulatory protein of Cyclin/CDKs complexes, $p27^{KIP1}$ (unpublished results), favouring the increased proliferation rate of melanoma cells (Fig. 2A). Notably, cyclin D1 expression is directly controlled by Ras/MAPK pathway and ROS (Burhans & Heintz, 2009).

#### 2.3.2.3 The Bcl-2/p53 apoptotic pathways

It has been shown that alterations within apoptotic pathways, as well as aberrant modulation by upstream signalling networks, such as MAPK and PI3K, contribute to the inherent chemoresistance observed in melanoma (Helmbach et al, 2001; Hocker et al, 2008). The protein p53 functions to initiate DNA repair and/or apoptosis when exposed to cellular stresses, such as UV radiation or high levels of ROS (Fig. 2B). The overall mutational rate in melanoma of this gene is near to 13% (Hocker & Tsao, 2007). As described in Section 2.3.1.5, direct mutation of TP53 is rare in sporadic melanoma, whereas p53 is frequently inactivated (Sekulic et al, 2008). Induction and activation of p53 play an essential role in halting cellular growth and repairing damaged DNA under conditions of substantial cellular stress. An important mediator of the cell cycle-inhibitory function of p53 is the cell cycle inhibitor $p21^{CIP1}$, which is induced by p53 and inhibits the cyclin E-CDK2 complex. This leads to decreased phosphorylation of Rb protein with the consequent cell cycle arrest at the G1/S transition point. Thus, melanoma cells can increase their proliferation rate taking advantage of their high levels of ROS and the defective function of p53 (Fig. 4).

The Bcl-2 network is one of the most crucial regulators of melanoma cell apoptosis (Soengas & Lowe, 2003). The Bcl-2 family is formed by both antiapoptotic and proapoptotic members. Bcl-2 protein has a physiologic role in the skin: in response to UV radiation, keratinocytes secrete NGF, which binds to melanocyte receptors and leads to increased Bcl-2 expression and resistance to apoptosis (Zhai et al, 1996). Aberrations in various signaling pathways contribute to elevated Bcl-2 levels in melanoma. Particularly, oncogenic NRAS and MITF favour the enhanced expression of this antiapoptotic protein in melanoma (Hocker et al, 2008). Alterations in others antiapoptotic members of the Bcl-2 family, such as Mcl-1, may play a role in decreasing the dependence on Bcl-2 for cell survival. Indeed, Mcl-1 has emerged as potentially critical melanoma survival gene and is highly expressed in primary as well as advanced melanoma (Tang et al, 1998). Various growth factor receptors on the melanoma cell surface signal through AKT to increase the levels of the Bcl-2 family proteins that can block apoptosis and this could be mediated by ROS (Fruehauf & Trapp, 2008)

#### 2.3.2.4 Melanocyte developmental pathways alterations

The genetic factors involved in the coordinated balance of proliferation, migration and survival required for melanocyte homing to the cutaneous surface may be usurped by melanoma cells during tumorigenesis.

KIT is an essential gene for melanocyte survival and development, which encodes a receptor tyrosine kinase (RTK) for the stem cell factor (SCF) ligand and functions as an upstream activator of the MAPK signalling pathway (Berger & Garraway, 2009). The role of KIT in melanoma tumorigenesis is rather controversial (Hocker et al, 2008). The fact that KIT alterations are associated with certain less common types of melanoma, would explain the relatively low frequency of mutations of this gene in unselected cases (Hocker et al, 2008). However, in uveal melanoma, c-Kit expression is present in nearly 80% of cases (Berger & Garraway, 2009; Sekulic et al, 2008). It is generally accepted that ROS generated by these ligand/receptor-initiated pathways can function as true second messengers and mediate important cellular functions such as proliferation and programmed cell death (Valko et al, 2006). Indeed, ROS act as second messengers in the MAPK pathway activated by KIT and they can mediate uveal melanoma cell proliferation through this signalling.

The MITF gene has emerged as a master regulator of melanocyte development (Hocker et al, 2008). As described in section 2.3.1.6, its product is a transcription factor involved in multiple processes, such as the regulation of pigment cell phenotype and melanocyte proliferation and survival (Widlund & Fisher, 2003). Interestingly, MITF amplifications are coincident with mutations in BRAF (Berger & Garraway, 2009). Unlike oncogenic NRAS and BRAF, which acquire new and tumour-specific cellular functions through nucleotide mutations, MITF becomes oncogenic via deregulation, affecting survival mechanisms that are also present in the normal melanocyte lineage (Berger & Garraway, 2009).

MiTF is a downstream target of β-catenin, a critical regulator of melanoma cell growth (Widlund et al, 2002) which, in turn, is an important downstream mediator of Wnt pathway signalling (Hocker et al, 2008). Thus, melanomas often show constitutive activation of the Wnt signalling as revealed by nuclear accumulation of β-catenin (Rimm et al, 1999). Wnts are secreted proteins with important developmental functions, particularly in neural crest cells such as melanocytes (Sekulic et al, 2008). The Wnt signalling pathway is also regulated by ROS (Fig. 4). A thioredoxin-related protein, nucleoredoxin (NRX), governs ROS-stimulated Wnt signalling in a temporal manner (Funato & Miki, 2010). NRX usually interacts with Dishevelled (Dvl), an essential adaptor protein for Wnt signalling, and blocks the activation of the Wnt pathway (Funato & Miki, 2010). Oxidative stress causes dissociation of NRX from Dvl, which enables Dvl to activate the downstream Wnt signalling pathway (Funato & Miki, 2010).

Gene transcription and post-translational modifications of MiTF are strongly influenced by multiple upstream pathways, some of which are modulated by ROS, such as RTK, MAPK and PI3K pathways (Fig. 4). Therefore, some authors linked the involvement of ROS in these signalling pathways to the progression of melanoma by the term reactive oxygen-driven tumour (Fried & Arbiser, 2008). In this sense, the overexpression of APE-1, a transcriptional target for MiTF, protected melanoma cells from $H_2O_2$-induced cell death (Yang et al, 2005). Interestingly, Liu *et al.* demonstrated that MiTF regulates cellular ROS response by upregulating APE-1. Thus, MiTF-positive melanoma cells are more resistant to $H_2O_2$-induced cell death as compared to MiTF-negative cells. MiTF accumulation in advanced melanoma may increase APE-1 levels and other survival factors such as Bcl-2, which in turn lead to better survival outcome for tumour cells (Liu et al, 2009). This is associated to the fact that high MiTF levels were correlated with poor outcome of patients with melanoma (Koyanagi et al, 2006).

As we can see so far, the melanoma network is highly interconnected with a great deal of functional redundancy built into it. The signalling pathways active in melanoma cells are interconnected through multiple feedback loops, and ROS are involved in the regulation of many of them (Fig. 4).

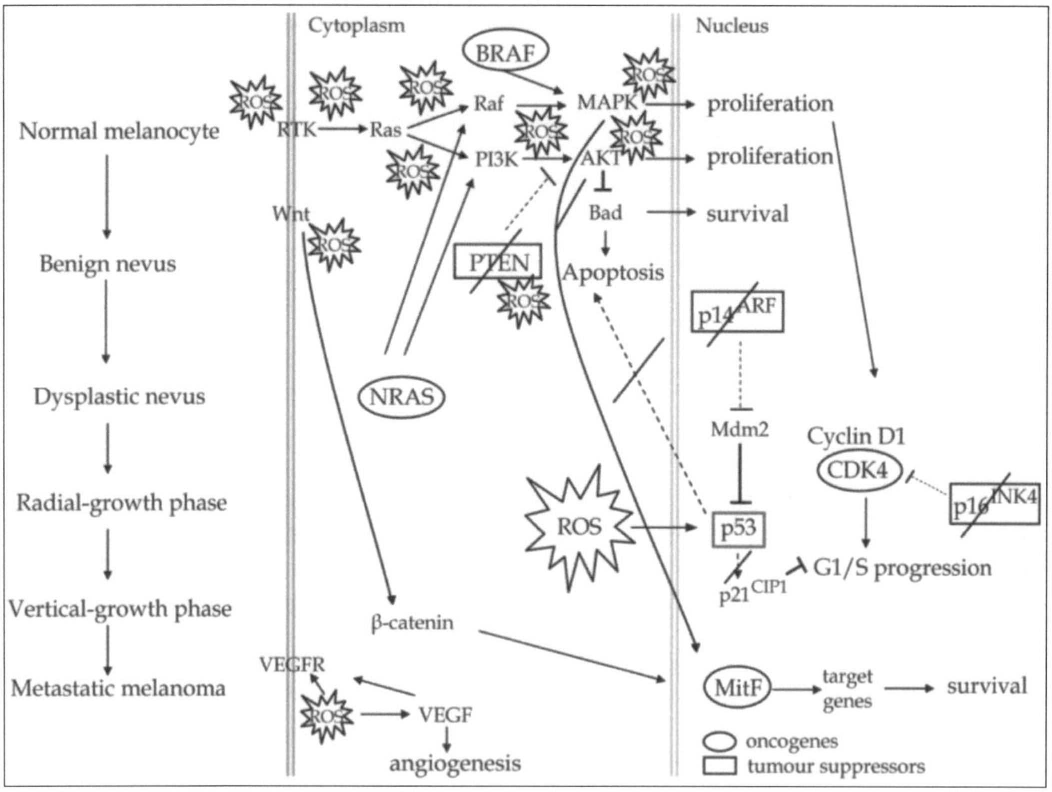


Fig. 4. ROS and the altered signalling pathways involved in the different steps of promotion and progression of melanoma.

### 2.4 ROS in invasion and metastasis of melanoma

Regarding the involvement of ROS in metastatic melanomas, several proteins related to different steps of migration, invasion and metastasis have been found to be induced by transcription factors or activated by signalling pathways described as mediated by ROS. For example, connexin 43 (Cx-43), which participates in tumour cell diapedesis and attachment to endothelial cells (Villares et al, 2009) along with a chondroitin sulfate proteoglycan of the extracellular matrix that favours the detachment of cells and the metastatic dissemination (Domenzain-Reyna et al, 2009), i.e. versican, are overexpressed in melanomas and are regulated by the redox-responsive transcription factor AP-1. Another mechanism that relates high ROS levels of melanoma cells to metastatic potential would be the cytoplasmic mislocalization of $p27^{KIP1}$ (unpublished results), since reduced nuclear levels of this protein increases proliferation and cytoplasmic localization would drive tumour cell invasion by other functions of this protein not related to cell cycle regulation (Wander et al, 2010).

NEDD9 has been supported as a melanoma gene important for invasion and metastasis (Kim et al, 2006). The overexpression of this gene induces malignant features related to metastatic potential in primary melanocytes and in nonmetastatic melanoma cells. This increased invasiveness is conferred by a functional and physical interaction between NEDD9 and focal adhesion kinase (FAK) at the cell periphery (Berger & Garraway, 2009). Hef1 (encoded by NEDD9) positively regulates the Src-FAK-Crk "migratory switch". Hef1 overexpression also induces the activation of ERK, p38, and JNK kinases through interactions with intermediary signalling effectors. As previously explained, these proteins that interact with Hef1 can be modulated by ROS (O'Neill et al, 2007).

Angiogenesis signalling in melanoma is mediated by growth factor receptors, including the VEGF, platelet-derived growth factor (PDGF), and basic-fibroblast growth factor (b-FGF) pathways. VEGF activation of VEGF receptors (VEGFR) is likely to play an important role in melanoma growth, survival, and invasiveness through autocrine loop formation (Graells et al, 2004; Lacal et al, 2005). As described above, ROS can modulate these pathways involved in angiogenesis (Fig. 4). In this sense, it has been well described that the expression of VEGF is induced by ROS and in particular it is most strongly activated by $H_2O_2$ (Valko et al, 2006).

## 3. Therapeutics approaches for melanoma based on reactive oxygen species levels

It is widely accepted that melanoma is resistant to all therapeutic modalities once the metastatic process started. Current treatment protocol for early-stage melanomas consists in surgical tumour excision, while in advanced stages, the adjuvant treatment including chemotherapy, unspecific immunotherapy and interferon offers poor results regarding free disease terms rate of survival. Thus, none of the currently available FDA approved therapies clearly alter the natural history of the disease for the population as a whole.

On the other hand, advanced personalized therapeutic procedures like golden nanospheres and gene therapy are recently being studied and represent an alternative for future treatment of melanoma. Despite all new knowledge and technological support the advanced stage melanoma management still remains an unsolved problem.

### 3.1 Use of ROS as therapeutic agents

The cytotoxic nature of ROS has been widely used to kill tumour cells in many cancer treatments. Various anti-cancer agents in clinical use today—including anthracyclines, cisplatin, bleomycin and ionizing radiation—generate ROS within the cells (Nishikawa, 2008). However, around a decade ago, the concept of taking advantage of the increased oxidative stress of cancer cells was proposed as a strategy to induce preferential cancer cell death based on the different redox states in normal and malignant cells. Different approaches exploit the fact that increased ROS may induce cell death by apoptosis.

Arsenic trioxide (ATO) is studied as an anticancer agent whose use originated in traditional Chinese medicine. In several tumour types, it is an established cell growth inhibitor and apoptosis inducer (Baysan et al, 2007; Han et al, 2008). In patients with acute promyelocytic leukemia, for example, low concentrations of ATO (less than or equal to micromolar concentrations) induce longlasting remission without significant myelosuppressive side effects. The ability of ATO to induce apoptosis in leukemic cells depends on the activity of the enzymes that regulate cellular $H_2O_2$ content (Jing et al, 1999). Regarding melanoma and ATO, in several melanoma cell lines a study demonstrates that a combination of treatments of melanoma cells with ATO and the antibiotic thiostrepton results in significant growth inhibitory effects, reversed when the cells are also treated with the free radical scavenger NAC, indicating an increase in intracellular ROS as part of the mechanism. Thiostrepton is commercially available as part of a topical antibiotic mixture used to treat bacterial infections in animals. It has also been used to effectively treat murine bacterial systemic infections (Bowling et al, 2008). However, to date, it has not been approved for human use.

Other drugs are studied alone or in combination with ATO to induce apoptosis. Disulfiram (DSF), an agent used to treat alcoholism for the past few decades, has been shown to induce apoptosis in thymocytes. It has been demonstrated that redox regulations in melanoma cells are aberrant and metal chelators (such as dithiocarbamate) alter the redox status and induce apoptosis in melanoma cells. Cen *et al.* have explored the effect of disulfiram (DSF), a member of the dithiocarbamate family, on apoptosis in melanoma cells, founding that DSF caused a 3 to 5-fold increase in apoptosis in all three melanoma cell strains being tested at a very low dose (25-50 ng/ml). The same dose of DSF did not have significant apoptotic effect on melanocytes (Cen et al, 2002). Disulfiram in combination with ATO were selected for a study based on their ability to alter GSH redox balance. They were chosen because ATO has been reported to be synergistic against various solid tumour cell lines *in vitro* and *in vivo* when given with buthionine sulfoximine (BSO), another agent that acts as DSF, both modulating GSH metabolism (Wu et al, 2004); and the effect of Disulfiram (DSF), has recently been explored on apoptosis in melanoma cells.

Another compound that showed therapeutic activity in malignant melanoma is Elesclomol (STA_4783), that was able to prolong the progression-free survival time in a Phase II clinical trial (Kirshner et al, 2008). The mechanism underlying proapoptotic activity of elesclomol is through the induction of ROS and oxidative stress. Elesclomol rapidly induced ROS in cancer cells, generating a transcription profile characteristic of an oxidative stress response. Moreover, pretreatment of cells with antioxidants blocked all *in vitro* activities associated with elesclomol, including ROS production and the induction of apoptosis. Unfortunately, the Phase III clinical trials of elesclomol were suspended in 2008 due to safety concerns.

Finally, Taxol (paclitaxel) is a chemotherapeutic agent that has shown promise in the treatment of previously unresponsive breast, ovary, and non-small cell lung carcinoma (Crown & O'Leary, 2000). It interferes with mitosis during the G2/M phase of the cell cycle. Besides, it was demonstrated that taxol mediated activation of MAPK signalling pathways is linked to the activation of the cell death machinery in human melanoma cell lines. The same study demonstrates that the downregulation of a protein UCP2 and subsequent induction of ROS are essential parts in this mechanism (Selimovic et al, 2008).

ROS are capable of exerting different effects according to their nature, localization and levels (Davies, 2000). Although classically they are thought of as cytotoxic and mutagenic or as inducers of oxidative stress, evidence show that ROS play a role in signal transduction. ROS can be implicated in stimulation or inhibition of cell proliferation, apoptosis, and cell senescence (Chen, 2000; Sundaresan et al, 1995). In BHK-21 and human prostate cells, a low concentration of exogenously added $H_2O_2$ caused a modest increase in proliferation, whereas higher levels resulted in slowed growth, cell cycle arrest, and/or apoptosis (Burdon, 1996; Wartenberg et al, 1999).

Furthermore, considering the relationship between ROS and metastasis, reviewed in the literatures, it indicates that ROS accelerate adhesion (Orr et al, 2000), invasion (Orr et al, 2000), migration (Wu, 2006; Wu et al, 2008) and angiogenesis (Ushio-Fukai & Nakamura, 2008). Therefore, ROS scavengers, such as catalase and superoxide dismutase, have been examined to inhibit tumour metastasis, although their effects are not very marked. Targeted delivery of these enzymes to the sites where ROS are generated is necessary to obtain sufficient inhibition of tumour metastasis.

Thus, an increase in ROS levels is not the only alternative for a possible cancer therapy. Scavenging of $H_2O_2$ in several tumour cells inhibits cell proliferation (Arnold et al, 2001). The inhibition of lung metastatic tumour growth of melanoma cells has been reported to occur in a mouse model by sustained delivery of catalase (Hyoudou et al, 2009). In that sense, a recent study of our group demonstrates that $H_2O_2$ scavenging impedes nuclear exportation of $p27^{KIP1}$ allowing cell cycle arrest through the accumulation of this protein in the nucleus (unpublished data).

Interleukin (IL)-2 has been shown to have clinical activity in metastatic melanoma. Nevertheless, *in vitro* studies have demonstrated that ROS generated by monocyte/macrophage populations may inhibit cytotoxic activity within the tumour, leading to the hypothesis that cytokine-based immunotherapy may be more effective if the generation of ROS were inhibited (Hansson et al, 1999; Kono et al, 1996). Clinical evidence in support of this hypothesis came from phase II studies that combine histamine, a potent inhibitor of ROS formation, with cytokine-based therapies for metastatic melanoma, acute myelogenous leukemia, and renal cell carcinoma (Hellstrand et al, 1997; Hellstrand et al, 1994).

Manipulating ROS levels by redox modulation is a way to selectively kill cancer cells without causing significant toxicity to normal cells. It is worth noting that redox alterations in cancer cells are very complex because of the multiple factors involved in the redox regulation and stress response, and that the simple addition of ROS-generating agents may not always lead to a preferential killing of cancer cells. This explains the importance of understanding the complex redox alterations in cancer cells.

### 3.2 Gene therapy

Gene Therapy is a relatively new paradigm for treatment of human diseases and is becoming a rationale area for the development of new therapeutic agents for cancer treatment. One major strategy of gene therapy to provide effective and specific activation of medical products inside the tumour mass implicates the control of the therapeutic agent activity by a Tumour Specific Promoter (TSP). TSPs corresponding to genes differentially activated in cancer cells have been used to control viral replication inside the tumour or the antitumour activity of therapeutic genes in melanoma (Cao et al, 1999; Diaz et al, 1998; Schoensiegel et al, 2004). Selection of a TSP is central for the design of a well defined medical product for gene transfer. Since solid tumours are highly heterogeneous it is more tempting to drive gene expression by designing promoters that include transcriptional regulatory elements responsive to the tumour environment conditions (Laurent et al, 2005).

Recently, we described a novel approach of gene therapy, which takes advantage of the prooxidant state of melanoma cells. (Policastro et al, 2009). This therapeutic strategy is based on a ROS-responsive chimeric promoter, containing a ROS-response motif located in the VEGF gene promoter and a second ROS-response motif obtained from the EGR1 gene promoter. This chimeric promoter was based on a ROS-response motif located in the VEGF gene promoter placed and a second ROS-response motif obtained from the EGR1 gene promoter. The activity of the chimeric promoter (named E6(40)VE) was largely dependent on variations in intracellular ROS levels and showed a high inducible response to exogenous $H_2O_2$. Transient expression of the Herpes Simplex virus thymidine kinase therapeutic gene (TK) driven by the chimeric promoter, followed by gancyclovir administration, inhibited human melanoma cells growth *in vitro* and *in vivo*. Moreover, electrotransfer of the TK gene followed by GCV administration exerted a potent therapeutic effect on melanoma established tumours. This response was improved when combined with chemotherapeutic drugs such as doxorubicin, which act by themselves by increasing ROS levels (Policastro et al, 2009).

## 4. Conclusion

Throughout this review, we summarized the updated knowledge about the involvement of ROS in the biology of melanoma, analyzing the alterations in both, specific pathways of melanocytes development and general ROS-regulated signalling pathways common to different types of tumours. Moreover, we provided a glimpse of the state-of-the-art advances in relation to therapeutic approaches for melanoma treatment in view of the high levels of ROS characteristic of melanoma cells as a differential feature that may be exploited to develop selective treatments with low toxicity for normal tissues.

Further studies on the biology of melanoma and ROS regulation in the context of recent new advances in genomics, proteomics and bioinformatics will allow a better comprehension of the complex signalling network in response to the high oxidative stress of melanoma. This approach will help to characterize individual patient tumour specimens identifying vulnerable targets and preventing deleterious damage in normal tissues.

## 5. Acknowledgements

The authors gratefully acknowledge Andrea C. Cruz for proofreading our work and advising us on the use of English language.

## 6. References

Arnold RS, Shi J, Murad E, Whalen AM, Sun CQ, Polavarapu R, Parthasarathy S, Petros JA, Lambeth JD (2001) Hydrogen peroxide mediates the cell growth and transformation caused by the mitogenic oxidase Nox1. *Proc Natl Acad Sci U S A* 98(10): 5550-5555

Bastian BC, Kashani-Sabet M, Hamm H, Godfrey T, Moore DH, 2nd, Brocker EB, LeBoit PE, Pinkel D (2000) Gene amplifications characterize acral melanoma and permit the detection of occult tumor cells in the surrounding skin. *Cancer Res* 60(7): 1968-1973

Baysan A, Yel L, Gollapudi S, Su H, Gupta S (2007) Arsenic trioxide induces apoptosis via the mitochondrial pathway by upregulating the expression of Bax and Bim in human B cells. *Int J Oncol* 30(2): 313-318

Bedogni B, Powell MB (2009) Hypoxia, melanocytes and melanoma - survival and tumor development in the permissive microenvironment of the skin. *Pigment Cell Melanoma Res* 22(2): 166-174

Bensaad K, Vousden KH (2007) p53: new roles in metabolism. *Trends Cell Biol* 17(6): 286-291

Berger MF, Garraway LA (2009) Applications of genomics in melanoma oncogene discovery. *Hematol Oncol Clin North Am* 23(3): 397-414, vii

Borovansky J, Mirejovsky P, Riley PA (1991) Possible relationship between abnormal melanosome structure and cytotoxic phenomena in malignant melanoma. *Neoplasma* 38(4): 393-400

Bowling BD, Doudican N, Manga P, Orlow SJ (2008) Inhibition of mitochondrial protein translation sensitizes melanoma cells to arsenic trioxide cytotoxicity via a reactive oxygen species dependent mechanism. *Cancer Chemother Pharmacol* 63(1): 37-43

Box NF, Terzian T (2008) The role of p53 in pigmentation, tanning and melanoma. *Pigment Cell Melanoma Res* 21(5): 525-533

Brar SS, Kennedy TP, Quinn M, Hoidal JR (2003) Redox signaling of NF-kappaB by membrane NAD(P)H oxidases in normal and malignant cells. *Protoplasma* 221(1-2): 117-127

Brune B, Zhou J (2007) Nitric oxide and superoxide: interference with hypoxic signaling. *Cardiovasc Res* 75(2): 275-282

Brunet A, Bonni A, Zigmond MJ, Lin MZ, Juo P, Hu LS, Anderson MJ, Arden KC, Blenis J, Greenberg ME (1999) Akt promotes cell survival by phosphorylating and inhibiting a Forkhead transcription factor. *Cell* 96(6): 857-868

Burch PM, Heintz NH (2005) Redox regulation of cell-cycle re-entry: cyclin D1 as a primary target for the mitogenic effects of reactive oxygen and nitrogen species. *Antioxid Redox Signal* 7(5-6): 741-751

Burdon RH (1996) Control of cell proliferation by reactive oxygen species. *Biochem Soc Trans* 24(4): 1028-1032

Burhans WC, Heintz NH (2009) The cell cycle is a redox cycle: linking phase-specific targets to cell fate. *Free Radic Biol Med* 47(9): 1282-1293

Cao G, Zhang X, He X, Chen Q, Qi Z (1999) A safe, effective in vivo gene therapy for melanoma using tyrosinase promoter-driven cytosine deaminase gene. *In Vivo* 13(2): 181-187

Cen D, Gonzalez RI, Buckmeier JA, Kahlon RS, Tohidian NB, Meyskens FL, Jr. (2002) Disulfiram induces apoptosis in human melanoma cells: a redox-related process. *Mol Cancer Ther* 1(3): 197-204

Cerutti PA (1985) Prooxidant states and tumor promotion. *Science* 227(4685): 375-381

Cohen C, Zavala-Pompa A, Sequeira JH, Shoji M, Sexton DG, Cotsonis G, Cerimele F, Govindarajan B, Macaron N, Arbiser JL (2002) Mitogen-actived protein kinase activation is an early event in melanoma progression. *Clin Cancer Res* 8(12): 3728-3733

Crown J, O'Leary M (2000) The taxanes: an update. *Lancet* 355(9210): 1176-1178

Curtin JA, Fridlyand J, Kageshita T, Patel HN, Busam KJ, Kutzner H, Cho KH, Aiba S, Brocker EB, LeBoit PE, Pinkel D, Bastian BC (2005) Distinct sets of genetic alterations in melanoma. *N Engl J Med* 353(20): 2135-2147

Chandel NS, Maltepe E, Goldwasser E, Mathieu CE, Simon MC, Schumacker PT (1998) Mitochondrial reactive oxygen species trigger hypoxia-induced transcription. *Proc Natl Acad Sci U S A* 95(20): 11715-11720

Chang SH, Worley LA, Onken MD, Harbour JW (2008) Prognostic biomarkers in uveal melanoma: evidence for a stem cell-like phenotype associated with metastasis. *Melanoma Res* 18(3): 191-200

Chen QM (2000) Replicative senescence and oxidant-induced premature senescence. Beyond the control of cell cycle checkpoints. *Ann N Y Acad Sci* 908: 111-125

Chinenov Y, Kerppola TK (2001) Close encounters of many kinds: Fos-Jun interactions that mediate transcription regulatory specificity. *Oncogene* 20(19): 2438-2452

Davies H, Bignell GR, Cox C, Stephens P, Edkins S, Clegg S, Teague J, Woffendin H, Garnett MJ, Bottomley W, Davis N, Dicks E, Ewing R, Floyd Y, Gray K, Hall S, Hawes R, Hughes J, Kosmidou V, Menzies A, Mould C, Parker A, Stevens C, Watt S, Hooper S, Wilson R, Jayatilake H, Gusterson BA, Cooper C, Shipley J, Hargrave D, Pritchard-Jones K, Maitland N, Chenevix-Trench G, Riggins GJ, Bigner DD,

Palmieri G, Cossu A, Flanagan A, Nicholson A, Ho JW, Leung SY, Yuen ST, Weber BL, Seigler HF, Darrow TL, Paterson H, Marais R, Marshall CJ, Wooster R, Stratton MR, Futreal PA (2002) Mutations of the BRAF gene in human cancer. *Nature* 417(6892): 949-954

Davies KJ (2000) Oxidative stress, antioxidant defenses, and damage removal, repair, and replacement systems. *IUBMB Life* 50(4-5): 279-289

Davies MA, Stemke-Hale K, Tellez C, Calderone TL, Deng W, Prieto VG, Lazar AJ, Gershenwald JE, Mills GB (2008) A novel AKT3 mutation in melanoma tumours and cell lines. *Br J Cancer* 99(8): 1265-1268

de Keizer PL, Packer LM, Szypowska AA, Riedl-Polderman PE, van den Broek NJ, de Bruin A, Dansen TB, Marais R, Brenkman AB, Burgering BM (2010) Activation of forkhead box O transcription factors by oncogenic BRAF promotes p21cip1-dependent senescence. *Cancer Res* 70(21): 8526-8536

Demunter A, Stas M, Degreef H, De Wolf-Peeters C, van den Oord JJ (2001) Analysis of N- and K-ras mutations in the distinctive tumor progression phases of melanoma. *J Invest Dermatol* 117(6): 1483-1489

Denko NC (2008) Hypoxia, HIF1 and glucose metabolism in the solid tumour. *Nat Rev Cancer* 8(9): 705-713

Diaz RM, Eisen T, Hart IR, Vile RG (1998) Exchange of viral promoter/enhancer elements with heterologous regulatory sequences generates targeted hybrid long terminal repeat vectors for gene therapy of melanoma. *J Virol* 72(1): 789-795

Domenzain-Reyna C, Hernandez D, Miquel-Serra L, Docampo MJ, Badenas C, Fabra A, Bassols A (2009) Structure and regulation of the versican promoter: the versican promoter is regulated by AP-1 and TCF transcription factors in invasive human melanoma cells. *J Biol Chem* 284(18): 12306-12317

Duran HA, de Rey BM (1991) Differential oxidative stress induced by two different types of skin tumor promoters, benzoyl peroxide and 12-O-tetradecanoylphorbol-13-acetate. *Carcinogenesis* 12(11): 2047-2052

Eferl R, Wagner EF (2003) AP-1: a double-edged sword in tumorigenesis. *Nat Rev Cancer* 3(11): 859-868

Elledge SJ (1996) Cell cycle checkpoints: preventing an identity crisis. *Science* 274(5293): 1664-1672

Eychene A, Rocques N, Pouponnot C (2008) A new MAFia in cancer. *Nat Rev Cancer*

Felty Q, Singh KP, Roy D (2005) Estrogen-induced G1/S transition of G0-arrested estrogen-dependent breast cancer cells is regulated by mitochondrial oxidant signaling. *Oncogene* 24(31): 4883-4893

Finkel T (2006) Intracellular redox regulation by the family of small GTPases. *Antioxid Redox Signal* 8(9-10): 1857-1863

Fried L, Arbiser JL (2008) The reactive oxygen-driven tumor: relevance to melanoma. *Pigment Cell Melanoma Res* 21(2): 117-122

Fruehauf JP, Trapp V (2008) Reactive oxygen species: an Achilles' heel of melanoma? *Expert Rev Anticancer Ther* 8(11): 1751-1757

Funato Y, Miki H (2010) Redox regulation of Wnt signalling via nucleoredoxin. *Free Radic Res* 44(4): 379-388

Fung H, Demple B (2005) A vital role for Ape1/Ref1 protein in repairing spontaneous DNA damage in human cells. *Mol Cell* 17(3): 463-470

Ghosh S, Hayden MS (2008) New regulators of NF-kappaB in inflammation. *Nat Rev Immunol* 8(11): 837-848

Giatromanolaki A, Sivridis E, Kouskoukis C, Gatter KC, Harris AL, Koukourakis MI (2003) Hypoxia-inducible factors 1alpha and 2alpha are related to vascular endothelial growth factor expression and a poorer prognosis in nodular malignant melanomas of the skin. *Melanoma Res* 13(5): 493-501

Gidanian S, Mentelle M, Meyskens FL, Jr., Farmer PJ (2008) Melanosomal damage in normal human melanocytes induced by UVB and metal uptake--a basis for the pro-oxidant state of melanoma. *Photochem Photobiol* 84(3): 556-564

Govindarajan B, Sligh JE, Vincent BJ, Li M, Canter JA, Nickoloff BJ, Rodenburg RJ, Smeitink JA, Oberley L, Zhang Y, Slingerland J, Arnold RS, Lambeth JD, Cohen C, Hilenski L, Griendling K, Martinez-Diez M, Cuezva JM, Arbiser JL (2007) Overexpression of Akt converts radial growth melanoma to vertical growth melanoma. *J Clin Invest* 117(3): 719-729

Graells J, Vinyals A, Figueras A, Llorens A, Moreno A, Marcoval J, Gonzalez FJ, Fabra A (2004) Overproduction of VEGF concomitantly expressed with its receptors promotes growth and survival of melanoma cells through MAPK and PI3K signaling. *J Invest Dermatol* 123(6): 1151-1161

Gray-Schopfer V, Wellbrock C, Marais R (2007) Melanoma biology and new targeted therapy. *Nature* 445(7130): 851-857

Green DR, Kroemer G (2009) Cytoplasmic functions of the tumour suppressor p53. *Nature* 458(7242): 1127-1130

Guldberg P, thor Straten P, Birck A, Ahrenkiel V, Kirkin AF, Zeuthen J (1997) Disruption of the MMAC1/PTEN gene by deletion or mutation is a frequent event in malignant melanoma. *Cancer Res* 57(17): 3660-3663

Guyton KZ, Kensler TW (1993) Oxidative mechanisms in carcinogenesis. *Br Med Bull* 49(3): 523-544

Ha L, Ichikawa T, Anver M, Dickins R, Lowe S, Sharpless NE, Krimpenfort P, Depinho RA, Bennett DC, Sviderskaya EV, Merlino G (2007) ARF functions as a melanoma tumor suppressor by inducing p53-independent senescence. *Proc Natl Acad Sci U S A* 104(26): 10968-10973

Halliwell B (2007) Oxidative stress and cancer: have we moved forward? *Biochem J* 401(1): 1-11

Han YH, Kim SZ, Kim SH, Park WH (2008) Arsenic trioxide inhibits the growth of Calu-6 cells via inducing a G2 arrest of the cell cycle and apoptosis accompanied with the depletion of GSH. *Cancer Lett* 270(1): 40-55

Hansson M, Hermodsson S, Brune M, Mellqvist UH, Naredi P, Betten A, Gehlsen KR, Hellstrand K (1999) Histamine protects T cells and natural killer cells against oxidative stress. *J Interferon Cytokine Res* 19(10): 1135-1144

Harris AL (2002) Hypoxia--a key regulatory factor in tumour growth. *Nat Rev Cancer* 2(1): 38-47

Helmbach H, Rossmann E, Kern MA, Schadendorf D (2001) Drug-resistance in human melanoma. *Int J Cancer* 93(5): 617-622

Helton ES, Chen X (2007) p53 modulation of the DNA damage response. *J Cell Biochem* 100(4): 883-896

Hellstrand K, Mellqvist UH, Wallhult E, Carneskog J, Kimby E, Celsing F, Brune M (1997) Histamine and interleukin-2 in acute myelogenous leukemia. *Leuk Lymphoma* 27(5-6): 429-438

Hellstrand K, Naredi P, Lindner P, Lundholm K, Rudenstam CM, Hermodsson S, Asztely M, Hafstrom L (1994) Histamine in immunotherapy of advanced melanoma: a pilot study. *Cancer Immunol Immunother* 39(6): 416-419

Hempel N, Ye H, Abessi B, Mian B, Melendez JA (2009) Altered redox status accompanies progression to metastatic human bladder cancer. *Free Radic Biol Med* 46(1): 42-50

Hess J, Angel P, Schorpp-Kistner M (2004) AP-1 subunits: quarrel and harmony among siblings. *J Cell Sci* 117(Pt 25): 5965-5973

Hocker T, Tsao H (2007) Ultraviolet radiation and melanoma: a systematic review and analysis of reported sequence variants. *Hum Mutat* 28(6): 578-588

Hocker TL, Singh MK, Tsao H (2008) Melanoma genetics and therapeutic approaches in the 21st century: moving from the benchside to the bedside. *J Invest Dermatol* 128(11): 2575-2595

Hyoudou K, Nishikawa M, Ikemura M, Kobayashi Y, Mendelsohn A, Miyazaki N, Tabata Y, Yamashita F, Hashida M (2009) Prevention of pulmonary metastasis from subcutaneous tumors by binary system-based sustained delivery of catalase. *J Control Release* 137(2): 110-115

Ibanez IL, Bracalente C, Molinari BL, Palmieri MA, Policastro L, Kreiner AJ, Burlon AA, Valda A, Navalesi D, Davidson J, Davidson M, Vazquez M, Ozafran M, Duran H (2009) Induction and rejoining of DNA double strand breaks assessed by H2AX phosphorylation in melanoma cells irradiated with proton and lithium beams. *Int J Radiat Oncol Biol Phys* 74(4): 1226-1235

Ibanez IL, Policastro LL, Tropper I, Bracalente C, Palmieri MA, Rojas PA, Molinari BL, Duran H (2011) H(2)O(2) scavenging inhibits G1/S transition by increasing nuclear levels of p27(KIP1). *Cancer Lett*

Jackson AL, Loeb LA (2001) The contribution of endogenous sources of DNA damage to the multiple mutations in cancer. *Mutat Res* 477(1-2): 7-21

Jenkins NC, Liu T, Cassidy P, Leachman SA, Boucher KM, Goodson AG, Samadashwily G, Grossman D (2010) The p16(INK4A) tumor suppressor regulates cellular oxidative stress. *Oncogene*

Jimenez-Cervantes C, Martinez-Esparza M, Perez C, Daum N, Solano F, Garcia-Borron JC (2001) Inhibition of melanogenesis in response to oxidative stress: transient downregulation of melanocyte differentiation markers and possible involvement of microphthalmia transcription factor. *J Cell Sci* 114(Pt 12): 2335-2344

Jing Y, Dai J, Chalmers-Redman RM, Tatton WG, Waxman S (1999) Arsenic trioxide selectively induces acute promyelocytic leukemia cell apoptosis via a hydrogen peroxide-dependent pathway. *Blood* 94(6): 2102-2111

Kabe Y, Ando K, Hirao S, Yoshida M, Handa H (2005) Redox regulation of NF-kappaB activation: distinct redox regulation between the cytoplasm and the nucleus. *Antioxid Redox Signal* 7(3-4): 395-403

Kietzmann T, Gorlach A (2005) Reactive oxygen species in the control of hypoxia-inducible factor-mediated gene expression. *Semin Cell Dev Biol* 16(4-5): 474-486

Kim M, Gans JD, Nogueira C, Wang A, Paik JH, Feng B, Brennan C, Hahn WC, Cordon-Cardo C, Wagner SN, Flotte TJ, Duncan LM, Granter SR, Chin L (2006)

Comparative oncogenomics identifies NEDD9 as a melanoma metastasis gene. *Cell* 125(7): 1269-1281

Kirshner JR, He S, Balasubramanyam V, Kepros J, Yang CY, Zhang M, Du Z, Barsoum J, Bertin J (2008) Elesclomol induces cancer cell apoptosis through oxidative stress. *Mol Cancer Ther* 7(8): 2319-2327

Kono K, Salazar-Onfray F, Petersson M, Hansson J, Masucci G, Wasserman K, Nakazawa T, Anderson P, Kiessling R (1996) Hydrogen peroxide secreted by tumor-derived macrophages down-modulates signal-transducing zeta molecules and inhibits tumor-specific T cell-and natural killer cell-mediated cytotoxicity. *Eur J Immunol* 26(6): 1308-1313

Kopnin PB, Agapova LS, Kopnin BP, Chumakov PM (2007) Repression of sestrin family genes contributes to oncogenic Ras-induced reactive oxygen species up-regulation and genetic instability. *Cancer Res* 67(10): 4671-4678

Kops GJ, Dansen TB, Polderman PE, Saarloos I, Wirtz KW, Coffer PJ, Huang TT, Bos JL, Medema RH, Burgering BM (2002) Forkhead transcription factor FOXO3a protects quiescent cells from oxidative stress. *Nature* 419(6904): 316-321

Kops GJ, de Ruiter ND, De Vries-Smits AM, Powell DR, Bos JL, Burgering BM (1999) Direct control of the Forkhead transcription factor AFX by protein kinase B. *Nature* 398(6728): 630-634

Koyanagi K, O'Day SJ, Gonzalez R, Lewis K, Robinson WA, Amatruda TT, Kuo C, Wang HJ, Milford R, Morton DL, Hoon DS (2006) Microphthalmia transcription factor as a molecular marker for circulating tumor cell detection in blood of melanoma patients. *Clin Cancer Res* 12(4): 1137-1143

Kuphal S, Winklmeier A, Warnecke C, Bosserhoff AK (2010) Constitutive HIF-1 activity in malignant melanoma. *Eur J Cancer* 46(6): 1159-1169

Lacal PM, Ruffini F, Pagani E, D'Atri S (2005) An autocrine loop directed by the vascular endothelial growth factor promotes invasiveness of human melanoma cells. *Int J Oncol* 27(6): 1625-1632

Laurent A, Nicco C, Chereau C, Goulvestre C, Alexandre J, Alves A, Levy E, Goldwasser F, Panis Y, Soubrane O, Weill B, Batteux F (2005) Controlling tumor growth by modulating endogenous production of reactive oxygen species. *Cancer Res* 65(3): 948-956

Levy C, Fisher DE (2011) Dual roles of lineage restricted transcription factors: The case of MITF in melanocytes. *Transcr* 2(1): 19-22

Levy C, Khaled M, Fisher DE (2006) MITF: master regulator of melanocyte development and melanoma oncogene. *Trends Mol Med* 12(9): 406-414

Liu F, Fu Y, Meyskens FL, Jr. (2009) MiTF regulates cellular response to reactive oxygen species through transcriptional regulation of APE-1/Ref-1. *J Invest Dermatol* 129(2): 422-431

Maellaro E, Dominici S, Del Bello B, Valentini MA, Pieri L, Perego P, Supino R, Zunino F, Lorenzini E, Paolicchi A, Comporti M, Pompella A (2000) Membrane gamma-glutamyl transpeptidase activity of melanoma cells: effects on cellular H(2)O(2) production, cell surface protein thiol oxidation and NF-kappa B activation status. *J Cell Sci* 113 ( Pt 15): 2671-2678

Maiese K, Hou J, Chong ZZ, Shang YC (2009) A fork in the path: Developing therapeutic inroads with FoxO proteins. *Oxid Med Cell Longev* 2(3): 119-129

Maldonado JL, Fridlyand J, Patel H, Jain AN, Busam K, Kageshita T, Ono T, Albertson DG, Pinkel D, Bastian BC (2003) Determinants of BRAF mutations in primary melanomas. *J Natl Cancer Inst* 95(24): 1878-1890

Martinez-Outschoorn UE, Balliet RM, Rivadeneira DB, Chiavarina B, Pavlides S, Wang C, Whitaker-Menezes D, Daumer KM, Lin Z, Witkiewicz AK, Flomenberg N, Howell A, Pestell RG, Knudsen ES, Sotgia F, Lisanti MP (2010) Oxidative stress in cancer associated fibroblasts drives tumor-stroma co-evolution: A new paradigm for understanding tumor metabolism, the field effect and genomic instability in cancer cells. *Cell Cycle* 9(16): 3256-3276

Medema RH, Kops GJ, Bos JL, Burgering BM (2000) AFX-like Forkhead transcription factors mediate cell-cycle regulation by Ras and PKB through p27kip1. *Nature* 404(6779): 782-787

Menon SG, Sarsour EH, Spitz DR, Higashikubo R, Sturm M, Zhang H, Goswami PC (2003) Redox regulation of the G1 to S phase transition in the mouse embryo fibroblast cell cycle. *Cancer Res* 63(9): 2109-2117

Meyskens FL, Jr., Buckmeier JA, McNulty SE, Tohidian NB (1999) Activation of nuclear factor-kappa B in human metastatic melanomacells and the effect of oxidative stress. *Clin Cancer Res* 5(5): 1197-1202

Meyskens FL, Jr., Farmer P, Fruehauf JP (2001) Redox regulation in human melanocytes and melanoma. *Pigment Cell Res* 14(3): 148-154

Mooi WJ, Peeper DS (2006) Oncogene-induced cell senescence--halting on the road to cancer. *N Engl J Med* 355(10): 1037-1046

Munoz-Munoz JL, Garcia-Molina F, Varon R, Tudela J, Garcia-Canovas F, Rodriguez-Lopez JN (2009) Generation of hydrogen peroxide in the melanin biosynthesis pathway. *Biochim Biophys Acta* 1794(7): 1017-1029

Nishikawa M (2008) Reactive oxygen species in tumor metastasis. *Cancer Lett* 266(1): 53-59

O'Neill GM, Seo S, Serebriiskii IG, Lessin SR, Golemis EA (2007) A new central scaffold for metastasis: parsing HEF1/Cas-L/NEDD9. *Cancer Res* 67(19): 8975-8979

Onumah OE, Jules GE, Zhao Y, Zhou L, Yang H, Guo Z (2009) Overexpression of catalase delays G0/G1- to S-phase transition during cell cycle progression in mouse aortic endothelial cells. *Free Radic Biol Med* 46(12): 1658-1667

Orr FW, Wang HH, Lafrenie RM, Scherbarth S, Nance DM (2000) Interactions between cancer cells and the endothelium in metastasis. *J Pathol* 190(3): 310-329

Paik JH, Ding Z, Narurkar R, Ramkissoon S, Muller F, Kamoun WS, Chae SS, Zheng H, Ying H, Mahoney J, Hiller D, Jiang S, Protopopov A, Wong WH, Chin L, Ligon KL, DePinho RA (2009) FoxOs cooperatively regulate diverse pathways governing neural stem cell homeostasis. *Cell Stem Cell* 5(5): 540-553

Perkins ND (2007) Integrating cell-signalling pathways with NF-kappaB and IKK function. *Nat Rev Mol Cell Biol* 8(1): 49-62

Policastro L, Molinari B, Larcher F, Blanco P, Podhajcer OL, Costa CS, Rojas P, Duran H (2004) Imbalance of antioxidant enzymes in tumor cells and inhibition of proliferation and malignant features by scavenging hydrogen peroxide. *Mol Carcinog* 39(2): 103-113

Policastro LL, Ibanez IL, Duran HA, Soria G, Gottifredi V, Podhajcer OL (2009) Suppression of cancer growth by nonviral gene therapy based on a novel reactive oxygen species-responsive promoter. *Mol Ther* 17(8): 1355-1364

Rimm DL, Caca K, Hu G, Harrison FB, Fearon ER (1999) Frequent nuclear/cytoplasmic localization of beta-catenin without exon 3 mutations in malignant melanoma. *Am J Pathol* 154(2): 325-329

Sarsour EH, Kumar MG, Chaudhuri L, Kalen AL, Goswami PC (2009) Redox control of the cell cycle in health and disease. *Antioxid Redox Signal* 11(12): 2985-3011

Satyamoorthy K, Herlyn M (2002) Cellular and molecular biology of human melanoma. *Cancer Biol Ther* 1(1): 14-17

Sauter ER, Yeo UC, von Stemm A, Zhu W, Litwin S, Tichansky DS, Pistritto G, Nesbit M, Pinkel D, Herlyn M, Bastian BC (2002) Cyclin D1 is a candidate oncogene in cutaneous melanoma. *Cancer Res* 62(11): 3200-3206

Schallreuter KU, Kothari S, Chavan B, Spencer JD (2008) Regulation of melanogenesis--controversies and new concepts. *Exp Dermatol* 17(5): 395-404

Schallreuter KU, Wood JM (2001) Thioredoxin reductase - its role in epidermal redox status. *J Photochem Photobiol B* 64(2-3): 179-184

Schoensiegel F, Paschen A, Sieger S, Eskerski H, Mier W, Rothfels H, Kleinschmidt J, Schadendorf D, Haberkorn U (2004) MIA (melanoma inhibitory activity) promoter mediated tissue-specific suicide gene therapy of malignant melanoma. *Cancer Gene Ther* 11(6): 408-418

Sekulic A, Haluska P, Jr., Miller AJ, Genebriera De Lamo J, Ejadi S, Pulido JS, Salomao DR, Thorland EC, Vile RG, Swanson DL, Pockaj BA, Laman SD, Pittelkow MR, Markovic SN (2008) Malignant melanoma in the 21st century: the emerging molecular landscape. *Mayo Clin Proc* 83(7): 825-846

Selimovic D, Hassan M, Haikel Y, Hengge UR (2008) Taxol-induced mitochondrial stress in melanoma cells is mediated by activation of c-Jun N-terminal kinase (JNK) and p38 pathways via uncoupling protein 2. *Cell Signal* 20(2): 311-322

Serrano M, Lin AW, McCurrach ME, Beach D, Lowe SW (1997) Oncogenic ras provokes premature cell senescence associated with accumulation of p53 and p16INK4a. *Cell* 88(5): 593-602

Sharpless NE, Kannan K, Xu J, Bosenberg MW, Chin L (2003) Both products of the mouse Ink4a/Arf locus suppress melanoma formation in vivo. *Oncogene* 22(32): 5055-5059

Shattuck-Brandt RL, Richmond A (1997) Enhanced degradation of I-kappaB alpha contributes to endogenous activation of NF-kappaB in Hs294T melanoma cells. *Cancer Res* 57(14): 3032-3039

Shaulian E, Karin M (2002) AP-1 as a regulator of cell life and death. *Nat Cell Biol* 4(5): E131-136

Sherr CJ (1996) Cancer cell cycles. *Science* 274(5293): 1672-1677

Shinozaki M, Fujimoto A, Morton DL, Hoon DS (2004) Incidence of BRAF oncogene mutation and clinical relevance for primary cutaneous melanomas. *Clin Cancer Res* 10(5): 1753-1757

Shlomai J (2010) Redox control of protein-DNA interactions: from molecular mechanisms to significance in signal transduction, gene expression, and DNA replication. *Antioxid Redox Signal* 13(9): 1429-1476

Soengas MS, Lowe SW (2003) Apoptosis and melanoma chemoresistance. *Oncogene* 22(20): 3138-3151

Stahl JM, Sharma A, Cheung M, Zimmerman M, Cheng JQ, Bosenberg MW, Kester M, Sandirasegarane L, Robertson GP (2004) Deregulated Akt3 activity promotes development of malignant melanoma. *Cancer Res* 64(19): 7002-7010

Steingrimsson E, Copeland NG, Jenkins NA (2004) Melanocytes and the microphthalmia transcription factor network. *Annu Rev Genet* 38: 365-411

Stone JR, Yang S (2006) Hydrogen peroxide: a signaling messenger. *Antioxid Redox Signal* 8(3-4): 243-270

Sundaresan M, Yu ZX, Ferrans VJ, Irani K, Finkel T (1995) Requirement for generation of H2O2 for platelet-derived growth factor signal transduction. *Science* 270(5234): 296-299

Szatrowski TP, Nathan CF (1991) Production of large amounts of hydrogen peroxide by human tumor cells. *Cancer Res* 51(3): 794-798

Tang L, Tron VA, Reed JC, Mah KJ, Krajewska M, Li G, Zhou X, Ho VC, Trotter MJ (1998) Expression of apoptosis regulators in cutaneous malignant melanoma. *Clin Cancer Res* 4(8): 1865-1871

Tarpey MM, Wink DA, Grisham MB (2004) Methods for detection of reactive metabolites of oxygen and nitrogen: in vitro and in vivo considerations. *Am J Physiol Regul Integr Comp Physiol* 286(3): R431-444

Tassabehji M, Newton VE, Read AP (1994) Waardenburg syndrome type 2 caused by mutations in the human microphthalmia (MITF) gene. *Nat Genet* 8(3): 251-255

Toullec A, Gerald D, Despouy G, Bourachot B, Cardon M, Lefort S, Richardson M, Rigaill G, Parrini MC, Lucchesi C, Bellanger D, Stern MH, Dubois T, Sastre-Garau X, Delattre O, Vincent-Salomon A, Mechta-Grigoriou F (2010) Oxidative stress promotes myofibroblast differentiation and tumour spreading. *EMBO Mol Med* 2(6): 211-230

Toyokuni S, Okamoto K, Yodoi J, Hiai H (1995) Persistent oxidative stress in cancer. *FEBS Lett* 358(1): 1-3

Ushio-Fukai M, Nakamura Y (2008) Reactive oxygen species and angiogenesis: NADPH oxidase as target for cancer therapy. *Cancer Lett* 266(1): 37-52

Valko M, Rhodes CJ, Moncol J, Izakovic M, Mazur M (2006) Free radicals, metals and antioxidants in oxidative stress-induced cancer. *Chem Biol Interact* 160(1): 1-40

van der Horst A, Burgering BM (2007) Stressing the role of FoxO proteins in lifespan and disease. *Nat Rev Mol Cell Biol* 8(6): 440-450

van der Vos KE, Coffer PJ (2011) The extending network of FOXO transcriptional target genes. *Antioxid Redox Signal* 14(4): 579-592

van Elsas A, Zerp SF, van der Flier S, Kruse KM, Aarnoudse C, Hayward NK, Ruiter DJ, Schrier PI (1996) Relevance of ultraviolet-induced N-ras oncogene point mutations in development of primary human cutaneous melanoma. *Am J Pathol* 149(3): 883-893

Verde P, Casalino L, Talotta F, Yaniv M, Weitzman JB (2007) Deciphering AP-1 function in tumorigenesis: fra-ternizing on target promoters. *Cell Cycle* 6(21): 2633-2639

Verhaegen M, Bauer JA, Martin de la Vega C, Wang G, Wolter KG, Brenner JC, Nikolovska-Coleska Z, Bengtson A, Nair R, Elder JT, Van Brocklin M, Carey TE, Bradford CR, Wang S, Soengas MS (2006) A novel BH3 mimetic reveals a mitogen-activated protein kinase-dependent mechanism of melanoma cell death controlled by p53 and reactive oxygen species. *Cancer Res* 66(23): 11348-11359

Vesely PW, Staber PB, Hoefler G, Kenner L (2009) Translational regulation mechanisms of AP-1 proteins. *Mutat Res* 682(1): 7-12

Victor N, Ivy A, Jiang BH, Agani FH (2006) Involvement of HIF-1 in invasion of Mum2B uveal melanoma cells. *Clin Exp Metastasis* 23(1): 87-96

Villares GJ, Dobroff AS, Wang H, Zigler M, Melnikova VO, Huang L, Bar-Eli M (2009) Overexpression of protease-activated receptor-1 contributes to melanoma metastasis via regulation of connexin 43. *Cancer Res* 69(16): 6730-6737

Wan PT, Garnett MJ, Roe SM, Lee S, Niculescu-Duvaz D, Good VM, Jones CM, Marshall CJ, Springer CJ, Barford D, Marais R (2004) Mechanism of activation of the RAF-ERK signaling pathway by oncogenic mutations of B-RAF. *Cell* 116(6): 855-867

Wander SA, Zhao D, Slingerland JM (2010) p27: a barometer of signaling deregulation and potential predictor of response to targeted therapies. *Clin Cancer Res*

Wang HT, Choi B, Tang MS (2010) Melanocytes are deficient in repair of oxidative DNA damage and UV-induced photoproducts. *Proc Natl Acad Sci U S A* 107(27): 12180-12185

Wartenberg M, Diedershagen H, Hescheler J, Sauer H (1999) Growth stimulation versus induction of cell quiescence by hydrogen peroxide in prostate tumor spheroids is encoded by the duration of the Ca(2+) response. *J Biol Chem* 274(39): 27759-27767

Warters RL, Adamson PJ, Pond CD, Leachman SA (2005) Melanoma cells express elevated levels of phosphorylated histone H2AX foci. *J Invest Dermatol* 124(4): 807-817

Watabe H, Valencia JC, Yasumoto K, Kushimoto T, Ando H, Muller J, Vieira WD, Mizoguchi M, Appella E, Hearing VJ (2004) Regulation of tyrosinase processing and trafficking by organellar pH and by proteasome activity. *J Biol Chem* 279(9): 7971-7981

Wellbrock C, Marais R (2005) Elevated expression of MITF counteracts B-RAF-stimulated melanocyte and melanoma cell proliferation. *J Cell Biol* 170(5): 703-708

Widlund HR, Fisher DE (2003) Microphthalamia-associated transcription factor: a critical regulator of pigment cell development and survival. *Oncogene* 22(20): 3035-3041

Widlund HR, Horstmann MA, Price ER, Cui J, Lessnick SL, Wu M, He X, Fisher DE (2002) Beta-catenin-induced melanoma growth requires the downstream target Microphthalmia-associated transcription factor. *J Cell Biol* 158(6): 1079-1087

Wu H, Goel V, Haluska FG (2003) PTEN signaling pathways in melanoma. *Oncogene* 22(20): 3113-3122

Wu WS (2006) The signaling mechanism of ROS in tumor progression. *Cancer Metastasis Rev* 25(4): 695-705

Wu WS, Wu JR, Hu CT (2008) Signal cross talks for sustained MAPK activation and cell migration: the potential role of reactive oxygen species. *Cancer Metastasis Rev* 27(2): 303-314

Wu XX, Ogawa O, Kakehi Y (2004) Enhancement of arsenic trioxide-induced apoptosis in renal cell carcinoma cells by L-buthionine sulfoximine. *Int J Oncol* 24(6): 1489-1497

Yang S, Irani K, Heffron SE, Jurnak F, Meyskens FL, Jr. (2005) Alterations in the expression of the apurinic/apyrimidinic endonuclease-1/redox factor-1 (APE/Ref-1) in human melanoma and identification of the therapeutic potential of resveratrol as an APE/Ref-1 inhibitor. *Mol Cancer Ther* 4(12): 1923-1935

Yang S, Meyskens FL, Jr. (2005) Alterations in activating protein 1 composition correlate with phenotypic differentiation changes induced by resveratrol in human melanoma. *Mol Pharmacol* 67(1): 298-308

Zhai S, Yaar M, Doyle SM, Gilchrest BA (1996) Nerve growth factor rescues pigment cells from ultraviolet-induced apoptosis by upregulating BCL-2 levels. *Exp Cell Res* 224(2): 335-343

Zhou XP, Gimm O, Hampel H, Niemann T, Walker MJ, Eng C (2000) Epigenetic PTEN silencing in malignant melanomas without PTEN mutation. *Am J Pathol* 157(4): 1123-1128

2

# The Role of the Microenvironment – Models for the Study of Melanoma

Lucia Speroni[1], Victoria de los Angeles Bustuoabad[2], Julieta Gasparri[1], Nadia Silvia Chiaramoni[1] and Silvia del Valle Alonso[1]
[1]*Laboratorio de Biomembranas, Universidad Nacional de Quilmes, Roque Saenz Peña 352, 1876, Bernal, Buenos Aires,*
[2]*División Medicina Experimental, Instituto de Investigaciones Hematológicas, Academia Nacional de Medicina, Pacheco de Melo 3081,1425 Buenos Aires, Argentina*

## 1. Introduction

Melanoma is a progressive disease that claims many lives each year due to lack of therapeutics effective for the long-term treatment of patients. Currently, the best treatment option is early detection followed by surgical removal. Cutaneous melanoma continues to represent both a challenge and a big paradox among solid tumors: though considerable prognostic markers are available, little is known about their biological significance. Recent data on the effect of an anti-melanoma target therapy, ipilimumab (Hodi *et al*, 2010) and new anti-BRAF molecules (Flaherty, 2010) raised hope on the treatment of melanoma. However, although response rates with small molecule inhibitors are high, most are not durable. Moreover, for a large subset of patients, reliable predictive biomarkers especially for immunologic modulators have not yet been identified. Progress on the treatment of both early and advanced melanoma may depend on identifying additional molecular targets and on understanding the mechanisms leading to response or resistance.

Animal models have been critical in the study of the molecular mechanisms of cancer and in the development of new therapeutic agents; nevertheless, there is still much room for improvement. The most widely used *in vivo* model involves the injection of tumor cells in the flank of mice. The relevance of each particular model depends on how close it replicates the histology, physiological effects, biochemical pathways and metastatic pattern observed in the same human tumor type. Numerous models have been developed to study human tumorigenesis and its properties, such as proliferation, migration, invasion, neoangiogenesis, and metastasis, as well as for the study of anti-cancer treatments. Among others, these include *in vitro* systems such as focus formation in tumor cell culture explants and continuous cell lines grown on tissue culture plates, or, alternatively, anchorage-independent growth in soft agar. The foregoing experimental models are suitable for studying molecular pathways in cell-cell and cell-extracellular matrix interactions that would be difficult to dissect in the animal. However they will encounter their limitation in terms that they are not particularly amenable to the investigation of interactions of tumor cells with the surrounding microenvironment of adjacent normal human cell tissues and structures. It has been shown that tumor progression is associated with extensive remodeling of adjacent tissues to provide a supportive environment for tumor growth, angiogenesis, invasion, and metastasis of cancer cells (Hanahan & Weinberg, 2000; Bissell & Radisky, 2001; Fidler 2002; Chambers *et al*, 2002)

In this chapter we will discuss the role of the microenvironment in the development of melanoma. Finally we will discuss the design of *in vivo* and *in vitro* models as tools for understanding the biology of melanoma as well as their utility for the evaluation of new treatments.

## 2. Melanoma anatomic clinical types

There are mainly four types of cutaneous melanoma:

Superficial spreading melanoma. The most commonly occurring melanoma, it accounts for approximately 70% of melanoma cases. It arises at the site of a pre-existing nevus. It affects men and women equally but it appears more frequently on the lower extremities in women and on the upper back in men. Superficial spreading melanoma often evolves during a period of 1 to 7 years.

Nodular melanoma. Up 15% of the cases and is more common among older males, particularly in trunk, head and neck. It is an aggressive type of melanoma due to its tendency to grow in depth invading the dermis and giving early metastasis. It evolves in months to less than 5 years.

Lentigo maligna melanoma. Occurs in 5% of the cases. It is diagnosed in the elderly on regions of the skin that were overexposed to the sun such as head, neck, and the dorsum of hands. This melanoma grows slowly in a radial fashion over a period of 5-20 years.

Acral lentiginous melanoma. Makes up 8% of the melanoma cases, but it is the most common melanoma diagnosed in dark-skinned people.

Cutaneous head and neck melanomas constitute 12%–21% of melanomas diagnosed annually and they have poorer outcomes relative to melanomas of other sites. Among head and neck melanomas, scalp/neck melanomas have a greater risk of melanoma-specific mortality (Tseng & Martinez, 2010).

Malignant melanomas may also arise from the melanocytes present at extracutaneous sites (noncutaneous melanomas) namely eye, anogenital regions, mucosal surfaces, nail beds, conjunctivae, orbit, esophagus, and leptomeninges. Unlike cutaneous melanomas, there is lack of association with sun damage, family history and precursor nevi in these neoplasms. Noncutaneous melanomas are rare neoplasms with a poor prognosis, they can metastasize to lymph nodes, bone, lung, liver, spleen, gastrointestinal tract, kidneys, adrenals, and subcutaneous tissue (reviewed in Hussein, 2008). In this chapter we will focus only in cutaneous melanomas.

## 3. The role of the microenvironment in the development of cutaneous melanoma

The microenvironment is a key factor in tumor progression. Poorly aggressive melanoma cells acquired a vasculogenic phenotype when they were exposed to a microenvironment preconditioned by aggressive metastatic melanoma cells (Seftor *et al*, 2006). The opposite effect has also been studied long ago by Illmensee & Mintz (1976) who showed that teratocarcinoma cells could be normalized by the blastocyst environment. Melanoma metastatic cells could be reverted to its cell type of origin, the neural-crest-derived melanocyte using an embryonic chick model (Kasemeier-Kulesa *et al,* 2008). Thus this evidence shows that whether a melanocyte remains normal or progresses to a neoplastic state would depend on the microenvironment, indicating that clues to understand the etiology of melanoma should be found at the tissue level of organization (Sonnenschein & Soto, 1999)

The frequency of melanoma tumors appears to be site -specific but yet this phenomenon is not well understood. Thus, we will analyze whether the characteristics of the skin of various anatomic sites might account for the different types of melanoma. Particularly we will focus on the cellular components, reactivity and biomechanical properties of the skin in distinct anatomic sites.

The human skin consists of a stratified, cellular epidermis and an underlying dermis of connective tissue. The dermal–epidermal junction is undulating in section; ridges of the epidermis project into the dermis. The junction provides mechanical support for the epidermis and provides a partial barrier against exchange of cells and large molecules. A fatty layer underlies the dermis, the panniculus adiposus, usually designated as "subcutaneous". The major cellular components of the epidermis are keratinocytes, melanocytes, Langerhans cells, Merkel cells, and dendritic cells, and in the dermis, fibroblasts, mast cells, macrophages and micro-vascular cells (endothelial cells and smooth muscle cells) and adipocytes in the underlying layer (McGrath *et al,* 2010).

Skin fibroblasts from different anatomic sites have distinct phenotypes, a phenomenon called topographic differentiation, which is maintained even after fibroblasts are isolated and cultured *in vitro.* A differential expression of HOX proteins which are involved in site-specific organization and in the migration of epidermal cells through integrins and cadherins was described. HOXA13 was expressed in toe and foreskin fibroblasts while HoxD9 was expressed in upper arm fibroblasts (Chang *et al,* 2002). Fibroblasts derived from soles and palms differ from those at other body sites. Interestingly, expression of keratin 9 was not observed in cultured non-palmoplantar keratinocytes when cultured alone or with non-palmoplantar fibroblasts. However, those keratinocytes expressed keratin 9 mRNA when co-cultured with palmoplantar fibroblasts, indicating that the phenotype of keratinocytes is anatomically-dependent. Failed migration of melanocytes and pigmentation in palms and soles appears to be regulated by the fibroblasts (Yamaguchi *et al,* 1999, 2005). Indeed, melanocyte density in the trunk skin of Caucasians, Asians and African-Americans was found to be similar, but was five-fold lower in palmoplantar skin.

Fibroblasts and keratinocytes also seem to participate in the development of melanomas from pre existent nevi (Coleman & Lugo, 1998; Fiuraskova *et al,* 2005), such as in the case of superficial spreading melanomas.

A type of dendritic cells, the Langerhans cells, are thought to play an important role in skin immunity. Studies in inflammatory ear skin explants of mice showed that migrating Langerhans cells were able to stimulate CD8+ T cell responses (reviewed in Stoitzner 2010). Another study showed that the antigenic response was dependent on Langerhans cells when the antigen was applied to the flank, but not when applied to the ear skin of mice (Wang *et al,* 2008). In the human the number of Langerhans cells in hair-bearing skin (chest, scalp and abdomen) is higher compared to hairless skin (palm and sole). On the other hand, higher numbers of Langerhans cells were found in the dorsum of the hand and foot compared to palm and sole (Thomas *et al,* 1984). The role of Langerhans cells is still controversial, pointing out that it might be equally strongly dependent on both the anatomic site and the condition of the skin.

Mast cells play an active role in inflammatory and allergic reactions. They also participate in tissue remodeling; through the releasement of histamine they control the growth of the epidermis by inhibiting the growth of keratinocyte epithelium. Histamine induces the production of MMP-9 in keratinocytes thereby facilitating the migration of immune cells, such as T cells, across the vascular basement membrane or into the epidermis during skin inflammation (reviewed in Harvima, 2008). Morever, human skin mast cell extracts have proven to enhance gel contraction in 3-D cultures of skin fibroblasts possibly by inducing collagen production and organization (Garbuzenko *et al*, 2002). A study showed that mast cells distribution in normal adult skin is site dependent. Higher numbers were found in the distal extremities, forearm and lower leg, compared with those in the trunk, upper leg, and upper arm. Mast cells on the face were not counted (Janssens *et al*, 2005).

UV radiation and aging are factors known to predispose to the development of cutaneous melanomas. This could be attributed to the onset of an inflammatory condition, particularly in the case of UV radiation, as well as to changes in the biomechanical properties of the skin. The role of inflammatory reactions in the development of cutaneous melanoma was demonstrated in a recent study in volunteers older than 40 years of age. The results indicated that the use of aspirin for 5 years or more reduced the risk of cutaneous melanoma by almost half (Curiel-Lewandrowski *et al*, 2011). UVB is a key factor during extrinsic skin aging, it induces collagen cleveage changing the structure of the skin. Because the collagen network can not be completely reconstituted *de novo*, skin elasticity is impaired in the long term. Indeed, in a study where human dermal fibroblasts cultured in 3-D collagen gels were irradiated with UVB it was shown that collagen degradation inhibited the synthesis of hyalorunic acid by the fibroblasts (Röck *et al*, 2011). Thus it is most likely that photoaging alters the extracellular matrix, which in turn induces changes on the phenotype of the embedded cells such as keratinocytes, fibroblasts and dendritic cells.

The biomechanical properties of the skin such as thickness and extensibility decrease with age, most likely due to a degeneration of the collagen network and the loss of glycosaminoglicans. This is particularly true in sun exposed areas on the face and neck (Escoffier *et al*, 1989; Cua *et al*, 1990), coincidently with the site of preference of melanomas with poorer prognosis. In a different study shoulder skin resulted to be thicker than thighs and calves skin (Smalls *et al*, 2006).

## 4. Building models to study the biology of melanoma

### 4.1 *In vivo* models

Since the microenvironment plays a key role in cancer development, accurate models for the study of melanoma should take into account the differential features of the anatomic sites of the skin. The most widely used *in vivo* model for the study of melanoma is the inoculation of tumor cells in the flank of mice. In a previous work we investigated whether the dermis of a different anatomical site of mice would offer different characteristics than those of the flank. Thus, we chose the dorsal region of the foot and compared it to the flank in terms of cellular influx and reactivity (Speroni *et al*, 2009a). We further compared the acute and chronic inflammatory response in the selected areas of the skin in order to gain better understanding of the reactivity of both anatomic sites.

### 4.1.1 The inflammatory response in distinct anatomic sites of the skin of mice
### 4.1.2 Nonspecific inflammatory response

We tested the acute inflammatory response of the two anatomic sites induced by an extract of lung homogenate in Balb/c mice. The release of histamine and bradykinin by mast cells induces edema after 2-3 h that persists for up to 24 h post injection. A 0.1 mg/ml lung homogenate (Van den Brenk *et al*, 1974) was prepared and 0.05 ml of this suspension was intradermically injected in the dorsal region of the foot and in the flank of Balb/c mice. Swelling was recorded as skin thickness using a dial micrometer (Pocotest, GESSH) and 3 $mm^2$ of skin from the injected site were excised and weighted. Controls were inoculated with PS.

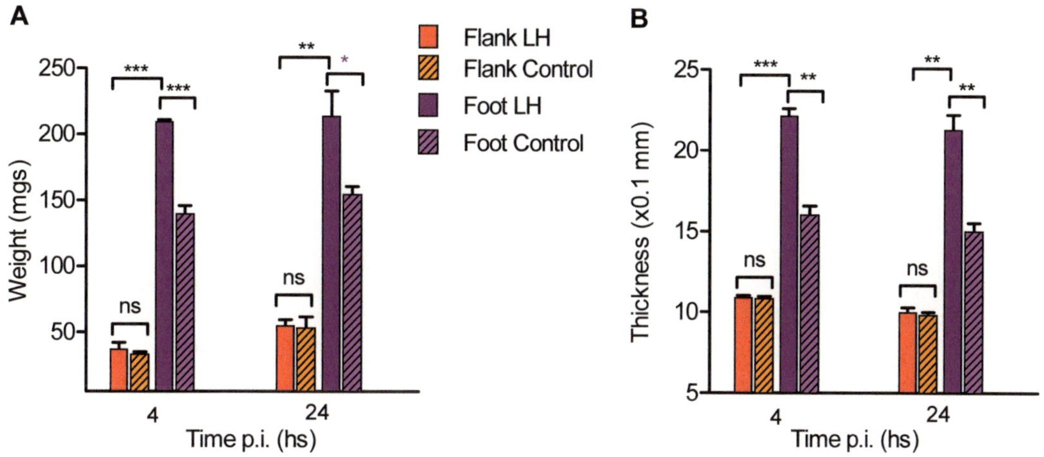


Fig. 1. Inflammatory response of the skin following lung homogenate (LH) injection. (A) weight and (B) thickness of the inoculated dermis of flank and dorsal region of the foot were recorded 4 and 24 h post injection (n=4). *, $p<0.05$; **, $p<0.005$; ***$p<0.001$ significant differences, ns, not significant; student t test

The injection of lung homogenate induced a significant inflammatory response in the dorsal region of the foot as evidenced by the significant increase in weight and thickness of the injected site. The edema persisted up to 24 h post injection. To the contrary, the skin from the flank did not show a significant response to the same inflammatory stimulus, weight and thickness were comparable to controls (Figure 1) (non published results).

The ability of the skin to respond to a chronic inflammatory stimulus was also tested. The injection of silica produces a granuloma due to a continuous lysis of macrophages in the injection site (Kessel *et al*, 1963). A suspension of 1 mg of silica in 0.05 ml of PS was intradermically injected in the flank and in the dorsal region of the foot of Balb/c mice. Local inflammation was recorded as thickness of the injected site using a dial micrometer (Pocotest, GESSH).

The response to silica (Figure 2) was significantly higher in the dermis of the dorsal region of the foot than in the dermis of the flank. Moreover in the dorsal region of the foot the response was sustained until 10 days after inoculation while in the flank was almost undetectable by that time. This result shows that the dermis of the dorsal region of the foot is more responsive to a chronic inflammatory stimulus than the dermis of the flank (non published results).

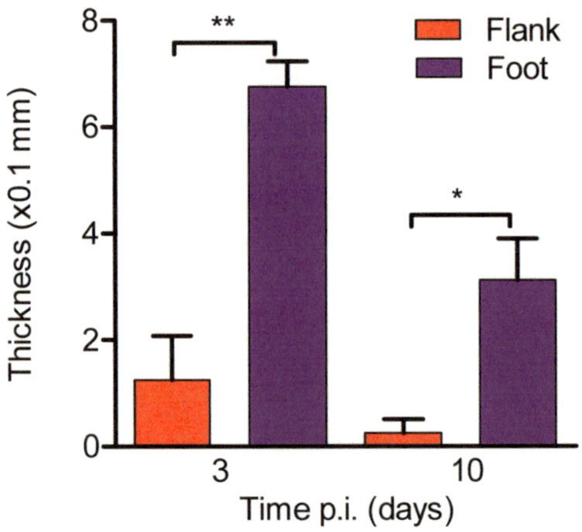


Fig. 2. Chronic inflammatory response to silica in the dermis of the flank and dorsal region of the foot (n=4) * $p<0.05$; ** $p<0.005$, Student t test between each group and control

#### 4.1.3 Specific immune response

In a previous work we tested the immune response in both anatomic sites after injection of sheep red blood cells (SRBC). Seven days after immunization with SRBC, sera was obtained and antibody titer was analyzed by hemagglutination assay. We found that a significantly higher antibody titer was obtained when SRBC were inoculated in the dorsal region of the foot than in the flank (Speroni *et al*, 2009a).

Since different levels of inflammatory and immune response were observed, we further evaluated the growth of B16F0 melanoma in both anatomic sites.

#### 4.1.4 Melanoma growth in different anatomic sites of the skin of mice

The development of B16F0 melanoma in the dorsal region of the foot showed a more malignant phenotype than when growing in the flank (Figure 3). The tumor in the flank (Figure 3A) showed large and numerous necrotic areas with leukocytic infiltration. Cells were disposed in an acinar-like structure, and intratumoral vascularization was scarce or absent. On the other hand, melanoma growing in the dorsal region of the foot (Figure 3B) showed a different architecture. Cells were distributed in irregular masses. High vascularization, and numerous inflammatory cells and hemosiderin deposits were observed. Another important difference with tumors growing in the flank was the absence of necrotic areas. Macroscopic and histological post-mortem examination of serial lung sections from hosts bearing B16F0 tumors showed neither macroscopic nor microscopic metastatic foci. Conversely, lung metastases were observed in 100% hosts bearing melanoma tumors in the dorsal region of the foot that survived beyond day 14 p.i. (mean) (Speroni *et al*, 2009a).

Importantly the hosts of tumors in the dorsal region of the foot had a poor survival compared to the hosts of flank tumors (Speroni *et al*, 2009a).

Our results clearly show that, even though the tumor cell line was the same, when injected in the mice, these cells originate remarkably different tumors which malignancy is dependent on the anatomic site of the skin. The skin of the dorsal region of the foot displayed a higher inflammatory and immune response most likely due to a higher cellular influx (Speroni *et al*, 2009a) than the flank skin. It is clear that several limitations exist with mouse models, particularly with the standard subcutaneous injection for the study of human cancer (Crnalic *et al*, 1997; Hirst & Balmain, 2004; Vitale *et al*, 2007). We have developed an alternative model to the standard inoculation of tumors into the flank of mice that, being equally easy to handle, might prove a better model for the study of melanoma progression and metastases (Speroni *et al*, 2009a; 2009b). Moreover, the model of tumor implantation in the dorsal region of the foot could be useful for the study of spontaneous metastases from tumors that do not originate metastases with the standard method of inoculating tumor cells in the flank.

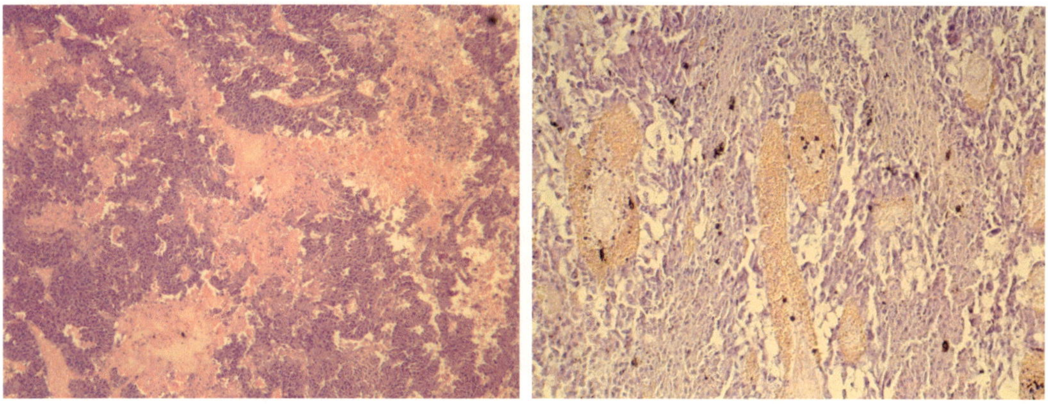

(a) (b)

Fig. 3. Histological analysis of tumors. Sections stained with hematoxylin-eosin from B16F0 tumor growing in the flank (a) and in the dorsal region of the foot (b). Original magnification 10X

### 4.2 *In vitro* models

Building more complex *in vitro* models of melanoma could improve our understanding on the initiation and different stages of the disease. Fibroblasts, one of the principle cell types of the stromal compartment, have shown to induce melanoma progression and invasion. The interaction between melanoma cells and fibroblasts creates a tumor promoting environment by the up-regulation of chemokines, cytokines, and growth factors. Factors secreted by fibroblasts and melanoma cells modulate collagen synthesis and promote tumor cell chemotaxis and invasion (Van Kempen *et al*, 2007). Moreover the invasive capacity of human melanoma cells is enhanced by the presence of fibroblasts (Bartolome *et al*, 2004; Li *et al*, 2009; Wandel *et al*, 2002). This culminates in an environment that supports growth and invasion. Cells growing in a 3D (three-dimensional) architecture resemble the *in vivo* situation more closely than do cells in conventional 2D cultures (monolayer). Because they can be finely tuned they offer the unique opportunity to dissect the molecular pathways and signaling between cell-cell and cell-extracellular matrix interaction. Moreover they could serve as a useful tool for the assessment of the drug efficacy in the treatment of melanoma in different stages.

## 5. Conclusion

The microenvironment plays a key role in tumor development to an extent that it poses the question whether a shift of paradigm in biology is needed in order to truly understand the phenomenon of cancer. The plasticity of cells is such that a cell adapts its phenotype according to what the systems imposes, i.e. the organization of the tissue and ultimately the self-organization of the system. In other words, the identity of a cell is not an intrinsic property of it but rather a condition dictated by spatio-temporal cues of the environment.

## 6. Acknowledgments

We would like to thank Dr. Oscar D. Bustuoabad for his help with experimental work and design and for critical discussions. This work was supported by grants from Consejo Nacional de Investigaciones Científicas y Técnicas and Universidad Nacional de Quilmes.

## 7. References

Bartolome, R.A.; Galvez, B.G.; Longo, N. Baleux, F.; Van Muijen, G.N.; Sanchez-Mateos, P.; Arroyo, A.G. & Teixido, J. (2004). Stromal cell-derived factor-1alpha promotes melanoma cell invasion across basement membranes involving stimulation of membrane-type 1 matrix metalloproteinase and Rho GTPase activities. *Cancer Res* 64(7):2534-43.

Bissell, M.J. & Radisky, D. (2001). Putting tumors in context. *Nat. Rev. Cancer* 1, 46-54.

Chambers, A.F.; Groom, A.C. & MacDonald, I.C. (2002). Dissemination and growth of cancer cells in metastatic sites. *Nat. Rev. Cancer* 2, 563-572.

Chang, H.Y.; Chi, J.T.; Dudoit, S.; Bondre, C.; van de Rijn, M.; Botstein, D. & Brown, P.O. (2002) Diversity, topographic differentiation, and in human positional memory fibroblasts. *Proc Natl Acad Sci USA* 99:12877–82.

Coleman, A.B. & Lugo, T.G. (1998) Normal human melanocytes that express a bFGF transgene still require exogenous bFGF for growth *in vitro*. *J Invest Dermatol* May; 110(5):793-9.

Crnalic, S. Häkansson, I.; Boquist, L.; Löfvenberg, R. & Brostrom L.A. (1997). A novel spontaneous metastasis model of human osteosarcoma developed using orthotopic transplantation of intact tumor tissue into tibia of nude mice. *Clin Exp Metastasis*; 15(2):164-72.

Cua, A.B.; Wilhelm, K.P. & Maibach, H.I. (1990). Elastic properties of human skin: relation to age, sex, and anatomical region. *Arch Dermatol Res*; 282: 283–288.

Curiel-Lewandrowski, C.; Nijsten, T.; Gomez, M.L.; Hollestein, L.M.; Atkins, M.B. & Stern, R.S. (2011). Long-Term Use of Nonsteroidal Anti-inflammatory Drugs Decreases the Risk of Cutaneous Melanoma: Results of a United States Case-Control Study. *J Invest Dermatol,* Mar 10. [Epub ahead of print].

Escoffier, C.; de Rigal, J.; Rochefort, A.; Vasselet, R.; Lévêque, J.L. & Agache, P.G. (1989) Age-related mechanical properties of human skin: an *in vivo* study. *J Invest Dermatol.* Sep;93(3):353-7.

Fidler, I.J. (2002). Critical determinants of metastasis. *Semin. Cancer Biol.* 12 , 89-96.

Fiuraskova, M.; Brychtova, S.; Sedlakova, E.; Benes, P.; Zalesak, B.; Hlobilkova, A.; Tichy, M. & Kolar, Z. (2005). Molecular changes in PDEGF and bFGF in malignant melanomas in relation to the stromal microenvironment. *Anticancer Res.* Nov-Dec; 25(6B):4299-303.

Flaherty, K.T. (2010). Narrative review: BRAF opens the door for therapeutic advances in melanoma. *Ann Intern Med.* Nov 2; 153(9):587-91.

Garbuzenko, E.; Nagler, A.; Pickholtz, D.; Gillery, P.; Reich, R.; Maquart, F.X. & Levi-Schaffer, F. (2002). Human mast cells stimulate fibroblast proliferation, collagen synthesis and lattice contraction: a direct role for mast cells in skin fibrosis. *Clin Exp Allergy* Feb; 32(2):237-46.

Hanahan, D. & Weinberg, R.A. (2000). The hallmarks of cancer. *Cell* 100, 57-70.

Harvima, I.T. (2008). Induction of matrix metalloproteinase-9 in keratinocytes by histamine. *J Invest Dermatol* Dec; 128(12):2748-50.

Hirst, G.L. & Balmain, A. (2004). Forty years of cancer modelling in the mouse *European Journal of Cancer*; 40:1974-1980.

Hodi, F.S.; O'Day, S.J.; McDermott, D.F.; Weber, R.W.; Sosman, J.A.; Haanen. J.B.; Gonzalez, R.; Robert, C.; Schadendorf, D.; Hassel, J.C.; Akerley, W.; van den Eertwegh, A.J.; Lutzky, J.; Lorigan, P.; Vaubel, J.M.; Linette, G.P.; Hogg, D.; Ottensmeier, C.H.; Lebbé, C.; Peschel, C.; Quirt, I.; Clark, J.I.; Wolchok, J.D.; Weber, J.S.; Tian, J.; Yellin, M.J.; Nichol, G.M.; Hoos, A. & Urba, W.J. (2010) Improved survival with ipilimumab in patients with metastatic melanoma. *N Engl J Med.* 2010 Aug 19; 363(8):711-23. Erratum in: *N Engl J Med.* Sep 23; 363(13):1290.

Hussein, M.R. (2008). Extracutaneous malignant melanomas. *Cancer Invest.* Jun; 26(5):516-34.

Illmensee, K. & Mintz, B. (1976) Totipotency and normal differentiation of a single teratocarcinoma cell cloned by injection into blastocysts. *Proc Natl Acad Sci USA;* 549-53.

Janssens, A.S.; Heide, R.; den Hollander, J.C.; Mulder, P.G.; Tank, B. & Oranje, A.P. (2005) Mast cell distribution in normal adult skin. *J Clin Pathol* Mar; 58(3):285-9.

Kasemeier-Kulesa, J.C.; Teddy, J.M.; Postovit, L.M.; Seftor, E.A.; Seftor, R.E.; Hendrix, M.J. & Kulesa, P.M. (2008). Reprogramming multipotent tumor cells with the embryonic neural crest microenvironment. *Dev Dyn.* Oct; 237(10):2657-66.

Kessel RW, Monaco L, Marchisio MA (1963) The specificity of the cytotoxic action of silica-a study *in vitro. Br J Exp Pathol.* Aug; 44:351-64.

Li, L.; Dragulev, B.; Zigrino, P.; Mauch, C.; and Fox, J.W. (2009). The invasive potential of human melanoma cell lines correlates with their ability to alter fibroblast gene expression *in vitro* and the stromal microenvironment *in vivo.* Int J Cancer 125(8):1796-804.

McGrath, J.A.; Eady, R.A.J.; and Pope, F.M. (2010). Anatomy and Organization of Human Skin. In: *Rook's Textbook of Dermatology,* Volume 1, Eighth Edition, chapter 3. Online ISBN 9781444317633.

Röck, K.; Grandoch, M.; Majora, M.; Krutmann, J.; and Fischer, J.W. (2011). Collagen fragments inhibit hyaluronan synthesis in skin fibroblasts in response to UVB: New insights into mechanisms of matrix remodelling. *J Biol Chem.* Mar 17. [Epub ahead of print].

Smalls, L.K.; Randall Wickett, R.; and Visscher, M.O. (2006). Effect of dermal thickness, tissue composition, and body site on skin biomechanical properties. *Skin Res Technol.* Feb; 12(1):43-9.

Seftor, E.A.; Meltzer, P.S.; Kirschmann, D.A.; Margaryan, N.V.; Seftor, R.E.B.; and Hendrix, M.J.C. (2006). The epigenetic reprogramming of poorly aggressive melanoma cells by a metastatic microenvironment. *J Cell Mol Med;* 10(1): 174-196.

Sonnenschein, C.; and Soto, A.M. (1999). *The Society of cells,* BIOS Scientific Publishers Limited, ISBN 1-85996-276-9, Oxford.

Speroni, L.; Bustuoabad, V. de los A.; Gasparri, J.; Chiaramoni, N.S.; Taira, M.C.; Ruggiero, R.A.; and Alonso, S. del V. (2009a). Alternative site of implantation affects tumor malignancy and metastatic potential in mice: Its comparison to the flank model. *Cancer Bio Ther*; 8:375-9.

Speroni, L.; Gasparri, J.; Bustuoabad, V. de los A.; Chiaramoni, N.S.; Smagur, A.; Szala, S.; Taira, M.C.; and Alonso, S. del V. (2009b). Antitumoral effect of IL-12 gene transfected via liposomes into B16F0 cells. *Acta Biochim. Pol.*, 56(2) 249-253.

Stoitzner, P. (2010). The Langerhans cell controversy: are they immunostimulatory or immunoregulatory cells of the skin immune system? *Immunol Cell Biol.* May-Jun; 88(4):348-50.

Thomas, J.A.; Biggerstaff, M.; Sloane, J.P.; and Easton, D.F. (1984). Immunological and histochemical analysis of regional variations of epidermal Langerhans cells in normal human skin. *Histochem J.* May; 16(5):507-19.

Tseng, W.H.; and Martinez, S.R. (2010). Tumor Location Predicts Survival in Cutaneous Head and Neck Melanoma. *J Surg Res.* 2010 Nov 10. [Epub ahead of print]

Van Den Brenk, H.A.; Stone, M.; Kelly, H.; Orton, C.; and Sharpington, C. (1974). Promotion of growth of tumour cells in acutely inflamed tissues. *Br J Cancer* Sep; 30(3):246-60.

Van Kempen, L.C.; Van Muijen, G.N.; and Ruiter, D.J. (2007). Melanoma progression in a changing environment. *Eur J Cell Biol* 86(2):65-7.

Vitale S.; Cambien. B.; Karimdjee, B.F.; Barthel, R.; Staccini, P.; Luci, C.; Breittmayer, V.; Anjuère, F.; Schmid-Alliana, A.; and Schmid-Antomarchi H (2007). Tissue-specific differential antitumour effect of molecular forms of fractalkine in a mouse model of metastatic colon cancer. *Gut*; 56:365-372.

Wandel, E.; Raschke, A.; Hildebrandt, G.; Eberle, J.; Dummer, R.; Anderegg, U.; and Saalbach, (2002). Fibroblasts enhance the invasive capacity of melanoma cells *in vitro*. *Arch Dermatol Res* Feb; 293(12):601-8.

Wang, L.; Bursch, L.S.; Kissenpfennig, A.; Malissen, B.; Jameson, S.C.; and Hogquist, K.A. (2008). Langerin expressing cells promote skin immune responses under defined conditions. *J Immunol* Apr 1; 180(7):4722-7.

Yamaguchi, Y.; Itami, S.; Tarutani, M.; Hosokawa, K.; Miura, H.; and Yoshikawa, K. (1999). Regulation of keratin 9 in nonpalmoplantar keratinocytes by palmoplantar fibroblasts through epithelial-mesenchymal interactions. *J Invest Dermatol* 112:483–8

Yamaguchi, Y.; Hearing, V.J.; Itami, S.; Yoshikawa, K.; and Katayama, I. (2005). Mesenchymal-epithelial interactions in the skin: aiming for site-specific tissue regeneration. *J Dermatol Sci* 40:1–9.

# 3

# Circulating Melanoma Cells

Mel Ziman[1, 2]
[1]School of Exercise, Biomedical and Health Science, Edith Cowan University;
[2]School of Pathology and Laboratory Medicine, University of Western Australia, Australia

## 1. Introduction

Cutaneous Melanoma is an aggressive cancer which accounts for 80% of skin cancer deaths. Australia has the highest incidence world-wide and rates are increasing annually (10,000 new cases and 1,700 deaths per year). Notably it is the most common cancer in 15-39 year olds and the leading cancer related cause of death in young males (WA Cancer Registry 2007). In the USA, incidence is rising faster than other cancers, with 60,000 new cases and 8,000 deaths in 2007 [1].

Mortality rates remain high due to metastasis of the tumour. Once melanoma has metastasised, survival is commonly 6 to 9 months, with 5-year survival rate less than 40% [2-4]. Several prognostic factors have been identified, based upon pathological evaluation of the primary tumour [5] and lymph node metastases [6]. However, metastatic disease particularly micrometastasis, is difficult to detect and occurs in over 30% of patients, including 8-30% of patients with *in situ* melanoma [7-9] and 15% of patients whose lymph nodes are negative at the time of surgical intervention [10,11]. In addition, metastasis can occur up to 35 years after diagnosis [12]. Effective therapies providing long term survival are very limited (<20%), often due to drug resistance associated with prevailing undetected mutations or acquisition of new mutations. Surprisingly few studies [13-15] have monitored circulating cells as a means of determining disease progression, and/or treatment efficacy or for design of personalised treatment strategies.

A great deal of information has been compiled in an attempt to identify prognostic factors that correlate with clinical outcomes. Current clinical staging is performed using measures of the pathological features of the primary tumour, lymph node and distant metastases [6], as well as LDH levels and now also, genetic changes in the primary tumour [16-19]. The inability to accurately predict melanoma progression, may be related to the fact that the majority of studies use primary and less often, metastatic tumour tissue to stratify patients and delineate prognostic markers. Very few studies analyse the circulating tumour cell (CTC) phenotype that gives rise to the metastases. There is therefore an unmet need for detailed analyses of CTCs to provide early identification of metastatic risk and prognosis and evaluation of adjuvant therapies.

## 2. Circulating tumour cells

Millions of cells are shed from a tumour every day (approx 4 × $10^6$ cells/g primary tumour) [20], and these cells invade lymphatic and/or venous circulatory systems. Once they have entered the blood stream they become a circulating melanoma cell population. The fact that metastasis can occur many years after surgery indicates that disseminated tumour cells may remain in the blood stream for decades, evading the immune system and apparently remaining quiescent. Interestingly, few establish clinically diagnosed metastasis [21,22]. Those that do, particularly after many years, must acquire some activating change [12].

Since most cancer patients die as a result of metastatic spread rather than from their primary tumours [22,23], metastatic inefficiency of the primary tumour is likely overcome by the large number of tumour cells that enter the systemic circulation daily, estimated to be up to $\sim 4 \times 10^6$ tumour cells released per gram of primary tumour [20,24]. Several studies have shown that the number of CTCs in patient peripheral blood increases with increasing stages of melanoma [25,26-29, 30]. Yet the variety and phenotype of these CTCs, their ability to remain in circulation for many years thus evading the immune system, and their activation causing metastasis, remain largely unexplored, particularly for melanoma.

## 3. Melanoma metastasis

When cancer cells detach from the primary tumour and enter into blood vessels (or the lymphatic system), they can do so actively or passively [7]. Passive cell intravasation, where cells are simply dislodged from the primary tumour, occurs as a result of increased hemodynamic flow [22,31,32]. By contrast, active migration occurs in cells which have separated from their neighbours and actively migrate. In addition, many circulating cells are apoptotic or necrotic and are unlikely to survive immune cell destruction [33-37].

The question remains then, is there a phenotypic and/or genotypic difference between cells that are able to survive in the circulation and metastasise from those that cannot? Fundamentally, gene expression signatures that prompt a melanoma cell to proliferate *in situ* must be different from those that permit a cell to actively migrate, and survive as a circulating cell, and then establish a secondary tumour. Several studies have documented the differential gene expression associated with malignant progression of melanoma. Pathways associated with initiation of melanoma metastasis include the transition from radial to vertical growth phase, epithelial to mesenchymal transitions, alterations in cell adhesion properties and suppression of apoptosis [38,39]. Included are several key steps; loss of adhesion, dermal invasion, migration from the primary site, intravasation followed by survival in the blood, migration into target tissues, and increased proliferation in the new tissue microenvironment followed by orchestration of angiogenesis at the new site [40].

Normal melanocyte cells in the epidermis are tethered tightly to other melanocyte cells and surrounding keratinocytes by cell surface molecules [41]. Once they become proliferative and malignant, melanoma cells lose many of the cell surface proteins that secure the tight epithelial cell–cell adhesive interactions [33]. One of the key cell surface proteins, CDH1 (Cadherin 1, E-cadherin), is bound via its cytoplasmic tail to α-catenin and β-catenin, and thus to the actin cytoskeleton to maintain close cell junctions [42]. Once melanoma cells become invasive, they no longer express CDH1, but express rather CDH5 (V-cadherin) or CDH2 (N-cadherin), proteins synonymous with the start of an epithelial to- mesenchymal transition (EMT) [43]. The EMT process, commonly utilised by migrating cells during embryonic development, involves switching of polarised epithelial cells to contractile, motile mesenchymal progenitor cells, and is triggered by secretion of growth factors (EGF (epithelial growth factor), FGF (fibroblast growth factor)) and chemotactic/pro-migratory factors SF/HGF (hepatocyte growth factor) and chemokines from stromal fibroblasts and macrophages. This secretion induces intracellular transduction pathways (Wnt, Notch) which in turn activate transcription factors (Twist and SNAI1 and 2) [44,45] bringing about the invasion of melanoma cells from the epidermal, dermal border to invasion of the dermis and entry of the cells into the circulation and metastasis [27,46]. The invasive process is also the result of activated signalling cascades such as the NEDD9-DOCK3-Rac (Neural precursor cell expressed developmentally down-regulated protein 9- Dorsocross3 - Rac) pathway. The movement of these cells through the extracellular matrix and their migration towards blood vessels is assisted by integrin and matrix metalloproteinases [27,47-49].

The next step in the active migration process is the attraction of tumour cells to lymph and blood vessels, a process mediated by ligand-receptor interactions between tumour cells and the stroma or endothelial cells. Tumour cells secrete CSF1 (colony stimulating factor 1) and growth factors such as EGF which activate the formation and proliferation of tumour-associated macrophages in the stroma. These cells in turn secrete chemokines including SDF-1 (stromal-cell-derived factor 1), SCL/CCL21 (chemokine C-C motif ligand 21) and I309/CCL1 (chemokine C-C motif ligand 1), which assist with chemotaxis of tumour cells expressing the appropriate receptors, CXCR4, CCR7 and CCR8, into blood vessels [27,50,51].

Whether cells actively move toward and into nearby blood vessels or whether the process is passive and coincidental may be of some significance. Expression of specific genes that assist entry into the circulation, either passively or actively, may determine cell survival and metastatic ability. That is cells expressing genes associated with EMT, or cell migration, may be more prone to tumourigenesis and metastasis.

Model systems that quantify circulating cells leaving the tumour, show, in fact, that $3–4\times10^6$ malignant cells/day are shed per gram of tumour suggesting that millions of cells may be shed from a tumour every day [24,52,53]. Characterisation of these circulating tumour cells in patients with metastatic prostate and breast cancer indicates that they are predominantly apoptotic [37] or necrotic and unlikely to survive [34,35,36]. Furthermore, circulating cells are often sheared and destroyed as they leave the tumour and enter the circulation. Moreover, immune cells in the circulation destroy the bulk of circulating cells and prevent all but the most active from producing metastases [33,54].

Some cells do however survive for long periods of time in the vasculature [55,33] where they are usually found in clumps or clusters known as circulating tumour microemboli, surrounded by a "cloak" of platelets and leukocytes which assists tumour cell survival for some time by evasion of the immune system [56-58]. Moreover, melanoma cell evasion of the immune system and thus survival in the blood stream is also due to the intracellular localisation of the ligand which typically activates NKD2D receptors on natural killer (NK) cells [59]. Thus evasion from attack by natural killer (NK) cells affords melanoma cells a powerful means of protection from NK cell mediated cytotoxicity. Metastatic melanoma cells also develop resistance to inhibitory cytokines through the modification of oncostatin M receptors [60,61]. With such an arsenal of survival mechanisms, melanoma cells may indeed survive in the circulation for long periods of time.

## 4. Detection of CTCs

Various methods have been used to quantify and characterise CTCs, including indirect methods, namely qRT-PCR [25,62-65], and direct analyses such as immunomagnetic bead capture, or fibre-optic array scanning technology [28,29,66,67,68]. From these results it is obvious that; a) CTCs are present at relatively low concentrations; one tumour cell per $10^6$ to $10^7$

normal blood cells or on average, 1 cell per ml of blood [69,70,71]; b) the number of cells appears to be related to stage [2,25,72]; c) melanoma cell markers differ with respect to stage [73]; and c) CTC gene expression differs from that of the primary tumour [28,29].
Quantitative RT-PCR has typically detected expression of melanocytic genes such as tyrosinase (TYR) [74, 75] since normal melanocytes are not thought to circulate in peripheral blood and therefore detection of transcripts from melanocytic genes should correlate to identification of CTCs [72,76]. The sensitivity and specificity of PCR for circulating melanoma cells is increased by analysis of multiple markers [76], and these commonly include melan-A (MLANA), beta-1,4-N-acetyl-galactosaminyl transferase 1 (B4GALNT1), silver homolog (SILV), melanoma cell adhesion molecule (MCAM), melanoma associated antigen p97 (MFI2), melanoma antigen family A3 (MAGEA3) and microphthalmia-associated transcription factor 4 (MITF4) [63,64,77,78]. Several studies have shown that levels of gene expression associated with melanoma CTCs in patient blood correlate to AJCC stage, survival and disease recurrence [2,25,72].
Alternately, CTCs can be positively selected from whole blood using immunomagnetic beads [66]. With this system, CTC numbers are shown to positively correlate with cell stage and be an independent prognostic indicator of progression-free and overall survival for breast cancer [79], melanoma [28] and many other cancers [71].

## 5. Differential gene expression profiles of circulating

The question remains then, how do we differentiate those cells that are able to survive in the circulation from those that cannot? Moreover, can we differentiate actively metastatic melanoma cells from those that are quiescent or apoptotic and is there a need to do so? It is thought that any cancer cell can acquire the ability to disseminate at any time, even early and prior to overt tumour formation [11,80]. For heterogeneous tumours such as melanoma, an unstable, genetically-variant, invasive cell may metastasise at any time [27]. Whether this is possible for all melanoma cells remains to be confirmed, but recent experiments suggest that all melanoma cells can initiate a new tumour when xenotransplanted into immunocompromised mice [81].
By contrast a plethora of information gathered over many decades indicates that melanoma cells express stage related markers that are associated with a more or less invasive tumour [73]. In Fig 1, for example, we have shows differential stage related expression of the melanoma cell adhesion molecule, MCAM. At early disease stages, MCAM is found in <50% cells of 4/10 primary tumours, as opposed to metastatic tissue, where all cells are MCAM+ (5/5, 93% cells).[82]. MCSP, on the other hand, is found on >80% of melanoma cells at all stages I-IV [14,83-85] so its expression is not stage related. CTCs are also likely to have differential gene expression signatures related to stage and these may differ relative to those of the primary tumour as previously demonstrated [28,29]. It is apparent that merely identifying the presence of CTCs using for example MCSP, does not necessarily provide evidence of disease progression. It may be necessary to analyse CTC phenotype or genotype to obtain more prognostic information.
In recent years a number of researchers have shown the existence of a sub-set of tumour initiating or melanoma stem cells within the primary tumour [86-90]. These cells are believed to be responsible for relapse and metastasis by virtue of their ability to survive treatment and initiate new tumour formation. Rare cancer stem cells would therefore be capable of effectively managing the metastatic process [91] and would act as stem cells for metastasis

formation at a new site [69]. Melanoma stem cell markers include JARID1B (jumonji, AT rich interactive domain 1B) [92], ABCB5 (ATP-Binding Cassette Subfamily B (MDR/TAP) Member 5), ABCG2 (ATP-binding cassette sub-family G member 2), MDR1 (Multi-Drug Resistance 1) [87,93-99] and more recently CD271 [100].

## 6. Markers of metastasis – Can they be identified in CTCs?

A plethora of studies have focused on identification of markers with sufficient specificity to accurately predict melanoma progression. Although many of these were identified using primary tissue or melanoma cell lines, they have been used for the multitude of CTC studies conducted thus far [72,101-103]. For qRT-PCR analysis of CTCs include SILV, MLANA, TYR, MAGEA3 and MAGE-A10 [25,62-64,72,104], or more recently, ABCB5 [86,87] [105]. From high throughput analyses of melanoma gene expression, several key progression pathways have been identified [38,39,103,106,107] but remain to be tested as informative for CTC analysis. Key amongst these pathways are: tyrosine kinase receptors (TKRs) (e.g. VEGFR, ERBB2, TGF-betaR), the Ras / Raf / MEK / ERK pathway, the PI3K / Akt / PTEN / mTOR pathway, cell cycle regulation pathways (Rb / p53 / p16INKA / p14ARF / HDM2), epigenetic gene expression regulation and DNA repair pathways (DNA methylation, histone acetylation, RNA interference), apoptotic pathways (e.g. death receptors: FAS, TRAILR, TNFR; mitochondrial pathway: Bcl2 family), common apoptosis effectors, protein chaperoning, degradation (HSP, proteasome) [25,108,109] and epithelial to mesenchymal transition (reviewed in [110]). A thorough screening of CTCs from metastatic melanoma patients for these activated pathways needs to be performed so as to establish their involvement in CTC survival, proliferation and intra- and extravasation. By detecting the presence and/or levels of genes associated with these activated / metastatic pathways, CTC analyses might be significantly enhanced.

Several reports also suggest that, in melanoma cells, altered regulation of melanocyte developmental pathways, are key to the acquisition of metastatic potential [111-116]. Indeed, melanoma metastasis reflects to some extent the migratory capacity of melanoblast developmental precursors, the neural crest cells. Moreover, genes that are critical for melanocyte development have been recognised as important factors of melanoma growth, for example MITF, DCT and SOX10 all function to maintain the stem or progenitor cell population of melanoblasts during migration from the neural crest and during melanoblast survival in the hair follicle niche [72,110,117-119] and may be equally important in melanoma cell maintenance and migration. It is important then to identify the expression of these developmental genes in CTCs and assess their association with metastasis.

## 7. Mutations in circulating melanoma cells

There is increasing evidence that melanoma metastasis is activated by mutations in multiple pathways including MAPK-ERK, PI3/AKT, PTEN and retinoblastoma pathways that regulate cyclin-dependent kinases (CDKs) (Table 1) [120,121]. MITF, a key transcription factor, is amplified in melanoma, and also regulated by c-KIT via MAPK/ERK and PI3/AKT pathways [122]. Differing mutations in multiple pathways have also now been identified for different melanoma subtypes [120,123,124]. It remains for stage and subtype related mutations to be profiled in CTCs.

There are currently eight defined subtypes of melanoma, based on mutations in key melanoma genes, but not all melanoma cases fit into these subtypes [125]. The majority of melanomas will have a mutation in either *BRAF* (57%) or NRAS (17%) but rarely have both [124]. Further details about known mutations are described below.

| | Pathway(s) activated by mutations |
|---|---|
| 1. | MAPK |
| 2. | c-KIT |
| 3. | GNAQ/GNA11 |
| 4. | NRAS |
| 5. | MITF |
| 6. | AKT/PI3K |
| 7. | CDK |
| 8. | P53/BCL |
| 9. | Undetermined |

Table 1. Melanoma subtypes - adapted from Vidwans et al. [125]

Many new treatments being developed for melanoma target these specific molecular pathways which are associated with tumour progression. Unfortunately the effectiveness of these potential treatments has so far been limited by drug resistance as a result of newly acquired mutations [126] or the inadequate analysis of existing additional mutations. Since the presence or absence of certain mutations can drastically effect the success of targeted treatments it would be of benefit to develop a detailed profile of mutations that exist in an individual patient to maximise efficacy of treatment. One possibility is to use CTCs for stage and subtype related mutation analysis.

## 8. Conclusion

From our own (Fig. 1) and many other reported studies [33-36,54], it is clear that positivity *per se* is not necessarily a prognostic indicator i.e. it is possible that not all circulating cells establish successful tissue metastases. Thus a more comprehensive set of experiments and additional markers are required to better understand the diagnostic and prognostic significance of circulating melanoma cells. These issues are best addressed by isolation, characterisation and quantification of circulating melanoma cells. Additionally, newly identified prognostic markers need to be measured in CTCs and assessed relative to patient outcome to delineate the metastatic potential of circulating melanoma cells and their usefulness as a prognostic indicator [72,127].

We hypothesise that the ability of circulating melanoma cells to become activated, proliferative and migratory from a quiescent cell depends on several key genes. An alternate hypothesis is that malignant cells disseminate from the primary tumour early in tumourigenesis and remain in a clinically latent state until either the cells themselves or the host environment is receptive to the development of metastases. Quintana and colleagues [81] and more recently Roesch et al., [92] show that single human melanoma cells with no specifically identifiable gene signature can re-establish melanoma tumours when xenotransplanted into severely immunocompromised mice. It is of paramount importance therefore that we identify pathways associated with metastasis of circulating cells, ie those pathways that confer metastatic properties on quiescent melanoma stem cells capable of evading human anti-tumour immune responses. Furthermore, it is necessary to identify whether CTC numbers, gene expression profiles, or a combination of both, are key factors in patient outcome. It also remains to be seen whether tumour related DNA mutations and the resultant activated proteins provide more accurate measures of melanoma progression. A combination of marker types is likely to be more accurate than measures that determine the presence and quantity of CTCs alone. Future studies in this field will need to be performed to address the multitude of issues alluded to in this chapter.

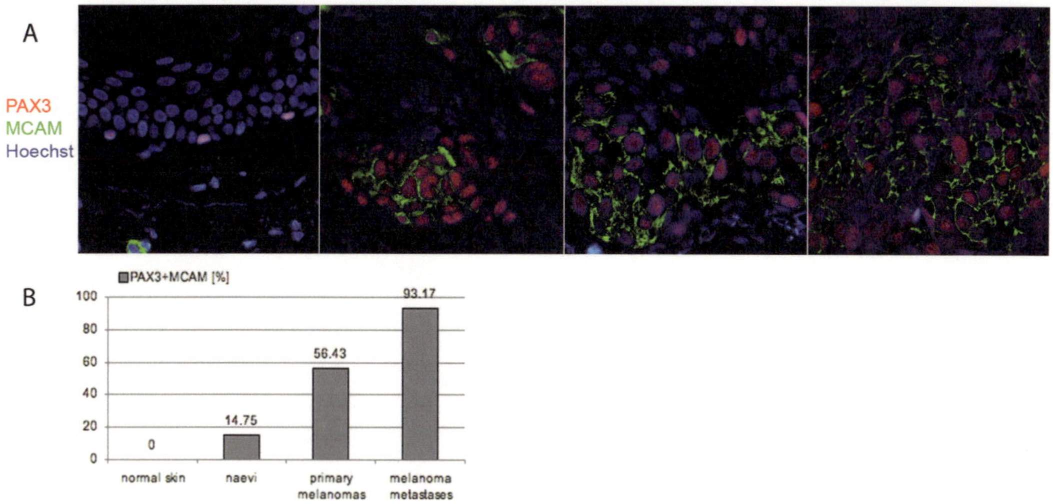


Fig. 1. A) Double immunofluorescent staining showing PAX3 (mouse monoclonal antibody, DSHB) and MCAM co-expression in normal skin (epidermal melanocytes), naevus, primary melanoma and melanoma metastasis respectively. Lines in (A) demarcate the epidermal-dermal border (EDB) or epidermal surface (ES). B) Graph showing the overall number of PAX3, MCAM double-labelled cells in normal skin, naevi, primary melanomas and melanoma metastases. Each column represents a percentage of PAX3-positive, MCAM-positive, averaged across all samples. Note: MCAM positive cells were all PAX3 positive (revised from [73])

## 9. References

[1] Lee KB, Weinstock MA, Risica PM. Components of a successful intervention for monthly skin self-examination for early detection of melanoma: the "Check It Out" trial. *J Am Acad Dermatol.* Jun 2008;58(6):1006-1012.

[2] Hoon DS, Bostick P, Kuo C, et al. Molecular markers in blood as surrogate prognostic indicators of melanoma recurrence. *Cancer Res.* Apr 15 2000;60(8):2253-2257.

[3] Postovit LM, Seftor EA, Seftor RE, Hendrix MJ. Targeting Nodal in malignant melanoma cells. *Expert Opin Ther Targets.* Apr 2007;11(4):497-505.

[4] Shivers SC, Wang X, Li W, et al. Molecular staging of malignant melanoma: correlation with clinical outcome. *JAMA.* Oct 28 1998;280(16):1410-1415.

[5] Breslow A. Tumor thickness, level of invasion and node dissection in stage I cutaneous melanoma. *Ann Surg.* Nov 1975;182(5):572-575.

[6] Balch CM, Buzaid AC, Soong SJ, et al. Final version of the American Joint Committee on Cancer staging system for cutaneous melanoma. *J Clin Oncol.* Aug 15 2001;19(16):3635-3648.

[7] Michaelson JS, Cheongsiatmoy JA, Dewey F, et al. Spread of human cancer cells occurs with probabilities indicative of a nongenetic mechanism. *Br J Cancer.* Nov 28 2005;93(11):1244-1249.

[8] Koyanagi K, Kuo C, Nakagawa T, et al. Multimarker quantitative real-time PCR detection of circulating melanoma cells in peripheral blood: relation to disease stage in melanoma patients. *Clin Chem.* Jun 2005;51(6):981-988.

[9] Zalaudek I, Horn M, Richtig E, Hodl S, Kerl H, Smolle J. Local recurrence in melanoma in situ: influence of sex, age, site of involvement and therapeutic modalities. *Br J Dermatol.* Apr 2003;148(4):703-708.

[10] Jack A, Boyes C, Aydin N, Alam K, Wallack M. The treatment of melanoma with an emphasis on immunotherapeutic strategies. *Surg Oncol.* Jul 2006;15(1):13-24.

[11] Weight RM, Viator JA, Dale PS, Caldwell CW, Lisle AE. Photoacoustic detection of metastatic melanoma cells in the human circulatory system. *Opt Lett.* Oct 15 2006;31(20):2998-3000.

[12] Singh AD, Rennie IG, Kivela T, Seregard S, Grossniklaus H. The Zimmerman-McLean-Foster hypothesis: 25 years later. *Br J Ophthalmol.* Jul 2004;88(7):962-967.

[13] Pinzani P, Mazzini C, Salvianti F, et al. Tyrosinase mRNA levels in the blood of uveal melanoma patients: correlation with the number of circulating tumor cells and tumor progression. *Melanoma Res.* Aug 2010;20(4):303-310.

[14] Kitago M, Koyanagi K, Nakamura T, et al. mRNA expression and BRAF mutation in circulating melanoma cells isolated from peripheral blood with high molecular weight melanoma-associated antigen-specific monoclonal antibody beads. *Clin Chem.* Apr 2009;55(4):757-764.

[15] Board RE, Ellison G, Orr MC, et al. Detection of BRAF mutations in the tumour and serum of patients enrolled in the AZD6244 (ARRY-142886) advanced melanoma phase II study. *Br J Cancer.* Nov 17 2009;101(10):1724-1730.

[16] Eton O, Legha SS, Moon TE, et al. Prognostic factors for survival of patients treated systemically for disseminated melanoma. *J Clin Oncol.* Mar 1998;16(3):1103-1111.

[17] Francken AB, Accortt NA, Shaw HM, et al. Prognosis and determinants of outcome following locoregional or distant recurrence in patients with cutaneous melanoma. *Ann Surg Oncol.* May 2008;15(5):1476-1484.

[18] Leiter U, Meier F, Schittek B, Garbe C. The natural course of cutaneous melanoma. *J Surg Oncol.* Jul 1 2004;86(4):172-178.

[19] Thompson JF, Scolyer RA, Kefford RF. Cutaneous melanoma in the era of molecular profiling. *Lancet.* Aug 1 2009;374(9687):362-365.

[20] Fidler IJ, Yano S, Zhang RD, Fujimaki T, Bucana CD. The seed and soil hypothesis: vascularisation and brain metastases. *Lancet Oncol.* Jan 2002;3(1):53-57.

[21] Chen Y, Clegg NJ, Scher HI. Anti-androgens and androgen-depleting therapies in prostate cancer: new agents for an established target. *Lancet Oncol.* Oct 2009;10(10):981-991.

[22] Bockhorn M, Jain RK, Munn LL. Active versus passive mechanisms in metastasis: do cancer cells crawl into vessels, or are they pushed? *Lancet Oncol.* May 2007;8(5):444-448.

[23] Chen LL, Blumm N, Christakis NA, Barabasi AL, Deisboeck TS. Cancer metastasis networks and the prediction of progression patterns. *Br J Cancer.* Sep 1 2009;101(5):749-758.

[24] Butler TP, Gullino PM. Quantitation of cell shedding into efferent blood of mammary adenocarcinoma. *Cancer Res.* Mar 1975;35(3):512-516.

[25] Mocellin S, Hoon D, Ambrosi A, Nitti D, Rossi CR. The prognostic value of circulating tumor cells in patients with melanoma: a systematic review and meta-analysis. *Clin Cancer Res.* Aug 1 2006;12(15):4605-4613.

[26] Ikuta Y, Nakatsura T, Kageshita T, et al. Highly sensitive detection of melanoma at an early stage based on the increased serum secreted protein acidic and rich in cysteine and glypican-3 levels. *Clin Cancer Res.* Nov 15 2005;11(22):8079-8088.

[27] Chiang AC, Massague J. Molecular basis of metastasis. *N Engl J Med.* Dec 25 2008;359(26):2814-2823.

[28] Ulmer A, Schmidt-Kittler O, Fischer J, et al. Immunomagnetic enrichment, genomic characterization, and prognostic impact of circulating melanoma cells. *Clin Cancer Res.* Jan 15 2004;10(2):531-537.

[29] Ulmer A, Beutel J, Susskind D, et al. Visualization of circulating melanoma cells in peripheral blood of patients with primary uveal melanoma. *Clin Cancer Res.* Jul 15 2008;14(14):4469-4474.

[30] Husemann Y, Geigl JB, Schubert F, et al. Systemic spread is an early step in breast cancer. *Cancer Cell.* Jan 2008;13(1):58-68.

[31] Dvorak HF. Tumors: wounds that do not heal. Similarities between tumor stroma generation and wound healing. *N Engl J Med.* Dec 25 1986;315(26):1650-1659.

[32] Liang S, Slattery MJ, Wagner D, Simon SI, Dong C. Hydrodynamic shear rate regulates melanoma-leukocyte aggregation, melanoma adhesion to the endothelium, and subsequent extravasation. *Ann Biomed Eng.* Apr 2008;36(4):661-671.

[33] Paterlini-Brechot P, Benali NL. Circulating tumor cells (CTC) detection: clinical impact and future directions. *Cancer Lett.* Aug 18 2007;253(2):180-204.

[34] Swartz MA, Kristensen CA, Melder RJ, et al. Cells shed from tumours show reduced clonogenicity, resistance to apoptosis, and in vivo tumorigenicity. *Br J Cancer.* Nov 1999;81(5):756-759.

[35] Larson CJ, Moreno JG, Pienta KJ, et al. Apoptosis of circulating tumor cells in prostate cancer patients. *Cytometry A.* Nov 2004;62(1):46-53.

[36] Mehes G, Witt A, Kubista E, Ambros PF. Circulating breast cancer cells are frequently apoptotic. *Am J Pathol.* Jul 2001;159(1):17-20.

[37] Glinsky GV. Apoptosis in metastatic cancer cells. *Crit Rev Oncol Hematol.* Apr 1997;25(3):175-186.

[38] Hoek KS, Schlegel NC, Brafford P, et al. Metastatic potential of melanomas defined by specific gene expression profiles with no BRAF signature. *Pigment Cell Res.* Aug 2006;19(4):290-302.

[39] Mandruzzato S, Callegaro A, Turcatel G, et al. A gene expression signature associated with survival in metastatic melanoma. *J Transl Med.* 2006;4:50.

[40] Mazzocca A, Carloni V. The metastatic process: methodological advances and pharmacological challenges. *Curr Med Chem.* 2009;16(14):1704-1717.

[41] Van Den Bossche K, Naeyaert JM, Lambert J. The quest for the mechanism of melanin transfer. *Traffic.* Jul 2006;7(7):769-778.

[42] Vogelmann R, Nguyen-Tat MD, Giehl K, Adler G, Wedlich D, Menke A. TGFbeta-induced downregulation of E-cadherin-based cell-cell adhesion depends on PI3-kinase and PTEN. *J Cell Sci.* Oct 15 2005;118(Pt 20):4901-4912.

[43] Moustakas A, Heldin CH. Signaling networks guiding epithelial-mesenchymal transitions during embryogenesis and cancer progression. *Cancer Sci.* Oct 2007;98(10):1512-1520.
[44] Peinado H, Portillo F, Cano A. Transcriptional regulation of cadherins during development and carcinogenesis. *Int J Dev Biol.* 2004;48(5-6):365-375.
[45] Cheng GZ, Chan J, Wang Q, Zhang W, Sun CD, Wang LH. Twist transcriptionally up-regulates AKT2 in breast cancer cells leading to increased migration, invasion, and resistance to paclitaxel. *Cancer Res.* Mar 1 2007;67(5):1979-1987.
[46] Hsu MY, Meier FE, Nesbit M, et al. E-cadherin expression in melanoma cells restores keratinocyte-mediated growth control and down-regulates expression of invasion-related adhesion receptors. *Am J Pathol.* May 2000;156(5):1515-1525.
[47] Egeblad M, Werb Z. New functions for the matrix metalloproteinases in cancer progression. *Nat Rev Cancer.* Mar 2002;2(3):161-174.
[48] Bartolome RA, Galvez BG, Longo N, et al. Stromal cell-derived factor-1alpha promotes melanoma cell invasion across basement membranes involving stimulation of membrane-type 1 matrix metalloproteinase and Rho GTPase activities. *Cancer Res.* Apr 1 2004;64(7):2534-2543.
[49] Sanz-Moreno V, Gadea G, Ahn J, et al. Rac activation and inactivation control plasticity of tumor cell movement. *Cell.* Oct 31 2008;135(3):510-523.
[50] Lewis CE, Pollard JW. Distinct role of macrophages in different tumor microenvironments. *Cancer Res.* Jan 15 2006;66(2):605-612.
[51] Pittet MJ. Behavior of immune players in the tumor microenvironment. *Curr Opin Oncol.* Jan 2009;21(1):53-59.
[52] Liotta LA, Kleinerman J, Saidel GM. Quantitative relationships of intravascular tumor cells, tumor vessels, and pulmonary metastases following tumor implantation. *Cancer Res.* May 1974;34(5):997-1004.
[53] Bockhorn M, Roberge S, Sousa C, Jain RK, Munn LL. Differential gene expression in metastasizing cells shed from kidney tumors. *Cancer Res.* Apr 1 2004;64(7):2469-2473.
[54] Holmgren L, O'Reilly MS, Folkman J. Dormancy of micrometastases: balanced proliferation and apoptosis in the presence of angiogenesis suppression. *Nat Med.* Feb 1995;1(2):149-153.
[55] Nguyen DX, Bos PD, Massague J. Metastasis: from dissemination to organ-specific colonization. *Nat Rev Cancer.* Apr 2009;9(4):274-284.
[56] Al-Mehdi AB, Tozawa K, Fisher AB, Shientag L, Lee A, Muschel RJ. Intravascular origin of metastasis from the proliferation of endothelium-attached tumor cells: a new model for metastasis. *Nat Med.* Jan 2000;6(1):100-102.
[57] Borsig L, Wong R, Hynes RO, Varki NM, Varki A. Synergistic effects of L- and P-selectin in facilitating tumor metastasis can involve non-mucin ligands and implicate leukocytes as enhancers of metastasis. *Proc Natl Acad Sci U S A.* Feb 19 2002;99(4):2193-2198.
[58] Laubli H, Stevenson JL, Varki A, Varki NM, Borsig L. L-selectin facilitation of metastasis involves temporal induction of Fut7-dependent ligands at sites of tumor cell arrest. *Cancer Res.* Feb 1 2006;66(3):1536-1542.
[59] Fuertes MB, Girart MV, Molinero LL, et al. Intracellular retention of the NKG2D ligand MHC class I chain-related gene A in human melanomas confers immune privilege and prevents NK cell-mediated cytotoxicity. *J Immunol.* Apr 1 2008;180(7):4606-4614.

[60] Lacreusette A, Nguyen JM, Pandolfino MC, et al. Loss of oncostatin M receptor beta in metastatic melanoma cells. *Oncogene.* Feb 8 2007;26(6):881-892.
[61] Zbytek B, Carlson JA, Granese J, Ross J, Mihm MC, Slominski A. Current concepts of metastasis in melanoma. *Expert Rev Dermatol.* Oct 2008;3(5):569-585.
[62] Koyanagi K, O'Day SJ, Gonzalez R, et al. Serial monitoring of circulating melanoma cells during neoadjuvant biochemotherapy for stage III melanoma: outcome prediction in a multicenter trial. *J Clin Oncol.* Nov 1 2005;23(31):8057-8064.
[63] Koyanagi K, Mori T, O'Day SJ, Martinez SR, Wang HJ, Hoon DS. Association of circulating tumor cells with serum tumor-related methylated DNA in peripheral blood of melanoma patients. *Cancer Res.* Jun 15 2006;66(12):6111-6117.
[64] Koyanagi K, O'Day SJ, Gonzalez R, et al. Microphthalmia transcription factor as a molecular marker for circulating tumor cell detection in blood of melanoma patients. *Clin Cancer Res.* Feb 15 2006;12(4):1137-1143.
[65] Voit CA, Schafer-Hesterberg G, Kron M, et al. Impact of molecular staging methods in primary melanoma: reverse-transcriptase polymerase chain reaction (RT-PCR) of ultrasound-guided aspirate of the sentinel node does not improve diagnostic accuracy, but RT-PCR of peripheral blood does predict survival. *J Clin Oncol.* Dec 10 2008;26(35):5742-5747.
[66] Krivacic RT, Ladanyi A, Curry DN, et al. A rare-cell detector for cancer. *Proc Natl Acad Sci U S A.* Jul 20 2004;101(29):10501-10504.
[67] Cools-Lartigue JJ, McCauley CS, Marshall JC, et al. Immunomagnetic isolation and in vitro expansion of human uveal melanoma cell lines. *Mol Vis.* 2008;14:50-55.
[68] Weight RM, Dale PS, Viator JA. Detection of circulating melanoma cells in human blood using photoacoustic flowmetry. *Conf Proc IEEE Eng Med Biol Soc.* 2009;2009:106-109.
[69] Pantel K, Brakenhoff RH, Brandt B. Detection, clinical relevance and specific biological properties of disseminating tumour cells. *Nat Rev Cancer.* May 2008;8(5):329-340.
[70] Pantel K, Otte M. Occult micrometastasis: enrichment, identification and characterization of single disseminated tumour cells. *Semin Cancer Biol.* Oct 2001;11(5):327-337.
[71] Allard WJ, Matera J, Miller MC, et al. Tumor cells circulate in the peripheral blood of all major carcinomas but not in healthy subjects or patients with nonmalignant diseases. *Clin Cancer Res.* Oct 15 2004;10(20):6897-6904.
[72] Medic S, Pearce RL, Heenan PJ, Ziman M. Molecular markers of circulating melanoma cells. *Pigment Cell Res.* Apr 2007;20(2):80-91.
[73] Medic S, Ziman M. PAX3 expression in normal skin melanocytes and melanocytic lesions (naevi and melanomas). *PLoS One.* 2010;5(4):e9977.
[74] Palmieri G, Ascierto PA, Perrone F, et al. Prognostic value of circulating melanoma cells detected by reverse transcriptase-polymerase chain reaction. *J Clin Oncol.* Mar 1 2003;21(5):767-773.
[75] Gradilone A, Cigna E, Agliano AM, Frati L. Tyrosinase Expression as a Molecular Marker for Investigating the Presence of Circulating Tumor Cells in Melanoma Patients. *Curr Cancer Drug Targets.* Apr 12 2010.
[76] Keilholz U, Goldin-Lang P, Bechrakis NE, et al. Quantitative detection of circulating tumor cells in cutaneous and ocular melanoma and quality assessment by real-time reverse transcriptase-polymerase chain reaction. *Clin Cancer Res.* Mar 1 2004;10(5):1605-1612.

[77] Reynolds SR, Albrecht J, Shapiro RL, et al. Changes in the presence of multiple markers of circulating melanoma cells correlate with clinical outcome in patients with melanoma. *Clin Cancer Res.* Apr 2003;9(4):1497-1502.
[78] Samija I, Lukac J, Maric-Brozic J, et al. Prognostic value of microphthalmia-associated transcription factor and tyrosinase as markers for circulating tumor cells detection in patients with melanoma. *Melanoma Res.* Mar 30 2010.
[79] Cristofanilli M, Budd GT, Ellis MJ, et al. Circulating tumor cells, disease progression, and survival in metastatic breast cancer. *N Engl J Med.* Aug 19 2004;351(8):781-791.
[80] Bernards R, Weinberg RA. A progression puzzle. *Nature.* Aug 22 2002;418(6900):823.
[81] Quintana E, Shackleton M, Sabel MS, Fullen DR, Johnson TM, Morrison SJ. Efficient tumour formation by single human melanoma cells. *Nature.* Dec 4 2008;456(7222):593-598.
[82] Rapanotti MC, Bianchi L, Ricozzi I, et al. Melanoma-associated markers expression in blood: MUC-18 is associated with advanced stages in melanoma patients. *Br J Dermatol.* Feb 2009;160(2):338-344.
[83] Pluschke G, Vanek M, Evans A, et al. Molecular cloning of a human melanoma-associated chondroitin sulfate proteoglycan. *Proc Natl Acad Sci U S A.* Sep 3 1996;93(18):9710-9715.
[84] Yang J, Price MA, Li GY, et al. Melanoma proteoglycan modifies gene expression to stimulate tumor cell motility, growth, and epithelial-to-mesenchymal transition. *Cancer Res.* Oct 1 2009;69(19):7538-7547.
[85] Erfurt C, Muller E, Emmerling S, et al. Melanoma-associated chondroitin sulphate proteoglycan as a new target antigen for CD4+ T cells in melanoma patients. *Int J Cancer.* May 15 2009;124(10):2341-2346.
[86] Schatton T, Frank MH. Cancer stem cells and human malignant melanoma. *Pigment Cell Melanoma Res.* Feb 2008;21(1):39-55.
[87] Schatton T, Murphy GF, Frank NY, et al. Identification of cells initiating human melanomas. *Nature.* Jan 17 2008;451(7176):345-349.
[88] Grichnik JM, Burch JA, Schulteis RD, et al. Melanoma, a tumor based on a mutant stem cell? *J Invest Dermatol.* Jan 2006;126(1):142-153.
[89] Monzani E, Facchetti F, Galmozzi E, et al. Melanoma contains CD133 and ABCG2 positive cells with enhanced tumourigenic potential. *Eur J Cancer.* Mar 2007;43(5):935-946.
[90] Zabierowski SE, Herlyn M. Melanoma stem cells: the dark seed of melanoma. *J Clin Oncol.* Jun 10 2008;26(17):2890-2894.
[91] Wicha MS. Cancer stem cells and metastasis: lethal seeds. *Clin Cancer Res.* Oct 1 2006;12(19):5606-5607.
[92] Roesch A, Fukunaga-Kalabis M, Schmidt EC, et al. A temporarily distinct subpopulation of slow-cycling melanoma cells is required for continuous tumor growth. *Cell.* May 14 2010;141(4):583-594.
[93] Herlyn M. Driving in the melanoma landscape. *Exp Dermatol.* Jun 2009;18(6):506-508.
[94] Passegue E, Rafii S, Herlyn M. Cancer stem cells are everywhere. *Nat Med.* Jan 2009;15(1):23.
[95] Smalley KS, Herlyn M. Integrating tumor-initiating cells into the paradigm for melanoma targeted therapy. *Int J Cancer.* Mar 15 2009;124(6):1245-1250.
[96] Vultur A, Herlyn M. Cracking the system: melanoma complexity demands new therapeutic approaches. *Pigment Cell Melanoma Res.* Feb 2009;22(1):4-5.

[97] Keshet GI, Goldstein I, Itzhaki O, et al. MDR1 expression identifies human melanoma stem cells. *Biochem Biophys Res Commun.* Apr 18 2008;368(4):930-936.
[98] Fang D, Nguyen TK, Leishear K, et al. A tumorigenic subpopulation with stem cell properties in melanomas. *Cancer Res.* Oct 15 2005;65(20):9328-9337.
[99] La Porta C. Cancer stem cells: lessons from melanoma. *Stem Cell Rev.* Mar 2009;5(1):61-65.
[100] Boiko AD, Razorenova OV, van de Rijn M, et al. Human melanoma-initiating cells express neural crest nerve growth factor receptor CD271. *Nature.* Jul 1 2010;466(7302):133-137.
[101] Bosserhoff AK. Novel biomarkers in malignant melanoma. *Clin Chim Acta.* May 2006;367(1-2):28-35.
[102] Bennett DC. How to make a melanoma: what do we know of the primary clonal events? *Pigment Cell Melanoma Res.* Feb 2008;21(1):27-38.
[103] Gogas H, Eggermont AM, Hauschild A, et al. Biomarkers in melanoma. *Ann Oncol.* Aug 2009;20 Suppl 6:vi8-13.
[104] Xi L, Nicastri DG, El-Hefnawy T, Hughes SJ, Luketich JD, Godfrey TE. Optimal markers for real-time quantitative reverse transcription PCR detection of circulating tumor cells from melanoma, breast, colon, esophageal, head and neck, and lung cancers. *Clin Chem.* Jul 2007;53(7):1206-1215.
[105] Ma J, Lin JY, Alloo A, et al. Isolation of tumorigenic circulating melanoma cells. *Biochem Biophys Res Commun.* Nov 26 2010;402(4):711-717.
[106] Talantov D, Mazumder A, Yu JX, et al. Novel genes associated with malignant melanoma but not benign melanocytic lesions. *Clin Cancer Res.* Oct 15 2005;11(20):7234-7242.
[107] Alonso SR, Tracey L, Ortiz P, et al. A high-throughput study in melanoma identifies epithelial-mesenchymal transition as a major determinant of metastasis. *Cancer Res.* Apr 1 2007;67(7):3450-3460.
[108] Winnepenninckx V, Lazar V, Michiels S, et al. Gene expression profiling of primary cutaneous melanoma and clinical outcome. *J Natl Cancer Inst.* Apr 5 2006;98(7):472-482.
[109] Kauffmann A, Rosselli F, Lazar V, et al. High expression of DNA repair pathways is associated with metastasis in melanoma patients. *Oncogene.* Jan 24 2008;27(5):565-573.
[110] Medic S, Ziman M. PAX3 across the spectrum: from melanoblast to melanoma. *Crit Rev Biochem Mol Biol.* Apr 28 2009:1-13.
[111] Gupta PB, Kuperwasser C, Brunet JP, et al. The melanocyte differentiation program predisposes to metastasis after neoplastic transformation. *Nat Genet.* Oct 2005;37(10):1047-1054.
[112] Gupta PB, Mani S, Yang J, Hartwell K, Weinberg RA. The evolving portrait of cancer metastasis. *Cold Spring Harb Symp Quant Biol.* 2005;70:291-297.
[113] White RM, Zon LI. Melanocytes in development, regeneration, and cancer. *Cell Stem Cell.* Sep 11 2008;3(3):242-252.
[114] Topczewska JM, Postovit LM, Margaryan NV, et al. Embryonic and tumorigenic pathways converge via Nodal signaling: role in melanoma aggressiveness. *Nat Med.* Aug 2006;12(8):925-932.
[115] McArdle L, Rafferty MM, Satyamoorthy K, et al. Microarray analysis of phosphatase gene expression in human melanoma. *Br J Dermatol.* May 2005;152(5):925-930.

[116] Carreira S, Goodall J, Denat L, et al. Mitf regulation of Dia1 controls melanoma proliferation and invasiveness. *Genes Dev.* Dec 15 2006;20(24):3426-3439.
[117] Kubic JD, Young KP, Plummer RS, Ludvik AE, Lang D. Pigmentation PAX-ways: the role of Pax3 in melanogenesis, melanocyte stem cell maintenance, and disease. *Pigment Cell Melanoma Res.* Dec 2008;21(6):627-645.
[118] Plummer RS, Shea CR, Nelson M, et al. PAX3 expression in primary melanomas and nevi. *Mod Pathol.* May 2008;21(5):525-530.
[119] Lang D, Lu MM, Huang L, et al. Pax3 functions at a nodal point in melanocyte stem cell differentiation. *Nature.* Feb 24 2005;433(7028):884-887.
[120] Whiteman DC, Zhou XP, Cummings MC, Pavey S, Hayward NK, Eng C. Nuclear PTEN expression and clinicopathologic features in a population-based series of primary cutaneous melanoma. *Int J Cancer.* May 1 2002;99(1):63-67.
[121] Duncan LM. The classification of cutaneous melanoma. *Hematol Oncol Clin North Am.* Jun 2009;23(3):501-513, ix.
[122] Levy C, Khaled M, Fisher DE. MITF: master regulator of melanocyte development and melanoma oncogene. *Trends Mol Med.* Sep 2006;12(9):406-414.
[123] Platz A, Egyhazi S, Ringborg U, Hansson J. Human cutaneous melanoma; a review of NRAS and BRAF mutation frequencies in relation to histogenetic subclass and body site. *Mol Oncol.* Apr 2008;1(4):395-405.
[124] Goel VK, Lazar AJ, Warneke CL, Redston MS, Haluska FG. Examination of mutations in BRAF, NRAS, and PTEN in primary cutaneous melanoma. *J Invest Dermatol.* Jan 2006;126(1):154-160.
[125] Vidwans SJ, Flaherty KT, Fisher DE, Tenenbaum JM, Travers MD, Shrager J. The Melanoma Disease Model: Subtypes. 2010; http://mmdm.cancercommons.org/smw/index.php/The_Melanoma_Disease_Model:_Subtypes. Accessed 7 February 2011.
[126] Ireland A, Millward M, Pearce R, Lee M, Ziman M. Genetic factors in metastatic progression of cutaneous melanoma: the future role of circulating melanoma cells in prognosis and management. *Clin Exp Metastasis.* Feb 11 2011.
[127] Fusi A, Collette S, Busse A, et al. Circulating melanoma cells and distant metastasis-free survival in stage III melanoma patients with or without adjuvant interferon treatment (EORTC 18991 side study). *Eur J Cancer.* Dec 2009;45(18):3189-3197.

4

# Regulation of the Glutathione S-Transferase P1 Expression in Melanoma Cells

Andrii Slonchak[1], Agata Chwieduk[2],
Joanna Rzeszowska-Wolny[3] and Maria Obolenskaya[1]
*[1]Institute of Molecular Biology and Genetics National Academy of Scienses of Ukraine*
*[2]Maria Sklodowska-Curie Memorial Cancer Center and Institute of Oncology*
*[3]Silesian University of Technology*
*[1]Ukraine*
*[2,3]Poland*

## 1. Introduction

Melanoma is a malignant tumor that results from DNA damage and related mutations in melanocytes (Rass & Reichrath, 2008). It usually occurs in result of collision of ultraviolet (UV) photon with a chromophore in a skin cell, production of reactive oxygen species which attack the melanocytes and induce oxidative stress with the DNA damage by oxidation. Conceptually, oxidative stress results from a change in the equilibrium between production of pro-oxidant and their consumption or deactivation, favoring an excess of pro-oxidant that have noxious consequences at the molecular and cellular levels (Ananthaswamy & Pierceall, 1990). There are several mechanisms and barriers that protect the body against ultraviolet radiation: the stratum corneum, the outermost layer of the skin, and melanin pigment attenuate penetration of UV into the skin; antioxidative enzymes detoxify and metabolize reactive oxygen species; DNA repair systems protect cells from UV-induced lesions (Hoeijmakers, 2001). The cellular antioxidant defense relies to the great extent on a powerful sulfur redox chemistry response in which glutathione S-transferases are active players.
Glutathione S-transferases (GSTs) comprise a multigene superfamily of enzymes that catalyze the conjugation of electrophilic toxic compounds with glutathione, playing a key role in phase II of detoxification (Hayes et al., 2005). GSTs are dimeric enzymes with subunit polypeptides organized into several cytosolic families ($\alpha$, $\mu$, $\pi$, $\sigma$, $\theta$, $\zeta$, $\omega$) and one microsomal form ($\kappa$) (Frova, 2006). The human Pi class isoform of GSTs (GSTP1-1) is widely expressed in epithelial tissues and is the dominant isoform in lung, brain, skin, esophagus, erythrocytes and also in fetal tissues including liver, lung, kidney, and placenta (Moscow et al., 1989). This isoform has been proposed to be a caretaker gene, protecting cells against genome damage mediated by oxidants and electrophiles from inflammation or environmental exposure. Besides its typical role in detoxification of electrophilic toxic compounds this enzyme carries out a wide range of other functions, such as removal of reactive oxygen species and generation of S-thiolated proteins during the oxidative stress (Hayes & Strange, 1995), binding and transfer of different ligands (Oakley et al., 1999), modulation of signaling pathways (Adler et al., 1999; Villafania et al., 2000; Wu et al., 2006; Zhao et al., 2006),

conjugation and transport of steroid hormones, dinitrosyl-diglutathionyl-iron complex storage and metabolism (De et al., 2003; Pedersen et al., 2007; Ricci et al., 2003; Turella et al., 2003).

The GSTP, GSTT and GSTM (GSTs) isoforms prevent carcinogenesis through inactivation of reactive electrophiles by conjugation to reduced glutathione. The human GSTP1 isoform also possesses selenium-independent peroxidase activity and restores organic hydro- and endoperoxides thus additionally protecting DNA from oxidative damage (Tan et al., 1988).

Therefore, it is biologically plausible that a deficiency in the activity of GSTs may contribute to the risk of UV-induced melanoma. There are many evidences that mutation-associated reduction of GST activity predisposes to melanoma (Bu et al., 2007; Dolzan et al., 2006). However, mutations are not the single cause of GSTP1 insufficiency. This phenomenon occurs in different tumors as a result of *GSTP1* gene repression by methylation of promoter or via specific set of transcription factors (Henderson et al., 1998).

Unlike down-regulation of *GSTP1* expression its overexpression is associated with the development of multidrug resistance (Harbottle et al., 2001). It is known that melanoma is the most aggressive form of skin cancer, which is notoriously resistant to all current modalities of anticancer therapy, including chemotherapy and γ-irradiation. Numerous genetic, functional and biochemical studies suggest that melanoma cells become insensitive to chemotherapeutic drugs by exploiting their resistance to apoptosis and by reprogramming their signaling pathways (Helmbach et al., 2001). It was demonstrated that *GSTP1* and multidrug resistance protein 1 (*MRP1*) are overexpressed in multi-drug resistant melanoma cells and responsible for resistance to chemotherapy (Depeille et al., 2005).

Thus, reactive oxygen species that damage melanocytes DNA, highly contribute to neoplastic transformation of melanocytes, what leads to the assumption that melanocytes should have reduced protection from electrophiles particularly due to reduced activity of corresponding detoxification enzymes. However, malignant melanoma is highly resistant to chemotherapy and γ-irradiation that points to the elevated detoxification and antioxidant activity in the tumor cells. This contradiction allowed us to suppose that activity of detoxification system, and particularly of GSTP1, may be down-regulated during neoplastic transformation, making the melanocytes sensitive to reactive oxygen species generated by UV-irradiation, and up-regulated by the therapeutic agents, conferring protection against them. To verify this assumption we decided to study the *GSTP1* expression and its regulation at transcriptional level in human malignant melanoma cell line Me45 before and after γ-irradiation. Due to the important role of GSTP1 in health and disease the regulation of *GSTP1* gene expression is in the focus of interests of numerous researchers and clinicians, but according to our knowledge, the potential role of *GSTP1* regulation in the etiology and the progress of melanoma were not studied before. Thereby we have addressed the following questions:

- What is the level of *GSTP1* expression in melanoma cells in comparison with the other malignant cell types and how does it change after γ-irradiation;
- Which cis-and trans-elements (transcription factors) participate in regulation of *GSTP1* transcription in melanoma cells;
- Which transcription factors may contribute to induction of this gene in response to γ-irradiation.

*GSTP1* gene expression is regulated at transcriptional, post-transcriptional, translational and post-translational levels (Daniel, 1993; Jhaveri et al., 1997; Moffat et al., 1997). We focused our attention on the regulation at transcriptional level particularly by transcription factors and cis-elements of the 5′-flanking region of the gene. Information about the structure of *GSTP1* promoter and transcription factors that were reported to interact with specific sites is summarized in Fig.1.

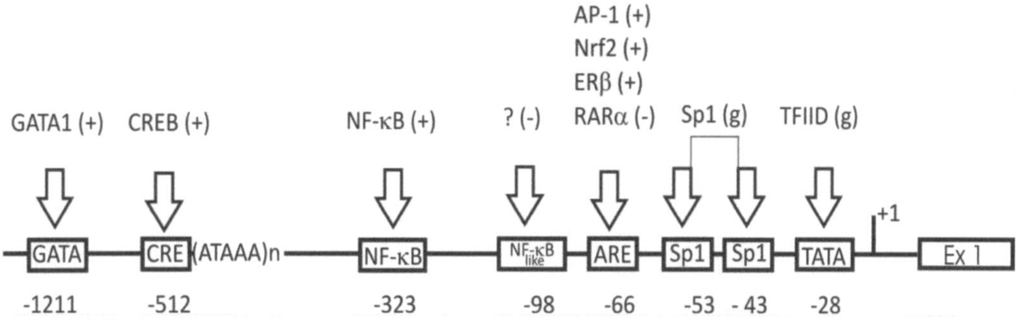


Fig. 1. Structure of the human *GSTP1* gene 5′-regulatorey region and transcription factors known to interact with the promoter elements (Slonchak et al., 2009): (+) – positive regulation, (-) – negative regulation, (g) – general transcription factors

The region spanning from – 80 to – 8 contains a TATA-box at – 28 to – 24, two Sp1 binding sites (G/C-boxes) located at – 43 to – 38 and – 53 to – 48 and antioxidant response element (ARE) at – 59 to – 66 (Cowell et al., 1988) and is essential for initiation of *GSTP1* transcription. Binding of Sp1 to the proximal G/C-box (Moffat et al., 1996a) and a transcription factor from AP-1 (Morrow et al., 1990) or NF-E2 family (Nishinaka et al., 2007) to ARE located in this minimal promoter are required to initiate the transcription. ARE is also responsible for gene induction by retinoic acid (Xia et al., 1996), estrogens (Montano et al., 2004), phorbol esters (Duvoix et al., 2004b), curcumin (Nishinaka et al., 2007) and doxorubicin (Duvoix et al., 2004a). The region spanning from – 1212 to – 90, which contains NF-κB-like element at – 98 to – 90 (Moffat et al., 1996b), NF-κB binding site at – 323 to – 314 (Morceau et al., 2004), cAMP response element (CRE) at – 512 to – 505 (Lo & li-Osman, 2002) and GATA-1 binding site at – 1212 to – 1207 (Morceau et al., 2000) is not essential for initiation of *GSTP1* transcription but mediates gene's responsibility to different stimuli. The NF-κB-like element mediates up-regulation of the *GSTP1* gene transcription in response to oxidative stress by binding NF-κB (Xia et al., 1996) and transcription silencing in MCF7 breast cancer cells (Moffat et al., 1996b). NF-κB binding site was reported to bind NF-κB and stimulate gene expression in response to TNFα treatment in leukemia cells (Morceau et al., 2004). CRE site binds CREB and mediates cAMP-dependent gene activation in lung cancer cells (Lo & li-Osman, 2002) and GATA-1 binds GATA-1 transcription factor and mediates the induction of *GSTP1* transcription during hemin-induced differentiation of K562 cells (Schnekenburger et al., 2003).

Despite the vast literature devoted to GSTP1 enzyme the functional characteristics of response elements in gene promoter and tissue-specific regulation of *GSTP1* transcription are poorly understood and were not studied in melanoma cells. To fill this gap we performed the functional analysis of *GSTP1* promoter in the human melanoma cell line. We examined *GSTP1* expression level in these cells, the functional role of cis-elements in *GSTP1* promoter and identified transcription factors binding with these elements. We also conducted the experiments to analyze the ability of *GSTP1* gene to be induced by γ-irradiation.

In this research we used cell line Me45, which is a human malignant melanoma cell line derived from a metastasis of skin melanoma into lymph node at 35 years old male. It was established in 1997 in the Department of Radiobiology of M. Sklodowska-Curie Cancer Centre and Institute of Oncology in Gliwice. Identity of melanoma cells was confirmed by immunocytochemical reaction with monoclonal antibodies to HMB50, S-100 and Melan A (Kumala et al., 2003; Przybyszewski et al., 2004; Rzeszowska-Wolny et al., 2009).

## 2. Materials and methods

### 2.1 Cell culture

Human melanoma cells Me45, mammary carcinoma cells MCF7, epithelial breast cells Hbl-100, bronchoalveolar carcinoma cells H358, alveolar carcinoma cells A549, erythroleukaemia cells K562, hepatocellular carcinoma cells HepG2, lung cancer cells Hct116, immortalized human bronchial epithelial cell BEAS2B, adrenal carcinoma cells FN-H296, mammary carcinoma cells MCF10A and choriocarcinoma cells BeWo were propagated in Dulbecco's modified Eagle's medium nutrient mixture F12 HAM (Sigma, USA) containing 12% fetal bovine serum (Gibco, USA) and 100 µg/ml gentamicine in tissue culture flasks. Culture medium for choriocarcinoma cells BeWo was also supplemented with MEM Non-Essential Amino Acid Solution 1x (MEM NEAA 100x, Gibco, USA). Incubation was performed at 37 °C in humidified atmosphere of air containing 5% $CO_2$.

### 2.2 γ-Irradiation of the cells

Me45 and BeWo cells grown to 80% confluence in 3 cm culture dishes were γ-irradiated at 1 Gy/min from a Clinac 600 GMV (Varian, Palo Alto, CA, USA) at room temperature to a total dose of 2 Gy corresponding to therapeutic dose and then incubated at 37 °C during 0.25-12 h. After incubation RNA was extracted from cells using RNA Mini kit (A&A Biotechnology, Poland).

### 2.3 Estimation of *GSTP1* expression

#### 2.3.1 RNA isolation and reverse transcription

Total RNA was isolated from cultured cells grown to 80% confluence in 6-well plates using Total RNA Mini kit (A&A Biotechnology, Poland). RNA (1µg/lane) was analyzed by electrophoresis in denaturing agarose gel. First strand cDNA was synthesized from 1 µg of total RNA using iScriptcDNA Synthesis kit (Bio-Rad, USA). The 20 µl reaction contained 4ul 5x iScript Reaction Mix, 1 µl iScriptReverce Transcriptase and 2 µg of total RNA. The reaction mixture was incubated 5 min at 25 °C, 30 min at 42 °C and 5 min at 85 °C. The resulted mixture was used directly for amplification by real-time PCR.

#### 2.3.2 Quantitative real-time PCR

*GSTP1* gene expression was determined by real-time PCR on DNA Engine Peltier Thermal Cycler with Chromo4 Real-Time PCR Detector (Bio-Rad, USA). PCR was performed in 20 µl reaction mixture contained 2 µl cDNA, 10 µl 2x Real Time PCR Master Mix SYBR Set A (A&A Biotechnology, Poland) and 10 pmole of each primer - *GSTP1L*: 5'-CCCAAGTTCCAGGACGGAGA-3' and *GSTP1R*: 5'-GCCCGCCTCATAGTTGGTGT-3'. Samples were denatured at 94 °C for 4 min, and cDNA products were amplified with 45 cycles of denaturation at 94 °C for 30 s, annealing at 60 °C for 30 s and extension at 72 °C for

30 s. The specificity of amplification was checked using post-PCR melting curves analysis. During exponential phase of PCR reaction, the crossing threshold ($C_T$) was determined for each amplification curve. MCF10A cell line was used as calibrator. Results were normalized to RPL41 ribosomal protein mRNA quantified with qRT-PCR performed under the same conditions. The relative quatification ratio was determined based on CT method with an efficiency correction using Opticon Monitor 3 Software (Bio-Rad, USA).

#### 2.3.3 Semi-quantitative western blot analysis

Cells grown to 80% confluence in 6-well plates were lysed in 500 µl of RIPA Buffer (Thermo Scientific, USA) supplemented with Complete Proteinase Inhibitor Cocktail (Roche, Switzerland). Protein concentration was determined using Bradford reagent (Bio-Rad, USA). Total proteins (25 µg) of each cell lysate were resolved in 12% SDS-PAGE according to Laemmli method (Laemmli, 1970), and electroblotted onto Immobilon-P Transfer Membrane (Millipore, USA). Immunodetection of GSTP1 protein was accomplished with rabbit polyclonal anti-GSTP1 antibody (StressGen, USA) diluted 1:1000 with 3% BSA in TBS following the procedure recommended by antibodies manufacturer. To detect the immunoreactive proteins, horseradish peroxidase-conjugated goat anti-rabbit IgG (Santa Cruz Biotechnology, USA) diluted 1:10000 with 3% BSA in TBS, and SuperSignal West Pico Chemiluminescent Substrate (Thermo Scientific, USA) was used. Visualization of the immunoreactive bands was achieved by exposing the membrane to the X-ray film. Films were developed and scanned. Band intensities were quantified with image analysis software GelPro 4.5 (Media cybernetics, USA). The amount of protein was normalized by Ponceau S staining of the membranes after electrotransfer.

### 2.4 Analysis of functional activity of cis-elements in *GSTP1* promoter and identification of transcription factors interacting with them

#### 2.4.1 Reporter constructs and transient transfection assay

Fragments of *GSTP1* gene promoter were prepared by PCR. The oligonucleotide 5′-ACTCACTGGTGGCGAAGACT-3′ (position +15 to +35) was used as the downstream primer for all constructions. Each of the following oligonucleotides was used as the upstream primers to amplify promoter fragments: 5′-CAT AAA CAC CAA CCT CTT CCC C-3′ (position -1379 to -1357) for pGSTP1415, 5′-ATA GCC TAA GGC ACA GCC AC-3′ (position -1162 to -1142) for pGSTP1197, 5′-TTT CCT TTC CTC TAA GCG GC-3′ (position -405 to -385) for pGSTP440, 5′-AGT CCG CGG GAC CCT CCA GA-3′ (position -105 to -85) for pGSTP140 and 5′-AGA GCG GCC GGC GCC GTG AC-3′ (position -85 to -64) for pGSTP120. Primers were designed by Vector NTI Advance 10.0 software (Invitrogen, USA) using *GSTP1* gene sequence AY324387. PCR was performed in 25 µl of reaction mixture containing 1x QIAGEN PCR Buffer, 1.5 mM $MgCl_2$, 200 µM each dNTP, 10 pmoles of each primer, 1x Q-solution, 500ng DNA and 2.5u Taq-DNA polymerase. DNA was denatured at 94 °C for 10 min, and promoter fragments were amplified with 30 cycles - denaturation at 94 °C for 30 s, annealing and extension at 60 °C for 120 s (for 1415bp fragment), 90 s (for 1197 bp fragment), 60 s (for 440 bp fragment) and 30 s (for 140 and 120 bp fragments). Final extension step was performed at 72 °C for 15 min. The amplified products were gel-purified using Gel-Out Kit (A&A Biotechnology, Poland) and subcloned into pCR2.1®-TOPO® vector (Invitrogen, USA), excised by KpnI and XhoI and religated into KpnI and XhoI linearized and dephosphorylated pGL3-basic plasmid (Promega, USA). DNA template for

PCR was isolated from human peripheral blood using Genomic Mini Kit (A&A Biotechnology, Poland). All PCR reagents and kits for plasmid isolation were obtained from Qiagen Inc. (USA). Plasmids for transfection were isolated using EndoFree Plasmid Maxi Kit (Qiagen Inc., USA). All enzymes were from MBI Fermentas (Lithuania). Sequences of relevant regions of the reporter constructs were confirmed by sequencing in both directions in OIigo.pl DNA IBB PAN Service (Poland).

Me45 cells were grown in 24-well plates to 60% confluence and transfected with 500 ng of pGSTP together with 25 ng of pRL-TK plasmid (Promega, USA) per well using Lipofectamine™ LTX and PLUS™ reagents (Invitrogen, USA). After 20h the culture medium was removed, cells were washed with PBS and lysed in 250 µl of Passive lysis buffer (Promega, USA). Firefly and *renilla* luciferase activities were assessed in 5 µl of the lysates using Dual Luciferase® Reporter Assay System (Promega, USA). Light emission resulting from luciferase activity was measured in Lumat LB 9506 luminometer (Berthold technologies, USA) by integration of peak light emission during 10 s at 25 °C. The ratio between arbitrary firefly and *renilla* luciferase light units was calculated for each probe. Each experiment was repeated three times with triplications in each one.

### 2.4.2 Electrophoretic mobility shift assay

Me45 cells were grown in T225 flasks to 80% confluence. After removal of culture medium cells were washed with PBS, harvested, and nuclear extracts were prepared according to Dignam's method (Dignam et al., 1983). A Bio-Rad Protein assay was used to determine protein concentration.

The following oligonucleotides and their complementary sequences were used as probes in EMSA experiment: ARE (ARE site of human *GSTP1* promoter) - 5′-CGC CGT GAC TCA GCA CTG GG-3′, NF-κB-like (NF-κB-like site of human *GSTP1* promoter) - 5′-TCC GCG GGA CCC TCC AGA AG-3′, NF-κB (NF-κB site of human *GSTP1* promoter) - 5′-CTT AGG GAA TTT CCC CCC GC-3′, CRE (CRE site of human *GSTP1* promoter) - 5′-GAG ACT ACG TCA TAA AAT AA-3′, GATA (GATA-1 binding site of human *GSTP1* promoter) - 5′-GAG ATCA ATA TCT AGA AAT AA-3′. Probes were prepared by denaturation of complementary oligonucleotides for 2 min at 95 °C, annealing for 20 min at 60 °C and 30 min at 22 °C. Probes (10 pmoles) were incubated for 30 min with 20 pmoles [γ-P32]-ATP 6000Ci/mmole (Hartmann Analytic, Germany) in 20 µl of reaction mixture containing 10 u PNK (Roche, Switzerland) and PNK Buffer. Unincorporated nucleotides were removed by gel-filtration through Bio-gel P-30 (Bio-Rad, USA).

Five micrograms of cell nuclear extracts were preincubated for 10 min at 25 °C with 1ug sonicated E. coli DNA and with or without 5-10 pmoles of unlabeled competitor in 20 mM Tris-HCl pH 7.4, 150 mM NaCl, 1.5 mM $MgCl_2$, 0.1 mM EDTA, 20% glycerol, 1 mM DTT. Then 0.1 pmole of [γ-P32]-ATP labeled probe was added to the mixture and incubated for a further 30 min at 25 °C. The reaction mixture was then loaded onto a prerun (200 V for 1 h at 4 °C) 6% native polyacrylamide gel (29:1 cross-linking ratio) containing 1x TBE. Electrophoresis was performed at 20 mA for 3h at 4 °C and the gel was then dried and radiographed. In supershift experiment the reaction mixture was preincubated for 20min at room temperature with 2 µg of antibody before the addition of radiolabeled probe. Consensus oligonucleotides for AP-1, NF-κB, CREB, GATA, ER and RAR, antibodies against human c-Jun (sc-44X crossreactive to JunB and JunD), c-Fos (sc-253X crossreactive to FosB and Fra2), MafF/G/K (sc-22831X), ERβ (sc-8974X), Nrf3 (sc-15460X), NF-κB1 p50 (sc-1191X),

NF-κBRelA/p65 (sc-7151) and normal rabbit IgG (sc-2027) were from Santa Cruz Biotechnology, USA.

## 3. Results

### 3.1 Me-45 melanoma cells reveal low level of *GSTP1*expression

At the first step of our study we examined *GSTP1* expression in Me45 cells in comparison with the other malignant cells including breast cancer cells MCF7, nonmalignant breast cells Hbl-100, bronchoalveolar carcinoma cells H358, alveolar carcinoma cells A549, myelogenous leukaemia cells K562, hepatocarcinoma cells HepG2, colon cancer cells Hct116, immortalized human bronchial epithelial cell BEAS2B, adrenal carcinoma cells FN-H296, choriocarcinoma cells BeWo and mammary carcinoma cells MCF10A. We estimated the amount of *GSTP1* mRNA in total RNA isolated from these cells (Fig. 2). The level of GSTP1 mRNA in Me45 cells was significantly lower than in majority of other cells and slightly higher than in BeWo cells. The GSTP1 mRNA content in MCF7 and HepG2 cells was below the level of detection.

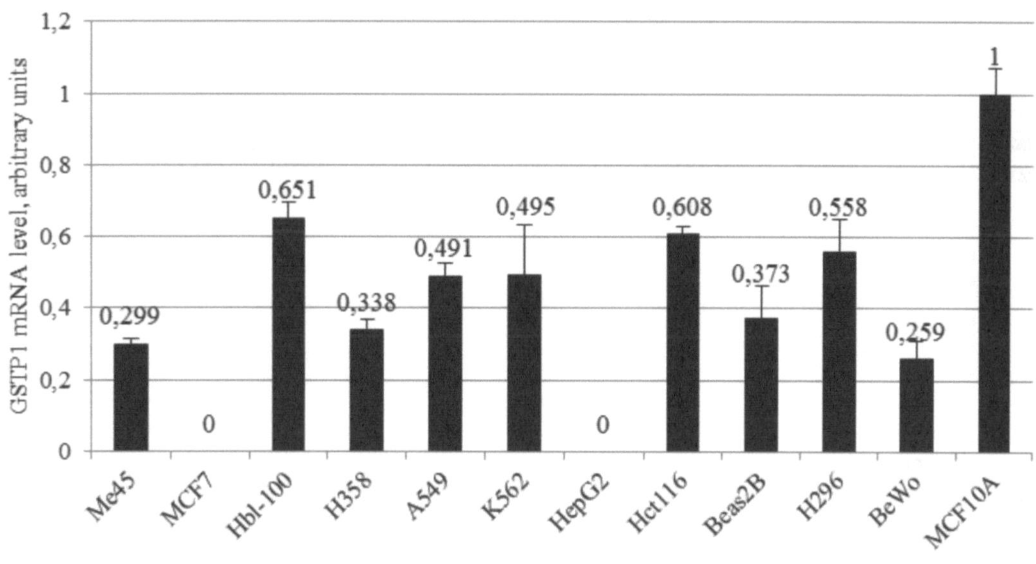


Fig. 2. Quantitative RT-PCR analysis of GSTP1 mRNA content in malignant cells (Slonchak et al, 2009). The values reflect the ratios of the normalized GSTP1 mRNA level in each cell type to the level in MCF10A cells that possess the highest *GSTP1* expression. The data were normalized to expression of RPL41 ribosomal protein gene and represented as the mean ± SD of three separate experiments with triplications in each

To verify whether the differences in GSTP1 mRNA content are persistent at the protein level, the semi-quantitative Western-blot analysis was undertaken. The GSTP1 protein content in Me45 cells was approximately 1.5-fold lower than in Hbl-100 cells and 1.9-fold higher than in BeWo cells (Fig. 3) that is compatible with the differences at mRNA level.

### 3.2 *GSTP1* expression in Me45 cells significantly elevates after γ-irradiation

The effect of ionizing radiation on *GSTP1* expression in Me45 melanoma cells was assessed by determination of GSTP1 mRNA content in total cellular RNA before irradiation and at

0.25 h, 1 h, 3 h, 5 h, 8 h and 12 h thereafter (Fig. 4). It increased beginning from 0.25 h after irradiation and reached a nearly 5-fold increase at 8 h i.e. *GSTP1* expression in Me45 cells is up-regulated by γ-irradiation.

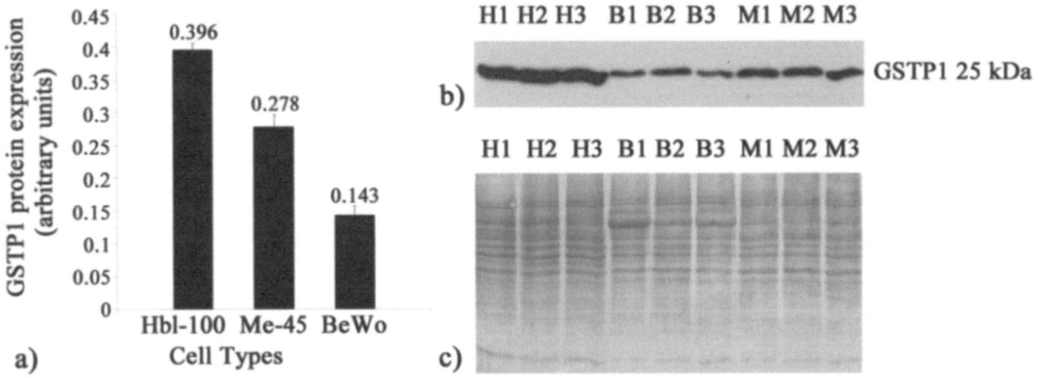


Fig. 3. GSTP1 protein level in Hbl-100, Me45 aand BeWo cells. a) The ratios of densitometry densities of GSTP1 bands to the densities of the whole lane on Ponceau S-stained membrane are represented as the mean ± SD of three separate experiments with triplications in each; b) The representative immunoblot probed with antibodies to GSTP1; c) The membrane stained with Ponceau S as a loading control. The letters H, B and M designate Hbl-100, BeWo and M45 cells correspondingly

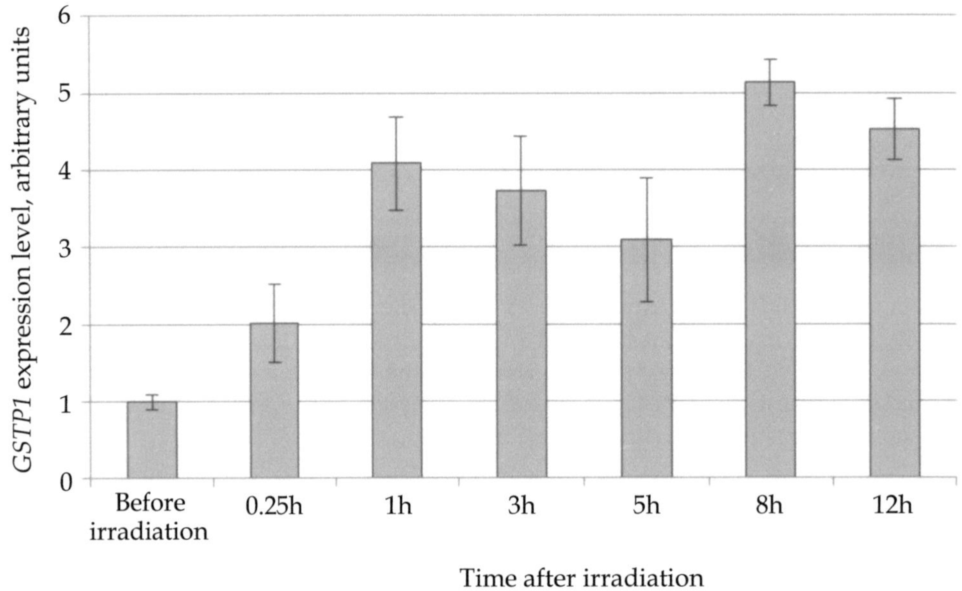


Fig. 4. Expression of *GSTP1* gene in Me45 cells before and after γ-irradiation. The values reflect the ratio of GSTP1 RNA in each time point to the value before irradiation. The data were normalized to content of RPL41 ribosomal protein mRNA and represented as the mean ± SD of three separate experiments with triplications in each

### 3.3 Regions of *GSTP1* promoter from – 1162 to – 405 and from – 105 to – 85 contain the negative regulatory elements and the region from – 405 to – 105 contains positive regulatory element in Me45 melanoma cells

The regulatory role of different regions of *GSTP1* promoter in Me45 cells was explored by transient transfection assay with the reporter constructs containing the firefly luciferase gene under the control of complete or truncated *GSTP1* promoter. We designed the reporter constructs each lacking the DNA fragment containing one transcription factor binding site. Transfection of the vector pGSTP1415 containing the complete *GSTP1* promoter (fragment from – 1379 to +35) resulted in relatively high level of *f-luc* gene expression (Fig. 5). Deletion of the flanking region from – 1379 to – 1162 with GATA-binding site did not change significantly the expression of the reporter gene. Further deletion of the region from – 1162 to – 405 with CRE resulted in increase of *f-luc* expression approximately 1.8-fold in comparison with previous construct. Deletion of the next region (from – 405 to – 105) containing NF-κB binding site, diminished expression of the reporter gene approximately 2.7-fold. Deletion of the region from – 105 to – 85, known as NF-κB-like element, heightened the *f-luc* expression 1.9-fold.

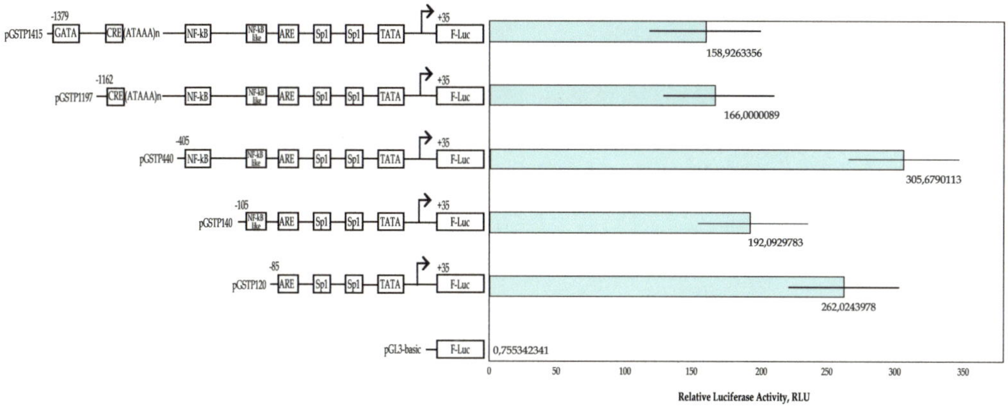


Fig. 5. Reporter constructs and relative luciferase activity in transfected Me45 cells. Data were normalized to expression of *renilla* luciferase from pRL-TK vector cotransfected together with the reporter constructs. Relative luciferase activity was calculated as a ratio of firefly to *renilla* luciferase light emission. Each bar in the figure represents the average ± SD of three independent transfection experiments with triplications in each

Thus transient transfection experiment revealed two negative regulatory elements located in the regions from – 1162 to – 405 and from – 105 to – 85 and the strong positive regulatory element located in the region from – 405 to – 105 in GSTP1 promoter in Me45 cells.

### 3.4 Nuclear proteins from Me45 cells specifically interact with ARE, NF-κB-binding site and CRE, but not with NF-κB-like and GATA sites

To test the ability of the regulatory elements identified in *GSTP1* promoter to interact with nuclear proteins from Me45 cells the electrophoretic mobility shift assay (EMSA) was performed. The ability of 20 bp promoter fragments, containing ARE, NF-κB-like, NF-κB, CRE and GATA sites to bind nuclear proteins from Me45 cells was examined in this experiment. Fig. 6 indicates that all oligonucleotides form complexes with Me45 nuclear proteins.

The specificity of protein binding was examined in a competition experiment, in which nuclear proteins were preincubated with 50- and 100-fold molar excess of unlabeled probe. This experiment demonstrated that CRE, NF-κB and ARE, but not NF-κB-like and GATA sites specifically bind nuclear proteins (Fig. 6B, C, Fig. 7). The complexes marked as non-specific were not eliminated by excess of any unlabeled oligonucleotide identical to that used as a probe.

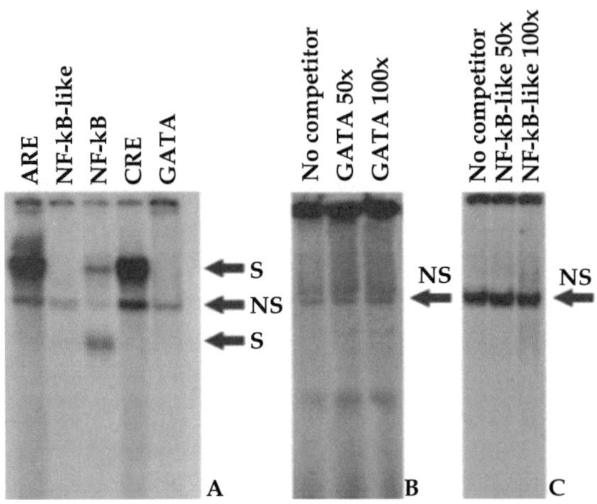


Fig. 6. In vitro binding of Me45 nuclear proteins to the *GSTP1* promoter sites. Electrophoretic mobility shift assay demonstrates that Me45 nuclear proteins form complexes with ARE, NF-κB, NF-κB-like, CRE and GATA sites. Results of competitive EMSA demonstrate that protein binding to NF-κB-like and GATA site is nonspecific. S – specific complex, NS – non-specific complex

### 3.5 Transcription factor NF-κB, and ERβ in complex with Fos or unidentified protein interact with *GSTP1* promoter elements in Me-45 cells

To identify the transcription factors that interact with *GSTP1* promoter in Me45 cells we used a competitive EMSA with the oligonucleotides of two types - those containing consensus cis-elements to the potential transcription factors and authentic cis-elements (fig. 7).

For identification of transcription factors that bind ARE site, a 50- and 100-fold molar excess of unlabeled oligonucleotides containing consensus binding sites for transcription factor AP-1, DNA-binding protein Maf (which mediates interaction of NF-E2 and related factors with DNA), estrogen receptor β (ER β) and retinoic acid receptor (RAR) were used. Neither of these consensus oligonucleotides competed for transcription factors with authentic ARE site (Fig. 7a). It means that DNA-binding domains of transcription factors that recognize consensus oligos do not interact with ARE site. This results were verified by supershift experiments with polyclonal antibodies to c-Jun (cross-reactive to JunB and JunD), c-Fos (cross-reactive to FosB, Fra1 and Fra2), MafF/G/K, ERβ and Nrf3. As indicated in Fig. 7b, neither Jun, Fos nor Maf and Nrf3 transcription factors are involved in formation of specific complex with ARE site. However, antibody to ERβ disrupted the original complex and the new complex with higher electrophoretic mobility was formed. Therefore it is plausible that ERβ binds to the *GSTP1* ARE site via another yet unidentified protein but not with its DNA-binding domain.

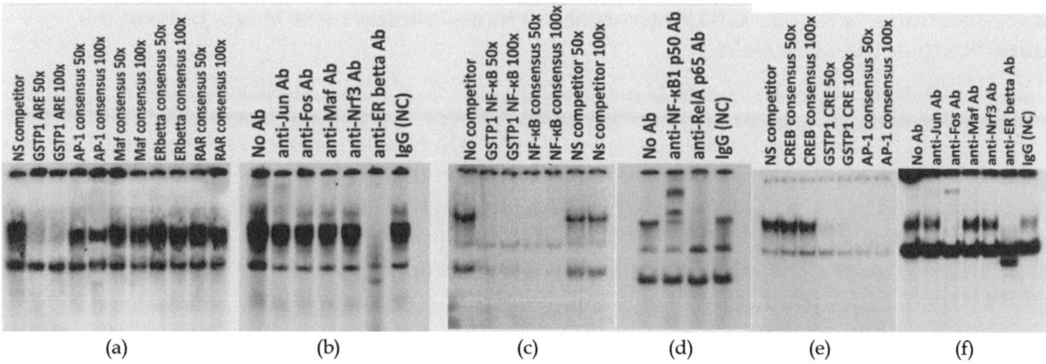


Fig. 7. Analysis of the complexes formed by ARE, NF-κB and CRE sites of *GSTP1* promoter with nuclear proteins. Formation of ARE-protein complex is inhibited by unlabeled authentic oligo with ARE site (a) and by ERβ antibody (b); NF-κB-site forms two complexes, both disrupted by the authentic corresponding oligo and oligo with NF-κB consensus (c); p50 antibody supershifts both complexes and p65 antibody disrupts the upper complex (d); The complex of CRE site with nuclear proteins is inhibited by authentic oligo, oligos with AP-1 consensus, but not CRE one compete with the CRE containing oligo (e); antibodies to Fos and ERβ supershift the complex (f)

The results of EMSA with oligonucleotide containing NF-κB site of *GSTP1* are represented in Fig. 7c. Two specific complexes were detected in the reaction with nuclear proteins. The unlabeled oligo with NF-κB consensus efficiently competed with the authentic oligo containing NF-κB response element for the nuclear proteins involved in formation of upper and lower complexes (Fig. 7c).

The composition of two different complexes with NF-κB response element was identified by supershift experiment with polyclonal antibodies to NF-κB1 p50 and RelA p65 subunits. Preincubation of nuclear proteins with antibody to p50 resulted in appearance of two supershifted bands (Fig. 7d). It means that both initial complexes contain p50 subunit of NF-κB. In the presence of p65 antibody the upper band disappeared pointing to the involvement not only p50 but also p65 subunit in this complex. Hence we provided the evidence that p50/p50 homodimer and p50/p65 heterodimer interact with *GSTP1* NF-κB binding site in Me45 cells.

To test the ability of CRE site to interact with CREB and AP-1 proteins, the corresponding oligonucleotides containing consensus binding sites for both transcription factors were used in the competition experiments. An autoradiograph in Fig. 7e indicates that oligo with consensus sequence to CREB did not compete with authentic oligo, while cold authentic probe and oligo with consensus to AP-1 competed successfully. Therefore it means that transcription factor AP-1 binds to CRE in Me45 cells.

The composition of CRE-protein complex was investigated by the supershift experiment with to Jun, Fos, MafF/G/K, ERβ and Nrf3. Incubation with antibodies antibodies to Fos and ERβ resulted in appearance of the new bands (Fig. 7f). Therefore both transcription factors take part in the complex formation with CRE in melanoma Me45 cells.

Thus, we demonstrated that positive regulatory element ARE interacts with ERβ in complex with another protein, negative regulatory element CRE interacts with Fos/ERβ-complex and positive regulatory element NF-κB binding site interacts with transcription factor NF-κB in the form of p50/p50 homodimer and p50/p65 heterodimer.

### 3.6 γ-Irradiation induces *GSTP1* expression in melanoma cells Me45, but not in choriocarcinoma cells BeWo

Transcription factor NF-κB (p65) is known to be activated during oxidative stress particularly that created by γ-irradiation and hydrogen peroxide (Gilmore, 1999). Taking this fact into account we have supposed that p50/p65-heterodimer of NF-κB, identified as a part of DNA-protein complex formed on *GSTP1* promoter in Me45 melanoma cells, may be responsible for *GSTP1* induction by γ-irradiation. To verify this assumption we used choriocarcinoma BeWo cells. The level of *GSTP1* expression in BeWo cells is very near to that in Me45 cells as it was shown in this study (Fig. 2). But as we have demonstrated previously the p50/p65-heterodimer is not involved in regulation of *GSTP1* transcription in BeWo cells while all other transcription factors are identical between two types of cells (Slonchak et al., 2009). As demonstrated in Fig. 8, GSTP1 mRNA content in BeWo cells in contrast to Me45 cells does not change significantly after γ-irradiation. It is quite possible that the sole difference between transcription factors regulating *GSTP1* transcription in two types of cells, the presence/absence of p65 subunit of NF-κB, mediates induction of *GSTP1* transcription in response to γ-irradiation in melanoma cells.

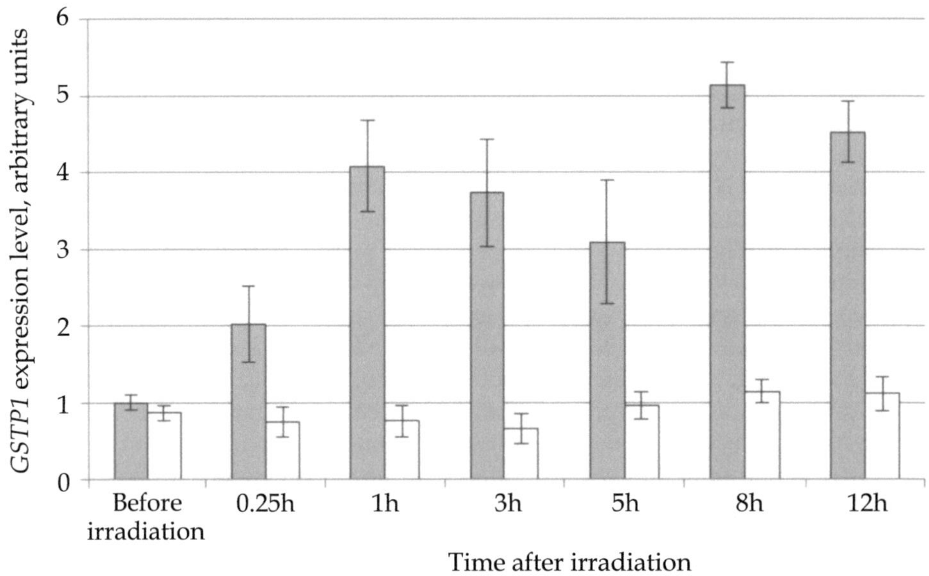


Fig. 8. Expression of *GSTP1* gene in Me45 and BeWo cells before and after γ-irradiation. Gray bars represent GSTP1 mRNA level in Me45 cells and white bars – in BeWo cells. The values were normalized to expression of RPL41 ribosomal protein gene and presented as the ratios to *GSTP1* expression in both cells before irradiation. The graphs represent the mean data ± SD of three separate experiments with triplications in each

## 4. Discussion

*GSTP1* is a caretaker gene as it detoxifies endogeneous and exogeneous toxic compounds and thus protects the organism against genome damage, oxidative stress (Hayes & Strange, 1995), cancer (Henderson et al., 1998), and degenerative diseases (Guven et al., 2011). Down-regulation of *GSTP1* expression with concomitant decrease of detoxification is a common precancerous event (Cookson et al., 1997; Meiers et al., 2007; Song et al., 2002) while its up-regulation at the later stages of tumor development causes multidrug resistance (Diah et al., 1999). The role of GSTP1 in development of malignant melanoma and its response to traditional therapy is far from being clear.

Nowadays it is known that *GSTP1* is expressed in normal human melanocytes and its expression is retained after malignant transformation (Hanada et al., 1991). Malignant melanocytes reveal resistance to the components of traditional therapy e.g. to etoposide, cis-platinum, γ-irradiation, which provoke the transition of the cells into apoptosis. In comparison with some other malignant cells (human leukemia cells HL-60, rat rhabdomyosarcoma cells R1) melanoma cells Me45 reveal greater resistance to each of these components and less quantity of cells are susceptible to apoptosis (Kumala et al., 2003). To unravel the potential role of *GSTP1* in the malignant transformation of melanocytes and their resistance to traditional treatment we have focused our attention on the *GSTP1* expression in malignant melanoma cells and molecular mechanisms of its regulation at transcriptional level. For this aim we examined the level of *GSTP1* expression in malignant melanoma cells Me45 before and after γ-irradiation and characterized cis-elements of *GSTP1* promoter and transcription factors interacting with them.

Among 12 malignant cell lines *GSTP1* expression in Me45 cells was at the low level (the cells MCF7 and HepG2 do not express *GSTP1* due to complete methlylation *of GSTP1* promoter and potent repression of gene transcription). The situation drastically changes after γ-irradiation. The Me45 and BeWo cells expressing *GSTP1* nearly at the same level before irradiation significantly differ from one another after irradiation. The *GSTP1* expression steadily rises in melanoma cells and remains at the same level in BeWo cells. It was known that *GSTP1* may inhibit pro-apoptotic signal transduction (Zhao et al., 2006; Zhou et al., 2005), conjugate etoposide to glutathione (Depeille et al., 2005) and by these ways protect the cells from apoptosis. Thereby the peculiarities of cell-specific regulation of *GSTP1* expression in melanocytes and its up-regulation after γ-irradiation may to some extent explain the development of melanoma and its extreme resistance to chemo- and radiotherapy.

Initiation of gene transcription in eukaryotes is a multistep process which includes chromatin remodeling, DNA demethylation, enchanseosome formation and the assembly of the general transcription machinery. Each event in this process is strictly controlled by cell- and state-specific coordinated interactions between transcription factors, coactivators and corepressors with chromatin and transcription machinery components. In this study we focused on the functional role of cis-elements of *GSTP1* promoter and corresponding transcription factors in regulation of gene transcription in human malignant melanoma cells. The interaction of cis-elements of *GSTP1* promoter with transcription factors were examined in different malignant cells (Duvoix et al., 2003; Henderson et al., 1998; Jhaveri & Morrow, 1998). All these studies have shown that in different kind of cells cell-specific transcription factors bind the same response elements. So far the regulation of *GSTP1* transcription in malignant melanocytes was not addressed. For the first time we have assessed the functional activity of *GSTP1* cis-elements in malignant melanocytes and identified two elements - antioxidant response element (ARE) and NF-κB binding site, that positively regulate *GSTP1* transcription, and cAMP response element (CRE), that regulates it negatively. The same was true for mammary epidermal cells Hbl-100 and choriocarcinoma BeWo cells (Slonchak et al., 2009). Therefore the different set of transcription factors may define either positive or negative regulation of *GSTP1* transcription in cell-specific manner.

In malignant melanocytes the positive regulatory element ARE interacts with ERβ through another yet not identified protein. This fact distinguishes Me45 cells among other malignant cells in which diverse transcription factors or in different way interact with this site. The diversity includes transcription factor AP-1 in breast cancer cells VCREMS (Moffat et al., 1994) and in leukemia cells K562 (Duvoix et al., 2004a); transcription factor NF-E2 in K562 cells (Borde-Chiche et al., 2001); RARα in HeLa cells (Xia et al., 1996) and ERβ in complex with Jun/Fos or with Nuclear Factor E2 related factor (Nrf2) in mammary carcinoma cells MDA-MB-231(Montano et al., 2004). It is interesting that transcription factors Jun and Fos in the latter complex cannot activate *GSTP1* transcription themselves but they recruit ERβ and the whole complex substantially activates transcription and mediates up-regulation of *GSTP1* expression by estradiol and antiestrogen tamoxifen (Montano et al., 2004).

It is also noteworthy that in Me45 cells ERβ indirectly interacts not only with antioxidant response element ARE, but also with cAMP response element CRE in complex with transcription factor Fos. In *GSTP1* promoter CRE was first identified in lung carcinoma cells Calu-6. In these cells it interacts with the transcription factor CREB-1 and mediates induction of *GSTP1* transcription by cAMP (Lo & li-Osman, 2002). In contrast to this communication we demonstrated that in Me-45 cells CRE acts as a negative regulatory element. Thus in one type of cells CRE acts as a positive element interacting with CREB and in the other type of cells as a negative element directly interacting with Fos in complex with ERβ. The similar phenomenon has been described for the gene encoding steroidogenic acute regulatory protein, which is up-regulated by CREB and down-regulated by Fos/Jun both interacting with CRE site (Manna & Stocco, 2007).

The role of ERβ in regulation of *GSTP1* expression was a disputable question until now. Possible implication of ER into regulation of *GSTP1* expression was demonstrated for the first time in 1988 by Moscow et al. who described the negative correlation between ER content and *GSTP1* expression in breast cancer cells (Moscow et al., 1988). Later Montano et al. demonstrated that ERβ acts as a positive regulator of *GSTP1* expression in the same cells (Montano et al., 2004). Here we found that ERβ indirectly interacts with two distinct sites of *GSTP1* promoter - positive regulatory element ARE and a negative regulatory element CRE and in both cases different transcription factors mediate the effect of ERβ. We believe that these data may explain the previous contradictions - the ability of ERβ to repress (Moscow et al., 1988) and induce (Montano et al., 2004) *GSTP1* transcription.

The region of *GSTP1* promoter from – 405 to – 105 which contains NF-κB response element acts as a strong positive regulatory element in Me45 cells. It interacts with p50 NF-κB1/p65 RelA heterodimer and with p50/p50 NF-κB1 homodimer in Me45 cells and only with p50/p50 NF-κB1 homodimers in BeWo cells (Slonchak et al., 2009). We suggest that activation of *GSTP1* transcription in Me45 cells by γ-irradiation and the insensitivity of BeWo cells to the influence of irradiation are connected with the differences in NF-κB dimers in both types of cells. Proteins from NF-κB family may be subdivided into two classes according to the sequence of their C-terminal domain, presence of transcription activation domain (TAD) and the sequence specificity of response elements with which they interact. Members of the class I (NF-κB1 p50 and NF-κB2 p52) do not contain TAD and have long C terminal domains with multiple copies of ankyrin repeats that inhibit the ability of the factors to activate transcription. The second class of NF-κB family includes c-Rel, v-Rel, RelB and RelA (p65). These proteins contain C-terminal activation domain TAD and can activate transcription (Schmid et al., 1994). The members of both classes in different combinations can form dimers with various regulatory potential. In different types of cells the homodimers p50/p50, p65/p65, c-Rel/c-Rel and heterodimers RelB/p50, RelB/p52, p65/c-Rel, RelB/p65 та RelB/c-Rel were identified (Neumann & Naumann, 2007).

The members of the first class bind preferably to GGGRN motif in promoters (R – purine base, N – any base). The members of the second class bind to YYCC motif (Y – pyrimidine base). Thereby p50/p50 homodimers bind to 11 bp sequence which contains two GGGRN repeats, separated by A/T-pair. The heterodimers consisting from the members of both classes bind GGRNWYYCC sequence (W – A or T) (Baldwin, Jr., 1996). The NF-κB binding site of *GSTP1* promoter is GGGAATTTCCCC sequence and it corresponds to typical binding site for NF-κB heterodimers. The homodimers p50/p50 may also interact with this site but this binding is weak and does not result in transcription activation (Neumann & Naumann, 2007). In this regard only the heterodimers containing either RelA, RelB or c-Rel with p50 or p52 are able to activate *GSTP1* transcription. In this study we found that p50/p65 RelA NF-κB heterodimer and p50/p50 homodimer interact with NF-κB binding site of *GSTP1* gene in Me45 cells in comparison with p50/p50 homodimers interacting with this site in BeWo cells. The obtained results together with the above mentioned characteristics of the members of both classes of NF-κB family explain very well the difference in response of Me45 and BeWo cells to γ-irradiation and the resistance of malignant melanoma cells to radiotherapy due to the activation of *GSTP1* expression. The important role of p50/p65 RelA NF-κB heterodimer in this process is highly expected. We have to note that γ-irradiation causes degradation of NF-κB inhibitor with which it is bound in the cytoplasm and translocation of NF-κB into the nucleus with its subsequent participation in regulation of gene transcription.

## 5. Conclusions

Melanoma is a malignant tumor of melanocytes that occurs in result of collision of UV photon with a chromophore in a skin cell, production of reactive oxygen species and oxidative stress with the DNA damage. Conceptually, oxidative stress results from a change in the equilibrium between production of pro-oxidant and their consumption or deactivation, favoring an excess of pro-oxidant that have noxious consequences at the molecular and cellular levels. The cellular antioxidant defense relies to the great extent on a powerful sulfur redox chemistry response in which glutathione S-transferases are active players. Therefore a deficiency in the activity of GSTs may contribute to the risk of UV-induced melanoma.

It is notorious that melanoma is the most aggressive form of skin cancer, which is resistant to all current modalities of anticancer therapy, including chemo- and radiotherapy. The overexpression of GST and multidrug resistance protein 1 may confer to the resistance of melanoma cells.

We demonstrated that the level of *GSTP1* expression in malignant melanoma cells Me45 was significantly lower than in eight other malignant cell lines and similar to that in choriocarcinoma cells BeWo. Despite the similarity of *GSTP1* expression in nonirradiated Me45 and BeWo cells their response to γ-irradiation was different - the level of GSTP1 steadily rises merely in Me45 cells, not in BeWo cells. To find out the clue for the difference in response of both types of cells to γ-irradiation we examined the regulation of *GSTP1* gene transcription. Two cis-elements, ARE and NF-κB binding site, positively regulate *GSTP1* transcription, and element CRE regulates it negatively in Me45 cells. The same is true for BeWo cells as we have shown previously. In both types of cells cis-element ARE interacts with ERβ through another yet not identified protein and cis-element CRE – with Fos/ERβ dimer. However in Me45 cells NF-κB binding site interacts with p50/p65 RelA and p50/p50 dimers of NF-κB while in BeWo cells – only with p50/p50 dimer. The induction of NF-κB in

response to γ-irradiation, the strong activating potential of p65 RelA subunit of NF-κB and subsequent up-regulation of *GSTP1* expression may stipulate the melanoma cells resistance to radiotherapy. However this cause may not be unique.
According to our results γ-irradiation induces activation of GSTP1 expression via transcription factor NF-κB. Therefore we suggest that inactivation of NF-κB may prevent melanoma resistance. Clinical trials with drugs that block NF-κB are currently in progress with promising results. As reviewed by Lee and Burckart, the NF-κB activation process can be inhibited by pharmacologic agents at each activation step: glucocorticoids inhibit NF-κB by up regulating IKB expression, cyclosporine and tacrolimus inhibit calcineurin, a phosphatase that indirectly induces IKB degradation, deoxyspergualin inhibits nuclear translocation of NF-κB, aspirin and salicylates inhibit IKB phosphorylation, tepoxalin and antioxidants inhibit NF-κB activation by influencing the redox state of the cell (Lee & Burckart, 1998). It's clear that development of specific inhibitory agents has to go in parallel with improvement of targeted drug delivery systems.

## 6. Acknowledgment

This work was supported by Polish Ministry of Science and Education grant #N40115732/3043 (R.-W.J) and by grant of the President of Ukraine for talented youth (S.A). The experimental part of the work was performed by the authors in the laboratory of Maria Sklodowska-Curie Memorial Cancer Center and Institute of Oncology (Poland). We thank Prof. Dr. hab. Anna El'skaya (Institute of Molecular Biology and Genetics NAS of Ukraine) for fruitful discussions and financial support of publication.

## 7. References

Adler, V., Yin, Z., Fuchs, S. Y., Benezra, M., Rosario, L., Tew, K. D., Pincus, M. R., Sardana, M., Henderson, C. J., Wolf, C. R., Davis, R. J., & Ronai, Z. (1999). Regulation of JNK signaling by GSTp. *EMBO Journal*, Vol.18, No.5, (March 1999), pp. 1321-1334, ISSN 0261-4189

Ananthaswamy, H. N. & Pierceall, W. E. (1990) Molecular mechanisms of ultraviolet radiation carcinogenesis. *Photochemistry and Photobiology*, Vol.52, No.6, (December 1990), pp. 1119-1136, ISSN 1751-1097

Baldwin, A. S., Jr. (1996). The NF-kappa B and I kappa B proteins: new discoveries and insights. *Annual Review of Immunology*, Vol.14, (1996), pp. 649-683, ISSN 0732-0582

Borde-Chiche, P., Diederich, M., Morceau, F., Wellman, M., & Dicato, M. (2001). Phorbol ester responsiveness of the glutathione S-transferase P1 gene promoter involves an inducible c-jun binding in human K562 leukemia cells. *Leukemia Research*, Vol.25, No.3, (March 2001), pp. 241-247, ISSN 0145-2126

Bu, H., Rosdahl, I., Holmdahl-Kallen, K., Sun, X. F., & Zhang, H. (2007). Significance of glutathione S-transferases M1, T1 and P1 polymorphisms in Swedish melanoma patients. *Oncology Reports*, Vol.17, No.4, (April 2007), pp. 859-864, ISSN 1791-2431

Cowell, I. G., Dixon, K. H., Pemble, S. E., Ketterer, B., & Taylor, J. B. (1988). The structure of the human glutathione S-transferase pi gene. *Biochemical Journal*, Vol.255, No.1, (October 1988), pp. 79-83, ISSN 0264-6021

De, M. F., Pedersen, J. Z., Caccuri, A. M., Antonini, G., Turella, P., Stella, L., Lo, B. M., Federici, G., & Ricci, G. (2003). The specific interaction of dinitrosyl-diglutathionyl-iron complex, a natural NO carrier, with the glutathione transferase superfamily:

suggestion for an evolutionary pressure in the direction of the storage of nitric oxide. *Journal of Biological Chemistry*, Vol.278, No.43, (October 2003), pp. 42283-42293, ISSN 0021-9258

Depeille, P., Cuq, P., Passagne, I., Evrard, A., & Vian, L. (2005). Combined effects of GSTP1 and MRP1 in melanoma drug resistance. *British Journal of Cancer*, Vol.93, No.2, (July 2005), pp. 216-223, ISSN 0007-0920

Dignam, J. D., Lebovitz, R. M., & Roeder, R. G. (1983). Accurate transcription initiation by RNA polymerase II in a soluble extract from isolated mammalian nuclei. *Nucleic Acids Research*, Vol.11, No.5, (March 1983), pp. 1475-1489, ISSN 0305-1048.

Dolzan, V., Rudolf, Z., & Breskvar, K. (2006). Genetic susceptibility to environmental carcinogenesis in Slovenian melanoma patients. *Acta Dermatovenerologica Alpina, Panonica, Et Adriatica*, Vol.15, No.2, (June 2006), pp. 69-78, ISSN 1318-4458

Duvoix, A., Schnekenburger, M., Delhalle, S., Blasius, R., Borde-Chiche, P., Morceau, F., Dicato, M., & Diederich, M. (2004a). Expression of glutathione S-transferase P1-1 in leukemic cells is regulated by inducible AP-1 binding. *Cancer Letters*, Vol.216, No.2, (December 2004), pp. 207-219, ISSN 0304-3835

Duvoix, A., Delhalle, S., Blasius, R., Schnekenburger, M., Morceau, F., Fougere, M., Henry, E., Galteau, M. M., Dicato, M., & Diederich, M. (2004b). Effect of chemopreventive agents on glutathione S-transferase P1-1 gene expression mechanisms via activating protein 1 and nuclear factor kappaB inhibition. *Biochemical Pharmacology*, Vol.68, No.6, (September 2004), pp. 1101-1111, ISSN 0006-2952

Frova, C. (2006). Glutathione transferases in the genomics era: new insights and perspectives. *Biomolecular Engeneering*, Vol.23, No.4, (September 2006), pp. 149-169, ISSN 1389-0344

Hanada, K., Ishikawa, H., Tamai, K., Hashimoto, I., & Sato, K. (1991). Expression of glutathione S-transferase-pi in malignant skin tumors. *Journal of Dermatological Science*, Vol.2, No.1, (January 1991), pp. 18-23, ISSN 0923-1811

Harbottle, A., Daly, A. K., Atherton, K., & Campbell, F. C. (2001). Role of glutathione S-transferase P1, P-glycoprotein and multidrug resistance-associated protein 1 in acquired doxorubicin resistance. *Internationa Journal of Cancer*, Vol.92, No.6, (June 2001), pp. 777-783, ISSN 0020-7136

Hayes, J. D. & Strange, R. C. (1995). Potential contribution of the glutathione S-transferase supergene family to resistance to oxidative stress. *Free Radical Research*, Vol.22, No.3, (March 1995), pp. 193-207, ISSN 1071-5762.

Hayes, J. D., Flanagan, J. U., & Jowsey, I. R. (2005). Glutathione transferases. *Annual Review of Pharmacology and Toxicology*, Vol.45, (2005), pp. 51-88, ISSN 0362-1642.

Helmbach, H., Rossmann, E., Kern, M. A., & Schadendorf, D. (2001). Drug-resistance in human melanoma. *International Journal of Cancer*, Vol.93, No.5, (September 2001), pp. 617-622, ISSN 0020-7136

Henderson, C. J., McLaren, A. W., Moffat, G. J., Bacon, E. J., & Wolf, C. R. (1998). Pi-class glutathione S-transferase: regulation and function. *Chemico-Biological Interactions*, Vol.111-112, (April 1998), pp. 69-82, ISSN 0009-2797

Hoeijmakers, J. H. (2001). Genome maintenance mechanisms for preventing cancer. *Nature*, Vol.411, No.6835, (May 2001), pp. 366-374, ISSN 0028-0836

Ivanov, V. N., Kehrl, J. H., & Ronai, Z. (2000). Role of TRAF2/GCK in melanoma sensitivity to UV-induced apoptosis. *Oncogene*, Vol.19, No.7, (February 2000), pp. 933-942, ISSN 0950-9232

Jhaveri, M. S. & Morrow, C. S. (1998). Contribution of proximal promoter elements to the regulation of basal and differential glutathione S-transferase P1 gene expression in human breast cancer cells. *Biochimica et Biophysica Acta*, Vol.1396, No.2, (March 1998), pp. 179-190, ISSN 0006-3002

Kumala, S., Niemiec, P., Widel, M., Hancock, R., & Rzeszowska-Wolny, J. (2003). Apoptosis and clonogenic survival in three tumour cell lines exposed to gamma rays or chemical genotoxic agents. *Cellular and Molecular Biology Letters*, Vol.8, No.3, (2003), pp. 655-665, ISSN 1425-8153

Laemmli, U. K. (1970). Cleavage of structural proteins during the assembly of the head of bacteriophage T4. *Nature*, Vol.227, No.5259, (August 1970), pp. 680-685, ISSN 0028-0836

Lee, J. & Burckart, G. (1998). Nuclear Factor Kappa B: Important Transcription Factor and Therapeutic Target. *The Journal of Clinical Pharmacology*, Vol.38, No.11, (November 1998), pp. 981-993, ISSN 0091-2700

Lo, H. W. & li-Osman, F. (2002). Cyclic AMP mediated GSTP1 gene activation in tumor cells involves the interaction of activated CREB-1 with the GSTP1 CRE: a novel mechanism of cellular GSTP1 gene regulation. *Journal of Cellular Biochemistry*, Vol.87, No.1, (2002), pp. 103-116, ISSN 0730-2312

Manna, P. R. & Stocco, D. M. (2007). Crosstalk of CREB and Fos/Jun on a single cis-element: transcriptional repression of the steroidogenic acute regulatory protein gene. *Journal of Molecular Endocrinology*, Vol.39, No.4, (October 2007), pp. 261-277, ISSN 0952-5041

Marino, M., Galluzzo, P., & Ascenzi, P. Estrogen signaling multiple pathways to impact gene transcription. Curr.Genomics, Vol.7, No.8, (November 2006), pp. 497-508,

Moffat, G. J., McLaren, A. W., & Wolf, C. R. (1994). Involvement of Jun and Fos proteins in regulating transcriptional activation of the human pi class glutathione S-transferase gene in multidrug-resistant MCF7 breast cancer cells. *Journal of Biological Chemistry*, Vol.269, No.23, (June 1994), pp. 16397-16402, ISSN 0021-9258

Moffat, G. J., McLaren, A. W., & Wolf, C. R. (1996a). Sp1-mediated transcriptional activation of the human Pi class glutathione S-transferase promoter. *Journal of Biological Chemistry*, Vol.271, No.2, (January 1996), pp. 1054-1060, ISSN 0021-9258

Moffat, G. J., McLaren, A. W., & Wolf, C. R. (1996b) Functional characterization of the transcription silencer element located within the human Pi class glutathione S-transferase promoter. *Journal of Biological Chemistry*, Vol.271, No.34, (August 1996), pp. 20740-20747, ISSN 0021-9258

Montano, M. M., Deng, H., Liu, M., Sun, X., & Singal, R. (2004). Transcriptional regulation by the estrogen receptor of antioxidative stress enzymes and its functional implications. *Oncogene*, Vol.23, No.14, (April 2004), pp. 2442-2453, ISSN 0950-9232

Moral, A., Palou, J., Lafuente, A., Molina, R., Piulachs, J., Castel, T., & Trias, M. (1997). Immunohistochemical study of alpha, mu and pi class glutathione S transferase expression in malignant melanoma. MMM Group. Multidisciplinary Malignant Melanoma Group. *British Journal of Dermatology*, Vol.136, No.3, (March 1997), pp. 345-350, ISSN 0007-0963

Morceau, F., Dupont, C., Palissot, V., Borde-Chiche, P., Trentesaux, C., Dicato, M., & Diederich, M. (2000). GTP-mediated differentiation of the human K562 cell line: transient overexpression of GATA-1 and stabilization of the gamma-globin mRNA. *Leukemia*, Vol.14, No.9, (September 2000), pp. 1589-1597, ISSN 0887-6924

Morceau, F., Duvoix, A., Delhalle, S., Schnekenburger, M., Dicato, M., & Diederich, M. (2004). Regulation of glutathione S-transferase P1-1 gene expression by NF-kappaB in tumor necrosis factor alpha-treated K562 leukemia cells. *Biochemical Pharmacology*, Vol.67, No.7, (April 2004), pp. 1227-1238, ISSN 0006-2952

Morrow, C. S., Goldsmith, M. E., & Cowan, K. H. (1990). Regulation of human glutathione S-transferase pi gene transcription: influence of 5'-flanking sequences and trans-activating factors which recognize AP-1-binding sites. *Gene*, Vol.88, No.2, (April 1990), pp. 215-225, ISSN 0378-1119

Moscow, J. A., Townsend, A. J., Goldsmith, M. E., Whang-Peng, J., Vickers, P. J., Poisson, R., Legault-Poisson, S., Myers, C. E., & Cowan, K. H. (1988). Isolation of the human anionic glutathione S-transferase cDNA and the relation of its gene expression to estrogen-receptor content in primary breast cancer. *Proceedings of the National Academy of Sciences of the United States of America*, Vol.85, No.17, (September 1988), pp. 6518-6522, ISSN 0027-8424

Moscow, J. A., Fairchild, C. R., Madden, M. J., Ransom, D. T., Wieand, H. S., O'Brien, E. E., Poplack, D. G., Cossman, J., Myers, C. E., & Cowan, K. H. (1989). Expression of Anionic Glutathione-S-transferase and P-Glycoprotein Genes in Human Tissues and Tumors. *Cancer Research*, Vol.49, No.6, (March 1989), pp. 1422-1428, ISSN 0008-5472

Neumann, M. & Naumann, M. (2007). Beyond IkappaBs: alternative regulation of NF-kappaB activity. *The FASEB Journal*, Vol.21, No.11, (September 2007), pp. 2642-2654, ISSN 0892-6638

Nguyen, T., Huang, H. C., & Pickett, C. B. (2000). Transcriptional regulation of the antioxidant response element. Activation by Nrf2 and repression by MafK. *Journal of Biological Chemistry*, Vol.275, No.20, (May 2000), pp. 15466-15473, ISSN 0021-9258

Nishinaka, T., Ichijo, Y., Ito, M., Kimura, M., Katsuyama, M., Iwata, K., Miura, T., Terada, T., & Yabe-Nishimura, C. (2007). Curcumin activates human glutathione S-transferase P1 expression through antioxidant response element. *Toxicology Letters*, Vol.170, No.3, (May 2007), pp. 238-247, ISSN 0378-4274

Oakley, A. J., Lo, B. M., Nuccetelli, M., Mazzetti, A. P., & Parker, M. W. (1999). The ligandin (non-substrate) binding site of human Pi class glutathione transferase is located in the electrophile binding site (H-site). *Journal of Molecular Biology*, Vol.291, No.4, (August 1999), pp. 913-926, ISSN 0022-2836

Pedersen, J. Z., De, M. F., Turella, P., Federici, G., Mattei, M., Fabrini, R., Dawood, K. F., Massimi, M., Caccuri, A. M., & Ricci, G. (2007). Glutathione transferases sequester toxic dinitrosyl-iron complexes in cells. A protection mechanism against excess nitric oxide. *Journal of Biological Chemistry*, Vol.282, No.9, (March 2007), pp. 6364-6371, ISSN 0021-9258

Pinkus, R., Weiner, L. M., & Daniel, V. (1996). Role of oxidants and antioxidants in the induction of AP-1, NF-kappaB, and glutathione S-transferase gene expression. *Journal of Biological Chemistry*, Vol.271, No.23, (June 1996), pp. 13422-13429, ISSN 0021-9258

Przybyszewski, W. M., Widel, M., Szurko, A., Lubecka, B., Matulewicz, L., Maniakowski, Z., Polaniak, R., Birkner, E., & Rzeszowska-Wolny, J. (2004). Multiple bystander effect of irradiated megacolonies of melanoma cells on non-irradiated neighbours. *Cancer Letters*, Vol.214, No.1, (October 2004), pp. 91-102, ISSN 0304-3835

Rass, K. & Reichrath, J. (2008). UV damage and DNA repair in malignant melanoma and nonmelanoma skin cancer. *Advances in Experimental Medicine and Biology*, Vol.624, (2008), pp. 162-178, ISSN 0065-2598

Ricci, G., Caccuri, A. M., Lo, B. M., Parker, M. W., Nuccetelli, M., Turella, P., Stella, L., Di Iorio, E. E., & Federici, G. (2003). Glutathione transferase P1-1: self-preservation of an anti-cancer enzyme. *Biochemical Journal*, Vol.376, No.Pt 1, (November 2003), pp. 71-76, ISSN 0264-6021

Rzeszowska-Wolny, J., Herok, R., Widel, M., & Hancock, R. (2009) X-irradiation and bystander effects induce similar changes of transcript profiles in most functional pathways in human melanoma cells. *DNA Repair (Amst)*, Vol.8, No.6, (June 2009), pp. 732-738, ISSN 1568-7864

Schiff, R., Reddy, P., Ahotupa, M., Coronado-Heinsohn, E., Grim, M., Hilsenbeck, S. G., Lawrence, R., Deneke, S., Herrera, R., Chamness, G. C., Fuqua, S. A., Brown, P. H., & Osborne, C. K. (2000) Oxidative stress and AP-1 activity in tamoxifen-resistant breast tumors in vivo. *Journal of the National Cancer Institute*, Vol.92, No.23, (December 2000), pp. 1926-1934, ISSN 0027-8874

Schmid, R. M., Liptay, S., Betts, J. C., & Nabel, G. J. Structural and functional analysis of NF-kappa B. (1994). Determinants of DNA binding specificity and protein interaction. *Journal of Biological Chemistry*, Vol.269, No.51, (December 1994), pp. 32162-32167, ISSN 0021-9258

Schnekenburger, M., Morceau, F., Duvoix, A., Delhalle, S., Trentesaux, C., Dicato, M., & Diederich, M. Expression of glutathione S-transferase P1-1 in differentiating K562: role of GATA-1. *Biochemical and Biophysical Research Communications*, Vol.311, No.4, (November 2003), pp. 815-821, ISSN 0006-291X

Slonchak, A. M., Chwieduk, A., Rzeszowska-Wolny, J., & Obolenska, M. Yu. (2009a). Transcription regulation in differential expression of the human GSTP1 gene in breast and choriocarcinoma cells. *Ukrainian biochemical journal*, Vol.81, No.4, (July 2009), pp. 48-58, ISSN 0201-8470

Slonchak, A. M., Chwieduk, A., Rzeszowska-Wolny, J. & Obolenskaya, M. Yu. (2009b). Crosstalk between transcription factors in regulation of the human glutathione S-transferase P1 gene expression in Me45 melanoma cells. *Biopolymers and Cell*, Vol.25, No.3, (May 2009), pp. 27-30, ISSN 0233-7657

Tan, K. H., Meyer, D. J., Gillies, N., & Ketterer, B. (1988). Detoxification of DNA hydroperoxide by glutathione transferases and the purification and characterization of glutathione transferases of the rat liver nucleus. *Biochemical Journal*, Vol.254, No.3, (September 1988), pp. 841-845, ISSN 0264-6021

Turella, P., Pedersen, J. Z., Caccuri, A. M., De, M. F., Mastroberardino, P., Lo, B. M., Federici, G., & Ricci, G. (2003). Glutathione transferase superfamily behaves like storage proteins for dinitrosyl-diglutathionyl-iron complex in heterogeneous systems. *Journal of Biological Chemistry*, Vol.278, No.43, (October 2003), pp. 42294-42299, ISSN 0021-9258

Villafania, A., Anwar, K., Amar, S., Chie, L., Way, D., Chung, D. L., Adler, V., Ronai, Z., Brandt-Rauf, P. W., Yamaizumii, Z., Kung, H. F., & Pincus, M. R. (2000). Glutathione-S-Transferase as a selective inhibitor of oncogenic ras-p21-induced mitogenic signaling through blockade of activation of jun by jun-N-terminal kinase. *Annals of Clinical and Laboratory Science*, Vol.30, No.1, (January 2000), pp. 57-64, ISSN 0091-7370

Wu, Y., Fan, Y., Xue, B., Luo, L., Shen, J., Zhang, S., Jiang, Y., & Yin, Z. (2006). Human glutathione S-transferase P1-1 interacts with TRAF2 and regulates TRAF2-ASK1 signals. *Oncogene*, Vol.25, No.42, (September 2006), pp. 5787-5800, ISSN 0950-9232

Xia, C., Hu, J., Ketterer, B., & Taylor, J. B. (1996). The organization of the human GSTP1-1 gene promoter and its response to retinoic acid and cellular redox status. *Biochemical Journal*, Vol.313 ( Pt 1), (January 1996), pp. 155-161, ISSN 0264-6021

Zhao, X., Fan, Y., Shen, J., Wu, Y., & Yin, Z. (2006). Human glutathione S-transferase P1 suppresses MEKK1-mediated apoptosis by regulating MEKK1 kinase activity in HEK293 cells. *Moleculs and Cells*, Vol.21, No.3, (June 2006), pp. 395-400, ISSN 1016-8478

Zhou, L., Jing, Y., Styblo, M., Chen, Z., & Waxman, S. (2005). Glutathione-S-transferase pi inhibits $As_2O_3$-induced apoptosis in lymphoma cells: involvement of hydrogen peroxide catabolism. *Blood*, Vol.105, No.3, (February 2005), pp. 1198-1203, ISSN 0006-4971

# Changing the Nature of Melanoma Cells by Manipulation of Ganglioside Expression

Pu Wang[1], Sadako Yamagata[2] and Tatsuya Yamagata[1]
[1]*Department of Chemical and Biomolecular Engineering, The Johns Hopkins University, Baltimore, Maryland,*
[2]*Laboratory of Tumor Biology and Glycobiology, Shenyang Pharmaceutical University, Shenyang 110016,*
[1]*U.S.A*
[2]*People's Republic of China*

## 1. Introduction

Gangliosides, GSLs that contain sialic acid residues, are components of all animal cell membranes. It was first found by Klenk in 1935. He extracted something of new that was called substance X from the brain of a Niemann–Pick disease patient (Klenk, 1939b). In the following years, he understood (Klenk, 1939a) that substance X was a mixture of compounds and he named them "gangliosides". Gangliosides attracted immediately the interest of many investigators, but in spite of this, progresses in elucidating their structures were slow. In 1947, the structure of sphingosine was elucidated (Carter et al., 1947) and in 1955 that of sialic acid (Gottschalk, 1955). Finally, in 1963, the first ganglioside structure was described (Kuhn and Wiegandt, 1963). Following studies were extensively devoted to fully understand the ganglioside structural complexity, metabolism, cellular topology, biological functions, and pathobiological implications (Macher and Sweeley, 1978; Miller-Podraza et al., 1992; Sandhoff and Christomanou, 1979; Sandhoff and Conzelmann, 1984; Svennerholm et al., 1994). This research is still far to be considered concluded, but today there is a general agreement to consider gangliosides as functional molecules involved in the modulation of tumor metastasis and of cell signaling, cell invasive proliferation, adhesion, and motility (Bassi et al., 1991; Bremer et al., 1984; Caputto et al., 1977; Chan, 1988; Chan, 1989; Davis and Daly, 1980; Facci et al., 1984; Glebov and Nichols, 2004a; Glebov and Nichols, 2004b; Goldenring et al., 1985; Kim et al., 1986; Kreutter et al., 1987; Leon et al., 1981; Lin and Shaw, 2005; Morgan and Seifert, 1979; Partington and Daly, 1979; Roisen et al., 1981; Rybak et al., 1983; Tsuji et al., 1983; Yates et al., 1989).

In particular, systematic analysis of ganglioside antigens in various types of cancer was carried out. In these studies, ganglioside changes were observed based on the comparison of tumor tissues with corresponding normal tissues. Dramatic changes of ganglioside composition and metabolism were first shown using a cultured cell population after viral transformation (Hakomori and Murakami, 1968; Mora et al., 1969). In Balb/c 3T3 cells transformed with Kirsten strain of murine sarcoma virus (the tumor is called 3T3KiMSV), asialo-GM2 (Gg3) is greatly accumulated, with deletion of higher gangliosides. Rabbit antibodies directed to Gg3 specifically stained 3T3KiMSV tumor grown in Balb/c mice. The antibodies did not stain various normal tissues of Balb/c mice, except for a small population in spleen (Rosenfelder et al., 1977). In more critical experiments, rats and mice were immunized with tumors derived from genetically identical (syngeneic) animals. For example, mAb M2590 was established after immunization of C57/BL mice with syngeneic B16 melanoma cells followed by selection of hybridoma clones showing specific reactivity with melanoma. Thus, the mAb reacted only with melanoma cells (human and hamster as well as mouse) but not with normal mouse, hamster, or human tissues (Taniguchi and Wakabayashi, 1984). Surprisingly, the epitope structure was identified as GM3, which is widely distributed in normal cells and tissues (Hirabayashi et al., 1985). Further studies revealed that M2590 reacted only with GM3 with density above a threshold value (Nores et al., 1987), that is the mAb recognized not only GM3 but also density of GM3. In line with the above cases, metastatic and invasive abilities of mouse melanoma B16 cell variants, in the order BL6>F10>F1>>WA4, are closely correlated with level of GM3 surface expression (Otsuji et al., 1995), and also with degree of adhesion to cultured endothelial cells (ECs) (mouse SPE1l human umbilical vein ECs) in vitro (Kojima et al., 1992; Otsuji et al., 1995). In addition, GM3 as the dominant GSL in B16 cells (Vedralova et al., 1995), has also been implicated involving in differentiation (Nojiri et al., 1986) and growth regulation (Bremer et al., 1986). These results suggested that ganglioside, GM3, organized in B16 cell membrane differ from the same antigens present in normal cell membrane of B16 cells, involved in changing the nature of melanoma cells via modulating the characteristics of melanoma cells in growth, differentiation, adhesion, invasion and metastasis.

Taken the advantage of recent success in the molecular cloning of glycosyltransferase genes responsible for the synthesis of gangliosides (Lloyd and Furukawa, 1998; Nagata et al., 1992) has enabled us to modify the expression profiles of gangliosides in cultured cells and experimental animals by manipulating the cloned genes (Furukawa et al., 2001). Although many studies have been performed to clarify the roles of gangliosides with various approaches such as usage of metabolic inhibitors, glycosidase treatment, carbohydrate probes including lectins and antibodies, and carbohydrate mutant cells and animals, results obtained with the manipulation of glycosyltransferase genes are providing us with much more exciting and novel information on the biological function of individual enzyme products. Although glycol-remodeling experiments revealed novel and unexpected functions of complex carbohydrates (Furukawa et al., 2001), molecular mechanisms for the roles of gangliosides remain to be investigated in many cases.

This chapter reviews experimental aspects of GM3-mediated invasive growth, motility and adhesion, which in turn resulting in metastasis of melanoma cells. The biological functions of GM3 would be further focused in modulating the nature of melanoma, especially in the process of metastasis. Relationship between the gene manipulation to modify GM3 expression and B16 cell function was extended to be discussed in order to understand how GM3 regulates molecular signals, leading to the change of melanoma B16 cell phenotype. We conclude by discussing the *in vitro* model of melanoma, B16 cells, that gangliosdes expression changed the nature of melanoma cells.

## 2. Biological functions of gangliosides

Gangliosides are classified as acidic glycosphingolipids containing sialic acid. Gangliosides occur not only as well known ganglio-series but also as globo-series or lacto-series gangliosides. Each ganglioside series shows distinctive cell type or tissue type specificity, and they may play different functional roles in adhesion or signaling characteristics of cell types (Hakomori, 2003). Many subsequent extensive studies clarified functional roles of gangliosides as the following ways: 1) intracellular membrane trafficking, sorting, targeting and shedding; 2) functional receptors; 3) cell adhesion; 4) modulation of cell membranes to form gangliosides enriched microdomains (GSMs); 5) mediators or modulators of signal transduction.

In the view of the biological functions and given the strong amphiphilic characteristics of gangliosides, theoretical considerations and experimental data from artificial membranes suggest that gangliosides can cooperate in governing the membrane domain formation, existence, and organization according to the gangliosides physical-chemical properties, such as the lipid transition temperature, the hydrogen-bond network at the lipid-water interface, the geometry of the hydrophilic headgroups, and the carbohydrate-water interactions. This kind of interaction not only includes ganglioside itself but also recruit signal tranducer molecues to form glycosphingolipid enriched microdomains (GEMs), through which exerts its biological functions. The interest for GEMs, zones of the membrane with a peculiar composition different from that of the majority of bilayer, became very strong in the last 15 years. The concept of "GEMs" evolved, based on detergent-resistant properties (Brown and London, 1997; Okada et al., 1984) and three models of GEMs have been established after extensive experiments: 1) unique caveolar structures, which are also enriched in characteristic hydrophobic membrane protein caveolin (Anderson, 1998; Rothberg et al., 1992) are firstly identified by transmission electron microscopy with anti-GSL antibodies (Rahmann et al., 1994; Sorice et al., 1997); 2) similar composition, detergent-resistantce, and cholesterol-dependent properties (e.g. structure and function are disrupted by cholesterol-binding reagents β-cyclodextrin, filipin, and nystatin) were further found in not only caveolar but also non-caveolar region, the term "lipid raft" was proposed, representing "floating signaling platform" (Simons and Ikonen, 1997). 3) recently, a different microdomain was proposed, termed "immunological synapse" by the size, dynamic status, and detergent-resistance properties (Krummel and Davis, 2002) are different from the above two cell membrane microdomains.

Based on the above model of GEMs, some tumor-associated gangliosides antigens have been recovered as detergent-insoluble, low-density membrane fractions organized closely with various transducer molecules such as c-Src, Ras, Rho, and focal adhesion kinase (FAK). For example, >90% of c-Src, >90% of Ras, ~50% of Rho, and ~25% of FAK are enriched in GM3 microdomains of B16 cells (Iwabuchi et al., 1998). These observations indicate the possible presence of gangliosides enriched microdomains in cells and their involvement in signal transduction.

Upon thse findings, we have tried to construct a conceptual view with a focus on how the mechanistic process of GM3 is converted to signaling impulses affecting cellular phenotype, especially in influencing melanoma B16 cell metastasis, such as adhesion, invasive proliferation and motility.

## 3. GM3 changes the nature of melanoma B16 cells

A significant role of GM3 in defining membrane-based cell functions is indicated by quantitative and qualitative changes of GM3 associated genes exression, as shown in Table 1. Besides the "classic" function of gangliosides as antigens and toxin receptors, it is also

| Regulation Manner by GM3 | Gene Name | GM3(+) | GM3(-) | GM3(-) | Biological Functions |
|---|---|---|---|---|---|
| Positive | Caveolin-1 | 1.378 | 0.321 | 0.146 | (1) (Felicetti et al., 2009), (4) (Felicetti et al., 2009), (5) (Felicetti et al., 2009) |
| | Ly-GDI | 2.156 | 0.423 | 0.387 | (5) (Seftor et al., 2002) |
| | PKN-1 | 1.658 | 0.626 | 0.495 | (4) (Wang et al., 2006) |
| | E-cadherein | 1.875 | 0.695 | 0.721 | (1) (Lau et al., 2011), (3) (Tang et al., 1994), (5) (Wong and Gumbiner, 2003), (6) (Semb and Christofori, 1998) |
| | Gelsolin | 1.841 | 0.543 | 0.502 | (4) (Fujita et al., 2001) |
| | PTEN | 2.482 | 0.290 | 0.153 | (1) (Stahl et al., 2003) |
| | MMP-9 | 1.915 | 0.174 | 0.282 | (4) (Desai and Chellaiah, 2006), (5) (Wang et al., 2010) |
| | MMP-2 | 1.532 | 0.534 | 0.472 | (4) (Leotlela et al., 2007), (5) (Denkert et al., 2002) |
| | Apaf1 | 1.350 | 0.608 | 0.509 | (2) (Rockmann and Schadendorf, 2005) |
| | RhoB | 2.247 | 0.427 | 0.318 | (5) (Jiang et al., 2004), (6) (Jiang et al., 2004), (5) (Jiang et al., 2004) |
| | Midkine | 1.403 | 0.518 | 0.417 | (1) (Escalante et al., 2000) |
| | Lymphotoxin α | 2.245 | 0.475 | 0.497 | (6) (Dobrzanski et al., 2004) |
| | Tnf α | 2.188 | 0.349 | 0.292 | (4) (Katerinaki et al., 2003), (5) (Katerinaki et al., 2003) |
| | Plau | 1.453 | 0.397 | 0.750 | (5) (Lee et al., 2006), (6) (Lee et al., 2006) |
| | Plaur | 2.209 | 0.543 | 0.720 | (2) (Besch et al., 2007) |
| Negative | Integrin β5 | 0.783 | 1.465 | 1.754 | (1) (Taverna et al., 2005; Taverna et al., 2004),(2) (Cardo-Vila et al., 2003), (3) (Niu et al., 2007), (4) (Zhang et al., 2002) |
| | Vimentin | 0.111 | 1.984 | 2.089 | (5) (Leader et al., 1987) |
| | TGF β1 | 0.571 | 2.124 | 3.309 | (1) (Paterson et al., 2002), (4) (Xu et al., 2003), (5) (Xu et al., 2003) |
| | TGFBR 2 | 0.716 | 1.453 | 1.903 | (1) (Li et al., 2008) |
| | N-Cam | 0.282 | 2.901 | 2.223 | (3) (Anastassiou et al., 2000) |
| | Src | 0.639 | 1.347 | 1.925 | (1) (Frame, 2002), (3) (Frame, 2002), (4) (Bourguignon et al., 2001), (5) (Frame, 2002) |

Table 1. GM3 regulated tumor related genes expression in melanoma B16 cells. The numbers represent the fold changes of the corresponding genes in GM3 modulating cells compared with that of control cells. The biological functions of the genes in the process of metastasis are shown as (1) Invasive Proliferation; (2) Apoptosis; (3)Adhesion; (4) Motility; (5) Invasion; (6) Metastasis

responsible for the processes of tumor cell phenotype including invasive proliferation, apoptosis, adhesion, motility, invasion and metastasis coupled with signal transduction. To keep the discussion focused, we would respectively elucidate the mechanisms of GM3 regulating melanoma B16 cells adhesion, invasive proliferation and motility, which in turn mediate metastasis of melanoma B16 cells.

### 3.1 Adhesion

There may be many cell adhesion/recognition systems in which GSLs play an essential role. However, only the initiation of B16 melanoma metastasis has been elucidated to an appreciable extent. Adhesion of mouse B16 melanoma cells to LacCer, Gb4 or Gg3 coated plates is mediated by interaction of GM3 (expressed highly on B16 melanoma cells) with the above GSLs (Kojima and Hakomori, 1989; Kojima and Hakomori, 1991a; Kojima and Hakomori, 1991b). Since GM3 dependent adhesion of B16 cells to nonactivated mouse endothelial cells (which express LacCer, Gb4, and Gg3) is regarded as the initial step in metastasis of B16 cells (Kojima et al., 1992; Otsuji et al., 1995), GM3 dependent adhesion has been extensively investigated. In detail, the adhesion system based on carbohydrate-carbohydrate interaction has the following characteristics: 1) adhesion process is rapid (within <10 min, compared to >30 min for integrin-dependent adhesion); 2) specificity is high in some cases, low in others; 3) most require bivalent cation such as $Ca^{2+}$., but a few do not; 4) synergistic with other adhesion systems, e.g., integrins; 5) negative interaction (repulsion) occurs between certain pairs of carbohydrates, e.g., GM3-GM3.

In addition, our results demonstrated that GM3 is able to regulate the expression of adhesive genes, such as E-cadherin, N-Cam and Src, which in turn modulate the adhesion of melanoma B16 cells (Table 1). Although we could not provide further evidence to show that these signaling molecules reside in GEMs, it will be of great interest to see the results of further studies along this line.

### 3.2 Proliferation

Studies performed during the early 1970s suggested that GSLs may interact with unidentified functional membrane components, which in turn may cause changes in cellular proliferation. However, at that time, no realistic information on such functional components was available. It took almost 20 years for the development of the current concept of growth factor receptors with tyrosine kinases. For understanding GM3 effects on B16 cell growth in culture, basic knowledge on types of growth factors required for culturing specific types of cells was needed.

#### 3.2.1 Fibroblast growth factor receptor

Thus, the first experiment was undertaken to determine the effects of GM3 on BHK cell growth. Given the reason that BHK cells require fibroblast growth factor (FGF) but not epithelial growth factor (EGF) or platelet derived growth factor (PDGF), fibroblast growth factor (FGF) was used to observe the inhibitory effects of GM3 on BHK cell growth. Curiously, GM3-enriched BHK cells became refractive to growth stimulation by FGF, and internalization of FGF was completed blocked (Bremer and Hakomori, 1982). It was assumed that high GM3 level blocked function of FGFR (Bremer and Hakomori, 1982). However, at that time, there was no knowledge on tyrosine kinase associated with FGFR; studies along this line were not performed until 20 years later (Toledo et al., 2004).

### 3.2.2 EGF receptor

This line of studies was further extended to effects of gangliosides on EGF-dependent A431 cell growth, and on tyrosine kinase associated with epithelial growth factor receptor (EGFR). GM3, but no other GSLs, strongly inhibited EGF-dependent cell growth, and EGFR tyrosine kinase (Bremer et al., 1986). Since EGFR is highly expressed in various epidermal cancers, and its tyrosine kinase activity is closely associated with cancer malignancy, a possibility was investigated whether any ganglioside could have better inhibitory effect than GM3 (see below).

Hanai et al. (Hanai et al., 1988b) further found that lyso-GM3 showed much stronger inhibitory effect than GM3 on EGFR tyrosine kinase in vivo as well as in membrane extract *in vitro*. Furthermore, lyso-GM3 was detected in normal A431 cells. In contrast, exogenously added "de-N-acetyl-GM3" (GM3 having de-N-acetyl sialic acid) strongly promoted EGFR tyrosine kinase and promoted growth of A431 cells (Hanai et al., 1988a). Thus, effect of gangliosides on EGFR tyrosine kinase is more complicated than originally considered, i.e., 1) tyrosine kinase is modulated by GM3 when EGFR is activated by EGF under normal conditions; 2) trace quantity of lyso-GM3 present, which may result from GM3 by de-N-acylation, strongly inhibits receptor function; 3) de-N-acetylation of GM3 in resting A431 cells may promote cell growth, possibly through a channel different from simple activation of EGFR. Exogenous lyso-GM3 is highly cytotoxic, whereas lyso-GM3 dimer is not cytotoxic, but inhibits EGFR tyrosine kinase as strongly as lyso-GM3. Therefore, synthetic lyso-GM3 dimer has been studied for inhibition of EGFR activity and A431 cell growth, for the purpose of developing pharmacologically effective inhibitors of epidermal tumor cell growth (Murozuka et al., 2007).

### 3.2.3 GM3/Ly-GDI Arhgdib inhibits cell proliferation through modulation of phosphotidylinositol 3-kinase (PI3K)/Akt/mammalian target of rapamycin (mTOR)/regulatory associated protein of mTOR (Raptor) pathway under rigorous environment.

#### 3.2.3.1 GM3 suppresses B16 invasive proliferation

Given the key role of GM3 in regulating cell growth as the above discussion, several lines of evidence have shown that GM3 invovled in tumor cell invasive proliferation Anchorage-independent growth experiments were effective *in vitro* experiments to determine the characteristics of tumor cell invasive proliferation. For example, reduced expression of GM3 and GM3 synthase as a result of v-Jun transformation resulted in enhanced ability of anchorage-independent growth and re-expression of GM3 by introducing GM3 gene to the transfectants correlated with a reduced ability of the cells to form colonies in nutrient agar (Miura et al., 2004). Contrary to this observation, expression of GM3 in 3LL Lewis lung carcinoma cells endowed cells with ability of anchorage-independent growth (Uemura et al., 2003). Thus, the effects of GM3 expression on anchorage-independent growth are controversial in different cell lines and the mechanism still remained unknown.

Our recent results demonstrated that GM3 modulates B16 invasive growth under rigorous environment, such as serum free or anchorage-independent growth. A close association of GM3 with B16 invasive proliferation was found in the following series of studies, which will be discussed in more detail below: 1) in melanoma B16 cells, GM3 suppression cell lines CAH-2 and CAH-3 showed remarkably enhancing anchorage-independent growth in soft agar medium. This observation demonstrates that the cells seemed easier to proliferate in rigorous environment once knocking down the expression of GM3. 2) in this context, GM3 knocking down by siRNA targeting St3gal5 resulted in highly activated cell proliferation under serum free and soft agar medium. These results give further support to the notion that GM3 reduction enhances invasive proliferating ability of B16 cells in rigorous condition. It is also the characteristic of tumor cells that the proliferation was deregulated and the cells can escape the rigorous environment (Wang et al., 2011).

**3.2.3.2 GM3 inhibits B16 invasive proliferation via PI3K/Akt/mTOR/Raptor pathway**

In many contexts, the proliferation of mammalian cells depends upon PI3K activity. The strongest influences are probably exerted through activation of Akt (Vivanco and Sawyers, 2002). Although some growth factors do not directly activate PI3Ks, stimulation of Ras, an extremely potent mitogenic signal, leads directly to activation of phosphotidylinositol 3-kinases (PI3Ks) (Rodriguez-Viciana et al., 2004) and, in some cases, it is clear that PI3Ks, and not the MEK/ERK pathway, are the most important mediators of the transforming activity of oncogenic Ras (Li et al., 2004). Furthermore, it is a prevalently accepted notion that PI3K transduces signals via mammalian target of rapamycin (mTOR)/S6K pathway which directly regulates the synthesis of proteins and has intrinsic relationship with translation. Therefore, it is no doubt that cell proliferation is regulated by PI3K. In addition, several lines of evidence show that GM3 signals are transferred to downstream molecules via PI3K pathway. In human keratinocyte-derived squamous carcinoma cell line (SCC12F2), GM3 depletion concretely stimulates the phosphorylation of Akt at Ser473 and Thr308 sites (Sun et al., 2002). Treatment with GM3 antibody is able to increase phosphorylation of the Thr308 site, but not the Ser473 (Sun et al., 2002) site, indicating that GM3 is able to module PI3K activity. These findings are also consistent with the known concept that GM3 is capable to regulate PI3K activity by inhibiting EGF receptor phosphorylation (Bremer et al., 1986). On the other hand, GM3 also showed ability to modulate phosphatase and tensin homolog (PTEN) activity, a dual-specificity phosphatase that antagonizes PI3K/Akt signaling (Choi et al., 2006). Thus, PI3K is an important molecule that is responsible for GM3 signal transduction. However, although PI3K has shown its presence in GEMs (Liu et al., 1996), it is yet unclarified if it is located downstream of GM3 to mediate cell proliferation, especially under rigorous environment.

As a first step, we have to introduce the components of PI3K signaling pathway (Fig. 1). In the PI3K/Akt/mTOR pathway, Akt is flanked by two tumor suppressors: PTEN, which antagonizes PI3K and therefore inhibits Akt, and tuberous sclerosis complex (TSC)1/TSC2 heterodimer, which inhibits mTOR by inhibiting the activity of Rheb. Akt activates mTOR via direct phosphorylation of TSC2 and by the inhibition of AMP-activated protein kinase (AMPK), thereby activating Rheb and mTOR-Raptor activity. Upon activation, mTOR-Raptor (regulatory associated protein of mTOR) activates S6K and inhibits eIF4E binding protein (4E-BP1) to accelerate mRNA translation, and also initiates feedback inhibition of Akt, which is at least in part mediated by S6K.

Next, we established a different concept to explain the involvement of PI3K pathway in mediating GM3 signals to abnormal melanoma proliferation under rigorous environment. Just as described above, PI3K/Akt, 3-phosphoinositide dependent protein kinase-1 (PDK1, Pdpk1), Raptor and rapamycin-insensitive companion of mTOR (Rictor) play important role in cell proliferation. Our data further demonstrated that they are the key molecules in mediating GM3 signals to the invasive proliferation of B16 cell. 1) That GM3 suppression specifically decreased the expression of Pdpk1 and Raptor indicated that Pdpk1 and Raptor are involved in the invasive proliferating pathway of melanoma B16 cells in soft agar or serum-free medium. 2) Pdpk1 and Raptor siRNA silencing cells had a similar growth rate to B16 control or parental cells under serum-containing conditions; however, the growing rate of Pdpk1 and Raptor knocking down cells, but not Rictor knocking down cells, was faster compared with B16 control or parental cells under serum-free conditions. 3) Raptor or Pdpk1 knocking down cells, but not Rictor knocking down cells, resulted in the formation of colony in soft agar. Collectively, these results further confirmed that GM3 regulates B16 cell invasive proliferation via Pdpk1 and Raptor in soft agar or serum deprived medium (Wang et al., 2011).

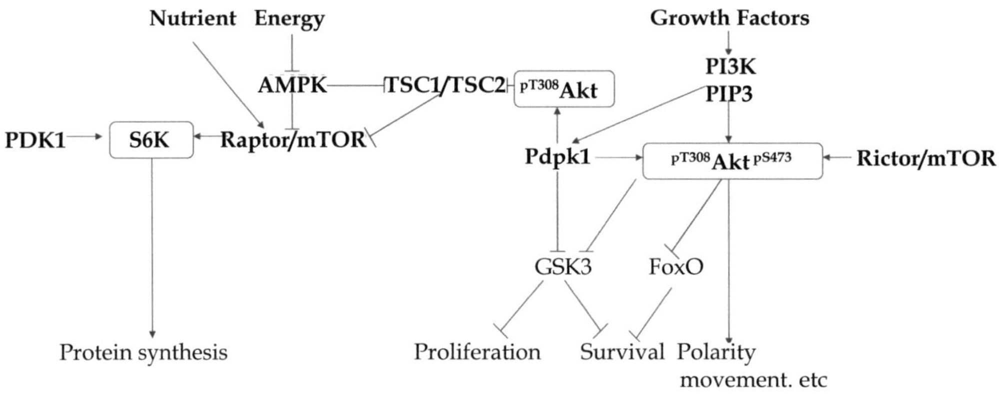


Fig. 1. PI3K signal transduction model. General concept of PI3K signaling pathway was summarized which involves in protein synthesis, proliferation, survival and polarity movement

### 3.2.3.3 Ly-GDI played a key role in mediating GM3 signals to inhibit B16 cell growth

Although it is confirmed that GM3 is capable to inhibit B16 melanoma cells proliferation via PI3K signaling pathway, it still seems to be conflicted with the universal accepted concept that PI3K is always hyper-activated in cancers, which drive the cells proliferation and avoid apoptosis (Luo et al., 2003). This controversy could not be resolved until we identified the Ly-GDI, which is located downstream of GM3 and acts as an effector of GM3 to change the nature of melanoma B16 cells. The proliferating characteristics would be changed once Ly-GDI expression was altered. Thus, it is not conflicting with the previously accepted concept since Ly-GDI would play a key role in mediating GM3 signals to inhibit B16 cell growth.

1. GM3 has been shown to regulate Ly-GDI expression at the transcriptional level in murine melanoma B16 cells. Ly-GDI expression was increased by addition of GM3 to the B16 transfectants and decreased after treatment with D-PDMP, an inhibitor of glucosyl-ceramide synthesis. These results clearly indicate that GM3 positively regulates Ly-GDI expression in B16 cells.
2. Phosphoinositide 3-kinase inhibitor, LY294002, suppressed the Ly-GDI expression that is stimulated by GM3 in B16 cells, suggesting that the GM3 signal is located upstream of the PI3K-Akt pathway. GM3 was shown to increase phosphorylation of Akt. Treatment of B16 cells with small interfering RNA (siRNA) targeted to Akt1/2 resulted in Ly-GDI suppression, indicating that Akt plays an important role in regulation of Ly-GDI expression. Suppression of Akt1/2 rendered cells insensitive to GM3, suggesting that

the GM3 signal may be transduced via Akt in view of the above reason, we further demonstrated that GM3 is located upstream of PI3K pathway to regulate Ly-GDI, by incubating B16 cells with GM3 in the presence or absence of PI3K inhibitors. As a result, PI3K inhibitor treatment thoroughly blocked the effects of GM3 in stimulating PI3K pathway, leading to overexpression of Ly-GDI. These results strongly demonstrated that GM3 regulates Ly-GDI expression via PI3K/Akt pathway, and $Akt^{Thr308}$ was identified as a key active form of Akt to mediate this process by Pdpk1 or Raptor knocking down.

3. Most importantly, Ly-GDI silenced B16 cells showed markedly enhanced invasive proliferation in soft agar or serum-free medium.

These results clearly revealed the important role of Ly-GDI in regulating the abnormal proliferation of melanoma B16 cells (Fig. 2) (Wang et al., 2011b) and provide a noteworthy theory to explain the effects of GM3 on melanoma invasive proliferation, though it is different from the previous theory that GM3 inhibits tumor cell proliferation via modulating different receptors.

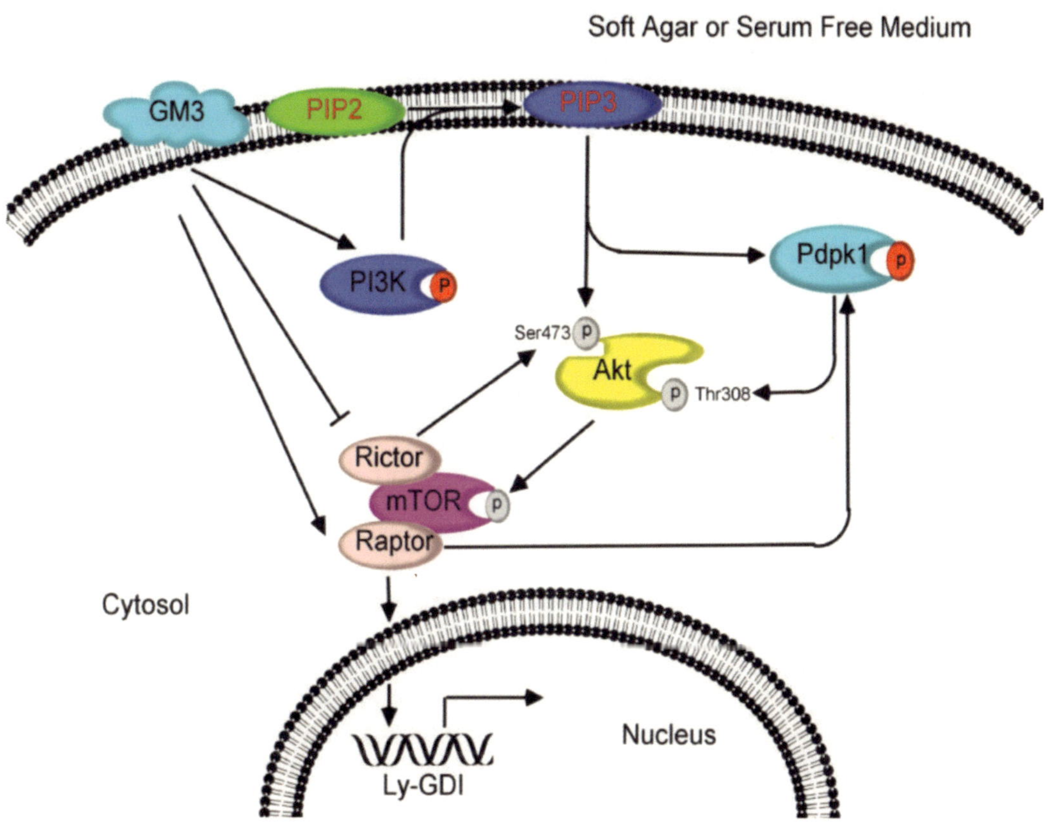


Fig. 2. Proposed cascade of signaling events regulating Ly-GDI expression by GM3, which in turn inhibits B16 cells proliferation under rigorous environment. GM3 signals are transduced in B16 cells through PI3K, Pdpk1, Akt, mTOR/Raptor pathway, leading to the enhanced expression of Ly-GDI mRNA, which in turn suppresses melanoma B16 cells proliferation under rigorous environment

### 3.3 Motility

Although there are several systems of GM3 mediated tumor cell motility in which GM3 plays an essential role, such as GSP/tetraspannin (TSP)/integrin and GM2/GM3/CD82 to explain the mechanism of cancer cell motility, there is no relative evidence to show the effects of GM3 on the motility of B16 cells. Based on the established theory, we found a new signal transduction pathway to mediate GM3 signals to the motility of B16 cells.

#### 3.3.1 GM3/TSP CD9 complex inhibits integrin-dependent cell motility

Both gangliosides and TSP are reported to locate at GEMs in association with integrins (Kawakami et al., 2002; Ono et al., 2001; Ono et al., 1999). Integrins have been implicated in regulating cellular processes such as adhesion, mobility, signaling, for review see (Hehlgans et al., 2007). Integrin function, including $\alpha/\beta$-subunit interaction, is affected by N-glycosylation status (for review see (Gu and Taniguchi, 2004)) and by interaction with TSP and/or gangliosides (Hakomori and Handa, 2002; Ono et al., 2001). TSP are palmitoylated and N-glycosylated and associate with integrin receptors, gangliosides and signaling molecules forming a membrane multi molecular complex referred as tetraspanin web (Ono et al., 2001); for review see (Hemler, 2005).

Since TSP CD9 inhibits cell motility and its expression is down-regulated in various human cancers (Cajot et al., 1997; Miyake et al., 1991), a possibility was opened that CD9 function was affected by glycosylation. ldlD mutant of Chinese Hamster Ovary cells, defective in UDPGlc: 4-epimerase, has been utilized for study of glycosylation of functional proteins (Kingsley et al., 1986; Krieger et al., 1989). ldlD cells with high CD9 expression were cloned after CD9 gene transfection. Motility of these ldlD/CD9 cells was greatly inhibited when cells were grown in serum-free medium (ITS: insulin/transferrin/selenium) containing galactose (Ono et al., 1999), allowing glycoproteins to be fully glycosylated and GM3 to be synthesized. A close association of GM3 with CD9 function was found in the following series of further studies, which will be discussed in more detail below:

1. CD9 and integrin $\alpha3$ were co-immunoprecipitated in ldlD/CD9 cells when GM3 was synthesized (+Gal condition), but not when GM3 synthesis did not occur (–Gal condition). Interaction of GM3 with CD9, and CD9 with $\alpha3$, were demonstrated by confocal microscopy. GM3/CD9/$\alpha3$ is associated in the same microdomain, which is resistant to 1% Brij 98 but soluble in Triton X-100 (Kawakami et al., 2002). Since CD9 is chloroform/methanol soluble, its complex with GM3 or other gangliosides was expected, similarly to proteolipid protein (Folch and Lees, 1951).
2. Various colorectal tumor cell lines whose motility was clearly inhibited by exogenous GM3 addition were all characterized by high CD9 expression. Motility of a CD9-non-expressing tumor cell line was unaffected by GM3 addition, but became inhabitable by GM3 when CD9 was expressed by its gene transfection (Ono et al., 2001).
3. Addition of $^3$H-labeled photoactivatable GM3 having $\omega$-phenylazido acyl group to HRT18 cells, followed by UV irradiation, caused specific $^3$H-labeling of CD9 but not other glycosynaptic proteins ($\alpha3$, $\alpha5$, or $\beta1$ integrin). However, other proteins were labeled by the probe (Ono et al., 2001).
4. Down regulation of GM3 synthesis is associated with oncogenesis in v-Jun transformation. Transfection of GM3 synthase gene resulted in reversion of oncogenic to normal phenotype in v-Jun-transformed chicken and mouse fibroblasts and inhibition of motility and invasiveness through formation of GM3/CD9/$\alpha5\beta1$ complex (Miura et al., 2004).

5. Human diploid embryonal lung WI38 fibroblasts are highly contact-inhibitable cells. They are biochemically unusual in having high level of CD9 and CD81, which are complexed with FGFR. GM3, the major ganglioside in these cells, interacts specifically with FGFR, whereas other gangliosides and glycophingolipids do not. Since FGFR is closely associated with c-Src and GM3, cell contact induced by interaction of GM3 with FGFR may inhibit tyrosine kinase associated with FGFR as well as c-Src (Toledo et al., 2004). The exact mechanism for GM3 interaction with FGFR remains to be elucidated.
6. In a typical case with bladder cancer cells, decrease or depletion of GM3 by D-threo-1-phenyl-2-palmitoylamino-3-pyrrolidino-1-propanol (P4) suppresses interaction of CD9 with integrin $\alpha3\beta1$, leading to enhanced motility and invasiveness (Mitsuzuka et al., 2005). Such conversion of less malignant to highly malignant cell phenotype was also caused by decrease of CD9 by RNAi. Besides, exogenous addition of GM3 resulted in inhibition of motility in YTS1 cells. These results suggest that integrin/CD9/GM3 organized in membrane, "glycosynapse 3" (for review see (Hakomori, 2002)), may define tumor cell invasiveness. This is also consistent with previous observations that highly invasive YTS1 is reverted to less-invasive phenotype by enhanced GM3 expression induced by brefeldin A (Satoh et al., 2001). Moreover, Mitsuzuka and coworkers (Mitsuzuka et al., 2005) demonstrated that GM3 levels, in bladder cancer cells, define glycosynapse function by controlling the interaction of CD9 with integrin $\alpha3$; and by modulating c-Src activity. Enhanced levels of GM3 induce csk translocation into glycosynapse resulting in phosphorylation on Tyr 527 of c-Src with consequent inhibition of c-Src activity and cell motility (Regina Todeschini and Hakomori, 2008).

### 3.3.2 GM2/GM3 complexed with CD82 inhibits cell motility

TSP CD82 was originally found as product of metastasis suppressing gene KAL-1, highly expressed in normal epithelial cells such as prostate, bladder, or colorectal epithelia and downregulated or depleted in their metastatic deposits (Adachi et al., 1996; Dong et al., 1995; Dong et al., 1996). CD82 is known to suppress cell invasiveness by inhibiting functional interaction of integrin with tyrosine kinase receptor for hypatocyte growth factor (HGF), hypatocyte growth factor receptor (Met) (Sridhar and Miranti, 2006). Met has been implicated in promotion of cancer cell motility and invasiveness; for review see (Birchmeier et al., 2003). In analogy with CD9, it is expected to observe an effect of glycosylation on CD82-dependent motility inhibition (Ono et al., 1999).

1. It is initially observed that GM2, but not GM3 or Gb4, specifically interacted with CD82 in normal bladder epithelial cell line HCV29, while GM3 showed specificity for CD9.
2. GM2/CD82 complex physically interacted with Met inhibiting functional interaction of integrin $\alpha3$ or $\beta1$ with Met, whereby HGF-induced Met tyrosine phosphorylation was strongly suppressed.
3. Treating normal cells with P4, which depleted GM2, or abrogating CD82 expression by RNAi method, greatly enhanced HGF-induced Met phosphorylation and cell motility. In contrast, highly invasive bladder cancer cells, YTS1 (lacking CD82), were characterized by HGF-independent Met activation and cell motility. Met activation and cell motility were inhibited by co-expression and mutual interaction of GM2 with CD82, as observed in YTS1 cells transfected with CD82 gene; or by the exogenous addition of GM2 (Illmensee and Mintz, 1976).
4. YTS-1 cells, when adhered on LN5-coated plate, showed strong activation of Met phosphorylation without stimulation by HGF, and this process was promoted when

gangliosides were depleted by P4 treatment of YTS-1 cells. These results indicated that highly malignant cells are characterized by enhanced cross-talk between integrin and Met kinase. Such cross-talk in normal cells is minimal, but was greatly enhanced when GM2 was depleted by P4; i.e., CD82/GM2 complex plays a major role in inhibiting not only HGF-induced Met kinase activity but also LN5-induced cross-talk between integrin and Met (Todeschini et al., 2007).

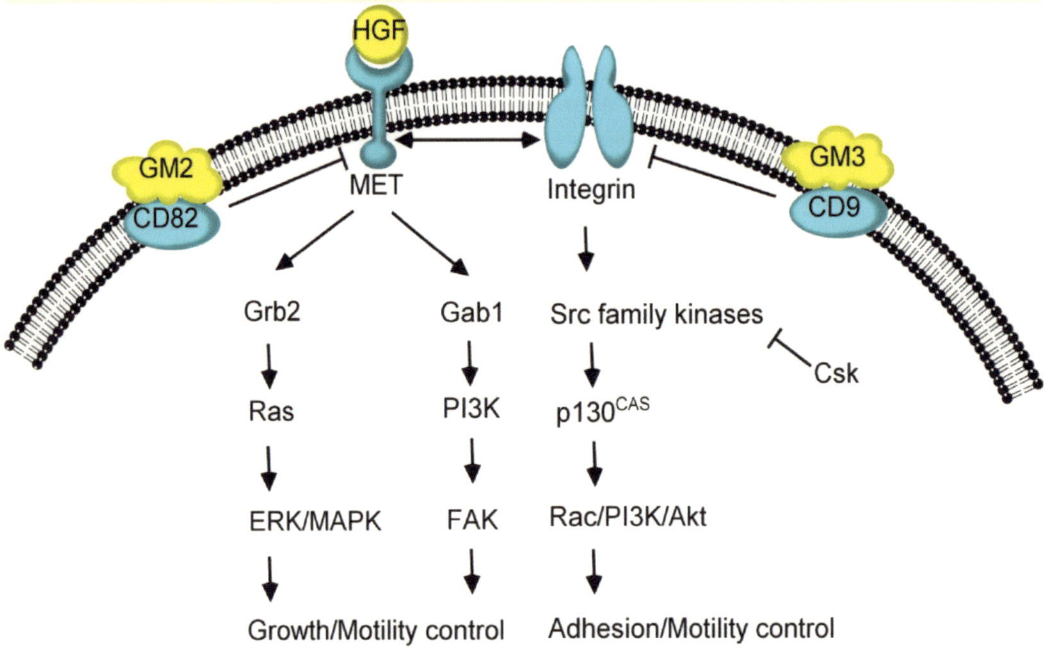


Fig. 3. Hypothetical associations among components of glycosynapse from bladder epithelial cells. Bladder epithelial cells express two major receptors as follows: 1) HGF receptor Met and its kinase (shown at left), which is inhibited by GM2-CD82 complex; 2) integrin receptor α3β1, which binds to extra cellular matrix component LN5/10-11 upon cell adhesion (shown at right). α3β1 activation is blocked by GM3-CD9 complex in bladder epithelial cells (Mitsuzuka et al., 2005). The functional interaction between systems 1 and 2 is blocked by GM2-CD82 complex. Signaling shown for both systems is arbitrary, based on a few previous reviews or studies by others and by our group (Birchmeier et al., 2003; Mitsuzuka et al., 2005). Grb2 and Gab1 are initial signaling molecules that may lead to activation of extra cellular signal-regulated kinase/mitogen-activated protein kinase (ERK/MAPK), PI3K, or FAK (Birchmeier et al., 2003), controlling cell growth and motility. α3β1 may act through Src family kinases (which are inhibitable by Csk) (Mitsuzuka et al., 2005; Toledo et al., 2004), and lead to Rak/PI3K/Akt signaling (Gu and Taniguchi, 2004), controlling cell adhesion and motility. From Todeschini et al.(Todeschini et al., 2007)

The molecular mechanism of GM2 inhibition of the HGF-Met signaling pathway leading to cell motility may be controlling the distribution of CD82 in- and outside of the glycosynapse; and interacting with CD82 in the glycosynapse forming the GM2/ CD82 complex which acts as a functional constituent of the microdomain. Fig. 3 shows a hypothetical scheme for this mechanism. Besides, inhibition of GM2/CD82 complex on Met activation, or on α3-to-Met interaction, may involve cis-carbonhydrate-carbonhydrate interaction (cis-CCI) between GM2 and N-linked glycan of CD82, since partial deletion of three N-linked glycans (at Asn129, 157, and 198) from mutant CD82 caused remarkable change in interaction with α3 and α5 integrins (Todeschini et al., 2007).

Further studies on effects of various gangliosides, and their combinations, on HCV29 cell motility, clearly indicate that GM2 together with GM3 (but not other gangliosides or GSLs, or their combinations) show stronger binding to CD82, compared to GM2 or GM3 alone, and based on the following observations:

1. GM2 binding to CD82 was greatly enhanced by addition of GM3, although GM3 per se did not bind to CD82 (Ono et al., 2000).
2. Cells expressing CD82, when cultured with silica nanospheres co-coated with GM2 and GM3, displayed much stronger inhibition of cell motility than those cultured with silica nanospheres coated with GM2 alone.
3. GM2/GM3 combination in the above process strongly inhibited phosphorylation of Src and MAPK.
4. ldlD mutant cells transfected with GM2 synthase gene showed greatly reduced motility when endogenous synthesis of both GM2 and GM3 occurred, as compared with cells grown under conditions in which only one of these gangliosides was synthesized.

In addition to functional changes 1) to 4) as above, a physical and chemical basis for interaction of GM2 and GM3 was provided by (a) electrospray ionization mass spectrometry (Ono et al., 2000), and (b) in situ cross-linking of cell surface GM2 and GM3 by periodate oxidation followed by succinyl dihydrazide (data not shown). Taken together, these results suggest the existence of heterotypic cis carbohydrate-to-carbohydrate interaction of GM2 and GM3, providing a basis for control of cell motility through inhibition of signal transduction (Regina Todeschini and Hakomori, 2008).

### 3.3.3 GM3 promotes cell motility via inducing matrix metalloproteinase (MMP-9) expression in melanoma B16 cells

As we know, the murine melanoma B16 cell line is characterized by its highly invasive and metastatic capacity. Growth factors, adhesion molecules, proteases, and other components are involved in the process of metastasis (Herlyn et al., 2002). MMP family members have been clearly shown to play an important role in this process (Hamilton et al., 1993; Tsuchida et al., 1987). Among the MMPs thus far studied, MMP-9 (gelatinase B) appears to have an important role in a wide array of physiological and pathophysiological processes, including pacental development, wound healing, angiogenesis, inflammation, tumor invasion, and metastasis (Van den Steen et al., 2002). Thus, studies of the mechanism(s) regulating the expression of MMP-9 are also important to the understanding of mechanisms underlying tumor metastasis.

MMP-9 secretion can be stimulated by interleukin 1β (IL-1B) (Librach et al., 1994), tumor necrosis factor (TNF) α (Meisser et al., 1999), HGF (Zhou and Wong, 2006), and EGF (Qiu et al., 2004). MMP-9 is stimulated in several cell lines via the PI3K/Akt signaling pathway (Shukla et al., 2007). Hyperactivated PI3K results in the activation of several transcriptional factors, such as nuclear factor (NF)-κB and activator protein (AP)-1, further leading to promotion of MMP-9 gene expression (Bancroft et al., 2002). Restoration of phosphatase and tensin homolog to hyperactivated PI3K cell lines reversibly suppresses MMP-9 expression. S6K located downstream of PI3K is involved in the regulation of MMP-9 expression following stimulation with hepatocyte growth factor (Zhou and Wong, 2006). These lines of evidence clearly show that PI3K signaling pathway plays an important role in MMP-9 regulation.

Reports from several laboratories have concluded that MMP-9 expression is modulated not only by cytokines but also by gangliosides (Hu et al., 2007; Moon et al., 2004; Zhang et al., 2006). GM1, present in the glycolipid-enriched microdomain, is one of the crucial factors regulating cancer metastatic potential via the modulation of MMP-9 localization and secretion, as well as suppression of tumor invasion potential (Zhang et al., 2006). Overexpression of the GD3 synthase gene suppresses MMP-9 expression by inhibiting the combination between the MMP-9 promoter and transcription factors (NF-κB and AP-1) in vascular smooth muscle cells (Moon et al., 2004). In murine FBJ cells, GD1a is found to suppress MMP-9 expression at the transcriptional level (Hu et al., 2007). On the other hand, overexpression of plasma membrane-expressed sialidase Neu3 inhibits MMP-9 expression in vascular smooth muscle cells; implying gangliosides promote MMP-9 (Moon et al., 2007). Thus, there is no definite concept as to whether gangliosides positively or negatively regulate MMP-9 expression.

Among tumor-associated glycolipids, ganglioside GM3 is the simplest ganglioside in structure that resides in the membrane of murine melanoma B16 cells (Iwabuchi et al., 1998).

1. GM3 has been shown to regulate TNF α both at the transcriptional and translational levels in murine melanoma B16 cells (Wang et al., 2007b; Wang et al., 2007c). TNF α expression was increased by addition of GM3 to the B16 transfectants and decreased after treatment with D-PDMP, an inhibitor of glucosyl-ceramide synthesis. These results clearly indicate that GM3 positively regulates TNF α expression in B16 cells.
2. PI3K inhibitors, wortmannin and LY294002, suppressed the TNF α expression that is stimulated by GM3 in B16 cells, suggesting that the GM3 signal is located upstream of the PI3K-Akt pathway. GM3 was shown to increase phosphorylation of Akt. Treatment of B16 cells with small interfering RNA (siRNA) targeted to Akt1/2 resulted in TNF α suppression, indicating that Akt plays an important role in regulation of TNF α expression. Suppression of Akt1/2 rendered cells insensitive to GM3, suggesting that the GM3 signal may be transduced via Akt (Wang et al., 2007a).
3. Rapamycin suppressed TNF α expression, indicating mammalian target of rapamycin (mTOR) to be involved in the pathway. Either siRNA Raptor or siRNA Rictor suppressed TNF α expression, but the latter suppressed the effects of GM3 on TNF α expression and Akt phosphorylation at Ser473, indicating the GM3 signal to be transduced via mTOR-Rictor and Akt (Ser473), leading to TNF α stimulation. Finally, Ly-GDI, the tumor suppressor gene, whose expression is associated with GM3, was shown to be upstream of TNF α (Wang et al., 2007b). Thus, the GM3 signal is transduced in B16 cells through a PI3K, mTOR-Rictor, Akt, Ly-GDI pathway, leading to stimulated expression of TNF α.
4. Since TNF α is known to stimulate MMP-9 synthesis, which is highly involved in tumor cell metastasis, we investigated the possibility that MMP-9 is regulated by GM3. In the present study, MMP-9, but not MMP-2, messenger RNA (mRNA) expression was found to be consistent with GM3 levels in every B16-derived cell variant. GM3 has been suggested to stimulate the PI3K/Akt signaling pathway in previous investigations (Bremer et al., 1986; Choi et al., 2006). GM3 signals are thus transduced via the PI3K/Akt pathway, leading to the regulation of MMP-9 expression.

5. Most importantly, cell migration tested by transwell experiments showed that the numbers of cells migrating were consistent with MMP-9 expression (Wu et al., 2011). These data strongly suggest that capacity of cell migration in B16 cells is proportional to MMP-9 expression, which is under the positive control of GM3 (Fig. 4).

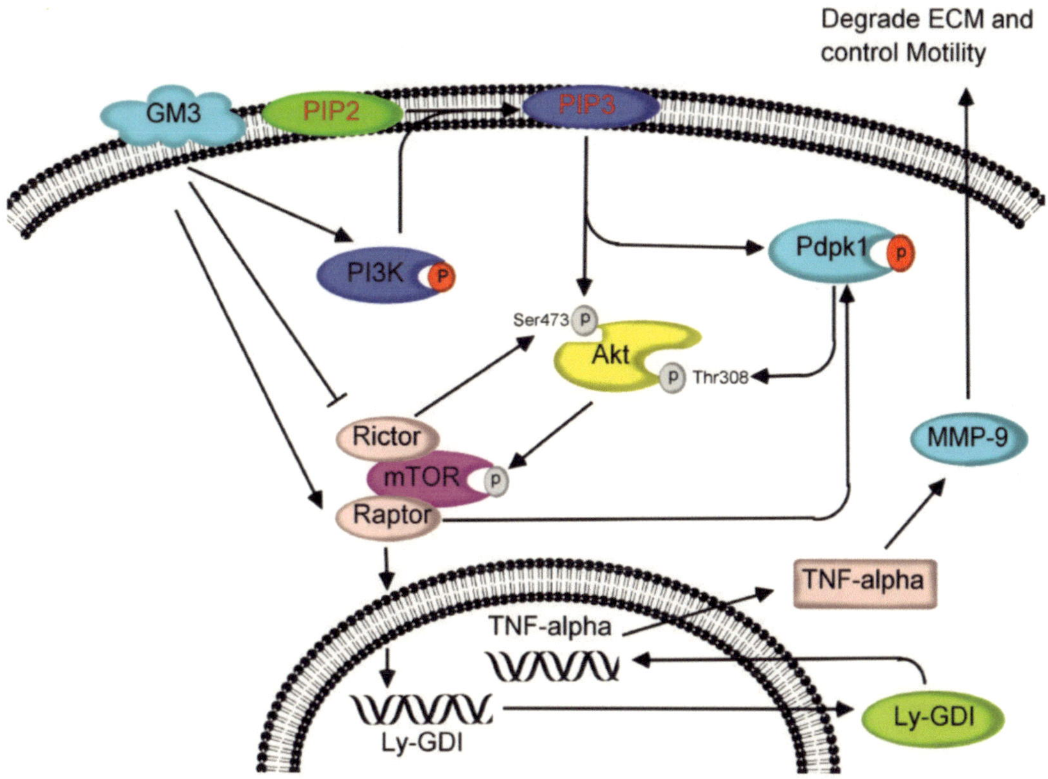


Fig. 4. Proposed cascade of signaling events regulating MMP-9 expression by GM3, which in turn promotes B16 cells motility via Ly-GDI. GM3 signals are transduced in B16 cells through PI3K, Pdk1, Akt, mTOR Raptor pathway, leading to the enhanced expression of Ly-GDI mRNA. Further data demonstrated that Ly-GDI located upstream of TNF α, which in turn regulate melanoma B16 cells motility via inducing MMP-9 secretion

### 3.4 Metastasis

Melanoma cells break the most basic rules of behavior by which multicellular organisms are built and maintained, and they exploit every kind of opportunity to do so. In studying the transgressions, we discover what the normal rules are and how they are enforced. Thus, in the context of cell biology, melanoma has a unique importance, and the emphasis given to melanoma research has profoundly benefited a much wider area of medical knowledge than that of melanoma alone.

Melanoma cells are defined by two heritable properties: they and their progeny (Hakomori, 1996) reproduce in defiance of the normal restraints on cell division and (Hakomori et al., 1998) invade and colonize territories normally reserved for other cells. It is the combination of these actions that makes cancers peculiarly dangerous. An isolated abnormal cell that does not proliferate more than its normal neighbors does not significant damage, no matter what other disagreeable properties it may have; but if its proliferation is out of control, it will give rise to a tumor, a relentlessly growing mass of abnormal cells. As long as the tumor cells remain clustered together in a single mass, however, the tumor is said to be benign. At this stage, a complete cure can usually be achieved by removing the mass surgically. A tumor is considered a cancer only if it is malignant, that is, only if its cells have acquired the ability to invade surrounding tissue. Invasiveness usually implies an ability to break loose, enter the bloodstream or lymphatic vessels, and form secondary tumors, called metastasis, at other sites in the body. The more widely a cancer spreads, the harder it becomes to eradicate.

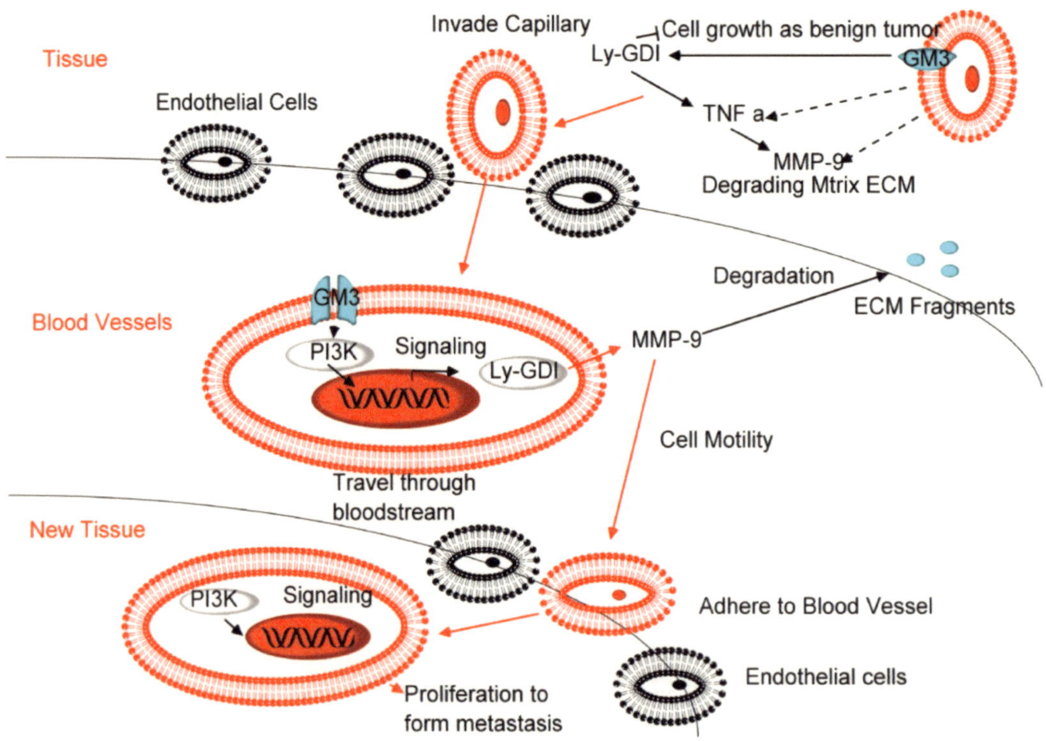


Fig. 5. Steps in the process of melanoma metastasis. This example illustrates the spread of a melanoma from an organ such as the lung or bladder to the skin. Tumor cells may invasively proliferate in the original tissue with inhibiting Ly-GDI expression. Then, tumor cells will enter the bloodstream directly by crossing the wall of a blood vessel, as diagrammed here, or, more commonly perhaps, by crossing the wall of a lymphatic vessel that ultimately discharges its contents (lymph) into the bloodstream. The motility of melanoma cells would be triggered by MMP-9 activation during this process. Finally, tumor cells that have entered a blood or lymphatic vessel will proliferate in a new tissue (skin) and finish the circle of metastasis

As discussed in this chapter, ganglioside GM3 is involved in every aspects of melanoma metastasis. Ly-GDI mediated melanoma invasive proliferation under rigorous conditions, which in turn benign tumor would form in tissues. At this stage, GM3 would concurrently modulate melanoma cell adhesion via gangliosides interaction or modulating adhesive genes expression, through which mediate melanoma cells getting loose from origninal tisse or adhere to the new locations. Once the activity of MMP-9 was stimulated by GM3 in melanoma cells, MMP-9 will trigger the motility of melanoma cells throughout the bloodstream or lymphatic vessels, and form secondary tumors (Fig. 5). That means a tumor is considered as a cancer with metastasis. Although these steps are not separate and are always combination of these actions, our *in vitro* experiments have partially revealed the metastatic mechanism of melanoma B16 cells. These results clearly indicated that GM3 changed the nature of melanoma B16 cells. In addition, elucidation of the molecular mechanism of gangliosides modulating tumor phenotype will help to find new therapeutic targets or critical genes in cancer therapy.

## 4. Conclusion

Our results along with others' investigations have shown that GM3 is invovled in each step of metastasis in melanoma B16 cells. 1) GM3 regulatea B16 cell adhesion via gangliosides interaction or modulating adhesive gene expression, such as E-cadherin, N-Cam and Src. 2) GM3 is able to inhibit B16 cells invasive proliferation under soft agar or serum deprived medium via stimulating Ly-GDI expression. 3) MMP-9 is identified to mediate B16 cell motility via Tnf α. Therefore, GM3, predominantly expressed ganglioside in B16 cells, is the key molecule responsible for the phenotype or nature of melanoma cells.

## 5. Abbreviations

| Abbreviations | Full Name |
|---|---|
| AMPK | AMP-activated protein kinase |
| AP-1 | activator protein-1 |
| CCI | carbonhydrate carbonhydrate interaction |
| ECs | endothelial cells |
| EGF | epithelial growth factor |
| EGFR | epithelial growth factor receptor |
| ERK/MAPK | Extracellular signal-regulated kinase/mitogen-activated protein kinase |
| 4E-BP1 | eIF4E binding protein |
| FAK | focal adhesion kinase |
| FGF | fibroblast growth factor |
| FGFR | fibroblast growth factor receptor |
| GEMs | glycosphingolipids enriched microdomains |
| HGF | hypatocyte growth factor |
| IL-1B | Interleukin-1β |
| MET | hypatocyte growth factor receptor |
| MMP-9 | matrix metalloproteinase 9 |
| mTOR | mammalian target of rapamycin |
| PDGF | platelet derived growth factor |
| Pdk1 | pyruvate dehydrogenase kinase |
| PI3K | phosphotidylinositol 3-kinase |

| | |
|---|---|
| PTEN | phosphatase and tensin homolog |
| P4 | D-threo-1-phenyl-2-palmitoylamino-3-pyrolidino-1-propanol |
| Raptor | regulatory associated protein of mTOR |
| Rictor | rapamycin-insensitive companion of mTOR |
| SCC12F2 | squamous carcinoma cell line |
| TNF α | Tumor necrosis factor alpha |
| TSC | tuberous sclerosis complex |
| TSP | tetraspannins |

## 6. References

Adachi, M. et al., 1996. Correlation of KAI1/CD82 gene expression with good prognosis in patients with non-small cell lung cancer. Cancer Res, 56(8): 1751-5.

Anastassiou, G. et al., 2000. Expression of the cell adhesion molecules ICAM-1, VCAM-1 and NCAM in uveal melanoma: a clinicopathological study. Oncology, 58(1): 83-8.

Anderson, R.G., 1998. The caveolae membrane system. Annu Rev Biochem, 67: 199-225.

Bancroft, C.C. et al., 2002. Effects of pharmacologic antagonists of epidermal growth factor receptor, PI3K and MEK signal kinases on NF-kappaB and AP-1 activation and IL-8 and VEGF expression in human head and neck squamous cell carcinoma lines. Int J Cancer, 99(4): 538-48.

Bassi, R., Chigorno, V., Fiorilli, A., Sonnino, S. and Tettamanti, G., 1991. Exogenous gangliosides GD1b and GD1b-lactone, stably associated to rat brain P2 subcellular fraction, modulate differently the process of protein phosphorylation. J Neurochem, 57(4): 1207-11.

Besch, R., Berking, C., Kammerbauer, C. and Degitz, K., 2007. Inhibition of urokinase-type plasminogen activator receptor induces apoptosis in melanoma cells by activation of p53. Cell Death Differ, 14(4): 818-29.

Birchmeier, C., Birchmeier, W., Gherardi, E. and Vande Woude, G.F., 2003. Met, metastasis, motility and more. Nat Rev Mol Cell Biol, 4(12): 915-25.

Bourguignon, L.Y., Zhu, H., Shao, L. and Chen, Y.W., 2001. CD44 interaction with c-Src kinase promotes cortactin-mediated cytoskeleton function and hyaluronic acid-dependent ovarian tumor cell migration. J Biol Chem, 276(10): 7327-36.

Bremer, E.G. and Hakomori, S., 1982. GM3 ganglioside induces hamster fibroblast growth inhibition in chemically-defined medium: ganglioside may regulate growth factor receptor function. Biochem Biophys Res Commun, 106(3): 711-8.

Bremer, E.G., Hakomori, S., Bowen-Pope, D.F., Raines, E. and Ross, R., 1984. Ganglioside-mediated modulation of cell growth, growth factor binding, and receptor phosphorylation. J Biol Chem, 259(11): 6818-25.

Bremer, E.G., Schlessinger, J. and Hakomori, S., 1986. Ganglioside-mediated modulation of cell growth. Specific effects of GM3 on tyrosine phosphorylation of the epidermal growth factor receptor. J Biol Chem, 261(5): 2434-40.

Brown, D.A. and London, E., 1997. Structure of detergent-resistant membrane domains: does phase separation occur in biological membranes? Biochem Biophys Res Commun, 240(1): 1-7.

Cajot, J.F., Sordat, I., Silvestre, T. and Sordat, B., 1997. Differential display cloning identifies motility-related protein (MRP1/CD9) as highly expressed in primary compared to metastatic human colon carcinoma cells. Cancer Res, 57(13): 2593-7.

Caputto, R., Maccioni, A.H. and Caputto, B.L., 1977. Activation of deoxycholate solubilized adenosine triphosphatase by ganglioside and asialoganglioside preparations. Biochem Biophys Res Commun, 74(3): 1046-52.

Cardo-Vila, M., Arap, W. and Pasqualini, R., 2003. Alpha v beta 5 integrin-dependent programmed cell death triggered by a peptide mimic of annexin V. Mol Cell, 11(5): 1151-62.

Carter, H.E., Glick, F.J., Norris, W.P. and Phillips, G.E., 1947. BIOCHEMISTRY OF THE SPHINGOLIPIDES. Journal of Biological Chemistry, 170(1): 285-294.

Chan, K.F., 1988. Ganglioside-modulated protein phosphorylation. Partial purification and characterization of a ganglioside-inhibited protein kinase in brain. J Biol Chem, 263(1): 568-74.

Chan, K.F., 1989. Ganglioside-modulated protein phosphorylation in muscle. Activation of phosphorylase b kinase by gangliosides. J Biol Chem, 264(31): 18632-7.

Choi, H.J. et al., 2006. Ganglioside GM3 modulates tumor suppressor PTEN-mediated cell cycle progression--transcriptional induction of p21(WAF1) and p27(kip1) by inhibition of PI-3K/AKT pathway. Glycobiology, 16(7): 573-83.

Davis, C.W. and Daly, J.W., 1980. Activation of rat cerebral cortical 3',5'-cyclic nucleotide phosphodiesterase activity by gangliosides. Mol Pharmacol, 17(2): 206-11.

Denkert, C., Siegert, A., Leclere, A., Turzynski, A. and Hauptmann, S., 2002. An inhibitor of stress-activated MAP-kinases reduces invasion and MMP-2 expression of malignant melanoma cells. Clin Exp Metastasis, 19(1): 79-85.

Desai, B.S. and Chellaiah, M., 2006. Bisphosphonates inhibit osteopontin induced prostate cancer cell motility by attenuating MMP-9 activity. AACR Meeting Abstracts, 2006(1): 774-b-.

Dobrzanski, M.J., Reome, J.B., Hollenbaugh, J.A., Hylind, J.C. and Dutton, R.W., 2004. Effector cell-derived lymphotoxin alpha and Fas ligand, but not perforin, promote Tc1 and Tc2 effector cell-mediated tumor therapy in established pulmonary metastases. Cancer Res, 64(1): 406-14.

Dong, J.T. et al., 1995. KAI1, a metastasis suppressor gene for prostate cancer on human chromosome 11p11.2. Science, 268(5212): 884-6.

Dong, J.T. et al., 1996. Down-regulation of the KAI1 metastasis suppressor gene during the progression of human prostatic cancer infrequently involves gene mutation or allelic loss. Cancer Res, 56(19): 4387-90.

Escalante, C.R., Aggarwal, A.K., Wilson, P.D. and Burrow, C.R., 2000. Monomeric Midkine Induces Tumor Cell Proliferation in the Absence of Cell-Surface Proteoglycan Binding. Biochemistry, 39(20): 5977-5987.

Facci, L. et al., 1984. Promotion of neuritogenesis in mouse neuroblastoma cells by exogenous gangliosides. Relationship between the effect and the cell association of ganglioside GM1. J Neurochem, 42(2): 299-305.

Felicetti, F. et al., 2009. Caveolin-1 tumor-promoting role in human melanoma. Int J Cancer, 125(7): 1514-22.

Folch, J. and Lees, M., 1951. Proteolipides, a new type of tissue lipoproteins; their isolation from brain. J Biol Chem, 191(2): 807-17.

Frame, M.C., 2002. Src in cancer: deregulation and consequences for cell behaviour. Biochimica et Biophysica Acta (BBA) - Reviews on Cancer, 1602(2): 114-130.

Fujita, H. et al., 2001. Gelsolin functions as a metastasis suppressor in B16-BL6 mouse melanoma cells and requirement of the carboxyl-terminus for its effect. Int J Cancer, 93(6): 773-80.

Furukawa, K., Takamiya, K., Okada, M., Inoue, M. and Fukumoto, S., 2001. Novel functions of complex carbohydrates elucidated by the mutant mice of glycosyltransferase genes. Biochim Biophys Acta, 1525(1-2): 1-12.

Glebov, O.O. and Nichols, B.J., 2004a. Distribution of lipid raft markers in live cells. Biochem Soc Trans, 32(Pt 5): 673-5.

Glebov, O.O. and Nichols, B.J., 2004b. Lipid raft proteins have a random distribution during localized activation of the T-cell receptor. Nat Cell Biol, 6(3): 238-43.

Goldenring, J.R., Otis, L.C., Yu, R.K. and DeLorenzo, R.J., 1985. Calcium/ganglioside-dependent protein kinase activity in rat brain membrane. J Neurochem, 44(4): 1229-34.

Gottschalk, A., 1955. Structural Relationship between Sialic Acid, Neuraminic Acid and 2-Carboxy-Pyrrole. Nature, 176(4488): 881-882.

Gu, J. and Taniguchi, N., 2004. Regulation of integrin functions by N-glycans. Glycoconj J, 21(1-2): 9-15.

Hakomori, S.-i., 2002. Inaugural Article: The glycosynapse. PNAS, 99(1): 225-232.

Hakomori, S., 1996. Tumor malignancy defined by aberrant glycosylation and sphingo(glyco)lipid metabolism. Cancer Res, 56(23): 5309-18.

Hakomori, S., 2003. Structure, organization, and function of glycosphingolipids in membrane. Curr Opin Hematol, 10(1): 16-24.

Hakomori, S. and Handa, K., 2002. Glycosphingolipid-dependent cross-talk between glycosynapses interfacing tumor cells with their host cells: essential basis to define tumor malignancy. FEBS Lett, 531(1): 88-92.

Hakomori, S., Handa, K., Iwabuchi, K., Yamamura, S. and Prinetti, A., 1998. New insights in glycosphingolipid function: "glycosignaling domain," a cell surface assembly of glycosphingolipids with signal transducer molecules,involved in cell adhesion coupled with signaling. Glycobiology, 8(10): xi-xix.

Hakomori, S.I. and Murakami, W.T., 1968. Glycolipids of hamster fibroblasts and derived malignant-transformed cell lines. Proc Natl Acad Sci U S A, 59(1): 254-61.

Hamilton, W.B., Helling, F., Lloyd, K.O. and Livingston, P.O., 1993. Ganglioside expression on human malignant melanoma assessed by quantitative immune thin-layer chromatography. Int J Cancer, 53(4): 566-73.

Hanai, N., Dohi, T., Nores, G.A. and Hakomori, S., 1988a. A novel ganglioside, de-N-acetyl-GM3 (II3NeuNH2LacCer), acting as a strong promoter for epidermal growth factor receptor kinase and as a stimulator for cell growth. J Biol Chem, 263(13): 6296-301.

Hanai, N., Nores, G.A., MacLeod, C., Torres-Mendez, C.R. and Hakomori, S., 1988b. Ganglioside-mediated modulation of cell growth. Specific effects of GM3 and lyso-GM3 in tyrosine phosphorylation of the epidermal growth factor receptor. J Biol Chem, 263(22): 10915-21.

Hehlgans, S., Haase, M. and Cordes, N., 2007. Signalling via integrins: implications for cell survival and anticancer strategies. Biochim Biophys Acta, 1775(1): 163-80.

Hemler, M.E., 2005. Tetraspanin functions and associated microdomains. Nat Rev Mol Cell Biol, 6(10): 801-11.

Herlyn, M. et al., 2002. New approaches to the biology of melanoma: a workshop of the National Institutes of Health Pathology B Study Section. Am J Pathol, 161(5): 1949-57.

Hirabayashi, Y. et al., 1985. Syngeneic monoclonal antibody against melanoma antigen with interspecies cross-reactivity recognizes GM3, a prominent ganglioside of B16 melanoma. J Biol Chem, 260(24): 13328-33.

Hu, D. et al., 2007. Ganglioside GD1a negatively regulates matrix metalloproteinase-9 expression in mouse FBJ cell lines at the transcriptional level. Connect Tissue Res, 48(4): 198-205.

Illmensee, K. and Mintz, B., 1976. Totipotency and normal differentiation of single teratocarcinoma cells cloned by injection into blastocysts. Proc Natl Acad Sci U S A, 73(2): 549-53.

Iwabuchi, K., Yamamura, S., Prinetti, A., Handa, K. and Hakomori, S., 1998. GM3-enriched microdomain involved in cell adhesion and signal transduction through carbohydrate-carbohydrate interaction in mouse melanoma B16 cells. J Biol Chem, 273(15): 9130-8.

Jiang, K. et al., 2004. Akt mediates Ras downregulation of RhoB, a suppressor of transformation, invasion, and metastasis. Mol Cell Biol, 24(12): 5565-76.

Katerinaki, E., Evans, G.S., Lorigan, P.C. and MacNeil, S., 2003. TNF-alpha increases human melanoma cell invasion and migration in vitro: the role of proteolytic enzymes. Br J Cancer, 89(6): 1123-9.

Kawakami, Y. et al., 2002. Tetraspanin CD9 is a "proteolipid," and its interaction with alpha 3 integrin in microdomain is promoted by GM3 ganglioside, leading to inhibition of laminin-5-dependent cell motility. J Biol Chem, 277(37): 34349-58.

Kim, J.Y., Goldenring, J.R., DeLorenzo, R.J. and Yu, R.K., 1986. Gangliosides inhibit phospholipid-sensitive Ca2+-dependent kinase phosphorylation of rat myelin basic proteins. J Neurosci Res, 15(2): 159-66.

Kingsley, D.M., Kozarsky, K.F., Hobbie, L. and Krieger, M., 1986. Reversible defects in O-linked glycosylation and LDL receptor expression in a UDP-Gal/UDP-GalNAc 4-epimerase deficient mutant. Cell, 44(5): 749-59.

Klenk, E., 1939a. Beitrdge zur Chemie der Lipiodosen. Z Phys Chem, 262: 128-143.

Klenk, E., 1939b. Uber die natur der phophatide und anderer lipoide des gehirns und der leber bei der niemann-pickschen krankheit. Z Phys Chem, 235: 24-36.

Kojima, N. and Hakomori, S., 1989. Specific interaction between gangliotriaosylceramide (Gg3) and sialosyllactosylceramide (GM3) as a basis for specific cellular recognition between lymphoma and melanoma cells. J Biol Chem, 264(34): 20159-62.

Kojima, N. and Hakomori, S., 1991a. Cell adhesion, spreading, and motility of GM3-expressing cells based on glycolipid-glycolipid interaction. J Biol Chem, 266(26): 17552-8.

Kojima, N. and Hakomori, S., 1991b. Synergistic effect of two cell recognition systems: glycosphingolipid-glycosphingolipid interaction and integrin receptor interaction with pericellular matrix protein. Glycobiology, 1(6): 623-30.

Kojima, N., Shiota, M., Sadahira, Y., Handa, K. and Hakomori, S.I., 1992. Cell adhesion in a dynamic flow system as compared to static system. Glycosphingolipid-

glycosphingolipid interaction in the dynamic system predominates over lectin- or integrin-based mechanisms in adhesion of B16 melanoma cells to non-activated endothelial cells. Journal of Biological Chemistry, 267(24): 17264-17270.
Kreutter, D. et al., 1987. Regulation of protein kinase C activity by gangliosides. J Biol Chem, 262(4): 1633-7.
Krieger, M. et al., 1989. Analysis of the synthesis, intracellular sorting, and function of glycoproteins using a mammalian cell mutant with reversible glycosylation defects. Methods Cell Biol, 32: 57-84.
Krummel, M.F. and Davis, M.M., 2002. Dynamics of the immunological synapse: finding, establishing and solidifying a connection. Curr Opin Immunol, 14(1): 66-74.
Kuhn, R. and Wiegandt, H., 1963. Die Konstitution der Ganglio-N-tetraose und des Gangliosids GI. Chemische Berichte, 96(3): 866-880.
Lau, M.T., Klausen, C. and Leung, P.C., 2011. E-cadherin inhibits tumor cell growth by suppressing PI3K/Akt signaling via beta-catenin-Egr1-mediated PTEN expression. Oncogene.
Leader, M., Collins, M., Patel, J. and Henry, K., 1987. Vimentin: an evaluation of its role as a tumour marker. Histopathology, 11(1): 63-72.
Lee, J., Duk Jung, I., Gyo Park, C., Han, J.W. and Young Lee, H., 2006. Autotaxin stimulates urokinase-type plasminogen activator expression through phosphoinositide 3-kinase-Akt-nuclear [corrected] factor kappa B signaling cascade in human melanoma cells. Melanoma Res, 16(5): 445-52.
Leon, A., Facci, L., Toffano, G., Sonnino, S. and Tettamanti, G., 1981. Activation of (Na+, K+)-ATPase by nanomolar concentrations of GM1 ganglioside. J Neurochem, 37(2): 350-7.
Leotlela, P.D. et al., 2007. Claudin-1 overexpression in melanoma is regulated by PKC and contributes to melanoma cell motility. Oncogene, 26(26): 3846-56.
Li, W., Zhu, T. and Guan, K.L., 2004. Transformation potential of Ras isoforms correlates with activation of phosphatidylinositol 3-kinase but not ERK. J Biol Chem, 279(36): 37398-406.
Li, X. et al., 2008. Prostate tumor progression is mediated by a paracrine TGF-beta/Wnt3a signaling axis. Oncogene, 27(56): 7118-30.
Librach, C.L. et al., 1994. Interleukin-1 beta regulates human cytotrophoblast metalloproteinase activity and invasion in vitro. J Biol Chem, 269(25): 17125-31.
Lin, J. and Shaw, A.S., 2005. Getting downstream without a Raft. Cell, 121(6): 815-6.
Liu, P., Ying, Y., Ko, Y.G. and Anderson, R.G., 1996. Localization of platelet-derived growth factor-stimulated phosphorylation cascade to caveolae. J Biol Chem, 271(17): 10299-303.
Lloyd, K.O. and Furukawa, K., 1998. Biosynthesis and functions of gangliosides: recent advances. Glycoconj J, 15(7): 627-36.
Luo, J., Manning, B.D. and Cantley, L.C., 2003. Targeting the PI3K-Akt pathway in human cancer: rationale and promise. Cancer Cell, 4(4): 257-62.
Macher, B.A. and Sweeley, C.C., 1978. Glycosphingolipids: structure, biological source, and properties. Methods Enzymol, 50: 236-51.
Meisser, A., Chardonnens, D., Campana, A. and Bischof, P., 1999. Effects of tumour necrosis factor-alpha, interleukin-1 alpha, macrophage colony stimulating factor and

transforming growth factor beta on trophoblastic matrix metalloproteinases. Mol Hum Reprod, 5(3): 252-60.

Miller-Podraza, H., Mansson, J.E. and Svennerholm, L., 1992. Isolation of complex gangliosides from human brain. Biochim Biophys Acta, 1124(1): 45-51.

Mitsuzuka, K., Handa, K., Satoh, M., Arai, Y. and Hakomori, S., 2005. A specific microdomain ("glycosynapse 3") controls phenotypic conversion and reversion of bladder cancer cells through GM3-mediated interaction of alpha3beta1 integrin with CD9. J Biol Chem, 280(42): 35545-53.

Miura, Y. et al., 2004. Reversion of the Jun-induced oncogenic phenotype by enhanced synthesis of sialosyllactosylceramide (GM3 ganglioside). Proc Natl Acad Sci U S A, 101(46): 16204-9.

Miyake, M., Koyama, M., Seno, M. and Ikeyama, S., 1991. Identification of the motility-related protein (MRP-1), recognized by monoclonal antibody M31-15, which inhibits cell motility. J Exp Med, 174(6): 1347-54.

Moon, S.K. et al., 2007. Overexpression of membrane sialic acid-specific sialidase Neu3 inhibits matrix metalloproteinase-9 expression in vascular smooth muscle cells. Biochem Biophys Res Commun, 356(3): 542-7.

Moon, S.K., Kim, H.M., Lee, Y.C. and Kim, C.H., 2004. Disialoganglioside (GD3) synthase gene expression suppresses vascular smooth muscle cell responses via the inhibition of ERK1/2 phosphorylation, cell cycle progression, and matrix metalloproteinase-9 expression. J Biol Chem, 279(32): 33063-70.

Mora, P.T., Brady, R.O., Bradley, R.M. and McFarland, V.W., 1969. Gangliosides in DNA virus-transformed and spontaneously transformed tumorigenic mouse cell lines. Proc Natl Acad Sci U S A, 63(4): 1290-6.

Morgan, J.I. and Seifert, W., 1979. Growth factors and gangliosides: a possible new perspective in neuronal growth control. J Supramol Struct, 10(2): 111-24.

Murozuka, Y., Watanabe, N., Hatanaka, K. and Hakomori, S.-i., 2007. Lyso-GM3, its dimer, and multimer: their synthesis, and their effect on epidermal growth factor-induced receptor tyrosine kinase. Glycoconjugate Journal, 24(9): 551-563.

Nagata, Y. et al., 1992. Expression cloning of beta 1,4 N-acetylgalactosaminyltransferase cDNAs that determine the expression of GM2 and GD2 gangliosides. J Biol Chem, 267(17): 12082-9.

Niu, J.X. et al., 2007. The role of adhesion molecules, alpha v beta 3, alpha v beta 5 and their ligands in the tumor cell and endothelial cell adhesion. Eur J Cancer Prev, 16(6): 517-27.

Nojiri, H., Takaku, F., Terui, Y., Miura, Y. and Saito, M., 1986. Ganglioside GM3: an acidic membrane component that increases during macrophage-like cell differentiation can induce monocytic differentiation of human myeloid and monocytoid leukemic cell lines HL-60 and U937. Proc Natl Acad Sci U S A, 83(3): 782-6.

Nores, G.A., Dohi, T., Taniguchi, M. and Hakomori, S., 1987. Density-dependent recognition of cell surface GM3 by a certain anti-melanoma antibody, and GM3 lactone as a possible immunogen: requirements for tumor-associated antigen and immunogen. J Immunol, 139(9): 3171-6.

Okada, Y., Mugnai, G., Bremer, E.G. and Hakomori, S., 1984. Glycosphingolipids in detergent-insoluble substrate attachment matrix (DISAM) prepared from substrate attachment material (SAM). Their possible role in regulating cell adhesion. Exp Cell Res, 155(2): 448-56.

Ono, M. et al., 2001. GM3 ganglioside inhibits CD9-facilitated haptotactic cell motility: coexpression of GM3 and CD9 is essential in the downregulation of tumor cell motility and malignancy. Biochemistry, 40(21): 6414-21.

Ono, M., Handa, K., Withers, D.A. and Hakomori, S., 1999. Motility inhibition and apoptosis are induced by metastasis-suppressing gene product CD82 and its analogue CD9, with concurrent glycosylation. Cancer Res, 59(10): 2335-9.

Ono, M., Handa, K., Withers, D.A. and Hakomori, S., 2000. Glycosylation effect on membrane domain (GEM) involved in cell adhesion and motility: a preliminary note on functional alpha3, alpha5-CD82 glycosylation complex in ldlD 14 cells. Biochem Biophys Res Commun, 279(3): 744-50.

Otsuji, E. et al., 1995. Inhibition of B16 melanoma metastasis by administration of G(M3)- or Gg3- liposomes: Blocking adhesion of melanoma cells to endothelial cells (anti-adhesion therapy) via inhibition of G(M3)-Gg3Cer or G(M3)LacCer interaction. International Journal of Oncology, 6(2): 319-327.

Partington, C.R. and Daly, J.W., 1979. Effect of gangliosides on adenylate cyclase activity in rat cerebral cortical membranes. Mol Pharmacol, 15(3): 484-91.

Paterson, I.C. et al., 2002. TGF-beta1 acts as a tumor suppressor of human malignant keratinocytes independently of Smad 4 expression and ligand-induced G(1) arrest. Oncogene, 21(10): 1616-24.

Qiu, Q., Yang, M., Tsang, B.K. and Gruslin, A., 2004. EGF-induced trophoblast secretion of MMP-9 and TIMP-1 involves activation of both PI3K and MAPK signalling pathways. Reproduction, 128(3): 355-63.

Rahmann, H., Rosner, H., Kortje, K.H., Beitinger, H. and Seybold, V., 1994. Ca(2+)-ganglioside-interaction in neuronal differentiation and development. Prog Brain Res, 101: 127-45.

Regina Todeschini, A. and Hakomori, S.I., 2008. Functional role of glycosphingolipids and gangliosides in control of cell adhesion, motility, and growth, through glycosynaptic microdomains. Biochim Biophys Acta, 1780(3): 421-33.

Rockmann, H. and Schadendorf, D., 2005. Role of Apaf-1 in Melanoma Drug Resistance and Apoptosis. J Investig Dermatol, 125(2): 386-387.

Rodriguez-Viciana, P., Sabatier, C. and McCormick, F., 2004. Signaling specificity by Ras family GTPases is determined by the full spectrum of effectors they regulate. Mol Cell Biol, 24(11): 4943-54.

Roisen, F.J., Bartfeld, H., Nagele, R. and Yorke, G., 1981. Ganglioside stimulation of axonal sprouting in vitro. Science, 214(4520): 577-8.

Rosenfelder, G., Young, W.W., Jr. and Hakomori, S.I., 1977. Association of the glycolipid pattern with antigenic alterations in mouse fibroblasts transformed by murine sarcoma virus. Cancer Res, 37(5): 1333-9.

Rothberg, K.G. et al., 1992. Caveolin, a protein component of caveolae membrane coats. Cell, 68(4): 673-82.

Rybak, S., Ginzburg, I. and Yavin, E., 1983. Gangliosides stimulate neurite outgrowth and induce tubulin mRNA accumulation in neural cells. Biochem Biophys Res Commun, 116(3): 974-80.

Sandhoff, K. and Christomanou, H., 1979. Biochemistry and genetics of gangliosidoses. Hum Genet, 50(2): 107-43.
Sandhoff, K. and Conzelmann, E., 1984. The biochemical basis of gangliosidoses. Neuropediatrics, 15 Suppl: 85-92.
Satoh, M. et al., 2001. Enhanced GM3 expression, associated with decreased invasiveness, is induced by brefeldin A in bladder cancer cells. Int J Oncol, 19(4): 723-31.
Seftor, E.A. et al., 2002. Molecular determinants of human uveal melanoma invasion and metastasis. Clin Exp Metastasis, 19(3): 233-46.
Semb, H. and Christofori, G., 1998. The tumor-suppressor function of E-cadherin. Am J Hum Genet, 63(6): 1588-93.
Shukla, S. et al., 2007. Activation of PI3K-Akt signaling pathway promotes prostate cancer cell invasion. Int J Cancer, 121(7): 1424-32.
Simons, K. and Ikonen, E., 1997. Functional rafts in cell membranes. Nature, 387(6633): 569-72.
Sorice, M. et al., 1997. Evidence for the existence of ganglioside-enriched plasma membrane domains in human peripheral lymphocytes. J Lipid Res, 38(5): 969-80.
Sridhar, S.C. and Miranti, C.K., 2006. Tetraspanin KAI1/CD82 suppresses invasion by inhibiting integrin-dependent crosstalk with c-Met receptor and Src kinases. Oncogene, 25(16): 2367-78.
Stahl, J.M. et al., 2003. Loss of PTEN promotes tumor development in malignant melanoma. Cancer Res, 63(11): 2881-90.
Sun, P., Wang, X.Q., Lopatka, K., Bangash, S. and Paller, A.S., 2002. Ganglioside loss promotes survival primarily by activating integrin-linked kinase/Akt without phosphoinositide 3-OH kinase signaling. J Invest Dermatol, 119(1): 107-17.
Svennerholm, L., Bostrom, K., Jungbjer, B. and Olsson, L., 1994. Membrane lipids of adult human brain: lipid composition of frontal and temporal lobe in subjects of age 20 to 100 years. J Neurochem, 63(5): 1802-11.
Tang, A. et al., 1994. E-cadherin is the major mediator of human melanocyte adhesion to keratinocytes in vitro. J Cell Sci, 107 ( Pt 4): 983-92.
Taniguchi, M. and Wakabayashi, S., 1984. Shared antigenic determinant expressed on various mammalian melanoma cells. Gann, 75(5): 418-26.
Taverna, D., Crowley, D., Connolly, M., Bronson, R.T. and Hynes, R.O., 2005. A direct test of potential roles for beta3 and beta5 integrins in growth and metastasis of murine mammary carcinomas. Cancer Res, 65(22): 10324-9.
Taverna, D. et al., 2004. Increased primary tumor growth in mice null for beta3- or beta3/beta5-integrins or selectins. Proc Natl Acad Sci U S A, 101(3): 763-8.
Todeschini, A.R., Dos Santos, J.N., Handa, K. and Hakomori, S.I., 2007. Ganglioside GM2-tetraspanin CD82 complex inhibits met and its cross-talk with integrins, providing a basis for control of cell motility through glycosynapse. J Biol Chem, 282(11): 8123-33.
Toledo, M.S., Suzuki, E., Handa, K. and Hakomori, S., 2004. Cell growth regulation through GM3-enriched microdomain (glycosynapse) in human lung embryonal fibroblast WI38 and its oncogenic transformant VA13. J Biol Chem, 279(33): 34655-64.
Tsuchida, T., Saxton, R.E., Morton, D.L. and Irie, R.F., 1987. Gangliosides of human melanoma. J Natl Cancer Inst, 78(1): 45-54.

Tsuji, S., Arita, M. and Nagai, Y., 1983. GQ1b, a bioactive ganglioside that exhibits novel nerve growth factor (NGF)-like activities in the two neuroblastoma cell lines. J Biochem, 94(1): 303-6.

Uemura, S., Kabayama, K., Noguchi, M., Igarashi, Y. and Inokuchi, J., 2003. Sialylation and sulfation of lactosylceramide distinctly regulate anchorage-independent growth, apoptosis, and gene expression in 3LL Lewis lung carcinoma cells. Glycobiology, 13(3): 207-16.

Van den Steen, P. et al., 2002. Biochemistry and molecular biology of gelatinase B or matrix metalloproteinase-9 (MMP-9). Crit Rev Biochem Mol Biol, 37: 376-536.

Vedralova, E., Borovansky, J. and Hach, P., 1995. Ganglioside profiles of experimental melanomas and of their melanosomal fractions. Melanoma Res, 5(2): 87-92.

Vivanco, I. and Sawyers, C.L., 2002. The phosphatidylinositol 3-Kinase AKT pathway in human cancer. Nat Rev Cancer, 2(7): 489-501.

Wang, L. et al., 2006. Ganglioside GD1a regulation of caveolin-1 and Stim1 expression in mouse FBJ cells: augmented expression of caveolin-1 and Stim1 in cells with increased GD1a content. Glycoconj J, 23(5-6): 303-15.

Wang, P. et al., 2007a. Positive regulation of tumor necrosis factor-alpha by ganglioside GM3 through Akt in mouse melanoma B16 cells. Biochem Biophys Res Commun, 356(2): 438-43.

Wang, P. et al., 2007b. GM3 signals regulating TNF-alpha expression are mediated by Rictor and Arhgdib in mouse melanoma B16 cells. Oncology, 73(5-6): 430-8.

Wang, P. et al., 2011. GM3 suppresses anchorage-independent growth via Rho GDP dissociation inhibitor beta in melanoma B16 cells. Cancer Sci, doi: 10.1111/j.1349-7006.2011.01963.x.Wang, X. et al., 2010. KLF8 promotes human breast cancer cell invasion and metastasis by transcriptional activation of MMP9. Oncogene.

Wong, A.S. and Gumbiner, B.M., 2003. Adhesion-independent mechanism for suppression of tumor cell invasion by E-cadherin. J Cell Biol, 161(6): 1191-203.

Wu, A.M. et al., 2011. GM3 upregulation of matrix metalloproteinase-9 possibly through PI3K, AKT, RICTOR, RHOGDI-2, and TNF-A pathways in mouse melanoma B16 cells. The Molecular Immunology of Complex Carbohydrates-3, Springer US, pp. 335-348.

Xu, Z., Shen, M.X., Ma, D.Z., Wang, L.Y. and Zha, X.L., 2003. TGF-beta1-promoted epithelial-to-mesenchymal transformation and cell adhesion contribute to TGF-beta1-enhanced cell migration in SMMC-7721 cells. Cell Res, 13(5): 343-50.

Yates, A.J., Walters, J.D., Wood, C.L. and Johnson, J.D., 1989. Ganglioside modulation of cyclic AMP-dependent protein kinase and cyclic nucleotide phosphodiesterase in vitro. J Neurochem, 53(1): 162-7.

Zhang, H., Li, Z., Viklund, E.K. and Stromblad, S., 2002. P21-activated kinase 4 interacts with integrin alpha v beta 5 and regulates alpha v beta 5-mediated cell migration. J Cell Biol, 158(7): 1287-97.

Zhang, Q., Furukawa, K., Chen, H.H., Sakakibara, T. and Urano, T., 2006. Metastatic potential of mouse Lewis lung cancer cells is regulated via ganglioside GM1 by modulating the matrix metalloprotease-9 localization in lipid rafts. J Biol Chem, 281(26): 18145-55.

Zhou, H.Y. and Wong, A.S., 2006. Activation of p70S6K induces expression of matrix metalloproteinase 9 associated with hepatocyte growth factor-mediated invasion in human ovarian cancer cells. Endocrinology, 147(5): 2557-66.

# 6

# Melanoma Cell Factory for Glycolipid Production

Maria Carmelita Z. Kasuya and Kenichi Hatanaka
*Institute of Industrial Science, The University of Tokyo*
*Japan*

## 1. Introduction

Glycolipids are ubiquitous in membranes of biological systems and play crucial roles in cell surface events including cell proliferation, differentiation, transmembrane signaling, cell-cell interactions, cell recognition, motility and cell - substrate interactions such as embryogenesis, inflammation and carcinogenesis (Hakomori, 1981; Kolter, 2002; Varki, 1999). Glycolipids, particularly gangliosides, mediate cell adhesion and modulate signal transduction. Gangliosides, cell surface glycolipids with at least one sialic acid residue, are located at the outer cell-surface of plasma membranes (Gervay et al., 1993). They are found predominantly in the nervous system where they constitute about 10% of all phospholipids. Gangliosides have also been detected in the liver of several species of shark, rat kidney, cerebelum of chicken, mouse erythrocytes, human brain and in human melanoma tumors (Li, 2002; Ozawa, 1993; Saito, 1982).

Gangliosides are involved in several diseases such as Tay-Sachs disease and Guillan-Barré syndrome. Impaired ganglioside metabolism is also relevant to Alzheimer's disease. Gangliosides bind specifically to virus such as influenza virus and various toxins such as tetanus, cholera and botulinum (Prichet & Paulson, 1989; Sun, 2000; Suzuki, 1990). Gangliosides are also implicated in skin cancer. Human melanoma cells overexpress ganglioside (Freeze et al., 1993). Normal melanocytes predominantly express GM3 (greater than 90%) and GD3 (less than 5%) (Hoon 1988, 1992). However, malignant melanoma expresses other types of gangliosides including GM2 and GD2. Human melanoma cells express the four major gangliosides (GM3, GD3, GM2 and GD2).

Considering the essential roles played by glycolipids in biochemical and cellular processes, development of methods for their rapid and efficient synthesis is necessary. Isolation from natural sources affords glycolipids but with very limited amounts. The conventional chemical synthetic approach gives glycolipids with high purity in good yield. However, the poor stereoselectivity and the multi-step operation involving tedious protection and deprotection schemes are among the many shortcomings. Enzyme synthesis promises high levels of regioselectivity and stereoselectivity but the availability and high cost have to be reckoned with.

As part of our continued interest in the synthesis of glycolipids, the saccharide primer strategy was employed as a viable alternative to existing methods (Kasuya, 2000, 2004, 2005, 2007, 2010a, 2010b, 2010c, 2010d; Sato, 2007). The saccharide primer method using animal cells and amphiphilic glycoside primers such dodecyl α- and β-lactoside, 12- and 2-azidododecyl lactosides, dodecyl α- and β-galactoside, dodecyl α- and β-glucoside, thiolactosides, glycosides with perfluoroalkyl chains and fluorinated galactoside was developed for the fast, simple and convenient synthesis of glycolipids. The saccharide primers were chemically synthesized and introduced into mouse melanoma B16 cells to generate GM3- and GM4-type gangliosides in fairly good yield.

For the production of ganglioside such as GM3 (NeuAcα3Galβ4Gluβ1Cer), mouse melanoma B16 cell is a good candidate to produce chemical quantities with homogeneity required for application since cancer cells proliferate even beyond confluency due to the absence of contact inhibition. Mouse melanoma B16 cells in culture could serve as the "cell factory" where the raw material (saccharide primer) is processed by endogenous donors and enzymes to generate products, biologically important glycolipids, with high stereo- and regioselectivity. By employing mouse melanoma B16 cells, production of desired ganglioside analogues, such as GM3 and GM4, via saccharide primer strategy is possible.

This chapter presents the versatiliy of melanoma B16 cells for the convenient production of glycolipids via saccharide primer strategy.

## 2. Saccharide primer method

The saccharide primer strategy (shown in figure 1) combines chemical synthetic methods with cellular biosynthetic processes for the synthesis of glycolipids. The basic building blocks, called saccharide primers, are synthetically accessible amphiphilic glycosides that resemble lactosyl ceramide, the intermediate in the biosynthetic pathway (Miura & Yamagata, 1997). When introduced to cells, the lactosyl ceramide analogues with a single lipophilic chain serve as substrate for cellular-mediated glycosylation to afford oligosaccharide with glycan structures exactly the same as those produced by the cells used (Sarkar 1995, 1997, 2000). By using different types of cells, a library of biologically important glycolipids can be generated from one kind of saccharide primer.

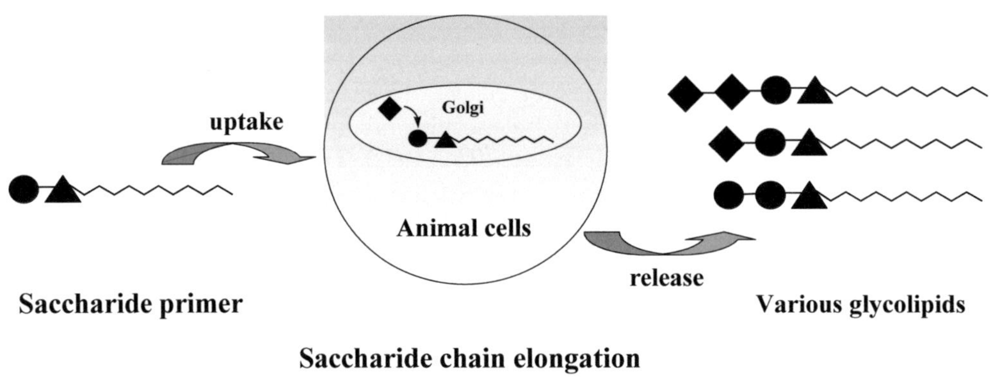


Fig. 1. Saccharide primer strategy

The basic requirements for the saccharide primer method are the appropriate cell line and the amphiphilic saccharide primer. Cells are treasuries of glycosyltransferases and glycosyl donors. Careful choice of cells is important because the kind of cells employed will determine the structure of the products formed. For mass production, the cell must be amenable to continuous culture for several days. The amphiphilic saccharide primer, substrate for cellular mediated glycosylation, consists of a saccharide head (hydrophilic moiety) and an alkyl tail (hydrophobic moiety). It is accessible in a few steps through simple chemical synthesis. Generally, the saccharide primers can be prepared by conventional methods of glycosylation of an alcohol with a glycoside derivative followed by deacylation under Zemplen conditions.

The cellular uptake of primer and release of glycosylated products by cells depend on the hydrophobic (aglycon moiety) and hydrophilic (saccharide moiety) balance. The appropriate chain length of the aglycon moeity is an important consideration to ensure the efficient uptake by cells, glycosylation and release of products to the culture medium for collection. A short aglycon unit such as an octyl group does not allow incorporation of the primer into the cells. On the other hand, a long aglycon unit such as a stearyl group allows entry into cells but the products are not released into the culture medium. The dodecyl aglycon is the most appropriate length to ensure uptake, elongation and release of product as shown in figure 2 (Nakajima et al., 1998).

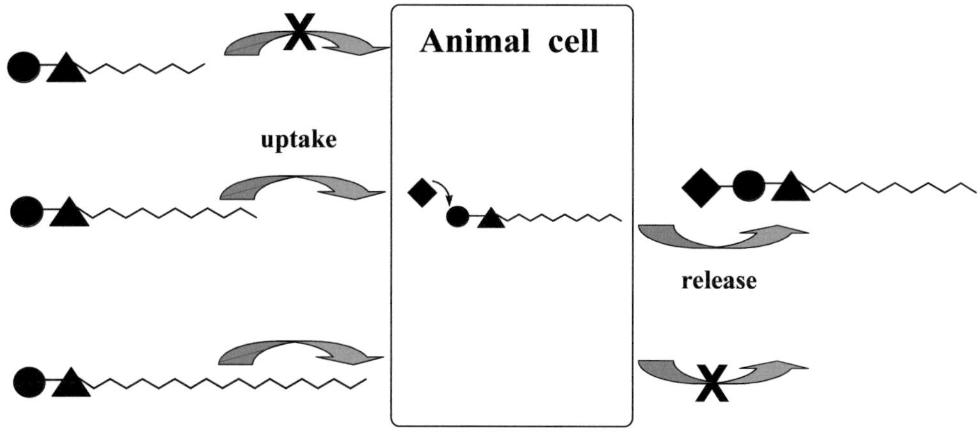


Fig. 2. Effect of alkyl chain length on saccharide primer uptake and release of product

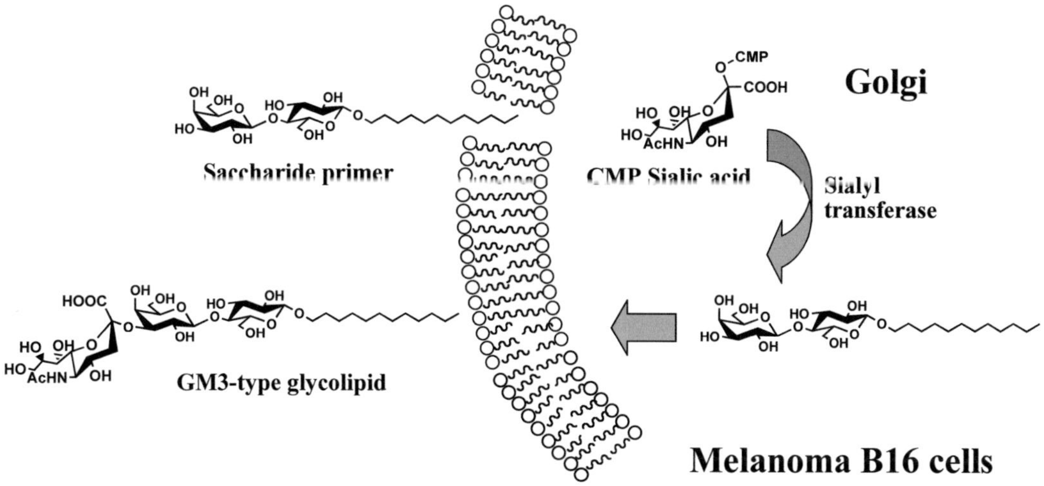


Fig. 3. Cellular enzyme-mediated glycosylation of saccharide primer

For priming to occur, the saccharide primers must pass through the plasma membrane and enter the Golgi, where the glycosyltransferases reside and where glycosylation takes place (Kolter et al., 2002). After diffusion through the cell membrane, the saccharide primers are assimilated into the glycosphingolipid biosynthetic pathway and function as acceptor for the glycosyl transferases. The sugar nucleotide donor and the glycosyl transferase are both endogenously prepared by the cells. When administered into animal cells such as mouse melanoma B16 cells, a lactoside primer functions as acceptor for the GM3 synthase, α-(2→3) sialyl transferase, resulting in sialylation of the terminal galactosyl residue of the lactosyl moiety to afford a GM3-type glycolipid as shown in figure 3.

### 2.1 Methodology

The important steps in glycolipid production using melanoma B16 cells via saccharide primer method include (1) chemical synthesis of saccharide primer, (2) administration, cellular uptake and glycosylation of saccharide primer, (3) lipid extraction, (4) analysis of products, and (5) structure elucidation of product (figure 4).

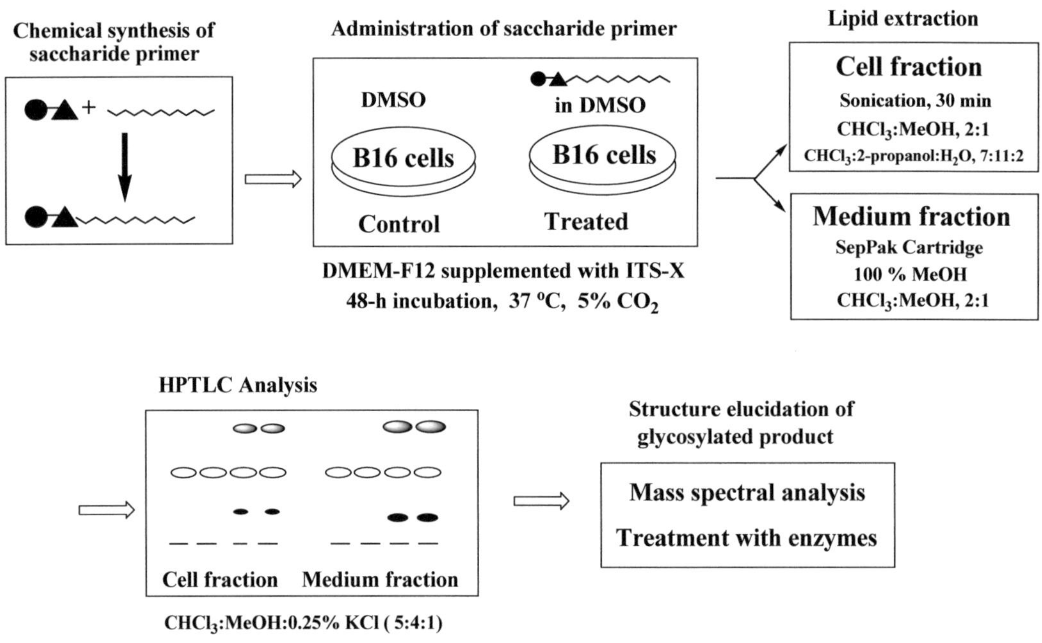


Fig. 4. General method for glycolipid production via saccharide primer strategy

#### 2.1.1 Chemical synthesis of saccharide primers

Generally, the saccharide primers are prepared in 2 steps: glycosylation of an alcohol with a monosaccharide (peracetylated galactose or glucose) or a disaccharide (peracetylated lactose) derivative followed by deacylation. Glycosylation is carried out using Lewis acid such as $BF_3 \cdot OEt_2$ as catalyst. The β-linked product is separated by column chromatography. Deacylation under Zemplen conditions using sodium methoxide and methanol affords the desired saccharide primers that could be purified by recrystallization using methanol. The structure of the saccharide primers is confirmed from the NMR and mass spectral results. A

50 mM stock solution is prepared by dissolving the saccharide primer in sterile dimethylsulfoxide ($Me_2SO$).

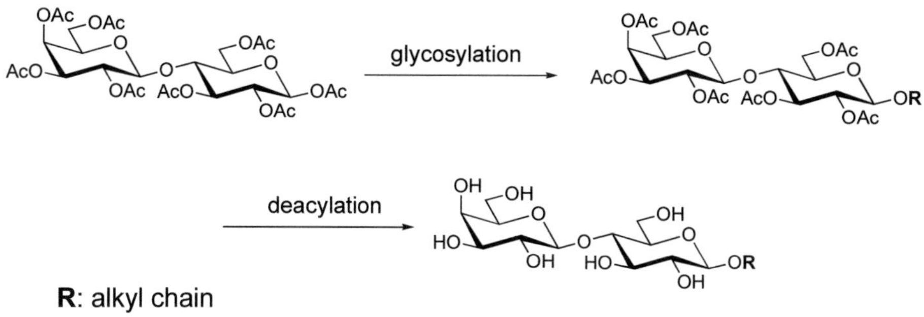


### 2.1.2 Administration, cellular uptake and glycosylation

Inocula of 2 x $10^6$ of mouse melanoma B16 cells are cultured in 100-mm dishes containing 7 mL of 1:1 DMEM-F12 supplemented with 10% fetal bovine serum (FBS) and maintained in humidified atmosphere of 5% $CO_2$ air at 37 °C for 48 h. Then, cells are washed twice with medium supplemented with insulin-transferrin-selenium X (ITS-X) solution to remove the serum, and then incubated with 50 μM of the saccharide primer for 48 h at 37 °C. During incubation of cells in the presence of primer, uptake and subsequent elongation by cellular enzymes take place to afford products that are released to the culture medium.

### 2.1.3 Extraction of lipids and structure elucidation of product

After incubation in the presence of primer, the culture media and cells are collected. The lipids are extracted from the cell pellet with $CHCl_3$ : MeOH (2 : 1, v/v), then with $CHCl_3$ : 2-propanol : water (7 : 11 : 2, v/v), in a sonicated bath. On the other hand, the lipids from the culture media are purified using SepPak C18 column. Lipids from the cell homogenate and culture medium fractions are analyzed by HPTLC with $CHCl_3$ : MeOH : 0.2 % aq KCl (5 : 4 : 1, v/v) as developing solvent. HPTLC plates are sprayed with resorcinol (Svennerholm, 1957), then with orcinol-$H_2SO_4$ reagent, and heated (120 °C) to detect the products of glycosylation. The putative bands corresponding to glycosylated primers are scraped from HPTLC plate, extracted with methanol and analyzed. The structure of the product is elucidated from the results of mass spectral analysis and enzyme hydrolysis.

## 3. Glycolipid production using various kinds of saccharide primers

### 3.1 Dodecyl glucoside, galactoside and lactoside primers

The saccharide primers are analogues of lactosyl ceramide, the natural precursor for the biosynthesis of glycolipids. Although the hydrophilic moieties are the same, the saccharide primers have a single hydrophobic tail, a dodecyl aglycon unit. Preliminary work focused on *n*-dodecyl β-lactoside primer that is structurally, the closest analogue to the natural precursor (Miura & Yamagata, 1997; Nakajima, 1998). *n*-Dodecyl β-lactoside primer does not have adverse effects on viability and morphology of melanoma B16 cells at an initial concentration of 50 μM. Cytotoxicity becomes prevalent at higher concentrations. Incubation of mouse melanoma B16 cells in the presence of dodecyl lactoside primer gave a GM3-type glycolipid (shown in Table 2) that was mostly found in the culture medium fraction. To determine whether primers with monosaccharide residue would have the same effect on B16 cells on glycolipid production, glucoside and galactoside primers with the same dodecyl aglycon unit were also prepared and administered into B16 cells (Kasuya et al., 2005).

| Saccharide primer | Cell Number[1] |
|---|---|
| 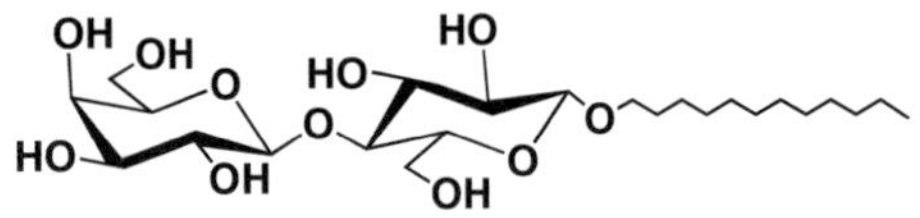 Dodecyl β-D-lactoside | $9.1 \times 10^6$ |
| 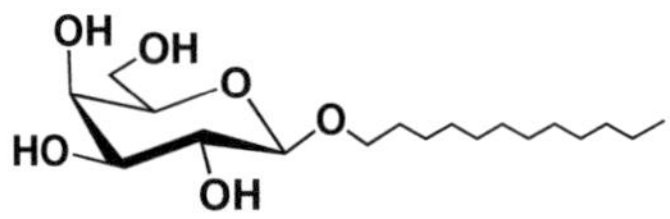 Dodecyl β-D-galactoside | $6.4 \times 10^6$ |
| 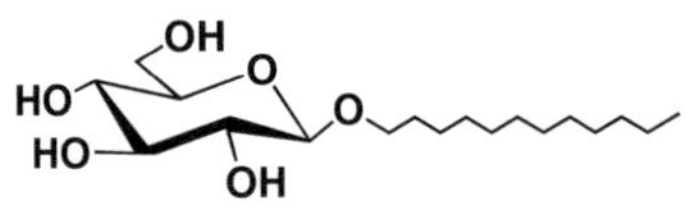 Dodecyl β-D-glucoside | cells died |

[1]Control: $10.8 \times 10^6$

Table 1. Cell number after 48-h incubation of cells with the saccharide primer.

As shown in table 1, the growth of melanoma B16 cells in the presence of β-lactoside was similar to that of control indicating that the lactoside primer does not express remarkable toxicity towards the cells at 50 μM concentration. However, the monosaccharide primers exhibited cytotoxicity to a certain extent. Relative to control, dodecyl galactoside primer reduced the cell number by almost half while dodecyl glucoside primer was cytotoxic. Although the galactoside primer exhibited moderate cytotoxicty, the galactoside primer passed through the plasma membrane and was assimilated in the glycosphingolipid biosynthetic pathway to function as acceptor for α-(2→3)-sialyl transferase, resulting in the direct glycosylation occurring at the galactosyl residue to afford a GM4-type glycolipid as shown in Table 2. Expectedly, the β-glucoside primer that expressed cytotoxicity (90 % of the cells died) was not elongated.

### 3.2 α- and β-linked saccharide primers

Whether or not the glycosidic linkage of the aglycon unit of saccharide primers affects the production of glycolipids by melanoma B16 cells was also investigated. Dodecyl α- and β- lactoside, dodecyl α- and β-galactoside, dodecyl α- and β-glucoside were chemically synthesized and introduced to mouse melanoma B16 cells (Kasuya et al., 2005).

The assimilation of primers into cells through the plasma membrane seemed to be unaffected by the anomeric linkage. Regardless of the α- or β-linkage to the aglycon unit,

| Saccharide primer | Product |
|---|---|
| 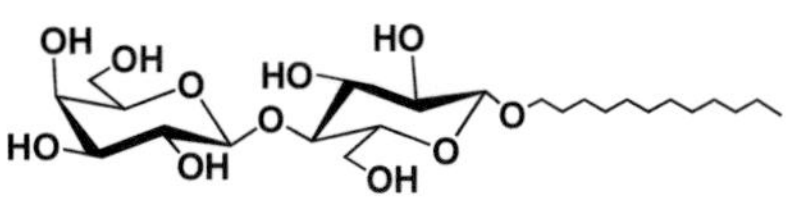 Dodecyl β-D-lactoside | 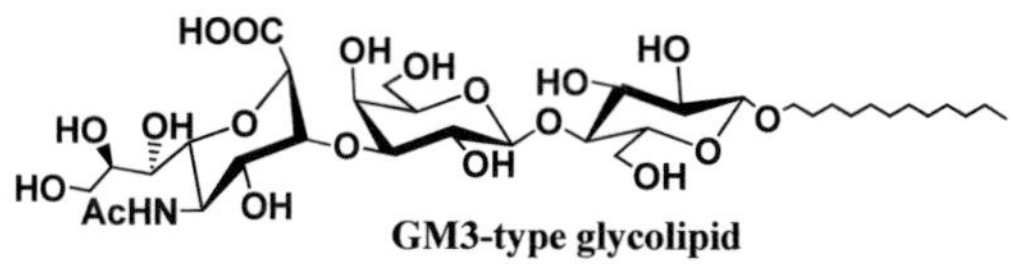 GM3-type glycolipid |
| 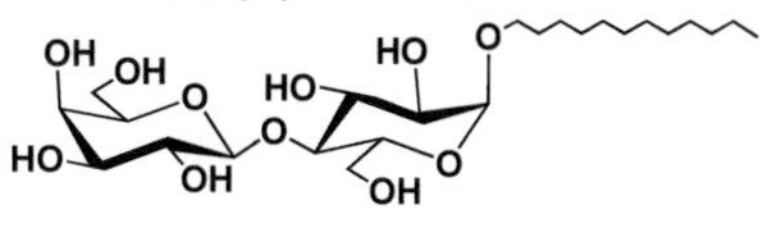 Dodecyl α-D-lactoside | 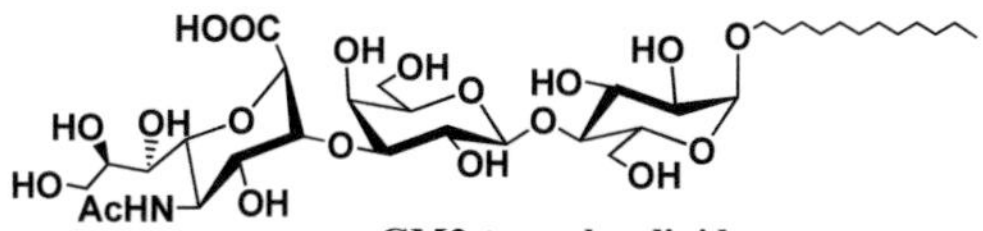 GM3-type glycolipid |
| 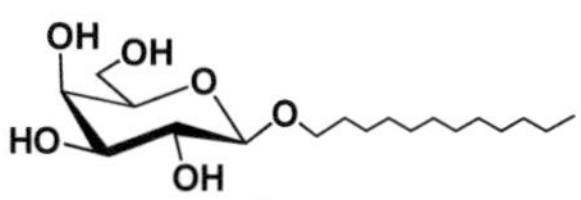 Dodecyl β-D-galactoside | 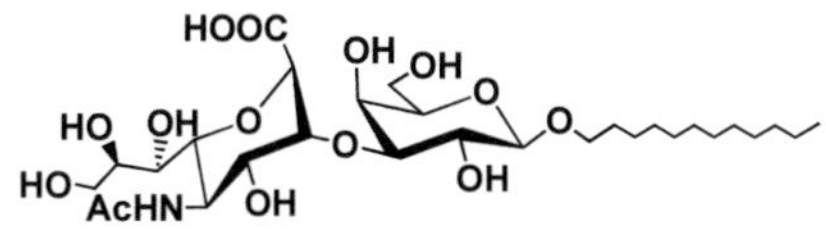 GM4-type glycolipid |
| 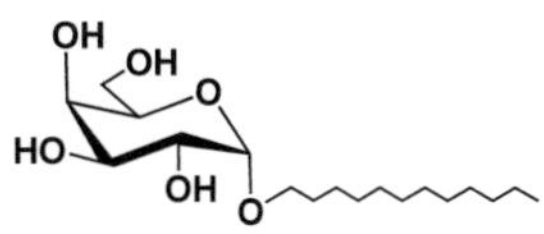 Dodecyl α-D-galactoside | No glycosylation product |
| 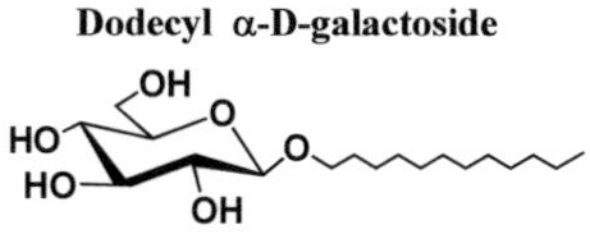 Dodecyl β-D-glucoside | No glycosylation product |
| 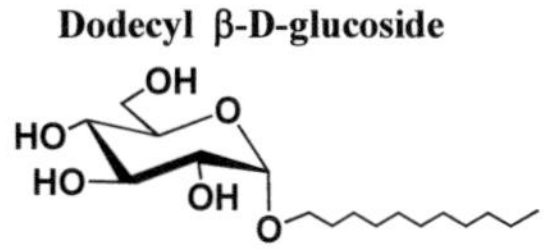 Dodecyl α-D-glucoside | No glycosylation product |

Table 2. Results after 48-h incubation of melanoma B16 cells with 50 μM α- or β- linked saccharide primers.

melanoma B16 cells take in the primers. However, elongation occurred only with dodecyl α- and β-lactoside, and dodecyl β-galactoside primers to afford GM3- and GM4-type oligosaccharides, respectively as shown in Table 2. In cellular sialylation, a terminal galactose residue that is β-linked to the adjacent saccharide or aglycon unit is necessary. Sialyltransferases reside in the Golgi compartment and transfer a sialic acid residue from CMP-sialic acid to the C-6 or C-3 hydroxyl group at the non-reducing Gal-, Gal NAc-, or GlcNAc residue. For glycosylation of primers by cells to occur, the glycoside must diffuse through the plasma membrane and enter the Golgi. The anomeric linkage of the aglycon unit seems irrelevant for primer incorporation into melanoma B16 cells. However, the anomeric β-linkage of the terminal galactoside residue that is the site for sialylation of the primers is significant for elongation.

### 3.3 Thiolactoside primers

Sulfur containing compounds have various applications in the pharmaceutical industry and in synthetic chemistry as glycosyl donors for the synthesis of complex oligisaccharides (Castaneda, 2007; Codee, 2005; Garegg, 1997; Krag, 2010; Witzak, 2005). Thiolactosides having a lactose moiety linked to a hydrophobic dodecyl aglycon unit via S-glycosidic bond have also been prepared and administered into mouse melanoma B16 cells (Mori et al., 2011).

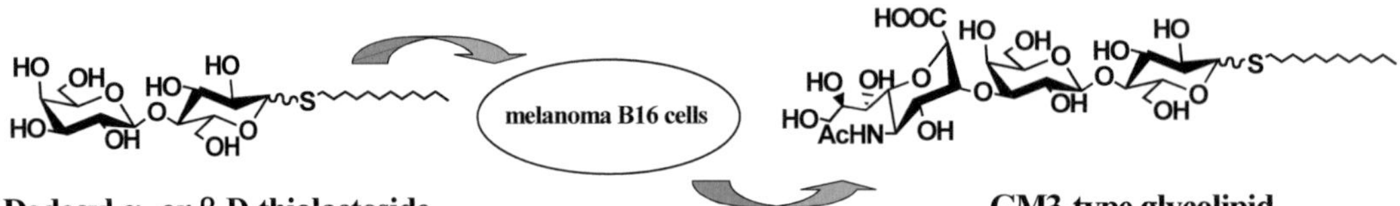


Cellular uptake of either *n*-dodecyl β-thiolactoside (β-LacSC12) or *n*-dodecyl α-thiolactoside (α-LacSC12) afforded GM3-type glycolipid. Noteworthy is that the sialyl transferases residing in the Golgi of melanoma B16 cells also recognized and elongated the primer with an S-glycoside linkage.

Interestingly, the addition of the thiolactoside primers resulted to a remarkable change on melanoma B16 cell morphology. Although B16 cells are epidermoid, cells became elongated and acquired a slender shape that is similar to fibroblast cells in the presence of thiolactoside primers (Figure 5). Significantly, increased melanin secretion was observed from B16 cells incubated in the presence of α-LacSC12 primer as evidenced by the brown coloration of the culture medium collected. The α-linked thiolactoside possibly inflicted stress on the melanoma B16 cells resulting to elevated production of the pigment melanin. As a natural response to stimuli, the skin produces melanin to protect from damage. Melanoma B16 cells increased production of the pigment to protect the cells from damage in the presence of the α-linked thiolactoside. Coloration of the culture medium was observed in the following order: α-LacSC12 > control > β-LacSC12.

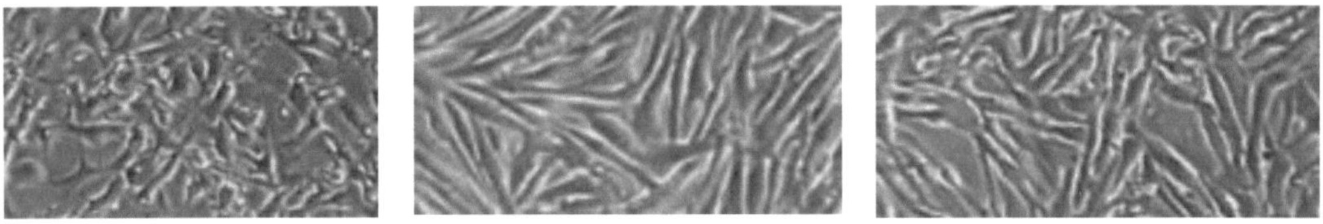

Control α-LacSC12 β-LacSC12

Fig. 5. Effect of thiolactoside primers on morphology of melanoma B16 cells.

### 3.4 2-Azido and 12-azido dodecyl lactoside primers

In view of the biological significance and potential application attached to the products obtained via saccharide primer method, it is essential that the saccharide primer should still be amenable to further modification after elongation. A functional group such as an azide is excellent for the preparation of glycopolymers and glycoconjugates. After internalization and glycosylation of saccharide primers by cells, the azido group at the aglycon can be selectively reduced to an amino group and conjugated for the synthesis of functional polymers.

Two types of saccharide primers, 12-azidododecyl β-lactoside and 2-azidododecyl β-lactoside were prepared and introduced to melanoma B16 cells (Kasuya, 2000; Murozuka, 2005). These primers were designed with the azido group at different positions in the aglycon unit to determine the effect of the position of the functional group on cellular uptake and glycolipid production.

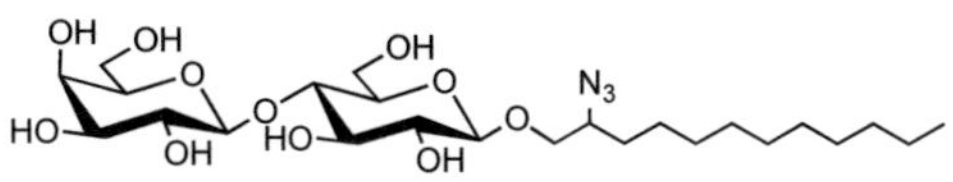

2-azidododecyl β-lactoside

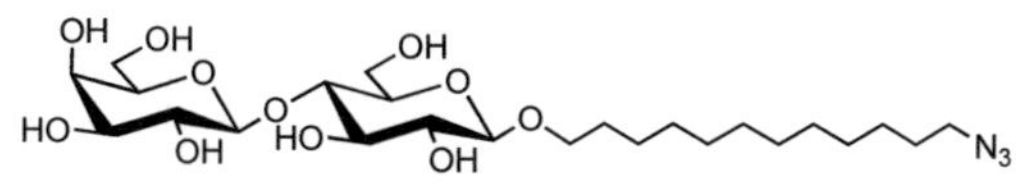

12-azidododecyl β-lactoside

Incubation with 50 μM of either 12-azidododecyl β-lactoside or 2-azidododecyl β-lactoside primers has no inherent damage to cells. Expectedly, melanoma B16 cells incorporated and elongated both primers to give GM3-type oligosaccharide that was mostly secreted in the culture medium. Like the rest of the primers used, the azidododecyl lactoside primers also inhibited the synthesis of endogenous GM3. The limited amount or capability of endogenous sialyltransferases possibly accounts for the inhibition.
Although both primers could be taken up by cells and transported to the Golgi, the glycosylation site, the relative ability to pass through the membrane and be recognized as substrate for sialyl transferases is different. The 2-azidododecyl β-lactoside could pass through the plasma membrane with relative ease than 12-azidododecyl β-lactoside. Consequently, the amount of product obtained from 2-azidododecyl β-lactoside (14% yield) was higher than the 12-azidododecyl β-lactoside (7.6% yield) under the same conditions.

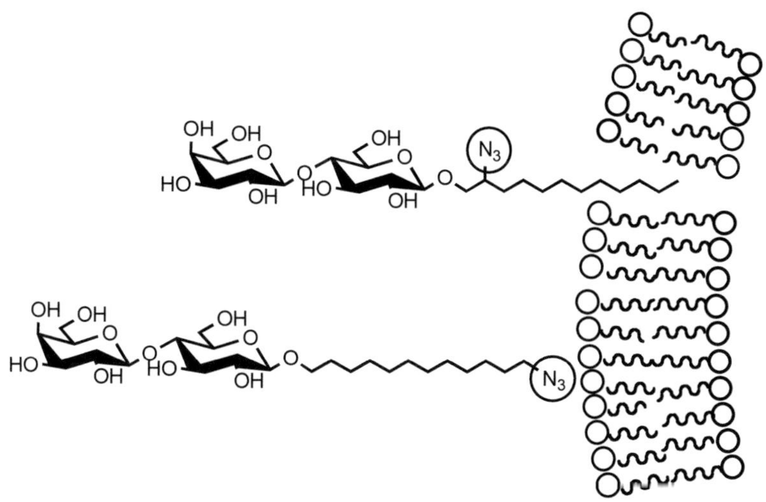

### 3.5 Fluorous-tagged saccharide primers

The interplay between the hydrophilic and hydrophobic balance brought about by the saccharide residue and the aglycon unit, respectively, is an important factor in glycolipid production using amphiphilic glycosides and melanoma B16 cells. This was demonstrated by using saccharide primers with various perfluoroalkyl aglycon units.
A series of lactosides with different perfluoroalkyl chain [LacH6F6 (each number indicates the number of $CH_2$ and $CF_2$, respectively), LacH2F8, LacH3F8, LacH2F10] were chemically synthesized and introduced to mouse melanoma B16 cells (Kasuya 2010a, 2010b, 2010c). After 48-h incubation, results showed that primers did not affect cell morphology and

viability at a concentration of 50 μM. Moreover, the numerous fluorine atoms did not pose a steric barrier to primer assimilation into cells. The fluorous-tagged lactoside primers were sialylated to afford GM3-type glycolipid that was mostly found in the culture medium.
Although the length of the aglycon unit subscribed to the recommended chain length, dodecyl (C12), to ensure efficient uptake and release of products, the amount of glycolipids produced and the amount of fluorous-tagged saccharides remaining in the cells varied depending on hydrophobicity that is attributed mainly on the fluorine content. Increasing the fluorine content renders the fluorous-tagged saccharide primers to be more hydrophobic (Kasuya et al., 2010). As shown in figure 6, as the fluorine content of the perfluoroalkyl tail increases, the amount of lactoside primer in the cells also increases. On the other hand, an increase in the fluorine content results to a decrease in the amount of product. Lac H2F10 with the highest fluorine content gave the least amount of product. Lac H6F6 having the least number of fluorine atoms gave the highest amount among the fluorous-tagged lactoside primers. Significantly, a relatively large amount of Lac H2F10, most hydrophobic among the fluorous-tagged primers used, was found in the cell fraction. Considering the immiscibility of fluorous layer with neither an aqueous nor an organic layer, it is noteworthy that the saccharide primers with perfluoroalkyl tail have a strong affinity for the lipid-rich cell membrane.

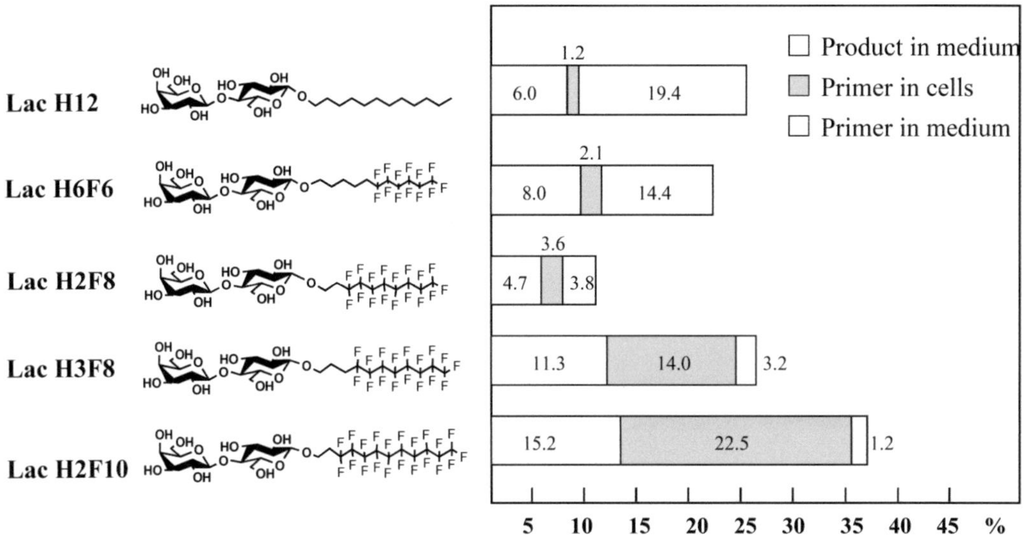


Fig. 6. Glycolipid production using saccharide primers with various perfluoroalkyl chains

### 3.6 Fluorinated galactoside primers

Ganglioside GM4 exhibits interesting biological activities. The challenging synthetic consideration that involves the regio- and stereoselective incorporation of sialic acid propelled the preparation of GM4 analogues by the saccharide primer strategy. This was achieved using dodecyl β-galactoside primer and mouse melanoma B16 cells. The replacement of a hydroxyl group by fluorine atom in the galactose residue was also pursued not only to prepare fluorinated GM4 analogues but also to establish the effect of the fluorine atom in the saccharide residue on melanoma B16 cells and glycosylation.

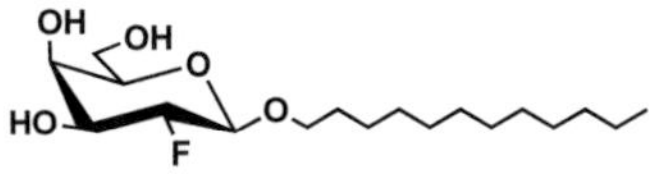

**2F Gal**

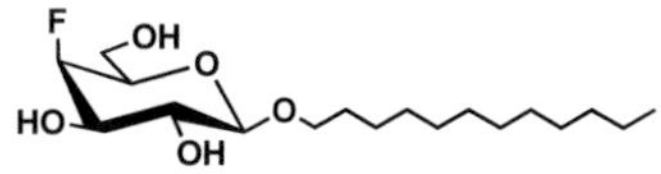

**4F Gal**

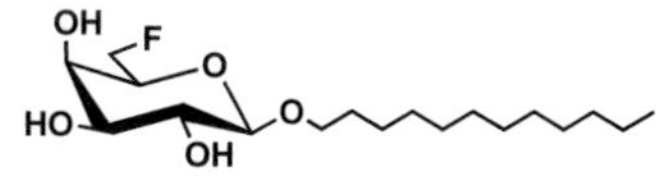

**6F Gal**

Fluorinated galactosides with dodecyl aglycon, 2F Gal, 4F Gal and 6F Gal, were chemically synthesized (Card & Reddy, 1983; Dax et al., 2000) and administered to mouse melanoma B16 cells to verify their potential as scaffolds for the synthesis of a GM4 analogue (Kasuya et al., 2007). Among the 3 kinds of primers, 2F Gal did not affect cell morphology and viability. In contrast, 4F Gal primer exhibited slight cytotoxicity and 6F Gal primer was cytotoxic at 50 μM concentration. The HPTLC results of the lipids obtained from the cell and culture medium fractions confirmed that the primers were taken-up by the cells but only the 2F Gal was glycosylated and the elongated product released to the culture medium. The MALDI TOF mass spectral results and treatment of the product with 2,3-sialidase (cloned from *S. typhimurium* LT2 and expressed in *E. coli*) confirmed the structure of the glycosylation product, a GM4 analogue.

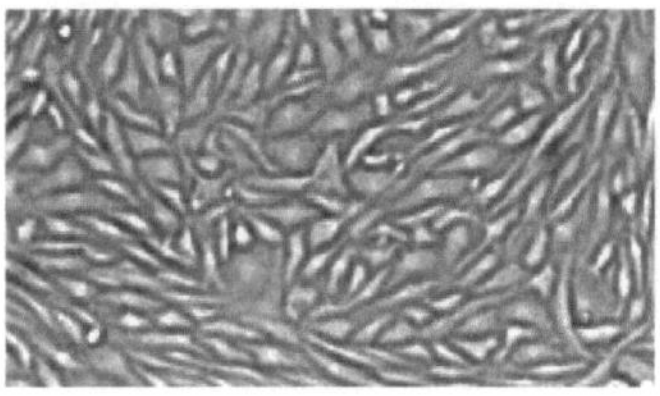

2F Gal

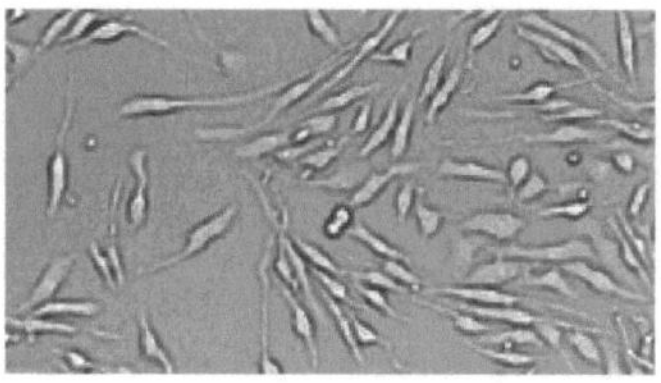

4F Gal

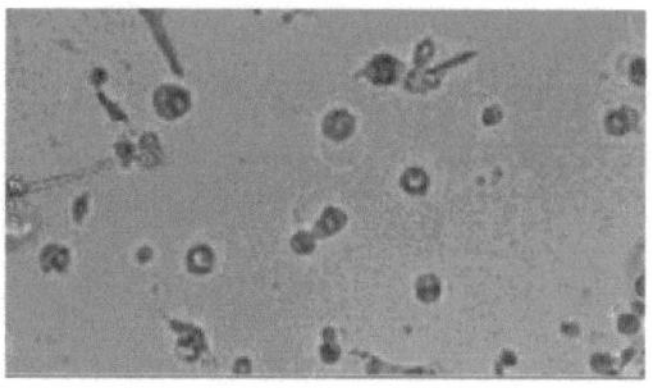

6F Gal

The presence of a fluorine atom was expected to have minimal effect on cell viability and primer assimilation into cells that may be attributed to the size and hydrophobicity of fluorine. However, replacement of one hydroxyl unit by a fluorine atom in different positions of the galactose residue elicited different cellular responses. A fluorine atom at 2 position of the galactose residue did not have adverse effects to the cell, and 2F Gal was glycosylated. However, a fluorine atom at 4 or 6 positions slightly, or greatly, affected cell viability. As a consequence, saccharide elongation of 4F and 6F Gal primers did not take place. Although sialyl transferases are amenable to substrate modifications, the type and position of substituent at the vicinity of the glycosylation site (C3 position) and their positive effect on cell viability are prerequisites for cellular enzyme glycosylation and substrate recognition by 2,3-sialyl transferase.

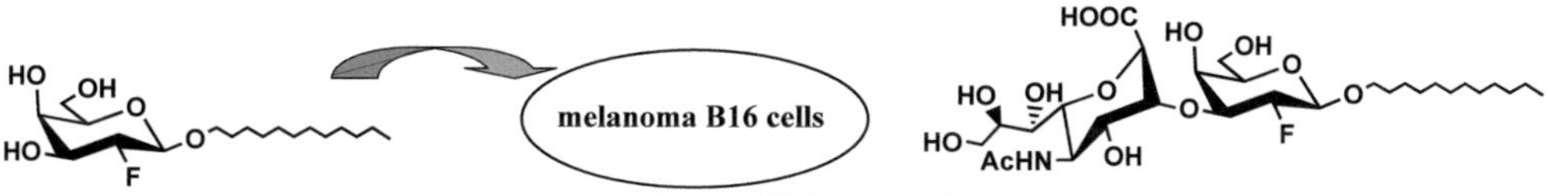


**Dodecyl 2-deoxy-2-fluoro-β-D-galactopyranoside** **GM4-type glycolipid**

## 4. Mass production

For the mass production of gangliosides via saccharide primer method, the choice of cell to be employed is crucial. The cells to be used should be amenable to continuous culture for several days that requires repeated administration of primer and harvest of culture medium. Moreover, cells should provide the desired glycolipid in fairly good yield. Mouse melanoma B16 cells meet these requirements for the production of ganglioside analogues. Other considerations for the mass production of gangliosides include optimization of seeded cell number, length of incubation time and primer concentration (Miyagawa et al., 2007).

Saccharide primers are cytotoxic when introduced to a small number of seeded cells as compared to a large number of cells due to the existence of stronger intercellular connection at the confluent state of cells. Generally, the higher the seeded cell number, the more product obtained.

The optimum length of incubation time is 48 h. Although the amount of glycosylated product increases linearly with respect to the length of incubation time, productivity does not significantly advance beyond 48-h incubation. Moreover, long exposure to saccharide primers affects cellular morphology.

The amount of sialylated primer increases linearly with increasing concentration while consequently inhibiting endogenous GM3 production. However, beyond the optimum concentration is cytotoxic.

### 4.1 GM4-type glycolipid

The simplest among the gangliosides is sialylgalactosyl ceramide GM4 (NeuAcα2→3GalCer) (Bazin, 1999; Gervay, 1993). GM4 is a minor ganglioside in human brain and has been detected in human myelin and human oligodendrocytes. However, the biological significance remains unknown. GM4 is scarce in natural sources so chemical and enzymatic synthesis remains to be the viable sources of quantitative amounts of GM4 (Otsubo, 2001; Satoh, 1996; Schnaar, 1998).

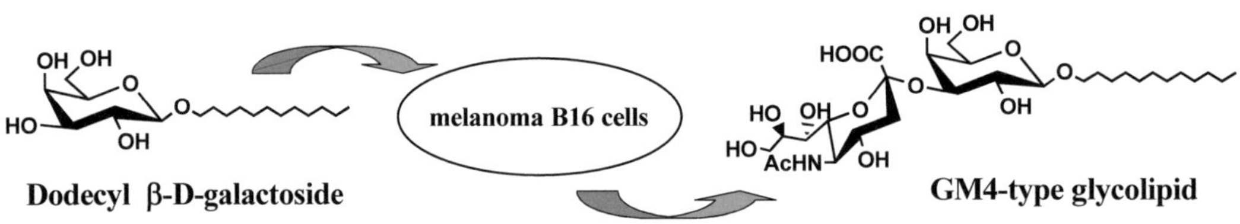


The utility of the saccharide primer method for the mass production of GM4-type ganglioside (Kasuya et al., 2010) was carried out. The optimum conditions for the mass production of GM4-type ganglioside by the saccharide primer method of employing mouse melanoma B16 cells and dodecyl β-galactoside primer (Gal C12) included: seeded cell number (5 x $10^6$, 15 cm dishes, 20 mL medium), concentration (50 μM) and incubation time (48 h or 72 h). Based on HPTLC results, more GM4 could be obtained from higher concentration of primer, 100 or 150 μM, but slight to moderate cytotoxicity was observed. Hence, 50 μM was administered to cells to ensure continuous culture requiring repeated administration of primer and harvest of culture medium.

GalC12 did not exhibit adverse effects on cell morphology and viability. However, formation of colonies became evident during the second week of incubation. Cells continue to glycosylate the primer but the amount produced decreased after repeated primer administration and harvest. The culture media containing the product from all the harvests were pooled and the glycolipids were adsorbed on HP20 resin and eluted with gradient MeOH. Purification of the products was accomplished using SepPak columns. Finally, purification by Centrifugal Partition Chromatography (CPC) (Kato et al., 2007) gave 4.0 mg of the GM4 analogue with high purity from 4.2 liters of culture medium.

## 5. Conclusion

In the production of glycolipids such as GM3- and GM4-type gangliosides, melanoma B16 cells could serve as the "cell factory" that processes the saccharide primers such dodecyl α- and β-lactoside, 2- and 12-azidododecyl lactosides, dodecyl β-galactoside, fluorinated galactoside, thiolactosides or glycosides with perfluoroalkyl chains and transforms them to GM3- and GM4-type gangliosides using endogenous enzymes and glycosyl donor. Generally, monosaccharide and disaccharide primers gave GM4- and GM3-type glycolipids, respectively.

**Production of GM4-type glycolipid**

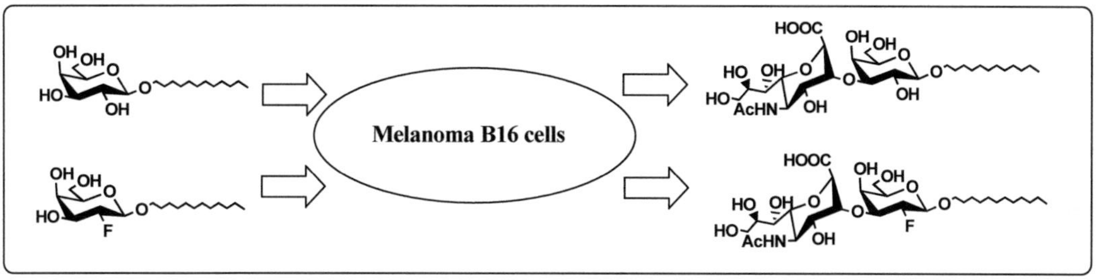


**Production of GM3-type glycolipid**

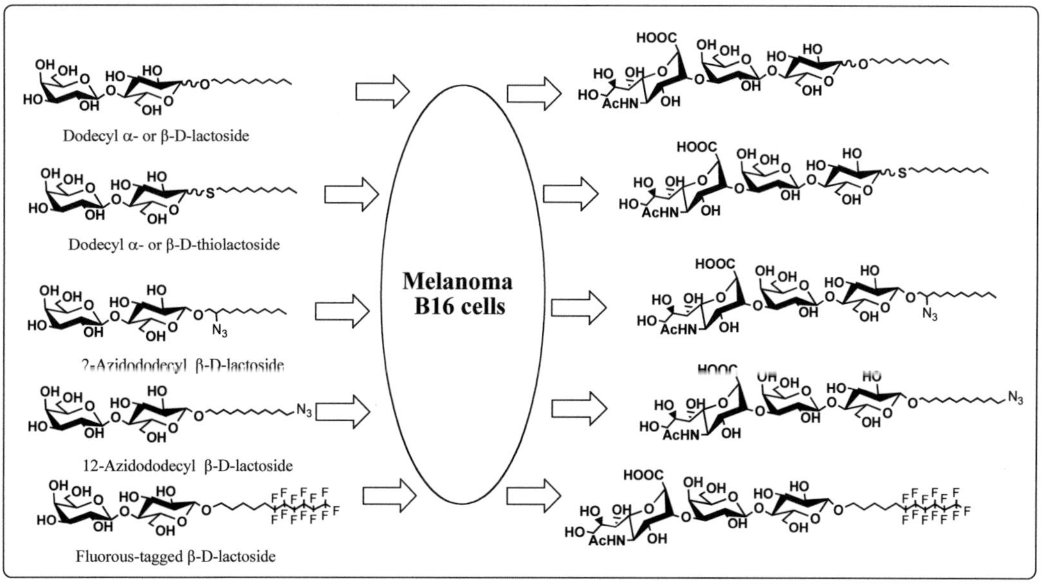


With a few exceptions, the galactoside and lactoside primers reported in this chapter (1) do not have adverse effects on morphology and viability of mouse melanoma B16 cells at 50 μM after incubation for 48 h, (2) are taken in by melanoma B16 cells and assimilated to the Golgi, the site of glycosylation, and (3) are recognized by cellular enzymes and elongated to afford glycolipids that are released to the culture medium for collection, purification and identification. By employing mouse melanoma B16 cells, production of biologically important glycolipids via saccharide primer method is fast, convenient and highly stereoselective. Significantly, expensive enzymes and glycosyl donor are no longer necessary since these are endogenous to melanoma B16 cells. Melanoma B16 cells is a good candidate in the mass production of glycolipids, particularly GM3- and GM4-type gangliosides, because it is amenable to continuous culture for several days.

Depending on the type of saccharide primer and the concentration administered into melanoma B16 cells, the various effects such as elevated pigmentation, alteration of cell morphology, and decreased production of endogenous glycolipids, the saccharide primer strategy offers a fresh approach to understanding the molecular and cellular mechanism underlying the pathogenesis of melanomas. Moreover, the saccharide primer strategy could open possibilities for new therapeutic options for melanoma.

## 6. Acknowledgements

This work was supported by a grant for "Development of Novel Diagnostic and Medical Applications through Elucidation of Sugar Chain Functions" from the New Energy and Industrial Technology Development Organization (NEDO).

## 7. References

Bazin, H., Du, Y., Polat, T., Lindhart, R. (1999) Synthesis of versatile neuraminic acid "*C*" disaccharide precursor for the synthesis of *C*-glycoside analogues of gangliosides, *Journal of Organic Chemistry,* Vol.64, pp. 7254-7259.

Card, P., Reddy, G. (1983) Fluorinated carbohydrates. 2. Selective fluorination of gluco- and mannopyranosides. Use of 2-D NMR for structural assignments. *Journal of Organic Chemistry*, Vol.48, pp. 4734-4743.

Castaneda, F., Burse, A., Boland, W., Kinne, R. K-H. (2007) Thioglycosides as inhibitors of hSGLT1 and hSGLT2: Potential therapeutic agents for the control of hyperglycemia in diabetes, *International Journal of Medical Sciences*, Vol.4, pp. 131-139.

Codee, J. D., Litjens, R. E., van den Bos, L. J., Overkleeft, H. S., der Marel, G. A. (2005) Thioglycosides in sequential glycosylation strategies, *Chemical Society Reviews* Vol.34, No.9, pp. 769-782.

Dax, K., Albert, M., Ortner, J., Paul, B. (2000), Synthesis of deoxyfluoro sugars from carbohydrate precursors, *Carbohydrate Research,* Vol.327, pp. 47-86.

Freeze, H., Sampath, D., Varki, A. (1993) Alpha-and beta-xylosides alter glycolipid synthesis in human melanoma and Chinese hamster ovary cells, *The Journal of Biological Chemistry* Vol.268, pp. 1618-1627.

Garegg, P. J. (1997) Thioglycosides as glycosyl donors in oligosaccharide synthesis, *Advances in Carbohydrate Chemistry and Biochemistry*, Vol.52, pp. 179-266.

Gervay, J., Peterson, J.M., Oriyama, T., Danishefsky, S. (1993) An unexpected sialylation: Total synthesis of GM4 and a positional Isomer, *Journal of Organic Chemistry*, Vol.58, pp. 5465-5468.

Hakomori, S. (1981) Glycosphingolipids in cellular interaction, differentiation, and oncogenesis. *Annual Reviews in Biochemistry*, pp. 733-764.

Hoon, DS., Irie, RF., Cochran, AJ., (1988) Gangliosides from human melanoma immonomodulate response of T cells to interleukin-2. *Cell Immunology*, Vol.111, No.2, pp. 410-419.

Hoon DS., Kaback, MM., Lim-Steele, J., Tsuchida. T., Morton, DL., Irie, RF. (1992) Ganglioside GN2 levels in human melanoma cells: inverse correlation with lysosomal beta-hexosaminidase A activity. *Biochemistry International.* Vol.27, No.2, pp. 343-352.

Kasuya, M.C.Z., Wang, L.; Lee, Y.C.; Mitsuki, M.; Nakajima, N.; Sato, T.; Hatanaka, K.; Yamagata, S.; Yamagata, T. (2000) Azido glycoside primer: a versatile building block for the biocombinatorial synthesis of glycosphingolipid analogues. *Carbohydrate Research,* Vol. 329, pp. 755-763.

Kasuya, M.C.Z.; Cusi, R.; Ishihara, O.; Miyagawa, A.; Hashimoto, K.; Sato, T.; Hatanaka, K. (2004) Fluorous-tagged compound: a viable scaffold to prime oligosaccharide synthesis by cellular enzymes. *Biochemical Biophysical Research Commununications,* Vol.316, No.3, pp. 599-604.

Kasuya, M.C.Z., Ikeda, M., Hashimoto, K., Hatanaka, K. (2005) Effect of anomeric linkage on the sialylation of glycosides by cells, *Journal of Carbohydrate Chemistry,* Vol.24, pp. 705-715.

Kasuya, M.C.Z.; Hatanaka, K. (2010) Production of GM4 analogue using animal cells in culture, *Chemistry and Biodiversity,* Vol.7, No.2, pp 440-446.

Kasuya, M.C.Z.; Tojino, M.; Mizuno, M.; Hatanaka, K.; (2010) Effect of fluorous tags on glycosylation of saccharide primers in animal cells, *Bulletin of the Chemical Society of Japan,* Vol.82, No.11, pp 1409-1415.

Kasuya, M.C.Z., Tojino, M., Mizuno, M., Hatanaka, K. (2010) Fluorous tag method for the simultaneous synthesis of different kinds of glycolipids, *Journal of Fluorine Chemistry,* Vol.131, pp.655-659.

Kasuya, M.C.Z., Nakano. S., Katayama, R., Hatanaka, K. (2010) Evaluation of the hydrophobicity of perfluoroalkyl chains in amphiphilic compounds that are incorporated into cell membrane, *Journal of Fluorine Chemistry,* Vol.131, pp.655-659.

Kasuya, M.C.Z., Ito, A., Hatanaka, K. (2007) Simple and Convenient Synthesis of a Fluorinated GM4 Analogue, *Journal of Fluorine Chemistry,* Vol.128, pp. 562-565.

Kato, T., Miyagawa, A., Kasuya, M.C.Z., Ito, A., Hatanaka, K. (2007) Purification by centrifugal partition chromatography of amphiphilic compounds, glycolipids and pseudo-glycolipids synthesized by using cells, *Journal of Chromatography,* Vol.178, pp. 154-159.

Kolter, T., R. Proia, K. Sandhoff. (2002) Combinatorial Ganglioside Biosynthesis, *Journal of Biological Chemistry,* Vol.277, pp 25859-25862.

Krag, J., Christiansen, M. S., Petersen, J. G., Jensen, H. H. (2010) Direct chemical glycosylation with pentenyl- and thioglycoside donors of N-acetylglucosamine, *Carbohydrate Research,* Vol.345, No.7, pp. 872-879.

Li, Y-T., Sugiyama, E., Ariga, T., Nakayama, J., Hayama, M., . Hama, Y., Nakagawa, H., Tai, T., Maskos, K., Li, S-C., Ksama, T. (2002) Association of GM4 ganglioside with the membrane surrounding lipid droplets in shark liver, *Journal of Lipid Research,* Vol.43, pp.1019-1025.

Miura, Y., Yamagata, T. (1997) Glycosylation of lactosylceramide analogs in animal cells: amphiphatic disaccharides primers for glycosphingolipid synthesis, *Biochemical and Biophysical Research Communications,* Vol.241, pp. 698-703.

Miyagawa, A., Kasuya, M.C.Z., Hatanaka. K. (2007) Alternative methods of globotrioside production using Vero cells: a microcarrier system procedure, *Chemistry Central Journal,* Vol.1, pp 26.

Mori, M.; Kasuya, M.C.Z., Mizuno, M., Hatanaka, K. (2011) Thiolactosides: Scaffolds for the synthesis of glycolipids in animal cells, *International Journal of Carbohyrate Chemistry.* In press.

Murozuka, Y., Kasuya, M.C.Z., Kobayashi, M., Watanabe, Y., Sato, T., Hatanaka, K. (2005) Efficient sialylation on azidododecyl lactosides by using B16 melanoma cells, *Chemistry and Biodiversity*, Vol.2, pp 1063-1078.

Nakajima, H., Miura, Y., Yamagata, T. (1998) Glycosylation of amphiphatic lactoside primers with consequent inhibition of endogenous glycosphingolipid synthesis, *Journal of Biochemistry,* Vol.124, pp. 148-156.

Otsubo, N., Ishida, H., Kiso., M., (2001) Synthesis of novel ganglioside GM4 analogues containing N- deacetylated and lactamized sialic acid: probes for searching new ligand structures for human L-selectin, *Journal of Carbohydrate Research,* Vol.330, pp 1-5.

Ozawa, H., Kotani, M., Kawashima, I., (1993) Generation of a monoclonal antibody specific for ganglioside GM4: Evidence for GM4 expression on astrocytes in chicken cerebellum, *Journal of Biochem*istry, Vol.114, pp. 5-8.

Pritchett, T.; Paulson, J. (1989) Basis for the potent inhibition of influenza virus infection by equine and guinea pig 2-macroglobulin, *Journal of Biological Chemistry,* Vol.264, No.17, pp. 9850-9858.

Saito, M., Rosenberg, A. (1982) Sialosylgalactosylceramide (GM4) is a major ganglioside in chicken embryonic liver. *Journal of Lipid Research,* Vol.23, pp.9-13.

Sarkar, A., Brown, J., Esko, J. (2000) Synthesis and glycan priming activity of acetylated disaccharides, *Carbohydrate Research*, Vol.329, pp. 287-300.

Sarkar, A., Rostand, S., Jain, R., Matta, K., Esko, J. (1997) Fucosylation of disaccharide precursors of sialyl LewisX inhibit selectin-mediated cell adhesion, *The Journal of Biological Chemistry,* Vol.272, pp. 25608-25616.

Sarkar, A., Fritz, T., Taylor, W., Esko, J. (1995) Disaccharide uptake and priming in animal cells: Inhibition of sialyl Lewis X by acetylated Galβ1→4GlcNAcβ-*O*-naphthalenemethanol, *Proceedings of the National Academy of Sciences of the United States of America,* Vol.92, pp. 3323-3327.

Sato, T., Hatanaka, K., Hashimoto, H., Yamagata, T. (2007) Synthesis of oligosaccharides using cell function, *Trends in Glycoscience and Glycotechnology*, Vol.19 pp.1-17.

Satoh, J., Tai, T., Kim, S.U. (1996) Differential expression of gangliosides and galactolipids in fetal human oligodendrocytes and astrocytes in culture, *Brain Research Development,* Vol.93, pp. 172-81.

Schnaar, R., Collins, B., Wright, L., Kiso, M., Tropak, M., Roder, J. Crocker, P. (1998.) Myelin N-associated glycoprotein binding to gangliosides: Structural specificity and functional implications. *Annals of the New York Academy of Science*, Vol.845, pp 92-105

Sun, X.-L.; Kanie, Y.; Guo, C.-H.; Kanie, O.; Suzuki, Y.; Wong, C.-H. (2000) Synthesis of C-3 modified sialylglycosides as selective inhibitors of influenza hemagglutinin and neuraminidase. *European Journal of Organic Chemistry,* pp 2643-2653.

Suzuki, Y., Sato, K., Kiso, M., Hasegawa, A. (1990) New ganglioside analogs that inhibit influenza virus sialidase, *Glycoconjugate Journal,* Vol.7, pp. 349-356.

Svennerholm, L. (1957) A colorimetric resorcinol - hydrochloric acid method, Biochimica et Biophysica Acta, Vol.24, pp. 604-611.

Varki, A.; Cummings, R.; Esko, J.D.; Freeze, H.H.; Hart, G.; Marth, J. (1999) *Essentials of Glycobiology*, Cold Spring Harbor Laboratory Press, New York.

Witzak, Z. J., Culhane, J.M. (2005) Thiosugars: new perspectives regarding availability and potential biochemical and medicinal applications, *Applied Microbiology and Biotechnology*, Vol.69, No.3, pp. 237-244.

# 7

# Melanoma-Induced Endothelial Cell Growth Involves Phospholipase $A_2$ and $COX_2$ Upregulation

Mario Alberghina, Carla Motta, Gabriella Lupo, Carmelina D. Anfuso and Renato Bernardini
*Department of Clinical and Molecular Biomedicine, University of Catania, Catania, Italy*

## 1. Introduction

Angiogenesis, the process of formation of new vessels, is fundamental in many biological processes including development, reproduction and wound repair. In tumor biology, key biochemical questions remain to be answered, in particular the molecular and cellular mechanisms responsible for establishing melanoma new vessels. The search of role for already identified soluble factors in experimental cell models encompassing brain endothelial cells, murine melanoma cell lines and pericytes could expand our molecular understanding of cerebral melanoma proliferation. The purpose of this chapter is to summarize existing knowledge of biochemical mechanisms of melanoma adhesion and angiogenesis, as well as new experimental data on the enzymatic and signaling cross-talk between tumor and microvascular cells.

## 2. Mechanisms of melanoma adhesion and transendothelial migration

During hematogeneous metastasis the blood borne malignant cells must successfully arrest in the microcirculation, invade the endothelium and escape from the vascular system. The process of extravasation (formation of dynamic, F-actin-rich pseudopodia that penetrate capillary endothelial walls) occurs when malignant cells, adherent to vascular endothelial cells (ECs), cause retraction of these cells and exposure of the underlying basal lamina. Models to studying the interaction between malignant cells and normal endothelium have been developed in vitro, using monolayers of vascular ECs, monolayers of vascular ECs on smooth muscle cell multilayers, or multicell biological membranes such as chorioallantoic or amniotic membranes (Nicholson, 1982).
Initial interactions of highly metastatic tumor cells with ECs cause morphological changes in ECs and involve mechanical contact and transient adhesion, mediated by endothelial selectins and their ligands on the neoplastic cells. This contact initiates a sequence of activation pathways that involves cytokines, growth factors, bioactive lipids, and reactive oxygen species produced by either the cancer cells or the endothelium. These molecules elicit expression of integrin adhesion molecules in cancer cells and ECs, matrix metalloproteinases, and chemotactic factors that promote, by gradient, the attachment of

tumor cells to the vessel wall and/or transvascular penetration. Induction of endothelial free radicals can be cytotoxic to cancer cells. Afterwards, the adhesion of tumor cells to endothelial basal lamina, where they rapidly spread by solubilizing the protein structure, appears to be mediated by specific cell molecules such as fibronectin, laminin, collagen and glycosaminoglycans. Considerable information on the regulation of the adhesive and migratory properties of melanoma cells on the endothelial floor is available (Cangara et al., 2010; Klemke et al., 2007).

### 2.1 Integrins

Several modes of integrin-mediated interaction between melanoma cells and ECs have been documented, e.g. between LFA-1 (αLβ2), VLA-4 (α4β1), and α4β7 on melanoma cells and their major receptors, ICAM-1, VCAM-1, and MAdCAM-1, respectively, on ECs. Adhesion of integrin/CD44 to hyaluronan is also important for the extravasation of melanoma cells into tissues. Therefore, not only the combination of chemokine receptors, but also adhesion molecules expressed on melanoma cells can determine their selective migration toward a particular site. Integrins are a superfamily of transmembrane heterodymeric (α and β subunits) surface receptors involved in cell-matrix and cell-cell adhesion. So far, at least, 18 α subunits and 8 β subunits have been isolated and characterized. Metastatic melanoma cells do express multiple adhesion receptors which can be either extremely specific for a single ligand or capable of binding multiple ligands. It is likely that the tumor cell's repertoire of adhesion receptors may influence not only its adhesive properties, but its metastatic characteristics as well. α6β1 integrin is expressed on the highly metastatic cell line B16/129 melanoma (Ruiz et al., 1993). It was suggested that α6 integrins play a dual role in the metastatic process, mediating the adhesion of tumor cells to the luminal surface of the endothelium and the adhesion to laminin in the subendothelial extracellular matrix (ECM) during extravasation. Malignant phenotype of melanoma cells expresses a melanoma-specific integrin (α7β1) that binds laminin and is not detectable in normal melanocytes (Kramer et al., 1991).

The expression of several cell adhesion molecules, notably vitronectin binding receptor αvβ3, has been associated with the metastatic potential of tumor cells. Confocal microscopy revealed the presence of the integrin αvβ3 on melanoma membrane protrusions and pseudopods penetrating the endothelial junction. αvβ3 was also enriched in heterotypic contacts between ECs and melanoma cells (Voura et al., 2001) (Fig. 1). However, many human melanoma cells do not express β3 integrins. Human melanoma cells with different metastatic potency, which do not express β2 or β3 integrins, express the VCAM-1 receptor α4β1. VCAM-1 is up-regulated on activated ECs and promotes transendothelial migration (Klemke et al., 2007). On the other hand, α6β1 and α6β4 integrins are present at a high level on the luminal and basolateral side of vascular endothelium. Human melanoma cell lines that express high constitutive levels of the metastasis-associated marker ICAM-1 were found to secrete IL-1 in vitro. The IL-1 present in melanoma-conditioned medium induced the expression of VCAM-1, endothelial-leukocyte adhesion molecule 1, and ICAM-1 on ECs in culture, and increased the rate at which melanoma cells and ECs adhered to each other (Burrows et al., 1991).

### 2.2 Signal transduction

Tumour cell transition from fluid to initial adhesive conditions to the endothelium involves an early polarization event and major rearrangements of the submembrane cytoskeleton that remain poorly understood. PKC is involved in the metastatic characteristics of melanoma cells. Among PKC isoforms, the $\alpha$ isoform is postulated to increase motility of melanoma cells (Oka & Kikkawa, 2005). Reduced PKC$\beta$ and increased PKC$\zeta$ and PKC$\iota$ expression, at both protein and mRNA levels in melanoma cell lines, was found (Voris et al., 2010). As a molecular mechanism for enhancement of invasion, PKC was proposed to mediate the signal of 12-(S)-hydroxyeicosatetraenoic acid (HETE), a 12-lipoxygenase metabolite of arachidonic acid, that upregulates expression of integrin molecules. In metastatic melanoma cells, misregulated expression of PKC$\alpha$ and PKC$\delta$, and elevated Src activity are required for efficient $\alpha v\beta 3$-mediated invasion.

Activation of signal transduction through the PKC/MEK/ERK during melanoma cell line B16BL6 cell invasion and metastasis has been reported (Tsubaki et al., 2007). In this context, results of Sandoval et al. (2001) suggest a critical role for $Ca^{2+}$ signaling and activation of PKC$\alpha$ in mediating the disruption of VE-cadherin junctions, and thereby in the mechanism of increased endothelial permeability (Fig. 1).

In integrin-ECM interactions, downstream signaling events include Ras, phosphatidylinositol-3 kinase (PI3K), MAP kinases, FAK, Src, Akt, Abl and Rac, Rho and cdc42 small GTPases. Signaling pathway via $\alpha 5\beta 1$ and $\alpha v\beta 3$ integrins may be mediated by cross-talk with receptor tyrosine kinases associated with growth factor ligands (Soung et al., 2010). Overexpression of the small GTPase, RhoC, in various human cancers has been correlated with high metastatic ability and poor prognosis. Rho-kinase (ROCK) is an important effector of Rho GTPases. The oncogenic serine/threonine kinase Akt is a downstream effector of PI3K. Akt activation contributes to the neoplastic phenotype by promoting cell cycle progression, increasing antiapoptotic functions, and enhancing tumor cell invasion. Using a human melanoma cell line WM35, results suggest that RhoC promotes invasion in part via activation of the PI3K/Akt pathway, in a manner independent of ROCK signaling (Ruth et al., 2006). In addition, PKC$\alpha$ and Src enhance $\alpha v\beta 3$-mediated invasion in part by increasing the GTPase activity of Rac relative to RhoA. PKC$\alpha$ influences focal adhesion formation, while PKC$\delta$ controls stress fibers (Putman et al., 2009). PKC interacts with Rho GTPases in the regulation of the actin cytoskeleton. The PKC-$\alpha$ isozyme binds the Rho GTPase cdc42, and both are coordinated with the Rac-PI3K signaling pathway in melanoma cell invasion and migration on extracellular matrix proteins (Byers et al., 2010).

Transendothelial migration (TEM) is blocked by pharmacological inhibitors of Src family protein-tyrosine kinases (PP2 and herbimycin A), PI3K (wortmannin), and phosphatidylinositol-specific phospholipase C (U73122). These data indicate that there are signaling pathways for TEM independent of chemokine attraction, but through adhesion molecules including CD44 (Katakai et al., 2002). Integrins regulate cell adhesion process partially through control of extracellular signal-regulated kinases 1 and 2 (ERK1/2). In mutant B-Raf-expressing melanoma cells (SKMEL-24 and SKMEL-28), the ERK1/2 pathway was constitutively active, and ECM adhesion-dependent regulation of ERK1/2 activity was by-passed. Furthermore, in melanoma cells, ERK1/2 translocates to the nucleus and regulated transcription events in an adhesion-independent manner (Conner et al., 2003). On the other hand, PI3 kinase/Akt pathway is downstream of the major vascular endothelial growth factor (VEGF) receptors in endothelial cells, and it is activated in EC migration process in response to tumor efferent stimulation (Anfuso et al., 2009; Brader & Eccles, 2004) (Fig. 1).

Contact of melanoma cells to HUVEC triggered rapid endothelial $[Ca^{2+}]_i$ response through PLC-IP3 pathway. In addition, alternation of endothelial adherens junctions following contact of melanoma cells was evidenced by changes in immunological staining patterns of vascular endothelial (VE)-cadherin. Inhibition of PI3K resulted in a reduction of melanoma cell transmigration (Peng et al., 2005).

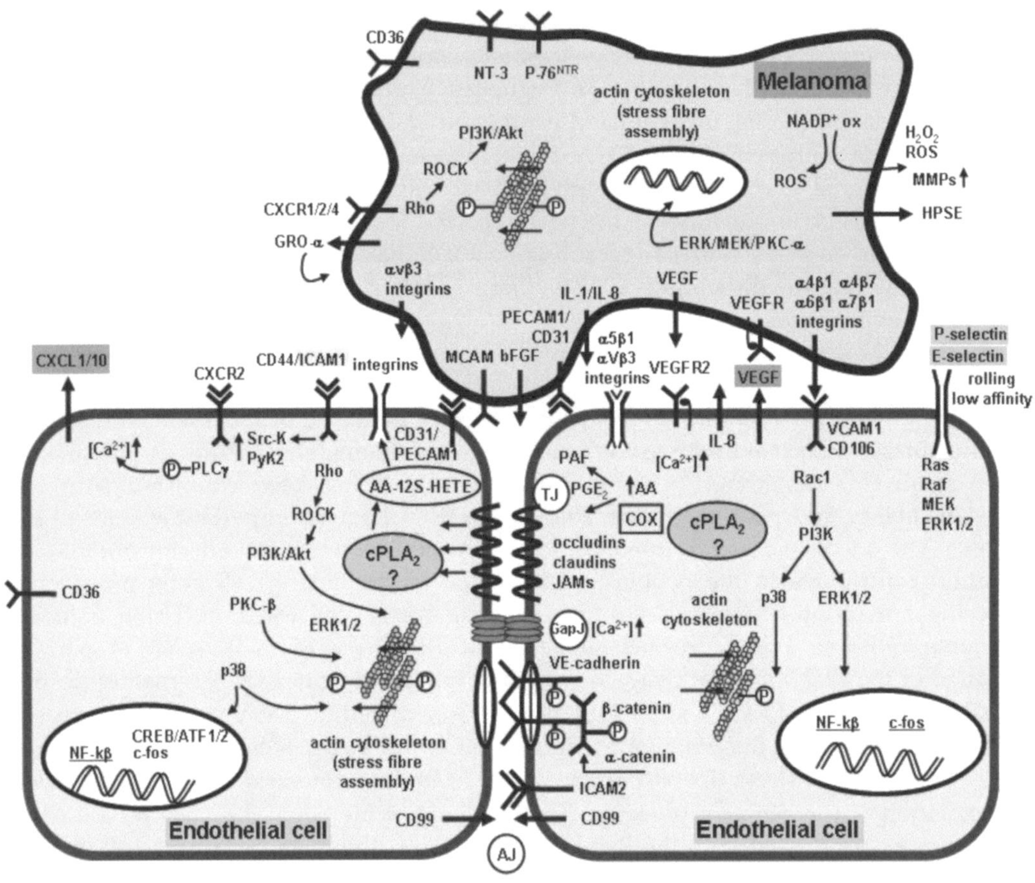


Fig. 1. Cell surface interactions and cellular responses between melanoma cells and endothelial cells (ECs), and ECs–ECs in blood vessels. During dissemination of malignant cells, the attachment of cancer cells to the ECs on microvasculature is considered to be an essential step. A spectrum of growth factors/chemokines is able to induce intracellular signaling responses in both ECs and melanoma cells which reciprocally secrete similar autocrine and paracrine growth factors and chemokines. Signaling responses include functional cross-talk between growth factor/growth factor receptors and integrins, and actin/myosin cytoskeleton reorganization. ECs exploit cytoskeletal elements to ensure the integrity of the cell monolayer in quiescent endothelium, and to enable the disintegration of the former barrier in response to various agonists. Functional association between VEGFR2 and integrin αvβ3 is of reciprocal nature since each receptor is able to promote activation of its counterpart. Potential tumor cell response includes enhanced cell proliferation, proteolytic activity, migration and invasion. Potential EC response contributes with tumor neovascularization and loosing of permeability properties of the microvascular barrier at the tight and gap junctions, and adherens junctions (cadherins)

### 2.3 Cadherins and selectins

E-cadherin is a protein with extracellular, transmembrane and cytoplasmic domains. The surface glycoprotein of E-cadherin acts to connect neighboring cells whereas the cytoplasmic tail is noncovalently linked to the actin cytoskeleton via catenins. E-cadherin not only acts as molecular glue, but also mediates intracellular signaling through β-catenin. Growth factor signaling pathways are important in regulating the cadherin-catenin complex through phosphorylation and dephosphorylation of β-catenin. Melanoma cells induce vascular VE-cadherin junction disassembly through heterotypic contact with human umbilical vein ECs (HUVEC) in co-culture. Melanoma-induced VE-cadherin disassembly and upregulation of p38 MAP kinase in ECs are regulated by both soluble factors from melanomas, particularly interleukin IL-8, IL-6, and IL-1β, VEGF, sVEGFR-1, bFGF, and through vascular cell adhesion molecule-1 (Khanna et al., 2010; Ruffini et al., 2011).

During cell-cell adhesion process, attachment of melanoma cells on the endothelium induces a twofold increase in transmembrane N-cadherin expression in melanoma cells and the redistribution of N-cadherin to the heterotypic contacts. Whereas N-cadherin and β-catenin colocalize in the contact regions between melanoma cells and HMVEC during the initial stages of attachment, β-catenin disappears from the heterotypic contacts during transmigration of melanoma cells. Immunolocalization and immunoprecipitation studies indicate that N-cadherin becomes tyrosine-phosphorylated, resulting in the dissociation of β-catenin from these contact regions. Concomitantly, an increase in the nuclear level of β-catenin occurs in melanoma cells, together with a sixfold increase in β-catenin-dependent transcription (Qi et al., 2005).

E-selectin and P-selectin, expressed on the EC surface, are considered to play also an important role in hematogenous metastasis, and are a marker for proliferating endothelium (Ludwig et al., 2004). E-selectin and P-selectin are barely expressed in unstimulated endothelial cells. Whereas E-selectin is not expressed in ECs in vivo, unless cells are stimulated by an inflammatory cytokine such as IL1β or tumor necrosis factor α, E-selectin is expressed in response to cytokines secreted by tumor cells in cancer patients (Kannagi et al., 1997). The adhesion of cancer cells to E-selectin expressed by ECs regulates the barrier function of these cells. An increase in the activity of endothelial ERK and p38 mitogen-activated protein kinases, with concomitant enhancement of TEM and migration of cancer cells has been observed (Tremblay et al., 2006).

On the other hand, activation of ERK by E-selectin modulates the opening of interendothelial spaces by initiating the activation of Src kinase activities and the dissociation of the VE-cadherin/β-catenin complex.

The adhesion of cancer cells to E-selectin expressed by ECs regulates the barrier function of these cells. An increase in the activity of endothelial ERK and p38 mitogen-activated protein kinases, with concomitant enhancement of TEM and migration of cancer cells, has been observed (Tremblay et al., 2006). On the other hand, the activation of ERK by E-selectin modulates the opening of interendothelial spaces by initiating the activation of Src kinase activities and the dissociation of the VE-cadherin/β-catenin complex.

Melanoma cellular adhesion molecule (MCAM), also known as MUC18, is a membrane glycoprotein that functions as a $Ca^{2+}$-independent adhesion molecule, and mediates homotypic and heterotypic adhesion between melanoma cells and ECs, respectively (McGary et al., 2002). Up-regulation of receptors and signaling molecules not found on melanocytes, but important for melanoma-melanoma and melanoma-EC interactions such as MCAM, N-cadherin and zonula occludens protein-1 (ZO-1), is operative in this context (Haass et al., 2005). In addition, transcription factors CREB/ATF-1 and ATF-2 are up-regulated in these cells. The expression of genes involved in angiogenesis, invasion and apoptosis such as bFGF, IL-8, EGF-R, PAR-1 correlates with higher metastatic potential of human melanoma cells (Melnikova et al., 2009) (Fig. 1).

### 2.4 Chemokines

Migration of melanoma cells into tissues occurs via a complex and sequential interaction between melanoma and ECs. If melanoma cells and the endothelium express pairs of tethering molecules such as L-, P-, and E-selectins and their sialylated carbohydrate ligands, melanoma cells flowing through the blood stream become tethered to a vessel wall and can roll along the endothelium. Subsequently, integrin activation and cell arrest in the endothelium are induced by chemokines, soluble or matrix-bound chemotactic factors produced by the surrounding tissue or ECs, and presented on the luminal surface of the vessel wall. EC-secreted chemoattractants can induce, in fact, melanoma cell chemotaxis.

A large number of chemokines have been discovered in recent decades. CXC chemokines are heparin-binding proteins that display unique disparate roles in the regulation of angiogenesis. Members (CXCL1-8) that contain the ERL motif bind to CXC chemokine receptor 2 (CXCR2) on endothelium and are angiogenic (Vandercappellen et al., 2008). For example, a serial mechanism for the maintenance of angiogenic microenvironment encompasses VEGF activation on ECs which can lead to upregulation of antiapoptotic molecule, Bcl-2, that in turn promotes the expression of EC-derived CXCL8; the upregulated expression of CXCL8 functions in an autocrine and paracrine manner to maintain the angiogenic EC phenotype. The growth-related oncogene (GRO) subgroup of chemokines (CXCL1/GROα, CXCL2/GROβ, CXCL3/GROγ) was originally identified from culture supernatant of melanoma cell lines (Richmond & Thomas, 1988), and acts as autocrine growth factor for the melanoma and other tumors (Fig. 1).

Some chemokines such as IL-8, RANTES (CCL5), MIP-1β (CCL4), and IP-10 (CXCL10) selectively attract melanoma cells. Chemotactic response to IL-8 is mediated by CXC-chemokine receptor CXCR1 (Ramjeesingh et al., 2003). CXCL1,2,3 are important mediators of tumorigenesis related to melanoma. CXCR1 or CXCR2 are stably overexpressed in human melanoma cell lines, and CXCR1- or CXCR2-induced modulation of the melanoma cell proliferation and migration was observed to be mediated through stimulated ERK1/2 phosphorylation (Singh et al., 2009) and PKA, PI3K/Akt, PKC, Ras/Raf/MEK/JNK/p38/ERK2 enhanced activities (Strieter et al., 2006). On the other hand, tumor ECs secrete high levels of CXCL9 in all, and CXCL10 in most melanoma metastases (Amatschek et al., 2011). In this context, tumor-derived chemokines further determine influx of ECs into the tumor. In HUVEC, GRO-α markedly increases metalloproteinase MMP-1 and -2, VEGF, angiopoietin-2, CD31, and receptor KDR and CXCr2 (Caunt et al., 2006).

Chemokines deliver downstream signals via heterotrimeric G-protein-coupled receptors, and not only increase the affinity of integrins for their ligands, but also stimulate cell motility. CXCL12/CXCR4 is the most commonly expressed chemokine/chemokine receptor pair in human cancers, in which it regulates cell adhesion, extravasation, metastatic colonization, angiogenesis, and proliferation. All of these processes require activation of signaling pathways that include G proteins, PI3K, JAK kinases, Rho GTPases, and focal adhesion-associated proteins.

In a human melanoma cell line, PI3Kγ regulates tumor cell adhesion in response to CXCL12 stimulation, through mechanisms different from those involved in cell invasion. Data indicate that, following CXCR4 activation after CXCL12 binding, the invasion and adhesion processes are regulated differently by distinct downstream events in these signaling cascades (Monterrubio et al., 2009).

## 3. Extracellular matrix degradative enzymes (heparanase, metalloproteinases) and oxidative stress

Heparan sulfate proteoglycans (HSPGs) are ubiquitous molecules present as cell surface components anchored in the plasma membrane, as ingredients of the insoluble ECM or as soluble molecules present in ECM and serum (Lander & Selleck, 2000). Cell surface HSPGs play a role in the cell signaling integration and influence biological processes by interacting with a large number of physiologically macromolecules (e.g., growth factors, chemokines) that regulate cell behavior in normal and pathological processes (Iozzo & San Antonio, 2001).

It has become increasingly clear that heparan sulfates (HSs) and HSPGs play important roles in regulating disease processes including tumor progression and invasion (Sasisekharan et al., 2002). Metastatic melanomas show aberrant modulation of several key HS biosynthetic enzymes such as 3-O-sulfotransferase and 6-O-sulfotransferase, and also catabolic enzymes such as HSulf-1, HSulf-2 and heparanase (HPSE), the mammalian endoglucuronidase whose promotion activity of aggressive tumor behavior has been widely implicated in cancer metastasis (Arvatz et al., 2011). In ECs, heparanase colocalizes with lysosomes predominately around the nucleus, and angiogenic factors cause its dispersion towards the plasma membrane for subsequent secretion. Extracellular heparanase, secreted by melanoma and ECs, is able to cleaving heparan sulfate side chains of HSPGs including syndecans, thus contributing to degradation of ECM and basement membrane underlying epithelial and ECs, and cell invasion. The enzyme produces HS fragments which are biologically active, for example, able to bind growth and angiogenic factors. On the other hand, heparanase contributes to melanoma metastasis and angiogenesis by generating bioactive HS from the cell-surface (Raman & Kuberan, 2010; Roy & Marchetti, 2009). Inhibition of HPSE-1 expression inhibits tumor cell invasion by metastatic melanoma cells (Roy et al., 2005).

HS sequence and length are regulators of fibroblast growth factor-2 (FGF-2) activity, an important mediator of melanoma angiogenesis and progression (Herlyn, 2005). HPSE is able to both enhance and inhibit FGF-2 binding and activity in an HPSE concentration-dependent manner. Cell exposure to HPSE or to HPSE-degraded HS modulates FGF-2-induced angiogenesis in melanoma (Reiland et al., 2006). In addition, heparin and HS have profound effects on $VEGF_{165}$ function (Robinson & Stringer, 2001). Two heparin-binding sites of the $VEGF_{165}$ dimer interact simultaneously with highly sulfated S-domain regions of the HS chain linked through a stretch of transition sequence (Robinson et al., 2006).

Treatment with exogenous heparanase downregulated brain metastatic melanoma (BMM) cell invasion. Extracellular HPSE modulates BMM cell signaling by involving syndecans (SDCs)1/4 carboxy terminal-associated proteins and downstream targets. Small GTPase guanine nucleotide exchange factor-H1 (GEF-H1) is a new component of a SDC signaling complex that is differentially expressed in BMM cells compared to corresponding nonmetastatic counterparts. Knockdown of GEF-H1, SDC1, or SDC4 decreased BMM cell invasiveness and GEF-H1 modulated small GTPase activity of Rac1 and RhoA in conjunction with heparanase treatment (Ridgway et al., 2010).

Notably, although heparanase inhibitors attenuated tumor progression and metastasis, other studies revealed that heparanase also functions in an enzymatic activity-independent manner. Thus, inactive heparanase was noted to improve adhesion and migration of primary ECs and to promote phosphorylation of signaling molecules such as Akt and Src, facilitating gene transcription (i.e. VEGF) and phosphorylation of selected Src substrates (i.e. VEGF receptors). The concept of enzymatic activity-independent function of HPSE had gained substantial support by the recent identification of the HPSE C-terminus domain as the molecular determinant behind its signaling capacity (Barash et al., 2010).

Among enzymatic-independent functions are the induction of Akt/PKB phosphorylation noted in endothelial- and tumor-derived cells, stimulation of PI3K- and p38-dependent EC migration, and upregulation of VEGF, all responses contributing to its potent pro-angiogenic activity. Protein domains of heparanase required for signaling are not identified to date, nor are identified heparanase binding proteins/receptors capable of transmitting heparanase signals. The possible function of mannose 6-phosphate receptor (MPR) and low-density lipoprotein-receptor related protein (LRP), recently implicated in cellular uptake of heparanase, as heparanase receptors mediating Akt phosphorylation, has been examined. HPSE addition to MPR- and LRP-deficient fibroblasts elicited Akt activation indistinguishable from control fibroblasts. In contrast, disruption of lipid rafts abrogated Akt/PKB phosphorylation following HPSE addition. These results suggest that lipid raft-resident receptor mediates heparanase signaling (Ben-Zaken et al., 2007).

Cancer metastasis is accompanied by orchestrated proteolytic activity executed by array of proteases such as matrix metalloproteases (MMP). The repertoire of the cellular molecules expressed on the cell surface (E-cadherin silencing, N-cadherin and VCAM-1, ICAM-1 overexpression, melanotransferrin and integrin $\alpha v\beta 3$ upregulation, CD9 tetraspanin redistribution) may promote invasion and metastasis through an interaction with increased MMP-2 (Fig. 1). This MMP plays a role in assisting melanoma cells to degrade type IV collagen in the basement membrane, an early step in metastasis cascade that promotes tumor cell disassociation and invasion. One of the mechanism by which integrins modulate tumor progression is the transduction of signals regulating expression of matrix-specific MMP (Munshi & Stack, 2006). $\alpha 5\beta 1$ integrin, a fibronectin-binding specific integrin, interacts with MMP-2 collagenase on the surface of SKMEL-147 human melanoma cells, suggesting that it controls cell invasion via regulation of MMP-2 collagenase expression. This control can occur either through signaling pathways involving PI3K, Akt, ERK protein kinases and the c-Jun, or via direct recruitment of MMP-2 to the cell surface (Morozevich et al., 2009).

While the importance of specific degradative proteases such as MMPs is well documented, there is some evidence that reactive oxygen species (ROS) are also involved in tumor-cell-endothelial interactions. Recent observations have demonstrated that neoplastic cells, in particular melanomas, produce increased levels of ROS and pyrrolic end products of lipid oxidation, and thus themselves have the capability to damage ECs (Sander et al., 2003; West et al., 2010; Wittgen & van Kempen, 2007).

## 4. Pericytes

In tumor vascular bed, proliferating ECs and pericytes are detected, but angiogenesis is present with characteristic and significant differences among the malignant tumor types. Particularly significant are the varying degrees of pericyte recruitment indicating differences in the functional status of the tumor vasculature. In addition, they show multiple abnormalities, i.e. loose association with ECs, extended cytoplasmic processes deep into the tumor tissue and altered expression of marker proteins (NG2, 3G5), vessel leakiness (Morikawa et al., 2002). The regulatory role of pericytes in angiogenesis is very poorly appreciated at molecular level, despite the fact that tumor metastasis invasion and intratumoral vessel growth need the perturbation of pericyte-EC cell-cell interactions and promotion of pericyte invasion during neovascularization by ECM degradation. Paracrine PDGF production by B16 mouse melanoma stimulates pericyte recruitment to tumor vessels, suggesting that pericyte abundance influences tumor cell apoptosis and tumor growth (Furuhashi et al., 2004).

## 5. Factors released by melanoma cells (VEGF, bFGF, PDGFα/β-TGF, IL-1, IL-8)

To promote angiogenesis, tumors secrete a variety of growth factors such as VEGF, bFGF, platelet-derived growth factor (PDGF) that induce EC activation in nearby vessels. VEGF is a major inducer of angiogenesis in tumors. In human melanoma cell lines, VEGF and bFGF expression, heterogeneous in levels, was observed (Danielsen & Rofstad, 1998). Melanoma and colorectal carcinoma cells express functional EGF/TGF- α receptors, and produce TGF-α, indicating that this growth factor is synthesized for autocrine stimulation. By screening a panel of 8 primary and 21 metastatic melanoma cell lines for constitutive secretion of cytokines, it was found that melanomas expressed bioactivity for transforming growth factor (TGF- β) (8/25 lines) and IFN (7/12), but not IL-2. Immunoassays detected interleukin IL-1α (4/25), IL-1β (12/25), IL-6 (13/29), IL-8 (29/29), TGF-β2 (5/12) and GM-CSF (11/29), but not IL-3, IL-4, TNF-α, or IFN-γ. IL-8 was produced by all lines tested. The data demonstrated that cultured melanoma cells produce a variety of cytokines which are potentially capable of influencing tumor growth in vivo (Bennicelli & Guerry, 1993). In tissue culture of choroidal melanomas and two established skin melanoma cell lines, high secretion of IL-6 was detectable in choroidal melanoma cultures, but not in the cell lines. IL-8 secretion was found in all melanoma cultures (Fig. 1). However, IL-10 was only secreted by one skin melanoma cell line and in choroidal melanoma cell cultures. Secretion of bFGF by choroidal melanomas was higher than by other cell lines. No differences were seen in the amount of TGF-β1 produced by melanoma cells (Enzmann et al., 1998). Secretion of interleukin-1 receptor antagonist (sIL-1ra), IL-6, IL-8, IL-10, TGF-α, TGF-β, VEGF, PDGF, bFGF, angiopoietin-1 and angiopoietin-2 was found in seven human uveal melanoma cell lines (Ijland et al., 1999).

In a study of a large number of uveal tumors, it was observed that while most tumor cells expressed bFGF at the protein level (89%), relatively few (22%) expressed VEGF. All 20 tumors tested by RT-PCR contained mRNA for both bFGF and VEGF. Co-culture experiments using an ATP based bioassay showed that uveal melanomas could support the growth of a rat brain endothelial cell line and HUVEC (Boyd et al., 2001). VEGF receptors VEGFR1, VEGFR2 and neurophilin-1 are expressed in A375 melanoma cells. Overproduction of $VEGF_{165}$ concomitantly expressed with its receptors favors cell growth and survival of melanoma cells through MAPK and PI3K signaling pathways (Graells et al., 2004).

PDGF receptor signaling participates in the stimulation of tumor angiogenesis. PDGF-BB is produced by ECs, and PDGFR-β is expressed by mural cells, including pericytes. PDGF-BB is produced by most types of solid tumors, and PDGF receptor signaling participates in various processes, including autocrine stimulation of tumor cell growth and recruitment of

tumor stroma fibroblasts. Furthermore, PDGF-BB-producing tumors are characterized by increased pericyte abundance and accelerated tumor growth (Suzuki et al., 2007).
By using an antibody-based proteomics strategy, galectin-1, a protein member of the group of lectins that bind to β-galactosides, was identified as protein with enhanced expression in cells from the melanocytic lineage and cancer tissues, and as a proangiogenic factor (Bolander et al., 2008). Indeed, in invasive B16 melanoma supernanants, proteomic analysis allowed the identification of 18 differential proteins, among which the proteins with a higher concentration, lactate dehydrogenase B, M2 pyruvate kinase, cathepsin D, and galectin-1 (Rondepierre et al., 2010). Uptake of galectin-1 by cultured endothelial cells specifically promotes H-Ras signaling to the Raf/MAP kinase/Mek/ERK cascade and stimulates EC proliferation and migration (Thijssen et al., 2010).

## 6. Cell co-culture models

The cross-talk between melanoma and ECs has been assessed in in vitro co-culture models in which signal transduction mechanisms can be closely studied. ECs are able to communicate with tumor cells through gap junctions, allowing cytosolic exchange of peptides and other small molecules (Saito-Katsuragi et al., 2007). Melanoma cells seeded on confluent lymphatic endothelial cells (LECs) were able to adhere by pseudopodia, and to induce endothelial junction dissolution and retraction. The passage of the tumor cells through the opened gap and the migration under LECs suggest that tumor cells could metastasize through the lymphatic vessel by destroying intercellular junctions (Ding Z. et al., 2005).
An interesting work demonstrated that B16 melanoma cells, together with Lewis lung carcinoma cells, produce the lipoxygenase metabolite 12(S)-HETE during in vitro interaction with CD3 microvascular ECs, which in turn induce EC retraction (Honn et al., 1994). These results suggest that 12(S)-HETE synthesis during tumor cell–endothelial cell interactions may represent a key contributory factor in cancer metastasis.
The supporting role of soluble pro-angiogenic cytokines such as bFGF and VEGF in the endothelial growth and their expression by co-cultured melanomas have been well described. Rat brain and human EC lines show significant enhancement of cell growth by 48–120 h of co-culture with melanoma cells without cell–cell contact (Boyd et al., 2002). In a co-culture system based on transwell indirect model, bone-marrow-derived mesenchymal stem cells (BMSCs) acquired endothelial phenotype and expressed VEGFR-1, VEGFR-2 and factor VIII after co-culture with B16 cells (Sun et al., 2008).
Treatments with angiogenesis inhibitors markedly suppressed in vitro tube formation by human endothelial cells and HUVEC, whereas tubular network formation by human melanoma MUM-2B and C8161 cells was relatively unaffected. The differential response of the two cell types was probably due to higher mRNA and protein endothelial expression for α5 integrin and heparin sulfate proteoglycan 2 than melanoma cells (van der Schaft et al., 2004). On the other hand, analyses of malignant melanomas in co-culture with microvascular ECs revealed a strong expression of bone morphogenic proteins and their capability to induce tube formation and migratory efficiency (Rothhammer et al., 2007).
A critical role in the regulation of melanoma-endothelial intercellular communication is interpreted by neuropilin-2 (NRP2), a co-receptor for VEGF and the semaphorin (SEMA) families. Overexpression of NRP2 in primary human ECs promoted cell survival induced by VEGF-A and VEGF-C. In contrast, SEMA3F, another ligand for NRP2, was able to inhibit

human EC survival and migration induced by VEGF-A and VEGF-C (Favier et al., 2006). In melanoma cells, NRP2 is upregulated in a two-dimensional co-culture systems of melanoma and ECs, suggesting that NRP2 assists melanoma cells in EC recruitment towards the development of a functional new vasculature, thus enhancing melanoma survival and providing potential routes for metastasis (Stine et al., 2011).

Studies using two-dimensional melanoma-EC cultures have greatly advanced our knowledge of angiogenesis, and will continue to be used extensively. Furthermore, results generated in two-dimensional cultures can be furthered by the use of three-dimensional model systems that mimic the natural tumor environment and may result in the development of treatments with better therapeutic outcomes. Collagen-implanted melanoma spheroid consists of cell aggregates grown in a collagen matrix. Melanoma spheres mimic an in vivo tumor with cells having differing access to oxygen and nutrients depending on position in the spheroid. Similar to a tumor in vivo, the proliferating cells are found on the outside of the spheroid, while the innermost cells have downregulated ERK and cyclin-dependent kinase activity (Haass et al., 2008).

In a 3-D co-culture system, human ECs and GFP-expressing melanoma cells formed distinct tumor clusters with integrated endothelial networks when seeded on tumor-derived extracellular matrix. In contrast, an entirely different phenotype was exhibited when the tumor matrix was replaced with collagen, suggesting that the extracellular matrix impinges on cellular function, possibly by an Akt-mediated mechanism (Sengupta et al., 2004). Furthermore, in melanoma cell lines co-cultured with vascular ECs in three dimensional spheroids, VEGF-induced angiogenesis was inhibited after treatment with resveratrol. This effect was associated with increased melanoma cell expression of p53 and matrix protein TSP1, as well as decreased hypoxia-driven expression of hypoxia inducible factor-1$\alpha$, and inhibition of VEGF production (Trapp et al., 2010).

## 7. Phospholipase $A_2$ activation

Cytosolic phospholipase $A_2$ (c$PLA_2$), which regulates the provision of arachidonic acid (AA), cyclooxygenase-2 (COX-2), and prostaglandin $E_2$ release, is highly upregulated in angiogenic ECs during tumor progression (Wendum et al., 2005), promoting integrin $\alpha v\beta 3$-mediated EC adhesion, spreading, and angiogenesis through prostaglandin cAMP-PKA dependent activation of the small GTPase Rac (Bogatcheva et al., 2005). Phospholipases $A_2$ are a diverse group of enzymes that catalyze the hydrolysis of the sn-2 substituent from glycerophospholipid substrates to yield a free fatty acid and 2-lysophospholipid acceptors (Balsinde et al., 2002). They are the rate limiting step for the AA production from membrane phospholipids, which in turn is the major precursor to prostaglandins, leukotrienes, and hydroxyeicosatetraenoic acids (via the cyclooxygenase, lipoxygenase, and epoxygenase pathways, respectively) that increase cell proliferation in response to various agonists in different cell types (Anfuso et al., 2007; Balsinde et al., 2002; Chakraborti, 2003; Lupo et al., 2002).

Among the $PLA_2$s is an 85 kDa c$PLA_2$ that requires $Ca^{2+}$ for catalysis, and a calcium independent $PLA_2$, i$PLA_2\beta$, for which several potential functions have been proposed, including a housekeeping role in phospholipid remodeling and a signaling role in cell growth, apoptosis, secretion, inflammation, and oxidant-induced cell injury (Chakraborti, 2003). A number of observations that i$PLA_2$ has a functional role in cellular signaling in addition to its roles in AA release and phospholipid remodeling have been reported (Akiba

& Sato, 2004). $iPLA_2$ mediates the phosphorylation of transcription factors through a PKA-dependent pathway (Martinson et al., 2003).

We recently demonstrated that human melanoma cells highly express $PLA_2$, COX-1/COX-2, and produce higher levels of prostaglandins than normal melanocytes; this response correlated with higher proliferation rate and was blocked by specific inhibitors of $PLA_2$ and cyclooxygenase (Scuderi et al., 2008). It was also demonstrated that in vitro ECs/ melanoma co-culture or EC cultures enriched with melanoma conditioned medium (CM) recapitulate the signals that arise from the relationship between these cell types in an intact vascularized tumor (Anfuso et al., 2009). In that study, it was performed cell culture experiments in which CMs prepared from two human melanoma lines, SKMEL-28 and OCM-1, were incubated with quiescent GP8.3 rat brain immortalized ECs, in order to study the CM effect on EC proliferation and migration and on the expression of phospholipases, and activation of the ERK1/2 and PI3K/AKT pathways. Melanoma CMs significant increased endothelial AA release versus control unstimulated cells. This result indirectly demonstrated that melanoma CM-stimulated AA release in ECs was mediated by activation of phospholipase $A_2$ enzymes. The use of the specific $iPLA_2$ inhibitor, bromoenol lactone, allowed to discriminate between the c- and $iPLA_2$ activity contribution. A major contribution of $cPLA_2$ enzyme activity in mediating AA release of melanoma CM-stimulated ECs was found.

Additional findings suggested that the mitogen-activated protein kinase ERK1/2 and PI3K are involved in the signaling pathways that mainly activate $cPLA_2$. Furthermore, it was observed, by confocal microscopy, activation of $cPLA_2$ in perinuclear and membrane regions of ECs grown in CM-stimulated cultures, suggesting that $cPLA_2$ and its downstream products, after long-lasting stimulation of ECs by melanoma CMs, play significant roles in nuclear functions such as regulation of gene expression and cell proliferation.

In order to clarify the roles of $cPLA_2$ and $iPLA_2$ in ECs stimulated by melanoma in in vitro models (Fig. 2), recently we were able to demonstrate that the non-contact presence of melanoma cells in EC co-cultures, in the absence (double co-cultures) or presence (triple co-cultures) of microvascular pericytes, increased $cPLA_2$ and $iPLA_2$ protein expression (Fig. 3). In cultured ECs, 48 hour exposure to melanoma cells significantly increased $cPLA_2$ expression, with a 2.7-fold ($p<0.01$) and 1.6-fold ($p<0.01$) increase in $iPLA_2$ total protein, respectively (Fig. 3 A,B). Furthermore, melanoma-stimulated GP8.3 ECs showed an increase in the constitutive phosphorylated form of $cPLA_2$ by 8.3-fold ($p<0.01$) compared to unstimulated control cells. Thus, the increase of $cPLA_2$ synthesis and phosphorylation (p-$cPLA_2$/$cPLA_2$ ratio from 0.20 to 1.66 for melanoma-stimulated ECs) may support an increase in $cPLA_2$ activity.

Since endothelial PKC$\alpha$ might be involved in stimulated endothelial $cPLA_2$ activity and p42/p44 MAPK phosphorylation by melanoma cells via the Raf-MEK pathway, we further evaluated the PKC$\alpha$ and ERK1/2 protein expression and activation. Tumor cells had no significant effect on total PKC$\alpha$ expression compared with unstimulated control ECs (Fig. 3C); however, the presence of melanoma did induce a 2.1-fold ($p<0.01$) increase in phosphorylated PKC$\alpha$ form expression in ECs, with basal phosphorylation levels around 70% in unstimulated ECs. In addition, as shown in Fig. 3D, the presence of melanoma cells in EC co-cultures did not induce changes or increases in endothelial total p42/p44 MAPK (ERK1/2, double band) protein expression. On the contrary, melanoma-stimulated GP8.3 cells showed an increase in phosphorylated form of ERK1/2 by 3.1-fold (p42, $p<0.01$), compared to control unstimulated ECs grown alone. These data indicate that in ECs the ERK kinase phosphorylation and $PLA_2$ activation are coincident. These results suggest that

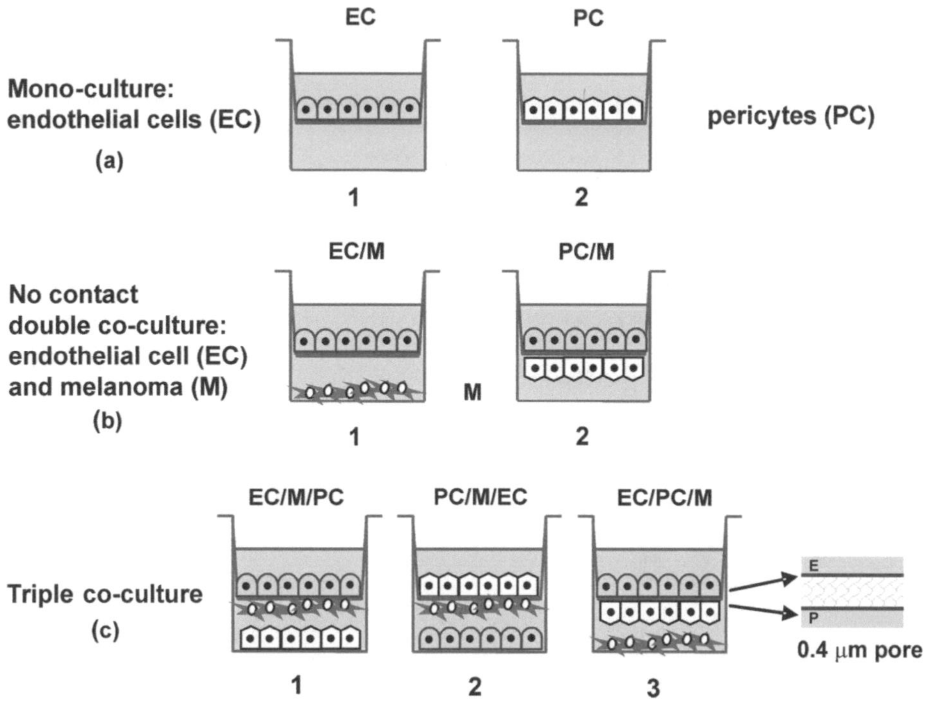


Fig. 2. Scheme of different Transwell systems for co-cultures of endothelial cells (ECs) and melanoma derived cells in monolayers. Immortalized rat brain endothelial cells (GP8.3) were fed with F10 HAM's medium supplemented with 10% FBS, 80 μg/ml heparin, 2 mM glutamine and antibiotics. Cultures of pericytes isolated from microvessels were prepared from bovine retinas as described previously (Lupo et al., 2001). The isolated cells were then cultured in DMEM supplemented with 2 mM glutamine, 10% FBS and antibiotics. COLO38 is a malignant melanoma cell line which expresses the MPG antigen and was grown in RPMI medium containing 2 mM glutamine, 10% FBS and antibiotics. Culture plates and inserts were coated on the upper and the bottom side with collagen. (a) EC or pericyte monolayers (1 and 2). (b) Melanoma cells are placed on the bottom of the wells, while ECs are present in the semipermeable filter insert (1). Pericytes are seeded on the lower side of the membrane insert, while ECs are present in the apical side of the filter insert (2). (c) Melanoma cells are seeded on the lower side of the membrane filter (1 and 2), and then ECs (1) or pericytes (2) are seeded in the upper compartment. In the third system, pericytes are seeded on the lower side of the filter, and then ECs are seeded in the upper compartment (3). In all systems, cells on both sides are exposed to conditioned medium from the cell type growing on the bottom of the wells. In panels (b)-2 and (c)-3, pericytes were first plated on the outside of the membrane filter (80,000 cells). 4 hour after, the inserts were placed into six-well plates with the culture medium. ECs were plated on the top surface of the same inserts (80,000 cells) on which pericytes have been plated two days before. Three days after, the inserts were placed into wells where COLO 38 melanoma cells have been already cultured for at least 2 days. As controls, ECs were also cultured with either COLO38 cells or pericytes alone (double co-culture) and without any other cell type. All control- and three cell type-cultures [panel (a)-1, panel (b)-1,2, panel (c)-3] were fed for 24 h in a serum-free DMEM-F10-HAM's (1:1) plus glutamine medium

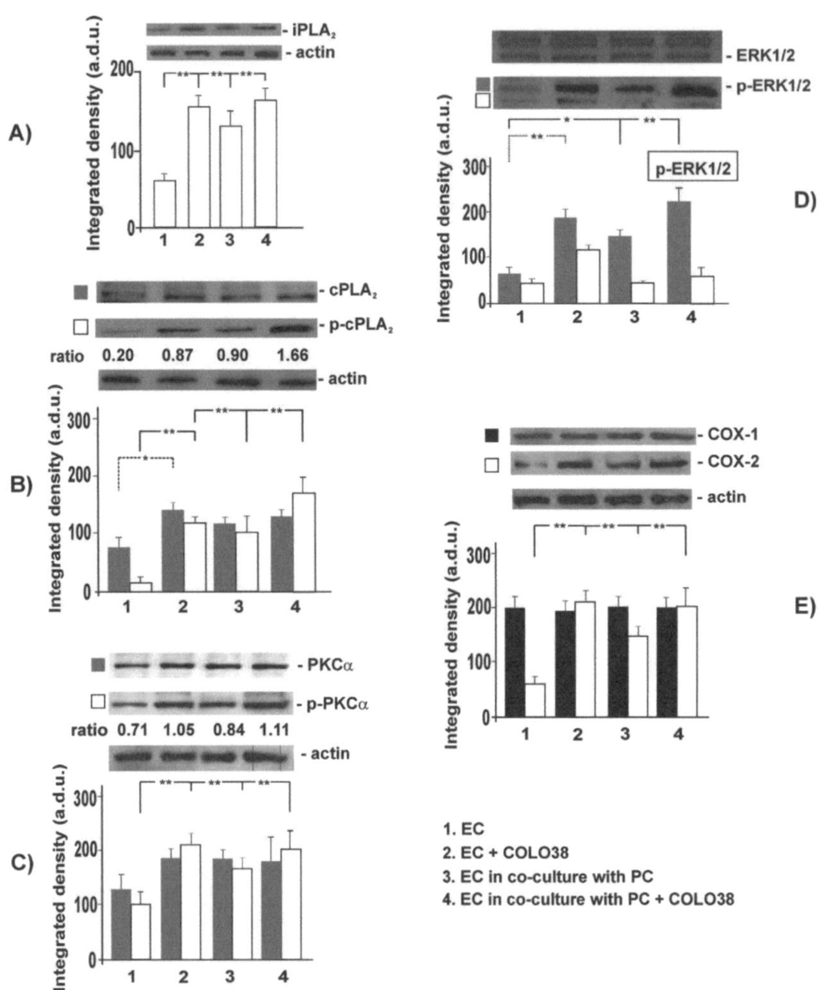


Fig. 3. Western blot analyses of $cPLA_2$, calcium-independent intracellular phospholipase $A_2$ ($iPLA_2$), total extracellular signal-regulated kinases (ERK1/2), PKCα, COX-1/-2 and phosphorylated forms of ERK1/2, $cPLA_2$ and PKCα protein expression in GP8.39 EC/bovine retinal pericyte (PC) co-cultures in the presence of COLO38 melanoma cells (triple co-culture). In the in vitro model of control blood brain barrier or tumor-conditioned blood brain barrier (see Fig. 2, panel b-2, c-3), 48 hours after incubation ECs were scraped from the insert with a rubber policeman, and lysates were resolved by SDS/PAGE (Lupo et al., 2005). Expressed proteins were independently revealed with $cPLA_2$, p-$cPLA_2$, PKCα, COX-2 or p-ERK monoclonal antibodies, and $iPLA_2$, p-PKCα, COX-1 or ERK1/2 polyclonal antibodies. The ratios of the band intensities, phospho-$cPLA_2$/total $cPLA_2$ and phospho-PKCα/total PKCα, are indicated. The values (bar graphs) expressed as arbitrary densitometric unit (a.d.u.), were obtained by the reading of blots using the Image J program, and are means ± S.E.M. from three independent experiments. Representative gels are shown; statistically significant differences by pairwise Student's *t*-test are indicated by asterisks (*$p<0.05$, **$p<0.01$), comparing EC/PC cultures in presence of COLO38 with EC monoculture or EC/PC co-cultures

ERK1/2 pathway is involved in enhanced AA liberation and GP8.3 EC proliferation (sequential activation of ERK1/2 and $cPLA_2$) induced by melanoma cell presence in the culture medium.

Because COX-1 and COX-2 govern the rate limiting step in the conversion of AA to its downstream prostanoid effectors, we also evaluated COX-1 and COX-2 expression in ECs in response to the presence of COLO38 cells in co-cultures. Melanoma-stimulated ECs, for 48 h, significantly expressed COX-2 total protein at levels higher (3.3-fold; $p<0.01$) than control unstimulated EC cultures (no additions) (Fig. 3E). Melanoma cells did not induce any change in COX-1 protein expression. These results indicate substantial contribution of COX-2 activity, chiefly stimulated by growth factors such as VEGF, to endothelial prostanoid synthesis, cell proliferation and motility in melanoma-conditioned ECs.

## 8. COX-2 and 12-lipoxygenase expression

COX-1 and COX-2 mediate the rate limiting step in arachidonic acid metabolism. Both in vitro and in vivo studies indicate that either COX-2 or COX-1 overexpression upregulates angiogenic factors in neoplastic cells and promotes tumor angiogenesis (Tsuji et al., 2001).

COX-2 promotes integrin $\alpha v\beta 3$-mediated EC adhesion, spreading, migration and angiogenesis through the prostaglandin-cAMP-PKA dependent activation of the small GTPase Rac (Ruegg et al., 2004).

There are several lines of evidence indicating that increased expression of COX-2 plays a functional role in the development and progression of malignant epithelial cancer (Kuźbicki et al., 2006). COX-2 is expressed in the vasculature of surgically resected human tumors. In tumor endothelial cells (TECs) from human melanoma, compared to normal endothelial cells (NECs), COX-2 mRNA was upregulated. Cell migration and proliferation were suppressed by COX-2 inhibitor NS398 in TECs but not in NECs. The number of $CD133^+/VEGF\text{-}2^+$ cells in the circulation was significantly suppressed by COX-2 inhibition. In addition, the number of progenitor marker-positive cells decreased in the tumor blood vessels after COX-2 treatment, which suggests that NS398 specifically targets both TECs and vascular progenitor cells without affecting NECs (Muraki et al., 2011).

COX-2 has also recently been reported as a marker of malignant melanoma (MM) in a study on 40 archival cases of MM and 35 cases of benign melanocytic lesions. The MM group and the benign melanocytic nevi group showed a highly statistically significant difference in the intensity of COX-2 expression. Staining intensity in the dermal component of MM cases also showed a tendency to increase with increasing tumor depth. By contrast, the intensity of the dermal component in the melanocytic nevi group decreased with increasing depth as the nevus cells matured from type A to type C cells (Minami et al., 2011). Furthermore, Kaplan-Meier curves illustrated a significant correlation between staining intensity and disease-specific survival (Becker, 2009).

In melanoma cell lines, A375 and Hs294, overexpression of COX-2 and its metabolite prostaglandin $E_2$ ($PGE_2$) receptors promotes cells migration. Treatment of A375 and Hs294 cells with berberine, an isoquinoline alkaloid, resulted in concentration-dependent inhibition of migration of these cells, which was associated with a reduction in the levels of COX-2 and $PGE_2$ receptors ($EP_2$ and $EP_4$). Treatment of the cells with 12-O-tetradecanoylphorbol-13-acetate (TPA), an inducer of COX-2 or $PGE_2$, enhanced cell migration, whereas berberine inhibited TPA- or $PGE_2$ promoted cell migration (Singh et al., 2011).

Specimens from dysplastic nevi, melanoma at different stages and melanoma metastasis lymphnodes overexpressed COX-2 compared to normal melanocytes. COX-2 was consistently observed in keratinocytes, dermal fibroblasts and inflammatory cells in regions adjacent to benign nevi and primary cutaneous melanomas (Goulet et al., 2003).

Omega-3 and omega-6 PUFA regulated COX-2 mRNA expression and $PGE_2$ production in 70W, a human melanoma cell line that metastasizes to the brain in nude mice. Additionally, $PGE_2$ increased in vitro Matrigel invasion, whereas exposure to $PGE_3$ significantly decreased invasion (Denkins et al., 2005).

12-Lipoxygenase (12-LOX), through its metabolite 12-HETE, has been demonstrated to play a pivotal role in experimental melanoma invasion and metastasis. Differences in 12-LOX protein expression during the progression of melanoma from human skin melanocytes to benign and dysplastic nevi have been found. Melanomas had higher levels of expression compared with dysplastic nevi, suggesting that 12-LOX may be an important marker of cancer progression (Winer et al., 2002).

## 9. Arachidonic acid metabolites: prostaglandins, 12(S)-HETE, leukotrienes

Lipid mediators derived from the arachidonic acid/5-LOX metabolism have a fundamental stimulatory role in melanoma progression associated with inflammation, whereas ω3 PUFA–derived metabolites have opposite effects (Bachi et al., 2009). Inhibitors of $cPLA_2$, 5-LOX and COX-2 reduced pulmonary metastasis formation by B16F10 melanoma cells in a dose-dependent manner. Importantly, all these inhibitors reduced PAF-induced angiogenesis in an in vivo mouse model employing Matrigel of basement membrane injected subcutaneously, and also reduced expression of MMP-2 and MMP-9 in the lungs (Jeong et al., 2010). Studies of adhesion of a highly metastatic melanoma cell line (WM-1617) demostrated that it contains at least two types of close intercellular adhesions: classic focal adhesions, and more extensive, irregularly shaped adhesions along lamellipodial edges. These adhesions are highly dynamic and highly sensitive to PKCε activation, for example, by the 12(S)-HETE. Eicosanoid-induced cell detachment seems to be triggered by myristoylated alanine-rich C-kinase substrate (MARCKS) phosphorylation (Estrada-Bernal et al., 2009). 12(S)-HETE stimulation of human epithelial carcinoma cell (A431) migration involved ERK1/2, PKC, PI3K and Src kinase. Focal adhesion kinase, a key organizer of focal cell adhesions, was tyrosine phosphorylated in response of 12(S)-HETE treatment, phosphorylation which required Src, but not PKC, PI3K or ERK1/2 enhanced activity (Szekeres et al., 2002).

Prostaglandins (PG) and arachidonic acid metabolites affect melanocyte dendricity, melanization, and proliferation (Kashiwagi et al., 2002; Parsad et al., 2002). PGD2, leukotriene (LT) B4, LTC4, LTD4, LTE4, thromboxane B2, and 12-(S)HETE increased dendricity and tyrosinase in human epidermal melanocytes whereas $PGE_1$, $PGF_{2a}$, and 6-keto$PGF_{1a}$ had no stimulatory effects (Tomita et al., 1992). In B16F10-induced melanoma metastasis, PGD2 reduced the protective effect of α-galactosylceramide, an effect depending on IFN-γ production by invariant NK T cells (Torres et al., 2008). Nimesulide, a selective inhibitor of COX-2 that causes the breakdown of proinflammatory 2-series prostaglandins, adversely affected the growth of B16F10 melanoma cells through the induction of differentiation, indicating that the antineoplastic activity observed for nimesulide may be ascribed to intracellular changes in PG level (Tabolacci et al., 2010).

## 10. Future research

The events that follow tumor cell adhesion to the endothelium and lead to either the estrablishment of secondary tumor colonies or angiogenesis are poorly understood. The availability of cell cultures of melanoma cell lines, endothelial cells, pericytes and astrocytes, and combinations in co-cultures of three or four cell types in an in vitro multicellular systems may greatly contribute to the elucidation of the interplay mechanisms during melanoma cell adhesion and migration through endothelial cells and surrounding pericytes in blood vessels. Although these triple or quadruple systems are still lacking, it is very likely that the use of them may allow in future to discover new and unexpected alterations of the gene and protein expression patterns during proinvasive, prometastatic melanoma migration as well as endothelial recruitment mediated by intracellular signaling. These findings may contribute to the development of new antivascular therapeutic agents that target both angiogenesis and tumor cell vasculogenic mimicry.

## 11. References

Akiba, S. & Sato, T. (2004). Cellular function of calcium independent phospholipase $A_2$. *Biol. Pharm. Bull.*, 27, 1174–1178

Amatschek, S., Lucas, R., Eger, A., Pflueger, M., Hundsberger, H., Knoll, C., Grosse-Kracht, S., Schuett, W., Koszik, F., Maurer, D., & Wiesner, C. (2011). CXCL9 induces chemotaxis, chemorepulsion and endothelial barrier disruption through CXCR3-mediated activation of melanoma cells. *Br. J. Cancer*, 104, 469-79

Anfuso, C.D., Lupo, G., Romeo, L., Giurdanella, G., Motta, C., Pascale, A., Tirolo, C., Marchetti, B. & Alberghina, M. (2007). Endothelial cell-pericyte cocultures induce $PLA_2$ protein expression through activation of PKCalpha and the MAPK/ERK cascade. *J. Lipid Res.*, 48, 782-93

Anfuso, C.D., Giurdanella, G., Motta, C., Muriana, S., Lupo, G., Ragusa, N. & Alberghina, M. (2009). PKCalpha-MAPK/ERK-phospholipase $A_2$ signaling is required for human melanoma-enhanced brain endothelial cell proliferation and motility. *Microvasc. Res.*, 78, 338-57

Arvatz, G., Shafat, I., Levy-Adam, F., Ilan, N. & Vlodavsky, I. (2011). The heparanase system and tumor metastasis: is heparanase the seed and soil? *Cancer Metastasis Rev.*, 30, 253-68

Bachi, A.L., Kim, F.J., Nonogaki, S., Carneiro, C.R., Lopes, J.D., Jasiulionis, M.G. & Correa, M. (2009). Leukotriene B4 creates a favorable microenvironment for murine melanoma growth. *Mol. Cancer Res.*, 7, 1117 1121

Balsinde, J., Winstead, M.V. & Dennis., E.A. (2002). Phospholipase $A_2$ regulation of arachidonic acid mobilization. *FEBS Lett.*, 531, 2-6

Barash, U., Cohen-Kaplan, V., Dowek, I., Sanderson, R.D., Ilan, N. & Vlodavsky, I. (2010). Proteoglycans in health and disease: new concepts for heparanase function in tumor progression and metastasis. *FEBS J.*, 277, 3890-903

Becker, M. R. (2009). COX-2 expression in malignant melanoma: a novel prognostic marker? *Melanoma Res.*, 19, 8-16

Bennicelli, J.L. & Guerry, D. (1993). Production of multiple cytokines by cultured human melanomas. *Exp. Dermatol.*, 2, 186-90

Ben-Zaken, O., Gingis-Velitski, S., Vlodavsky, I. & Ilan, N. (2007). Heparanase induces Akt phosphorylation via a lipid raft receptor. *Biochem. Biophys. Res. Commun.*, 361, 829-34

Bogatcheva N.V., Sergeeva, M.G, Dudek, S.M. & Verin, A.D. (2005). Arachidonic acid cascade in endothelial pathobiology. *Microvasc. Res.*, 69, 107–127

Bolander, A., Agnarsdóttir, M., Strömberg, S., Ponten, F., Hesselius, P., Uhlen, M. & Bergqvist, M. (2008). The protein expression of TRP-1 and galectin-1 in cutaneous malignant melanomas. *Cancer Genomics Proteomics*, 5, 293-300

Boyd, S.R., Tan, D.S., de Souza, L., Neale, M.H., Myatt, N.E., Alexander, R.A., Robb, M., Hungerford, J.L. & Cree, I.A. (2002). Uveal melanomas express vascular endothelial growth factor and basic fibroblast growth factor and support endothelial cell growth. *Br. J. Ophthalmol.*, 86, 440-7

Brader, S. & Eccles, S.A. (2004). Phosphoinositide 3-kinase signalling pathways in tumor progression, invasion and angiogenesis. *Tumori*, 90, 2-8

Burrows, F.J., Haskard, D.O., Hart, I.R., Marshall, J.F., Selkirk, S., Poole, S. & Thorpe, P.E. (1991). Influence of tumor-derived interleukin 1 on melanoma-endothelial cell interactions in vitro. *Cancer Res.*, 1, 4768-75

Byers, H.R., Boissel, S.J., Tu, C. & Park, H.Y. (2010). RNAi-mediated knockdown of protein kinase C-alpha inhibits cell migration in MM-RU human metastatic melanoma cell line. *Melanoma Res.*, 20, 171-8

Cangara, H.M., Ishida, T., Hara, T., Sun, L., Toh, R., Rikitake, Y., Kundu, R.K., Quertermous, T., Hirata, K. & Hayashi, Y. (2010). Role of endothelial cell-selective adhesion molecule in hematogeneous metastasis. *Microvasc. Res.*, 80, 133-41

Caunt, M., Hu, L., Tang, T., Brooks, P.C., Ibrahim, S. & Karpatkin, S. (2006). Growth-regulated oncogene is pivotal in thrombin-induced angiogenesis. *Cancer Res.*, 66, 4125-32

Chakraborti, S. (2003). Phospholipase $A_2$ isoforms: a perspective. *Cell Signal.*, 15, 637-65

Conner, S.R., Scott, G. & Aplin, A.E. (2003). Adhesion-dependent activation of the ERK1/2 cascade is by-passed in melanoma cells. *J. Biol. Chem.*, 278, 34548-54

Danielsen, T. & Rofstad, E.K. (1998). VEGF, bFGF and EGF in the angiogenesis of human melanoma xenografts. *Int. J. Cancer*, 76, 836-41

Denkins, Y., Kempf, D., Ferniz, M., Nileshwar, S., & Marchetti, D. (2005). Role of omega-3 polyunsaturated fatty acid on ciclooxygenase-2 metabolism in brain metastatic melanoma. *J. Lipid Res.*, 46, 1278-84

Ding, Z., Liu, Z., Bi, Y., Tian, H., Li, G. & Song, T. (2005). Morphological study of the interaction between M21 melanoma and lymphatic endothelium. *Lymphology*, 38, 87-91

Enzmann, V., Faude, F., Kohen, L. & Wiedemann, P. (1998). Secretion of cytokines by human choroidal melanoma cells and skin melanoma cell lines in vitro. *Ophthalmic Res.*, 30, 189-94

Estrada-Bernal, A., Gatlin, J.C., Sunpaweravong, S. & Pfenninger, K.H. (2009). Dynamic adhesions and MARCKS in melanoma cells. *J. Cell Sci.*, 122, 2300-2310

Favier, B., Alam, A., Barron, P., Bonnin, J., Laboudie, P., Fons, P., Mandron, M., Herault, J.P., Neufeld, G., Savi, P., Herbert, J.M. & Bono, F. (2006). Neuropilin-2 interacts with VEGFR-2 and VEGFR-3 and promotes human endothelial cell survival and migration. *Blood*, 108, 1243-50

Furuhashi, M., Sjöblom, T., Abramsson, A., Ellingsen, J., Micke, P., Li, H., Bergsten-Folestad, E., Eriksson, U., Heuchel, R., Betsholtz, C., Heldin, C.H. & Ostman, A. (2004). Platelet-derived growth factor production by B16 melanoma cells leads to increased pericyte abundance in tumors and an associated increase in tumor growth rate. *Cancer Res.*, 64, 2725-33

Goulet, A.C., Einsphar, J.G., Alberts, D.S., Beas, A., Burk, C., Bhattacharyya, A., Bangert, J., Harmon, J.M., Fujiwara, H., Koki, A. & Nelson, M.A. (2003). Analysis of ciclooxygenase 2 (Cox-2) expression during malignant melanoma progression. *Cancer Biol. Ther.*, 6, 713-718

Graells, J., Vinyals, A., Figueras, A., Llorens, A., Moreno, A. Marcoval, J., Gonzalez, F.J. & Fabra, A. (2004). Overproduction of VEGF concomitantly expressed with its receptors promotes growth and survival of melanoma cells through MAPK and PI3K signaling. *J. Invest. Dermatol.*, 123, 1151-61

Haass, N.K., Smalley, K.S., Li, L. & Herlyn, M. (2005). Adhesion, migration and communication in melanocytes and melanoma. *Pigment Cell Res.*,18, 150-9

Haass, N.K., Sproesser, K., Nguyen, T.K., Contractor, R., Medina, C.A., Nathanson, K.L., Herlyn, M. & Smalley, K.S. (2008). The mitogen-activated protein/extracellular signal-regulated kinase kinase inhibitor AZD6244 (ARRY-142886) induces growth arrest in melanoma cells and tumor regression when combined with docetaxel. *Clin. Cancer Res.*, 14, 230–239

Herlyn, M. (2005). Metastatic melanoma cells. Introduction. *Cancer Metastasis Rev.*, 24, 193-4

Honn, K.V., Tang, D.G., Grossi, I., Duniec, Z.M., Timar, J., Renaud, C., Leithauser, M., Blair, I., Johnson, C.R., Diglio, C.A., et al. (1994). Tumor cell-derived 12(S)-hydroxyeicosatetraenoic acid induces microvascular endothelial cell retraction. *Cancer Res.*, 54, 565-74

Ijland, S.A., Jager, M.J., Heijdra, B.M., Westphal, J.R. & Peek, R. (1999). Expression of angiogenic and immunosuppressive factors by uveal melanoma cell lines. *Melanoma Res.*, 9, 445-50

Iozzo, R. V. & San Antonio, J. V. (2001). Heparan sulfate proteoglycans: heavy hitters in the angiogenesis arena. *J. Clin. Invest.*, 108, 349-55

Jeong, W.C., Kim, K.J., Ju, H.W., Back, H.K., Kim, H.K., Im, S.Y. & Lee, H.K. (2010). Cytoplasmic phospholipase A2 metabolites play a critical role in pulmonary tumor metastasis in mice. *Anticancer Res.*, 30, 3421-7

Kannagi, R. (1997). Carbohydrate-mediated cell adhesion involved in hematogenous metastasis of cancer. *Glycoconj. J.*, 14, 577-584

Kashiwagi, K.,Tsukamoto, K., Suzuki, M. & Tsukahara, S. (2002). Effects of isopropyl unoprostone and latanoprost on melanogenesis in mouse epidermal melanocytes. *J. Glaucoma*, 11, 57–64

Katakai, T, Hara, T, Sugai, M, Gonda, H, Nambu, Y, Matsuda, E, Agata, Y. & Shimizu, A. (2002). Chemokine-independent preference for T-helper-1 cells in transendothelial migration. *J. Biol. Chem.*, 277, 50948-58

Khanna, P., Yunkunis, T., Muddana, H.S., Peng, H.H., August, A. & Dong, C. (2010). p38 MAP kinase is necessary for melanoma-mediated regulation of VE-cadherin disassembly. *Am. J. Physiol. Cell. Physiol.*, 298, C1140-50

Klemke, M., Weschenfelder, T., Konstandin, M.H. & Samstag, Y. (2007). High affinity interaction of integrin α4β1 (VLA-4) and vascular cell adhesion molecule 1 (VCAM-

1) enhances migration of human melanoma cells across activated endothelial cell layers. *J. Cell. Physiol.*, 212, 368-74

Kramer, R.H., Vu, M., Cheng, Y.F. & Ramos, D.M. (1991). Integrin expression in malignant melanoma. *Cancer Metastasis Rev.*, 10, 49-59

Kuźbicki, L., Sarnecka, A. & Chwirot, B.W. (2006). Expression of ciclooxygenase 2 in benign nevi and during human cutaneous melanoma progression. *Melanoma Res.*, 16, 29-36

Lander, A. D. & Selleck, S. B. (2000). The elusive functions of proteoglycans: in vivo veritas. *J. Cell. Biol.*, 148, 227-232

Ludwig, R.J., Boehme, B., Podda, M., Henschler, R., Jager, E., Tandi, C., Boehncke, W.H., Zollner, T.M., Kaufmann, R. & Gille, J. (2004). Endothelial P-selectin as a target of heparin action in experimental melanoma lung metastasis. *Cancer Res.*, 64, 2743-50

Lupo, G., Anfuso, C.D., Ragusa, N., Strosznajder, R.P., Walski, M. & Alberghina, M. (2001). t-Butyl hydroperoxide and oxidized low density lipoprotein enhance phospholipid hydrolysis in lipopolysaccharide-stimulated retinal pericytes. *Biochim. Biophys. Acta,* 1531, 143-55

Lupo, G., Assero, G., Anfuso, C.D., Nicotra, A., Palumbo, M., Cannavò, G., Renis, M., Ragusa, N., & Alberghina, M. (2002). Cytosolic phospholipase $A_2$ mediates arachidonoyl phospholipid hydrolysis in immortalized rat brain endothelial cells stimulated by oxidized LDL. *Biochim. Biophys. Acta*, 1585, 19-29

Lupo, G., Nicotra. A, Giurdanella, G., Anfuso, C.D., Romeo, L., Biondi, G., Tirolo, C., Marchetti, B., Ragusa, N. & Alberghina, M. (2005). Activation of phospholipase A(2) and MAP kinases by oxidized low-density lipoproteins in immortalized GP8.39 endothelial cells. *Biochim. Biophys. Acta,* 1735, 135-50

Martinson, B.D., Albert, C.J., Corbett, J.A., Wysolmerski, R.B. & Ford, D.A. (2003). Calcium-independent phospholipase $A_2$ mediates CREB phosphorylation in double-stranded RNA-stimulated endothelial cells. *J. Lipid Res.*, 44, 1686–1691

McGary, E.C., Lev, D.C. & Bar-Eli, M. (2002). Cellular adhesion pathways and metastatic potential of human melanoma. *Cancer Biol. Ther.*, 1, 459-65

Melnikova, V.O., Balasubramanian, K., Villares, G.J., Dobroff, A.S., Zigler, M., Wang, H., Petersson, F., Price, J.E., Schroit, A., Prieto, V.G., Hung, M.C. & Bar-Eli, M. (2009). Cross-talk between protease-activated receptor 1 and platelet-activating factor receptor regulates melanoma cell adhesion molecule (MCAM/MUC18) expression and melanoma metastasis. *J. Biol. Chem.*, 284, 28845-55

Minami S., Christopher, A., Lum, M.D., Kevin, M., Kitagawa, M.D., Thomas, S. & Namiki, M.D. (2011). Immunohistochemical expression of cyclooxygenage-2 in melanocytic skin lesions. *Int. J. Dermatol.*, 50, 24-29

Monterrubio, M., Mellado, M., Carrera, A.C. & Rodríguez-Frade, J.M. (2009). PI3Kgamma activation by CXCL12 regulates tumor cell adhesion and invasion. *Biochem. Biophys. Res. Commun.*, 388, 199-204

Morikawa, S., Baluk, P., Kaidoh, T., Haskell, A., Jain, R.K. & McDonald, D.M. (2002). Abnormalities in pericytes on blood vessels and endothelial sprouts in tumors. *Am. J. Pathol.*, 160, 985-1000

Morozevich, G., Kozlova, N., Cheglakov, I., Ushakova, N. & Berman, A. (2009). Integrin alpha5beta1 controls invasion of human breast carcinoma cells by direct and indirect modulation of MMP-2 collagenase activity. *Cell Cycle*, 8, 2219-25

Munshi, H.G. & Stack, M.S. (2006). Reciprocal interactions between adhesion receptor signaling and MMP regulation. *Cancer Metastasis Rev.*, 25, 45-56

Muraki, C., Ohga, N., Hida, Y., Nishihara, H., Kato, Y., Tsuchiya, K., Matsuda, K., Totsuka, Y., Shindoh, M. & Hida, K. (Feb 2011). Cyclooxygenase-2 inhibition causes antiangiogenic effects on tumor endothelial and vascular progenitor cells. *Int. J. Cancer*

Nicholson, G.L. (1982). Metastatic tumor cell attachment and invasion assay utilizing vascular endothelial cell monolayers. *J. Histochem. Cytochem.*, 30, 214-220

Oka, M. & Kikkawa, U. (2005). Protein kinase C in melanoma. *Cancer Metastasis Rev.*, 24, 287-300

Parsad, D., Pandhi, R., Dogra, S. & Kumar, B. (2002). Topical prostaglandin analog (PGE2) in vitiligo - a preliminary study. *Int. J. Dermatol.*, 41, 942–945

Peng, H.H., Hodgson, L., Henderson, A.J. & Dong, C. (2005). Involvement of phospholipase C signaling in melanoma cell-induced endothelial junction disassembly. *Front. Biosci.*, 10, 1597-606

Putnam, A.J., Schulz, V.V., Freiter, E.M., Bill, H.M. & Miranti, C.K. (2009). Src, PKCalpha, and PKCdelta are required for alphavbeta3 integrin-mediated metastatic melanoma invasion. *Cell Commun. Signal.*, 7, 10-28

Qi, J., Chen, N., Wang, J. & Siu, C.H. (2005). Transendothelial migration of melanoma cells involves N-cadherin-mediated adhesion and activation of the beta-catenin signaling pathway. *Mol. Biol. Cell*, 16, 4386-97

Raman, K. & Kuberan, B. (2010). Chemical tumor biology of heparan sulfate proteoglycans. *Current Chem. Biol.*, 4, 20-31

Ramjeesingh, R., Leung, R. & Siu, C.H. (2003). Interleukin-8 secreted by endothelial cells induces chemotaxis of melanoma cells through the chemokine receptor CXCR1. *FASEB J.*, 17, 1292-4

Reiland, J., Kempf, D., Roy, M., Denkins, Y. & Marchetti, D. (2006). FGF2 binding, signaling, and angiogenesis are modulated by heparanase in metastatic melanoma cells. *Neoplasia*, 8, 596-606

Richmond, A. & Thomas, H.G. (1988). Melanoma growth stimulatory activity: isolation from human melanoma tumors and characterization of tissue distribution. *J. Cell. Biochem.*, 36, 185-98

Ridgway, L.D., Wetzel, M.D. & Marchetti, D. (2010). Modulation of GEF-H1 induced signaling by heparanase in brain metastatic melanoma cells. *J. Cell. Biochem.*, 111, 1299-309

Robinson, C.J. & Stringer, S.E. (2001). The splice variants of vascular endothelial growth factor (VEGF) and their receptors. *J. Cell Sci.*, 114, 853-65

Robinson, C.J., Mulloy, B., Gallagher, J.T. & Stringer, S.E. (2006). VEGF165-binding sites within heparan sulfate encompass two highly sulfated domains and can be liberated by K5 lyase. *J. Biol. Chem.*, 281, 1731-40

Rondepierre, F., Bouchon, B., Bonnet, M., Moins, N., Chezal, J.M., D'Incan, M. & Degoul, F. (2010). B16 melanoma secretomes and in vitro invasiveness: syntenin as an invasion modulator. *Melanoma Res.*, 20, 77-84

Rothhammer, T. Bataille, F., Sprussm, T., Eissner, G. & Bosserhoff, A.K. (2007). Functional implication of BMP4 expression on angiogenesis in malignant melanoma. *Oncogene*, 26, 4158-4170

Roy, M., Reiland J., Murry, B.P., Chouljenko, V., Kousoulas, K.G. & Marchetti, D. (2005). Antisense-mediated suppression of heparanase gene inhibits melanoma cell invasion. *Neoplasia*, 7, 253-262

Roy, M. & Marchetti, D. (2009). Cell surface heparan sulfate released by heparanase promotes melanoma cell migration and angiogenesis. *J. Cell. Biochem.*, 106, 200-9

Rüegg, C., Dormond, O. & Mariotti, A. (2004). Endothelial cells integrin and Cox-2: mediators and therapeutic target of tumor angiogenesis. *Biochim. Biophys. Acta*, 1654, 51-67

Ruffini, F., Failla, C.M., Orecchia, A., Bani, M.R., Dorio, A.S., Fortes, C., Zambruno, G., Graziani, G., Giavazzi, R., D'Atri, S. & Lacal, PM. (2011). Expression of the soluble vascular endothelial growth factor receptor-1 in cutaneous melanoma: role in tumour progression. *Br. J. Dermatol.*, 164, 1061-70

Ruiz, P., Dunon, D., Sonnenberg, A. & Imhof, B.A. (1993). Suppression of mouse melanoma metastasis by EA-1, a monoclonal antibody specific for alpha 6 integrins. *Cell Adhes. Commun.*, 1, 67-81

Ruth, M.C., Xu, Y., Maxwell, I.H., Ahn, N.G., Norris, D.A. & Shellman, Y.G. (2006). RhoC promotes human melanoma invasion in a PI3K/Akt-dependent pathway. *J. Invest. Dermatol.*, 126, 862-8

Saito-Katsuragi, M., Asada, H., Niizeki, H., Katoh, F., Masuzawa, M., Tsutsumi, M., Kuniyasu, H., Ito, A., Nojima, H. & Miyagawa, S. (2007). Role for connexin 26 in metastasis of human malignant melanoma: communication between melanoma and endothelial cells via connexin 26. *Cancer*, 110, 1162–1172

Sander, C.S., Hamm, F., Elsen, P. & Thiele, J.J. (2003). Oxidative stress in malignat melanoma and non-melanoma skin cancer. *Br. J. Dermatol.*, 148, 913-922

Sandoval, R., Malik, A.B., Minshall, R.D., Kouklis, P., Ellis, C.A. & Tiruppathi, C. (2001). $Ca^{(2+)}$ signalling and PKCalpha activate increased endothelial permeability by disassembly of VE-cadherin junctions. *J. Physiol.*, 533(Pt 2), 433-45

Sasisekharan, R. Shriver, Z., Venkataraman, G. & Narayanasami, U. (2002). Roles of heparan-sulphate glycosaminoglycans in cancer. *Nature Rev. Cancer*, 2, 521-528

Scuderi, M.R., Anfuso, C.D., Lupo, G., Motta, C., Romeo, L., Guerra, L., Cappellani, A., Ragusa, N., Cantarella, G. & Alberghina, M. (2008). Expression of Ca(2+)-independent and Ca(2+)-dependent phospholipases A(2) and cyclooxygenases in human melanocytes and malignant melanoma cell lines. *Biochim. Biophys. Acta*, 1781, 635-42

Sengupta, S., Kiziltepe, T. & Sasisekharan, R. (2004). A dual-color fluorescence imaging-based system for the dissection of antiangiogenic and chemotherapeutic activity of molecules. *FASEB J.*, 18, 1565-7

Singh, T., Vaid, M., Katiyar, N., Sharma, S. & Katiyar, S.K. (2011). Berberine, an isoquinoline alkaloid, inhibits melanoma cancer cell migration by reducing the expressions of cyclooxygenase-2, prostaglandin $E_2$ and prostaglandin $E_2$ receptors. *Carcinogenesis*, 32, 86-92

Singh, S., Nannuru, K.C., Sadanandam, A., Varney, M.L. & Singh, R.K. (2009). CXCR1 and CXCR2 enhances human melanoma tumourigenesis, growth and invasion. *Br. J. Cancer*, 100, 1638-46

Soung, Y.H., Clifford, J.L. & Chung, J. (2010). Crosstalk between integrin and receptor tyrosine kinase signaling in breast carcinoma progression. *BMB Rep.*, 43, 311-8

Stine, M.J., Wang, C.J., Moriarty, W.F., Ryu, B., Cheong, R., Westra, W.H., Levchenko, A. & Alani, R.M. (Feb 2011). Integration of genotypic and phenotypic screening reveals molecular mediators of melanoma-stromal interaction, *Cancer Res.*

Strieter, R.M., Burdick, M.D., Mestas, J., Gomperts, B., Keane, M.P. & Belperio, J.A. (2006). Cancer CXC chemokine networks and tumour angiogenesis. *Eur. J. Cancer*, 42, 768-78

Sun, T., Sun, B.C., Ni, C.S., Zhao, X.L., Wang, X.H., Qie, S., Zhang, D.F., Gu, Q., Qi, H. & Zhao, N. (2008). Pilot study on the interaction between B16 melanoma cells-line and bone-marrow derived mesenchymal stem cells. *Cancer Lett.*, 263, 35-43

Suzuki, S., Heldin, C.H. & Heuchel, R.L. (2007). Platelet-derived growth factor receptor-beta, carrying the activating mutation D849N, accelerates the establishment of B16 melanoma. *BMC Cancer*, 7, 224-231

Szekeres, C.K., Trikha, M. & Honn, K.V. (2002). 12(S)-HETE, pleiotropic functions, multiple signaling pathways. *Adv. Exp. Med. Biol.*, 507, 509-15

Tabolacci, C., Lentini, A., Provenzano, B., Gismondi, A., Rossi, S., & Beninati, S. (2010). Similar antineoplastic effects of nimesulide, a selective COX-2 inhibitor, and prostaglandin E1 on B16-F10 murine melanoma cells. *Melanoma Res.*, 20, 273- 279

Thijssen, V.L., Barkan, B., Shoji, H., Aries, I.M., Mathieu, V., Deltour, L., Hackeng, T.M., Kiss, R., Kloog, Y., Poirier, F. & Griffioen, A.W. (2010). Tumor cells secrete galectin-1 to enhance endothelial cell activity. *Cancer Res.*, 70, 6216-24

Tomita, Y.,Maeda, K. & Tagami, H. (1992). Melanocyte-stimulating properties of arachidonic acid metabolites: possible role in postinflammatory pigmentation. *Pigment Cell Res.*, 5, 357-361

Torres, D., Paget, C., Fontaine, J., Mallevaey, T., Matsuoka, T., Maruyama, T., Narumiya, S., Capron, M., Gosset, P., Faveeuw, C. & Trottein, F. (2008). Prostaglandin D2 inhibits the production of IFN-gamma by invariant NK T cells: consequences in the control of B16 melanoma. *J. Immunol.*, 180, 783-92

Trapp, V., Parmakhtiar, B., Papazian, V., Willmott, L. & Fruehauf, J.P. (2010). Anti-angiogenic effect of resveratrol mediated by decreased VEGF and increase TSP1 expression in melanoma-endothelial cell coculture. *Angiogenesis*, 13, 305-315

Tremblay, P.L., Auger, F.A. & Huot, J. (2006). Regulation of transendothelial migration of colon cancer cells by E-selectin-mediated activation of p38 and ERK MAP kinases. *Oncogene*, 25, 6563-73

Tsubaki, M., Matsuoka, H., Yamamoto, C., Kato, C., Ogaki, M., Satou, T., Itoh, T., Kusunoki, T., Tanimori, Y. & Nishida, S. (2007). The protein kinase C inhibitor, H7, inhibits tumor cell invasion and and metastasis in mouse melanoma via suppression of ERK1/2. *Clin. Exp. Metastasis*, 24, 431-8

Tsuji, S., Tsujii, M., Kawano, S. & Hori, M. (2001). Ciclooxygenase-2 upregulation as a perigenetic change in carcinogenesis. *J. Exp. Clin. Cancer Res.*, 20, 117-29

van der Schaft, D.W., Seftor, R.E., Seftor, E.A., Hess, A.R., Gruman, L.M., Kirschmann, D.A., Yokoyama, Y., Griffioen, A.W. & Hendrix, M.J. (2004). Effect of angiogenesis inhibitors on vascular networks formation by human endothelial and melanoma cells. *J. Natl. Cancer Inst.*, 96, 1473-7

Vandercappellen, J., Van Damme, J. & Struyf, S. (2008). The role of CXC chemokines and their receptors in cancer. *Cancer Lett.*, 267, 226-44

Voris, J.P., Sitailo, L.A., Rahn, H.R., Defnet, A., Gerds, A.T., Sprague, R., Yadav, V., Caroline, Le Poole, I. & Denning, M.F. (2010). Functional alterations in protein kinase C beta II expression in melanoma. *Pigment Cell Melanoma Res.*, 23, 216-24

Voura, E.B., Ramjeesingh, R.A., Montgomery, A.M. & Siu, C.H. (2001). Involvement of integrin alpha(v)beta(3) and cell adhesion molecule L1 in transendothelial migration of melanoma cells. *Mol. Biol. Cell.*, 12, 2699-710

West, X.Z., Malinin, N.L., Merkulova, A.A,. Tischenko, M., Kerr, B.A., Borden, E.C., Podrez, E.A., Salomon, R.G. & Byzova, T.V. (2010). Oxidative stress induces angiogenesis by activating TLR2 with novel endogenous ligands. *Nature*, 467, 972-6

Winer, I., Normolle, D.P., Shureiqi, I., Sondak, V.K., Johnson, T., Su, L. & Brenner, D.E. (2002). Expression of 12-lipoxygenase as a biomarker for melanoma carcinogenesis. *Melanoma Res.*, 12, 429-34

Wittgen, H.G. & van Kempen, L.C. (2007). Reactive oxygen species in melanoma and its therapeutic implications. *Melanoma Res.*, 17, 400-9

Wendum, D., Comperat, E., Boelle, P.Y., Parc, R., Masliah, J., Trugnan, G. & Fléjou, J.F. (2005). Cytoplasmic phospholipase $A_2$ alpha overexpression in stromal cells is correlated with angiogenesis in human colorectal cancer. *Mod. Pathol.*, 18, 212–220

# 8

# Pigment Epithelium-Derived Factor – An Angiostatic Factor with a Broader Function in Melanoma

A. Fernández-Barral[1], J.L. Orgaz[1,2] and B. Jiménez[1]
[1]*Instituto de Investigaciones Biomédicas, CSIC-UAM-Departamento de Bioquímica UAM, Madrid,*
[2]*Present address: Randall Division of Cell & Molecular Biophysics, King's College London, London, SE1 1UL,*
[1]*Spain*
[2]*U.K.*

## 1. Introduction

Metastatic spread is achieved through changes in the tissue microenvironment driven by tumor cells that allow the formation of various dissemination routes using a variety of mechanisms; such as angiogenesis and vasculogenesis (hematogeneous routes), lymphangiogenesis (lymphatic routes), and in some particular cases like melanoma, vasculogenic mimicry (vasculogenic channels lined by melanoma cells) (Carmeliet, 2005; Hendrix *et al.*, 2003; Kopp *et al.*, 2006; Tammela and Alitalo, 2010). Building of dissemination routes has to be coordinated with the acquisition of new capabilities by tumor cells that enable them to locally invade, intravasate into dissemination channels, survive in the circulation, extravasate, and ultimately adapt to a foreign territory. All this complex cascade of events is orchestrated by multiple cell types and diverse families of factors and signaling circuits controlling intracellular as well as intercellular key communication events (Nguyen *et al.*, 2009b).

Interestingly, a particular subset of extracellular factors have the dual capacity to simultaneously impinge on the formation of the dissemination routes and to modulate many of the properties that the tumor cells themselves have to acquire in order to fulfill all steps required to successfully colonize a foreign territory starting from a primary lesion in a drastically different environment. This chapter focuses on an angiostatic factor, pigment epithelium derived factor (PEDF), with a broader function in melanoma that allows it to dually impinge on destroying some of the more relevant dissemination routes and on counteracting key tumor cell properties that enable the metastatic spread of melanoma cells. Understanding of the molecular and cellular mechanisms controlling melanoma progression has become an active field of research over the last five years unveiling a complex intertwined relationship between melanoma cells and the diverse cell types present in the tumor microenvironment, as well as a number of key molecular mediators (Shackleton and Quintana, 2010; Villanueva and Herlyn, 2008). Plasticity of melanoma cells allows them for appropriate reprogramming underlying the decision making process that arbitrates proliferation and migration as mutually exclusive cellular responses that need to alternate in the course of tumor progression (Hendrix *et al.*, 2007; Hoek *et al.*, 2008). We have recently interrogated the role of PEDF, an angiostatic factor produced at high levels by skin melanocytes, in controlling the switch between proliferative and invasive states of melanoma cells and its contribution to restrict the metastatic cascade. Our results demonstrate that loss of PEDF expression enables melanoma cells to acquire an invasive state and therefore its reprogramming is critical for the malignant progression of melanoma (Orgaz *et al.*, 2009).

## 2. Angiogenesis and melanoma. The role of endogenous inhibitors of angiogenesis

As in every tissue of our body angiogenesis is finely tuned in the skin by the balance of endogenous angiogenic growth factors and endogenous angiogenic inhibitors (Jimenez and Volpert, 2001). Although the pattern of skin vascularization established during development renders the skin a mildly hypoxic microenvironment ($pO_2$ in the dermal/epidermal junctions ranging from 0.5% to 10%) (Bedogni and Powell, 2009), a number of physiological processes like skin wound healing and cycles of hair follicle growth, and an increasingly recognized number of cutaneous pathologies (Laquer *et al.*, 2009; Nguyen *et al.*, 2009a) require new vessel formation to respectively achieve proper tissue homeostasis in physiological contexts or to chronically activate angiogenesis in the pathological settings.
Angiogenesis is a hallmark of cancer and it is of significant relevance for the life threatening stage of the disease, the metastatic spread (Hanahan and Weinberg, 2000; Hanahan and Weinberg, 2011). Angiogenesis is a pivotal process required to effectively deliver oxygen and nutrients and to eliminate waste products in lesions beyond 1-2mm of diameter (Folkman, 2006). Unlimited growth of primary lesions, activation of dormant micrometastases (Goss and Chambers, 2010), as well as the growth of micrometastases to macrometastases (Gao *et al.*, 2008), all require neovascularization. The so called tumor angiogenic switch refers to the mechanisms responsible for shifting the balance toward predominance of angiogenic growth factors accompanied by loss of angiogenesis inhibitors. Activation of tumor angiogenic switch triggers the transition from the avascular to the vascular phase of tumor growth, which is characterized by uncontrolled, excessive and aberrant neovascularization. The vascular phase sustains unlimited neoplastic growth and provides diverse vascular routes for the metastatic dissemination of the primary lesion. There is significant evidence supporting that cancer metastasis can be determined by the angiogenic potential of the primary tumor cells (Kerbel, 2008). Also, preclinical studies using mouse models, as well as clinical studies using biopsies have shown that there is a direct association between incidence of metastases and the microvascular density in vascular hot spots in the tumor periphery (Nico *et al.*, 2008).
Based on the relevance of tumor neovascularization for the progression of the disease and patient outcome, there has been over the last four decades an explosion of the cellular and molecular knowledge of the mechanisms and key molecules involved in the creation of the diverse types of vessels networks that allow for tumor cell dissemination. All this knowledge also led to a rapid and fruitful translation to the clinic of the first generation of antiangiogenic drugs (Ellis and Hicklin, 2008; Ferrara and Kerbel, 2005; Jain, 2008; Jubb *et al.*, 2006; Loges *et al.*, 2009; Orgaz *et al.*, 2008) which have been used up to now in the context of advanced disease and as a general rule in combination with a wide range of

chemotherapeutic agents or radiation therapy. Also, the general principle of antiangiogenic therapy of cancer in the clinic has been almost exclusively based on the use of single antiangiogenic agents or drugs. Although most of these studies have obtained reasonably encouraging results, further evaluation of more complex therapeutic regimens targeting simultaneously multiple angiogenesis pathways should be warranted in patients with advanced melanoma and other cancers; or when required to overcome resistance to first line antiangiogenic drugs (Bergers and Hanahan, 2008). Notwithstanding, the broad armory of identified antiangiogenic drugs should allow designing optimum combinations of antiangiogenic drugs that hopefully will be: (i) more efficient and of greater benefit for each particular type of cancer, (ii) used as second line antiangiogenic therapies in cases of resistance to first line antiangiogenic drugs, or (iii) useful to suitably design the most likely effective strategy considering the characteristics of each patient's type of tumor vascular bed.

The mildly hypoxic microenvironment of the skin significantly contributes to melanocyte transformation, as the result of hypoxia effects promoting both proliferation and survival. Thus, hypoxia has emerged as a relevant tumor-promoting environmental factor in melanoma (Bedogni and Powell, 2009). Additionally, hypoxia is one of the main regulators of angiogenic growth factors and angiogenic inhibitors, which contributes to tilt the balance toward inducers of angiogenesis and to impose the loss of relevant angiostatic factors during tumor progression (Rey and Semenza, 2010).

Studies with human melanoma xenograft models in nude mice as well as with human melanoma biopsies demonstrated that melanoma cells are an important source of angiogenic growth factors like vascular endothelial growth factor (VEGF), basic fibroblast growth factor (bFGF), placenta growth factor (PlGF), transforming growth factors-$\alpha$ and $\beta$ (TGF- $\alpha$ and $\beta$), platelet derived growth factor-B (PDGF-B) and interleukin-8 (IL-8), among others (Basu *et al.*, 2009; Mahabeleshwar and Byzova, 2007). A number of studies have correlated melanoma neovascularization with poor patient prognosis, overall survival, ulceration and increase rate of relapse; as it is the case in many other types of cancers (Ria *et al.*, 2010). However, production of angiogenesis inhibitors by melanoma cells and their regulation in the course of melanoma progression has remained poorly explored.

We have recently focused on the study of the angiostatic factor pigment epithelium derived factor (PEDF) in human melanocytes and melanoma progression (Fernandez-Garcia *et al.*, 2007; Garcia *et al.*, 2004; Orgaz *et al.*, 2009). PEDF was originally described as the most potent angiostatic factor in the eye that plays a relevant role in ensuring the correct pattern of vascularization of diverse eye compartments (Bouck, 2002). PEDF is produced at high levels by retinal pigment epithelial (RPE) cells, and it counteracts a number of potent angiogenic growth factors in the retina like VEGF, insulin growth factor-1 (IGF-1), bFGF, etc; ensuring the right balance of angiogenic regulators that leads to an optimum physiological pattern of blood vessels for correct retinal function. Importantly, avascular eye compartments like the vitreous and cornea are rich in PEDF. To further support the relevance of PEDF in the eye, a number of eye pathologies like diabetic retinopathy and eye related macular degeneration are associated with loss of PEDF expression and therefore predominance of the action of angiogenic growth factors, leading to excessive and aberrant vascularization patterns associated with loss of vision (Tombran-Tink, 2010).

We have recently shown that melanocytes are also among the cell types in our body that produce and secrete the highest levels of PEDF (Orgaz *et al.*, 2009), which are comparable to the levels produced by RPE cells, neural cells or retinoblastoma cells. However, endothelial cells, one of the main targets of PEDF's action, produce very low levels of this angiostatic factor and therefore rely on other cell types to bring PEDF to many scenarios where proper tissue homeostasis requires halting the angiogenic cascade to render the vasculature to a quiescent state. If PEDF is highly produced by melanocytes the following questions arise: (i) is there an autocrine role of PEDF on pigment cells? It has been recently described that PEDF is stored in melanosomes, although its putative role in the regulation of pigment production and secretion remains to be explored (Chi *et al.*, 2006). Furthermore, PEDF directly modulates the proliferative and migratory capability of normal melanocytes (Orgaz *et al.*, 2009), (ii) is PEDF expression regulated during melanoma progression?, and which are the functional consequences of its modulation? Our insights about these questions will be addressed in the following section.

Primary melanoma biopsies are characterized by high PEDF expression in the vast majority of human biopsies analyzed, although a significant degree of heterogeneity exists (Orgaz *et al.*, 2009; and unpublished data). Conversely, PEDF expression is lost in cutaneous metastases of human melanoma (Orgaz *et al.*, 2009).

When is angiogenesis switched on during melanoma progression and its relevance for the metastatic spread of human melanoma is still a matter of certain debate (Basu *et al.*, 2009; Helfrich *et al.*, 2010). Lack of consensus most probably reflects difficulty on adequately defining staging and progression of melanoma, together with limitations of currently available models to explain how melanoma evolves and malignizes (see Section 3.1). It seems plausible that acquisition of angiogenic potential and increase in microvascular density occur gradually as melanoma lesions progress from the radial growth phase (RGP) to the vertical growth phase (VGP) and to the metastatic phase (M). In our studies we found that the most dramatic regulation of PEDF levels corresponds to the transition from primary melanoma to cutaneous metastases of melanoma (described in more detail in Section 3.3). Also most likely melanomas progressively develop a more profuse network of blood vessels from RGP to VGP, but due to the extreme heterogeneity of human melanoma biopsies we were unable to find important differences on the level of PEDF when comparing RGP to VGP biopsies, although there was a tendency to a decrease from RGP to VGP (unpublished data).

We have directly explored by means of global gene expression analysis using microarrays the consequences of PEDF overexpression on the angiogenic potential of human melanoma cells. Importantly, exogenous PEDF overexpression abrogates the ability of aggressive melanoma cells to produce potent angiogenic growth factors like VEGF or IL-8, tilting the balance toward inhibition of melanoma angiogenesis (Orgaz *et al.*, 2011). Given the role of VEGF and IL-8 as highly potent angiogenic growth factors in melanoma, together with their role in directly promoting melanoma cell migration and invasion; the abrogation of their production by melanoma cells upon PEDF's action is of special relevance. Additionally, both VEGF and IL-8 increase vascular permeability and therefore, by eliminating these angiogenic growth factors PEDF normalizes to a certain extent tumor vascular leakiness and thereby impedes melanoma intravasation/extravasation. Finally, a number of extracellular matrix proteins (like collagen IV A2 (COL4A2) and fibronectin 1 (FN1)), matrix enzymes and matrix metalloproteinases (such as tissue inhibitors of metalloproteinases (TIMPs), a disintegrin and metalloproteinase domain (ADAMs), a disintegrin-like and metalloprotease (reprolysin type) with thrombospondin type 1 motif (ADAMTs)) or serine (or cysteine) proteinase inhibitor (SERPINs) and integrins (like integrin β3) relevant in different steps of the angiogenic cascade were modulated by PEDF, with a trend corresponding to halting the angiogenic process (Orgaz *et al.*, 2011).

Finally, as melanoma cells become more aggressive they acquire the ability to mimic molecularly and functionally the endothelial cells. This specific reprogramming, characteristic of highly aggressive melanoma cells, is called vasculogenic mimicry, and endows them with the ability to form vascular channels lined by melanoma cells; which represent a unique escape route for the spread of melanoma (Hess *et al.*, 2007). We found that PEDF is able to impede the formation of melanoma vasculogenic channels in the lungs of nude mice in colonization assays of human melanoma cell lines (Orgaz *et al.*, 2009); which adds another mechanism of antimetastatic action for this multifunctional factor. The molecular basis by which PEDF abrogates melanoma vasculogenic mimicry are still unknown and would be extremely interesting to explore in view of the relevance of this mechanism in the context of melanoma dissemination.

Another relevant aspect of the tumor vasculature that distinguishes it from normal vasculature is the degree of vessel maturation (Baluk *et al.*, 2005; Jain, 2003). Over the last decades it was demonstrated that the efficacy of antiangiogenic strategies in solid tumors is inversely correlated to the degree of maturation of the tumor vascular bed (Helfrich and Schadendorf, 2011; Jimenez and Volpert, 2001). This was the case not only for strategies based on interference with angiogenic growth factors and their receptors, but also for angiostatic factors like PEDF. We demonstrated that PEDF only induces vessel regression of immature vessels poorly covered by pericytes, while those tumor vessels that are covered with pericytes over the course of time of tumor establishment remain invulnerable to PEDF's angiostatic action (Garcia *et al.*, 2004). This important mechanistic observation opened up the following therapeutic windows: (i) use of antiangiogenic strategies at very early stages of tumor progression, when presumably a larger proportion of the vessels are still immature; (ii) use of antiangiogenic strategies in tumor types in which the majority of vessels remain immature; and (iii) design combination therapies in which antiangiogenic strategies directed to endothelial cells are concomitantly used with drugs directed to pericytes aimed to destabilize the tumor vasculature by depriving it of the interactions with pericytes, and therefore rendering it immature. Notwithstanding the limitation on the angiostatic action of PEDF, which is restricted to immature vessels, all direct PEDF's effects on melanoma cells contribute to halt melanoma metastases, and strongly support the development of novel therapeutic strategies based on knowledge of the diverse actions of this biological modifier of melanoma.

The mechanism by which PEDF induces immature blood vessel regression has been studied in detail over the last years by us and others. A common characteristic in the mechanism of action of PEDF and all the endogenous inhibitors of angiogenesis so far described (thrombospondin-1, angiostatin, endostatin, canstatin, tumstatin, etc) is that they are capable of inducing apoptosis in endothelial cells present in immature, remodeling vessels, thus causing selective regression of the expanding aberrant tumor vasculature without affecting normal vessels (Jimenez and Volpert, 2001; Volpert, 2000). Angiogenic growth factors like VEGF act like essential survival factors in this pathological scenario, but the action of endogenous inhibitors of angiogenesis is dominant over that of inducers. PEDF induces apoptosis in remodeling endothelial cells by inducing Fas ligand (CD95L) expression on the surface of activated endothelial cells via nuclear factor kappa-light-chain-enhancer of activated B cells (NFKB) (Aurora *et al.*, 2010; Volpert *et al.*, 2002), which initiates an extrinsic cell death cascade. In concert, PEDF hampers endothelial cells survival by reducing the expression of pro-survival factor caspase-8 FLICE-inhibitory protein (c-FLIP) through the Nuclear Factor of Activated T-cells (NFAT) (Zaichuk *et al.*, 2004). Besides, we have also

demonstrated that under stress conditions like serum withdrawal or lack of extracellular matrix attachment, PEDF has a certain capacity to induce melanoma cell apoptosis although with a weaker potency than in endothelial cells (Garcia *et al.*, 2004). Reduced survival of melanoma cells caused by the absence of attachment in the presence of high PEDF circulating levels has important consequences for the outcome of tumor cells in transit to the metastatic site.
There are still a number PEDF's putative actions on the various tumor vascularization mechanisms described so far that remain to be explored and that are of critical importance: (i) does PEDF affect haematopoyetic precursor cells recruitment?, (ii) does PEDF block vasculogenesis (formation of new vessels from endothelial progenitor cells)?, (iii) does PEDF induce lymphatic vessels regression? There is no report linking PEDF to vasculogenesis, but it has recently been described that PEDF decreases lymph node metastasis of prostate cancer, while paradoxically increases extratumoral lymphangiogenesis by unknown mechanisms (Halin *et al.*, 2010).
In the context of spread of the disease an attractive benefit of antiangiogenic strategies is their potential to keep micrometastases in a dormant state (Gao *et al.*, 2008; Goss and Chambers, 2010). Thrombospondin-1 has been proven to be effective in preventing the growth of dormant pulmonary micrometastases in human melanoma xenografts after surgical resection or curative radiation of the primary tumor (Rofstad *et al.*, 2004; Rofstad *et al.*, 2003). PEDF's capability to maintain dormant micrometastases in check, preventing their growth to macrometastases remains to be evaluated, but it could be of relevant therapeutic interest.
Moreover, it has been shown that PEDF is also produced by a wide variety of epithelial cell types in different tissues and its role in controlling primary tumor growth, angiogenesis and metastatic spread has been explored in a wide range of tumors using diverse mouse models, and analysis of human biopsies. Levels of angiostatic PEDF decrease during the progression of a number of cancers, such as hepatocelular carcinoma (Matsumoto *et al.*, 2004), prostate cancer (Halin *et al.*, 2004; Qingyi *et al.*, 2009), breast adenocarcinoma (Cai *et al.*, 2006), glioblastoma (Guan *et al.*, 2003) and Wilm´s tumors (Abramson *et al.*, 2003). A number of recent excellent reviews cover the antitumor and antimetastatic action of PEDF on several tumor types (Broadhead *et al.*, 2009; Fernandez-Garcia *et al.*, 2007; Hoshina *et al.*, 2010).

## 3. Halting melanoma progression. The role of pigment epithelium-derived factor

### 3.1 Cutaneous melanoma. Current models of melanoma progression

Melanoma cells arise from melanocytes, normal cells specialized in the production of pigment melanin, which reside in the basal layer of the epidermis, among other locations, and whose homeostasis is tightly controlled by epidermal keratinocytes (Gray-Schopfer *et al.*, 2007).The classical model of melanoma progression describes melanoma development as a series of histopathological steps regarding the thickness and the grade of invasion of the lesion (Clark, 1991). Nevi are relatively benign lesions that rarely progress to melanoma, in part because most of melanocytes in nevocytic lesions are in a state of senescence-associated growth arrest (Michaloglou *et al.*, 2005). RGP, melanomas have high proliferative potential but null or very low invasive ability, being confined to the epidermis (Gray-Schopfer *et al.*, 2007). In contrast, VGP, melanomas are competent for metastasis, fully invade the upper part of the epidermis as well as the dermis and the subcutaneous tissue, being able to reach blood or lymph circulation and eventually colonize and develop secondary tumors at distant organs (Chin *et al.*, 2006; Gray-Schopfer *et al.*, 2007). This model is in agreement with the tumor clonal evolution model (Nowell, 1976), which hypothesizes that cancer evolves from a poorly to a highly metastatic phase through accumulation of molecular alterations (mutations and/or epigenetic changes) that enhance proliferative and invasive potential of tumor cells, and that would promote lineal progression from RGP to VGP to metastasis (Miller and Mihm, 2006).

Even though the classification of melanomas according to the thickness of the lesion is one of the most widely used methods for the diagnosis and prognosis of melanoma (Fecher *et al.*, 2007), frequently there are lesions whose thickness does not correlate with their actual aggressiveness and metastatic outcome (Lomuto *et al.*, 2004; Slingluff *et al.*, 1988). Besides, this model does not offer either convincing explanations for the heterogeneity found in metastatic melanoma cells, nor for the persistent failure of anti-melanoma therapies. Consequently, in the last decade researchers have aimed to establish a molecular classification of melanoma utilizing gene expression profiling tools (Fecher *et al.*, 2007; Hoek, 2007; Hoek, 2009). A number of studies have been able to classify collections of melanoma cell lines or biopsies into groups differing in their aggressiveness and metastatic potential, confirming the large heterogeneity of melanoma and the importance of the microenvironment in determining gene expression programs of melanoma cells and progression to metastasis (Bittner *et al.*, 2000; Haqq *et al.*, 2005; Hoek, 2007; Pavey *et al.*, 2004).

One of these studies, by means of genome-wide gene expression analysis and functional assays, described that most melanoma cell lines could be categorized according to their gene expression profile into two extreme phenotypes, proliferative or invasive (Hoek *et al.*, 2006). The proliferative gene signature encompasses a number of melanocytic lineage genes such as microphthalmia-associated transcription factor (MITF) and some of its targets, while the invasive phenotype signature is defined by suppressed expression of proliferative genes in favor of others related to the modification of the tumor microenvironment (Hoek *et al.*, 2006). Based on this and other studies a new melanoma progression model was proposed, which takes into account the heterogeneous nature of melanoma and the key role of the tumor microenvironment (Carreira *et al.*, 2006; Goodall *et al.*, 2008; Hoek, 2009; Hoek *et al.*, 2008; Hoek *et al.*, 2006). This new model, referred to as phenotype switching, considers metastatic potential split into two mutually exclusive and reversible states, proliferative and invasive, and hypothesizes that melanoma progression is driven by the reversible switching between these two phenotypes (Hoek, 2009). A primary lesion would be initially composed of proliferative phenotype cells. Signals from the microenvironment, such as hypoxia or inflammation, would make some cells switch their gene signature to become invasive, which would allow them to escape from the primary tumor and eventually reach and colonize a foreign distant organ. There, signals from the new environment would reprogram cells back to the proliferative signature, ultimately developing metastases (Carreira *et al.*, 2006; Goodall *et al.*, 2008; Hoek *et al.*, 2008).

The phenotype switching model also relies on human melanoma high plasticity and ability to be reprogrammed. As mentioned before, an example of the high plasticity of melanoma cells is vasculogenic mimicry (Seftor *et al.*, 2002). Some aggressive melanoma cells have been found to express molecular markers typical of other cell types, such as endothelial cells, which presumably allow melanoma cells to form vasculogenic networks that mimic blood vessels, and that could serve as an alternative route of escape for melanoma cells. This phenomenon has also been reported to occur *in vivo* in aggressive human melanoma samples, and correlates with poor outcome (Folberg *et al.*, 2000; Hendrix *et al.*, 2003; Maniotis *et al.*, 1999). Furthermore, poorly aggressive melanoma cells can be reprogrammed to highly aggressive and invasive by exposing them to matrices preconditioned by more aggressive melanoma cells, highlighting the importance of the tumor microenvironment in driving melanoma progression (Postovit *et al.*, 2006; Seftor *et al.*, 2006).

### 3.2 Melanoma invasion

Primary melanoma patients can be usually cured by surgical removal of the tumor when detected early, but most of the times melanoma rapidly metastasizes with a poor outcome (Gray-Schopfer *et al.*, 2007). Therefore it is essential to understand the mechanisms by which melanoma cells escape from the primary tumor and spread and invade other organs, in order to develop improved therapies that increase patient survival rates. Following there is a brief summary detailing some key molecules involved in melanoma migration/invasion and metastasis; interested readers are suggested to read topic reviews elsewhere (Gaggioli and Sahai, 2007; Uong and Zon, 2010).

MITF plays a pivotal role in melanocyte and melanoma biology, as it is involved not only in the control of migration and invasion, but also in proliferation, survival, and differentiation of melanocytic cells (Levy *et al.*, 2006). The fine tuning of MITF activity enables melanoma cells to switch between a proliferative (high MITF) or invasive (low MITF) state, while very high levels promote differentiation and complete absence of MITF is incompatible with survival (Carreira *et al.*, 2006; Gray-Schopfer *et al.*, 2007).

Additionally, a number of growth factors and cytokines are upregulated as melanoma becomes more invasive, such as hepatocyte growth factor (HGF), TGF-β, IL-8, Nodal and several members of fibroblast growth factor (FGF) family (al-Alousi *et al.*, 1996; Albino *et al.*, 1991; Topczewska *et al.*, 2006). In addition to the autocrine effect on melanoma cells themselves upregulating cell motility genes, these factors are thought to have also paracrine pro-invasive effects, since they can signal to other cell types of the microenvironment, such as fibroblasts, to produce more pro-invasive molecules, like tenascin C and HGF (De Wever *et al.*, 2004). On the other hand, HGF receptor c-Met has also been shown to have pro-invasive effects in melanocytes and melanoma cells (McGill *et al.*, 2006).

Melanoma inhibitory activity (MIA) protein is highly expressed in malignant melanomas but not in melanocytes (Bosserhoff, 2005). Several studies have shown that MIA enhances melanocyte and melanoma migration and invasion (Tatzel *et al.*, 2005), and additionally have suggested a central role for MIA in early melanoma development by regulating important melanoma-related pathways (Bosserhoff, 2005).

The Snail family transcription factors Snail and Slug have also increased activity in melanoma, since they downregulate the expression of keratinocyte-interacting surface molecules, such as E-cadherin and occluding, while upregulate N-cadherin, favoring interaction with stromal cells and not keratinocytes (Gaggioli and Sahai, 2007; Kajita *et al.*, 2004). Furthermore, Snail co-ordinately upregulates the expression of cell motility genes including matrix metalloproteinase (MMP)- 2, secreted protein acidic and rich in cysteine (SPARC), tissue inhibitor of metalloproteinases 1 (TIMP-1) and RhoA (Kuphal *et al.*, 2005).

Recently several studies have highlighted that melanoma cells also display a high plasticity regarding their cell motility. Melanoma cells can migrate and invade with different modes of movement that presumably allow them to adapt to varying microenvironments (Sahai and Marshall, 2003; Sanz-Moreno *et al.*, 2008). The main switches of these melanoma cell motility programs are Rho-GTPases family members Rac and Rho (Sanz-Moreno et al., 2008), which are overexpressed in cancer (Sahai, 2005). Rac promotes a more elongated shape that requires matrix metalloproteinases in order to invade, while RhoA favors a rounded morphology and a movement less dependent on proteases (Sanz-Moreno *et al.*, 2008). On the other hand, MMPs are upregulated in invasive melanoma and they are thought to promote melanoma dissemination, probably through different mechanisms since different MMPs are thought to have pro- or anti-invasive effects (Overall and Lopez-Otin, 2002).

### 3.3 PEDF as a brake for melanoma progression

As previously mentioned, the antiangiogenic activity of PEDF prompted the study of its potential antitumor effects. We (Fernandez-Garcia *et al.*, 2007; Garcia *et al.*, 2004) and others (Abe et al., 2004; Doll et al., 2003; Ek et al., 2006b) described a complex mechanism underlying the potent inhibition of melanoma metastasis by PEDF. PEDF's antitumor activity in melanoma and other tumors is based on its dual action on the tumor microenvironment and on the tumor cells themselves (Fernandez-Garcia *et al.*, 2007). PEDF inhibits tumor angiogenesis by means of induction of apoptosis on endothelial cells and modulation of the angiogenic profile of melanoma cells, eventually destroying the main source of nutrients to the primary tumor as well as one of the main routes of dissemination to distant organs. Additionally, PEDF exerts a potent inhibitory action on melanoma cells, inducing apoptosis under stress conditions (such as absence of growth factors or detachment from the extracellular matrix) and abrogating migration and invasion. As a whole, PEDF overexpression in melanoma cells leads to a decrease in primary tumor growth and an inhibition of lung metastasis formation (Fernandez-Garcia *et al.*, 2007; Filleur *et al.*, 2009).
In the previous section we described that PEDF is produced by low aggressive melanomas. Given that cutaneous melanoma develops from skin melanocytes, two questions soon arise: i) are normal melanocytes expressing this factor endogenously?, ii) if so, which could be the role of PEDF in normal melanocytic cells? By means of assessing a large collection of primary cultures of cutaneous melanocytes and other cell types of the skin we found that melanocytes secrete very high levels of PEDF comparable to other cell types known to express this factor (Orgaz *et al.*, 2009). In agreement with previous reports, dermal fibroblasts also express high levels of PEDF, which has been described to be involved in the control of their proliferative potential (Francis *et al.*, 2004; Tresini *et al.*, 1999); additionally, PEDF secreted by fibroblasts could also play a role in maintaining a correct vascularization of the skin. In contrast, PEDF is expressed at very low levels by epidermal keratinocytes or microvascular endothelial cells (Orgaz *et al.*, 2009).
In melanocytes, PEDF is one of the players involved in the regulation of their proliferation and migratory ability (Fig. 1). PEDF silencing in primary melanocytes leads to an increase in their migration and invasion, as well as a moderate augment in their growth rate (Orgaz *et al.*, 2009). Melanocytes arise from highly migratory embryonic neural crest progenitors, and therefore display an enormous migratory potential (Gupta *et al.*, 2005; Zbytek *et al.*, 2008) that must be tightly controlled in the skin (Hsu *et al.*, 2002). In addition to the regulatory signals from adjacent keratinocytes, an additional brake to their uncontrolled dissemination could be self-imposed within melanocytes by expressing high levels of PEDF themselves. As suggested for the fibroblasts, melanocytes could be also participating in the maintenance of appropriate angiogenesis in the skin by secreting this potent antiangiogenic factor, taking into account previous studies reporting an excessive vascularization of multiple organs upon PEDF knockdown (Doll *et al.*, 2003). Additional paracrine actions on other cell types, keratinocytes for instance, remain to be investigated.

Importantly, recent evidence points to a possible role of PEDF in melanocytic lineage-specific functions, such as pigment production. Melanocytes utilize specialized membrane vesicles called melanosomes to synthesize, store and deliver melanin to the cell membrane, eventually being transferred to surrounding keratinocytes (Barral and Seabra, 2004; Lin and Fisher, 2007). In a recent study we have found that PEDF overexpression in melanoma cell lines modulates the expression of Rab27A and melanophilin, two regulators of melanosome trafficking and melanin transfer (Orgaz *et al.*, 2011). Accordingly, previous reports had proposed the involvement of PEDF in pigment production, as PEDF was found in immature melanosomes of melanoma cells (Chi *et al.*, 2006) and it was also shown to induce tyrosinase expression (Abul-Hassan *et al.*, 2000) and melanosome maturation in RPE cells (Malchiodi-Albedi *et al.*, 1998). However, further studies are warranted in order to elucidate the functional role of PEDF in melanin production and/or secretion.

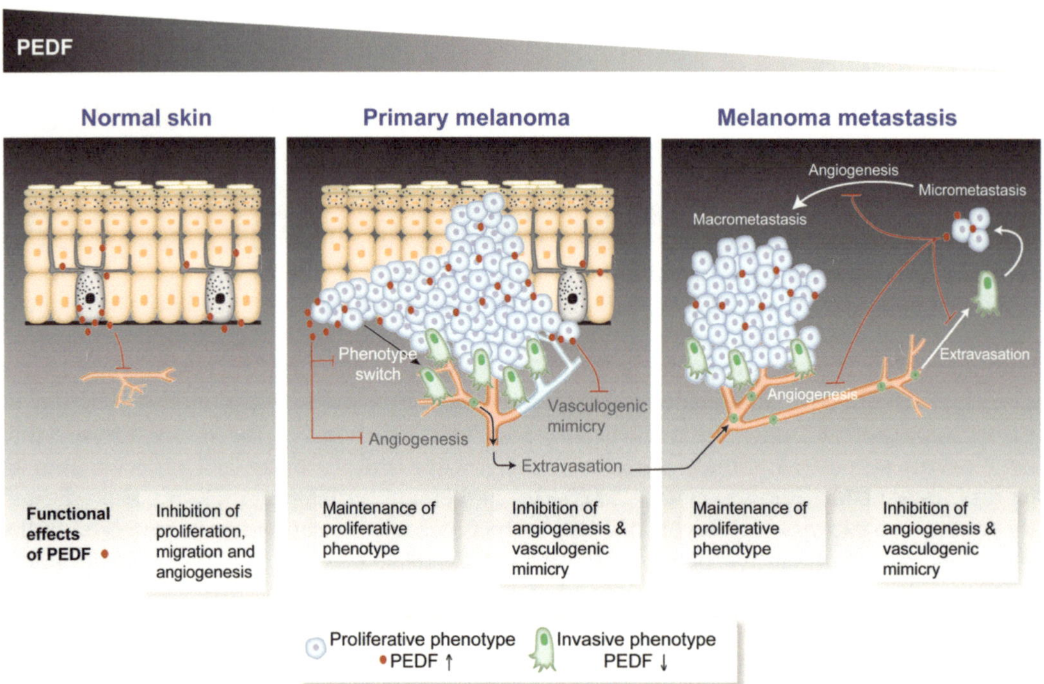


Fig. 1. Regulation of expression of PEDF during melanoma progression and functional effects in melanocytes and melanoma cells. Skin melanocytes express high levels of PEDF, which contribute to restrict their migratory and proliferative ability, and to regulate skin vascularization. In melanoma, PEDF expression is regulated by yet unidentified mechanisms that determine high levels in proliferative phenotype cells, and low levels in invasive phenotype cells. Melanoma progression is driven by switching between proliferative and invasive phenotypes, which involves reprogramming of PEDF and heterogeneous expression of this factor in primary and metastatic melanomas

The high expression of PEDF in skin melanocytes and its antitumor effects in melanoma raise the question whether PEDF expression could be modulated during melanoma development as it takes place in other types of cancer. However, defining melanoma progression is a complex task. Therefore, we utilized different approaches in order to interrogate levels of PEDF during melanoma malignization (Orgaz *et al.*, 2009). When taking into account histopathological criteria (classical model of melanoma progression), PEDF expression is greatly diminished or lost in metastasis-derived melanoma cell lines compared to cell lines established from RGP or VGP tumors, even though we found a significant variability in PEDF levels across melanoma cell lines. Accordingly, PEDF expression is lower in metastatic melanoma biopsies compared to primary melanomas (Orgaz *et al.*, 2009; and unpublished data) (Fig. 1).

This first analysis was expanded taking advantage of the vast collection of publicly available gene expression data from large series of melanoma cell lines and primary cultures of melanocytes. Firstly, we confirmed the downregulation of PEDF expression in melanoma compared to primary melanocytes (Fig. 1) (Hoek, 2007; Orgaz *et al.*, 2009). When classifying a number of series of melanoma cell lines regarding their gene expression profile into proliferative or invasive phenotype, we found that there is a significant decrease of PEDF expression in invasive phenotype melanoma cell lines. This suggests again an inverse correlation between melanoma aggressiveness and invasiveness, and expression levels of PEDF (Orgaz *et al.*, 2009).

Furthermore, expression of PEDF is subject to certain plasticity and can be reprogrammed during the metastatic progression of melanoma. We utilized paired cell lines isolated from the same metastasis of a cutaneous melanoma patient, and that display extreme phenotypes, poorly or highly aggressive (Seftor *et al.*, 2005). Only the poorly aggressive melanoma cell line expresses PEDF at high levels comparable to those of melanocytes, while it is undetectable in the highly aggressive cell line. The heterogeneity of PEDF expression is also found *in vivo* when analyzed in biopsies from dermal or lymph node melanoma metastases. Most of the biopsies from metastases are negative for PEDF, but when positive they display a heterogeneous staining pattern of PEDF expression (Orgaz *et al.*, 2009). Both observations strongly suggest that PEDF expression could be reprogrammed during the metastatic process in melanoma, in the context of the phenotype switching model, being expressed only by the poorly aggressive subpopulation of tumor cells (Fig. 1). Regulatory signals from the tumor microenvironment could be responsible, at least in part, for this switching in PEDF expression. As an example, primary melanocytes grown on collagen matrix preconditioned by a highly aggressive melanoma cell line display decreased PEDF expression levels compared to melanocytes grown on untreated matrix (Seftor *et al.*, 2005).

The inverse correlation between melanoma aggressiveness and PEDF expression raises additional important questions. Firstly, what is the functional significance of PEDF modulation during melanoma progression? We addressed this by silencing endogenous PEDF expression in several melanoma cell lines utilizing short hairpin RNAs specific to PEDF delivered by lentiviral transduction. As in melanocytes, endogenous PEDF restricts the migratory and invasive ability of melanoma cells, which greatly translates *in vivo*: we found that PEDF inhibits spontaneous lung colonization by melanoma cells as well as formation of spontaneous lung metastases from a primary tumor (Orgaz *et al.*, 2009). Inhibition of spontaneous metastases formation by PEDF is particularly noteworthy, since it highlights that this factor also restricts the initial steps of the metastatic cascade, local invasiveness from the primary tumor and intravasation. Additionally, PEDF impinges on vasculogenic mimicry ability of melanoma cells (Fig. 1), diminishing the formation of vasculogenic networks by melanoma cells both *in vitro* on collagen matrices and *in vivo* in the lung parenchyma after tail vein injection into immunocompromised mice (Orgaz *et al.*, 2009).

Therefore, in the model that we propose reprogramming of PEDF expression is important for the switching between proliferative and invasive phenotypes that are thought to drive metastatic progression of melanoma. Unknown mechanisms so far determine that PEDF expression is high in proliferative phenotype primary tumor cells, where it restricts migratory and invasive abilities, angiogenic potential and vasculogenic mimicry, as a whole leading to a diminished metastatic potential. However, loss of PEDF helps melanoma cells to acquire an invasive phenotype essential to disseminate and colonize distant organs. There, some metastatic cells would be reprogrammed by signals from the new microenvironment toward proliferative phenotype cells, switching back to express PEDF again. Eventually these cells will develop micrometastases and macrometastases, where additional reprogramming events will take place leading to a metastatic lesion heterogeneous for PEDF expression. Additionally, mechanisms yet to be described determine a loss of PEDF expression in fully developed melanoma metastases (Fig. 1).

Despite the knowledge we have gathered regarding PEDF modulation in melanoma, important questions still remain to be resolved. First of all, which are the regulators of PEDF during melanoma progression? Elucidating the mechanisms that promote or repress PEDF expression would help better understand how PEDF changes in the course of transformation and malignant progression of melanoma. Our results suggest that PEDF expression could be modulated by two general types of mechanisms, reprogramming events and loss of expression.

Assessing PEDF expression during maturation and migration of neural crest precursors toward epidermis could allow investigating the relationship between migratory potential and differentiation state and PEDF expression in a physiological context. Eventually this could also help identify possible factors involved in reprogramming PEDF in the different environments that neural crest precursors encounter in their way toward epidermis. Some of these factors are likely to be responsible for modulating PEDF expression in melanoma cells, given that tumor cells frequently activate signaling pathways and utilize regulatory mechanisms typical of progenitor cells.

Signals from the microenvironment such as hypoxia and inflammation are thought to reprogram and switch melanoma cells toward an invasive phenotype, and therefore, could be responsible for the downregulation of PEDF during melanoma progression. As a matter of a fact, earlier reports described that PEDF expression is decreased by hypoxia in retinoblastoma (Dawson *et al.*, 1999) and RPE (Notari *et al.*, 2005). Additionally, transcription factors that drive and are at the core of each phenotype gene signature could be direct regulators of PEDF expression. MITF is an appealing candidate, since it is a key factor in melanoma and melanocyte biology (Levy *et al.*, 2006) with anti-invasive effects and whose expression is tightly associated with the proliferative phenotype (Carreira *et al.*, 2006; Hoek *et al.*, 2008). Similar to PEDF, some studies have reported a trend toward loss of MITF expression in metastases compared to primary melanomas (Carreira *et al.*, 2006; Goodall *et al.*, 2008).

Additionally, genetic and epigenetic mechanisms could lead to a loss of PEDF expression as melanoma evolves to metastatic. The expression of a number of angiogenesis regulators in cancer is controlled by gain of expression of oncogenes and loss of tumor suppressors (Bouck, 1990). PEDF is a direct target of p53-related p63 and p73 proteins in colorectal carcinoma (Sasaki *et al.*, 2005). In melanoma, TA-p73 isoform has been recently described to inhibit anchor independent growth through KCNK1 protein, whose expression decreases in melanoma compared to normal skin (Beitzinger *et al.*, 2008). Therefore it would be interesting to assess whether p73 is implicated in regulating PEDF expression during melanoma progression. Human melanomas display either oncogenic NRAS (20% melanomas) or BRAF (50-70%), thought to be responsible of the initial transformation of melanocytes, uncoupling cell growth from external mitogenic stimuli (Chin, 2003; Chin *et al.*, 2006). However, by means of an analysis of publicly available microarray data from melanoma cell lines, we did not observe a significant correlation between PEDF expression levels and BRAF or NRAS mutation status (unpublished data). Finally, loss of expression of PEDF could occur upon epigenetic silencing of its promoter. Maspin, another member of Serpin family with anti-invasive and anti-tumor activities, is expressed at high levels in melanocytes but it is silenced in naevi and melanomas by epigenetic mechanisms (Denk *et al.*, 2007).

Although molecular aspects of the mechanism of action of PEDF on endothelial cells or neural derived cells have been described little is known about the molecular mechanisms underlying PEDF´s actions in melanoma, particularly in the inhibition of invasion and metastasis.

Interestingly, a recent study by us utilizing a gene expression analysis upon PEDF overexpression in melanoma cell lines has started to reveal some factors and pathways that could be mediating PEDF antimetastatic effects (Orgaz *et al.*, 2011). PEDF downregulates several key promigratory and proangiogenic factors such as IL-8, TGF-α and TGF-β, as well as a number of proteases and extracellular matrix proteins, like collagen IV, that could account for the lesser invasive ability and angiogenic potential of melanoma cells expressing PEDF. Additionally, PEDF modulates genes previously involved in melanoma progression toward a trend in agreement with decreased aggressiveness and invasiveness, such as factors from the Notch (Pinnix and Herlyn, 2007) or Wnt (Weeraratna, 2005) pathways, as well as FGF13 (Hoek *et al.*, 2004), insuling-like growth factor binding protein 3 (IGFBP3) (Xi *et al.*, 2006) or inhibin beta A (INHBA) (Hoek *et al.*, 2006), among many others. Interestingly, a number of melanoma markers with increased levels upon melanoma malignization are predominantly downregulated by PEDF overexpression, such as MIA or S100-β (Deichmann *et al.*, 1999; Utikal *et al.*, 2007).

## 4. Therapeutic applications of pigment epithelium derived-factor

### 4.1 Biochemical features of PEDF

Therapeutic applications of PEDF are closely related to the cellular niches where this factor is produced and to the multiplicity of cellular functions and activities ascribed to this secreted serpin family member.

SERPINs are a large superfamily of genes that codes for serine protease inhibitors in mammals (Tombran-Tink *et al.*, 2005). These proteins are able to control several processes such as blood coagulation, complement activation and extracellular matrix remodelling (Filleur *et al.*, 2009; Tombran-Tink *et al.*, 2005). However, there is a small number of serpin family members with non-inhibitory protease activity, among which is included PEDF (*SERPINF1*) (Becerra *et al.*, 1995; Lawrence *et al.*, 1990; Steele *et al.*, 1993). The inhibitory activity against proteinases resides in a domain called reactive centre loop (RCL). The reason why PEDF lacks protease inhibitory capability is due to the presence in the RCL of several proline residues preceding the cleavage site (Simonovic *et al.*, 2001).

Amino acid analyses indicate that PEDF shares considerable sequence homology with other members of the serpin family (Steele *et al.*, 1993); however, residues 40-67, at the N-terminal

(N-ter) region, and residues 277-301 at C-terminal (C-ter) are specific to PEDF. This feature suggests that these residues could be involved in maintaining the distinct structure of PEDF in these regions or in determining specific functions of this non-inhibitory serpin (Tombran-Tink *et al.*, 2005; Xu *et al.*, 2006). Tombran-Tink and collaborators also compared sequence homology of PEDF protein among different species and analyzed structural homology. They found a high degree of conservation in the leader sequence, responsible for protein secretion, a C-ter glycosilation site, and four specific regions: two domains present at N-ter region, corresponding to residues 40-67 and 78-95; and other two regions, 277-301 and 384-415, located at C-ter of the protein (Tombran-Tink *et al.*, 2005).

PEDF was initially isolated from conditioned medium of human fetal RPE cells and identified as a neurotrophic factor (Tombran-Tink and Johnson, 1989), although further studies showed that it is widely expressed throughout fetal and adult tissues (Ek *et al.*, 2006b). This broad expression is suggestive of a general and relevant function of PEDF in mammals. PEDF is also known as EPC-1 (early population doubling cDNA-1), and has been shown to participate in cell cycle regulation, initially in fibroblasts (Pignolo *et al.*, 1993; Tombran-Tink and Johnson, 1989; Tombran-Tink *et al.*, 1995) and later in other cell types like endothelial cells (Duh *et al.*, 2002; Hutchings *et al.*, 2002). PEDF's cell cycle regulatory function requires the presence of a putative nuclear localization sequence (residues 141-151) that is highly conserved in *SERPINF1* among different species, and could mediate PEDF translocation to the nucleus (Tombran-Tink *et al.*, 2005). One of the most relevant functional characteristics of PEDF is its antiangiogenic activity, being considered as the most potent natural inhibitor of physiological and pathological angiogenesis (Dawson *et al.*, 1999). PEDF is also a very effective neurotrophic factor that induces cell differentiation, cell survival, and protection from cell death in many cell types of the nervous system. PEDF prevents degeneration of retinal neurons that are exposed to transient ischemic reperfusion (Ogata *et al.*, 2001), and also protects other regions of the brain and spinal cord from the damaging effects caused by oxidative stress and glutamate toxicity (Bilak *et al.*, 1999; Cao *et al.*, 1999; DeCoster *et al.*, 1999; Taniwaki *et al.*, 1995). It has been shown the implication of NFkB in all these processes, which induces the expression of neurotrophic factors and anti-apoptotic genes that participate in the control of cell survival, proliferation and death (Barnstable and Tombran-Tink, 2004; Yabe *et al.*, 2001). Neurotrophic activity has been mapped to the N-ter region of PEDF, encompassing residues $Val^{58}$-$Thr^{101}$ (Simonovic *et al.*, 2001). This region is involved in binding to a putative plasma membrane receptor in cerebellar granule neurons and retinoblastoma cells (Alberdi *et al.*, 1999). PEDF is also secreted by ependymal and endothelial cells from the subventricular zone of the brain, where it promotes the self-renewal of adult neural stem cells (Andreu-Agullo *et al.*, 2009; Ramirez-Castillejo *et al.*, 2006). Furthermore, PEDF presents three phosphorylation sites located in $Ser^{24}$, $Ser^{114}$ and $Ser^{227}$, and the regulation of their phosphorylation state modulates the switch of PEDF's function from neurotrophic ($Ser^{24}$ and $Ser^{114}$ phosphorylated) to angiangiogenic ($Ser^{227}$ phosphorylated) (Becerra, 2006).

In order to better understand the mechanism of action of PEDF, it was necessary to identify the structural domains responsible for each of its described biological functions. Two major epitopes were identified at the N-ter region of PEDF: 34-mer peptide (residues 24-57) responsible of the antiangiogenic and pro-apoptotic actions of PEDF; and a second epitope, 44-mer peptide (residues 58-101), which induces neuronal differentiation of retinoblastoma cells (Filleur *et al.*, 2005) and plays a neurotrophic role in many neuronal cell types (Bilak *et al.*, 2002). There are another two highly conserved smaller epitopes, one upstream 34-mer, the TGA epitope, and an internal fragment of 44-mer, referred to as ERT. Filleur and collaborators showed *in vivo* that the epitopes TGA and the complete 34-mer inhibit tumor angiogenesis in prostate adenocarcinoma by inducing apoptosis of endothelial cells and blocking endothelial cell migration. Curiously, ERT despite of being located inside the neurotrophic 44-mer peptide, also presents antiangiogenic activity in prostate adenocarcinoma. Complete 44-mer is able to induce neurite outgrowth in Y-79 retinoblastoma cell line and causes apoptosis of endothelial cells, blocking migration and angiogenesis (Filleur *et al.*, 2005). In a more recent study, smaller regions of 34-mer epitope (named P14, P18 and P23, according to their respective length) were tested for angioinhibitory activity *in vitro* and *in vivo*. P14 and P23 display antiangiogenic activity *in vitro* (both blocking endothelial chemotaxis, and inducing apoptosis in the case of P23), but not *in vivo*; while P18 is a more potent antiangiogenic peptide than 34-mer in prostate cancer, being able to block bFGF and VEGF-dependent angiogenesis in the *in vivo* cornea neovascularisation assay (Mirochnik *et al.*, 2009). Another study by Ek and colleagues identified other small peptides with antitumoral activity in an orthotopic osteosarcoma model. They generated six 25-mer peptides along the functionally distinct regions of PEDF characterized so far. Residues 78-102 inhibit proliferation, whereas residues 90-114 stimulate adhesion of PEDF to type I collagen. Furthermore, residues 387 to 411 inhibit invasion of osteosarcoma cells *in vitro* and residues 40-64 promote osteogenic differentiation (Ek *et al.*, 2007).

The multifunctional character of PEDF and the evidence of the different roles displayed depending on the cell type, suggest that PEDF could be acting through distinct domains recognized by several specific receptors. The identification of these putative receptors and the characterization of the binding affinity of each functionally identified peptide toward them could make a breakthrough in the understanding of PEDF's mechanism of action and, therefore, the possibility of its therapeutic use in multiple pathological contexts.

### 4.2 PEDF receptors

Several studies have characterized the affinity of PEDF for the surface of human retinoblastoma cells, cerebellar granular neurons (Alberdi *et al.*, 1999), motor neurons (Bilak *et al.*, 2002), neural retina (Aymerich *et al.*, 2001) and endothelial cells (Yamagishi *et al.*, 2004). PEDF could be sequestered in the extracellular matrix based on ionic interactions with sulphated (heparin, heparin sulfate and condroitin sulfate) (Alberdi *et al.*, 1998), and non-sulfated (hyaluronan) (Becerra *et al.*, 2008) glycosaminglycans and type I collagen (Meyer *et al.*, 2002). In order to identify the potential receptor(s) of PEDF, Simonovic and collaborators carried out a three-dimensional study of PEDF, and identified an asymmetric charge distribution, with a high acidic region located at C-ter and basic amino acids at opposite region of PEDF protein (Simonovic *et al.*, 2001). This basic region is involved in the binding of PEDF to heparin through three clustered basic amino acid residues, $Lys^{146}$, $Lys^{147}$ and $Arg^{149}$. Moreover, $Asp^{256}$, $Asp^{258}$ and $Asp^{300}$ residues present in the acidic region of PEDF are crucial to type I collagen binding (Meyer *et al.*, 2002; Yasui *et al.*, 2003).

Using the 34-mer and 44-mer epitopes it was possible to propose the existence of two distinct putative receptors for PEDF. These epitopes are able to bind the surface of endothelial and prostate cells, but they do not compete for receptor binding (Filleur *et al.*, 2005). This result suggests the existence of two PEDF receptors with different functions: PEDF-$R^N$, that interacts with 44-mer epitope and regulates the neurotrophic and neuroprotective activities of PEDF; and PEDF-$R^A$, which is involved in blocking angiogenesis by binding to 34-mer epitope (Fig. 2). The differential expression of these two putative PEDF receptors in the diverse cell types analyzed supports the idea of distinct functions for each receptor type. PEDF-R^N^ is an 80-kDa receptor, which is located on the surface of human retinoblastoma cells, neural retina, cerebellar granular and motor neurons, whereas PEDF-R^A^ is a 60-kDa receptor specifically present on endothelial cells (Filleur *et al.*, 2009).

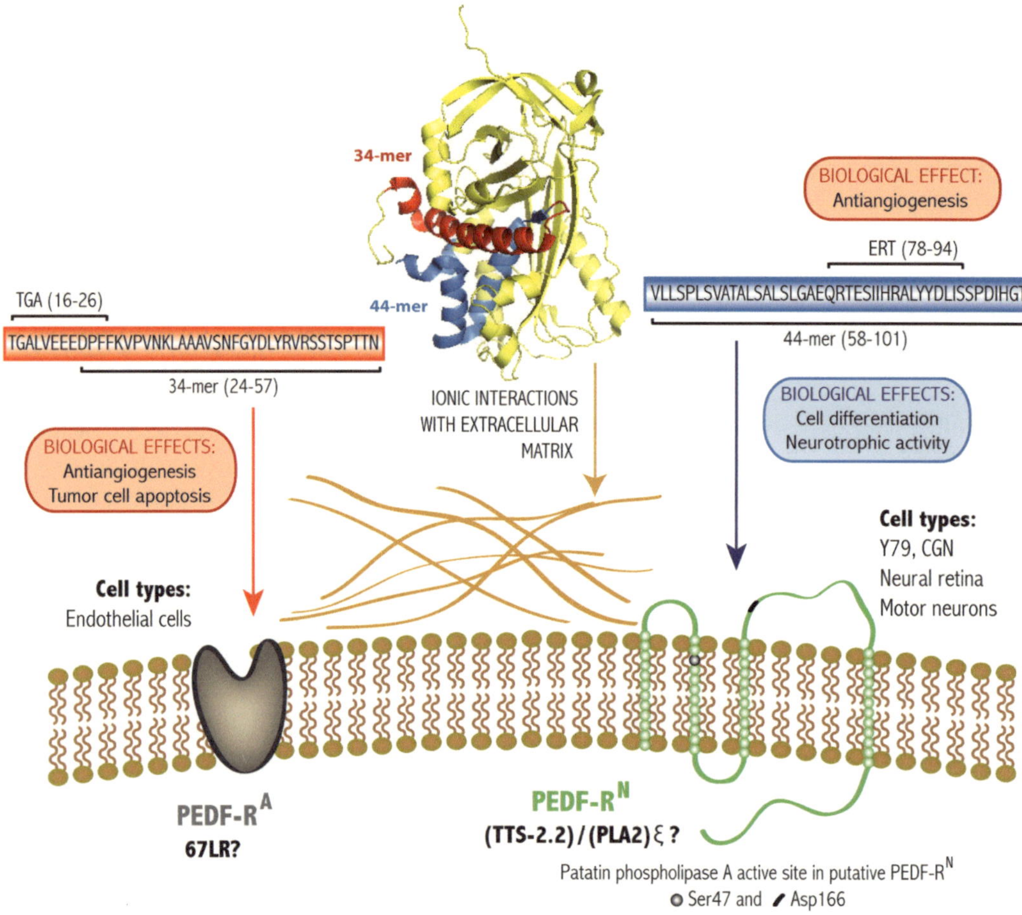


Fig. 2. Three-dimensional structure of PEDF, small peptides derived from PEDF and receptors. Crystal structure of PEDF molecule showing the location of 34-mer and 44-mer peptides. PEDF could be sequestered in the extracellular matrix by ionic interactions with type I collagen and glycosaminglycans. 34-mer, TGA and ERT peptides display antiangiogenic action through their bind to 60-kDa receptor (PEDF-R$^A$, proposed as the non-integrin 67-kDa laminin receptor) in endothelial cells. 34-mer also has the capability to induce apoptosis in tumor cells. 44-mer and ERT peptides present a neurotrophic action through their binding to the TTS-2.2/ (PLA2) ξ receptor (putatively identified as the PEDF-R$^N$) in several cell types. Abbreviations: 67LR: Non-Integrin 67-kDa laminin receptor; TTS-2.2/(PLA2)ξ: Transport secretion protein 2.2/Independent phospholipase $A_2$; Y79: human retinoblastoma cell line; CGN: cerebellar granular neurons

Further studies identified on the surface of the retina and human immortalized retinoblastoma cells (ARPE-19) the human Transport Secretion Protein 2-2 (TTS-2.2) /Independent phospholipase $A_2$ ($PLA_2$)ξ (also known in mice as adipose triglyceride lipase-ATGL, desnutrin, and patatin-like phospholipase domain containing protein-PNPLP2), an important lipase involved in triglyceride metabolism, as a specific PEDF receptor (Notari *et al.*, 2006). The phospholipase $A_2$ domain of this receptor releases bioactive fatty acids that function as second messengers. Therefore, depending on the lipid released, this receptor could activate different signal transduction pathways. It is still not fully demonstrated if the 80-kDa (PLA2)ξ receptor is the previously identified PEDF-$R^N$ receptor (Fig. 2).
Recently, a new receptor for PEDF has been identified, the non-integrin 67-kDa laminin receptor (67LR) (Bernard *et al.*, 2009), which may be related to the 60-kDa receptor previously reported in endothelial cells (Yamagishi *et al.*, 2004). This hypothesis is supported by the observation of antiangiogenic effects (inhibition of endothelial cell migration and induction of endothelial cell apoptosis) when 34-mer epitope binds to 67LR and the previously described 60-kDa receptor.
However, whether these characterized receptors are expressed on the surface of melanocytes and melanoma cells to mediate multiple PEDF's biological activities, and whether other unknown melanocytic lineage-specific receptors could play a role in translating PEDF's effects, remains to be investigated.

### 4.3 Therapeutic prospects for PEDF

During the last two decades many groups have described PEDF as a multifunctional protein that plays effective neuroprotective and antiangiogenic activities. The wide diversity of PEDF functions, along with the fact that it is an endogenous molecule, makes PEDF a unique candidate for a therapeutic agent in many diseases.
Several studies have already shown the role of PEDF in various pathological conditions such as ocular and chronic inflammatory diseases, atherosclerosis and diabetes. Moreover, several groups have demonstrated, *in vivo* and *in vitro*, the antitumor and antimetastatic potential of PEDF. They described the capability of PEDF to induce tumor cell differentiation in neuroblastoma (Crawford *et al.*, 2001) and prostate cancer (Filleur *et al.*, 2005); a direct tumor suppression action in osteosarcoma (Takenaka *et al.*, 2005), melanoma (Abe *et al.*, 2004; Garcia *et al.*, 2004) and prostate cancer (Filleur *et al.*, 2005; Guan *et al.*, 2007); and its angiostatic action in a wide number of tumor types that include, among others, melanoma (Abe *et al.*, 2004; Garcia *et al.*, 2004; Orgaz *et al.*, 2009; Yang and Grossniklaus, 2010).
The use of PEDF as a therapeutic agent in the clinic requires deeper knowledge of its biological effects and underlying molecular mediators. An important feature is the development of effective therapeutic agents based on the optimum combination of biological activities beneficial for each specific pathological context, together with the development of optimum delivery systems to allow proper targeting and stability during treatment. One of the possibilities is the use of recombinant full-length PEDF protein (rPEDF) produced in human embryonic kidney cells. Also, as PEDF is secreted at high levels by RPE cells, endogenous PEDF protein can be purified from the conditioned medium of RPEs. rPEDF has been successfully tested *in vitro* and *in vivo* in osteosarcoma (Takenaka *et al.*, 2005), prostate cancer (Doll *et al.*, 2003) and neuroblastoma (Crawford *et al.*, 2001). Due to its endogenous nature, short-term treatment would not lead to any immune response after systemic administration. However, the main disadvantage of this strategy is the susceptibility of rPEDF to cleavage by proteases, and therefore a limited bioavailability.

PEDF is a protein that is 418 amino acids in length. Filleur and collaborators elucidated that two small fragments of PEDF, 34-mer and 44-mer, were able to display the antiangiogenic and neurotrophic roles (respectively) as the complete protein (Filleur *et al.*, 2005). Shorter peptides improve the stability and delivery, and reduce the possibility of being recognized by the immune system. However, the use of rPEDF or small peptides derived from functionally active regions requires a systemic distribution; and therefore due to the antiangiogenic activity of this factor or derived peptides, its presence in plasma could have unexplored side effects on physiologic vascularization during the menstrual cycle and wound healing (Ek *et al.*, 2006a).

An alternative strategy that has been widely tested by a number of groups in mouse models of cancer is the use of viral vectors for the delivery of either full length PEDF or small peptides derived from the diverse functional regions identified. Gene transfer using viral or plasmid vectors is an attractive tool for human cancer gene therapy. Several studies have used this strategy in different types of cancer, such as pancreatic cancer (Hase *et al.*, 2005), neuroblastoma (Streck *et al.*, 2005), prostate cancer (Guan *et al.*, 2007) and melanoma (Abe *et al.*, 2004; Garcia *et al.*, 2004; Orgaz *et al.*, 2009; Yang and Grossniklaus, 2010), with a reduction of primary tumor size and number of metastases after PEDF delivery.

In melanoma, Abe's group and us were the first to describe the antitumor effect of PEDF *in vitro* and *in vivo* in malignant melanoma cell lines (Abe *et al.*, 2004; Garcia *et al.*, 2004). To this aim, Abe and collaborators overexpressed PEDF by transfection of G361 melanoma cell line and observed in nude mice a reduction of tumor angiogenesis and an almost complete inhibition of G361 growth in melanoma xenografts. These effects are the result of suppression of tumor angiogenesis and induction of Fas ligand-dependent apoptosis in tumor cells (Abe *et al.*, 2004). We used a retroviral strategy to transduce the human melanoma cell line UCD-Mel-N, which does not express significant levels of endogenous PEDF. We observed a considerable inhibition of primary tumor growth in subcutaneous xenotransplants in immunocompromised mice and a complete abrogation of lung metastases formation in the tail vein injection model. We demonstrated that the inhibition of primary melanoma tumor growth by PEDF is based on selective destruction of immature vessels, together with a significant direct induction of apoptosis in melanoma cells. Although it was first demonstrated that PEDF inhibits endothelial cell migration and induces apoptosis in remodelling endothelium, we showed that PEDF also has direct effects on melanoma cells, inhibiting melanoma cell migration and inducing apoptosis under stress conditions like absence of growth factors or detachment from the extracellular matrix (Garcia *et al.*, 2004). In a recent work we also used a lentiviral transduction strategy to silence PEDF in poorly aggressive melanoma cell lines with high expression of endogenous PEDF. PEDF knockdown in these melanoma cell lines enables the acquisition of an invasive phenotype, showing the critical importance of PEDF for the malignant progression of human melanoma (Orgaz *et al.*, 2009).

Retroviral and lentiviral vectors are attractive tools for human cancer gene therapy and, based on their ability to integrate into the genome, they have the potential to achieve long-term stable expression and maintain therapeutic levels of secreted peptides (Hase *et al.*, 2005). Both types of virus are able to transduce proliferating cells, although only lentiviruses present the advantage of transducing non-dividing cells. This feature is of great advantage for gene transfer as a complementary treatment in cancer, due to the fact that chemotherapy is only effective in actively proliferative cells, allowing non-dividing cells to be resistant to treatment and enabling the development of metastasis. Although viral systems seem to be a promising therapy for cancer and other diseases, there are still some problems and patient risks that have to be solved, such as (i) obtaining clinically effective viral titres, (ii) stable transgene expression in individuals requiring long-term treatment, and (iii) the risk of *de novo* cancer initiation via recombination within the patient's cell genome.

The biological effect of small peptides derived from PEDF retaining different functional activities has not yet been explored in melanoma, although it would be very relevant for the therapeutic development of PEDF in the context of aggressive melanoma. Also, characterization of PEDF's receptors expressed in melanoma cells is very important in order to understand the molecular mechanism of action underpinning the multiple biological actions of PEDF on melanoma cells, as well as to develop new therapeutic strategies based on the receptors and pathways that mediate PEDF's actions in aggressive melanoma.

## 5. Conclusions

Collectively, our findings strongly support PEDF as a potent biological modifier that effectively halts the metastatic spread of human melanoma by combining distinct functional epitopes respectively impinging on the vascular component of the tumor microenvironment and on the set of capabilities that a melanoma cell must acquire in order to successfully leave its primary site to colonize distant foreign environments.

## 6. Acknowledgment

Supported by grants Ministerio de Educacion y Ciencia SAF2007-62292 and SAF2010-19256 to BJ. AFB has been supported by a CSIC-JAE fellowship and JLO by a SAF2007-62292 contract.

## 7. References

Abe R., Shimizu T., Yamagishi S., Shibaki A., Amano S., Inagaki Y., Watanabe H., Sugawara H., Nakamura H., Takeuchi M., Imaizumi T., & Shimizu H. (2004). Overexpression of pigment epithelium-derived factor decreases angiogenesis and inhibits the growth of human malignant melanoma cells in vivo. *Am J Pathol* 164: 1225-32.

Abramson LP., Stellmach V., Doll JA., Cornwell M., Arensman RM., & Crawford SE. (2003). Wilms' tumor growth is suppressed by antiangiogenic pigment epithelium-derived factor in a xenograft model. *J Pediatr Surg* 38: 336-42; discussion 336-42.

Abul-Hassan K., Walmsley R., Tombran-Tink J., & Boulton M. (2000). Regulation of tyrosinase expression and activity in cultured human retinal pigment epithelial cells. *Pigment Cell Res* 13: 436-41.

al-Alousi S., Carlson JA., Blessing K., Cook M., Karaoli T., & Barnhill RL. (1996). Expression of basic fibroblast growth factor in desmoplastic melanoma. *J Cutan Pathol* 23: 118-25.

Alberdi E., Hyde CC., & Becerra SP. (1998). Pigment epithelium-derived factor (PEDF) binds to glycosaminoglycans: analysis of the binding site. *Biochemistry* 37: 10643-52.

Alberdi E., Aymerich MS., & Becerra SP. (1999). Binding of pigment epithelium-derived factor (PEDF) to retinoblastoma cells and cerebellar granule neurons. Evidence for a PEDF receptor. *J Biol Chem* 274: 31605-12.

Albino AP., Davis BM., & Nanus DM. (1991). Induction of growth factor RNA expression in human malignant melanoma: markers of transformation. *Cancer Res* 51: 4815-20.

Andreu-Agullo C., Morante-Redolat JM., Delgado AC., & Farinas I. (2009). Vascular niche factor PEDF modulates Notch-dependent stemness in the adult subependymal zone. *Nat Neurosci* 12: 1514-23.

Aurora AB., Biyashev D., Mirochnik Y., Zaichuk TA., Sanchez-Martinez C., Renault MA., Losordo D., & Volpert OV. (2010). NF-kappaB balances vascular regression and angiogenesis via chromatin remodeling and NFAT displacement. *Blood* 116: 475-84.

Aymerich MS., Alberdi EM., Martinez A., & Becerra SP. (2001). Evidence for pigment epithelium-derived factor receptors in the neural retina. *Invest Ophthalmol Vis Sci* 42: 3287-93.

Baluk P., Hashizume H., & McDonald DM. (2005). Cellular abnormalities of blood vessels as targets in cancer. *Curr Opin Genet Dev* 15: 102-11.

Barnstable CJ., & Tombran-Tink J. (2004). Neuroprotective and antiangiogenic actions of PEDF in the eye: molecular targets and therapeutic potential. *Prog Retin Eye Res* 23: 561-77.

Barral DC., & Seabra MC. (2004). The melanosome as a model to study organelle motility in mammals. *Pigment Cell Res* 17: 111-8.

Basu B., Biswas S., Wrigley J., Sirohi B., & Corrie P. (2009). Angiogenesis in cutaneous malignant melanoma and potential therapeutic strategies. *Expert Rev Anticancer Ther* 9: 1583-98.

Becerra SP., Sagasti A., Spinella P., & Notario V. (1995). Pigment epithelium-derived factor behaves like a noninhibitory serpin. Neurotrophic activity does not require the serpin reactive loop. *J Biol Chem* 270: 25992-9.

Becerra SP. (2006). Focus on Molecules: Pigment epithelium-derived factor (PEDF). *Exp Eye Res* 82: 739-40.

Becerra SP., Perez-Mediavilla LA., Weldon JE., Locatelli-Hoops S., Senanayake P., Notari L., Notario V., & Hollyfield JG. (2008). Pigment epithelium-derived factor binds to hyaluronan. Mapping of a hyaluronan binding site. *J Biol Chem* 283: 33310-20.

Bedogni B., & Powell MB. (2009). Hypoxia, melanocytes and melanoma - survival and tumor development in the permissive microenvironment of the skin. *Pigment Cell Melanoma Res* 22: 166-74.

Beitzinger M., Hofmann L., Oswald C., Beinoraviciute-Kellner R., Sauer M., Griesmann H., Bretz AC., Burek C., Rosenwald A., & Stiewe T. (2008). p73 poses a barrier to malignant transformation by limiting anchorage-independent growth. *Embo J* 27: 792-803.

Bergers G., & Hanahan D. (2008). Modes of resistance to anti-angiogenic therapy. *Nat Rev Cancer* 8: 592-603.

Bernard A., Gao-Li J., Franco CA., Bouceba T., Huet A., & Li Z. (2009). Laminin receptor involvement in the anti-angiogenic activity of pigment epithelium-derived factor. *J Biol Chem* 284: 10480-90.

Bilak MM., Corse AM., Bilak SR., Lehar M., Tombran-Tink J., & Kuncl RW. (1999). Pigment epithelium-derived factor (PEDF) protects motor neurons from chronic glutamate-mediated neurodegeneration. *J Neuropathol Exp Neurol* 58: 719-28.

Bilak MM., Becerra SP., Vincent AM., Moss BH., Aymerich MS., & Kuncl RW. (2002). Identification of the neuroprotective molecular region of pigment epithelium-derived factor and its binding sites on motor neurons. *J Neurosci* 22: 9378-86.

Bittner M., Meltzer P., Chen Y., Jiang Y., Seftor E., Hendrix M., Radmacher M., Simon R., Yakhini Z., Ben-Dor A., Sampas N., Dougherty E., Wang E., Marincola F., Gooden C., Lueders J., Glatfelter A., Pollock P., Carpten J., Gillanders E., Leja D., Dietrich K., Beaudry C., Berens M., Alberts D., & Sondak V. (2000). Molecular classification of cutaneous malignant melanoma by gene expression profiling. *Nature* 406: 536-40.

Bosserhoff AK. (2005). Melanoma inhibitory activity (MIA): an important molecule in melanoma development and progression. *Pigment Cell Res* 18: 411-6.

Bouck N. (1990). Tumor angiogenesis: the role of oncogenes and tumor suppressor genes. *Cancer Cells* 2: 179-85.

Bouck N. (2002). PEDF: anti-angiogenic guardian of ocular function. *Trends Mol Med* 8: 330-4.

Broadhead ML., Dass CR., & Choong PF. (2009). In vitro and in vivo biological activity of PEDF against a range of tumors. *Expert Opin Ther Targets* 13: 1429-38.

Cai J., Parr C., Watkins G., Jiang WG., & Boulton M. (2006). Decreased pigment epithelium-derived factor expression in human breast cancer progression. *Clin Cancer Res* 12: 3510-7.

Cao W., Tombran-Tink J., Chen W., Mrazek D., Elias R., & McGinnis JF. (1999). Pigment epithelium-derived factor protects cultured retinal neurons against hydrogen peroxide-induced cell death. *J Neurosci Res* 57: 789-800.

Carmeliet P. (2005). Angiogenesis in life, disease and medicine. *Nature* 438: 932-6.

Carreira S., Goodall J., Denat L., Rodriguez M., Nuciforo P., Hoek KS., Testori A., Larue L., & Goding CR. (2006). Mitf regulation of Dia1 controls melanoma proliferation and invasiveness. *Genes Dev* 20: 3426-39.

Chi A., Valencia JC., Hu ZZ., Watabe H., Yamaguchi H., Mangini NJ., Huang H., Canfield VA., Cheng KC., Yang F., Abe R., Yamagishi S., Shabanowitz J., Hearing VJ., Wu C., Appella E., & Hunt DF. (2006). Proteomic and bioinformatic characterization of the biogenesis and function of melanosomes. *J Proteome Res* 5: 3135-44.

Chin L. (2003). The genetics of malignant melanoma: lessons from mouse and man. *Nat Rev Cancer* 3: 559-70.

Chin L., Garraway LA., & Fisher DE. (2006). Malignant melanoma: genetics and therapeutics in the genomic era. *Genes Dev* 20: 2149-82.

Clark WH, Jr. (1991). Human cutaneous malignant melanoma as a model for cancer. *Cancer Metastasis Rev* 10: 83-88.

Crawford SE., Stellmach V., Ranalli M., Huang X., Huang L., Volpert O., De Vries GH., Abramson LP., & Bouck N. (2001). Pigment epithelium-derived factor (PEDF) in neuroblastoma: a multifunctional mediator of Schwann cell antitumor activity. *J Cell Sci* 114: 4421-8.

Dawson DW., Volpert OV., Gillis P., Crawford SE., Xu H., Benedict W., & Bouck NP. (1999). Pigment epithelium-derived factor: a potent inhibitor of angiogenesis. *Science* 285: 245-8.

De Wever O., Nguyen QD., Van Hoorde L., Bracke M., Bruyneel E., Gespach C., & Mareel M. (2004). Tenascin-C and SF/HGF produced by myofibroblasts in vitro provide convergent pro-invasive signals to human colon cancer cells through RhoA and Rac. *FASEB J* 18: 1016-8.

DeCoster MA., Schabelman E., Tombran-Tink J., & Bazan NG. (1999). Neuroprotection by pigment epithelial-derived factor against glutamate toxicity in developing primary hippocampal neurons. *J Neurosci Res* 56: 604-10.

Deichmann M., Benner A., Bock M., Jackel A., Uhl K., Waldmann V., & Naher H. (1999). S100-Beta, melanoma-inhibiting activity, and lactate dehydrogenase discriminate progressive from nonprogressive American Joint Committee on Cancer stage IV melanoma. *J Clin Oncol* 17: 1891-6.

Denk AE., Bettstetter M., Wild PJ., Hoek K., Bataille F., Dietmaier W., & Bosserhoff AK. (2007). Loss of maspin expression contributes to a more invasive potential in malignant melanoma. *Pigment Cell Res* 20: 112-9.

Doll JA., Stellmach VM., Bouck NP., Bergh AR., Lee C., Abramson LP., Cornwell ML., Pins MR., Borensztajn J., & Crawford SE. (2003). Pigment epithelium-derived factor regulates the vasculature and mass of the prostate and pancreas. *Nat Med* 9: 774-80.

Duh EJ., Yang HS., Suzuma I., Miyagi M., Youngman E., Mori K., Katai M., Yan L., Suzuma K., West K., Davarya S., Tong P., Gehlbach P., Pearlman J., Crabb JW., Aiello LP., Campochiaro PA., & Zack DJ. (2002). Pigment epithelium-derived factor suppresses ischemia-induced retinal neovascularization and VEGF-induced migration and growth. *Invest Ophthalmol Vis Sci* 43: 821-9.

Ek ET., Dass CR., & Choong PF. (2006a). PEDF: a potential molecular therapeutic target with multiple anti-cancer activities. *Trends Mol Med* 12: 497-502.

Ek ET., Dass CR., & Choong PF. (2006b). Pigment epithelium-derived factor: a multimodal tumor inhibitor. *Mol Cancer Ther* 5: 1641-6.

Ek ET., Dass CR., Contreras KG., & Choong PF. (2007). PEDF-derived synthetic peptides exhibit antitumor activity in an orthotopic model of human osteosarcoma. *J Orthop Res* 25: 1671-80.

Ellis LM., & Hicklin DJ. (2008). VEGF-targeted therapy: mechanisms of anti-tumour activity. *Nat Rev Cancer* 8: 579-91.

Fecher LA., Cummings SD., Keefe MJ., & Alani RM. (2007). Toward a molecular classification of melanoma. *J Clin Oncol* 25: 1606-20.

Fernandez-Garcia NI., Volpert OV., & Jimenez B. (2007). Pigment epithelium-derived factor as a multifunctional antitumor factor. *J Mol Med* 85: 15-22.

Ferrara N., & Kerbel RS. (2005). Angiogenesis as a therapeutic target. *Nature* 438: 967-74.

Filleur S., Volz K., Nelius T., Mirochnik Y., Huang H., Zaichuk TA., Aymerich MS., Becerra SP., Yap R., Veliceasa D., Shroff EH., & Volpert OV. (2005). Two functional epitopes of pigment epithelial-derived factor block angiogenesis and induce differentiation in prostate cancer. *Cancer Res* 65: 5144-52.

Filleur S., Nelius T., de Riese W., & Kennedy RC. (2009). Characterization of PEDF: a multi-functional serpin family protein. *J Cell Biochem* 106: 769-75.

Folberg R., Hendrix MJ., & Maniotis AJ. (2000). Vasculogenic mimicry and tumor angiogenesis. *Am J Pathol* 156: 361-81.

Folkman J. (2006). Angiogenesis. *Annu Rev Med* 57: 1-18.

Francis MK., Appel S., Meyer C., Balin SJ., Balin AK., & Cristofalo VJ. (2004). Loss of EPC-1/PEDF expression during skin aging in vivo. *J Invest Dermatol* 122: 1096-105.

Gaggioli C., & Sahai E. (2007). Melanoma invasion - current knowledge and future directions. *Pigment Cell Res* 20: 161-72.

Gao D., Nolan DJ., Mellick AS., Bambino K., McDonnell K., & Mittal V. (2008). Endothelial progenitor cells control the angiogenic switch in mouse lung metastasis. *Science* 319: 195-8.

Garcia M., Fernandez-Garcia NI., Rivas V., Carretero M., Escamez MJ., Gonzalez-Martin A., Medrano EE., Volpert O., Jorcano JL., Jimenez B., Larcher F., & Del Rio M. (2004). Inhibition of xenografted human melanoma growth and prevention of metastasis development by dual antiangiogenic/antitumor activities of pigment epithelium-derived factor. *Cancer Res* 64: 5632-42.

Goodall J., Carreira S., Denat L., Kobi D., Davidson I., Nuciforo P., Sturm RA., Larue L., & Goding CR. (2008). Brn-2 represses microphthalmia-associated transcription factor expression and marks a distinct subpopulation of microphthalmia-associated transcription factor-negative melanoma cells. *Cancer Res* 68: 7788-94.

Goss PE., & Chambers AF. (2010). Does tumour dormancy offer a therapeutic target? *Nat Rev Cancer* 10: 871-7.

Gray-Schopfer V., Wellbrock C., & Marais R. (2007). Melanoma biology and new targeted therapy. *Nature* 445: 851-7.

Guan M., Yam HF., Su B., Chan KP., Pang CP., Liu WW., Zhang WZ., & Lu Y. (2003). Loss of pigment epithelium derived factor expression in glioma progression. *J Clin Pathol* 56: 277-82.

Guan M., Jiang H., Xu C., Xu R., Chen Z., & Lu Y. (2007). Adenovirus-mediated PEDF expression inhibits prostate cancer cell growth and results in augmented expression of PAI-2. *Cancer Biol Ther* 6: 419-25.

Gupta PB., Kuperwasser C., Brunet JP., Ramaswamy S., Kuo WL., Gray JW., Naber SP., & Weinberg RA. (2005). The melanocyte differentiation program predisposes to metastasis after neoplastic transformation. *Nat Genet* 37: 1047-54.

Halin S., Wikstrom P., Rudolfsson SH., Stattin P., Doll JA., Crawford SE., & Bergh A. (2004). Decreased pigment epithelium-derived factor is associated with metastatic phenotype in human and rat prostate tumors. *Cancer Res* 64: 5664-71.

Halin S., Rudolfsson SH., Doll JA., Crawford SE., Wikstrom P., & Bergh A. (2010). Pigment epithelium-derived factor stimulates tumor macrophage recruitment and is downregulated by the prostate tumor microenvironment. *Neoplasia* 12: 336-45.

Hanahan D., & Weinberg RA. (2000). The hallmarks of cancer. *Cell* 100: 57-70.

Hanahan D., & Weinberg RA. (2011). Hallmarks of cancer: the next generation. *Cell* 144: 646-74.

Haqq C., Nosrati M., Sudilovsky D., Crothers J., Khodabakhsh D., Pulliam BL., Federman S., Miller JR, 3rd., Allen RE., Singer MI., Leong SP., Ljung BM., Sagebiel RW., & Kashani-Sabet M. (2005). The gene expression signatures of melanoma progression. *Proc Natl Acad Sci U S A* 102: 6092-7.

Hase R., Miyamoto M., Uehara H., Kadoya M., Ebihara Y., Murakami Y., Takahashi R., Mega S., Li L., Shichinohe T., Kawarada Y., & Kondo S. (2005). Pigment epithelium-derived factor gene therapy inhibits human pancreatic cancer in mice. *Clin Cancer Res* 11: 8737-44.

Helfrich I., Scheffrahn I., Bartling S., Weis J., von Felbert V., Middleton M., Kato M., Ergun S., & Schadendorf D. (2010). Resistance to antiangiogenic therapy is directed by vascular phenotype, vessel stabilization, and maturation in malignant melanoma. *J Exp Med* 207: 491-503.

Helfrich I., & Schadendorf D. (2011). Blood vessel maturation, vascular phenotype and angiogenic potential in malignant melanoma: One step forward for overcoming anti-angiogenic drug resistance? *Mol Oncol.*

Hendrix MJ., Seftor EA., Hess AR., & Seftor RE. (2003). Vasculogenic mimicry and tumour-cell plasticity: lessons from melanoma. *Nat Rev Cancer* 3: 411-21.

Hendrix MJ., Seftor EA., Seftor RE., Kasemeier-Kulesa J., Kulesa PM., & Postovit LM. (2007). Reprogramming metastatic tumour cells with embryonic microenvironments. *Nat Rev Cancer* 7: 246-55.

Hess AR., Margaryan NV., Seftor EA., & Hendrix MJ. (2007). Deciphering the signaling events that promote melanoma tumor cell vasculogenic mimicry and their link to embryonic vasculogenesis: role of the Eph receptors. *Dev Dyn* 236: 3283-96.

Hoek K., Rimm DL., Williams KR., Zhao H., Ariyan S., Lin A., Kluger HM., Berger AJ., Cheng E., Trombetta ES., Wu T., Niinobe M., Yoshikawa K., Hannigan GE., & Halaban R. (2004). Expression profiling reveals novel pathways in the transformation of melanocytes to melanomas. *Cancer Res* 64: 5270-82.

Hoek KS., Schlegel NC., Brafford P., Sucker A., Ugurel S., Kumar R., Weber BL., Nathanson KL., Phillips DJ., Herlyn M., Schadendorf D., & Dummer R. (2006). Metastatic potential of melanomas defined by specific gene expression profiles with no BRAF signature. *Pigment Cell Res* 19: 290-302.

Hoek KS. (2007). DNA microarray analyses of melanoma gene expression: a decade in the mines. *Pigment Cell Res* 20: 466-84.

Hoek KS., Eichhoff OM., Schlegel NC., Dobbeling U., Kobert N., Schaerer L., Hemmi S., & Dummer R. (2008). In vivo switching of human melanoma cells between proliferative and invasive states. *Cancer Res* 68: 650-6.

Hoek KS. (2009). Melanoma progression, gene expression and DNA microarrays. *G Ital Dermatol Venereol* 144: 39-49.

Hoshina D., Abe R., Yamagishi SI., & Shimizu H. (2010). The role of PEDF in tumor growth and metastasis. *Curr Mol Med* 10: 292-5.

Hsu MY., Meier F., & Herlyn M. (2002). Melanoma development and progression: a conspiracy between tumor and host. *Differentiation* 70: 522-36.

Hutchings H., Maitre-Boube M., Tombran-Tink J., & Plouet J. (2002). Pigment epithelium-derived factor exerts opposite effects on endothelial cells of different phenotypes. *Biochem Biophys Res Commun* 294: 764-9.

Jain RK. (2003). Molecular regulation of vessel maturation. *Nat Med* 9: 685-93.

Jain RK. (2008). Lessons from multidisciplinary translational trials on anti-angiogenic therapy of cancer. *Nat Rev Cancer* 8: 309-16.

Jimenez B., & Volpert OV. (2001). Mechanistic insights on the inhibition of tumor angiogenesis. *J Mol Med* 78: 663-72.

Jubb AM., Oates AJ., Holden S., & Koeppen H. (2006). Predicting benefit from anti-angiogenic agents in malignancy. *Nat Rev Cancer* 6: 626-35.

Kajita M., McClinic KN., & Wade PA. (2004). Aberrant expression of the transcription factors snail and slug alters the response to genotoxic stress. *Mol Cell Biol* 24: 7559-66.

Kerbel RS. (2008). Tumor angiogenesis. *N Engl J Med* 358: 2039-49.

Kopp HG., Ramos CA., & Rafii S. (2006). Contribution of endothelial progenitors and proangiogenic hematopoietic cells to vascularization of tumor and ischemic tissue. *Curr Opin Hematol* 13: 175-81.

Kuphal S., Palm HG., Poser I., & Bosserhoff AK. (2005). Snail-regulated genes in malignant melanoma. *Melanoma Res* 15: 305-13.

Laquer V., Hoang V., Nguyen A., & Kelly KM. (2009). Angiogenesis in cutaneous disease: part II. *J Am Acad Dermatol* 61: 945-58; quiz 959-60.

Lawrence DA., Strandberg L., Ericson J., & Ny T. (1990). Structure-function studies of the SERPIN plasminogen activator inhibitor type 1. Analysis of chimeric strained loop mutants. *J Biol Chem* 265: 20293-301.

Levy C., Khaled M., & Fisher DE. (2006). MITF: master regulator of melanocyte development and melanoma oncogene. *Trends Mol Med* 12: 406-14.

Lin JY., & Fisher DE. (2007). Melanocyte biology and skin pigmentation. *Nature* 445: 843-50.

Loges S., Roncal C., & Carmeliet P. (2009). Development of targeted angiogenic medicine. *J Thromb Haemost* 7: 21-33.

Lomuto M., Calabrese P., & Giuliani A. (2004). Prognostic signs in melanoma: state of the art. *J Eur Acad Dermatol Venereol* 18: 291-300.

Mahabeleshwar GH., & Byzova TV. (2007). Angiogenesis in melanoma. *Semin Oncol* 34: 555-65.

Malchiodi-Albedi F., Feher J., Caiazza S., Formisano G., Perilli R., Falchi M., Petrucci TC., Scorcia G., & Tombran-Tink J. (1998). PEDF (pigment epithelium-derived factor) promotes increase and maturation of pigment granules in pigment epithelial cells in neonatal albino rat retinal cultures. *Int J Dev Neurosci* 16: 423-32.

Maniotis AJ., Folberg R., Hess A., Seftor EA., Gardner LM., Pe'er J., Trent JM., Meltzer PS., & Hendrix MJ. (1999). Vascular channel formation by human melanoma cells in vivo and in vitro: vasculogenic mimicry. *Am J Pathol* 155: 739-52.

Matsumoto K., Ishikawa H., Nishimura D., Hamasaki K., Nakao K., & Eguchi K. (2004). Antiangiogenic property of pigment epithelium-derived factor in hepatocellular carcinoma. *Hepatology* 40: 252-9.

McGill GG., Haq R., Nishimura EK., & Fisher DE. (2006). c-Met expression is regulated by Mitf in the melanocyte lineage. *J Biol Chem* 281: 10365-73.

Meyer C., Notari L., & Becerra SP. (2002). Mapping the type I collagen-binding site on pigment epithelium-derived factor. Implications for its antiangiogenic activity. *J Biol Chem* 277: 45400-7.

Michaloglou C., Vredeveld LC., Soengas MS., Denoyelle C., Kuilman T., van der Horst CM., Majoor DM., Shay JW., Mooi WJ., & Peeper DS. (2005). BRAFE600-associated senescence-like cell cycle arrest of human naevi. *Nature* 436: 720-4.

Miller AJ., & Mihm MC, Jr. (2006). Melanoma. *N Engl J Med* 355: 51-65.

Mirochnik Y., Aurora A., Schulze-Hoepfner FT., Deabes A., Shifrin V., Beckmann R., Polsky C., & Volpert OV. (2009). Short pigment epithelial-derived factor-derived peptide inhibits angiogenesis and tumor growth. *Clin Cancer Res* 15: 1655-63.

Nguyen A., Hoang V., Laquer V., & Kelly KM. (2009a). Angiogenesis in cutaneous disease: part I. *J Am Acad Dermatol* 61: 921-42; quiz 943-4.

Nguyen DX., Bos PD., & Massague J. (2009b). Metastasis: from dissemination to organ-specific colonization. *Nat Rev Cancer* 9: 274-84.

Nico B., Benagiano V., Mangieri D., Maruotti N., Vacca A., & Ribatti D. (2008). Evaluation of microvascular density in tumors: pro and contra. *Histol Histopathol* 23: 601-7.

Notari L., Miller A., Martinez A., Amaral J., Ju M., Robinson G., Smith LE., & Becerra SP. (2005). Pigment epithelium-derived factor is a substrate for matrix metalloproteinase type 2 and type 9: implications for downregulation in hypoxia. *Invest Ophthalmol Vis Sci* 46: 2736-47.

Notari L., Baladron V., Aroca-Aguilar JD., Balko N., Heredia R., Meyer C., Notario PM., Saravanamuthu S., Nueda ML., Sanchez-Sanchez F., Escribano J., Laborda J., & Becerra SP. (2006). Identification of a lipase-linked cell membrane receptor for pigment epithelium-derived factor. *J Biol Chem* 281: 38022-37.

Nowell PC. (1976). The clonal evolution of tumor cell populations. *Science* 194: 23-8.

Ogata N., Wang L., Jo N., Tombran-Tink J., Takahashi K., Mrazek D., & Matsumura M. (2001). Pigment epithelium derived factor as a neuroprotective agent against ischemic retinal injury. *Curr Eye Res* 22: 245-52.

Orgaz JL., Martinez-Poveda B., Fernandez-Garcia NI., & Jimenez B. (2008). Following up tumour angiogenesis: from the basic laboratory to the clinic. *Clin Transl Oncol* 10: 468-77.

Orgaz JL., Ladhani O., Hoek KS., Fernandez-Barral A., Mihic D., Aguilera O., Seftor EA., Bernad A., Rodriguez-Peralto JL., Hendrix MJ., Volpert OV., & Jimenez B. (2009). 'Loss of pigment epithelium-derived factor enables migration, invasion and metastatic spread of human melanoma'. *Oncogene* 28: 4147-61.

Orgaz JL., Benguria A., Sanchez-Martinez C., Ladhani O., Volpert O., & Jimenez B. (2011). Changes in the gene expression profile of A375 human melanoma cells induced by over-expression of multifunctional pigment epithelium-derived factor. *Melanoma Res* In Press.

Overall CM., & Lopez-Otin C. (2002). Strategies for MMP inhibition in cancer: innovations for the post-trial era. *Nat Rev Cancer* 2: 657-72.

Pavey S., Johansson P., Packer L., Taylor J., Stark M., Pollock PM., Walker GJ., Boyle GM., Harper U., Cozzi SJ., Hansen K., Yudt L., Schmidt C., Hersey P., Ellem KA., O'Rourke MG., Parsons PG., Meltzer P., Ringner M., & Hayward NK. (2004). Microarray expression profiling in melanoma reveals a BRAF mutation signature. *Oncogene* 23: 4060-7.

Pignolo RJ., Cristofalo VJ., & Rotenberg MO. (1993). Senescent WI-38 cells fail to express EPC-1, a gene induced in young cells upon entry into the G0 state. *J Biol Chem* 268: 8949-57.

Pinnix CC., & Herlyn M. (2007). The many faces of Notch signaling in skin-derived cells. *Pigment Cell Res* 20: 458-65.

Postovit LM., Seftor EA., Seftor RE., & Hendrix MJ. (2006). Influence of the microenvironment on melanoma cell fate determination and phenotype. *Cancer Res* 66: 7833-6.

Qingyi Z., Lin Y., Junhong W., Jian S., Weizhou H., Long M., Zeyu S., & Xiaojian G. (2009). Unfavorable prognostic value of human PEDF decreased in high-grade prostatic intraepithelial neoplasia: a differential proteomics approach. *Cancer Invest* 27: 794-801.

Ramirez-Castillejo C., Sanchez-Sanchez F., Andreu-Agullo C., Ferron SR., Aroca-Aguilar JD., Sanchez P., Mira H., Escribano J., & Farinas I. (2006). Pigment epithelium-derived factor is a niche signal for neural stem cell renewal. *Nat Neurosci* 9: 331-9.

Rey S., & Semenza GL. (2010). Hypoxia-inducible factor-1-dependent mechanisms of vascularization and vascular remodelling. *Cardiovasc Res* 86: 236-42.

Ria R., Reale A., Castrovilli A., Mangialardi G., Dammacco F., Ribatti D., & Vacca A. (2010). Angiogenesis and progression in human melanoma. *Dermatol Res Pract* 2010: 185687.

Rofstad EK., Henriksen K., Galappathi K., & Mathiesen B. (2003). Antiangiogenic treatment with thrombospondin-1 enhances primary tumor radiation response and prevents growth of dormant pulmonary micrometastases after curative radiation therapy in human melanoma xenografts. *Cancer Res* 63: 4055-61.

Rofstad EK., Galappathi K., & Mathiesen B. (2004). Thrombospondin-1 treatment prevents growth of dormant lung micrometastases after surgical resection and curative radiation therapy of the primary tumor in human melanoma xenografts. *Int J Radiat Oncol Biol Phys* 58: 493-9.

Sahai E., & Marshall CJ. (2003). Differing modes of tumour cell invasion have distinct requirements for Rho/ROCK signalling and extracellular proteolysis. *Nat Cell Biol* 5: 711-9.

Sahai E. (2005). Mechanisms of cancer cell invasion. *Curr Opin Genet Dev* 15: 87-96.

Sanz-Moreno V., Gadea G., Ahn J., Paterson H., Marra P., Pinner S., Sahai E., & Marshall CJ. (2008). Rac activation and inactivation control plasticity of tumor cell movement. *Cell* 135: 510-23.

Sasaki Y., Naishiro Y., Oshima Y., Imai K., Nakamura Y., & Tokino T. (2005). Identification of pigment epithelium-derived factor as a direct target of the p53 family member genes. *Oncogene* 24: 5131-6.

Seftor EA., Meltzer PS., Schatteman GC., Gruman LM., Hess AR., Kirschmann DA., Seftor RE., & Hendrix MJ. (2002). Expression of multiple molecular phenotypes by aggressive melanoma tumor cells: role in vasculogenic mimicry. *Crit Rev Oncol Hematol* 44: 17-27.

Seftor EA., Brown KM., Chin L., Kirschmann DA., Wheaton WW., Protopopov A., Feng B., Balagurunathan Y., Trent JM., Nickoloff BJ., Seftor RE., & Hendrix MJ. (2005). Epigenetic transdifferentiation of normal melanocytes by a metastatic melanoma microenvironment. *Cancer Res* 65: 10164-9.

Seftor EA., Meltzer PS., Kirschmann DA., Margaryan NV., Seftor RE., & Hendrix MJ. (2006). The epigenetic reprogramming of poorly aggressive melanoma cells by a metastatic microenvironment. *J Cell Mol Med* 10: 174-96.

Shackleton M., & Quintana E. (2010). Progress in understanding melanoma propagation. *Mol Oncol* 4: 451-7.

Simonovic M., Gettins PG., & Volz K. (2001). Crystal structure of human PEDF, a potent anti-angiogenic and neurite growth-promoting factor. *Proc Natl Acad Sci U S A* 98: 11131-5.

Slingluff CL, Jr.., Vollmer RT., Reintgen DS., & Seigler HF. (1988). Lethal "thin" malignant melanoma. Identifying patients at risk. *Ann Surg* 208: 150-61.

Steele FR., Chader GJ., Johnson LV., & Tombran-Tink J. (1993). Pigment epithelium-derived factor: neurotrophic activity and identification as a member of the serine protease inhibitor gene family. *Proc Natl Acad Sci U S A* 90: 1526-30.

Streck CJ., Zhang Y., Zhou J., Ng C., Nathwani AC., & Davidoff AM. (2005). Adeno-associated virus vector-mediated delivery of pigment epithelium-derived factor restricts neuroblastoma angiogenesis and growth. *J Pediatr Surg* 40: 236-43.

Takenaka K., Yamagishi S., Jinnouchi Y., Nakamura K., Matsui T., & Imaizumi T. (2005). Pigment epithelium-derived factor (PEDF)-induced apoptosis and inhibition of vascular endothelial growth factor (VEGF) expression in MG63 human osteosarcoma cells. *Life Sci* 77: 3231-41.

Tammela T., & Alitalo K. (2010). Lymphangiogenesis: Molecular mechanisms and future promise. *Cell* 140: 460-76.

Taniwaki T., Becerra SP., Chader GJ., & Schwartz JP. (1995). Pigment epithelium-derived factor is a survival factor for cerebellar granule cells in culture. *J Neurochem* 64: 2509-17.

Tatzel J., Poser I., Schroeder J., & Bosserhoff AK. (2005). Inhibition of melanoma inhibitory activity (MIA) expression in melanoma cells leads to molecular and phenotypic changes. *Pigment Cell Res* 18: 92-101.

Tombran-Tink J., & Johnson LV. (1989). Neuronal differentiation of retinoblastoma cells induced by medium conditioned by human RPE cells. *Invest Ophthalmol Vis Sci* 30: 1700-7.

Tombran-Tink J., Shivaram SM., Chader GJ., Johnson LV., & Bok D. (1995). Expression, secretion, and age-related downregulation of pigment epithelium-derived factor, a serpin with neurotrophic activity. *J Neurosci* 15: 4992-5003.

Tombran-Tink J., Aparicio S., Xu X., Tink AR., Lara N., Sawant S., Barnstable CJ., & Zhang SS. (2005). PEDF and the serpins: phylogeny, sequence conservation, and functional domains. *J Struct Biol* 151: 130-50.

Tombran-Tink J. (2010). PEDF in angiogenic eye diseases. *Curr Mol Med* 10: 267-78.

Topczewska JM., Postovit LM., Margaryan NV., Sam A., Hess AR., Wheaton WW., Nickoloff BJ., Topczewski J., & Hendrix MJ. (2006). Embryonic and tumorigenic pathways converge via Nodal signaling: role in melanoma aggressiveness. *Nat Med* 12: 925-32.

Tresini M., Pignolo RJ., Allen RG., & Cristofalo VJ. (1999). Effects of donor age on the expression of a marker of replicative senescence (EPC-1) in human dermal fibroblasts. *J Cell Physiol* 179: 11-7.

Uong A., & Zon LI. (2010). Melanocytes in development and cancer. *J Cell Physiol* 222: 38-41.

Utikal J., Schadendorf D., & Ugurel S. (2007). Serologic and immunohistochemical prognostic biomarkers of cutaneous malignancies. *Arch Dermatol Res* 298: 469-77.

Villanueva J., & Herlyn M. (2008). Melanoma and the tumor microenvironment. *Curr Oncol Rep* 10: 439-46.

Volpert OV. (2000). Modulation of endothelial cell survival by an inhibitor of angiogenesis thrombospondin-1: a dynamic balance. *Cancer Metastasis Rev* 19: 87-92.

Volpert OV., Zaichuk T., Zhou W., Reiher F., Ferguson TA., Stuart PM., Amin M., & Bouck NP. (2002). Inducer-stimulated Fas targets activated endothelium for destruction by anti-angiogenic thrombospondin-1 and pigment epithelium-derived factor. *Nat Med* 8: 349-57.

Weeraratna AT. (2005). A Wnt-er wonderland--the complexity of Wnt signaling in melanoma. *Cancer Metastasis Rev* 24: 237-50.

Xi Y., Nakajima G., Hamil T., Fodstad O., Riker A., & Ju J. (2006). Association of insulin-like growth factor binding protein-3 expression with melanoma progression. *Mol Cancer Ther* 5: 3078-84.

Xu X., Zhang SS., Barnstable CJ., & Tombran-Tink J. (2006). Molecular phylogeny of the antiangiogenic and neurotrophic serpin, pigment epithelium derived factor in vertebrates. *BMC Genomics* 7: 248.

Yabe T., Wilson D., & Schwartz JP. (2001). NFkappaB activation is required for the neuroprotective effects of pigment epithelium-derived factor (PEDF) on cerebellar granule neurons. *J Biol Chem* 276: 43313-9.

Yamagishi S., Inagaki Y., Nakamura K., Abe R., Shimizu T., Yoshimura A., & Imaizumi T. (2004). Pigment epithelium-derived factor inhibits TNF-alpha-induced interleukin-6 expression in endothelial cells by suppressing NADPH oxidase-mediated reactive oxygen species generation. *J Mol Cell Cardiol* 37: 497-506.

Yang H., & Grossniklaus HE. (2010). Constitutive overexpression of pigment epithelium-derived factor inhibition of ocular melanoma growth and metastasis. *Invest Ophthalmol Vis Sci* 51: 28-34.

Yasui N., Mori T., Morito D., Matsushita O., Kourai H., Nagata K., & Koide T. (2003). Dual-site recognition of different extracellular matrix components by anti-angiogenic/neurotrophic serpin, PEDF. *Biochemistry* 42: 3160-7.

Zaichuk TA., Shroff EH., Emmanuel R., Filleur S., Nelius T., & Volpert OV. (2004). Nuclear factor of activated T cells balances angiogenesis activation and inhibition. *J Exp Med* 199: 1513-22.

Zbytek B., Carlson JA., Granese J., Ross J., Mihm MC., & Slominski A. (2008). Current concepts of metastasis in melanoma. *Expert Rev Dermatol* 3: 569-585.

# 9

# The Influence of the Skin Microenvironment Air-Liquid Interface on Melanoma

Shuji Toda[1], Shigehisa Aoki[1], Kazuyoshi Uchihashi[1], Aki Matsunobu[1], Mai Yakushiji[1], Akifumi Ootani[2], Eisuke Koike[3] and Nobuhisa Yonemitsu[4]
[1]*Department of Pathology & Microbiology, Faculty of Medicine & Graduate School of Medicine, Saga University, Saga 849-8501,*
[2]*Department of Internal Medicine Faculty of Medicine & Graduate School of Medicine, Saga University, Saga 849-8501,*
[3]*Department of Surgery, Koike Hospital, Saga 840-0861,*
[4]*Department of Pathology, Sasebo Chuo Hospital, Nagasaki 857-1195*
*Japan*

## 1. Introduction

The skin that is exposed to atmospheric air is situated at an air–liquid interface (ALI) through its contact with gas phase. Thus, ALI is an essential microenvironment of the skin. In fact, ALI promotes the growth and differentiation of normal keratinocytes (Sugihara et al., 1991). In cutaneous squamous cell carcinoma cells, ALI also accelerates their invasive growth more greatly than submerged condition without ALI (Inoue et al., 2001). ALI is thus considered to be a critical factor for both normal and neoplastic subjects of the skin.

The critical skin neoplasm melanoma is still at present responsible for about 80% of all skin cancer-related deaths (Miller et al., 2006). This tumor is considered to originate from epidermal melanocytes or their precursor cells (Bennett, 1993). Thus, the epidermal microenvironments seem crucial for the initiation and progression of melanoma cells. Furthermore, the prognosis of melanoma with ulcer formation is worse than that of melanoma without ulcer formation (Grande et al., 2006). Given that skin ulcer causes cutaneous cell types under the epidermis to situate at ALI by the ulcer-induced exposure of them to atmospheric air, ALI may be related to the growth and invasion of melanoma cells. However, it has been unclear whether the skin microenvironment ALI directly affects the biological behavior of melanoma cells.

On the basis of the background above, we have recently demonstrated that ALI promotes the growth of melanoma cells, but not their apoptosis and invasion, through mitogen-activated protein kinase (MAPK) activation (Chong et al., 2010). In this article, we introduce ALI culture system and describe the effects of ALI on the biological behavior of melanoma cells.

## 2. Effects of ALI on melanoma cell behavior

Air-liquid interface (ALI) is a common microenvironment of the skin. However, the influences of ALI on the biological behavior of melanoma cells have been poorly understood. To well understand the interesting issue, we first introduce ALI culture system. Next we show that ALI promotes the growth of melanoma cells, but not their invasion and apoptosis, through the activation of mitogen-activated protein kinase (MAPK), using the ALI culture system of two melanoma cell lines of KHm-1 (King et al., 1978) and HMY-1 (Ojima et al., 1998). Finally, we discuss the mechanisms underlining ALI-induced overgrowth of melanoma cells.

### 2.1 Air-liquid interface (ALI) culture system

By application of a double dish-culture method, ALI culture system is organized, as described previously (Toda et al., 2005). Briefly, 2 ml type I collagen gel solution (Nitta Gelatin, Osaka, Japan) was poured into a 30-mm inner dish with a nitrocellulose bottom (Millicell-CM, Millipore, Bedford, MA) and incubated at 37 °C for 30 min to solidify the gel. This inner dish was placed into a 90-mm outer dish, and the complete medium was added to both dishes. Then, $1 \times 10^6$ melanoma cells were spread onto the gel and they grew confluent within 2 days. At 3 days in culture, the media of the inner and outer dishes were removed, and 10 ml fresh complete medium was added to only the outer dish to create ALI. The cells were exposed to a humidified air supplemented with 5% $CO_2$ at 37 °C. In this way, the cells were situated at ALI. In this system, the cells were kept moist and fed by the culture

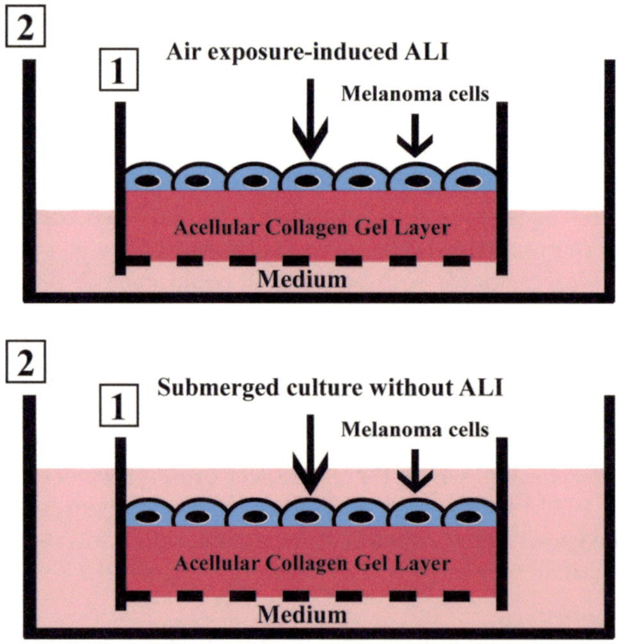


Fig. 1. Collagen gel invasion assay system with (upper panel) or without ALI (lower panel). Upper panel, Melanoma cells are seeded on the acellular gel layer in inner dish (1). The inner dish (1) is put in outer dish (2) with culture medium. In this way, the cells on the gel layer are localized under air exposure-induced ALI. The cells are kept in moist and fed by culture medium that percolates by capillary action from the medium-containing outer dish. Lower panel indicates submerged culture without ALI (control). In these systems, the invasion of melanoma cells into collagen gel is analyzed by the method described in Materials and Methods

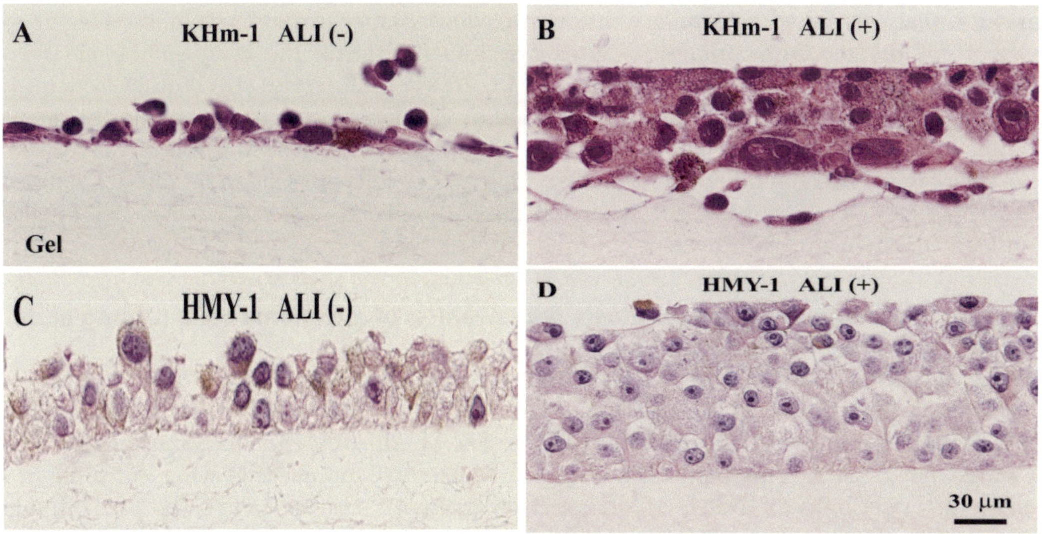


Fig. 2. Histology of two melanoma cell types of KHm-1 (A and B) and HMY-1 (C and D) with (B and D) or without ALI (A and C). ALI promotes the stratification of KHm-1 and HMY-1 melanoma cell types more greatly than submerged condition without ALI. In all conditions, the infiltration of these melanoma cell types into the gel was not observed. Brown pigments indicate melanin pigments

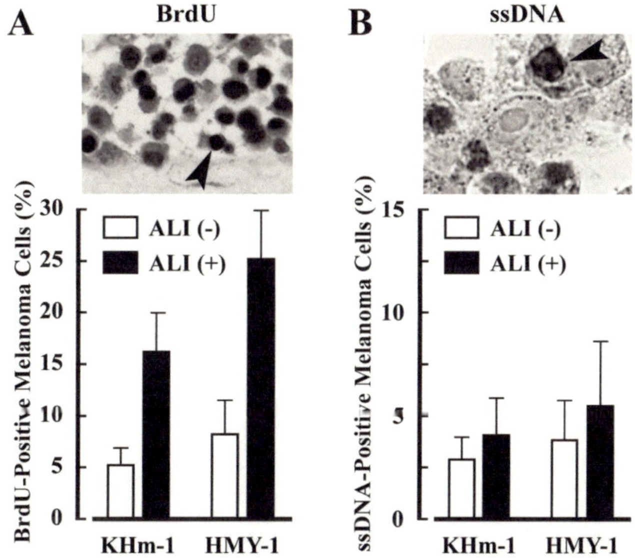


Fig. 3. Growth (A) and apoptosis (B) of melanoma cells with or without ALI, using immunohistochemistry of BrdU (growth marker) and ssDNA (apoptosis marker). BrdU (upper panel in A) and ssDNA (upper panel in B) are clearly detected in the nuclei of KHm-1 melanoma cells in black (arrowhead). The BrdU uptake of melanoma cells with ALI was about 3 times that of the cells without ALI ($p<0.001$), while melanoma cells with or without ALI showed no significant change in the apoptotic rate ($p>0.05$)

medium that percolated by capillary action into cellular layer through acellular collagen gel layer from the medium-containing outer dish. As a control, the cells on the gel were cultured in a submerged condition without ALI. Figure 1 illustrates this culture system. In this system, we can also determine the invasion of various cancer cell types into the gel. In addition, cancer-stromal cell interaction such as the growth and infiltration of cancer cells can be analyzed in the modified system, in which cancer cells are seeded on the stromal cell-embbeded or -nonembedded gel (Inoue et al., 2001). Thus, this system has been called "collagen gel invasion assay system".

### 2.2 Effects of ALI on growth, apoptosis and invasion of melanoma cells (Chong et al., 2010)

ALI accelerates the stratification of melanoma cells more prominently than submerged condition without ALI (Fig. 2), suggesting that ALI promotes the proliferation of melanoma cells. In fact, the bromodeoxyuridine (BrdU) uptake of ALI-treated melanoma cells is about 3 times that of ALI-nontreated cells (Fig. 3A). When melanoma cells were cultured in a submerged condition for 2 days following treatment with ALI for 7 days, the BrdU uptake of the cells decreased to that of ALI-nontreated cells. Thus, ALI-promoted growth of melanoma cells is considered to be reversible, supporting our previous study that ALI reversibly promotes fibroblast growth (Toda et al, 2000).

On the other hand, melanoma cells with or without ALI show no significant change in the apoptotic rate that is assayed by immunohistochemistry with single stranded DNA (ssDNA) antibody (Fig. 3B). Interestingly, melanoma cells with or without ALI do not undergo their invasion into collagen gel (Fig. 2). Namely, ALI promotes the growth of melanoma cells, but not their apoptosis and invasion. In addition, dermal fibroblasts accelerate the invasion of melanoma cells cultured on the fibroblast-embedded gel (Fig. 4). The invasion of melanoma cells into the gel is more prominently enhanced by the treatment of ALI than by the non-treatment of ALI. Thus, the combination of dermal fibroblasts with ALI seems critical for the invasion of melanoma cells. Furthermore, adipose tissue stromal cells (ATSCs) as well as dermal fibroblasts promote the invasion of melanoma cells in the same system with or without ALI , supporting our previous study that ATSCs enhance the invasion of gastric adenocarcinoma cells (Nomoto-Kojima et al., 2011). Therefore, subcutaneous ATSCs also seem critical for the spread of melanoma cells.

During the ALI-induced overgrowth of melanoma cells, mitogen-activated protein kinase (MAPK) pathway (Raf-1, MEK-1 and p-ERK-1/2) is activated (Fig. 5).

In addition, the MEK inhibitor PD-98059 that leads to the inactivation of ERK-1/2 (MAPK) inhibits the stratification of melanoma cells even with ALI, although the agent induces a spindle-shaped morphology in the cells (Fig. 6). PD-98059 also abolishes the ALI-promoted the expression of BrdU and pERK-1/2 of melanoma cells (Fig. 6).

Thus, the ALI-affected overgrowth seems to be closely related to the MAPK activation. In our previous study (Toda et al., 2000), ALI-treated fibroblasts proliferate more extensively than the ALI-nontreated cells, while the treated fibroblasts express the MAPK pathway signals more greatly than the nontreated cells. The MAPK pathway may be involved in the mechanisms of ALI-induced cellular overgrowth. As described above, ALI does not induce the infiltration of melanoma cells into collagen gel. In fact, ALI does not promote the expression of the following invasion- and motility-related molecules: MMP-1, MMP-9, laminin 5 and filamin A. Thus, ALI alone may not be involved in the mechanisms of melanoma cell invasion. However, ALI enhances the dermal fibroblast- and ATSC-induced invasion of melanoma cells, as described above. This suggests that ALI in combination with these mesenchymal stromal cell types is closely associated with the invasion of melanoma cells. Figure 7 illustrates the effects of ALI and its combination with dermal fibroblasts and ATSCs on the growth and invasion of melanoma cells. Finally, the PI3K-AKT, $p16^{INK4A}$-CDK4/6-RB and β-catenin pathways, which are suggested to be critical for melanoma cell growth (Smalley, 2009), yet remain to be elucidated. In our laboratory, these molecule regulations by ALI are under investigation.

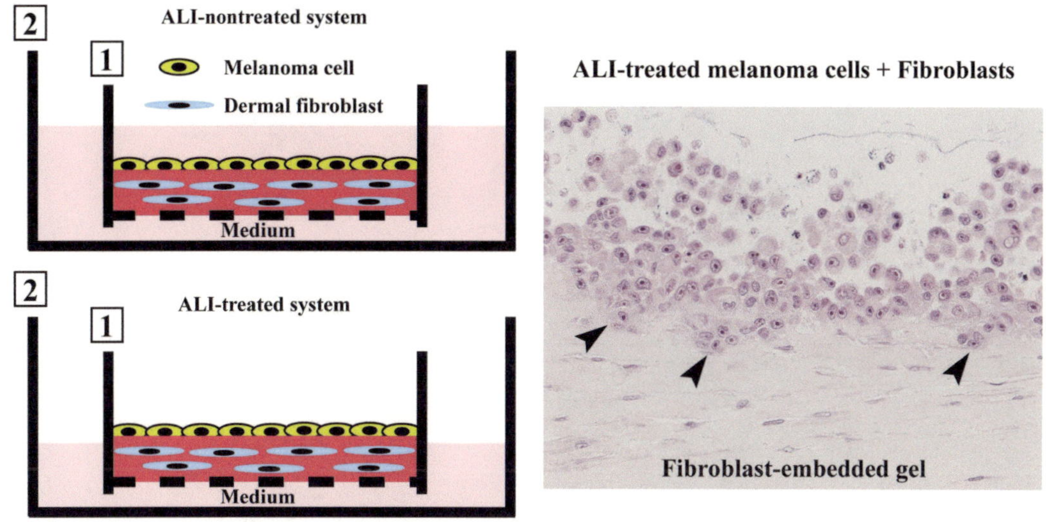


Fig. 4. Culture model with or without ALI for analyzing melanoma cell-dermal fibroblast interaction (left panels), and histology of ALI-treated melanoma cells cultured on dermal fibroblast-embedded collagen gel at 7 days (right panel). Left upper panel, Melanoma cells are seeded on a dermal fibroblast-embedded collagen gel layer in an inner dish with a nitrocellulose membrane as its base. The inner dish is placed in a larger outer dish, and then the complete medium is added to both dishes. Cells are fed by a sufficient medium from both the inner and outer dishes because of the permeability of the nitrocellulose membrane. In this way, melanoma cells are cultured in a submerged condition without ALI under a cancer-stromal interaction. Left lower panel, Melanoma cells are seeded on a dermal fibroblast-embedded collagen gel layer in the inner dish. The inner dish is placed in a larger outer dish, and then the complete medium is added to the outer dish only. In this way, melanoma cells are cultured in an ALI-treated condition under a cancer-stromal interaction. Right panel, ALI-treated melanoma cells undergo stratification on the fibroblast-embedded gel, and then they infiltrate into the gel. Arrowheads indicate the invasion of melanoma cells into the gel

### 2.3 Mechanisms of ALI-related behavior of melanoma cells

ALI is suggested to exert its effects by causing cells to increase their own oxygen availability, which is important for cellular respiration (Bebok, et al., 2001). Therefore, oxygen itself and oxidative stress molecules may be involved in the ALI-promoted overgrowth and MAPK activation. Furthermore, the following possible mechanisms of ALI-promoted growth of melanoma cells may be considered : (1) intracellular diffusion of

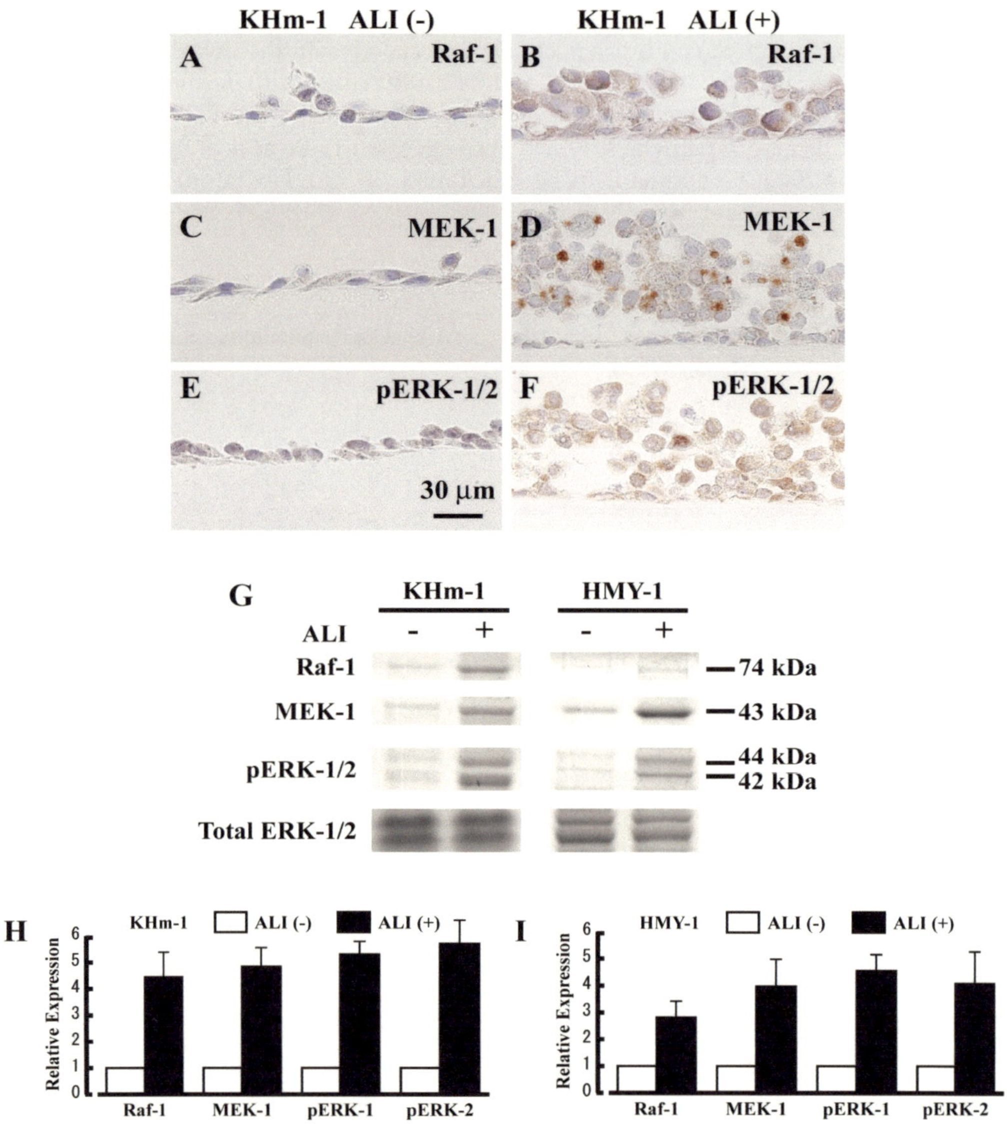


Fig. 5. Expression of MAPK pathway (Raf-1, MEK-1 and ERK-1/2) of melanoma cells with or without ALI. In immunohistochemistry (A-F), KHm-1 melanoma cells with ALI (B, D and F) express Raf-1 (A and B), MEK-1 (C and D) and ERK-1/2 (E and F) more extensively than those without ALI (A, C and D). Western blotting (G) confirmed the immunohistochemical results. Analyses by Densitometry (H and I) show that ALI significantly enhances Raf-1, MEK-1 and ERK-1/2 expression of KHm-1 (H) and HMY-1 (I) melanoma cells (all values, $p<0.001$)

oxygen through cell membrane may take place more easily in a fluid-less microenvironment of ALI than in a fluid-rich counterpart of submerged condition without ALI; (2) cell growth-related molecules may be more concentrated within a fluid-less microenvironment of ALI; and (3) ALI may specifically activate cell membrane microdomains (rafts), which regulate a variety of signal transduction molecules (Brown, 2002; Kim et al., 2004). To evaluate these possibilities in more detail, further studies are needed. In particular, gas molecules and signaling pathway regarding cell growth, invasion and locomotion should be investigated in the context of ALI-cell membrane interaction.

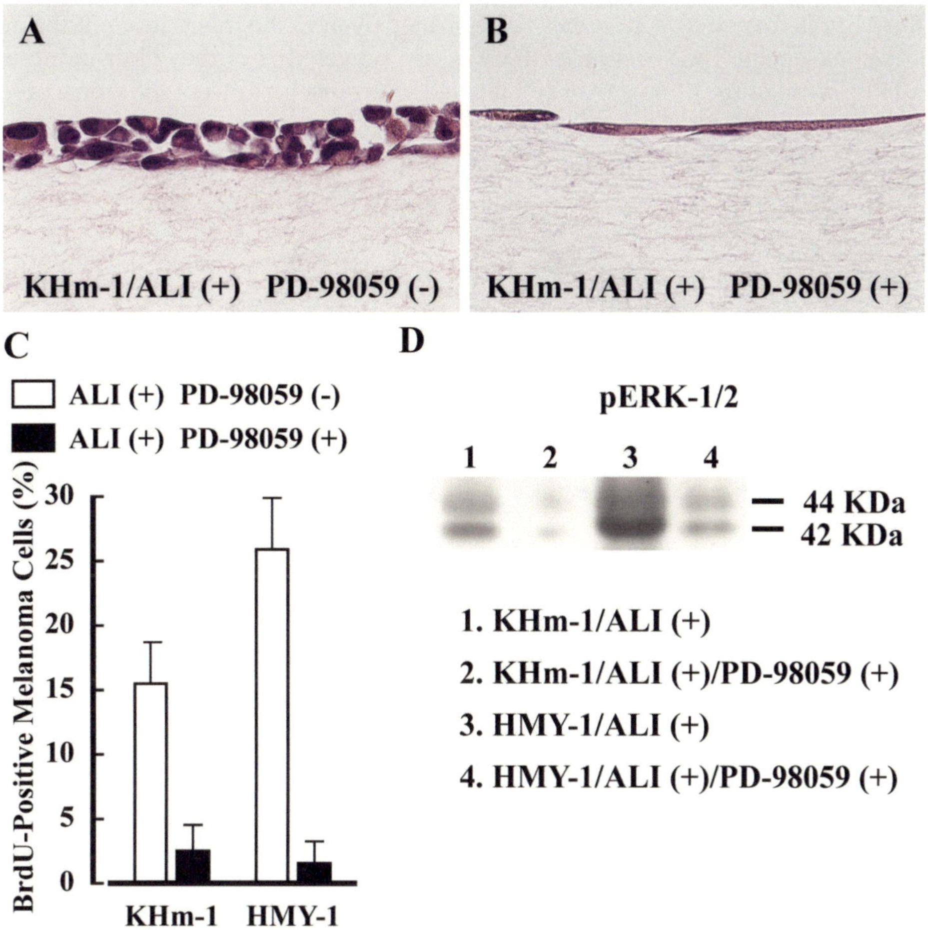


Fig. 6. Effects of the MEK inhibitor PD-98059 on the morphology, BrdU uptake and MAPK (ERK-1/2) expression of melanoma cells with ALI. ALI-treated KHm-1 melanoma cells without PD-98059 (A) undergo cellular stratification on the gel. In contrast, the melanoma cells with PD-98059 show no stratification and they become spindle-shaped (B). In ALI-treated KHm-1 and HMY-1 melanoma cell types, PD-98059 significantly inhibits both BrdU uptake (C, $p<0.0001$) and pERK-1/2 expression (D) of the cell types

The prognosis of melanoma with ulcer formation is worse than that of melanoma without ulcer formation (Grande et al., 2006). Skin ulcer seems to cause the cutaneous cell types of the dermis under the epidermis to situate at ALI by the ulcer-induced exposure of them to atmospheric air. In general, normal and cancer cell types are supported by the interstitum that has two major types of solid structures: (1) collagen fiber bundles and (2) proteoglycan filaments (Guyton and Hall, 2000). The interstitial fluid, which is derived by filtration and diffusion from capillaries, is entrapped mainly in the minute spaces among proteoglycan filaments. This combination of proteoglycan filaments and the fluid entrapped within them (gel water) organizes a moist tissue gel of the interstitum, while intravascular space has rich fluid (free water) due to both the existence of much serum and the lack of the matrix meshwork. In the moist gel, oxygen and nutrients are also supplied from capillaries. In this way, the ALI microenvironment seems to be created even in the interstitium of the dermis. Thus, the melanoma cell overgrowth that is activated by the ulcer-induced ALI microenvironment of the dermis may be involved in the mechanisms of the worse prognosis of melanoma cells with ulcer formation.

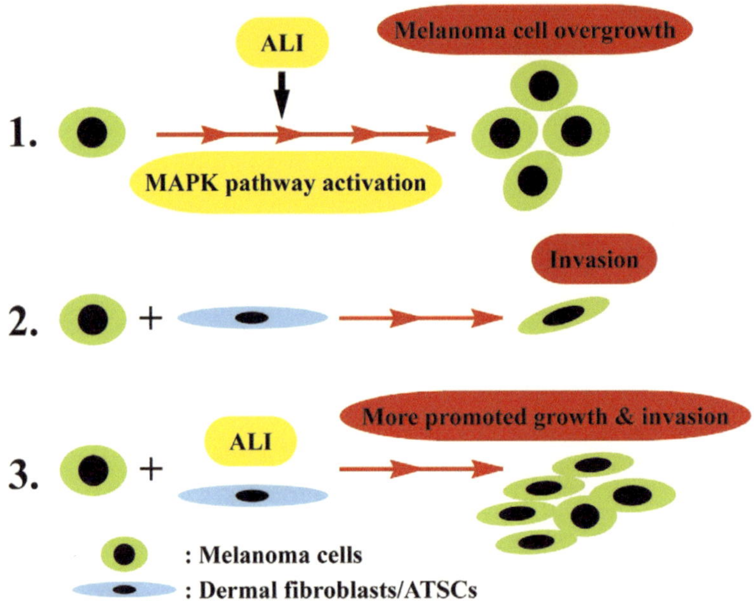


Fig. 7. Scheme of the effects of ALI and its combination with dermal fibroblasts and adipose tissue stromal cells (ATSCs) on the growth and invasion of melanoma cells. 1., ALI induces the overgrowth of melanoma cells, but not their invasion, through the activation of MAPK pathway. 2., Dermal fibroblasts as well as ATSCs induce the invasion of melanoma cells. 3., ALI in combination with dermal fibroblasts as well as ATSCs enhances the growth and invasion of melanoma cells

## 3. Conclusion

Here we have shown that the skin microenvironment ALI promotes the proliferation of melanoma cells, but not their apoptosis and invasion, through MAPK activation. Given that advanced melanoma is not responsive to chemotherapy, immunologic therapy and radiotherapy, ALI may be taken into account for the biology and therapeutic strategy of melanoma. The device that abolishes ALI microenvironment within melanoma tissue may be a promising tool for the treatment of advanced melanoma in combination with the conventional and molecular-targeted therapies. For example, water-rich nano-particles that lead to the abolishment of ALI within the tumor tissue may be created.

## 4. Acknowledgment

This work was supported in part by Grants-in-Aid from Japanese Ministry of Education, Culture, Sports, Science and Technology for Scientific Research Nos. 18591871, 20592023 and 23591050 (to Prof. Shuji Toda), and personal Grants from Koike Hospital, Sasebo Chuo Hospital and Yamada Clinic (to Prof. Shuji Toda). We thank Messrs. H. Ideguchi, F. Mutoh, S. Nakahara, and Mrs. M. Nishida for their excellent technical assistance.

## 5. References

Bebok, Z., Tousson, A., Schwiebert, L.M. and Venglarik, C.J. (2001) Improved oxygenation promotes CFTR maturation and trafficking in MDCK monolayers. Am. J. Physiol. Cell Physiol. 280; C135-C145.

Bennett, D.C. (1993) Genetics, development, and malignancy of melanocytes. Int. Rev. Cytol. 146; 191-260.

Brown, D. (2002) Structure and function of membrane rafts. Int. J. Med. Microbiol. 291; 433-437.

Chong, H.Y., Aoki, S., Uchihashi, K., Matsunobu, A., Yamasaki, F., Misago, N., Piao, M., Tetsuji, U., Yonemitsu, N., Sugihara, H. and Toda, S. (2010) The air-liquid interface, a skin microenvironment, promotes growth of melanoma cells, but not their apoptosis and invasion, through activation of mitogen-activated protein kinase. Acta. Histochem. Cytochem. 43: 1-7.

Grande Sarpa, H., Reinke, K., Shaikh, L., Leong, S.P., Miller, J.R. 3rd., Sagebiel, R.W. and Kashani-Sabet, M. (2006) Prognostic significance of extent of ulceration in primary cutaneous melanoma. Am J Surg Pathol. 30; 1396-400.

Guyton, A.C. and Hall, J.E. (2000) Textbook of medical physiology. 10th, W.B. Saunders, Philadelphia.

Inoue, T., Toda, S., Narisawa, Y. and Sugihara, H. (2001) Subcutaneous adipocytes promote the differentiation of squamous cell carcinoma cell line (DJM-1) in collagen gel matrix culture. J. Invest. Dermatol. 117; 244-250.

Kim, J., Adam, R.M., Solomon, K.R. and Freeman, M.R. (2004) Involvement of cholesterol-rich lipid rafts in interleukin-6-induced neuroendocrine differentiation of LNCaP prostate cancer cells. Endocrinology 145; 613-619.

King, L.E. Jr, Solomon, S.S. and Hashimoto, K. (1978) Characterization of a human melanoma cell line (KHm-1) containing phosphodiesterase activity only for cyclic adenosine 3':5'-monophosphate. Cancer Res. 38; 3879-3885

Miller, A.J. and Mihm, M.C. Jr. (2006) Melanoma. N. Engl. J. Med. 355; 51-65.

Nomoto-Kojima, N., Aoki, S., Uchihashi, K., Matsunobu, A., Koike, E., Ootani, A., Yonemitsu, N., Fujimoto, K., and Toda, S. (2011) Interaction between adipose tissue stromal cells and gastric cancers in vitro. Cell Tissue Res. 344: 287-298.

Ojima, F., Ido, T., Kijima-Suda, I. and Nakagawa, Y. (1998) Biodistribution study of murine monoclonal anti-GD3 antibody in nude mice bearing human melanoma xenografts for development of immunoscintigraphy. Tohoku J. Exp. Med. 185; 89-100.

Smalley, K.S.M. (2010) Understanding melanoma signaling networks as the basis for molecular targeted therapy. J. Invest. Dermatol. 130: 28-37.

Sugihara, H., Toda, S., Miyabara, S., Kusaba, Y. and Minami, Y. (1991) Reconstruction of the skin in three-dimensional collagen gel matrix culture. In Vitro Cell. Dev. Biol. 27A; 142-146.

Toda, S., Yokoi, F., Yamada, S., Yonemitsu, N., Nishimura, T., Watanabe, K., Sugihara, H. (2000) Air exposure promotes fibroblast growth with increased expression of mitogen-activated protein kinase cascade. Biochem. Biophys. Res. Commun. 270: 961-966.

Toda, S., Yamada, S., Aoki, S., Inokuchi, A. and Sugihara, H. (2005) Air-liquid interface promotes invasive growth of laryngeal squamous cell carcinoma with or without hypoxia. Biochem Biophys Res Commun.326; 866-872.

# Part 2

## Pigmentation

# 10

# Melanocyte Pygmentation – Friend or Foe on the Route to Melanoma

Baldea Ioana
*Department of Physiology, University of Medicine and Pharmacy, Cluj-Napoca Romania*

## 1. Introduction

The epidermis forms the top protective covering of normal human skin and is itself composed of multiple layers from the stratum corneum at the top, to proliferating cells in the deep/basal layer (Liu & Fisher, 2010).

The epidermal cell population is mainly constituted of two cell types: keratinocytes and melanocytes. Keratinocytes constitute the majority of the epidermis; they have a "supporting" and regulatory role for the melanocytes. Keratinocytes are linked through tight desmosomal intercellular junctions and also anchored into the basal membrane through hemidesmosomes, but melanocytes remain as singly scattered, unattached cells.

Each single, well-differentiated, melanocyte interacts with 36 viable keratinocytes at various stages of progression to the upper cornified layer of the epidermis (Fitzpatrick & Breathnach, 1963) to form epidermal units. These structural and functional cellular units exhibit complex, life-long, cellular interactions originally laid down during embryonic life.

There are considerable interindividual and intraindividual variations in melanocyte population densities, with more than twice as many melanocytes located in head and forearm skin compared with elsewhere on the body, as well as darker skin in the folded areas of axillae and perineum, traits that remain remarkably consistent between races (Szabo, 1967).

Despite significant variation in skin pigmentation, the density of melanocytes at the epidermal-dermal junction is very similar across different skin types (Yamaguchi & Hearing, 2009). Thus the main contributor to racial differences in skin pigmentation is cellular activity rather than absolute melanocyte numbers (Szabo, 1967).

Melanocytes play a central role in the response of skin to sunlight exposure. They are directly involved in UV-induced pigmentation as a defense mechanism. People with different skin color possess varied sensitivity to ultraviolet (UV) exposure, with darker skinned individuals being less susceptible to sun-induced skin alterations, including cancer, than fair skinned ones (Elwood & Diffey 1993).

Such a difference can be explained in terms of protective UV filtering by epidermal pigmentation, because the skin color is also related to the type of melanin, the number, size, type, distribution and degradation of melanosomes, and the tyrosinase activity of melanocytes (Nordlund & Ortonne 1998, Yamaguchi & Hearing 2009).

The decreased photocarcinogenesis seen in individuals with darker skin may also be attributed to the more efficient removal of UV-damaged cells (Yamaguchi & Hearing 2009, Alonso & Fuchs, 2003, Fuchs, 2008).

The melanocytes, when differentiated, assume the highly dendritic phenotype that facilitates closer contact and transfer of the melanosomes to nearby keratinocytes where they shield nuclei from ultraviolet (UV) irradiation.

At least four theories have been proposed to be involved in the transfer of the melanosomes (Slominski et al., 2004): 1) the "cytophagic" theory, where the keratinocyte, as active partner, phagocytoses the tips of dendrites that contain stage IV mature melanosomes (Garcia, 1979); 2) the "discharge" theory, where mature melanosomes are released into the intercellular space to be internalized by adjacent keratinocytes; 3) the "fusion" theory, where mature melanosomes pass from melanocyte to keratinocyte via fusion of their respective plasma membranes (Okazaki et al., 1976.); and 4) the "cytocrine" theory, whereby melanocytes would inject melanin into recipient keratinocytes (Masson, 1948).

Epidermal melanocytes rarely collect mature melanosomes intracytoplasmically; instead, they translocate them to keratinocytes. This is in contrast to bulbar follicular melanocytes, which are commonly heavily laden with fully mature stage IV melanosomes. When melanocytes were cocultured with keratinocytes, a highly dendritic phenotype was induced through filopodia, many of which contained melanosomes (Scott et al., 2002).

Keratinocytes in coculture with melanocytes can also suppress melanogenic proteins such as the TRP1 (Phillips et al., 2001). Besides this, melanocyte growth, dendricity, spreading, cell-cell contacts, and melanization can all be regulated by keratinocyte-secreted factors (Tenchini et al., 1995). Interestingly, the regulatory role exercised by keratinocytes is restored in melanoma cells if expression of E-cadherin is induced, permitting their adhesion to keratinocytes (Hsu et al., 2000).

An increase in melanogenically active melanocytes is seen following UV irradiation (Rosdahl et al., 1978), but it is not clear if these additional cells are truly derived from division of already functioning melanocytes.

In contrast, melanocytes in the hair follicle divide during the hair cycle. Melanocyte loss (mostly probably via apoptosis) occurs in both sun-exposed and covered skin with an 10% reduction per decade after 30 years of age until 80 years, followed by more dramatic cell loss thereafter (Nordlund, 1989).

Melanocyte alteration can lead to melanoma, a tumor that has become one of the most rapidly increasing malignancies in the Caucasian population with 2.5-3% more cases each year in the US. It shows a relatively high incidence among young people compared to most other cancer types. (Wang et al., 2001).

## 2. Melanin and melanogenesis

Cutaneous melanin pigment plays a critical role in camouflage, mimicry, social communication, and protection against harmful effects of solar radiation. In the epidermis, melanin is synthesized by melanocytes. Besides skin, melanin can also be found in hair, retinal pigment epithelium, iris, and certain parts of the central nervous system.

The primary function of skin melanin has not yet been established. A number of roles have been proposed that include photoprotection, thermoregulation, antibiotic, cation chelator, free radical sink, and by-product of the scavenging of the superoxide radical in the skin by tyrosinase (Giacomoni, 1995; Hill & Hill, 2000; Morisson, 1985).

Melanins are synthesized, matured, and stored within melanosomes. Melanogenesis includes: melanosome biogenesis, melanin synthesis and transfer of the melanosomes to the surrounding keratinocytes (Chen et al., 2009).

Melanosome biogenesis can be classified into four distinct stages of maturation (I, II, III, IV) based on melanosomal morphologies (Hearing, 2005; Raposo et al., 2002). Stage I and II melanosomes are termed premelanosomes, as melanin synthesis has not yet begun. Stage I melanosomes are closely related to lysosomes because they share a lysosomal lineage (Hearing, 2005; Orlow, 1995; Raposo et al., 2001, 2002; Valencia et al., 2006). Typical stage II melanosomes are ovoid in shape, containing elongated and highly organized fibrillar - matrics. Active melanin synthesis occurs in stage III melanosomes and results in the deposition of black electron-dense pigment on the fibrillar matrix. When the internal matrix of a melanosome is completely filled with melanin, it no longer has discernable internal filaments at the electron microscope level, and the melanosome reaches a mature stage (i.e., stage IV). More detailed staging of melanosomes can be obtained from electron microscope images when melanosomes undergo inter-stage transitions from stage I to IV. These additional stages are I-II, II-III, and III-IV (Chen et al., 2006, 2009a, 2009b).

Late-stage melanosomes (III and IV) are transferred to keratinocytes in normal skin. However, that process may be impaired in melanoma cells. Stage IV melanosomes frequently have damaged membranes and leak melanin into the cytoplasm, a morphological indicator of endogenous melanogenic cytotoxicity (Chen et al., 2006, 2009 a, 2009b).

There are two categories of melanin: black-brown eumelanin and yellow-reddish pheomelanin.

The availability of L-tyrosine for enzymatic oxidation is a central component for the initiation of melanogenesis. In the melanosomes L-tyrosine comes either from the hydroxylation of L-phenylalanine to L-tyrosine by phenylalanine hydroxylase (PAH) or is actively transported inside the organnells from cytoplasm (Schallreuter et al., 2008).

Tyrosine uptake is largely through system L -transport, which supplies the tyrosine for both protein synthesis and melanogenesis, as shown in a melanoma cell line (SK-mel 23) (Jara et al., 1991). Tyrosine uptake by cells was inhibited by the analog substrate 4-S-cysteinylphenol and by tryptophan as well as the specific system L -inhibitor 2-amino-bicyclo-2,2,1-heptane-2-carboxylic acid. (Pankovich & Jimbow 1991) Although this mechanism is responsible for the cellular uptake of tyrosine, there may be separate permeases to regulate the access of tyrosine to the melanosome because the process is analogous to amino acid export (Land et al., 2006).

L-tyrosine is then hydroxylated to L-dihydroxyphenylalanine (L-DOPA), a reaction catalyzed by either the tyrosine hydroxylase activity of tyrosinase (TYR) or tyrosine hydroxylase (THI) (Simon et al., 2009). Thus, the three enzymes, i.e. phenylalanine hydroxilase, tyrosine hydrolase and tyrosinase are crucial for the initiation of melanogenesis, supporting the concept of a "three enzyme theory" (Schallreuter et al., 2008).

The next step, oxidation of L-DOPA to dopaquinone (DQ) is common to both eu and pheomelanin synthesis. Orthoquinines such as dopaquinone (DQ), are extremely reactive molecules (Ito & Wakamatsu, 2008) and can be formed directly during the initial stage of melanogenesis (Cooksey et al., 1997).

The first step in eumelanogenesis is a relatively slow process involving the intramolecular addition of the amino group to produce cyclodopa (Land & Riley, 2000; Land et al., 2003). However, as cyclodopa is formed, it is rapidly oxidized to dopachrome through a redox exchange (Land et al., 2003).

Production of dopachrome, an orange red pigment is faster than the production of cyclodopa, when the cyclodopa concentration is above 0.7μM, leading to dopachrome accumulation during the early phase of eumelanogenesis. Dopachrome spontaneously decomposes by decarboxylation at neutral pH to give di-hydro indol (DHI) and di-hydro indol carboxylic acid (DHICA) in a 70: 1 ratio (Palumbo et al., 1987). However, in the presence of dopachrome tautomerase (DCT), also termed tyrosinase-related protein-2 (TYRP2), dopachrome undergoes tautomerization to preferentially produce DHICA (Palumbo et al., 1991). The ratio of DHICA to DHI in natural eumelanins is thus determined by the activity of DCT (Tsukamoto et al., 1992). DHICA synthesis seems to protect melanocytes against cytotoxic effects of melanogenesis, thus DCT was reported to be essential for melanocyte survival (Hearing, 2000).

Metal cations, especially $Cu^{2+}$ also accelerate the dopachrome rearrangement and affect the DHICA/DHI ratio, but DCT seems to be more effective in catalyzing the tautomerization (Palumbo et al., 1987, 1991). During eumelanogenesis, DHI oxidation takes place by redox exchange with DQ (Edge et al., 2006), although such a reaction is likely to be less efficient for DHICA. Thus, DHICA may require its oxidation to the quinone form by a direct action of tyrosinase in humans (Olivares et al., 2001) or by TYRP1 in mice (Jimenez-Cervantes et al., 1994; Kobayashi et al., 1994). Human TYRP1 is unable to catalyze the DHICA oxidation (Boissy et al., 1998).

The initial step of pheomelanogenesis is the conjugation of dopaquinone to cysteine or glutathione to yield cysteinyldopa (CD) and glutathionyldopa (Simon, 2009). The reaction of DQ and cysteine produces the 5-5 and 2-5-CD isomers in a ratio of 5.3:1 (Ito and Prota, 1977). Cysteinyldopas are further transformed into dihydrobenzothiazine-3-carboxylic acid (DHBTCA). (Greco et al., 2009). In the later stages of pheomelanogenesis, benzothiazine groups are slowly converted to the benzothiazole (BZ) and thus the polymeric structure of the pheomelanin pigment contains both benzothiazine and benzothiazole units (Wakamatsu et al., 2009).

Trichochromes are dimeric and trimeric intermediates that have a bi (l,4) benzothiazine chromophore. The close similarity in structural features of trichochromes and pheomelanin and their coexistence in pigmented tissues suggest that they are formed oxidatively from the same monomer units and differ only in their mode of polymerization (Simon, 2009).

In vivo melanogenesis produces mixtures of eumelanin and pheomelanin. The total amount of melanin produced is proportional to DQ production, which is in turn proportional to tyrosinase activity.

A mixed melanogenesis three-step pathway has been proposed (Ito & Wakamatsu, 2008; Simon et al., 2009). The initial stage is the production of CD isomers, which continues as long as the cysteine concentration is above 0.13 μM. The second stage is the oxidation of CDs to produce pheomelanin as long as CDs concentrations are above 9 μM. The last stage is the production of eumelanin, which begins only after most CDs and cysteine are depleted. Therefore, the ratio of eumelanin to pheomelanin is determined by tyrosinase activity and the availability of tyrosine and cysteine in melanosomes (Land et al., 2003).

Human epidermal and uveal melanocytes in culture produce pheomelanin at rather constant levels regardless of the degree of pigmentation while they produce eumelanin at levels proportional to pigmentation (Ito & Wakamatsu, 2008; Wakamatsu et al., 2006, 2008).

The most important enzyme which regulates the velocity and specificity of the melanogenesis is tyrosinase (Slominski et al., 2004). Tyrosinase catalyzes three distinct reactions in the melanogenic pathway: hydroxylation of monophenol (L-tyrosine), dehydrogenation of L-DOPA, and dehydrogenation of DHI; L-DOPA serves as cofactor in the first and third reactions (Hearing & Tsukamoto, 1991; Korner & Pawelek, 1982; Pawelek & Korner, 1982; Wood & Schallreuter, 1991; Ros et al., 1993). L-DOPA is the most efficient electron donor necessary to start tyrosine hydroxylation, although ascorbic acid, dopamine, and superoxide anion radicals can potentially activate the enzyme (Wood & Schallreuter, 1991).

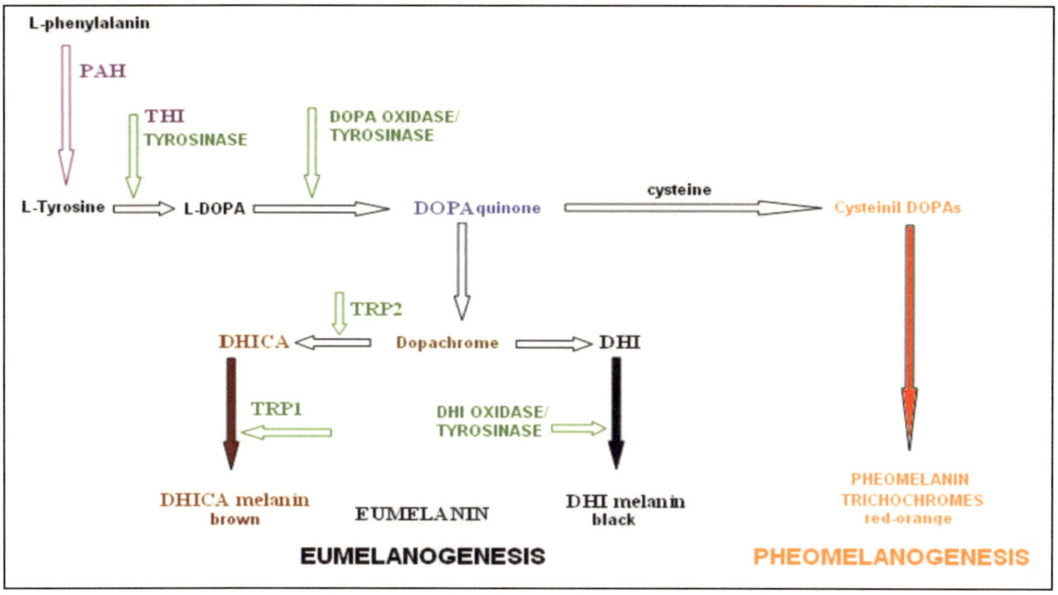


Fig. 1. Biochemical reactions of melanin synthesis; Abbreviations: DHI- di hydro indol, DHICA- di hydro carboxylic acid, DOPA -dihydroxyphenylalanine, PAH- phenylalanine hydroxilase, THI- tyrosine hydroxilase, TRP- tyrosinase related proteins. The initial step in the melanin biosynthesis is the hydroxylation of tyrosine to DOPA, which is then converted to DOPAquinone. Pheomelanogenesis takes place in the presence of cysteine and leads to the red-orange pigments, pheomelanins and trichochromes, while eumelanogenesis pathway needs the participation of tyrosinase and related proteins to produce either brown DHICA melanin of black DHI melanin

The effect of ascorbic acid on the monophenolase activity of tyrosinase has been explained by its reducing action on enzymatically generated quinines, thus inducing accumulation of L-DOPA, the main electron donor to the $Cu^{2+}$ enzyme active site (Ros et al., 1993).

Tyrosine related protein TRP1/TYRP1 share structural similarities with tyrosinase and originated by the duplication of the ancestral tyrosinase gene (Olivares et al., 2001, 2009). The activities of these tyrosinase-related proteins, TYRP1 and TYRP2, greatly affect the quantity and quality, the ratio of DHI to DHICA and the degree of polymerization of eumelanins produced (Lamoreux et al., 2001; Ozeki et al., 1995, 1997a, 1997b).

Both of them are important for the eumelanogenic pathway; they also act as stabilizers and regulators of the tyrosinase activity. Tyrp1 appears to control the molecular size of eumelanin produced in mice. Brown mice that lack Tyrp1 activity produce eumelanin with lower molecular weights than wild type, black mice (Ozeki et al., 1997a, 1997b). In humans, TYRP1 has tyrosine hydroxylase activity (Jackson et al., 1991; Jimenez-Cervantes et al., 1994; Kobayashi et al., 1994) and TYRP2 acts as dopachrome tautomerase (Jackson et al, 1992; Tsukamoto et al., 1992; Yokoyama et al., 1994). An additional function of TYRP1 may be the securing of appropriate processing of tyrosinase and stabilization of its enzymatic activity and, possibly, maintenance of melanosomal structure integrity (Hearing, 2000; Le Poole et al., 2000; Sarangarajan & Boissy, 2001; Sarangarajan et al., 2000). TYRP2 is important for melanocyte survival by implication in endogenous melanogenesis cytotoxicity homeostasis (Hearing, 2000).

## 3. Regulation of melanogenesis – internal factors

Cutaneous pigmentation plays a crucial role in defending the body against harmful UV rays and other environmental challenges (Costin & Hearing, 2007). This process is under a complex genetic control: in mammals, over 350 loci associated with pigmentation have been cloned or mapped (Olivares & Solano, 2009; Hearing, 2000; Montoliu et al., 2009).

Protein products of these loci acting as enzymes, structural proteins, transcriptional regulators, transporters, receptors and growth factors have a wide array of functions and cellular targets (Hearing, 1999; Nordlund et al., 2006). Among them are the important enzymatic melanosomal proteins coded by the albino(c)/TYR (Kwon et al., 1991, 1993), brown (b)/TYRP1 (Jackson et al., 1991) and slaty(slt)/TYRP2/DCT (Jackson et al., 1992) silver (slt)/SILV (Kwon et al., 1991, 1993), pink-eyed dilute (p)/P/OCA2 (Box et al., 1998; Oetting & King, 1999; Silvers, 1979; Simoncini et al., 2000), underwhite (uw)/LOC51151, MART1 (Carlson et al., 2003; Slominski, 2002; Slominski et al., 2001; Wankowicz-Kalinska et al., 2003) and OA1 (Orlow & Brilliant, 1999) loci.

The behavior of the melanocytes in vitro is different than in vivo, as a part of the epidermal melanin unit. The pheomelanin / eumelanin ratio is regulated by keratinocytes (Duval et al., 2002). Key elements in the regulation of melanogenesis are represented by tyrosinase and TYRPs. Their activities are also involved in the type of melanin pigment produced in melanosomes and also in controlling the endogenous citotoxicity of the melanogenesis process to the melanocytes.

The most important positive regulator of melanogenesis is the melanocortin (MC1) receptor with its ligands, melanocortins, other proopiomelanocortin (POMC) products, adrenocorticotropic hormone (ACTH) (Eberle et al., 1988; Lerner, 1993; Pawelek, 1976, 1985; Pawelek et al., 1988, 1992), whereas among the negative regulators, agouti protein stands out, determining the intensity of melanogenesis and the type of melanin synthesized.

α-MSH, which binds the MC1 receptor is an important regulator of skin pigmentation and the UV response of melanocytes and stimulates eumelanin synthesis (Abdel-Malek et al., 2009).

In vivo α-MSH injected to pubertal viable yellow mice producing a mixed-type melanin increased tyrosinase activity twofold with a concomitant increase in total melanin and more eumelanic hair was produced (Burchill et al., 1986).

Decreased α-MSH secretion following bromocriptine led to reduced tyrosinase activity and pheomelanic hair production along with a total melanin decrease. In vitro treatment of human melanocytes with the synthetic α-MSH resulted in an increase of eumelanin content in all the seven cell lines of different ethnic origins examined (Hunt et al., 1995).

Treatment with phenylthiourea (a tyrosinase inhibitor) resulted in a reduction of eumelanin content to a half with a concomitant twofold increase of pheomelanin content in melanocytes (Le Pape et al., 2008).

The main antagonist for the MC1R is the agouti signaling protein (ASP) (Lu et al., 1994). ASP acts within the microenvironment of the hair follicle during hair growth, switching eumelanin synthesis into pheomelanin synthesis.

The human agouti gene is expressed in adipose tissue, testis, ovary, and heart and at lower levels in liver, kidney, and foreskin (Wilson et al., 1995). Expression in transgenic mice of the human agouti protein produced a yellow coat (Wilson et al., 1995), although human hair does not show the agouti pattern.

When treated with agouti protein combined with phenylthiourea and extra cysteine to induce tyrosinase inhibition, non agouti melan-a (ala) mouse melanocytes (mainly eumelanic) produced over 200-fold increases in the pheomelanin to eumelanin ratio (Hida et al., 2009). Expression of ASP in cell culture blocks the α-MSH-stimulated accumulation of cAMP in mouse melanoma cells (Wilson et al., 1995).

In lower vertebrates, melanin concentrating hormone (MCH) induces melanosome aggregation within melanophores (whitening of the color). In mammals, MCH expression was detected in cultured human endothelial cells but not in human keratinocytes, melanocytes, and fibroblasts (Hoogduijn et al., 2002).

MCHR1, but not MCHR2, expression was detected in human melanocytes and melanoma cells (Hoogduijn et al. 2001, 2002; Saito et al., 2001). Stimulation of cultured human melanocytes with MCH reduced the α-MSH-induced increase in cAMP production (Hoogduijn et al., 2002). Furthermore, the melanogenic actions of α-MSH were inhibited by MCH. MCHR1 has also been identified as a novel autoantigen in patients affected with vitiligo (Kemp et al., 2002).

MC1 and MC2 receptors are coupled to pathways that have the cAMP as a second messenger (Coneet al., 1996; Nordlund et al., 1998). Their main ligand, α-MSH stimulates the processing of tyrosinase and tyrosinase-related proteins and the formation of melanosomes (Hearing, 1999, 2000; Nordlund et al., 1998).

Regulation by α-MSH of transcription and translation of tyrosinase and melanin related proteins (MRPs) could be mediated indirectly through microphthalmia-associated transcription factor (MITF) or directly through activation of PKA-or PKC-dependent pathways. Nevertheless, there is a consensus that MSH stimulates production and activity of MRPs at the transcriptional, translational, and posttranslational levels. Furthermore, MSH stimulates delivery of tyrosine to melanosomes (Potterf & Hearing, 1998).

Besides circulating MSH and other POMC products, the final POMC peptides can potentially be produced in all cutaneous compartments (epidermis, dermis, and adnexa) by epithelial and melanocytic cells and cells of mesenchymal origin such as immune cells, fibroblasts, and endothelial cells and also by release from sensory nerve endings (Slominski et al., 2000). Local POMC gene expression and production of POMC peptides can be modulated with UVR, cytokines, growth factors and cAMP and varies according to phase of the hair cycle (Slominski et al., 2000). Thus locally produced melanocortins and adrenocorticotropin could regulate melanogenesis though para-, auto-, or intracrine mechanisms (Slominski et al., 2000). Melanocytes produce, process POMC and express intracellular MSH receptors (Slominski et al., 2000), and a POMC processing system has been identified in human melanosomes (Peters et al., 2000). Cultured normal epidermal melanocytes treated with β-endorphin show increased melanogenesis, dendricity and proliferation and β-endorphin and μ-opiate antigens have been colocalized in melanosomes (Kauser et al., 2003).

Factors known to raise intracellular cAMP levels such as MSH itself, ACTH, dibutyryl cAMP, cholera toxin, forskolin (Simon et al., 2009) and phosphodiesterase inhibitors also stimulate MC receptors expression and activity (Slominski et al., 2004), leading to an activation of melanogenesis.

Topical application of forskolin to K14-stem cell factor transgenic mice with $Mclr^{e/e}$ background (producing mostly pheomelanin) resulted in a dramatic shift to eumelanogenesis (Spry et al., 2009).

In normal and malignant melanocytes, interleukin (IL-1α, IL-1β, endothelin-1, adult T-cell leukemia-derived factor/thioredoxin (ADF/TRX), interferons (IFN-α, IFN-β, IFN-γ), dibutyryl cAMP, and the hormones MSH and ACTH can stimulate expression of the MC-1 gene and of functional cell surface MSH receptors (Slominski et al., 2004).

Endothelin (ET) is secreted by keratinocytes and stimulated by UVB radiation (Imokawa et al., 1992; Yada et al., 1991); it is a potent stimulator of proliferation and differentiation of human melanocytes (Yada et al., 1991), it increases tyrosinase activity and TYRP1 mRNA expression (Imokawa et al., 1995), also it increases melanocyte dendricity (Hara et al., 1995).

IL-1 can also stimulate MC-1 receptor expression in normal and malignant human keratinocytes (Birchall et al., 1991). A similar effect was described for thymidine dimers and small single-stranded DNA fragments (ssDNA) that are produced intracellulary after UV-induced damage (Eller & Gilchrest 2002; Gilchrest & Eller, 1999).

Tumor necrosis factor (TNF-α) inhibits MC1 expression in melanocytes (Funasaka et al., 1998).

The c-kit/SCF interaction is critical for melanocyte survival (Steel et al., 1992) as shown by the induction of apoptosis in murine melanocytes after injection of a c-kit-blocking antibody (ACK2) (Ito et al., 1999). C-kit is also required for melanocyte activation during the murine hair cycle (Botchkareva et al., 2001; Peters et al., 2002). Epithelial-derived SCF may be the physiological regulator in the c-kit-expressing melanoblasts and melanocyte of mammalian skin by modulating migration and melanocyte cytoskeleton (Botchkareva et al., 2001), differentiation (Lahav et al., 1994; Luo et al., 1995), melanogenesis (Costa et al., 1996; Luo et al., 1995), and cell survival/apoptosis (Ito et al., 1999).

Studies performed on cultured melanoma cells have shown that epinephrine or norepinephrine as well as other adrenergic agonists can stimulate moderately tyrosinase activity and melanin production (Slominski et al., 2004).

Other positive intrinsic regulators of skin pigmentation are endocrine factors (estrogens, androgens), vitamin D, growth factors (fibroblast growth factor - β-FGF), inflammation related factors (eicosanoids, histamine), bone morphogenic proteins; while amongst negative regulators are endocrine factors (glucocorticoids, melatonin), melanocortin antagonists, neural factors (acetylcholine, serotonin, dopamine), cytokines (IL-1, IL-6, IFN-α, IFN-γ, TNF-α, TNF-β), growth factors (TGF-β1), retinoids (Slominski et al., 2004).

Many of the factors described previously that increase melanogenesis are upregulated upon UV irradiation (Yamaguchi & Hearing, 2009).

The aminoacids L-tyrosine and L-DOPA increase melanogenesis through increasing MC1R expression and activity, besides being the substrate for tyrosinase activity (Slominski et al., 2004). L-Tyrosine and L-DOPA act through related but distinct mechanisms (Slominski et al., 2004), with L-tyrosine inducing both melanosomes synthesis and tyrosinase translocation to melanosomes, while L-DOPA primarily increased tyrosinase. Their effects on tyrosinase gene transcription differ, e.g., L-tyrosine has no effect on tyrosinase mRNA, while L-DOPA produces an initial increase in tyrosinase mRNA followed by a decrease below control levels (Slominski & Costantino, 1991). The latter effect could be due to tyrosinase mediated oxidation of L-DOPA generating toxic intermediates of melanogenesis, which would in turn shut-off tyrosinase gene expression as protective mechanism against self-destruction (Slominski & Costantino, 1991).

The ratio of tyrosine to cysteine have also been involved in controlling melanogenesis. By decreasing the extracellular concentration of cystine in cultures of human melanoma cells, a shift to more eumelanic cells was obtained (del Marmol et al., 1996). When cells were cultured at a higher concentration of tyrosine it was found a twofold increase in melanin production in human melanocytes with a decreased ratio of pheomelanin to total melanin (Smit et al. 1997).

High levels of tyrosine are known to reduce the proliferative effect of $\alpha$-MSH and forskolin (Schwan, 2001) and also alter melanocytes morphology (Schwan, 2001); tyrosine also stimulates the activity of tyrosinase and melanogenesis. (Baldea et al., 2009; Smit et al., 1997, 1998, 2008; Wenczl et al., 1998)

The concentration of cysteine in melanosomes is genetically regulated. The subtle gray *(sut)* pigment mutation in mice arose due to a mutation in the Slc7a 11 gene that encodes the plasma membrane cystine/glutamate exchanger xCT. The resulting low rate of extracellular cystine transport into sut melanocytes reduced pheomelanin production with minimal or no effect on eumelanin production (Chintala et al., 2005).

Melanosomal pH in melanosomes is involved in switching between eu and pheomelanogenesis (Simon et al., 2009). Melanosomes in melanocytes from white/fair skin are acidic while those from black/dark skin are near neutral (Smith et al., 2004). Furthermore, the great diversity in normal human skin pigmentation appears to stem from mutations in only several genes, including P, MATP and SLC24A5 (Lamason et al., 2005; Norton et al., 2007).

Mutations in those genes may result in changing the melanosomes ph (Ancans et al. 2001). The effects of more acidic ph on mixed melanogenesis are twofold: a lower activity of tyrosinase and a slower rate of dopaquinone cyclization (the first step in eumelanogenesis) while the CD-quinone cyclization (yielding the first bicyclic intermediate in pheomelanogenesis) proceeds faster (Thompson et al., 1985). Thus, pheomelanogenesis is kinetically favored under more acidic environment in melanosomes.

Effects of metal ions on mixed melanogenesis might have a role in regulating melanogenesis because some metal ions are present at certain levels in melanosomes (Liu et al., 2005).

In eumelanogenesis, DCT plays an important role in promoting the production of DHICA in tautomerization of dopachrome, a reaction also catalyzed by $Cu^{2+}$.

Pheomelanosomes isolated from red human hair contain $Fe^{3+}$, $Zn^{2+}$, and $Cu^{2+}$ at 98, 25, and 20 μmol/g melanin, respectively, in addition to 141 μmol/g of $Mg^{2+}$ (Liu et al., 2005). In pheomelanogenesis, these metal ions have been shown to modify the course of melanogenesis at the monomer level. During oxidation of 5SCD by a chemical oxidant, the presence of $Zn^{2+}$ protects the carboxyl group of QI through chelate formation to preferentially form BTCA in place of BT (Di Donato et al., 2002; Napolitano et al., 2001). Under the same conditions, $Fe^{3+}$ ions appear to form chelates with intermediates to accelerate the ring contraction leading to BZ (Di Donato et al., 2002). $Cu^{2+}$ ions are also involved in modification of the reaction pathway, with a greater yield of the 3-oxo-derivative ODHBT.

At the intracellular level, the major regulatory pathway is cyclic adenosine monophosphate (cAMP) through the activation of protein kinase A (PKA) (reviewed in Slominski et al., 2004) and involves phosphorylation of cAMP responsive element binding protein (CREB) and CREB binding protein (CBP). At the intracellular level, the major regulatory pathway is cyclic adenosine monophosphate (cAMP) through the activation of protein kinase A (PKA) and involves phosphorylation of cAMP responsive element binding protein (CREB) and CREB binding protein (CBP). Phosphorylated CREB interacts with CBP to activate the expression of MITF throughout the CRE in the promoter region of the gene. MITF in turn regulates transcription of genes coding MRPs. Because CRE is absent from the promoter of tyrosinase and TYRP1 genes, the transcriptional control of melanogenesis by cAMP is coordinated predominantly by MITF. However, transcription of TYRP2 can potentially be activated through direct activation of CRE by CREB (reviewed in Slominski et al., 2004).

MITF is one of the most critical factors for the regulation of melanocyte function. In addition to serving as an essential regulator for expression of enzymes and structural proteins involved in melanin production (such as tyrosinase, TYRP2/DCT), MITF is also an essential regulator of genes involved in melanocyte development, proliferation, replenishment during feather and hair cycles, survival (such as BCL2, p21, p16, CDK2, TBX2) and malignant transformation. (Arnheiter, 2010; Liu & Fisher, 2010)

In addition, PH and TH hydroxylation phenylalanine to tyrosine and tyrosine to DOPA, respectively, are controlled by the PKA-dependent phosphorylation of regulatory serine residues (Stryer, 1988).

cAMP also modifies other pathways controlling melanocyte differentiation and proliferation, for example, the phosphatidylinositol (PI) 3-kinase pathway with its downstream regulatory element p70S6 kinase (Busca & Ballotti, 2000; Haddad et al., 1999). Inhibition of this pathway stimulates melanogenesis, and the pathway can be partially inhibited by cAMP (Busca & Ballotti, 2000).

cAMP may also regulate dendritogenesis and possibly melanogenesis through activation of the Rho family of small GTP-binding proteins (Busca & Ballotti, 2000).

cAMP can also inhibit melanogenesis through PKA-independent p21Ras activation (Busca & Ballotti, 2000). Ras would activate Braf kinase and consequently mitogen-activated protein (MAP) kinases ERK1 and ERK2. MAP kinases phosphorylate MITF leading to its ubiquitination and degradation, thus removing a major transcriptional regulator of MRP genes expression (Busca & Ballotti, 2000; Englaro et al., 1998; Jordan & Jackson, 2000). In addition, activation of ras oncogene inhibits melanogenesis in normal and malignant melanocytes (Englaro et al., 1998).

Another signal transduction pathway important in the regulation of melanogenesis is represented by protein kinase C (PKC). Thus diacylglycerol (endogenous activator of PKC) can stimulate melanin synthesis both in cell culture and in vivo, while melanogenesis is blocked by PKC inhibitors or cellular depletion of PKC (Slominski et al., 2004).

Additional pathways that have been involved in the positive regulation of melanogenesis include those activated by nitric oxide (NO) and cGMP (Romero-Graillet et al., 1996) as well as thymidine dimers (Romero-Graillet et al., 1996; Eller et al., 2002) and small single-stranded DNA fragments (ssDNA) (Eller et al., 2002).

These pigmentary effects of small oligonucleotides could follow a pathway functionally similar to the SOS response system of bacteria (Eller et al., 2002).

## 4. Biologic roles of ultraviolet light in melanocytes

The detrimental effects of solar UVR (295-400nm) on the skin are well established and are usually categorized as: acute or chronic. Acute effects include DNA and oxidative damage, mutation, immunosuppression, erythema (sunburn) and tanning. The chronic effects include skin cancers, which are thought to be a consequence of mutation, immunosuppression and photoaging, which is thought to be a consequence of the induction of matrix metalloproteinases (MMPs) (Young, 2006).

The emission spectrum of the sun is rich in UVA radiation with UVB radiation accounting for less than 5% of total UVR content. However, because most skin chromophores are primarily UVB absorbers, it is that part of the solar spectrum that causes most of the biological effects.

UV radiation from sunlight increases the risk of developing three types of skin cancer: basal cell carcinoma (BCC), squamous cell carcinoma (SCC), and malignant melanoma, in order of frequency (Liu & Fisher, 2010). While melanoma arises from the pigment-producing melanocytes in skin, BCC and SCC arise from keratinocytes.

UV is a powerful extrinsic regulator of skin pigmentation. As a first line of defense, melanin produced by melanocytes within the epidermis filters UV light, preventing UV-induced DNA damage upon sun exposure. Hence, individuals with fairer/lighter skin suffer more frequently from skin cancers, as darker skin prevents photocarcinogenesis more efficiently (Miyamura et al., 2007; Yamaguchi, 2006).

Although direct evidence is lacking, it is assumed that solar ultraviolet A (UVA) radiation (320–400 nm) may play a significant role relative to ultraviolet B (UVB) radiation (290–320 nm) in melanoma etiology (Wang et al., 2001). When UV radiation damages a cell, it mutates the cellular DNA with distinctive mutational patterns.

The major UVB lesions produced are cyclobutane-type pyrimidine dimers (CPDs) due to direct absorption of UVB radiation in DNA. CPDs are quite mutagenic, especially in mammalian cells, initiating primary base substitutions in DNA. UVB induces cytosine to thymine transitions at the dipyrimidine sites, creating a UV-specific mutation signature that is ubiquitously observed in multiple organisms (Liu & Fisher, 2010).

In contrast, UVA radiation is very weakly absorbed by DNA. Most of the studied biologic effects of UVA radiation, like lipid peroxidation and membrane damage are mediated by reactive oxygen species (ROS) and they are probably the major contributors to UVA-induced cell death (Tyrell, 1994; Girotti et al., 2001; Schmitz et al., 1995). Failure to eliminate UV-damaged cells through control led apoptosis may result in disease states such as skin cancer or lead to faster aging of the skin (Brash et al., 1991).

Repair of DNA photolesions requires cell cycle arest prior to replication and mitosis (Murray, 1992). It has been hypothesized that the DNA photodamage to the telomere 3' overhang (TTAGGG) may be a specific trigger for the cellular defense responses to UVR (Eller et al., 2003) and that this is the reason why oligonucleotides with homology (i.e. TT) to this sequence are able to induce such responses as p53 activation.

Skin darkening in response to solar UVR occurs via two distinct mechanisms: Immediate pigment darkening (IPD) and delayed tanning (DT). Both processes are influenced by genetic factors and are more pronounced with darker constitutive pigmentation. They are mechanistically different processes, and their exact biological role remains to be discovered. IPD starts during UV irradiation as a grayish coloration that gradually fades to a brown color over a period of minutes to days depending on UVR dose and individual complexion. These changes are due to oxidation of pre-existing melanin and redistribution of melanosomes from a perinuclear to a peripheral dendritic location (Routaboul et al., 1999). The color change may be so subtle as to be almost undetectable in fair-skinned individuals but is easily observed in skin types IV (or darker). IPD was not showed so far to have a photoprotective effect; hence, its biological function remains unknown.

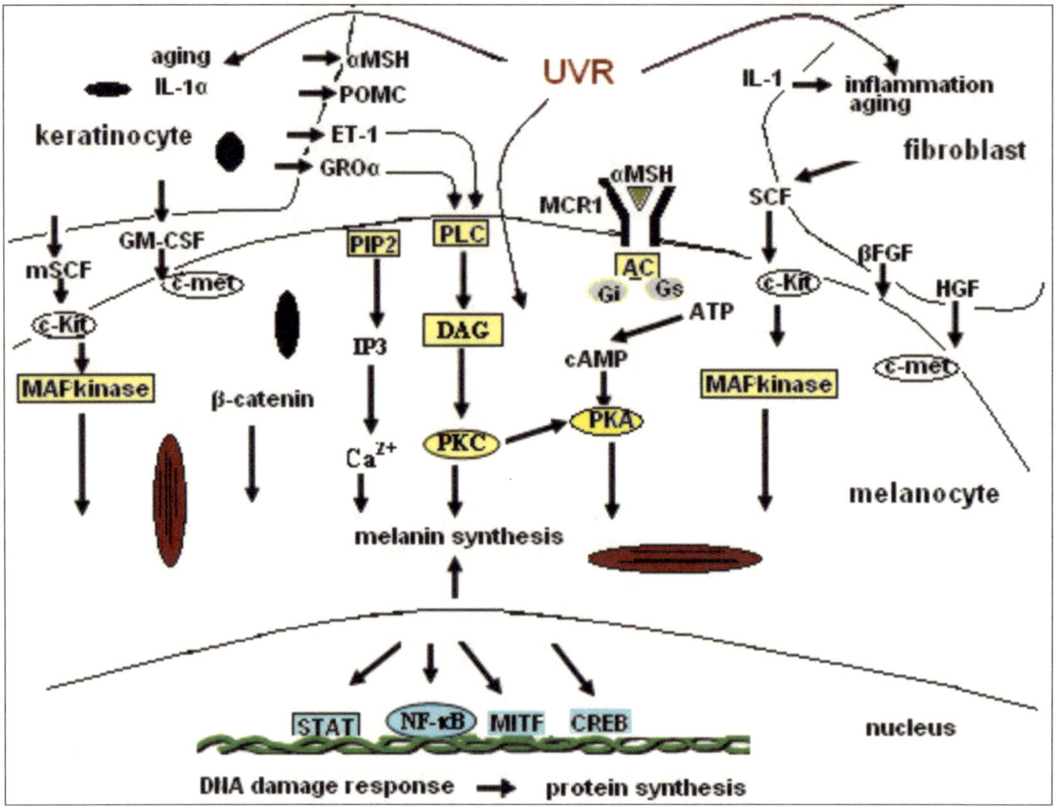


Fig. 2. Mechanisms of ultraviolet radiation - induced pigmentation in the skin cells; Abbreviations: AC- adenilate cyclase, αMSH- α melanocyte stimulating hormone, cAMP- cyclic adenosine monophosphate, βFGF-βfibroblast growth factor, DAG- diacilglycerol, ET-1- endothelin-1, GROα- growth related oncogene α, GM-CSF- granulocyte-macrophage colony-stimulating factor, HGF- hepatocyte growth factor, IL-1- interleukin -1, IP3- inositol-tri-phosphate, MAPkinase- mitogen activated phosphokinase, MC1R- melanocortin receptor 1, mSCF- membrane bound stem cell factor, PIP2-phospho inositol di-phosphate, PKA, PKC- protein kinase A & C, PLC- phospholipase C, POMC- proopiomelanocortin, SCF -m stem cell factor, transcription factors (STAT, MITF, CREB, NF-kβ), UVR- ultraviolet radiation. The keratinocytes and fibroblasts stimulate the melanocyte melanogenesis through paracrine secretion of the above factors and activation of their subsequent receptors. The most important mechanisms rely on PLC-DAG-PKC, respective AC-cAMP-PKA activation of the transcription factors. Also $Ca^{2+}$increase in cytoplasm through the PIP2-IP3 pathway, stimulates the synthesis of the enzymes involved in melanogenesis (e.g. tyrosinase and related proteins)

DT, which results from melanogenesis, is associated with increased melanocyte activity and proliferation. It is evident 3-4 days after UVR exposure and is maximal from 10 days to 3-4 weeks depending on complexion and UVR dose. It may take several weeks for the skin to return to its base constitutive color. UVA-induced DT is two or three orders of magnitude less efficient per unit than the UVB induced, has an earlier onset and is oxygen dependent (Eller & Gilchrest; 2000).

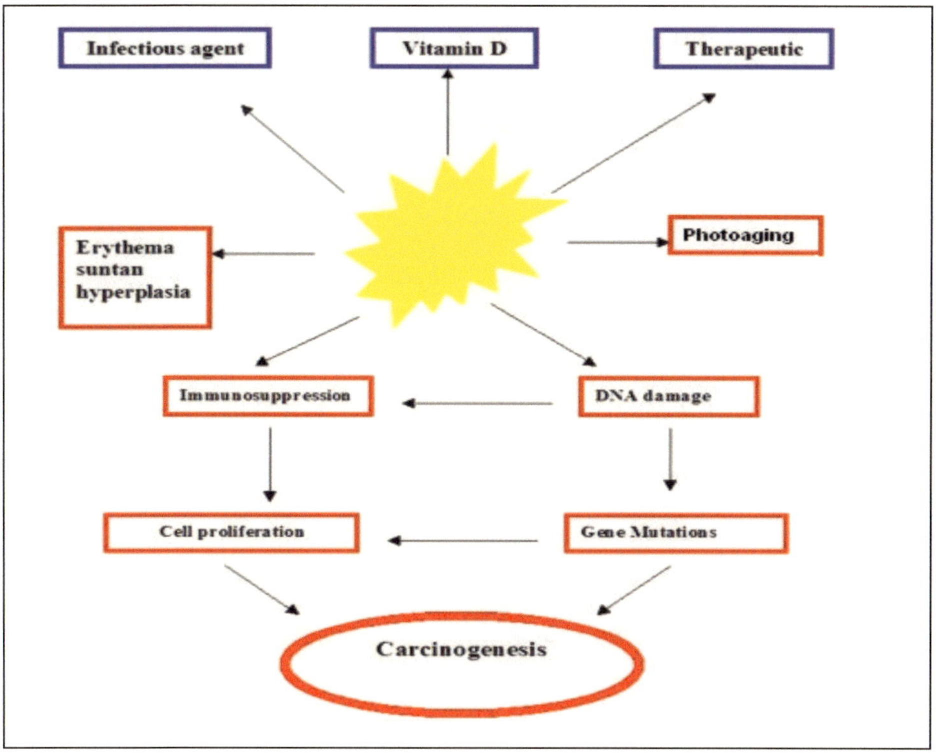


Fig. 3. Biological effects of solar irradiation on the skin (source WHO, 2006)

In response to UV induced DNA damage, the p53 expression in keratinocytes is activated, initiating the pigment synthesis in melanocytes via the p53-dependent cAMP- MITF tanning pathway (Cui et al., 2007), although this protection is probably not as effective as constitutive epidermal pigmentation. P53 binds directly to the POMC promoter, initiating POMC transcription and $\alpha$-MSH production; $\alpha$-MSH binds with its receptor MC1 R, activating the cAMP pathway in melanocytes. MITF activation leads to activation of melanogenesis through enhanced transcription of the pigment enzyme genes TYR, TYRP1, and DCT/TYRP2. Besides melanin synthesis, the expression of the genes necessary for melanosome biogenesis, melanosome transport and dendritogenesis is control led coordinately by MITF (Cheii et al., 2010).

UVR modulates the process of melanosome transfer from the melanocytes to the keratinocytes through upregulated expression of PAR-2 and lectin-binding receptors and increase phagocytic activity of cultured keratinocytes (Boissy, 2003). UVR also decreases the cytoplasmic dynein levels resulting in augmented melanosomal anterograde transport (Randolph et al., 2000). The melanosomes are redistributed to supranuclear areas, thus shielding the nuclei of skin cells and eventually transported to the superficial epidermis during epidermal keratinocyte maturation.

UV radiation has also been implicated in modulating the proliferation and differentiation state of melanocytes (Kawaguchi et al., 2001). Normal epidermis contains TYRP1-positive mature melanocytes, KIT-positive precursors, and few MITF-positive cells. In addition, UV appears to contribute to melanocyte maturation and development through a MITF-activation-dependent pathway (Kawaguchi et al., 2001). Upon UV irradiation, SCF has been observed to be released by keratinocytes and activates KIT on melanocytes (or their precursors), which first differentiate into MITF-positive and TYRP2 (DCT)-positive melanoblasts, and then mature into TYRP1-positive melanocytes. Pre-existing TYRP1-positive mature melanocytes may be incapable of proliferating and differentiating further and thus may enter alternative pathways upon UV irradiation (Kawaguchi et al., 2001).

Another biologic role for UV in skin is stimulating the production of vitamin D from cholesterol-derived precursors, but it destroys folate through photolysis. Maximum production of vitamin D can be achieved after exposure to suberythemal doses of UVB.

Many factors that increase melanogenesis (POMC, α-MSH, β-FGF, endothelins, and inflammation mediators) are upregulated upon UV irradiation (Yamaguchi & Hearing, 2009). α-MSH is an important regulator of the response of melanocytes to UV and stimulates eumelanin synthesis (Abdel-Malek et al., 2009).

UVR also upregulates the expression of MSH receptors, amplifying the melanogenic effect of exogenous MSH in a dose-dependent manner in vivo and in cell culture systems (Slominski et al., 2004). In murine melanoma, UVR action appeared to involve arrest of the cell cycle at the G2 phase, when cultured melanocytes express maximal MSH receptor activity and responsiveness to MSH (Pawelek et al., 1992). The G2 phase coupling of increased MSH receptor expression was associated with increased cellular responsiveness to the ligand (Pawelek et al., 1992). Nevertheless, G2 restricted expression and activity of MSH receptors appears to be specific for rodent melanocytes, since it has not been observed in a human model.

UV also activates DNA damage response pathways within minutes of a single exposure, regulating damaged cells via UV-induced apoptosis, cell cycle arrest, DNA repair, or pathways linked to oxidative stress (Liu & Fisher, 2010).

There is considerable variation between the ability of human populations to efficiently tan. This variation has been clinically classified by Fitzpatrick in six skin phototypes (Fitzpatrick, 1988).

Phototype I has pale, white skin, blue eyes, blond/red hair, it never tans, phototype II has fair skin, light colored eyes, it tans poorly, both of them have a high risk of sunburn; phototype III has darker white skin, it has a good ability to tan and a moderate risk of sunburn; phototype IV has olive skin, it tans easily and has a low risk of sunburn; phototype V has brown skin, and phototype VI has dark brown or black skin, they both have an excellent ability to tan and a very low risk of sunburn (Fitzpatrick, 1988). The variations in human skin inducible pigmentation by UVR are partially due to the existence of the redhead/MC1 R allele (Liu & Fisher, 2010). Epidemiological studies found a strong association between MC1R loss-of-function allele and the risk for malignant transformation of epidermal melanocytes (Abdel-Malek et al., 2009), thus implying that MC1R functions as a melanoma susceptibility gene (Cui et al., 2007).

Exposure of cultured melanocytes to T-oligonucleotides, which activated the DNA damage response, resulted in increased melanogenesis via increasing MClR expression. Moreover, forskolin activation of the cAMP pathway, had the same effects as α-MSH on the UV response of human melanocytes, and reduced the extent of DNA photoproducts in UV-irradiated mouse skin as well as human skin substitutes (D'Orazio et al., 2006; Passeron et al., 2009). Besides increasing pigmentation, α-MSH reduces UV-induced oxidative DNA damage by inhibiting the generation of hydrogen peroxide and enhances the repair of DNA photoproducts (Bohm et al., 2005; Kadekaro et al., 2005). Activation of MC1R upregulates the expression of DNA repair genes (Smith et al., 2008).

| Skin phototype | Constitutive skin color | Ability to tan (facultative skin color) | Susceptibility to sunburn | Susceptibility to skin cancer |
|---|---|---|---|---|
| I | White | Very poor/none | High | High |
| II | White | Poor | High | High |
| III | White | Moderate/Good | Moderate | Moderate |
| IV | Olive | Very good | Low | Low |
| V | Brown | Very good | Very low | Very low |
| VI | Black | Very good | Very low | Very low |

Table 1. Classification of human skin types with respect to their ability to tan and UV-induced carcinogenesis (adapted after Fitzpatrick, 1988)

## 5. Cytotoxicity of melanins and their precursors

The transformation process whereby UV damage may result in melanoma initiation is poorly understood, especially in terms of UV-induced genotoxicity in pigmented cells, where melanin can act either as a sunscreen or as a photosensitizer (Picardo et al., 1999). Patients with OCA1, (who do not present tyrosinase activity) develop nonmelanoma skin cancers but not melanoma (Streutker et al., 2000).

It seems that melanogenesis, especially pheomelanogenesis, is more potent in inducing oxidative damage in the melanocytes and surrounding cells than melanin itself. Also, the synthesis of pheomelanin, consumes cysteine and this may further limit the capacity of the cellular antioxidative defense (Smith et al., 2008). In fact, in cultured normal melanocytes, stimulation of melanogenesis leads to the suppression of proliferation, cell senescence and eventually to cell death (Hirobe et al., 2003). Melanogenesis process generates highly toxic melanin intermediates and byproducts. Those intermediates are usually small molecules, such as 5,6-dihydroxyindole, 5,6-dihydroxyindole-2-carboxylic acid, quinones, indole-quinones, 5-S-cysteinyldopa and hydrogen peroxide (Hearing, 2005). Amongst them, some are the result of tyrosinase activity: ortho-quinones including dopaquinone, dopachrome, DHI-quinone, and DHICA-quinone (Hearing, 2005). Orthoquinines can also be formed directly during the initial stage of melanogenesis (Cooksey et al., 1997).

Ectopic expression of tyrosinase in the absence of TYRP1 or DCT may cause severe cytotoxicity to nonmelanocytic cells in which no melanosomal compartmentalization is present (Singh & Jimbow, 1998). The mechanism of cytotoxicity of DHI and DHICA, and also of 5-S-cysteinyldopa, involves the production of reactive oxygen species, but their toxicity seems to be less important in melanocytes due to melanosomal containment (Singh & Jimbow, 1998).

The escape of those toxic substances from melanosomes into the cytoplasm, nucleus, and mitochondria induces cytotoxic effects that are deleterious to melanocytes and melanoma cells (Chen et al., 2009a, 2009b). One of the roles of melanosomes in normal melanocytes is to provide an environment where these chemical reactions can occur and to permit the formation of melanin biopolymers, which in turn inactivate the process and keep the cytotoxic effects under control (Chen et al., 2009a).

Dopachrome, although less reactive, is able to inactivate important sulfhydryl enzymes, eventually leading to cell death. Thus, TYRP2/DCT who catalysis the transformation of dopachrome to DHICA is considered to be a "rescue" enzyme, essential for melanocyte survival (Hearing, 2005). DHICA sensitizes DNA SSB with 313 nm exposure, especially in the presence of oxygen (Routaboul et al., 1995). Mutations in DCT that decrease catalytic function affect DHICA production and are generally quite cytotoxic to melanocytes. Melanocytes typically express DCT before any of the other melanogenic enzymes, presumably to minimize such toxicity (Steel et al., 1992).

Melanin precursors may have protective roles in melanocytes. DHI and to a less extent, DHICA can contribute significantly to the skin protection from damaging UV radiation by quenching oxygen species and providing an additional amount of photoprotective pigment. Upon photoexcitation, DHI can react with oxygen and related species, giving rise to hydroxylated oligomer species that can polymerize to eumelanic pigments (Ito & Wakamatsu, 2008).

Hence, detoxification of endogenous melanogenic cytotoxicity appears to be a double edged sword. In the case of melanomas, the detoxifying functions of melanosomes might render cells resistant to anticancer drugs. It has been shown that the melanogenic system is involved in the regulation of drug sensitivity. Melanosomes are involved in drug trapping and export (Chen et al., 2006) and in the regulation of drug sensitivity through the melanosome biogenesis pathway (Chen et al., 2009a, 2009b).

The cytotoxicity of ortho-quinones could potentially lead to chemotherapeutic approaches to treat melanoma; 4-S-cysteaminylphenol and its derivatives appear to be the most promising antimelanoma agents (Ito & Wakamatsu, 2008).

The end product of eumelanogenesis, eumelanin acts as a redox pigment with both reducing and oxidizing capabilities towards oxygen radicals and other chemical redox systems, it mainly functions like a pseudosuperoxidedismutase. Also, the pigment has free radical scavenger activity since it binds redox active metals and initiates photon/phonon conversion (Ito & Wakamatsu, 2008).

In contrast to eumelanin, pheomelanin is hypothesized to play a role in melanomas. Some hypothesize that there is a link between the increased cancer risk in pacients with lower phototype and the increased phototoxicity of pheomelanin (Simon, 2009). The pheomelanin pigment is synthesized starting from a combination of 5-5 and 2-5-CD isomers in different ratio. The pigment derived from 5-5-CD is more photoreactive than that derived from 2-5-CD, the later being resistant to photochemical damage by natural sunlight (Greco, 2009).

Studies of UVB-induced cyclobutane dimerization and apoptosis of keratinocytes in congenic black, yellow and albino mice showed that pheomelanin sensitizes apoptosis (via caspase-3 activation) (Brash et al., 1991; Takeuchi et al., 2004).

There remains the need to understand the molecular composition of pheomelanins to determine what chromophores activate oxygen (Simon, 2009).

In vitro studies showed that 5-SCD photobinds to native DNA after exposure to UVB radiation and also induced single-strand breaks (SSB) in DNA (Chedekel and Zeize, 1988). 5-SCD is photochemically unstable in the presence of UVA radiation and oxygen (Costantini et al., 1994), leading to superoxide anion production (Chedekel and Zeize, 1988). UV irradiation of pheomelanin can also lead to the formation of hydroxyl radicals, and hydrogen peroxide capable of affecting important biological targets such as DNA (Chedekel and Zeize, 1988) or membrane lipids (Schmitz et al., 1995), acting as UVB and UVA photosensitizer in mammalian skin in vivo (Takeuchi et al. 2004).

Melanogenesis, but not melanin itself, was associated with oxidative based damage in human melanoma cells (Kvam & Tyrrell 1999, Kvam & Dahle, 2003). Melanocyte "autodestruction" by intermediates of melanin metabolism has been implicated in the etiology of vitiligo (Le Poole et al., 1994).

Tyrosine-induced melanogenesis in melanocytes was accompanied by increased production of ROS (Baldea et al., 2009) and decreased concentration of intracellular glutathione (Smit et al., 2008); it also increased early induction of Heme Oxygenase 1 gene, a typical response to oxidative stress, after UVA irradiation (Marrot et al., 2005). The ratio of pheomelanin to total melanin in melanocyte cultures from skin type 1 and skin type IV, after tyrosine stimulation remained the same in skin type IV, but relatively more pheomelanin was induced in skin type 1. This was associated with an increase in UVA-induced SSB in DNA (Wenczl et al., 1998). The hypothesis of melanocyte carcinogenesis states that an essential part of melanocytes' malignant transformation is a change in the redox state of melanin from a mostly antioxidant state to a prooxidant state (Meyskens et al., 2001). This is supported by data that show that melanoma cells have a remarkably abnormal content of antioxidants, including vitamin E, polyunsaturated fatty acids, and catalase (Picardo et al, 1996; Briganti & Picardo, 2003; Kwan & Dahle, 2003). Also, clinical displastic nevi, recognized precursors of melanoma, suffer from chronic oxidative stress, even without the influence of UV radiation, due to increased pheomelanin synthesis. (Smit et al., 2008)

Melanin precursors have genotoxic and mutagenic effects, which may be amplified by the free radicals and reactive oxygen species generated during melanogenesis. This mutagenic environment in melanoma cells may lead to genetic instability and appearance of new, more aggressive cell populations resistant to therapy (Slominski et al., 1998).

Diffusion of potentially cytotoxic products of melanogenesis from melanosomes is thought to be minimal in normal melanocytes. There are several cytosolic processes that are invoked as cytoprotective mechanisms (Smith et al., 2008). The intermediates that may reach the cytosol consist essentially of quinones liberated directly or generated by oxidation from hydroquinones that leak through the melanosomal membrane. Quinone detoxification can be done by quenching by glutathione with the formation of S-glutathionyl adducts, by quinone reductases (DT-diaphorase), inactivation of dihydroxyindoles by O-methylation catalyzed by the enzyme catechol-O-methyl transferase (Axelrod & Lerner, 1963), glucuronidation and sulfonation mainly due to hepatic metabolism of the methylated derivatives formed in mellanogenic cells (Pavel et al., 1986).

## 6. Oxidative stress defence in melanocytes

Melanogenesis and stratum corneum thickening occur concurrently during the normal tanning response. Although photoprotection may be considered to be a passive physical process, e.g. the attenuation of UVR by melanin and/or stratum corneum thickening, it may also be considered as an active enzymatic process, e.g. as a means by which DNA repair is enhanced or ROS are inactivated. Chimeric epidermal reconstructs with melanocytes from one skin type added to keratinocyte cultures of a different skin type suggest keratinocyte/melanocyte interaction with both cell types regulating antioxidant defense in a skin type-dependent way (Bessou-Touya et al., *1998).*

Melanocytes seem to be extremely susceptible to free radicals, either in the activation of their physiologic role or in deleterious effects (Shindo et al., 1993; Picardo et al., 1991; Romero-Graillet et al., 1996). One reason is low catalase levels in these cells (Maresca et al., 2006). Therefore, antioxidants are considered to be among the physiologic photoprotective compounds of the skin (Applegate & Frenck 1995; Briganti & Picardo, 2003).

The initial free radical scavenging machinery involves superoxide dismutase (SOD), which catalyzes the dismutation of two molecules of the superoxide radical anion into hydrogen peroxide and diatomic oxygen. Then, hydrogen peroxide is converted by catalase (Cat) and peroxidases into water (Steenvoorden & van Henegouwen, 1997).

Thioredoxin reductase together with its electron acceptor thioredoxin, thioredoxin peroxidases, glutathione reductase/glutathione coupled to glutathione peroxidase - present in small amounts in melanocytes (Yohn et al., 1991) are involved in the removal of $H_2O_2$ deriving from enzymatic dismutation of superoxide anion ($O^{2-}$) catalyzed by SOD (Nordberg & Arner, 2001; Schallreuter & Wood, 2001). The high SOD/Cat ratio, can lead to an increased intracellular production of hydrogen peroxide, thus is considered as a parameter of the cells susceptibility to external oxidative stress (Maresca et al., 2006).

UVA irradiation is depleting the skin of antioxidants (Sanders et al., 2004), among which Cat is the most sensitive. Low levels of Cat activity were previously observed in different cutaneous experimental models (which contained lightly pigmented melanocytes) and they were always associated with a stress-prone status (Maresca et al., 2006; Bessou-Touya et al., 1998; Gramatico et al., 1998; Picardo et al., 1999, Kadekaro et al., 2003; Kvam E & Dahle, 2004). In melanocytes, the role of Cat is critical because it is the first enzyme devoted to the neutralization of $H_2O_2$ (Yohn et al., 1991) a byproduct of the melanogenic pathway (Nappi & Vass, 1996). Cat oxidative damage is detrimental, because when damaged it recovers slowly (Shindo et al., 1994; Shindo & Hashimoto, 1997). This results in accumulation of $H_2O_2$ in the cell and damaged several structures, including Cat (Shindo et al., 1994; Shindo & Hashimoto, 1997) and tyrosinase (Schallreuter et al., 2008).

Overall, UVA was also more effective than UVB in inducing impairment in Cat activity (Zigman et al., 1996; Rhie et al., 2001; Hellemans et al., 2003) .

In the melanocytes, the dominant skin pigment melanin and its precursors are complex redox systems, the resultant properties of which are modified by ph, temperature, illumination with ultraviolet and visible light. Melanins act as a filter absorbing UV photons as well as a quencher of free radicals generated in the skin after UV exposure.

Eumelanin is capable of scavenging the superoxide anion and hydrogen peroxide, whereas pheomelanin acts as a photosensitizing agent (Prota, 1997), amplifying ROS production and increasing DNA damage after UVA (Menon et al., 1983; Ranadive et al., 1986; Prota, 1997; Kvam & Dahle, 2004).

The overall scheme proposed for auto-oxidation of melanin consists of one electron reduction of molecular oxygen to superoxide anion, followed by SOD reduction of superoxide to $H_2O_2$, degraded by catalase and oxidation of superoxide to $O_2$, and spontaneous dismutation of superoxide to equimolar $H_2O_2$ and $O_2$. Autooxidation of melanin may be important, rate limiting process in coupled reactions where melanin functions as an electron transfer agent (Sarna & Swartz, 2006).

Oxygen radicals, and in particular hydrogen peroxide, are considered as intracellular second messengers since they have major roles in cell survival and integrity (Schalreuter et al, 2008). Their level is increased by extracellular ligands such as cytokines (Schreck & Bauerle 1991), ROS act as biologic mediators of UV-induced phosphorylation of membrane receptors (Tyrell, 1994; Schmitz et al, 1995, Peus et al., 1999; Girotti, 2001, Kvam & Dahle, 2003); $H_2O_2$ is a normal byproduct of the melanogenic pathway (Nappi & Vass, 1996); in several cellular systems, $H_2O_2$ acts as an intracellular second messenger for TNF$\alpha$ and TGF$\beta$ (Thannickal & Fanburg, 1995; Chen et al., 1995; Lo et al., 1996); it activates growth factor receptors and in particular those of epidermal growth factor (EGFR) and initiates multiple signaling responses associated with mitogenesis and cell growth regulation (Ulrich & Schlessinger 1990).

$H_2O_2$, in micromolar concentrations can be deleterious to many proteins and peptides leading to deactivation / disruption of many important proteins and peptides involved in melanogenesis including tyrosinase (deactivation of the enzyme active site due to a methionine residue in position 374) (Schweikardt et al., 2007), POMC derived peptides (α-MSH, β-endorphin) (Spencer et al., 2007), 6R-l-erythro 5,6,7,8-tetrahydrobiopterin (6BH4), acetylcholinesterase (Schallreuter, 2005), the prohormone convertases PC1, PC2, Furin, PACE4 and, even the antioxidant mechanism including catalase, thioredoxin reductase and the methionine sulfoxide reductases A&B (Schallreuter, 2005; Spencer et al., 2007; Gibbons et al, 2006). However, $H_2O_2$ is upregulating multiple transcription factors including p53, MITF and NFkB (nuclear factor kappa B), epidermal growth factor (EGFR), and the antioxidant enzymes catalase, thioredoxin reductase, glutathione reductase and the methionine sulfoxide reductases A & B (Schallreuter et al, 2001; Schallreuter, 2005; Gibbons et al, 2006). Enzyme activities are directly controlled by $H_2O_2$ in a concentration dependent manner. This is also the case for PAH, THI and tyrosinase, (Wood et al., 2004; Schallreuter et al, 2008) thus being involved in melanocyte mitogenesis, melanogenesis and cell growth regulation. Regulation and protection of tyrosinase against a ROS burst is also provided by both tyrosinase related proteins TYRP1 and TRP2. TYRP1 has been recognised as a peroxidase (Halaban et al., 1990), while TRP2 has an additional function as dopachrome tautomerase (Prota, 1992). In addition to TYRP1 and TRP2 the calcium binding protein calnexin is present in the melanosomal membrane adding another force for redox homeostasis in the melanosome (Jimbow et al., 2001).

## 7. Melanocyte senescence – defence against carcinogenesis

Senescence is a checkpoint response due to DNA activation by the disfunctional telomeres after exposure to oncogenic stress (such as UV radiation). Senescence blocks proliferation (and the resultant oncogenic threat), but allows the cell to live on and perform its physiologic function (Mooi & Peeper, 2006).

As activation of BRAF, or NRAS, alone induces senescence in melanocytes, melanoma progression must be accompanied by compensating events, for example inactivation of the CDKN2A locus encoding p161NK4a via genetic lesions (Bennett, 2008), epigenetic silencing (Richards and Medrano, 2009; Rothhammer and Bosserhoff, 2007), or repression of p161NK4a expression through activation of Wnt/β-catenin signalling (Delmas et al., 2007). Consistent with senescence representing a major barrier to melanoma initiation is the observation that benign nevi, as well as carrying frequent activating mutation of BRAF or NRAS, include a mass of senescent melanocytes (Gray-Schopfer et al., 2006; Michaloglou et al., 2005). If the initial senescence barrier is overcome, melanomas can progress to a radial growth phase. For the majority of melanomas that do not arise from a pre-existing nevus, senescence bypass via bi-allelic loss of p161NK4a would occur prior to activation of BRAF/ NRAS. By contrast, nevi may be generated by monoallelic loss of p161NK4a prior to BRAF/NRAS mutation, with subsequent inactivation of the second p16INK4a allele leading to melanoma. Thus, the order in which mutations occur will determine whether melanoma arises de novo or from a pre-existing nevus (Hoek & Goding, 2010).

Normal, adult skin melanocytes are long lived cells with a very low, if any, proliferation rate in vivo that produce abundant levels of the antiapoptotic protein Bcl2 (McGill et al, 2002) and Slug (Gupta, 2005). These factors protect cells from p53-dependent apoptosis and promote melanocyte survival, even at the cost of entering senescence after mutagenic stimuli induced damage (Hoek & Goding, 2010). It is possible that melanoma originates from differentiated melanocytes by a process of de-differentiation arising from "phenotype-switching", sustained by the observation that differentiated melanocytes can be induced to proliferate in culture (Hoek & Goding, 2010).

The most important factor that regulates the choice between a proliferation-type response in melanocytes or a differentiation, pigment production and senescence/apoptosis response seems to be MITF. MITF is implicated in differentiation through the activation of pigmentation genes and is the key regulator of cell division, driving a differentiation-associated cell cycle arrest via up-regulation of p16 and p21 (Goding, 2010). MITF can also promote cell division by suppressing p27 expression and senescence and inhibit proliferation via up-regulation of p21 Cipl and p 161NK4a. Thus in addition to its role in survival and differentiation, MITF is also charged with suppressing senescence and coordinating cell cycle entry and exit depending on its levels and activity (Hoek & Goding, 2010).

MITF was also identified as a lineage-addiction oncogene, being amplified to varying degrees in about one-sixth of melanomas (Garraway et al., 2005).

## 8. Conclusions

UV exposure alone or through induced melanin synthesis, generates cytotoxic compounds that might trigger oxidative damage of important biological targets such as DNA and membranes, but it also activates the defense mechanisms of the cell. However, how much these phototoxic and photoprotective events are functionally important in vivo requires further studies.

There is an intimate relationship between pigmentation, senescence, apoptosis and cell division, and the key role in regulating these mechanisms is attributed to MITF. A better understanding of the skin responses to oncogenic threats, and especially UV radiation could be beneficial in improving the prevention of skin carcinogenesis and photo-aging.

## 9. References

Abdel-Malek Z A, Ruwe A, Kavanagh-Starner R, Kadekaro A L, Swope V, Haskeli-Luevano C, Koikov L & Knittel J J. α-MSH tripeptide analogs activate the melanocortin 1 receptor and reduce UV-induced DNA damage in human melanocytes *Pigment Cell Melanoma Res.* 2009; 22: 635-644

Alonso L & Fuchs E. Stem cells of the skin epithelium. *Proc. Natl. Acad. Sci. USA.* 2003; 100: 11830-11835

Ancans J, Tobin D J, Hoogduijn M J, Smit N P, Wakamatsu K & Thody A J. Melanosomal pH controls rate of melanogenesis, eumelanin/phaeomelanin ratio and melanosome maturation in melanocytes and melanoma cells. *Exp. Cell Res.* 2001; 268: 26-35

Applegate L N & Frenk E. Cellular defense mechanisms of the skin against oxidant stress and in particular UVA radiation. *Eur. J. Dermatol.* 1995; 5: 97–103

Arnheiter H. The discovery of the microphthalmia locus and its gene, *Mitf Pigment Cell Melanoma Res.* 2010; 23: 729-735

Axelrod J., & Lerner A B, O-methylation I the conversion of tyrosine to melanin. *Biochim. Biophys. Acta* 1963: 71; 650-655

Baldea I, Mocan T, Cosgarea R. The role of ultraviolet radiation and tyrosine stimulated melanogenesis in the induction of oxidative stress alterations in fair skin melanocytes. *Exp Oncol* 2009; 31(4): 200-208

Bennett D C. How to make a melanoma: what do we know of the primary clonal events? *Pigment Cell Melanoma Res.* 2008; 21: 27-38.

Bessou-Touya S, Picardo M, Maresca V, Surlève Bazeille JE, Pain C & Taieb A. Chimeric human epidermal reconstructs to study the role of melanocytes and keratinocytes in pigmentation and photoprotection. *J Invest Dermatol* 1998; 111: 1103–1108

Birchall N, Orlow SJ, Kupper T & Pawelek J. Interactions between ultraviolet light and interleukin-1 on MSH binding in both mouse melanoma and human squamous carcinoma cells. *Biochem Biophys Res Commun.* 1991; 175: 839–845

Bohm M, Wolff I, Scholzen T E, Robinson S J, Healy E, Luger T A & Schwartz A. alpha-Melanocyte stimulating hormaone protects from ultraviolet radiataion induced apoptosis and DNA damage. *J. Biol. Chem.* 2005; 280: 5795-5802

Boissy R E, Sakai C, Zhao H, Kobayashi T & Hearing VJ. Human tyrosinase-related protein-1 (TRP-1) does not function as a DHICA oxidase activity in contrast to murine TRP-1. *Exp. Dermatol.* 1998; 7: 198-204.

Boissy R E. Melanosome transfer to and translocation in the keratinocyte. *Exp Dermatol.* 2003; 12: Suppl 2, 5–12

Botchkareva N V, Khlgatian M, Longley B J, Botchkarev V A & Gilchrest B A. SCF/c-kit signaling is required for cyclic regeneration of the hair pigmentation unit. *FASEB J.* 2001; 15: 645–658

Box N F, Wyeth J R, Mayne C J, O'Gorman L E, Martin N G & Sturm R A. Complete sequence and polymorphism study of the human TYRP1 gene encoding tyrosinase-related protein 1. Mamm Genome. 1998; 9: 50–53

Brash, D.E., Rudolph, JA, Simon, J.A., Lin, A., Mckenna, G.J., Baden, H.P., Halperin, AJ, & Ponten, J. A role for sunlight in skin cancer: UV-induced p53 mutations in squamous cell carcinoma. *Proc Natl. Acad. Sci. USA*; 1991; 88: 10124-10128

Briganti S & Picardo M. Antioxidant activity, lipid peroxidation and skin diseases. What's new? *J Eur Acad Dermatol* 2003; 17: 663–669

Burchill S A, Thody A J & Ito S. Melanocyte stimulating hormone, tyrosinase activity and the regulation of eumelanogenesis and phaeomelanogenesis in the hair follicular melanocytes of the mouse. *J Endocrinol.* 1986;109: 15-21

Busca R and Ballotti R. Cyclic AMP a key messenger in the regulation of skin pigmentation. *Pigment Cell Res.* 2000; 13: 60 –69

Carlson J A, Slominski A, Linette G P, Mihm M C Jr & Ross J S. Biomarkers in melanoma: predisposition, screening and diagnosis. *Expert Rev Mol Diagn* 2003; 3: 163–184

Chedekel M R & Zeise L. Sunlight, melanogenesis and radicals in the skin. *Lipids.* 1988; 23: 587-591

Cheii Y, Ohanna M, Ballotti R, & Bertolotto, C. Fifteen-year quest for microphthalmia - associated transcription factor target genes. *Pigment Cell Melanoma Res.* 2010; 23, 27-40

Chen K G, Valencia J C, Lai B, Zhang G, Paterson JK, Rouzaud F, Berens W, Wincovitch S M, Garfield S H, Leapman R D, Hearing V J & Gottesman M M. Melanosomal sequestration of cytotoxic drugs contributes to the intractability of malignant melanomas. *Proc Natl Acad Sci. USA* , 2006; 103: 9903-9907

Chen K G., Valencia J C, Gillet J-P, Hearing V J & Gottesman M M. Involvement of ABC transporters in melanogenesis and the development of multidrug resistance of melanoma. *Pigment Cell Melanoma Res.* 2009a; 22: 740-749

Chen K G, Leapman R D, Zhang G , Lai B ,Valencia J C , Cardarelli C O , Vieira W D , Hearing V J & Gottesman M M. Influence of the melanosome dynamics on melanoma drug sensitivity. *J Natl Cancer Inst.*, 2009b; 101, 1259-1271

Chen Q, Olashaw N & Wu J. Participation of reactive oxygen species in the lysophosphatidic acid-stimulated mitogen-activated protein kinase kinase activation pathway. *J. Biol. Chem.* 1995; 270: 28499-28502

Chintala S, Li W, Lamoreux M L. et al. Stc7all gene controls production of pheomelanin pigment and proliferation of cultured cell. *Proc. Natl. Acad. Sci. USA;* 2005: 102, 10964-10969

Cone R D, Lu D, Koppula S, Vage D I, Klungland H, Boston B, Chen W, Orth D N, Pouton C & Kesterson RA. The melanocortin receptors: agonists, antagonists, and the hormonal control of pigmentation. *Recent Prog Horm Res* 51: 287–318, 1996.

Cooksey C J, Garratt P J, Land E J, Pavel S, Ramsden C A, Riley P A & Smit N P M. Evidence for the indirect formation of the catecholic intermediate substrate responsible for the autoactivation kinetics of tyrosinase. *J Biol Chem* 1997; 272: 26226-26235

Costa J J, Demetri G D, Harrist T J, Dvorak A M, Hayes D F, Merica E A, Menchaca D M, Gringeri A J, Schwartz L B & Galli S J. Recombinant human stem cell factor (kit ligand) promotes human mast cell and melanocyte hyperplasia and functional activation in vivo. *J. Exp. Med.* 183: 2681–2686, 1996.

Costantini C M, d'Ischia A, Palumbo A &, Prota G. Photochemistry of 5-S-cysteinildopa. *Photochem. Photobiol.*1994; 60:33-37

Costin G E & Hearing V J. Human skin pigmentation: melanocytes modulate skin color in response to stress. *FASEB J.* 2007; 21:976-994

Cui R, Widlund H R, Feige E. et al. Central role of p53 in the suntan response and pathologic hyperpigmentation. *Cell.* 2007; 128, 853-864.

del Marmol V, Ito S, Bouchard B, Libert A, Wakamatsu K, Ghanem G & Solano F. Cysteine deprivation promotes eumelanogenesis in human melanoma cells. *J Invest Dermatol* 1996; 107: 698 - 702

Delmas V, Beermann F, Martinozzi S. et al. Beta-catenin induces immortalization of melanocytes by suppressing p161NK4a' expression and cooperates with N-Ras in melanoma development. *Genes Dev.* 2007; 27: 2923-2935.

Di Donato P A, Napolitano A, Prota G Metal ions as potential regulatory factors in the biosynthesis of red hair pigments: a new benzothiazole intermediate in the iron or copper assisted oxidation of 5-S-cysteinildopa. *Biochim. Biophys. Acta.* 2002; 1571:157-166

D'Orazio J A, Nobuhisa T, Cui R, Arya M, Spry M, Wakamatsu K, Igras V, Kunisada T, Granter S R, Nishimura E K, Ito S & Fisher D E. Topical drug rescue strategy and skin protection based on the role of Mc1r in UV-induced tanning. *Nature.* 2006; 21: 443(7109):340-4

Duval C, Smit N P, Kolb A M, Regnier M, Pavel S & Schmidt R. Keratinocytes control the pheo/eumelanin ratio in cultured normal human melanocytes. *Pigment Cell Res.* 2002; 15: 440-446

Eberle AN. The Melanotropins: Chemistry, Physiology and Mechanism of Action. New York: Karger, 1988.

Edge R, d'Ischia M, Land E J, Napolitano A, Navarantnam S, Panzella L, Pezzella A, Ramsden C A & Riley P A. Dopaquinone redox exchange with dihydroxyindole and dihydroxyindole-2-carboxilic acid. *Pigment Cell Res.* 2006; 19: 443-450

Eller M S, Li G Z, Firoozabaldi R, Puri N & Gilchrest B A. Induction of a p95/Nbs1-mediated S phase checkpoint by telomere 3' overhang specific DNA. *FASEB J.* 2003; 17: 152-162

Eller M S & Gilchrest BA. Tanning as part of the eukaryotic SOS response. *Pigment Cell Res.* 2000; 13 Suppl 8: 94 -97

Eller M S, Hadshiew I M & Gilchrest BA. The role of DNA damage and telomeres in melanogenesis. In: Mechanisms of Sun-tanning, edited by Ortonne JP and Ballotti R. London: Martin Dunitz, 2002, p. 239 -245.

Elwood, J M & Diffey B L. A consideration of ambient solar ultraviolet radiation in the interpretation of studies of studies of aetiology of melanoma. *Melanoma Res.* 1993; 3:113–122

Englaro W, Bertolotto C, Busca R, Brunet A, Pages G, Ortonne JP & Ballotti R. Inhibition of the mitogen-activated protein kinase pathway triggers B16 melanoma cell differentiation. *J. Biol. Chem.* 1998; 273: 9966 -9970

Fitzpatrick T B & Breathnach A S. Das epidermale melanineinheit system. *Dermatol Wochenschr.* 1963; 147: 481–489

Fitzpatrick T B. The validity and practicality of sun reactive skin type I through VI. *Arch Dermatol* 1988; 124: 869–871

Fuchs, E. Skin stem cells: rising to the surface. *J. Cell Biol.* 2008; 180, 273-284.

Funasaka Y, Chakraborty AK, Hayashi Y, Komoto M, Ohashi A, Nagahama M, Inoue Y, Pawelek J, and Ichihashi M. Modulation of melanocyte-stimulating hormone receptor expression on normal human melanocytes: evidence for a regulatory role of ultraviolet B, interleukin-1alpha, interleukin-1 beta, endothelin-1 and tumour necrosis factor-alpha. Br *J. Dermatol* 139: 216 -224, 1998.

Garcia RI. Ultrastructure of melanocyte-keratinocyte interactions. *Pigment Cell Res* 4: 299 - 310, 1979. 203

Garraway LA, Widlund H.R., Rubin, MA et al. Integrative genomic analyses identify MITF as a lineage survival oncogene amplified in malignant melanoma. *Nature* 2005; 436: 117-122.

Giacomoni P U. Open questions in photobiology III. Melanin and photoprotection. *J Photochem. Photobiol.* 1995; B29: 87-89

Gibbons N C J, Wood J M, Rokos H & Schallreuter K U. Computer Simulation of Native Epidermal Enzyme Structures in the Presence and Absence of Hydrogen Peroxide ($H_2O_2$): Potential and Pitfalls. *J. Invest. Dermatol.* 2006; 126: 2576–2582

Gibbons N C, Wood J M, Rokos H & Schallreuter K U. Computer simulation of native epidermal enzyme structures in the presence proopiomelanocortin peptides directly in the epidermis of patients with vitiligo. *J Invest Dermatol* 2007; 127: 411-420

Gilchrest BA & Eller MS. DNA photodamage stimulates melanogenesis and other photoprotective responses. *J Invest Dermatol Symp Proc* 1999; 4: 35–40

Girotti AW. Photosensitized oxidation of membrane lipids: Reaction pathways, cytotoxic effects, and cytoprotective mechanisms. *J Photochem Photobiol* B 2001; 63: 103–113.

Goding C R. Dicing with death: Mitf regulates DICER. *Pigment Cell Res.* 2010: 23-24

Grammatico P, Maresca V, Roccella F, Roccella M, Biondo L, Catricalà C et al. Increased sensitivity to peroxidizing agents is correlated with an imbalance of antioxidants in normal melanocytes from melanoma patients. *Exp. Dermatol.* 1998; 7:205–212

Gray-Schopfer V C, Cheong S C, Chong H, Chow J, Moss L, Abdel-Malek Z A, Marais R, Wynford-Thomas, D & Bennett D C. Cellular senescence in naevi and immortalisation in melanoma: a role for p16? Br. *J. Cancer.* 2006; 95, 496-505.

Greco G, Wakamatsu K, Panzella L, Ito S, Napolitano A & d'lschia, M. Isomeric cysteinyldopas provide a (photo) degradable bulk component and a robust structural element in red human hair pheomelanin. *Pigment Cell Mel. Res.* 2009; 22: 319-327

Gupta PB, Kuperwasser C, Brunet JP, et al. The melanocyte differentiation program predisposes to metastasis after neoplastic transformation. *Nat.Genet.* 2005; 37:1047-1054

Haddad MM, Xu W, Schwahn DJ, Liao F & Medrano EE. Activation of a cAMP pathway and induction of melanogenesis correlate with association of p16 (INK4) and p27 (KIP1) to CDKs, loss of E2F-binding activity, and premature senescence of human melanocytes. *Exp. Cell. Res.* 1999; 253: 561–572

Halaban R, Moellmann G. Murine and human b locus pigmentation genes encode a glycoprotein (gp75) with catalase activity. *Proc Natl Acad Sci USA.* 1990; 87(12):4809-13.

Hara M, Yaar M & Gilchrest BA. Endothelin-1 of keratinocyte origin is a mediator of melanocyte dendricity. *J. Invest. Dermatol.* 1995; 105: 744 –748

Hearing V J. Biochemical control of melanogenesis and melanosomal organization. *J. Invest. Dermatol. Symp. Proc.* 1999; 4: 24 –28

Hearing V J. The melanosome: the perfect model for cellular responses to the environment. *Pigment Cell Res.* 2000; 13: 23–34

Hearing V J. Biogenesis of pigment granules: a sensitive way to regulate melanocyte function. J Dermatol Sci. 2005; 37, 3-14

Hearing V J & Tsukamoto K. Enzymatic control of pigmentation in mammals. *FASEB J.* 1991; 5: 2902–2909

Hellemans L, Corstjens H, Neven A, Declercq L & Maes D. Antioxidant enzyme activity in human stratum corneum shows seasonal variation with an age-dependent recovery. *J Invest Dermatol* 2003; 120: 434–439

Hida T, Wakamatsu K, Sviderskaya E V, Donkin A J, Montoliu L, Lamoreux L M, Yu B, Millhauser GL, Ito S, Barsh G S, Jimbow K & Bennett D C. Agouti protein, mahogunin, and attractin in pheomelanogenesis and melanoblast-like alteration of melanocytes: a cAMP-independent pathway, *Pigment Cell Melanoma Res.* 2009; 22:623-634

Hill H Z & Hill G H. UVA, pheomelanin and the carcinogenesis of melanoma. *Pigment Cell Res.* 13 Suppl. 2000; 8:140-144

Hirobe T, Wakamatsu K & Ito S. Changes in the proliferation and differentiation of neonatal mouse pink-eyed dilution melanocytes in the presence of excess tyrosine. *Pigment Cell Res.* 2003; 16: 619-628

Hoek K S. & Goding C R. Cancer stem cells versus phenotype-switching in melanoma. *Pigment Cell Melanoma Res.* 2010: 23; 746-759

Hoogduijn M J, Ancans J & Thody A J. Melanin-concentrating hormone may act as a paracrine inhibitor of melanogenesis. Br *J Dermatol* 2001; 144: 651–677

Hoogduijn M J, Ancans J, Suzuki I, Estdale S & Thody A J. Melanin-concentrating hormone and its receptor are expressed and functional in human skin. *Biochem. Biophys. Res.* Commun 2002; 296: 698–701

Hsu M Y, Meier F E, Nesbit M, Hsu J Y, Van Belle P, Elder D E & Herlyn M. E-cadherin expression in melanoma cells restores keratinocyte-mediated growth control and down-regulates expression of invasion-related adhesion receptors. *Am. J. Pathol.* 2000; 156: 1515- 1525

Imokawa G, Miyagishi M, and Yada Y. Endothelin-1 as a new melanogen: coordinated expression of its gene and the tyrosinase gene in UVB-exposed human epidermis. *J. Invest. Dermatol.* 1995; 105: 32–37

Imokawa G, Yada Y & Miyagishi M. Endothelins secreted from human keratinocytes are intrinsic mitogens for human melanocytes. *J Biol Chem* 1992; 267: 24675–24680

Ito S & Prota G. A facile one-step synthesis of cysteinildopas using mushroom tyrosinase. *Experientia,* 1977; 33: 1118-1119

Ito S, Kawa Y, Ono H, Okura M, Baba T, Kubota Y, Nishikawa S I & Mizoguchi M. Removal of stem cell factor or addition of monoclonal anti-c-KIT antibody induces apoptosis in murine melanocyte precursors. *J Invest Dermatol* 1999; 112: 796–801

Ito S & Wakamatsu K. Chemistry of mixed melanogenesis-pivotal role of dopaquinone-review. *Photochem. Photobiol.* 2008; 84: 582-592

Jackson J J, Chambers D M, Budd P S & Johnson R. The tyrosinase-related protein-1 gene has a structure and promoter sequence very different from tyrosinase. *Nucleic Acids Res* 1991; 19: 3799–3804

Jackson J J, Chambers D M, Tsukamoto K, Copeland N G, Gilbert D J, Jenkins N A & Hearing V J. A second tyrosinase related protein, TRP-2, maps to and is mutated at the mouse slaty locus. *EMBO J.* 1992; 11: 527–535,

Jara J R, Martinez-Liarte J H & Solano F. Inhibition by analogues of L-tyrosine transport by B16/F10 melanoma cells. *Melanoma Res.* 1991; 1:15-21

Jimbow K, Chen H, Park J S & Thomas P D. Increased sensitivity of melanocytes to oxidative stress and abnormal expression of tyrosinase- active site accounting for loss of function mutations. *Pigment Cell Res* 2007; 20: 394–401

Jimenez-Cervantes C, Solano F, Kobayashi T, Urabe K, Hearing V J, Lozano J A, Garcia-Boron J C. A new enzymatic function in the melanogenic pathway. The 5,6-dihydroxyindole-2-carboxilic acid oxidase activity of tyrosinase related protein-1 (TRP1). *J Biol Chem.* 1994; 269: 17993-18001

John D. Simon Seeing red: pheomelanin synthesis uncovered. *Pigment Cell Melanoma Res.* 2009; 22: 382-383

Jordan S A & Jackson J J. MGF (KIT ligand) is a chemokinetic factor for melanoblast migration into hair follicles. Dev. Biol. 2000; 225: 424–436

Kadekaro A L, Kavanagh R J, Wakamatsu K, Ito S, Pipitone M A, Abdel-Malek Z A. Cutaneous photobiology. The melanocytes vs, the sun: who will win the final round? *Pigment Cell Res* 2003; 16: 434–447

Kadekaro A L, Kavanagh R, Kanto H, Terzieva S, Hauser J, Kobayashi N, Schwemberger S, Cornelius J, Babcock G, Shertzer HG, Scott G & Abdel-Malek Z A. α-Melanocortin and endothelin-1 activate anti-apoptotic pathways and reduce DNA damage in human melanocytes. *Cancer Res.* 2005; 65: 4292-4299

Kauser S, Schallreuter KU, Thody AJ, Gummer C, and Tobin DJ. Regulation of human epidermal melanocyte biology by beta-endorphin. *J. Invest. Dermatol.* 2003; 120: 1073–1080

Kawaguchi Y, Mori N, & Nakayama A. Kit(+) melanocytes seem to contribute to melanocyte proliferation after UV exposure as precursor cells. *J. Invest. Dermatol* 2001; 116: 920-925

Kemp E H, Waterman E A, Hawes B E, O'Neill K, Gottumukkala R V, Gawkrodger D J, Weetman A P & Watson P F. The melanin-concentrating hormone receptor 1, a novel target of autoantibody responses in vitiligo. *J. Clin. Invest.* 2002; 109: 923–930

Kevin G, Chen J, Valeneia C, Gillet J P, Hearing V J, Gottesman M M, Involvement of ABC transporters in melanogenesis and the development of multidrug resistance of melanoma. *Pigment Cell Melanoma Res.* 2009; 22: 740-749

Kobayashi T, Urabe K, Winder A J, Jimenez-Cervantes C, Imokawa G, Brewington T, Solano F, Garcia-Boron J C, Hearing V J. Tyrosinase related protein 1 (TRP1) functions as a DHICA oxidase in melanin biosynthesis. *EMBO J.* 1994; 13: 5818-5825

Koch W H & Chedekel M R. Photoinitiated DNA damage by melanogenic intermediates in vitro. *Photochem. Photobiol.* 1986; 44: 703-710

Korner A & Pawelek J. Mammalian tyrosinase catalyzes three reactions in the biosynthesis of melanin. *Science* 1982; 217: 1163–1165

Kvam E & Dahle J. Pigmented Melanocytes Are Protected Against Ultraviolet-A-Induced Membrane Damage. *J Invest Dermatol* 2003; 121: 564–569

Kvam E & Dahle J. Melanin synthesis may sensitize melanocytes to oxidative DNA damage by ultraviolet A radiation and protect melanocytes from direct DNA damage by ultraviolet B radiation. *Pigment Cell Res.* 2004; 17: 549–550

Kvam E & Tyrrell R M. The role of melanin in the induction of oxidative DNA base damage by ultraviolet A irradiation of DNA or melanoma cells. *J. Invest. Dermatol.* 1999; 113: 209–213

Kwon B S, Chintamaneni C, Kozak C A, Copeland N G, Gilbert D J, Jenkins N, Barton D, Francke U, Kobayashi Y & Kim K K. A melanocyte-specific gene, Pmel 17, maps near the silver coat color locus on mouse chromosome 10 and is in a syntenic region on human chromosome 12. *Proc Natl Acad Sci USA* 1991; 88: 9228 -9232

Kwon B S. Pigmentation genes: the tyrosinase gene family and the pmel 17 gene family. *J. Invest. Dermatol.* 1993; 100: 134S–140S

Lahav R, Lecoin L, Ziller C, Nataf V, Carnahan J F, Martin F H & Le Douarin N M. Effect of the Steel gene product on melanogenesis in avian neural crest cell cultures. Differentiation 1994; 58: 133–139

Lamason R L, Mohideen M A, Mest J R, et al. SLC24A5, a putative cation exchanger affects pigmentation in zebrafish and humans. *Science* 2005; 310: 1782-1786

Lamoreux M L, Wakamatsu K, & Ito S. Interaction of major coat color gene functions in mice as studied by chemical analysis of eumelalanin and pheomelanin. *Pigment Cell Res.* 2001;14: 23-31

Land E J, Ito S, Wakamatsu K & Riley P A. Rate constants for the first two chemical steps of eumelanogenesis. *Pigment Cell Res.* 2003; 16: 487-493

Land E J, Ramsden C A, Riley P A. Toxicological aspects of melanins and melanogenesis. In: Nordlund J J, Boissy R E, Hearing V J, King R A, Williams S, Oetting S, Ortonne J P, eds. The Pigmentary System, Second Edition. Blackwell Publishing, 2006; 354-394

Land E J, Riley P A. Spontaneous redox reactionsof dopaquinone and the balance between the eumelanic and phaeomelanic pathways. *Pigment Cell Res.* 2000;13: 273-277

Le Pape E, Wakamatsu K, Ito S, Wolber R & Hearing V J. Regulation of eumelanin/ pheomelanin synthesis and visible pigmentation in melanocytes by ligands of the melanocortin 1 receptor. *Pigment Cell Melanoma Res.* 2008; 21: 477-486

Le Poole IC, van den Wijngaard RM, Smit NP, Oosting J, Westerhof W, and Pavel S. Catechol-O-methyltransferase in vitiligo. *Arch. Dermatol. Res.* 1994; 286: 81–86

LePoole I C, Boissy R, Sarangarajan R, Chen J, Forristal J, Sheth P, Westerhof W, Babcock G, Das P & Saelinger C. PIG3V, an immortalized human vitiligo melanocyte cell line, expresses dilated endoplasmic reticulum. In Vitro Cell Dev. Biol. Anim. 2000; 36: 309 -319

Lerner AB. The discovery of the melanotropins. A history of pituitary endocrinology. Ann NY Acad Sci 1993; 680: 1–12

Liu J J & Fisher D E. Lighting a path to pigmentation: mechanisms of MITF induction by UV *Pigment Cell Melanoma Res.* 2010: 23; 741-745

Liu Y, Hong L, Wakamatsu K, Ito S, Adhyaru B, Cheng C Y, Bowers C R, & Simon J D. Comparison of structural and chemical properties of balck and red human hair melanosomes. *Photochem. Photobiol.* 2005; 81: 135-144

Lo Y Y C, Wong J M S & Cruz T F. Reactive oxygen species mediate cytokine activation of c-Jun $NH_2$-terminal kinases. *J. Biol. Chem.* 1996; 271: 15703-15707

Lu D, Willard D, Patel I R, Kadwell S, Overton L, Kost T, Luther M, Chen W, Woychik R P, Wilkison W O & Cone R D. Agouti protein is an antagonist of the melanocyte-stimulating-hormone receptor. *Nature* 1994; 371: 799–802

Luo D, Chen H, Searles G & Jimbow K. Coordinated mRNA expression of c-Kit with tyrosinase and TRP-1 in melanin pigmentation of normal and malignant human melanocytes and transient activation of tyrosinase by Kit/SCF-R. *Melanoma Res* 1995; 5: 303–309

Maresca V, Flori E, Briganti S, Camera E, Cario-André M, Taïeb A & Picardo M. UVA-induced modification of catalase charge properties in the epidermis is correlated with the skin phototype *J Invest Dermatol* 2006: 126; 182–190

Marrot L, Belaïdi J P, Jones C, Perez P, Meunier Jr. Molecular responses to stress induced in normal human caucasian melanocytes in culture by exposure to simulated solar UV. *Photochem Photobiol* 2005; 81(2): 367-375

Marrot L, Belaidi JP, Meunier JR, Perez P, Agapakis-Causse C. The human melanocyte as a target for UVA radiation and an endpoint for photoprotection assessment. *Photochem Photobiol.* 1999; 69:686–693

Masson P. Pigment cells in man. In: Biology of Melanosomes, edited by Miner RW and Gordon M. New York: NY Acad Sci, 1948, p. 15–24.

McGill GG, Horstmann M, Widlund HR, Du J, Motyckova G, Nishimura E K, Lin Y L, Ramaswamy S, Avery W, Ding H F.et al. Bcl2 regulation by the melanocyte master regulator Mitf modulates lineage survival and melanoma cell viability. *Cell* 2002; 109:707-718

Menon I A, Persad S, Ranadive N S & Haberman H F. Effect of ultraviolet–visible irradiation in the presence of melanin isolated from human black or red hair upon Ehrlich ascites carcinoma cells. *Cancer Res.* 1983; 43: 3165–3169

Meyskens Jr, Farmer P & Fruehauf J P. Redox regulation in human melanocytes and melanoma. *Pigment Cell Res* 2001; 14: 148–154

Michaloglou C, Vredeveld, L E, Soengas, M S, Denoyelle E, Kuilman L, van der Horst E M, Majoor D M, Shay J W, Mooi W J, & Peeper D S. BRAFV600-associated senescence-like cell cycle arrest of human naevi. *Nature* 2005; 436, 720-724.

Miyamura Y, Coelho S G, Wolber R, Miller S A, Wakamatsu K, Zmudzka B Z, Ito S, Smuda C, Passeron T, Choi W, Batzer J, Yamaguchi Y, Beer J Z & Hearing V J. Regulation of human skin pigmentation and responses to ultraviolet radiation. *Pigment Cell Res.* 2007; 20: 2–13

Montoliu L, Oetting W S & Bennet D C. Color Genes. European Society for *Pigment Cell Res*earch. 2009 (URL: http//www.espcr.org/micemut)

Mooi W.J. Peeper D.S. Oncogene-Induced Cell Senescence — Halting on the Road to Cancer, *N Engl J Med* 2006; 355:1037-1046

Morisson W L. What is the function of melanin? Arch Dermatol 1985; 121: 1160-1163

Murray A W. Creative blocks: cell-cycle checkpoints and feedback controls. *Nature.* 1992; 359: 599-604

Napolitano A, Di Donato P, Prota G. Zinc–catalysed of 5-S-cysteinildopa to 2,2'-bi(2H-1,4,benzothiazine): tracking the biosynthetic pathway of tricochromes, the characteristic pigments of red haie. *J Org. Chem.* 2001; 66: 6958-6966

Nappi A J & Vass E. Hydrogen peroxide generation associated with the oxidations of the eumelanogenic precursors 5,6-dihydroxyindole and 5,6-dihydroxyindole-2-carboxylic acid. *Melanoma Res.*1996; 6: 341-349

Nordberg J & Arnér E S J. Reactive oxygen species, antioxidants and the mammalian thioredoxin system. *Free Radical Biol. Med.* 2001; 31:1287–1312

Nordlund J J, Amornsiripanitch S, Rheins L A, Abdel-Malek Z A, Boissy R E & Bell M. Role of the melanocyte in epidermal inflammatory and immune responses. *Pigment Cell Res.* Suppl 1988; 1: 101–112

Nordlund JJ. The lives of pigment cells. Clin Geriatr Med 1989; 5: 91–108

Nordlund, JJ, Ortonne, JP: The normal colour of human skin. In: JJ Nordlund, Re Boissy, Vj Hearing, JP. Ortonne (eds). The Pigmentary System 1998; Oxford University Press, 475–487

Nordlund J J, Boissy R E, Hearing V J, King R A, Ortonne J P & Oetting W S. The pigmentary System. Physiology and physiopathology, 2nd edn. 2006. (Maiden, Ma: Wiley-Blackwell)

Norton H L, Kittles R A, Parra E, McKeigue P, Mao X, Cheng K, Canfield V A, Bradley D G, McEvoy B & Shriver M D. Genetic evidence for the convergent evolution of light skin in Europeans and East Asians, *Mol Biol. Evol.* 2007; 24: 710-722

Oetting W S & King R A. Molecular basis of albinism: mutations and polymorphisms of pigmentation genes associated with albinism. Hum. Mutat. 1999; 13: 99 –115

Okazaki K, Uzuka M, Morikawa F, Toda K & Seiji M. Transfer mechanism of melanosomes in epidermal cell culture. *J. Invest. Dermatol.* 1976; 67: 541–547

Olivares C, Jimenez-Cervantes C, Lozano J A, Solano F & Garcia-Boron J C. The 5,6-dihydroxyindole-2-carboxilic acid (DHICA) oxidase activity of human tyrosinase, *Biochem J*, 2001; 354:131-139

Olivares C, Solano F. New insights into the active site structure and catalytic mechanism of tyrosinase and its related proteins. *Pigment Cell Melanoma Res.* 2009; 22: 750-760

Orlow S J. Melanosomes are specialized members of the lysosomal lineage of organelles. *J Invest Dermatol.* 1995; 105, 3-7

Orlow S J & Brilliant M H. The pink-eyed dilution locus controls the biogenesis of melanosomes and levels of melanosomal proteins in the eye. *Exp. Eye Res.* 1999; 68: 147–154

Ozeki H, Ito S, Wakamatsu K, & Hirobe T. Chemical characterization of hair melanins in various coat-color mutants of mice. *J Invest Dermatol* 105: 361–366, 1995.

Ozeki H, Ito S, Wakamatsu K & Isiguro I. Chemical characterization of pheomelanogenesis starting from dihydroxyphenilalanine and cysteine. Effects of tyrosinase and cysteine concentrations and reaction time. *Biochim Biophys Acta* 1997a; 1336:539-548

Ozeki H, Ito S, Wakamatsu K., & Isiguro I. Chemical characterization of eumelanins with special emphasis on 5,6-dihydroxyindole-2-carboxylic acid content and molecular size. *Anal Biochem.*1997b; 248: 149-157

Palumbo A, d'Ischia M, Misuraca G & Prota G. Effect of metal ions the rearrangement of dopachrome. *Biochim. Biophys. Acta*, 1987; 925, 203-209

Palumbo A, Solano F, Misuraca G, Aroca P, Garcia-Boron J C, Lozano J A, Prota G. Comparative action of dopachrome tautomerase and metal ions on the rearrangement of dopachrome. *Biochim. Biophys. Acta*, 1991; 1115:1-5

Pankovich J M & Jimbow K. Tyrosine transport in a human melanoma cell line as a basis for selective transport of cytotoxic analogues. *Biochem J.* 1991; 280:721-725

Passeron T, Namiki T, Passeron H J, Le Pape E & Hearing V J. Forskolin protects keratinocytes from UVB-induced apoptosis and increases DNA repair independent of its effects on melanogenesis. *J Invest Dermatol*, 2009; 129: 162-166

Pavel S, Elzinga H, Muskiet F A J, Smit J M, Mulder N H & Schraffordt Koops H. Eumelanin-related indolic compounds in the urine of treted melanoma patients. *J Clin Chem Biochem.* 1986; 24: 173-176

Pawelek J M. Factors regulating growth and pigmentation of melanoma cells. *J. Invest. Dermatol.* 1976; 66: 201–209

Pawelek J. Studies on the Cloudman melanoma cell line as a model for the action of MSH. Yale *J. Biol. Med.* 1985; 58: 571–578

Pawelek J M & Korner A M. The biosynthesis of mammalian melanin. *Am. Sci.* 1982; 70: 136 -145

Pawelek J, Bolognia J, McLane J, Murray M, Osber M & Slominski A. A possible role for melanin precursors in regulating both pigmentation and proliferation of melanocytes. *Prog Clin. Biol. Res.* 1988; 256: 143–154

Pawelek J, Chakraborty A, Osber M P, Orlow S J, Min K K, Rosenzweig K E & Bolognia J L. Molecular cascades in UV-induced melanogenesis: a central role for melanotropins? *Pigment Cell Res.* 1992; 5: 34 –356

Peters E M, Tobin D J, Botchkareva N, Maurer M & Paus R. Migration of melanoblasts into the developing murine hair follicle is accompanied by transient c-Kit expression. *J. Histochem. Cytochem.* 2002; 50: 751–766

Peters EM, Tobin D J, Seidah N G & Schallreuter K U. Proopiomelanocortin-related peptides, prohormone convertases 1 and 2 and the regulatory peptide 7B2 are present in melanosomes of human melanocytes. *J. Invest. Dermatol.* 2000; 114: 430–437

Peus D, Vasa R A, Meves A, Pott M, Beyerle A, Squillace K & Pittelkow M R. H2O2 is an important mediator of UVB-Induced EGF-receptor phosphorilation in cultured keratinocytes. *J Invest Dermatol* 1998; 110:966–971

Phillips J, Gawkrodger D J, Caddy C M, Hedley S, Dawson R A, Smith-Thomas L, Freedlander E & MacNeil S. Keratinocytes suppress TRP-1 expression and reduce cell number of co-cultured melanocytes: implications for grafting of patients with vitiligo. *Pigment Cell Res.* 2001; 14: 116 –125

Picardo M, Grammatico P, Roccella F, Roccella M, Grandinetti M, Del Porto G & Passi S. Imbalance in the antioxidant pool in melanoma cells and normal melanocytes from patients with melanoma. *J Invest Dermatol* 1996; 107: 322–326

Picardo M, Maresca V, Eibenschutz L, De Bernardo C, Rinaldi R& Grammatico P. Correlation between antioxidants and phototypes in melanocyte cultures. A possible link of physiologic and pathologic relevance. *J Invest Dermatol* 1999; 113: 424–425

Picardo M, De Zompetta C, Luca C, Cirone M, Faggioni A, Passi S, & Prota G. Skin surface lipoperoxides as mediators of UV-induced epidermal cell changes. *Arch. Dermatol Res.* 1991; 283:191–197

Potterf S B & Hearing V J. Tyrosine transport into melanosomes is increased following stimulation of melanocyte differentiation. *Biochem. Biophys. Res. Commun* 1998; 248: 795–800

Prota G. Melanins and Melanogenesis. San Diego: *Academic Press*, 1992.

Prota G. *Pigment Cell Res*earch: what directions? *Pigment Cell Res.* 1997; 10:5–11

Ranadive N S, Shirwadkar S, Persad S & Menon I A. Effect of melanin-induced free radicals on the isolated rat peritoneal mast cells. *J. Invest. Dermatol.* 1986; 86:303–307

Randolph Byers H, Yaar M Eller, Mark S , Jalbert N L & Gilchrest B A. Role of Cytoplasmic Dynein in Melanosome Transport in Human Melanocytes. *J. Invest. Dermatol.* 2000; 114, 990–997

Raposo G, Fevrier B, Stoorvogel W & Marks M S. Lysosome related organelles: a view from immunity and pigmentation. *Cell Struct. Funct.* 2002; 27,443-456

Raposo G, Tenza D, Murphy D M, Berson J F & Marks M. Distinct protein sorting and localization to premelanosomes, melanosomes and lysosomes in pigmented melanocitic cells. *J Cell Biol.* 2001; 152, 809-824

Rhie G, Seo J Y & Chung J H. Modulation of catalase in human skin in vivo by acute and chronic UV radiation. *Mol. Cells* 2001; 11: 399–404

Richards H.W & Medrano EE. Epigenetic marks in melanoma. *Pigment Cell Melanoma Res.* 2009; 22: 14-29.

Roméro-Graillett C, Aberdam E, Biagioli M, Massabni W, Ortonne JP, & Ballotti R, Ultraviolet B Radiation acts through the nitric oxide and cGMP signal transduction pathway to stimulate melanogenesis in human melanocytes. *J. Biol. Chem.* 1996; 271: 28052–28056

Ros J R, Rodriguez-Lopez J N & Garcia-Canovas F. Effect of L-ascorbic acid on the monophenolase activity of tyrosinase. *Biochem J.* 1993; 295: 309–312

Rosdahl I K & Szabo G. Mitotic activity of epidermal melanocytes in UV-irradiated mouse skin. *J. Invest. Dermatol.* 1978; 70: 143–148

Rothhammer L & Bosserhoff AX. Epigenetic events in malignant melanoma. *Pigment Cell Res.* 2007; 20, 92-111

Routaboul C, Denis A & Vinche A. Immediate pigment darkening: description, kinetic and biological function. *Eur. J. Dermatol.* 1999; 9:95–99

Saito Y, Wang Z, Hagino-Yamagishi K, Civelli O, Kawashima S & Maruyama K. Endogenous melanin-concentrating hormone receptor SLC-1 in human melanoma SK-MEL-37 cells. *Biochem. Biophys. Res. Commun* 2001; 289: 44 –50

Sanders C S, Chang H, Hamm F, Elsner P, Thiele J J. Role of oxidative stress and the antioxidant network in cutaneous carcinogenesis. *Int. J. Dermatol.* 2004; 43:326–335

Sarangarajan R & Boissy R E. Tyrp1 and oculocutaneous albinism type 3. *Pigment Cell Res.* 2001; 14: 437–444

Sarangarajan R, Zhao Y, Babcock G, Cornelius J, Lamoreux M L & Boissy R E. Mutant alleles at the brown locus encoding tyrosinase-related protein-1 (TRP-1) affect proliferation of mouse melanocytes in culture. *Pigment Cell Res.* 2000; 13: 337–344

Sarna T, Swartz H A. The physical properties of melanin, In: Nordlund J J, Boissy R E, Hearing V J, King R A, Williams S, Oetting S, Ortonne J P, eds. The Pigmentary System, Second Edition. Blackwell Publishing, 2006; 311-342

Schallreuter K U, Wazir U, Kothari S, Gibbons N C, Moore J & Wood J M. Human phenylalanine hydroxylase is activated by H2O2: a novel mechanism for increasing the L-tyrosine supply for melanogenesis. *Proc Natl Acad Sci USA* 1990; 87: 4809–4813.

Schallreuter KU & Wood J M. Thioredoxin reductase: its role in epidermal redox status. *J. Photochem. Photobiol.* 2001; 64:179–184

Schallreuter K U. Oxidative stress in the human epidermis. *G Ital Dermatol Venereol* 2005; 140: 505–514.

Schallreuter K U, Rubsam K, Chavan B, Zothner C, Gillbro J M, Spencer J D & Wood J M. Functioning methionine sulfoxide reductases A and B are present in human epidermal melanocytes in the cytosol and in the nucleus *Biochem Biophys Res Commun* 2006: 342: 145–152.

Schallreuter K U, Kotharil S, Chavan B & Spencer J D. Regulation of melanogenesis – controversies and new concepts. *Exp. Dermatol.* 2008; 17: 395–404

Schmitz S, Thomas PD & Allen TM et al. Dual role of melanins and melanin precursors as photoprotective and phototoxic agents: Inhibition of ultraviolet radiation-induced lipid peroxidation. *Photochem Photobiol.* 1995; 61: 650–655.

Schreck R & Baeuerle P A. A role for oxygen radicals as second messengers. *Trends Cell Biol* 1991; 1:39–42

Schwahn D J. Tyrosine levels regulate the melanogenic response to alpha- melanocyte stimulating hormone in human melanocytes: implication for pigmentation and proliferation. *Pigment Cell Res* 2001; 14: 32-39

Schweikardt T, Olivares C, Solano F, Jaenicke E, Garcia-Borron J C, Decker H. A three-dimensional model of mammalian tyrosinase related protein in vitiligo. Br. *J. Dermatol.* 2001; 144: 55–65.

Scott G, Leopardi S, Printup S, and Madden BC. Filopodia are conduits for melanosome transfer to keratinocytes. *J. Cell Sci.* 2002; 115: 1441–1451

Shindo Y& Hashimoto T. Time course of changes in antioxidant enzymes in human skin fibroblasts after UVA irradiation. *J. Dermatol. Sci*. 1997; 14: 225–232

Shindo Y, Witt E & Packer L. Antioxidant defence mechanisms in murine epidermis and dermis and their responses to ultraviolet light. *J. Invest. Dermatol*. 1993; 100:260–265

Silvers W. The Coat Colors of Mice. A Model for Mammalian Gene Action and Interaction. 1979. edn. Springer Verlag New York

Simon J D, Peles D, Wakamatsu K & Ito S. Current challenges in understanding melanogenesis: bridging chemistry, biological control, morphology, and function *Pigment Cell Melanoma Res*. 2009; 22: 563-579

Simoncini T, Hafezi-Moghadam A, Brazil D P, Ley K, Chin W W & Liao J K. Interaction of oestrogen receptor with the regulatory subunit of phosphatidylinositol-3-OH kinase. *Nature* 2000; 407: 538–541

Singh M V & Jimbow K. Tyrosinase transfection produces melanin synthesis and growth retardation in glioma cells. *Melanoma Res*. 1998; 8: 493-498

Slominski A & Costantino R. Molecular mechanism of tyrosinase regulation by L-dopa in hamster melanoma cells. *Life Sci*. 1991; 48: 2075–2079

Slominski A, Carlson A, Worstman J & Mihm M Jr. The role of molecular biology in diagnostic pathology of melanoma. *Methods Mol. Med*. 2001; 61: 123–163

Slominski A, Paus R & Mihm M. Inhibition of melanogenesis as an adjuvant strategy in the treatment of melanotic melanomas: selective review and hypothesis. *Anticancer Res*. 1998; 18: 3709–3716

Slominski A, Tobin DJ., Shibahara S & Wortsman J. Melanin Pigmentation in Mammalian Skin and Its Hormonal Regulation. *Physiol Rev* 2004; 84: 1155–1228

Slominski A, Wortsman J, Luger T, Paus R & Salomon S. Corticotropin releasing hormone and proopiomelanocortin involvement in the cutaneous response to stress. *Physiol Rev* 80: 979–1020, 2000.

Slominski A. Coming of age of melanogenesis-related proteins. *Arch. Pathol. Lab. Med*. 2002; 126: 775–777

Smit N P, Kolb RM, Lentjes E G, Noz K C, van der Meulen H, Koerten H K, Vermeer B-J & Pavel S. Variations in melanin formation by cultured melanocytes from different skin types, *Arch. Dermatol. Res*. 1998; 290:342–349

Smit N P, van der Meulen H, Koerten H K, Kolb R M, Mommaas A M, Lentjes E G & Pavel S, Melanogenesis in Cultured Melanocytes can be Substantially Influenced by L-Tyrosine and L-Cysteine. *J. Invest. Dermatol*. 1997; 109: 796–800

Smit NP, van Nieuwpoort F A, Marrot L, Out C, Poorthuis B, van Pelt H, Meunier J-R & Pavel S. Increased Melanogenesis is a Risk Factor for Oxidative DNA Damage-Study on Cultured Melanocytes and Atypical Nevus Cells. *Photochem. Photobiol*. 2008, 84: 550–555

Smith A G, Luk N, Newton R A, Roberts D W, Sturm R A & Muscat G E. Melanocortin-1 receptor signaling markedly induces the expression of the NR4A nuclear receptor subgroup in melanocytic cells. *J. Biol. Chem*. 2008; 283: 12564-12570

Spencer J D, Gibbons N C, Rokos H, Peters E M, Wood J M & Schallreuter K U. Oxidative stress via hydrogen peroxide affects melanocytes. *Biochem Biophys Res Commun*. 2004: 322: 88–92.

Spry M L, Vanover J C, Scott T, Abona-Ama O, Wakamatsu K, Ito S, & D'Orazio J A. Prolonged treatment of fair skinned mice with topical forskolin causes persistent tanning and UV protection. *Pigment Cell Melanoma Res.* 2009; 22: 219-229

Steel K P, Davidson D R & Jackson J J. TRP 2/Dt is a new early melanoblast marker, shows that steel growth factor (c-kit ligand) is a survival factor. *Development* 1992; 115: 1111-1119

Steenvoorden D P T & van Henegouwen B. The use of endogenous antioxidants to improve photoprotection. *Photochem. Photobiol. B* 1997; 41:1–10

Streutker C J, McCready D, Jimbow K, From L. malignant melanoma in a patient with oculocutaneous albinism. *J Cutan med Surg.* 2000; 4:149-152

Stryer L. Biochemistry. 1988; New York: Freeman

Sturm R A, Teasdale R D & Box N F. Human pigmentation genes: identification, structure and consequences of polymorphic variation. *Gene* 2001; 277: 49 –62

Szabo G. The regional anatomy of the human integument with special reference to the distribution of hair follicles, sweat glands and melanocytes. *Philos. Trans. R. Soc. Lond. Ser. B* 1967; 252: 447–489

Takeuchi H, Morton D L, Kuo C, Turner R R, Elashoff D, Taback B, Fujimoto A & Hoon D S. Prognostic significance of molecular upstaging of paraffin-embedded sentinel lymph nodes in melanoma patients. *J Clin Oncol* 2004; 22: 2671–2680.

Tenchini ML, Morra F, Soranzo C & Malcovati M. Effects of keratinocyte-secreted soluble factors on spreading, number of dendrites and cell-cell contacts of human epidermal melanocytes and dermal fibroblasts: a quantitative analysis. *Epithelial Cell Biol.* 1995; 4: 143–155

Thannickal V J & Fanburg B L. Activation of an $H_2O_2$-generating NADH oxidase in human lung fibroblasts by transforming growth factor-ß1 *J. Biol. Chem.* 1995; 270, 30334-30338

Thompson A E, Land J, Chedekel M R, Subbarao K V & Truscott T G. A pulse radiolysis investigation of the oxidation of the melanin precursors 3,4-dihydroxyphenylalanine (dopa) and the cysteinyldopas. *Biochim. Biophys. Acta.* 1985; 843: 49-57

Tsukamoto K, Jackson J J, Urabe K, Montague P M & Hearing V J. A second tyrosinase related protein, TRP-2 is a melanogenic enzyme termed DOPAchrome tautomerase. *EMBO J*, 1992; 11: 519-526

Tyrrell R M. The molecular and cellular pathology of solar ultraviolet radiation. *Mol Aspects Med* 1994; 15: 1–77

Urlich A & Schlessinger J. Signal transduction by receptors with tyrosine kinase activity. *Cell* 1990; 61:203–212

Valencia J C, Watabe H, Chi A Rouzaud F, Chen K G, Vieira W D, Takahashi K, Yamaguchi Y, Berens W, Nagashima K, Shabanowitz J, Hunt D F, Appella E & Hearing V J. Sorting of Pmel 17 to melanosomes through the plasma membrane by AP1 and AP2: evidence for the polarized nature of melanocytes. *J Cell Sci.* 2006; 119: 1080-1091

Wakamatsu K, Kavanagh R, Kadekaro A L, Terzieva S, Sturm R A, Leachman S, Abdel-Malek Z & Ito S. Diversity of pigmentation in cultured melanocytes is due to differences in the type as well as quantity of melanin. *Pigment Cell Res.* 2006; 19:154-162

Wakamatsu K, Hu D N, MaCormick S A, & Ito S. Characterisation of human iridal and choroidal melanocytes from eyes with various colored irides. *Pigment Cell Melanoma Res.* 2008; 21: 97-105

Wakamatsu, K., Ohtara, K., and Ito, S. Chemical analysis of late stages of pheomelanogenesis; conversion of dihydrobenzothiazine to a benzothiazole structure. *Pigment Cell Mel. Res.* 2009; 22:(4) 474-486

Wang SQ, Setlow R, Berwick M Polsky D, Ashfaq A. Marghoob MD, Kopf A W & Bart R S. Ultraviolet A and melanoma: *A review. J. Am. Acad. Dermatol* 2001; 44: 837–846

Wankowicz-Kalinska A, Le Poole C, van den Wijngaard R, Storkus W J & Das PK. Melanocyte-specific immune response in melanoma and vitiligo: two faces of the same coin? *Pigment Cell Res.* 2003; 16: 254 -260

Wenczl E, Van der Schans G P, Roza L, Kolb R M, Timmerman A J, Smit N P, Pavel S & Schothorst AA (Pheo) melanin photosensitizes UVA-induced DNA damage in cultured human melanocytes. *J Invest Dermatol* 1998; 111: 678–682

Wilson B D, Ollmann M M, Kang L, Stoffel M, Bell G I & Barsh G S. Structure and function of ASP, the human homolog of the mouse agouti gene. *Hum. Mol. Genet.* 1995; 4: 223–230

Wood J M, Chavan B, Hafeez I & Schallreuter K U. Regulation of tyrosinase by tetrahydropteridines and H2O2. *Biochem. Biophys. Res. Commun* 2004: 325: 1412–1417

Wood J M & Schallreuter K U. Studies on the reactions between human tyrosinase, superoxide anion, hydrogen peroxide and thiols. Biochim. *Biophys. Acta* 1991; 1074: 378 -385

Yada Y, Higuchi K & Imokawa G. Effects of endothelins on signal transduction and proliferation in human melanocytes. *J. Biol. Chem.* 1991; 266: 18352–18357

Yamaguchi Y, Takahashi K, Zmudzka B Z, Kornhauser A, Miller S A, Tadokoro T, Berens W, Beer J Z & Hearing V J. Human skin responses to UV radiation: pigment in the upper epidermis protects against DNA damage in the lower epidermis and facilitates apoptosis. *FASEB J.* 2006; 20:1486–1488

Yamaguchi, Y & Hearing, V. J. Physiological factors that regulate skin pigmentation. *BioFactors* 2009; 35: 193–199

Yohn J, Norris D, Yrastorza D, Buno I, Leff J, Hake S & Repine J. Disparate antioxidant enzyme activities in cultured cutaneous fibroblasts, keratinocytes and melanocytes. *J Invest. Dermatol.* 1991; 97: 405–410

Yokoyama K, Suzuki H, Yasumoto K, Tomita Y & Shibahara S. Molecular cloning and functional analysis of a cDNA coding for human DOPAchrome tautomerase/tyrosinase-related protein-2. *Biochim. Biophys. Acta* 1994; 1217: 317–321

Young A. R. Photobiology of melanins. In: Nordlund J J, Boissy R E, Hearing V J, King R A, Williams S, Oetting S, Ortonne J P, eds. The Pigmentary System, Second Edition. Blackwell Publishing, 2006; 342-353

Zigman S, Reddan J, Schultz J B & McDaniel T. Structural and functional changes in catalase by near-UV radiation. *Photochem Photobiol* 1996; 63: 818–824

11

# Melanin and Its Role in Hyper-Pigmentation – Current Knowledge and Future Trends in Research

Manyatja Brenda Mapunya and Namrita Lall
*Medicinal Plant Science, Department of Plant Science, University of Pretoria, Pretoria 0002, South Africa*

## 1. Introduction

The use of plants as medicines is dated back to early man (Phillipson, 2001). Humans relied on nature for their basic needs such as food, shelter, clothing, fertilizers, flavours, fragrances and last but not least medicines. Plants have formed the sophisticated traditional medicine systems that have been in existence for thousands of years (Anon, 1998, Yelisida, 2005; Cunningham, 1993).

Traditional medicine refers to the health practices, approaches, knowledge and beliefs incorporating plants, animals and mineral based medicines, spiritual therapies, manual techniques and exercises, applied singularly or in-combination to treat, diagnose and prevent illnesses or maintain well-being of individuals. Medicine, in several developing countries, using local traditions and beliefs, is still the mainstay health care till to date. The practice of traditional medicine is widespread in China, India, Japan, Pakistan, Sri Lanka and South Africa etc (Hoareau and Dasilva, 1999; Coetzee et al, 1999; Diederichs, 2002, Nair, 2005). In China 40% of the total medicinal consumption is attributed to traditional tribal medicines. In Japan, herbal medicine preparations are more in demand than mainstream pharmaceutical products (Hoareau and Dasilva, 1999).

Africa is a rich source of medicinal plants (Hoareau and Dasilva, 1999). They are an integral part of African culture, which is the oldest and most diverse in the world. Plants have been used in African medicine to treat fever, asthma, constipation, hypertension, skin diseases etc (Medical news press). About 80% of the black population uses traditional medicine as the primary healthcare system (Bussman and Sharon, 2006, Van wyk et al 1997).

### 1.1 Uses of plants

Plants are a source of fuel, building material, craft material, dyes, food supplements and medicine all over the world. Approximately 80% of black population make use/ rely on plants for these services (Light, 2005). Traditional medicine can be viewed as a parallel system to western health care. Approximately 3000 species are used by an estimated 200,000 indigenous traditional healers (Van wyk et al. 1997). Plants can be used for different purposes, some of them are mentioned below:

### 1.2 Plants as a source of food

Food is any substance composed primarily of carbohydrates, fats, water, and /or proteins that can be drunk or eaten by human beings or animals for nutrition or pleasure (figure 1.1). Food sources include plants, animals or other categories such as fungus or fermented products like alcohols (Davidson, 2006).

Many plant or plant parts are eaten as food. There are around 2000 plants species which can be cultivated for food, and many have several distinct cultivars (Davidson, 2006; Mander, 1999). Fruits are ripened extensions of plants including seeds within. Many plants have evolved fruits that are attractive as a food source to animals as well. Fruits, therefore, make up a significant part of the diets of most cultures. Some botanical fruits such as tomatoes, pumpkin etc are eaten by humans as vegetables.

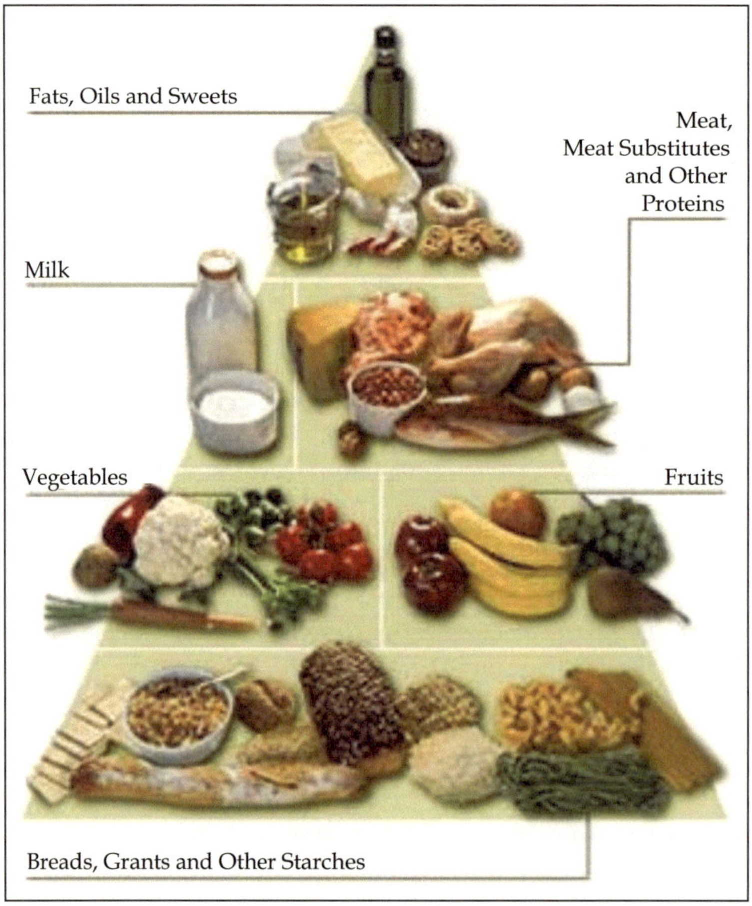


Fig. 1. Food pyramid (http://dietmotion.com/images/food-pyramid.jpg)

### 1.3 Drug discovery

Although natural products, particularly secondary metabolites, have formed the basis of medicines, the presence of these compounds in the biochemistry of the plant is very often difficult to justify. It has been suggested that these compounds may have been synthesized by the plant as part of the defence system of the plant, e.g. plants are known to produce phytoalexins as a response to attack by bacteria and fungi (Louw et al, 2002). The presence of highly toxic natural products has also been highlighted in some animals namely the Amazonian frogs so as to deter predation by other animals. Whatever the reasons for the presence of these compounds in nature could be, it is needless to state that they provide invaluable resources that have been used to find new drug molecules. Table 1.1 gives an indication of the development of new drugs from natural products. Spectroscopic methods coupled with good extraction techniques like chromatography, have contributed to the phenomenal success of natural product chemistry over the past 50 years. A sound isolation strategy has helped in the isolation and characterisation of many bioactive molecules. Nowadays, bioassay-guided fractionation of medicinal plants is a feature of routine in the attempt to isolate components from natural sources. These techniques are not only being restricted to plant sources but they are also being applied to microbial and even fungal sources of metabolites. In practice as soon as the material is collected, in the case of plants, it needs to be identified by a taxonomist so as to ascertain the correct identity of the material. Voucher specimens for herbarium specimens are kept. Various parts of the plant are collected separately (leaves, flowers, stem, wood, bark, root, root bark etc.) and are dried quickly in drying cabinets preparing them for isolation of active compounds (Gurib-Fakim, 2006).

| **Drugs/ chemical** | **Action** | **Plant source** |
|---|---|---|
| Acetyldigoxin | Cardiotonic | *Digitalis lanata*<br>(Grecian foxglove, woolly foxglove) |
| Adoniside | Cardiotonic | *Adonis vernalis*<br>(pheasant's eye, red chamomile) |
| Caffeine | CNS stimulant | *Camellia sinensis*<br>(tea, also coffee, cocoa and other plants) |
| Camptothecin | Anticancerous | *Camptotheca acuminate* |
| Colchicine | Antitumor, antigout | *Colchicum autumnale*<br>(autumn crocus) |
| Galanthamine | Cholinesterase inhibitor | *Lycoris squamigera*<br>(magic lily, resurrection lily, naked lady) |
| Glycyrrhizin | Sweetener, treatment for Addison's disease | *Glycyrrhiza glabra*<br>(licorice) |
| Irinotecan | Anticancer, antitumor agent | *Camptotheca acuminate* |
| Lapachol | Anticancer, antitumor | Tabebuia species<br>(trumpet tree) |
| Monocrotaline | Topical antitumor agent | *Crotalaria sessiliflora* |

Table 1.1 Plant based drugs and medicines (Taylor, 2000)

### 1.4 Plants as a source of cosmetics

Cosmetic product refers to any substance or preparation intended for application to any external surface of the human body (i.e. the epidermis, hair system nails, lips and external genitals organs) or teeth or buccal mucosa wholly or mainly for the purpose of cleaning, perfuming or protecting them or keeping them in good conditions or changing their appearance or combating body odour or perspiration except where such cleaning, perfuming, protecting, keeping and changing is wholly for the purpose of treating or preventing diseases (Aburjai and Natsheh, 2003; Dweck, 1996). Novel bioactive ingredients for cosmetics are derived from sea, earth and plant kingdom. Popular ingredients include Chinese herbs, Vitamins, minerals, antioxidants, enzymes, hormones and naturals.

Plants have been used for cosmetic purposes since time immemorial. They have once been the main source and foundation of all cosmetics before various methods were discovered of synthesizing substances with similar properties (Aburjai and Natsheh, 2003). The first cosmetic derived from plant is dated about 3100-2907 BC which was used in Egypt (Dold and Cocks, 2002; Cocks et al, 2003).

There are many plants which are being used for cosmetics. Ginseng is a traditional drug used for more than 2000 years. It activates the skin metabolism (Tanaka and Okada, 1991), reduces keratinisation (Kim et al, 1989), provides moisture and softens, alleviate wrinkling and enhance skin whiteness (Dweck, 1997). Other plants that have been used in cosmetics preparations are *Artemisia vulguris* and *Artemisia absinthum* which are used for skin diseases. The entire plant is made into decoction and is used as a wash for many kinds of wounds and skin ulcers (Dweck, 1997). *Salvia officinalis* (L) also called common sage, true sage or garden sage is used as a lotion to improve the condition of hair and skin. The major *S. officinalis* constituents responsible for the effect of hair are tannins, saponins as well as borneol and camphor (Aburjah and Natsheh, 2003; Boiceanu et al, 1986). Majority of South African plants such as *Calodendrum capensis*, are being used traditionally as cosmetics but they have not been scientifically validated.

## 2. Hyper-pigmentation

Hyper-pigmentation of skin is a common problem that is prevalent in middle aged and elderly people. Hyper-pigmentation can be caused by excessive exposure to UV light, drug reaction and can also occur during ageing. Dermatological disorders associated with hyper-pigmentation include age spots, melasma and site of actinic damage to mention the few (Pandya and Guevera, 2000).

Melanin is the pigment responsible for the colour of skin in humans. It also occurs in bacteria, fungi and plants. Tyrosinase is known to be the key enzyme in melanin biosynthesis (Nerya et al, 2003). Over-activity of this enzyme leads to overproduction of melanin leading to hyper-pigmentation of the skin and under-activity leads to disorders such as vitiligo (depigmentation spots that occurs on the skin) and whitening of hair. Overproduction of melanin can be prevented by avoiding excessive UV light exposure and can be treated with skin-lightening agents such as bleaching hydroquinone, kojic acid and retinoids (Halder et al, 2004). Inhibition of tyrosinase can also lead to reduced melanin production. Some commercially available chemical and fungal derived skin-lightening agents have been proven to have chronic, cytotoxic, mutagenic effects in humans (Nerya et al, 2003; Wang et al, 2006; Wu et al, 2003). Therefore, there is a need for alternative herbal derived and pharmaceutical agents for the treatment of hyper-pigmentation of human skin.

## 2.1 Structure and function of the skin

The skin is one of the heaviest body organs. It covers between 1.5 and 2 m, comprising about one sixth of the body's total weight. The skin performs several important physiological functions; this includes regulation of body temperature and metabolism, excretion (via sweat glands), synthesis of vitamin D in the epidermal layer when exposed to UV rays, uses specialised cells to protect us from UV rays of the sun etc (Murphy, 1995). The skin consists of three layers (figure 2.1) namely:

i. **Epidermis**- It is the outer layer of the skin which also consists of several layers- the basal cell layer, the spinous cell layer, the granular cell layer and the stratum corneum. Cells in the epidermis include the keratinocytes which are the most abundant cells in this layer, melanocytes which constitutes about 5% of the living cells in this layer (Murphy, 1995).
ii. **Dermis**- This layer is just below the epidermis. It consists of fats, collagen and also elastin fibres that provide strength and flexibility to the skin. In older persons the elastin fibres fragments and much of the skin's elastic quality is lost. This, along with the loss of subcutaneous fat, results in wrinkles (Murphy, 1995).
iii. **Subcutaneous layer or hypodermis**- This is the inner most layer of the skin. It serves as storage for fats. The fats stored in this layer represent an energy source for the body and helps to insulate the body against changes in the outside temperature (Murphy, 1995).

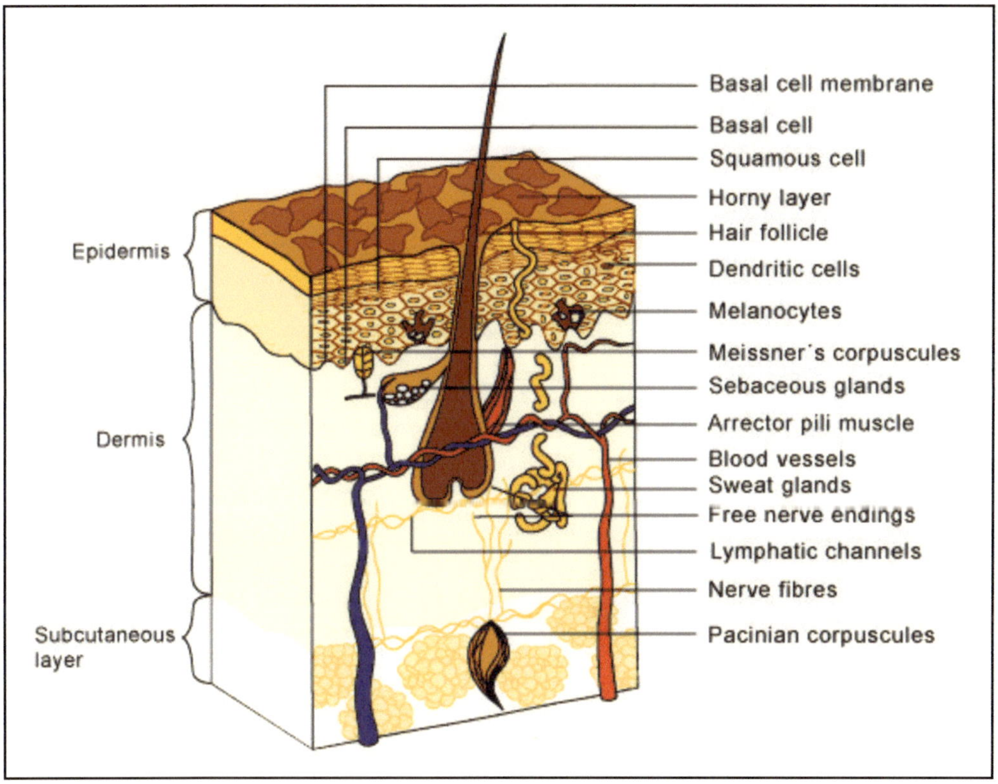


Fig. 2. Structure of the normal skin
(http://skincare.dermis.net/content/e01aufbau/e660/e661/e700/013_haut_aufbau_eng.gif)

### 2.2 Melanin biosynthesis and its importance

Melanin is a class of compounds found in the plant, animal and protista kingdoms, where it serves predominantly as a pigment (Kim and Uyama, 2005). In humans, melanin is the primary determinants of the color of the skin, hair and eyes. It is synthesized within melanosomes, membrane-bound granules, from melanocytes and is then transferred to keratinocytes through a physiological process called melanogenesis (figure 2.2) (Ancans et al, 2003; Kim and Uyama, 2005). Tyrosinase is known to be the key enzyme in melanin biosynthesis (figure 2.2). It catalyses two distinct reactions: hydroxylation of the amino acid tyrosine to 3,4 dihydroxyphenylalanine (DOPA) by monophenolase action and oxidation of DOPA in to o-dopaquinone by diphenolase action. This o-quinone is transformed into melanins in a series of non-enzymatic reactions (Baurin et al, 2002; Wang et al, 2006). There are two types of melanin pigments that can be produced by the melanocytes cells namely: 'eumelanin' (black or brown) and 'pheomelanin' (red or yellow) (figure 2.3) (Commo et al, 2004; Summers, 2006). The color of hair, skin etc in human is determined by the type, distribution and degree of melanin pigment synthesized. Each individual of different racial

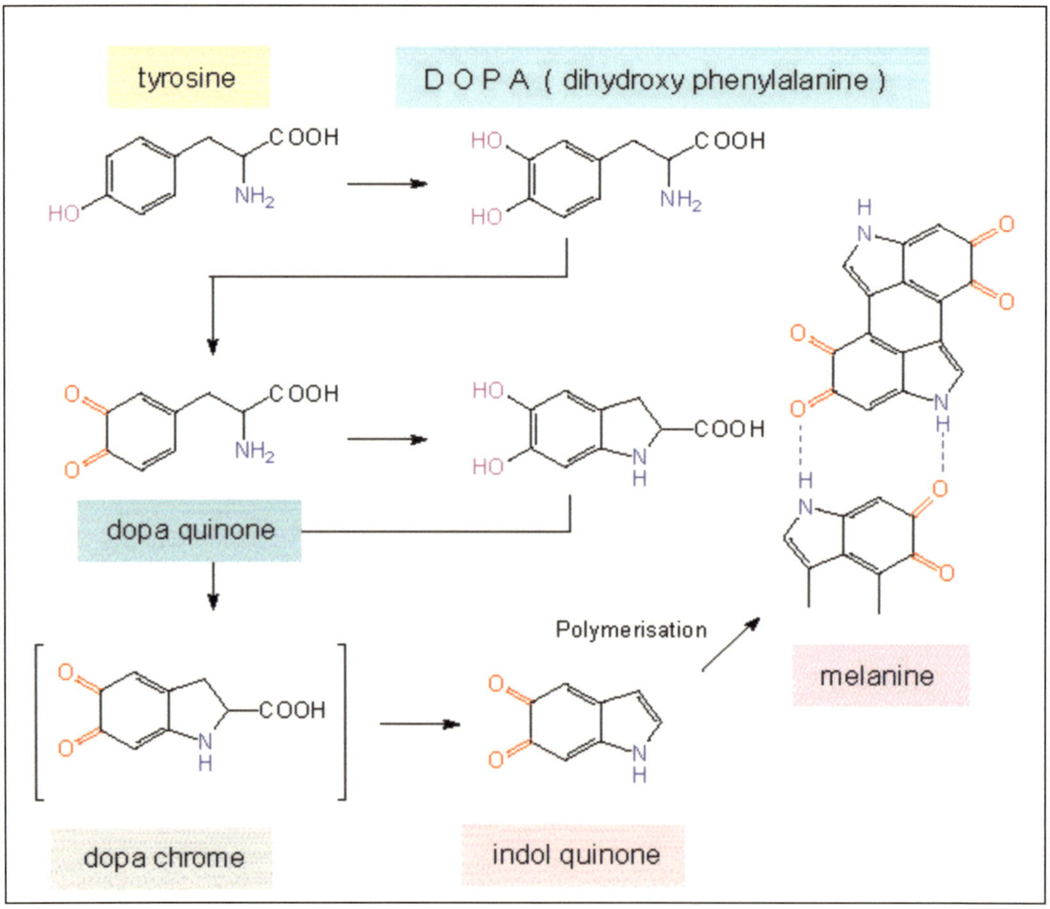


Fig. 3. Melanin biosynthesis pathway (Moss, 2005)
(http://www.chem.qmul.ac.uk/iubmb/enzyme/reacqwa tion/AminoAcid/melanin.html)

group have more or less the same number of melanocytes cells, thus the type of melanin produced depends on the functioning of the melanocytes e.g. people with darker skin are just genetically programmed to constantly produce higher levels of melanin even without exposure to UV light and the melanosomes remains singular (figure 2.4) (Commo et al, 2004; Baurin et al, 2002; Kim and Uyama, 2005; Summers, 2006; Sturm et al, 1998). In individuals with fair or lighter skin colour, melanosomes cluster in membrane bound organelles (figure 2.4) (Sturm et al, 1998). The role of melanin is to protect the skin against UV light damage by absorbing UV sunlight and by removing reactive oxygen species (Kim and Uyama, 2005; Summers, 2006).

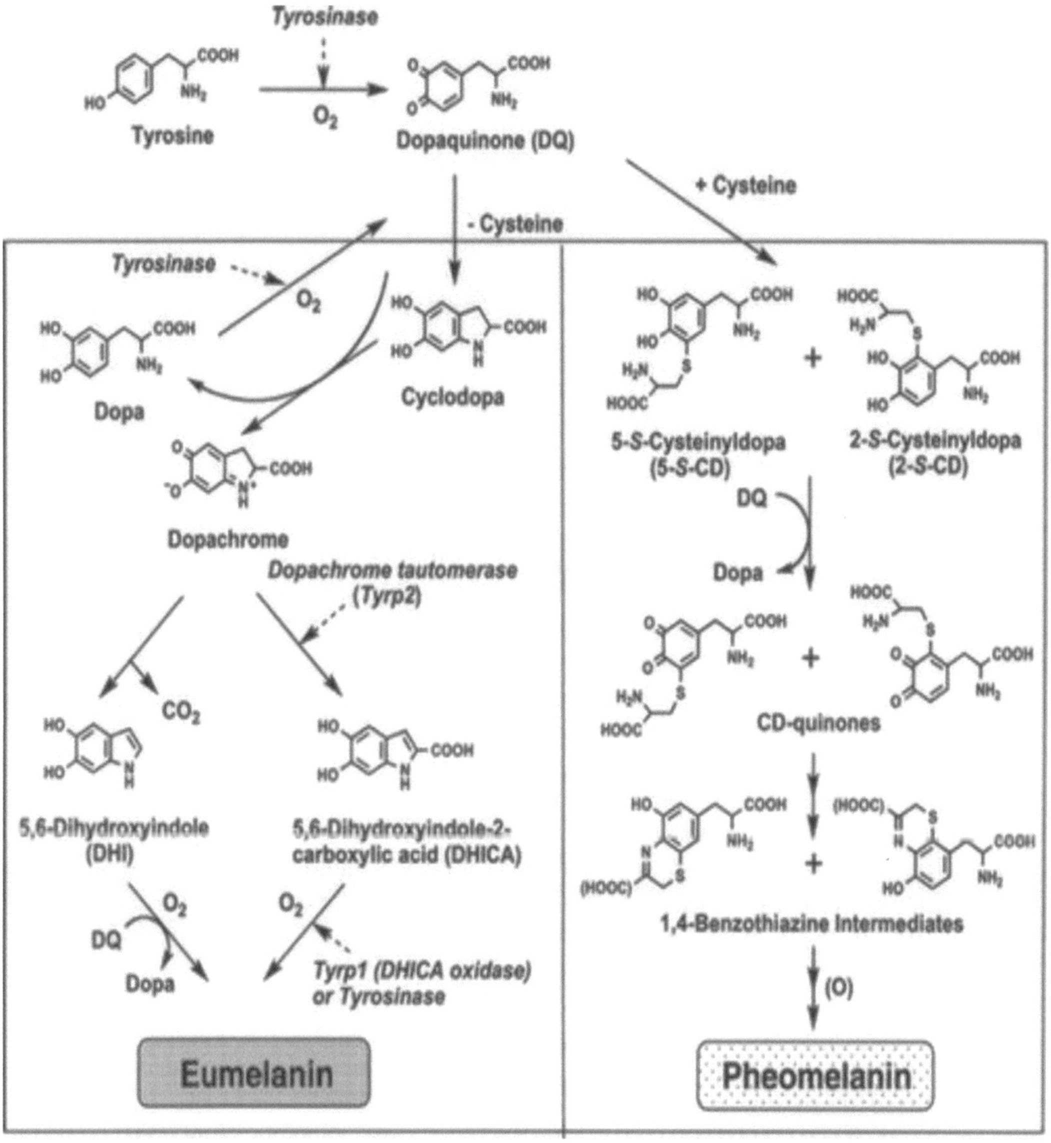


Fig. 4. Production of different pigments by melanosomes (Simon et al, 2008)

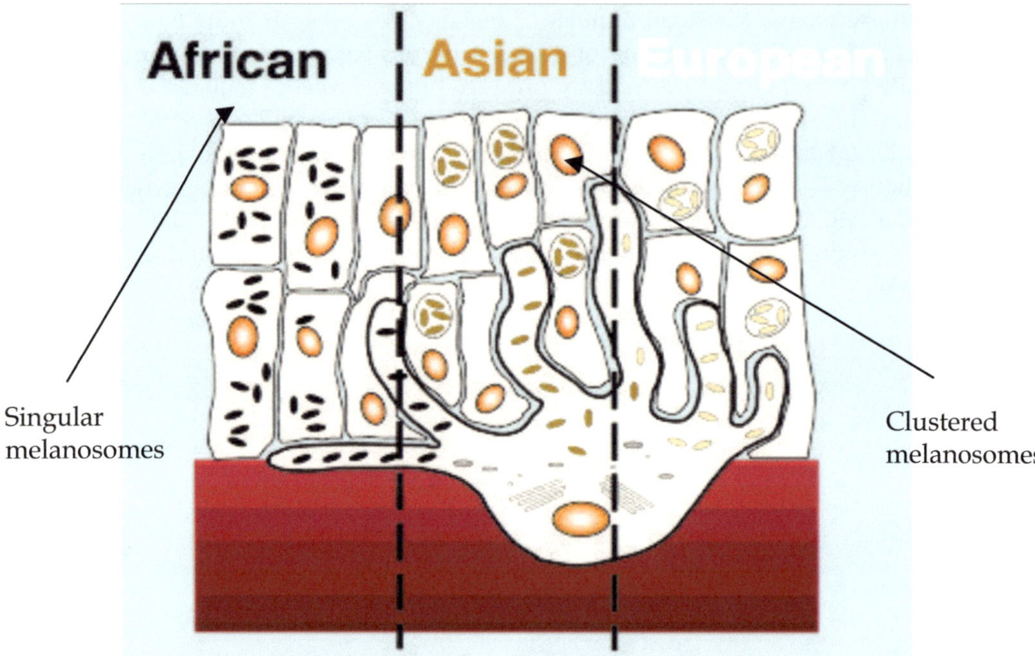


Fig. 5. Structure of melanosome distribution for different racial groups (Sturm et al, 1998)

### 2.3 Factors affecting skin pigmentation

The process of melanogenesis is affected by a variety of environmental, hormonal and genetic factors. Environmental factors include excessive exposure to UV light, which induces immediate pigment-darkening due to swelling and re-alignment of melanosomes (Rendon, 2003, Schulleuter et al, 1998; Simon et al, 2008). Example for hormonal factors is evident in pregnant women whereby during this period, dark brown patches occur on the forehead, face, cheeks and it can occur due to reactions caused by usage of drugs. Genetic factors are evident in cases like albinism whereby individuals loses the TPR1 gene which disrupts the correct formation of the melanosomal complex and thereby inhibits melanin synthesis, resulting in hypopigmented phenotype (Sturm et al, 1998)

### 2.4 Hyper-pigmentation disorders

Hyper-pigmentation is a common and distressing problem. Females report more often, although not rare in males. These disorders have a tremendous psychological impact especially in females. There are different kinds of hyper-pigmentation disorders that are encountered during life. Some of them are as follows:

#### 2.4.1 Age spots

This is also known as brown spots, lentigines or liver spots. They usually appear on the hands, but can also appear on the face, arm and feet as brown patches. They are harmless and are caused by excessive exposure of the skin to the sun. It may also be caused by nutritional deficiency, impaired liver function dietary and ageing (Moss, 2005, Murphy, 1995).

### 2.4.2 Melasma

Melasma appears as blotchy, brownish pigmentation on the face of adults. Both sides of the face are usually affected. The most common sites of involvement are the cheeks, bridge of nose, forehead, and upper lip. The precise cause of melasma is unknown. People with a family history of melasma are more likely to develop melasma themselves. A change in hormonal status may trigger melasma. It is commonly associated with pregnancy and is also called chloasma, or the "mask of pregnancy." Birth control pills may also cause melasma, however, hormone replacement therapy used after menopause has not been shown to cause the condition. Sun exposure also contributes to melasma. While there is no cure for melasma, many treatments have been developed. Melasma may disappear after pregnancy; it may remain for many years, or a lifetime. Sunscreens are essential in the prevention of melasma (American Academy of Dermatologists press 2008; Montemarano, 2008; Daniel et al, 2003).

### 2.4.3 Freckles

Freckles are clusters of concentrated melanin which are most often visible on people with a fair complexion. A freckle is also called an "ephelis". They can be found on anyone no matter the background; however, having freckles is genetic and is related to the presence of the dominant melanocortin-1 receptor (MC1R) gene variant. The formation of freckles is triggered by exposure to sunlight. The exposure to UV-B radiation activates melanocytes to increase the melanin production, which causes freckles to become darker. Freckles are predominantly found on the face, although they may appear on any skin exposed to the sun. Freckles are rare on infants and more common on children before puberty; they are less common on adults (Hanson et al, 2006; Daniel et al, 2003).

### 2.4.4 Melanoma

Excessive exposure to the sun is the most common cause of skin darkening. The darkening is due to the skin's increased production of melanin, which is a protective mechanism against the sun's harmful ultraviolet rays. In the last few decades, a suntan has been equated with a healthy, outdoor look, and large numbers of ordinarily fair-skinned people have deliberately exposed their skin to the sun to acquire suntans. This practice has led to an alarming rise in skin cancer, including **malignant melanoma,** which is often fatal. Fortunately, fashion is beginning to change, and deeply tanned skin is no longer considered chic.

Melanoma, also referred to as "malignant melanoma," is the most serious form of skin cancer because - with the exception of some rare forms of skin cancer - it is the skin cancer most likely to spread to lymph nodes and internal organs. Today, melanoma accounts for 77% of all deaths from skin cancer.

Dermatologists believe that the number of deaths from melanoma could be significantly reduced if more people were able to recognize melanoma in its earliest stages. It is important to know that there are different types of melanoma. This article describes the four most common types of melanoma, which accounts for about 100% of diagnosed cases. Below you will find an explanation of what each of these four types of melanoma looks like and important points to remember. Here are a few of these key points:

- With early detection and treatment, the cure rate for melanoma is about 95%.

- Not all melanoma develops from a changing mole. Melanoma also can appear where there was not a previous lesion and look like a non-pigmented scar or cyst.
- Melanoma can appear as a nail streak or non-healing bruise.

Four types of melanoma

1. Superficial spreading melanoma (about 70% of diagnosed cases)
2. Nodular melanoma (about 15% of diagnosed cases)
3. Lentigo maligna melanoma (about 10% of diagnosed cases)
4. Acral lentiginous melanoma (about 5% of diagnosed cases)

#### 2.4.4.1 Superficial spreading melanoma

Superficial spreading melanoma (SSM) is the most common type of melanoma in the United States, accounting for about 70% of all diagnosed melanoma cases. This type of melanoma can strike at any age and occurs slightly more often in females than males. SSM is the leading cause of death from cancer in young adults.

When SSM occurs in females, it most commonly appears on the legs. In males, it is more likely to develop between the neck and pelvis. However, this does not mean that females do not get SSM on their trunks or that males do not see SSM on their legs. This melanoma can occur anywhere on the skin's surface.

A typical SSM lesion has:

- Irregular borders
- Various shades of black, brown, gray, blue, pink, red, or white. Within the lesion there can be a remarkable variation in color involving white, pink, brown, and black.

In the early stages, SSM usually appears as a flat spot that looks like a freckle that is spreading sideways on the skin. Over time, the pigmentation in the lesion may darken, and the lesion may grow, develop increasingly irregular borders, and have areas of inflammation within the lesion. The area around the lesion may begin to itch. Occasionally, a SSM may become "less" pigmented as a person's immune responses try to destroy it. If a lesion becomes less pigmented, this does not mean that the lesion no longer requires treatment. It definitely needs to be examined by a dermatologist.

Superficial spreading melanoma can progress rapidly. If you see a lesion that you suspect could be melanoma, have it examined by a dermatologist.

#### 2.4.4.2 Nodular melanoma

Nodular melanoma (NM) is the most aggressive type of melanoma and accounts for about 15% of all melanomas diagnosed in the United States. It can appear anywhere on the body and occurs more often in males than females. It can develop at any age; however, it is most often seen in people aged 60 and older.

NM differs from other types of melanoma in three ways:

- Tends to grow more rapidly in thickness (penetrate the skin) than in diameter
- May not have a readily visible phase of development
- Instead of arising from a pre-existing mole, it may appear in a spot where a lesion did not previously exist

Since NM tends to grow deeper more quickly than it does wide and can occur in a spot that did not have a previous lesion, the prognosis is often worse because it takes longer for a person to be aware of the changes.

NM is most often darkly pigmented; however, some NM lesions can be light brown or even colorless (non-pigmented). A light-colored or non-pigmented NM lesion may escape detection because the appearance is not alarming. An ulcerated and bleeding lesion is common.

The following photos show diagnosed cases of NM, which often appears as a dome-shaped, darkly pigmented lesion.

If a lesion appears where none existed before, have it examined as soon as possible by a dermatologist.

#### 2.4.4.3 Lentigo maligna melanoma

Lentigo maligna melanoma (LMM) typically occurs on sun-damaged skin in the middle-aged and elderly, especially on the face. This melanoma may be mistaken in its early, and most treatable, stages for a benign "age spot" or "sun spot." LMM accounts for about 10% of the melanomas diagnosed in the United States. Since LMM is so easily mistaken, it can go undetected for years. This can be quite dangerous.

LMM begins as a spreading, flat, patch with irregular borders and variable colors of brown. This lesion is called "lentigo maligna." This spreading brownish patch may grow slowly for years and is often mistaken for lentigo simplex — a benign (non cancerous) brownish patch that can develop in the elderly after years of sun exposure.

As the lesion grows and evolves, both the pigmentation and borders tend to become more irregular. This often occurs slowly over a period of 10 to 15 years. It also can happen rapidly — in a matter of weeks or months. As the lesion grows deeper into the skin (thickness increases), it may become various shades of black and brown. Dark nodules may appear within the irregular borders. These nodules are the invasive tumor, and if large enough to be felt by touch, will feel lumpy.

If you have a large pigmented patch of skin, especially one with an irregular border, see a dermatologist as soon as possible.

#### 2.4.4.4 Acral lentiginous melanoma

In the United States, acral lentiginous melanoma (ALM) accounts for about 5% of all diagnosed melanomas. It also is the most common form of melanoma in Asians and people with dark skin, accounting for 50% of melanomas that occur in people with these skin types.

ALM is sometimes referred to as a "hidden melanoma" because these lesions occur on parts of the body not easily examined or not thought necessary to examine. ALM develops on the palms, soles, mucous membranes (such as those that line the mouth, nose, and female genitals), and underneath or near fingernails and toenails.

ALM is often overlooked until it is well advanced because in the early stages, it often looks like a bruise or nail streak. Here is what it usually looks like on each area of the body:

- Palm or sole - Melanoma usually begins as an irregularly shaped tan, brown, or black spot. It is often mistakenly attributed to some recent injury — that is, the patient recalls a relatively recent bruise or blow in the general area of the pigmented spot.
- Mucous membranes - When melanoma develops on a mucus membrane, it is most likely to develop inside the nose or mouth. Early symptoms include nosebleeds and nasal stuffiness and a pigmented mass inside the mouth. Melanomas also can develop on the mucous membranes of the anus, urinary tract, and female genitalia.

- Under a nail - The first sign may be a "nail streak" — a narrow, dark stripe under the nail. ALM usually develops on the thumb or big toe; however, it can occur under any fingernail or toenail. Many individuals, especially dark-skinned people, have fixed nail streaks that are completely benign. A new nail streak not associated with recent trauma, an enlarging nail streak, a wide or very darkly pigmented streak, or a nail that is separating or lifting up from the nail bed should be examined by a dermatologist. A possible indication of advanced ALM is a nail streak with associated pigmentation in the nail fold skin or destruction of the nail plate.

ALM of the fingers or toes also can develop without an obvious nail streak — particularly the non-pigmented variety. ALM may, for example, look very much like a chronic infection of the nail bed. As an ALM tumor increases in size, it usually becomes more irregular in shape and color. However, some ALM lesions can be lightly colored or colorless. The surface of the ALM lesion may remain flat, even as the tumor invades deeply into the skin. Thickening ALM on the sole of the foot can make walking painful and be mistaken for a plantar wart.

The second photo shown above depicts an advanced tumor. This patient believed he had a long-standing bruise on his toe and refused to be examined by a physician. By the time ALM was finally diagnosed and surgically removed, it had invaded deeply into tissue and spread to other organs. The patient died of metastatic melanoma.

Be sure to see a dermatologist as soon as possible if you notice a:

- Bruise that does not fade or comes and goes
- Nail lifts up or separates from the nail bed
- New nail streak not associated with recent trauma
- Enlarging nail streak
- Wide or very darkly pigmented nail streak
- Pigmented mass in the mouth
- Nosebleeds and nasal stuffiness

#### 2.4.4.5 Non-pigmented subtypes

While uncommon, melanoma occasionally does not have brown or black pigmentation. An uncommon subtype called **amelanotic melanoma** usually appears as a pink or red nodule (lump). Another uncommon subtype, **desmoplastic neutrotrophic melanoma** (DNM), usually looks like a non-pigmented scar. When a scar or keloid appears on the skin and the skin has not been injured, DNM is suspected. The lesion also can appear as a cyst that may or may not be pigmented. DNM tends to appear on sun-damaged skin in elderly patients, occurring mostly on the head and neck.

## 3. Treatment of hyper-pigmentation

Like other disorders hyper-pigmentation of the skin can be treated. Depending on the type and depth of pigmentation different treatment procedures are followed. The use of sun screens is important and this helps to reduce the development of pigmentation disorders. Skin lighteners are also used for the treatment of hyper-pigmentation this includes chemicals such as bleaching hydroquinone, retinoid etc which are available commercially (Cayce et al, 2004, Tiedtke et al, 2004).

### 3.1 Commercially available skin-lighteners

There are different types of skin-lightening agents that are available commercially to combat dark marks or skin hyper-pigmentation. Some of these chemically derived compounds have shown to have poor penetration of the skin and shows some cytotoxic and mutagenic effect on people. Among treatments the use of chemicals such as 'Kojic acid', 'Hydroquinone', 'Arbutin', 'Aloesin' etc are the most common ones. Descriptions of some of these chemicals are as follows:

#### 3.1.1 Hydroquinone (HQ)

It is a hydroxyphenolic chemical that inhibits the conversion of L-DOPA to melanin by inhibiting the tyrosinase enzyme. Some of the possible mechanisms of action are the destruction of melanocytes, degradation of melanosomes and inhibition of the synthesis of DNA and RNA (Mashhood, 2006). Concentrations of HQ in commercially available formulations vary from 2% to 4%. Clinically and historically evaluation demonstrated clear improvements in most patients during the study done by Pandya and Guevara 2003. However, during this study 72% of the patients showed to develop irritant dermatitis over time, despite the low frequency of application.

#### 3.1.2 Kojic acid (5-hydroxy-2-[hydroxyl methyl]-4-pyrone)

It is a naturally occurring hydrophilic, 'fungal derivative', evolved from certain species of *Acetobater, Aspergillus* and *Penicillin*. It acts by inhibiting the production of free tyrosinase with efficacy similar to hydroquinone. In Japan, kojic acid has been increasingly used in skin products. This is because until recently, topically applied kojic acid at 1% concentration had not exhibited any sensitizing activity. However, more recent long term Japanese studies have shown that kojic acid has a potential of causing 'contact dermatitis' and 'erythema' (Nakagawa et al, 1995; Mashhood, 2006).

#### 3.1.3 Arbutin (b-D-glucopyranoside derivative of hydroquinone)

It is a naturally occurring plant derived compound that has been used for post-inflammatory hyper-pigmentation. The action of arbutin depends on its concentration (Maeda and Fukuda, 1996). Higher concentrations are more efficacious than lower concentrations. A dose-dependent reduction in tyrosinase activity, as well as melanin content in melanocytes, is demonstrated. It was reported that it may cause paradoxical hyper-pigmentation (Mashhood, 2006).

#### 3.1.4 Aloesin

It is a natural derivative of *Aloe vera* that inhibits tyrosinase at noncytotoxic concentrations. Aloesin acts as an inhibitor of DOPA oxidation. It is an experimental product and thus it is not available clinically (Rendon & Gaviria, 2005).

## 4. Cosmeceutical formulations from plants

Due to instability, poor penetration of the skin, irritation and mutagenic effects of chemical and fungal derived compounds in cosmetical applications, humans opt for herbal products for the treatment of different types of skin problems. There are many South African plants which are being used in herbal cosmetics. Rooibos (*Aspalathus linearis*) is famous for being naturally caffeine free (Morton, 1983) and its low tannin content minimizes the risk of reduced iron absorption, a phenomena frequently found in tea drinkers due to iron-tannin complexation. Rooibos is rich in flavonoids, polyphenols, phenolic acids, oligosaccharides and polysaccharides (Dos et al, 2005). The major flavonoids found in Rooibos tea are aspalathin, iso-orientin, orientin and rutin (Shimamura et al, 2006).

The skin is the largest organ of the body and is exposed to environmental oxidative stress. The incorporation of Rooibos extracts in topical cosmetic formulations has become very popular in recent years because it can target the site of action to reduce ultraviolet radiation damage and photo-aging (Mavon et al, 2005; Van Niekerk and Viljoen, 2008). Rooibos proved to exhibit anti-inflammatory and antimicrobial properties in cosmetic applications. According to earlier reports, hair growth was found to improve with the use of hair care products containing Rooibos. There are many herbal products derived from rooibos (fig 2.5).

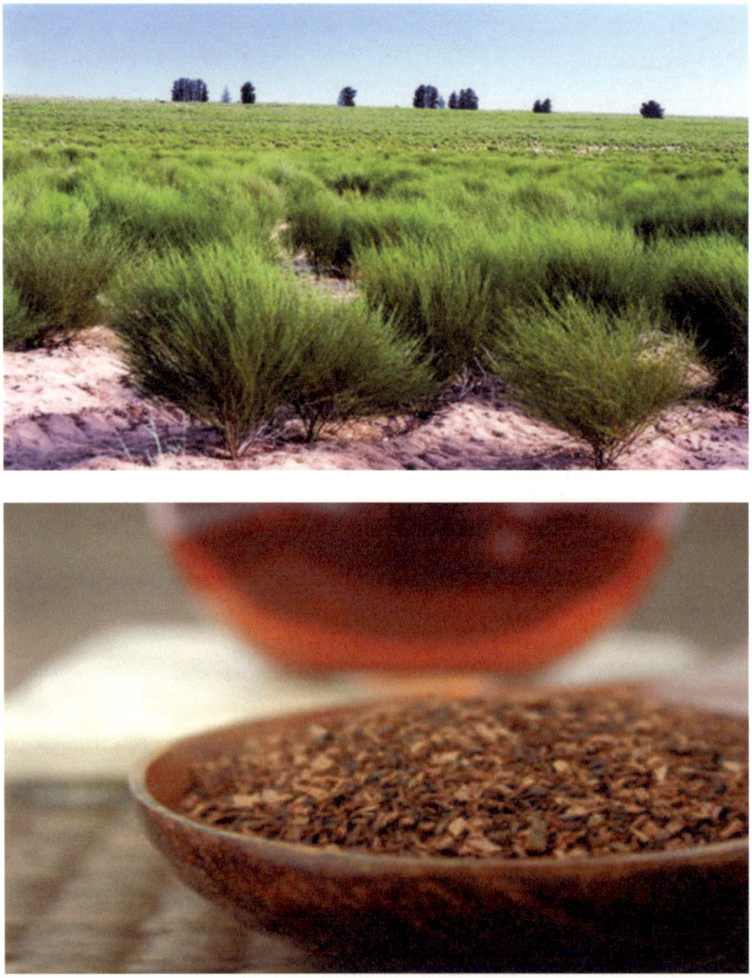

Fig. 6. Rooibos (*Aspalathus linearis*) (http://www.inheritanceskincare.com/)

*Artemisia afra* is also popular for skin ailments. An infusion or decoction is used as a lotion by natives in South Africa to bathe hemorrhoids, herpes and venereal sores, while a hot bath in the decoction is used to bring out the rash in measles, mumps and chickenpox. The plant is also held in the mouth to ease the pain of boils and to hasten their bursting. It also has similar uses to *Artemisia herba-alba* and used externally on boils, carbuncles, and large acne pimples. A poultice of the leaf is applied locally to relieve neuralgia, to the swellings in mumps, and to any glandular or skin inflammation. A lotion is also made from the plant for washing the body and rejuvenating the skin (Dweck, 1996). Due to the above mentioned side effects and poor skin penetration ability of the existing agents which are used for the treatment of hyper-pigmentation, it is imperative to find alternative agents from plants.

## 5. References

American Academy of Dermatologists press 2008 melasma (http://www.aad.org/public/publications/pamphlets/common_melasma.html)

Ancans, J., Tobin, D.J., Hoogduijn, M.J., Smit, N.P., Wakamatsu, K., Thody, A.J., 2003. Melanosomal pH controls rate of melanogenesis, Eumelanin/Phaeomelanin Ratio and Melanosome maturation in melanocytes and melanoma cells. Experimental cell research 268:26-35

Baurin, N., Arnoult, E., Scior, T., Do, Q. T., Bernard, P., 2002. Preliminary screening of some tropical plants for antityrosinase activity. Journal of Ethnopharmacology 82: 155-158

Commo, S., Gaillard, O., Bernard, B.A., 2004. Human hair graying linked to a specific depletion of hair follicle melanocytes affecting both the bulb and the outer root sheath. British Journal of Dermatology, 150, 435-443

Cayce, K.A., Feldman, S. R., McMichael, A. J., 2004. Hyperpigmentation: a review of common treatment options. Journal of Drugs in Dermatology 5:1-8

Daniel, L., Stulberg, M.D., Nicole-Clark, M.D., 2003. Common hyperpigmentation disorders in adults: Part 1. Diagnostic approach, café au latí Macules, Diffuse hyperpigmentaion, Sun exposure, and phototoxity reactions. American Family Physician 68:1956-1960

Daniel, L., Stulberg, M.D., Nicole-Clark, M.D., 2003. Common hyperpigmentation disorders in adults: Part 2. Melanoma, Seborrheic Keratoses, Acanthosis Nigricans, Melasma, Diabetic Dermopathy, Tinea Versicolor, and Postinflammatory hyperpigmentation. American Family Physician 68:1963 1968

Dos, A., Ayhan, Z., Sumnu, G., 2005. Effects of different factors on sensory attributes, overall acceptance and preference of Rooibos (Aspalathus linearis) tea. Journal of Sensory Studies, 20:228-242.

Dweck, A.C., 1996. Ethnobotanical plants from South Aftrica part 2. Cosmetics and Toiletries Magazine. 114-119

Halder, R.M., Richards, M.D., Richards, G.M., 2004. Topical agents used in the management of hyperpigmentation, 9, 453

Hanson, K.M., Gratton, E., Bardeen., C.J., 2006. Sunscreen enhauncement of UV-induced reactive oxygen species in the skin. Free Radicalbiology and medicine 41(8): 1205-1212

Kim, Y-J., Uyama, H., 2005. Tyrosinase inhibitors from natural and synthetic sources: structure, inhibition mechanism and perspective for the future. Cell Molecular Life Sciences 62: 1707-1723

Maeda, K., Fukuda, M., 1996. Arbutin: mechanism of its depigmenting action in human melanocytes culture. Journal of Pharmacology 276: 765-769.

Mashhood, A. A., 2006. Treatment of hyperpigmentation disorders. Journal of Pakistan association of Dermatologists 16: 65-68

Mavon, A., Raufast, V., Redoulès, D., 2004. Skin absorption and metabolism of a new vitaminE prodrug, ´-tocopherol-glucoside: in vitro evaluation in human skin model. Journal of Controlled Release, 100: 221-231.

Moss, G. P., 2005 (http://www.chem.qmul.ac.uk/iubmb/enzyme/reacqwation/AminoAcid/melanin.html)

Montemarano, A., 2008. Melasma. Medscape Journal. Page 1-10

Morton, J.F., 1983. Rooibos Tea, Aspalathus linearis, a caffeinless, low-tannin beverage. Economic Botany, 37(2):164-173.

Murphy, G F., 1995. Dermatopathology, A practical guide to common disorders. 1st edition. W.B. Sanders Company, Philadelphia, Pennyslavania

Nakagawa, M., Kawai, K., Kawai, K., 1995. Contact allergy to kojic acid in skin care products. Contact Dermatitis 32: 9-13

Nerya, O., Vaya, J., Musa, R., Izrael, S., Ben-Arie, R., Tamir, S., 2003. Glabrene and Isoliquiritigen as tyrosinase inhibitors from licorice roots. Journal of Agricultural food chemistry 51: 1201-1207

Pandya, A. G., 2000. Disorders of hyper-pigmentation. Dermatological Clinics 18: 91-98

Rendon, M., Jorge, I., Gaviria, M. D., 2003. Procedures in cosmetic Dermatological Series.

Rendon, M.I., Gaviria, J.R., 2005. Review of skin-lightening agents. Dermatol Surgery 31: 886-889

Schulleuter, K., Slominski A., Pawelek, J.M., Jimbow, K., Gilcrest, B.A., 1998. What controls melanogenesis? Experimental Dermatology. 143-150

Shimamura, N., Miyase, T., Umehara, K., Warashina, T., Fuji, S., 2006. Phytoestrogensfrom Aspalathus linearis. Biological and Pharmaceutical Bulletin, 29(6):1271-1274.

Simon, J. D., Hong, L., Peles, D.N., 2008. Insights into Melanosomes and Melanin from Some Interesting Spatial and Temporal Properties. Journal of Physical Chemistry 112 (42): 13201–13217

Sturm, R.A., Box, N.F., Ramsay, M., 1998. Human pigmentation genetics: the difference is only skin deep. Review article. BioEssays 20: 712-721

Summers, B., 2006. A lightening tour of skin-brightening options. South African Pharmaceutical and Cosmetic Review 33: 29-30

Tiedtke, J., Morel, J., Marks, O., 2004. Depigmentation factor bioflavonoids- A safe and effective skin lightener based on encapsulated citrus bioflavonoids. Cosmetochem 2: 12-17

Van Niekerk, C., Viljoen, A., 2008. Indigenous South African medicinal plants part II Aspalanthus linearis (Rooibos). South African Pharmaceutical Journal. 41-42

Wang, K-H., Lin, R-D., Hsu, F-L., Huang, Y-H., Chan, H-C., Lee, M-H., 2006. Cosmetic applications of selected traditional Chinese herbal medicines. Journal of Ethnopharmacology 106: 353-359

Wu, L-C., Chen, Y-C., Ho, J-A., Yang, C-S., 2003. Inhibitory effect of Red kojic extracts on mushroom tyrosinase. Journal of Agriculture and food Chemistry 51: 4240-4246

Aburjai, T., Natsheh, F.M., 2003. Plants used in cosmetics, Phytotherapy Research 17: 987-1000

Anon, 1998. Enviromental guidelines to practical forest management. Forest and Park Edita. Helesinki

Boiceanu, S., Constantinescu, D., Dumitrescu, E., Paraschiv, V., Teodorescu, E., 1986. Hair preparation. Rom 2: RO88523

Bussmann, R. W, Sharon, D., 2006. Traditional medicinal plant use in Northern Peru: tracking two thousand years healing culture. Journal of Ethnobiology and Ethnomedicine 2: 47-52

Cocks, M.L., Dold, T, Wiersum, F., 2003. The cost of culture: the role of natural resources in maintaining Xhosa customs in the Eastern Cape. Veld and flora 89: 146-149

Cotzee, C., Jefthas, E., Reinten, E., 1999. Indigenous plant genetic resources of South Africa. ASHS press, Alexandria, VA. Pp 160-1663

Cunningham, A. B., 1993. African medicinal plants: setting priorities at the interface between conservation and primary health care. Working paper 1. UNESCO Paris.

Davidson, A., 2006. The Oxford Companion to Food 2nd edition. United Kingdom: Oxford University Press, 11-15

Dold, A. P., Cocks, M. L., 2002. The trade in medicinal plants in the Eastern Cape Province, South Africa. The Journal of Science 98: 589-597

Diederichs, N., Geldenhuys, C., Mitchell, D., 2002. The first legal harvesters of protected medicinal plants in South Africa. Science in Africa on-line magazine

Dweck, A.C., 1996. Botanicals – research of actives. Cosmet Toiletries 111: 45–57.

Dweck, A.C., 1997a. African fragranced plants. Cosmet Toiletries 112: 47–54.

Gurib-Fakim, A., 2006. Medicinal plants: Traditions of yesterday and drugs of tomorrow. Molecular Aspects of Medicine 27: 1-93

Hoareau, L., Dasilva, E. J., 1999. Medicinal plants: a re-emerging health aid. Journal of Biotechnology 2: 1-6

Kim, H.Y., Jin, S.H., Kim, S.I., 1989. Effect of 13-cis-retinoic acid and ginseng saponin on hyperkeratinization of guinea pig skin. Koryo Insam Hakhoechi 13: 248–253.

Light, M. E., Sparg, S. G., Stafford, G. I., van Staden, J., 2005. Riding the wave: South Africa's contribution to ethnopharmacological research over the last 25 years. Journal of Ethnopharmacology 100: 127-130

Louw, C. A. M., Reigner, T. J. C., Korsten, L., 2002. Medicinal bulbous plants of South Africa and their traditional relevance in the control of infectious diseases. Journal of Ethnopharmacology 82: 147-154

Mander, M., 1999. Marketing of indigenous Medicinal Plants in South Africa: A case study in KwaZulu-Natal. Food and Agriculture Organisation of the United Nations, Forest Product Division. 1-2

Nair, M. D., 2005. Traditional medicines and medicinal plants, and their protection modalities from an intellectual property rights perspective. Plant Genetic Resource 3 (2): 314-319

Phillipson, J. D., 2001. Phytochemistry and medicinal plants. Phytochemistry 56: 237-243

Tanaka, H., Okada, T., 1991. Effect of Panax ginseng on the production of glycosaminoglycans in cultured human skin fibroblast. Frag Journal 19: 90–91.

Yesilada, E., 2005. Past and the future contributions to traditional medicine in the health care system of the Middle-East. Journal of Ethnopharmacology 100: 135-137
Van Wyk, B.-E., Van Oudtshoorn, B., Gericke, N., 1997. *Medicinal* Plants of South Africa (first ed.), Eriza, Pretoria, South Africa.

# Part 3

## Pathway

# 12

# Genomics of Human Malignant Melanoma

Margit Balázs, Szilvia Ecsedi, Laura Vízkeleti and Ágnes Bégány
*University of Debrecen Department of Preventive Medicine,*
*Hungarian Academy of Sciences University of Debrecen*
*Public Health Research Group*
*University of Debrecen Department of Dermatology*
*Hungary*

## 1. Introduction

Malignant melanoma is considered the most aggressive form of skin cancer. The incidence rate of the disease has steadily risen over the past few decades throughout the world. If melanoma is diagnosed early, it can be cured by surgical resection, but as soon as the first distant metastasis appears, the disease becomes one of the most aggressive types of metastatic, chemoresistant lesions. Cutaneous melanocytes originate from highly motile neural crest progenitors that migrate to the skin during embryonic development. They are pigment-producing skin cells that reside between keratinocytes in the basal layer of the epidermis, producing melanin in response to a variety of external stimuli, such as ultraviolet (UV) radiation. Although UV radiation is the main exogenous etiological risk factor for the development of the disease, other presently unknown factors are also involved. As estimated by the World Health Organization worldwide number of newly diagnosed skin cancer cases is between 2 and 3 million each year, of which 132,000 are melanoma. Additionally, in most western countries, the incidence of melanoma doubles roughly every decade.

Malignant melanoma progresses through a series of well-defined clinical and histopathological stages, advancing in a stepwise manner from either a common acquired or a dysplastic nevus through the primary radial growth phase (RGP) and the vertical growth phase (VGP) to distant metastasis [Welch et al., 1997]. Different subtypes of the disease represent diverse entities, as there are marked differences in their biological behaviours. While the most common superficial spreading subtype (SSM) is characterised by a prolonged RGP, nodular melanoma (NM) begins to grow vertically from its onset. Clinical staging of primary cutaneous melanoma is based on measurements of tumour thickness (in millimetres), the presence or absence of ulceration, penetration through cutaneous layers, mitotic rate and evidence of lymph node, cutaneous or distant metastasis [Chin et al., 2006]. The vertical progression of lesions is representative of the degree of tumour progression and is measured by the Breslow thickness, which was first used in the early 1970s and measures the thickness of the tumour from the top of the epidermal granular layer (or from the ulcer base if the tumour is ulcerated) to the innermost depth of invasion. Ulceration of the tumour surface of melanoma covering the epidermis is one of the most sensitive parameters of metastatic potential. The currently used diagnostic and prognostic approaches to recognise the disease at an early stage are based on morphological observations supplemented by sentinel lymph node biopsy, which can define the prognosis of melanoma and assist in choosing the optimal surgical treatment. However, despite the extensive research approaches that have been employed to study this disease, current prognostic biological markers, either alone or in combination, are not adequate for accurately performing individualised assessment of the predicted risk of melanoma progression and are often not helpful in defining the most effective therapy [Chin et al., 2006]. Similar to other solid tumours, it is assumed that the morphologic heterogeneity of melanoma originates from distinct genetic alterations that lead to diverse pathways of melanoma development and progression. To design effective therapeutic approaches, it is of critical importance to identify the genetic determinants of disease initiation and progression. Additionally, it is crucial to define the functionally important genetic/genomic alterations that result in melanoma initiation and progression [Ghosh & Chin, 2009]. Advances in genetic and genomic methodologies during the past decade have exponentially increased our understanding of the molecular genetic alterations associated with this disease.

## 2. Molecular pathways involved in melanoma initiation and progression

The genomic heterogeneity of melanoma and the complexity of the molecular pathways involved in disease development and progression suggest that no individual genetic or molecular alteration is crucial in these processes per se. The accumulation of and interactions between such alterations in combination with the interactions between the tumour cells and the microenvironment are involved in the generation of a specific set of biological outcomes [Palmieri et al., 2009].

Current knowledge about the main molecular pathways at the DNA level and their interactions during melanomagenesis are summarised below. However, many other drivers of melanomagenesis remain to be discovered.

### 2.1 Main genes involved in melanomagenesis and related signalling pathways

#### 2.1.1 CDKN2A and CDK4 in familial melanoma

In addition to recognised heritable traits, such as skin, hair and eye colour, and the presence of a large number of nevi (benign, atypical or giant congenital), a familial history of melanoma (at least 3 affected relatives) is a significant risk factor for disease development [Chin et al., 2006; Sekulic et al., 2008]. Approximately 10% of individuals diagnosed with melanoma have a familial predisposition associated with a 2.24-fold increase in the risk of tumour development [Igbokwe & Lopez-Terrada, 2011]. Single-base mutations and deletions of the *CDKN2A* (cyclin-dependent kinase inhibitor 2A) gene at the 9p21 locus have been found to be the major germline alterations involved in these tumours, contributing to 10% to 40% of familial melanoma cases. The penetrance of *CDKN2A* mutations appears to be influenced by geographical location [Meyle & Guldberg, 2009]. Other melanoma-prone families harbour mutations in different genes, including germline mutations in *CDK4* (cyclin-dependent kinase 4) or unidentified genes on chromosomes 1p22 and 20q11.22 [Meyle & Guldberg, 2009; Sekulic et al., 2008].

*CDKN2A* encodes 2 overlapping, but distinct tumour-suppressor proteins, $p16^{INK4a}$ and $p14^{ARF}$, utilising alternative promoters and first exons (1$\alpha$ for INK4a and 1$\beta$ for ARF) [Chin et al., 2006]. As most pathogenic mutations occur in exon 2 of these genes, they are often simultaneously altered in multiple tumours [Palmieri et al., 2009].

**p16$^{INK4a}$-CDK4/6-RB pathway**

RB1 (retinoblastoma 1) is an essential gatekeeper at the G1/S transition point of the cell cycle. In its underphosphorylated form, RB1 binds to the E2F transcription factor, preventing induction of the expression of genes crucial for the G1/S transition. However, when RB1 is phosphorylated by the activation of the CCND1 (cyclin D1) - CDK4/6 complex, E2F is released, leading the cell cycle to progress through the G1/S transition [Sekulic et al., 2008]. The key regulatory molecule involved in this mechanism is p16$^{INK4a}$, which inhibits the activity of CDK4/6 kinases in a dose-dependent manner and consequently causes cell cycle arrest [Chin et al., 2006]. Recently, it has been shown that p16$^{INK4a}$ functions as an alternate RB-independent regulator and suppressor of UV-induced DNA damage by reactive oxygen species and reduces the effect of oxidative stress in melanocytes via the p38 stress-activated protein kinase [Jenkins et al., 2011].

Frequent point mutations in the coding region of the *CDKN2A* locus typically target and inactivate p16$^{INK4a}$, while preserve p14$^{ARF}$ in 25% to 40% of melanoma-prone families and 0.2% to 2% of sporadic melanomas [Chin et al., 2006; Meyle & Guldberg, 2009]. Additionally, *CDKN2A* appears to be homozygously deleted in approximately 50% of melanomas or silenced by promoter hypermethylation in 20% to 75% of tumours [Moore et al., 2008; Sekulic et al., 2008].

Other members of the pathway rarely harbour mutations. Germline mutations in **CDK4**, an RB kinase inhibited by INK4a, have been only found in 15 melanoma-prone families [Meyle & Guldberg, 2009]. Most of these rare mutations target a conserved arginine residue at position 24 and substitute it with cysteine (R24C). Therefore, the mutant protein lacks the ability to bind to INK4a, but the CDK4-CCND1 interaction is preserved, resulting in the constitutive activation of this complex [Chin et al., 2006; Sekulic et al., 2008]. It is important to note that inactivating *p16$^{INK4a}$* mutations and activating *CDK4$^{R24C}$* mutations are not observed simultaneously, which suggests that they are mutually exclusive [Chin et al., 2006; Sekulic et al., 2008]. Alterations of *CDK4* are also observed in sporadic melanomas (more commonly in the acral and mucosal types) in the form of focal gene amplification without *p16$^{INK4a}$* deletion [Sekulic et al., 2008]. Other molecular alterations that are sometimes observed are **CDK6** overexpression, rare mutations in **CCND1** (approximately 4% of tumours) and inactivating mutations in **RB1** in approximately 6% of sporadic melanomas, but germline mutation in **RB1** is also observed, with an increased risk of tumour development [Sekulic et al., 2008].

**p14$^{ARF}$-MDM2-p53 pathway**

Inactivation of the p53 pathway is a common trait of cancers. The p53 protein is often referred to as the guardian of the genome because as a transcription factor, it regulates several genes involved in cell cycle arrest, senescence, DNA repair and apoptosis [Sekulic et al., 2008]. This broad set of functions entails precise control of the intracellular protein level by a complex network of positive and negative regulators. The main negative regulator is the MDM2 protein, which by binding to p53, promotes its ubiquitination and consequent proteosomal degradation. MDM2 is inhibited by p14$^{ARF}$, which leads to the stabilisation of p53 [Sekulic et al., 2008]. Following DNA damage, p53 activates p21$^{WAF1/CIP1}$, which blocks the CCNDE-CDK2 complex, causing cell cycle arrest at the G1/S transition point through the decreased phosphorylation of RB1, thus allowing DNA repair or apoptosis to occur [Sekulic et al., 2008].

*p53* is one of the most commonly mutated genes in human cancers. However, in contrast to most solid tumours, in which the pathway is inactivated at the level of p53 itself, point mutations in this gene are very rare in melanoma (occurring in approximately 9% of cases) and appear to rely on the inactivation of *CDKN2A* [Chin et al., 2006]. Although most mutations affect $p16^{INK4a}$ with or without $p14^{ARF}$ alterations, some melanoma-prone families exhibit mutations in $p14^{ARF}$ alone, which suggests that the loss of this gene itself could be sufficient for melanoma formation, and both $p16^{INK4a}$ and $p14^{ARF}$ are essential for melanoma suppression [Meyle & Guldberg, 2009; Sekulic et al., 2008]. Some data suggest that the tumour suppressor function of $\mathrm{p14^{ARF}}$ might be fulfilled by other, unidentified p53-independent mechanisms, which could also have important clinical implications [Sekulic et al., 2008].

### 2.1.2 Receptor tyrosine kinases (RTKs)

RTKs are important targets of molecular alterations in various cancers. Although most of these changes occur at the expression level, several RTKs localise to regions affected by DNA copy number gains or amplifications [Chin et al., 2006]. In malignant melanoma, the most frequently altered RTKs are EGFR (epidermal growth factor receptor), c-MET (the oncogenic form of the hepatocyte growth factor receptor) and c-KIT (stem cell factor receptor) [Ghosh & Chin, 2009].

**EGFR** (7p12) can be activated by EGF family ligands, such as EGF, TGF-α, amphiregulin or heparin-binding EGF [Ghosh & Chin, 2009]. Amplification, usually via copy number gains of the entire chromosome 7, and overexpression of EGFR have been frequently observed in late-stage melanomas and in association with the nodular subtype, which suggests that EGFR may support metastatic potential [Chin et al., 2006; Ghosh & Chin, 2009; Rother & Jones, 2009; Timar et al., 2010]. However, no focal *EGFR* amplification or mutation has been reported in melanoma [Chin et al., 2006; Ghosh & Chin, 2009]. Additionally, the EGFR signalling loop plays an important role in the RAS-driven tumourigenecity of melanoma cells. Animal models have suggested that autocrine EGFR signalling is essential for RAS-mediated transformation by promoting survival through PI3K activation of AKT [Chin et al., 2006; Ghosh & Chin, 2009].

The **c-MET** receptor (7q31) is normally expressed on epithelial cells and melanocytes and is activated by its ligand, HGF (hepatocyte growth factor). Similar to EGFR, c-MET overexpression and copy number gains of the locus are late-stage events in tumour progression that contribute to the metastatic character of skin melanomas, but no focal gene amplification and/or activating mutations have been demonstrated [Chin et al., 2006; Ghosh & Chin, 2009; Timar et al., 2010]. Oncogenic c-MET activation mainly occurs in an autocrine manner with the establishment of a HGF-MET autocrine loop, which drives the development of metastatic disease rather than the initial steps of melanomagenesis [Chin et al., 2006; Ghosh & Chin, 2009]. Finally, it was recently shown that c-MET can be a direct target of microphthalmia-associated transcription factor (MITF), which can be itself amplified in a subset of melanomas [Chin et al., 2006; Ghosh & Chin, 2009].

The **c-KIT** gene (4q12) encodes an RTK that binds stem cell factor (SCF). Interestingly, c-KIT does not represent a typical RTK in malignant melanoma, as a progressive loss of its expression can frequently be observed during tumour progression. Furthermore, c-KIT-expressing metastatic melanomas exhibit increased sensitivity to SCF-mediated apoptosis [Chin et al., 2006; Ghosh & Chin, 2009]. It has recently been reported that in some melanomas, *c-KIT* harbours a known GIST-associated point mutation, L576P, which maps to the 5′ juxtamembrane domain, where most activating *c-KIT* mutations cluster [Chin et al., 2006; Ghosh & Chin, 2009]. A recent analysis showed that approximately 21% of mucosal, 11% of acral and 28% of melanoma developing on chronic sun-damaged skin exhibited an alteration in *c-KIT*. This suggests that the mutational and amplification status of *c-KIT*, which is usually mutually exclusive with *BRAF* and *NRAS* status, might have a significant clinical impact and may identify a patient subpopulation that would benefit from imatinib (c-KIT inhibitor) therapy [Ghosh & Chin, 2009; Igbokwe & Lopez-Terrada, 2011; Rother & Jones, 2009; Ko & Fisher, 2011].

### 2.1.3 Main pathways involved in melanoma: RAS/MAPK and PI3K signalling

Two major signalling cascades exist in melanoma: the RAS/MAP kinase pathway, which is mainly responsible for cellular proliferation, and the PI3 kinase pathway, which plays an important role in tumour cell survival. However, these regulatory functions are not exclusive, as interactions between the members of the two cascades enhance tumourigenesis, cell growth, chemoresistance, invasion, migration and cell cycle dysregulation [Sekulic et al., 2008].

#### 2.1.3.1 RAS/MAPK pathway

The RAS/MAPK signalling cascade is carried out through various RTKs, including FGFR, c-KIT, c-MET or EGFR, and is strongly affected during tumourigenesis and progression. A receptor-ligand interaction initiates the phosphorylation cascade through RAS-RAF-MEK-MAPK kinases and finally activates enzymes (involved in metabolic regulation), cytoskeletal components (affecting cell shape and migration) and specific transcription factors, such as ETS1/2, that are essential for the initiation of the expression of target genes related to cell proliferation and survival [Chin et al., 2006; Sekulic et al., 2008]. Hyperphosphorylated ERKs are common features of human cancers, including melanoma (approximately 90% of cases). This enforced activation is usually achieved through activating mutations related to upstream mediators, such as *RAF* and *RAS* [Chin et al., 2006; Igbokwe & Lopez-Terrada, 2011; Palmieri et al., 2009].

Activating mutations in the **RAS** proto-oncogene family (*HRAS*, *NRAS* and *KRAS*) are detected in melanoma with an incidence of between 10% and 15%. Point mutations in **NRAS** (Q61L) are the most common type of these mutations and are found in 56% of congenital nevi (but are rare in dysplastic and benign acquired nevi), as well as 33% of primary and 26% of metastatic melanomas correlated with a nodular subtype and intermittent sun exposure [Chin et al., 2006; Ghosh & Chin, 2009; Rother & Jones, 2009; Sekulic et al., 2008]. **HRAS** point mutations, together with genomic 11p amplifications, are rarely associated with melanomas. However, they are more frequent in Spitz nevi and indicate benign behaviour, whereas *KRAS* activations have not been observed in melanocytic lesions [Blokx et al., 2010; Chin et al., 2006; Ghosh & Chin, 2009]. Mouse models have revealed that RAS family members have distinct roles in melanocyte biology: *HRAS* mutations in combination with the inactivation of $p16^{INK4a}$, $p14^{ARF}$ and/or *p53* promote the development of nonmetastatic melanoma, whereas *NRAS* activations together with $p16^{INK4a}$ and $p14^{ARF}$ deficiencies cause cutaneous melanoma with a high penetrance and short latency [Chin et al., 2006; Ghosh & Chin, 2009].

The **RAF** proto-oncogene family consists of *ARAF*, *BRAF* and *CRAF*. Activating mutations in **BRAF** are the most widespread genetic alterations observed in human melanoma, with up to a 70% incidence, and they are associated with intermittent sun exposure and influence the pattern of metastasis. In contrast, mutations in *ARAF* and *CRAF* have not been observed in human melanomas [Chin et al., 2006; Ghosh & Chin, 2009; Ko & Fisher, 2011; Meyle & Guldberg, 2009; Palmieri et al., 2009; Sekulic et al., 2008; Viros et al., 2008]. Among these point mutations, the most common is V600E (a valine to glutamic acid substitution), which accounts for >90% of all *BRAF* mutations [Meyle & Guldberg, 2009]. The *BRAF*$^{V600E}$ mutation is induced by UV damage, but its specific relationship with UV exposure has not yet been identified. It has recently been suggested that because *MC1R* variants are strongly associated with *BRAF* activation, they may modify the connection between *BRAF* mutation, nevus burden and melanoma risk, indicating that activating mutations for *BRAF* are somehow indirectly induced by UV radiation [Ko & Fisher, 2011; Palmieri et al., 2009]. *BRAF* mutations are common in nodular and superficial spreading melanomas arising in skin in association with intermittent sun exposure (59%), in contrast to the lentigo maligna melanomas that occur in chronically sun-exposed areas (11%) and acral (23%) and mucosal (11%) melanomas, and they are absent in uveal melanomas [Chin et al., 2006; Ghosh & Chin, 2009; Rother & Jones, 2009]. Activating mutations are also seen in benign and dysplastic nevi, which often remain growth-arrested throughout an individual's life time and rarely progress into melanoma, suggesting a role in the early neoplastic stages of melanoma and that there may be a *BRAF*$^{V600E}$-induced checkpoint for malignant transformation [Chin et al., 2006; Ghosh & Chin, 2009]. Congenital nevi are often positive for the senescence marker SA-β-Gal and for p16$^{INK4a}$. In vitro studies have shown that in normal cells, BRAF$^{V600E}$ can induce p16$^{INK4a}$, SA-β-Gal and cell cycle arrest, resulting in oncogene-induced senescence [Chin et al., 2006; Ghosh & Chin, 2009; Palmieri et al., 2009]. However, p16$^{INK4a}$ positivity is not 100% correlated with SA-β-Gal positivity, suggesting the presence of other factors involved in cell senescence, such as those regulated by IGFBP7 (IGF-binding protein 7). Benign nevi contain both BRAF$^{V600E}$ and high levels of IGFBP7, while BRAF$^{V600E}$ melanomas do not [Ghosh & Chin, 2009]. Additionally, BRAF can also cooperate with the p14$^{ARF}$-MDM2-p53 pathway because in p53-deficient zebrafish, mutant BRAF can induce invasive melanoma [Ko & Fisher, 2011; Palmieri et al., 2009].

*BRAF* and *NRAS* mutations are mutually exclusive at the single-cell level in melanoma, but they can be found in the same tumour with different segregation into neoplastic cells, potentially resulting in distinct biological properties and heterogeneous responses to therapy [Palmieri et al., 2007]. These alterations are also found in benign and dysplastic nevi, indicating that their activation is an early event in melanoma and is sufficient for initiation but is not involved in progression; therefore, additional genetic alterations are necessary for malignant transformation [Conway et al., 2010; Igbokwe & Lopez-Terrada, 2011]. This exclusion may be based on the ability of melanoma cells carrying an *NRAS* mutation to bypass BRAF and signal via CRAF [Rother et al., 2009]. *BRAF* or *NRAS* mutations and concurrent genetic aberrations in *BRAF* and *PTEN* or *MC1R* are highly associated with intermittent sun exposure, whereas in acral melanomas or melanomas arising from chronic sun-exposed skin, wild-type *BRAF* and *N-RAS* can usually be found and are associated with copy number gains of *CCND1* and *CDK4*, indicating the greater importance of the p16$^{INK4a}$-RB cascade in these melanocytic lesions [Palmieri et al., 2007]. Finally, *RAF-RAS* mutations, possibly in association with mutant *c-KIT* and p16$^{INK4a}$ alterations, might be useful in distinguishing secondary new and metastatic melanomas, which could have considerable prognostic and clinical significance, as these melanomas are prone to systemic spread and are often incurable [Blokx et al., 2010].

#### 2.1.3.2 PI3K/AKT pathway

The PI3 kinase signalling cascade is activated by a number of extracellular signals in both paracrine and autocrine manners, such as signals from integrins, extracellular matrix proteins, HGF and insulin-like growth factors. This pathway is often hyperactive in melanoma and antagonises the intrinsic apoptotic pathway [Chin et al., 2006; Ghosh & Chin, 2009; Sekulic et al., 2008]. Genetic alterations targeting members of the PI3K pathway are not as frequent as in the case of the RAS/MAPK pathway. PI3 kinase mutation occurs at a low frequency in melanoma (5%) [Palmieri et al., 2009]. The major genetic alteration observed is the deletion of **PTEN** (phosphatase and tensin homologue) at the 10q23 locus, which encodes a lipid and protein phosphatase. Loss of a *PTEN* allele or a change in its expression have been observed in approximately 20% and 40% of lesions, respectively; however, homozygous deletion and point mutations are rare in melanomas [Chin et al., 2006; Ghosh & Chin, 2009; Igbokwe & Lopez-Terrada, 2011; Timar et al., 2010]. As a negative regulator of the PI3 kinase pathway, PTEN reduces the intracellular level of $PIP_3$ induced by PI3K and consequently blocks AKT activation and phosphorylation of the mTOR transcription factor, which promotes the expression of target genes involved in cellular division, cell migration and survival. Loss of *PTEN* may represent an essential aberration in the formation of invasive melanomas [Ko & Fisher, 2011].

Another important member of the PI3 kinase pathway is **AKT**, which exists in three isoforms: AKT1, AKT2 and AKT3. Although the complexity of this signalling pathway is not fully understood, it appears that the activation of different AKT isoforms may play distinct roles in tumour cell proliferation and survival and is associated with *in situ* melanomas and lesions arising from sun-exposed skin [Chin et al., 2006; Ghosh & Chin, 2009; Rother & Jones, 2009]. Following $PIP_3$ formation, AKT becomes phosphorylated by PDK1 (pyruvate dehydrogenase kinase isozyme 1, mitochondrial) and consequently inactivates proapoptotic proteins, such as BAD, and activates the NFκB and FOXO1 transcription factors, which promote the expression of genes involved in survival [Sekulic et al., 2008]. Constitutive activation of **AKT3** through DNA copy number gains may be present in 40% to 60% of sporadic melanomas and stimulates a vertical growth phenotype, survival, migration, angiogenesis, glycolytic metabolism and cell cycle progression through the upregulation of CCND1 [Ghosh & Chin, 2009; Ko & Fisher, 2011; Palmieri et al., 2009; Sekulic et al., 2008]. However, it has been shown that **AKT1** activation inhibits tumour cell migration and the invasion of particular cell lines, including melanomas [Chin et al., 2006; Ghosh & Chin, 2009].

PTEN can also regulate RAS/MAPK signalling and promotes cell cycle arrest at the G1/S transition point through the upregulation of $p27^{KIP1}$. Moreover, activating mutant RAS can phosphorylate PI3K, resulting in increased AKT activity. Therefore, *PTEN* loss and the presence of oncogenic *RAS* are redundant [Rother & Jones, 2009; Sekulic et al., 2008].

### 2.1.4 Other important pathways in melanoma: WNT and MSH signalling

#### 2.1.4.1 WNT pathway

WNT (wingless-type MMTV integration site family) signalling has significant developmental functions, especially in neural crest cells, such as melanocytes [Chin et al., 2006; Sekulic et al., 2008]. Activation of the canonical WNT pathway inactivates GSK3β (glycogen synthase kinase 3 beta), which normally promotes the proteosomal degradation of β-catenin via phosphorylation and results in an increased level of β-catenin that enhances the expression of target genes, such as *MITF* and *CCND1*, through activation of the TCF-LEF transcriptional complex [Chin et al., 2006; Sekulic et al., 2008]. Despite the frequent stabilising β-catenin mutations that occur in melanoma cell lines, the incidence of these genetic alterations is much lower in primary melanoma samples. However, immunohistochemical studies have provided evidence of nuclear accumulation of β-catenin, which reflects the activation of the canonical WNT pathway and the contribution of MITF as an important upstream regulator of melanoma survival/proliferation [Chin et al., 2006]. Overexpression of **WNT5a** is often observed in melanomas; nevertheless, its function is associated with protein kinase C activation rather than β-catenin [Chin et al., 2006; Timar et al., 2010]. Furthermore, upregulation of **WNT2** has also been found in melanomas, contributing to the inhibition of normal apoptotic progress, and determination of its protein level can be useful in distinguishing between melanoma and nevi [Palmieri et al., 2009].

#### 2.1.4.2 MSH pathway

MSH signalling is a key regulator of pigmentation through binding to its specific receptor, MC1R (melanocortin 1 receptor). **MC1R,** which is highly polymorphic, is expressed on epidermal melanocytes and determines the UV-induced skin response through modulating the induction efficiency of intracellular cAMP production [Chin et al., 2006; Meyle & Guldberg, 2009; Sekulic et al., 2008]. People with a red-hair-colour phenotype are unable to tan and exhibit more freckles; therefore, they display a 2.7 to 16.0-fold increase in risk of developing melanoma [Sekulic et al., 2008]. Some investigators have suggested that certain *MC1R* alleles have a pigment-independent effect on melanomagenesis [Chin et al., 2006; Meyle & Guldberg, 2009]. MSH-MC1R binding activates the canonical PKA (protein kinase A) response by inducing adenylate cyclase to produce cAMP, phosphorylates Rsk and/or PKA, which finally stimulate the CREB/ATF1 transcription factors. This complex both induces the expression of specific genes involved in pigmentation through direct regulation and activates the *MITF* promoter, which defines the tissue-specific expression of genes involved in pigmentation. The expression level of *MITF* affects the resulting phenotype; a low level defines pheomelanin, red-blond pigments, whereas a high level defines eumelanin, brown-black pigments [Chin et al., 2006]. In addition to PKA phosphorylation, activation of the RAS/MAPK pathway and inactivation of the PI3K pathway also appear to be consequences of cAMP stimulation. The general nature of cAMP and CREB/ATF1 activation, compared to the highly tissue restricted nature of MITF activation, suggests the presence of a cooperating site that maps to the Sox10 consensus element in the *MITF* promoter [Chin et al., 2006].

### 2.1.5 Novel pathways in melanoma: Notch1 and iNOS signalling

#### 2.1.5.1 Notch1 pathway

The Notch signalling pathway plays key roles in tissue homeostasis and the regulation of cell fate [Bedogni & Powell, 2009]. Depending on cell-cell interactions and the extracellular environment, Notch can act as either a tumour suppressor or an oncogene [Palmieri et al., 2009]. Upon activation, the Notch receptor undergoes two consecutive enzymatic cleavages, which result in the formation of $N^{ICD}$, a truncated variant of the receptor. $N^{ICD}$ translocates to the nucleus and forms a complex with the CBF1 transcription factor and other co-activators, which influences the intensity and duration of Notch signals and consequently induces transcription from promoters containing CBF1-responsive elements [Bedogni &

Powell, 2009; Palmieri et al., 2009]. Normally, Notch1 signalling induces growth arrest and differentiation in keratinocytes via $p21^{WAF1/CIP1}$ induction and blocking WNT signalling. In melanomas and atypical nevi, Notch1 and 2 and their ligands are significantly upregulated. Notch1 exerts its effects through interactions with several pathways [Bedogni & Powell, 2009; Palmieri et al., 2009]. Binding to β-catenin mediates oncogenic activity either via the WNT pathway or by regulating N-cadherin. Notch1 also exhibits cross-talk with and inhibits the MAPK and PI3K pathways, contributing to the vertical growth phase. Furthermore, direct interactions between $N^{ICD}$ and NFκB cause the nuclear retention of NFκB transcription factor and enhance melanoma cell survival (late Notch-dependent activation). $N^{ICD}$ can also directly regulate IFNγ expression by creating a complex with both NFκB and IFNγ promoters. Finally, RAS-mediated malignant transformation also requires intact Notch signalling [Palmieri et al., 2009]. Taken together, these data suggest that *Notch* may represent a novel target involved in melanomagenesis.

#### 2.1.5.2 iNOS pathway

NO (nitric oxide) free radical production by NOS (nitric oxide synthase) plays an important role in immune responses. Three isoforms can be distinguished: nNOS/NOS I (neuronal) and eNOS/NOS III (endothelial) are constitutively expressed, and iNOS/NOS II (inducible) is transcriptionally regulated by several mediators [Palmieri et al., 2009]. In normal melanocytes, free radicals are completely inactivated via the redox function of eumelanin. Both reactive oxygen species (ROS) and reactive nitrogen species (RNS) have been identified in melanoma [Jenkins et al., 2011]. The effect of NO in tumour progression is dose dependent; a high NO concentration can lead to apoptosis via its effect on multiple apoptosis-related proteins, such as p53 and Bcl-2, and growth inhibition, whereas a low NO concentration may contribute to tumour growth and angiogenesis [Palmieri et al., 2009]. However, the role of **iNOS** in melanoma progression is still controversial. A higher level of iNOS has been found in subcutaneous and lymph node metastases of nonprogressive melanomas compared to that in progressive tumours, but the degree of iNOS expression is lower in metastases than in nevi or primary melanomas [Palmieri et al., 2009]. Finally, **nNOS** may also have an impact on melanomagenesis because approximately 82% of primary tumours, 72% of atypical nevi and 49% of benign nevi have been reported to express this protein, whereas normal melanocytes do not exhibit nNOS expression. Therefore, *de novo* expression of nNOS may be a marker for early stage tumours [Palmieri et al., 2009].

Currently, the most effective therapy against melanoma is surgical resection of primary tumours, followed by observation of a sentinel lymph node [Gerami et al., 2009]. The cytogenetic heterogeneity of human melanomas results in significant problems in the classification of histologically ambiguous primary tumours and in differentiation between melanomas and other lesions, such as Spitz nevi, blue nevi or proliferating congenital nevi [Braun-Falco et al., 2009; Scolyer et al., 2010]. Understanding these alterations (Figure 1) and evaluating all of the known molecular targets in melanoma through the application of new molecular biological techniques, such as FISH, PCR, sequencing and microarrays, in addition to the gold standard of histopathologic examination, will be crucial in predicting subsets of patients with particular biological and clinical characteristics who may respond favourably to a therapy that specifically targets a characteristic molecular signature [Gerami et al., 2009; Ghosh & Chin, 2009; Palmieri et al., 2007].

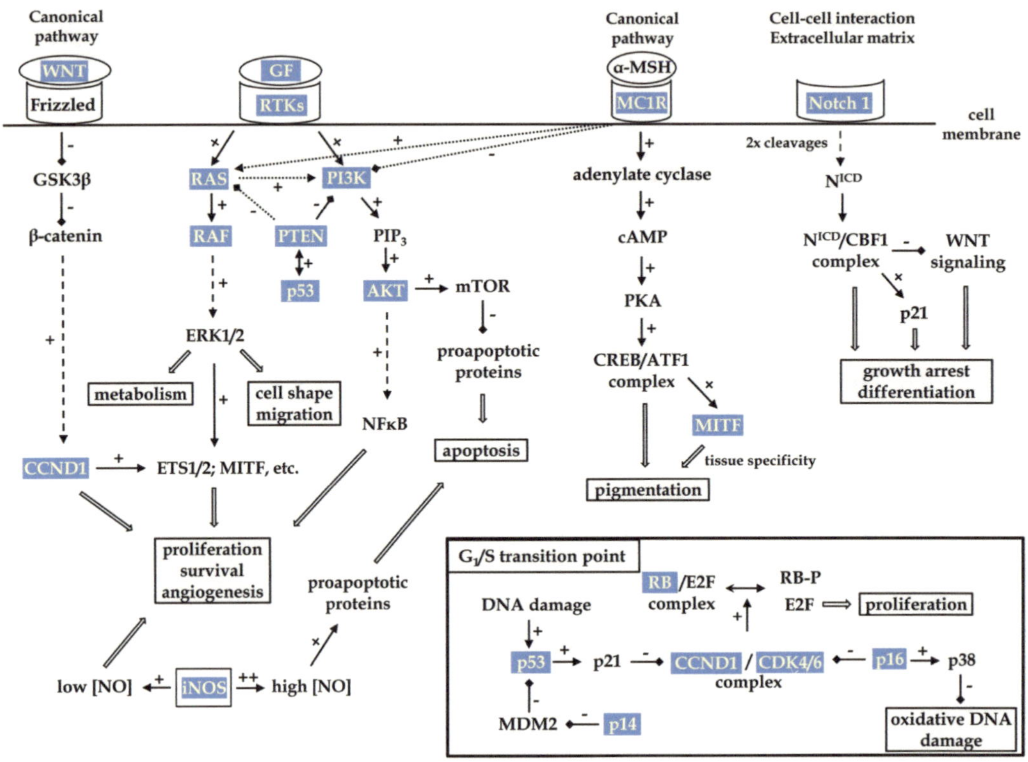


Fig. 1. Schematic representation of the signalling pathways affected in melanoma progression. Members showed (epi)genetic and/or expressional alterations are highlighted with blue

## 3. Genetic alterations in malignant melanoma

Molecular biological techniques developed during the last two decades have greatly improved our understanding of the genetic background of malignant melanoma. A number of studies using classical chromosome banding, fluorescence *in situ* hybridisation (FISH) and chromosomal and array comparative genomic hybridisation (CGH) have been performed to define the genetic alterations that underlie the development and progression of melanoma [Trent et al., 1991; Bastian et al., 1998; Chin et al., 2006]. These studies have identified a large number of non-random alterations on chromosomes 1p, 6, 7, 8q, 9, 10q, 11q and 17, the frequencies of which are reflective of the malignant potential of the sporadic form of the disease. As a result of detailed analysis, a number of tumour suppressors and oncogenes have been implicated as key factors in melanoma pathogenesis, including *CDKN2A*, *PTEN*, *BRAF*, *NRAS*, *MITF*, *AIM1*, *CCND1*, and *MYC* [Poetch et al., 2003; Casarso et al., 2005; Rákosy et al., 2008; Lázár et al., 2009; Dalton et al. 2010].

### 3.1 Non-random copy number alterations

Comparative genomic hybridisation represents the best approach for searching for DNA sequence copy number alterations in cancer genomes. Improvement of the resolution and sensitivity of CGH during the last decade has allowed the discovery of recurrent copy number alterations and new genetic targets in different cancer types, including malignant melanoma. Although chromosomal and array CGH have revealed a large number of common non-random alterations (DNA sequence amplifications and deletions, Figure 2), no obvious or validated melanoma-relevant molecular targets have yet been identified [Gosh & Chin, 2009]. The non-random nature of melanoma-specific copy number alterations may allow the segregation of melanomas into subtypes based on distinct clinical and biological behaviours. The array CGH investigation of primary melanoma producing the greatest number of findings was reported by Curtin et al. [Curtin et al., 2005]. At the beginning of this study, it was hypothesised that the clinical heterogeneity of the disease could be explained by genetically distinct types of melanomas with different susceptibilities to ultraviolet light.

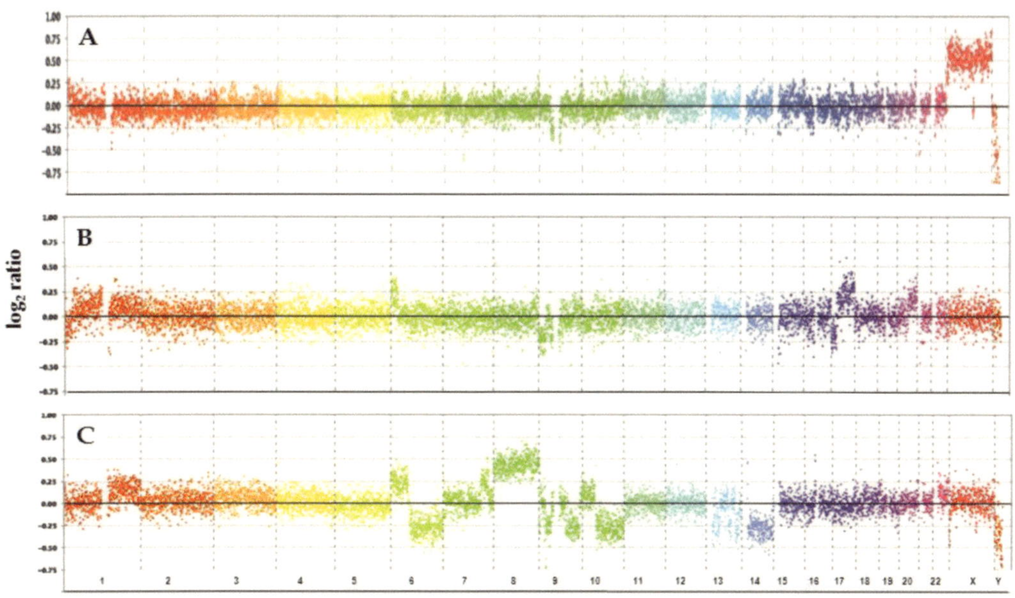


Fig. 2. Array CGH profiles of malignant melanoma. A.) Control sample without copy number alteration. B.) Array CGH profile of a primary malignant melanoma sample. C.) melanoma metastasis

Chromosome copy number alterations and the mutational status of the *BRAF* and *NRAS* genes were compared in 126 primary melanomas, and melanoma tissue samples were grouped based on their degree of exposure to ultraviolet light. The four types of melanoma included in these groupings were as follows: acral melanoma (melanoma occurring on the non-hair-bearing skin of the palms or soles), mucosal melanoma (tumours arising on mucosal membranes), tumours arising from skin with chronic sun-induced damage and lesions arising from skin without chronic sun-induced damage. Melanomas without chronic sun-induced damage frequently showed mutations in the *BRAF* oncogene, together with losses of chromosome 10q (site of *PTEN*), or mutations in the *NRAS* gene alone. In contrast, melanomas arising from skin with chronic sun-induced damage (mucosal and acral melanomas) did not exhibit *BRAF* or *NRAS* mutations but instead displayed an increased number of copies of the *CCND1* or *CDK4* genes. The different genetic alterations were identified in different anatomical sites of the skin and with varying levels of ultraviolet exposure indicate that distinct molecular pathways are involved in the development and progression of the disease [Curtin et al., 2005].

### 3.1.1 Genetic differences between benign and malignant melanocytic lesions

The cytogenetic heterogeneity of the different subtypes of benign and malignant skin lesions were recently summarised by Blokx et al. [2010]. Some of the important DNA copy number alterations that distinguish melanomas from nevi can be successfully detected by interphase FISH [Bauer & Bastian, 2006; Gerami et al., 2010]. Based on previous array CGH observations, four DNA regions were selected, targeting 3 loci on chromosome 6 (*MYB1*: 6q23, *RREB1*: 6p25 and centromere 6) and *CCND1* on chromosome 11q13 as being the most powerful discriminators between melanomas and nevi that can assist in the diagnostic classification of melanocytic tumours that cannot be consistently classified by other currently available methods. The sensitivity of the four DNA probes was further tested by FISH in 110 nevi and 123 melanomas, and it was found that the overall sensitivity of the tested probes was 83%, and the specificity was 94% [Gerami et al., 2010]. In another study, the same group reported that copy number changes at 11q13 (*CCND1*) and 8q34 (harbouring the *MYC* oncogene) were highly associated with prognosis and could discriminate between metastasising and no metastasising melanomas [Gerami et al., 2011].

The histopathologic subtypes of cutaneous melanomas (superficial spreading, nodular, acral lentiginous and lentigo maligna melanomas) are characterised based on the growth pattern of the radial growth phase of melanoma. Using interphase cytogenetics, several groups have showed that the different subtypes exhibit differences in chromosomal aberrations [Poetsch et al., 1998; Bastian et al., 2000; Treszl et al., 2004; Bastian et al., 2006] that may also contribute to distinct outcomes. Comparing the CGH profiles of AMs (acral melanomas) and SSMs, a significant difference was seen between the amplified loci/samples and between the two subtypes of melanomas. While all AMs exhibited at least one gene amplification, less than 15% of SSM samples showed amplification [Bastian, 2000]. The most frequently amplified region was 11q13, harbouring the *CCND1* oncogene, which probably arises early in the progression of AM. The biological relevance of the *CCND1* amplification was further investigated, and the results showed that *CCND1* amplification was strongly correlated with protein expression and indicated that *CCND1* is an oncogene involved in malignant melanoma [Bastian, 2002]. Recently, we reported that coamplification of *CCND1* with other genes (especially *TAOS1*) within the 11q13 amplicon could contribute to a more aggressive phenotype than that of *CCND1* alone [Lazar et al., 2009].

Targeting a combination of these loci using FISH may become a useful standardised prognostic test for melanoma skin cancer in the future. However, it is important to note that FISH analysis should be performed in combination with standard clinical and histopathological evaluations [Gerami et al., 2010].

### 3.1.2 New melanoma genes discovered by high-resolution array CGH

A systematic analysis of the melanoma genome led to the discovery of a new lineage survival oncogene, *MITF* (3p14), which is amplified or shows copy number gains in 10% of primary and 15% to 20% of metastatic melanomas [Garraway et al., 2005]. Based on FISH analysis, the *MITF* copy number fluctuates between 4 and 13 copies per cell. However, no amplification can be detected in nevi samples. Comparing *MITF* copy number alterations and clinical parameters, it was found that patients presenting tissue carrying the amplified gene exhibited survival of less than five years. A similar correlation was seen for MITF protein expression, which implicates *MITF* gene amplification in the progression and lethality of a subset of melanomas. It was clearly demonstrated that MITF plays a crucial role in melanocyte biology and melanoma progression [Hoek et al., 2008] and potentially acts as a dominant oncogene. *MITF* regulates the expression of a large variety of genes, including genes involved in pigmentation, cell cycle regulation, differentiation, survival and migration. In addition to amplification, altered *MITF* function during melanomagenesis can be achieved by single-base substitutions or by mutation of its regulator, SOX10 [Cronin et al., 2009]. Targeting MITF in combination with BRAF or cyclin-dependent kinase inhibitors may offer a rational therapeutic opportunity to successfully treat this aggressive, chemoresistant disease.

The discovery of new targets by array CGH was also reported by Gast et al. [2010]. In this study, SNP arrays with 250,000 targets were applied to 60 cell lines derived from metastasised melanomas. Amplifications were found to be more common than deletions in these cell lines. Similar to the findings of other studies, homozygous and heterozygous deletions of the *CDKN2A* gene were the most frequent type of deletion found at the 9p21 locus, and these alterations were associated with a lack of gene expression. In addition to the common alterations described above, it was observed that melanoma cell lines without *BRAF* and *NRAS* oncogenic mutations exhibited losses of the entire 13q and 16q chromosome regions. These data further confirm that distinct molecular pathways are involved in malignant melanomas, driving melanoma initiation and progression in association with either oncogenic *BRAF* or *NRAS* mutations complemented mainly by the loss of tumour suppressor genes, including *CDKN2A* and *PTEN*. Alternatively, they may implicate the amplification of *CCDN1* (11q13) and *CDK4*, together with deletions of the 13q and 16q chromosome arms, which contain two major players, the *RB1* and *MC1R* genes respectively [Gast et al., 2010]. Losses of the entire chromosome 13q region have been predominantly observed in melanoma cell lines without *BRAF* and *NRAS* oncogenic mutations. Uncovering the potential role of the deletion of the q arms of both chromosomes 13 and 16 requires further investigations in primary melanomas.

A chromosome 6p gain is one of the most frequent alterations found in melanomas, as determined by CGH and classical cytogenetic studies. A novel melanoma metastasis gene on 6p25-p24 (*NEDD9*: neural precursor cell expressed, developmentally downregulated 9) showing recurrent focal amplification in 35% of human melanomas and melanoma cell lines was discovered by a cross-species comparison [Kim et al., 2006]. The expression of *NEDD9* is significantly upregulated relative to nontransformed melanocytes and benign melanocytic neoplasia, and this gene is overexpressed in 52% of melanomas, but only 14% of nevi. It was found that *NEDD9* amplification and overexpression were strongly associated with enhanced invasion and metastasis formation related to malignant melanomas. The large regional gain on chromosome 6p and the high recurrence of the alteration likely indicate the presence and synergistic activities of multiple oncogenes on 6p, in addition to *NEDD9*. The observation that more than 50% of human primary melanomas exhibit higher NEDD9 expression relative to benign nevi suggests the possibility that the amplification or overexpression of NEDD9 in a regional/focal manner may identify a subset of primary melanoma tumours with increased risk of metastasis [Kim et al., 2006].

## 4. Gene expression profiling of melanoma

Molecular classification of cutaneous malignant melanoma by gene expression profiling was first described in 2000 [Bittner et al., 2000]. Based on the obtained gene expression data, two major clusters were identified, but no correlation was found between the cluster groups and any clinical variable associated with their tumour sets. Another group investigated the relationship between the gene expression profiles and clinical outcomes of 58 primary melanomas; 254 genes were found whose expression might have a role in predicting the clinical outcome of melanoma patients [Winnepenninckx et al., 2006]. A study was recently conducted with the major aim of identifying new prognostic markers and therapeutic targets that might aid clinical cancer diagnosis and management [Jeffs et al., 2009]. Global transcript profiling identified a signature characterised by decreased expression of developmental and lineage specification genes, including MITF, EDNRB, DCT, and TYR, and increased expression of genes involved in interactions with the extracellular environment, such as PLAUR, VCAN, and HIF1a. Migration assays showed that the gene signature was correlated with the invasive potential of the cell lines, and external validation using publicly available data indicated that tumours with the invasive gene signature were less melanocytic and might be more aggressive. It is significant that the invasion signature could be detected in both primary and metastatic tumours, suggesting that gene expression conferring increased invasive potential in melanoma may occur independently of tumour stage [Jeffs et al., 2009].

The impact of genomics on understanding human melanoma progression and metastasis was summarised by Ren et al. [2008]. Several groups have found distinct differences in gene expression patterns along the spectrum of melanoma tumour progression, with many showing distinct sets of over- and underexpressed genes that have been validated as having distinct, key roles in melanoma progression. Several research groups have attempted to develop large gene classifier sets composed of several hundreds or often thousands of genes. A critical analysis of gene expression studies relating to malignant melanoma progression was performed recently by Timár et al. [2010]. Despite the stunning success of genomics in defining genomic markers or gene signatures for breast cancer prognosis and for predicting therapies, there has been virtually no similar progress related to malignant melanoma. In summarising the microarray studies that have been performed on skin melanomas, it is noticeable that different groups used different microarray platforms in highly heterogeneous patient cohorts and pathological sample collections. Additionally, the investigated tumours may be heterogeneous even within a single study, containing sometimes limited numbers of primary melanomas or cutaneous, lymphatic or visceral metastases. Furthermore, the biological behaviour and histological appearance of the tumours were not taken into account in some studies, although some authors concluded that the gene expression signatures of superficial spreading and nodular melanomas are considerably different from each other [Jaeger et al., 2007]. Underlying the discrepancies in these data the problem is that the defined prognostic gene sets have not been validated in independent cohorts or datasets, with the exception of one study performed in primary tumours [Winnepenninckx et al., 2009].

The most recent systematic approach to characterise the spectrum of cancer-associated mRNA alterations through the integration of transcriptomic and structural genomic data has revealed new insights into melanoma biology and will likely lead to a new era of discovery in melanoma genomics that promises to reveal molecular mechanisms associated with the disease [Berger et al., 2010]. More than 700 non-synonymous coding variants have been identified. However, only a subset of these was validated to clarify whether they were bona fide somatic mutations. Based on the results described above, it is expected that most of these variants are inherited SNPs and that approximately 30% are somatic mutations. The most interesting variants include a mutation observed in the melanoma cell line 501 Mel (*CTNNB1, chr3:41241117, C/T*), which was noted 135 times in the COSMIC database of somatic mutations in cancer. A new approach, paired-end massively parallel sequencing of cDNA, together with analyses of high-resolution chromosomal copy number data was used, as a result 11 novel melanoma gene fusions were identified, that produced by underlying genomic rearrangements and 12 novel read-through transcripts. These chimeric transcripts were mapped at base-pair resolution and traced to their genomic origins using matched chromosomal copy number information. Furthermore, these data were used to discover and validate base-pair mutations that accumulated in these melanomas, revealing a surprisingly high rate of somatic mutations and lending support to the notion that point mutations constitute the major driver of melanoma progression. Taken together, these results may indicate new avenues for target gene discovery related to melanoma, while also providing a template for large-scale transcriptome studies across diseases associated with many tumour types [Berger et al., 2010].

## 5. Epigenetic events: an explanation for altered gene expression in melanoma

Over the past two decades, gene expression studies have revealed a relatively large number of genes that show altered expression at both the mRNA and protein levels. Despite some contradictory results that are probably due to the genetic variability and heterogeneity of primary melanomas, the altered expression of a group of transcripts can be affirmed to play a crucial role in the carcinogenesis and progression of melanomas. In addition to the success of mutation and copy number variation studies related to certain genes, the demonstration of gene deregulation has prompted scientists to explore other alterations that could be the cause of altered expression and that could further act as biomarkers for early diagnosis and represent a characteristic of less favourable clinical outcomes. The commonly used term "epigenetics" has been rapidly spreading over the last decade. It emerged to define heritable changes in genome function that cannot be explained by direct influence over DNA sequences. As epigenetic mechanisms affect gene expression, resulting in different phenotypes without directly altering the underlying DNA sequence, it is reasonable that they should have an impact on cancer development. Because the importance of epigenetic processes in gene regulation is currently a topic of doubt and discussion, standard nomenclature for different types of epigenetic modifications is not available in the literature, although it is reasonable to distinguish between them based on the phase during which a specific event influences gene expression (Figure 3). There are two types of such alterations that are known to occur at the transcriptional level: DNA methylation and chromatin modification (post-transcriptional covalent change and chromatin rearrangement without chemical alteration). The third type of epigenetic alteration that has been discovered to date is RNA interference, which only affects a phenotype later, at the post-transcriptional level, as it directly cleaves mRNA, resulting in disrupted or no translation.

### 5.1 DNA methylation

#### 5.1.1 Methyltransferases: potential epigenetic drug candidates

The best described factor involved in epigenetic inheritance is DNA methylation, a covalent modification of cytosines (mainly at position 5, but also at position 4 or 6) that results in 5-methyl-cytosine occurs in CpG dinucleotides that are part of CpG islands that can most commonly be found at or near promoter regions in mammals. This process is accomplished through specific molecules: DNA methyltransferases (DNMTs), which are responsible for establishing and maintaining the unique methylation pattern on DNA. Three different types of DNMT have been reported to date. DNMT2 has rather low activity and functions only in tRNA methylation. DNMT1 and DNMT3 play essential roles in both mammalian development and in cancer biology, as they catalyse the addition of a methyl group to cytosines from the donor S-adenosyl-methionine. However, they require different substrates. Because DNMT1 is methylation dependent, it predominantly methylates hemimethylated CpGs. Therefore, DNMT1 is responsible for maintaining the methylation pattern, which is extremely important in cell division. DNMT3a and DNMT3b are referred to as *de novo* methylases because they act independently of previous methylation of the complementary strand. Both DNMT3a and DNMT3b could be important factors in establishing a new CpG methylation pattern, though DNMT3 exhibits a preference for centromeric regions [Cheng & Blumental, 2008]. Additionally, if a methyl group has already been

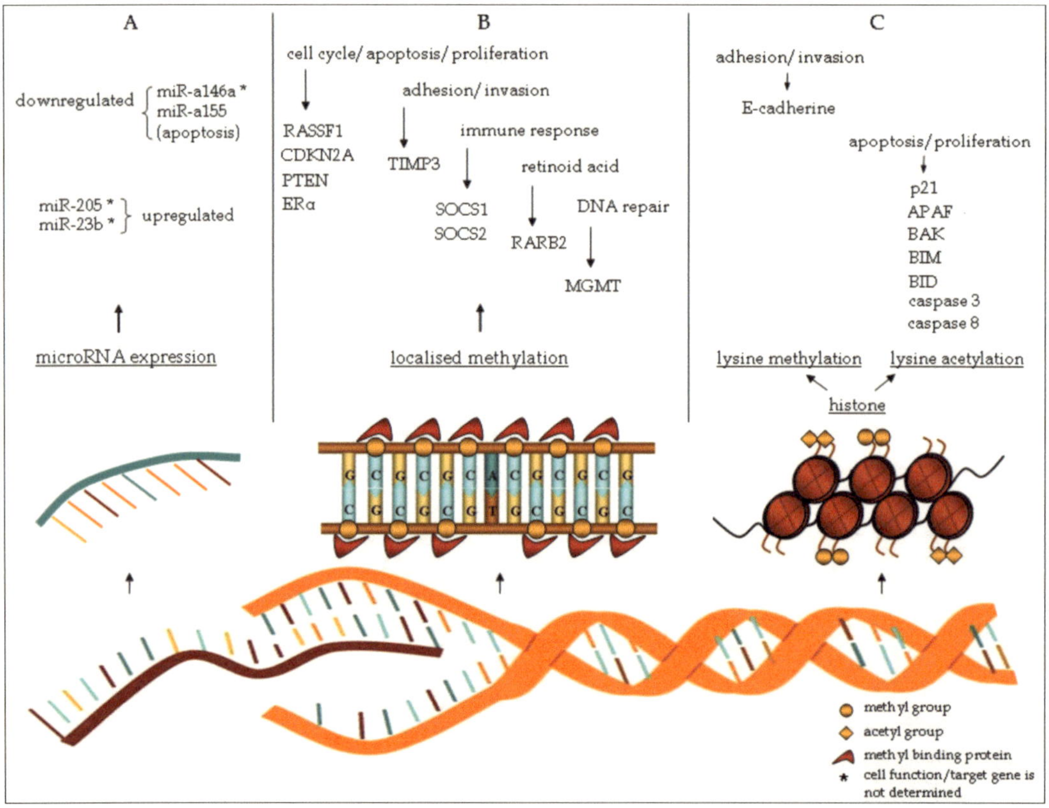


Fig. 3. Main regulatory elements and pathways involved in the three main epigenetic mechanisms in melanoma. A: microRNA regulation at post-transcriptional level results in decreasing in gene expression. B: localised methylation occuring at the promoter regions attracts methyl-CpG-binding proteins to construct transcriptionally silent heterochromatin and cause direct downregulation of genes involved in various pathways. C: histone post-transcriptional modifications alter gene expression of invasion and proliferation related molecules

added to a cytosine residue, methyl-CpG-binding proteins can attach to methylated regions. Therefore, a specific signature is constructed in assembling transcriptionally silent heterochromatin. It is widely accepted that DNA methylation of promoter regions, which are the main site of CpGs, can cause direct inactivation of specific genes [Howell et al., 2009; Sigalotti et al., 2010].

Because DNA methylation is described as a reversible mechanism, inhibition of promoter hypermethylation might represent the most promising therapeutic target for the treatment of melanoma. DNMT inhibitors are compounds that are able to demethylate 5-methyl-cytosines by the direct obstruction of DNMT enzymes. To date, 3 types of DNMT inhibitors have been characterised. 1. Nucleoside analogues were the first of these inhibitors to be developed and include 5-azacitidine (Vidaza) and 5-aza-2'-deoxycytidine (Decitabin). The common feature of these two drugs is their incorporation into DNA strands; because they contain an amino group instead of carbon at the 5 position of cytosine, they cannot be methylated. Currently, both molecules are undergoing phase I or phase II clinical trials in combination with either interferon α-2b or temozolomide. 2. Zebularine, a new type of nucleoside analogue, is less toxic compared to others because it does not contain an amino group. To date, only one study conducted on murine B16 melanoma has suggested a positive effect of Zebularine resulting in an increase in life span. 3. Non-nucleoside analogue DNMT inhibitors currently include procainamide and procaine. However, there are no data available related to their effect on melanoma. 4. Antisense oligonucleotides are substitute molecules for the DNMT1 enzyme (DNMT1 ASO), and they are currently undergoing preclinical drug testing [Howell et al., 2009; Sigalotti et al., 2010].

### 5.1.2 Localised hypermethylation

Given the existence of relatively easy approaches that require even minute amounts of tumour DNA, there are currently substantial amounts of data available that refer to gene silencing associated with the localised CpG hypermethylation of a specific gene promoter. There are two options for investigating this epigenetic phenomenon: it can be estimated indirectly or measured directly. Indirect assessment consists of three steps: first, measuring mRNA or protein expression; next, treating samples with a specific drug that acts against the process of methylation, mainly by inactivating DNMT3a (see above); and finally, measuring gene expression again. Powerful arguments have been presented in the literature that support direct experiments as being less ambiguous; additionally, because treatment is only possible in cell lines, tumour tissues are not appropriate for this purpose. In spite of the existence of a large dataset that has revealed more than 80 genes downregulated by promoter methylation, to allow their clinical utilisation, the detected elements must be distinguished based on the number of primary tumour samples involved in the study and the frequency of positive results as eligibility criteria for diagnosis or to determine whether they are a candidate therapeutic target. Promoter hypermethylation of two molecules involved in the cell cycle, Ras association domain-containing protein 1 (*RASSF1A*) and the cyclin-dependent kinase inhibitor 2A-coding gene (*CDKN2A*), has been confirmed by multiple, substantive experiments; these findings have also been confirmed in melanoma cell lines [Furuta et al., 2004; Marini et al., 2006; Sigalotti et al., 2010]. A higher level of methylation of oestrogen receptor alpha (*ERα*) compared to normal tissues has also been revealed in both tumour specimens and cell lines [Furuta et al., 2004; Mori et al., 2006]. Gaining 5-methyl-cytosines in the promoter regions of suppressor of cytokine signalling molecules (*SOCS1* and *SOCS2*) has been demonstrated simultaneously with *MGMT*, which plays an essential role in DNA repair, and with *TIMP3*, which encodes a protein that protects the extracellular matrix from enzymatic degradation [Liu et al., 2008].

Downregulation of *RARB2* (retinoic acid receptor B2) has been validated in repeated studies: 6 groups have investigated the methylation level of the *RARB2* promoter, but their results are still inconsistent: some of these investigators have recorded high levels methylation in most of the examined specimens, while others have reported promoter methylation in only a few melanomas [Furuta et al., 2004; Liu et al., 2008]. One of the most remarkable studies concluded that *PTEN* methylation was a predictor for patient survival, even though it had not been associated with other clinical records. This study involved 230 primary melanomas [Lahtz et al., 2009].

In addition to the rapid progress that has been made in studying promoter hypermethylation at the single-gene level, only one group has attempted to conduct an array-based experiment, having chosen the most powerful and high-throughput bead array technology, to provide valuable information on the methylation pattern of the 1505 gene promoter. It is important to note that previous studies have given irrefutable proof of the reproducibility of this approach. It is regrettable that researchers have focused on only comparing the methylation level of primary invasive melanomas with benign melanocytes; therefore, no data are available on the methylation markers of diverse melanomas with different clinical behaviours. However, the findings of these investigators support the claim that a covalent change from cytosine to 5-methyl-cytosine in the promoter region occurs as an early aberration event in melanomas. The group's results have clearly identified a group of genes in a statistically powerful interpretation that can be used to discriminate nevi from melanomas considering their methylation signature. Furthermore, they adapted this high-throughput methylation profiling to FFPE samples, which are generally prepared by pathologists, abundantly available and appropriate for further routine screening [Conway et al., 2011].

### 5.1.3 Methylation patterns of cell-free DNA

It is notable that efforts are now under way to develop methods to measure the methylation of genes in body fluids that are easy to obtain. Additionally, it is firmly believed that the methylation pattern of a specific gene in cell-free DNA (serum or urine) should resemble the markings of that gene in tumour tissue. Regarding early diagnosis, this represents a rapidly growing field, and a blood test aimed at quantifying tumour suppressor genes has already been made commercially available for colon cancer samples. Similar attempts have also been made in melanomas: hypermethylation of *RASSF1A* in serum has been demonstrated, although 3 conflicting publications have reported that it occurs to a lesser (19%) or a greater (63%) extent in melanomas [Furuta et al., 2004; Liu et al., 2008]. In serum, *CDKN2A* has also exhibited hypermethylation to a considerably higher level than in tumour tissues [Marini et al., 2006].

Because one of the most notable previous investigations demonstrated the prognostic relevance of *PTEN* methylation (as described above), studies were extended to quantify its methylation pattern in serum. A significant correlation was found between the methylation level of tumour tissue specimens and blood serum. Moreover, *PTEN* methylation might function as an early event in carcinogenesis, rather than a progression-related mechanism, based on experiments that compared the methylation levels of tumours and melanocytes

[Mirmohammadsadegh et al., 2006]. As it has been firmly demonstrated that *PTEN* silencing is due to an epigenetic event [Furuta et al., 2004], although it may have little impact on tumour progression, *PTEN* appears to be the most relevant candidate for the early diagnosis of melanoma by non-invasive tools.

### 5.1.4 Genome-wide hypomethylation

While most groups are studying extensively promoter-related hypermethylation, the importance of genome-wide demethylation or hypomethylation remains underestimated. However, these phenomena might also reflect important epigenetic alterations due to their ability to cause genetic instability. Genome-wide hypomethylation is characterised by the overall loss of 5-methyl-cytosines, which is believed to correspond to the loss of methylcytosines of repetitive transposable elements. During evolution, these elements integrated into the human genome and became protected from transcription due to their higher levels of methylcytosines. Considering the abundance of repetitive elements, it is clear why scientists generalise the loss of their 5-methyl-cytosine content to the 'whole genome'. Repetitive elements constitute 40% of the human genome and mainly consist of two different types: among *SINE* (short interspersed nucleotide element) sequences, only the Alu family is known, ranging from 400 to 500 bp, and it can be found in $10^5$ copies across the human genome; *LINE* (long interspersed nucleotide element) sequences are longer than 5000 to 6000 bp, and $10^4$ copies of these elements are spread throughout the genome [Howell et al., 2009].

Investigations of demethylation in carcinogenesis have raised a crucial question: how can genome-wide hypomethylation contribute to genetic instability? As described above, the overall loss of 5-methyl-cytosines can be explained by the modification of repetitive elements exhibiting strong homology. As these elements are reactivated by hypomethylation, they can recombine with each other, causing karyotypic instability [Wild &Flanagan, 2010].

The cause of their demethylation remains in question, as current evidence is divided between two hypotheses: hypomethylation could be an important early cancer-causing aberration, or it might occur as a passive inconsequential side effect of carcinogenesis. Both theories have gathered supporting data. Based on animal experiments, DNMTs have a higher affinity for recognising and affecting damaged DNA; therefore, their normal function of maintaining methylation patterns during replication might fail, suggesting passive demethylation as a subsequent genetic alteration. For many years, it has been hypothesised that indirect proof of active demethylation is provided by the imprinting of gametes and early embryos, which undergo massive epigenetic reprogramming involving demethylation followed by remethylation [James et al., 2003; Wild & Flanagan, 2010]. Regrettably, studies on melanomas have been unable to give evidence of active demethylation. However, results from breast cancer studies are promising: oestrogen receptor-alpha-responsive genes show remarkable demethylation followed by remethylation under the influence of oestrogen treatment. These encouraging results might prompt scientists to extend their experiments to investigate the active demethylation of *ERa*-responsive elements in melanoma cell lines. As previous studies in melanoma have detected promoter hypermethylation of *ERa*, suggesting an important role of *ERa* epigenetics, in addition to hypermethylation, *ERa* might provide a significant contribution to the field of active demethylation [Méteiver et al., 2008].

To date the existence of genome-wide hypermethylation has been demonstrated in 16 melanoma cell lines compared to melanocytes via repetitive elements. We are unable to conclude what the actual clinical effects of genome-wide methylation as the above-mentioned study focused only on comparing cell lines to controls, instead of drawing a demethylation-based distinction between cell lines with different characteristics. Our unpublished data also suggest a significant difference between normal tissues (nevus and skin) and melanoma specimens. However, aberrant hypomethylation may be the best marker for early diagnosis, as the results of a number of studies agree on the relevance of *LINE* hypomethylation in both cell lines and tissues [Tellez et al., 2009].

It is important to note that single-copy DNA regions can also feature hypomethylation, accompanied by mRNA and protein upregulation, as has been shown in colorectal, hepatocellular and breast cancers, although there is currently no evidence to suggest the same characteristics for melanomas.

### 5.2 Histone modification and microRNA regulation of melanoma

Eukaryotic DNA is packed into chromatin consisting of nucleosome units, each of which contains two copies of H2A, H2B, H3 and H4, as well as 146 bp of DNA. Each histone contains flexible N-terminal tails that can be a target for various post-translational modifications that determine the electrostatic power between DNA and histones and, therefore, contribute to determining transcriptionally active euchromatin or inactive heterochromatin. Histone modifications uniquely define the "histone code" that is read by multi-protein chromatin remodelling complexes to finally determine the transcriptional status of a target gene by modulating the chromatin compaction grade. While most studies rely on cell lines, there are preliminary results that show the importance of histone methylation in advance staged melanomas: a type of histone methyl-transferase (H3K27 HMT EZH2) has been found to be upregulated in tumours, and as it has an inhibitory effect on the transcription of *E-cadherin*, it could contribute to invasion [O'Neill et al., 2001; Sigalotti et al., 2010]. In addition to histone methylation, losses of histone lysine acetylation have also been reported. The hypoacetylation-related suppression of CDKN1A/P21 and the pro-apoptotic proteins (APAF-1, BAX, BAK, BID, BIM, caspase 3 and caspase 8) have also been described in melanoma cell lines [Feinberg et al., 2006].

Another promising field of melanoma epigenetics is related to gene regulation by microRNAs (miRNAs). These are small, non-coding RNAs transcribed in the nucleus into primary transcripts, followed by further cleavage by a complex of Drosha and its cofactor into precursor miRNAs (pre-miRNAs). Pre-miRNAs are exported to the cytoplasm, where Dicer protein reduces them to short double strands, which are then incorporated into RNA-induced silencing complexes that recognise target mRNA sequences, causing sequence-specific degradation and thus impairing their translation.

Only a single high-throughput experiment involving a relatively large set of samples has been performed on this topic [Levati et al., 2009]. However, the results of this study demonstrated inconsistency between cell lines and tumour tissues; moreover, the microarray results could not be confirmed by qPCR. Despite the high discrepancy in many cases, this group found that miRNA-205 and miRNA-23b were notably reduced, whereas miR-146a and miR-155 were upregulated only in tumour specimens compared to melanocytes and melanoma cell lines. Further functional studies have demonstrated the role of miRNA-155 in cell proliferation and survival [Levati et al., 2011].

Although strenuous efforts have been made to characterise the epigenetic changes involved in melanoma, studies have more often focused on elucidating alterations in DNA methylation than on estimating the functions of microRNAs and the realignment of histone molecules in melanomas. Despite the availability of a huge amount of data regarding promoter-related hypermethylation, the function of this phenomenon related to progression is still controversial. Some experiments have shown that tumours associated with different clinical stages exhibit a characteristic methylation signature, while others have found that the patterns of 5-methyl-cytosine gains in promoter regions are rather homogeneous in melanomas, or exhibit minimal differences between various clinical subgroups of tumours. However, some studies have suggested that differential methylation patterns have a greater impact in driving melanocytic lesions to melanoma. According to the literature, the current state of our knowledge about genome-wide hypomethylation seems to be clearly outlined. Studies have already shown that hypomethylation of repetitive elements occurs as an early event in melanomas. Therefore, hypomethylation can offer a new facility that emphasises early detection in the case of applying a technical approach that may make rapid, systematic screening possible.

Despite the strong progress in this field, it is still difficult to provide a concise summary about the importance of epigenetic changes in melanomas, although it can be asserted that promising findings will prompt further efforts in designing additional studies to obtain better insights into how melanoma progression is controlled by epigenetic events. Long-term follow-ups of epigenetic drug treatments will be indispensable to characterise possible adverse effects of general demethylation.

Finally, it should be noted that epigenetic mechanisms do not act separately but represent different utility in an integrated apparatus: the results of most recent studies indicate more challenges for the design of future experiments, as they have revealed that DNA methylation can influence histone modification to maintain altered gene expression, and miRNAs could also be a target of DNA methylation, besides representing a unique epigenetic mechanism.

Although the genomic methods described above are mainly used in research laboratories, they are also employed in the clinical field as methods for patient selection in clinical trials and as predictive tests for the selection of treatments for some malignancies (e.g., Oncotype DX; Genomic Health, Redwood City, CA; MammaPrint, Agendia, Amsterdam, Netherlands). Integration of genomic datasets from different platforms, such as gene copy number and expression profiling data, represents a powerful method for the identification of functionally relevant molecular aberrations. However, genomic techniques do not supplant more targeted analytical methods. The complementary use of both of these approaches will be essential to identify and exploit molecular changes in cancer for improved diagnosis and treatment.

## 6. Acknowledgements

Supported by the Hungarian National Research Fund (OTKA K75191), the Hungarian Academy of Sciences (grant number 2006TKI247) and the TÁMOP 4.2.1./B-09/1/KONV-2010-0007 project, the project is implemented through the New Hungary Development Plan, co-financed by the European Social Fund and the European Regional Development Fund and the Hungarian Medical Research Council (grant number 193/09-ETT).

## 7. References

Bastian, B.C., LeBoit, E.P., Hamm, H., Brocker, B.E., and Pinkel, D. (1998). Chromosomal gains and losses in primary cutaneous melanomas detected by comparative genomic hybridization. Cancer Res. 58, 2170–2175., ISSN: 1557-3265

Bastian, B.C., Kashani-Sabet, M., Hamm, H., Godfrey, T., Moore, D.H. 2nd, Bröcker, B.E., LeBoit, E.P., and Pinkel, D. (2000). Gene amplifications characterize acral melanoma and permit the detection of occult tumour cells in the surrounding skin. Cancer Res. 60(7), 1968-1973., ISSN: 1557-3265

Bastian, B. Genetic progression from melanocytes malignant melanoma. in From melanocytes to melanoma. The progression to malignancy Eds: Hearing VJ and Leong SPLL. 197-204., eISBN:1-58829-459-5

Bauer, J., and Bastian, B. (2006). Distinguishing melanocytic nevi from melanoma by DNA copy number changes: comparative genomic hybridization as a research and diagnostic tool. Dermatol Ther. 19(1), 40-49., ISSN: 1529-8019

Bedogni, B., and Powell, M.B. (2009). Unique transforming properties of Notch1 in human melanocytes. Pigment Cell Melanoma Res. 22(6), 702-703., ISSN: 1755-148X

Bittner, M., Meltzer, P., Chen, Y., Jiang, Y., Seftor, E., Hendrix, M., Radmacher, M., Simon, R., Yakhini, Z., Ben-Dor, A., Sampas, N., Dougherty, E., Wang, E., Marincola, F., Gooden, C., Lueders, J., Glatfelter, A., Pollock, P., Carpten, J., Gillanders, E., Leja, D., Dietrich, K., Beaudry, C., Berens, M., Alberts, D., and Sondak, V. (2000). Molecular classification of cutaneous malignant melanoma by gene expression profiling. Nature. 406(6795), 536-540., ISSN: 1476-4687

Blokx, W.A., van Dijk, M.C., and Ruiter, D.J. (2010). Molecular cytogenetics of cutaneous melanocytic lesions - diagnostic, prognostic and therapeutic aspects. Histopathology. 56(1), 121-132., ISSN: 1365-2559

Braun-Falco, M., Schempp, W., and Weyers, W. (2009) Molecular diagnosis in dermatopathology: what makes sense, and what doesn't. Exp Dermatol. 18(1), 12-23., ISSN: 1600-0625

Casorzo, L., Luzzi, C., Nardacchione, A., Picciotto, F., Pisacane, A., and Risio, M. (2005). Fluorescence in situ hybridization (FISH) evaluation of chromosomes 6, 7, 9 and 10 throughout human melanocytic tumourigenesis. Melanoma Res. 15(3), 155-160., ISSN: 1755-148X

Cheng, X., and Blumenthal, R.M. (2008). Mammalian DNA methyltransferases: a structural perspective. Structure. 16(3), 341-350., ISSN: 1878-4186

Chin, L., Garraway, L.A., and Fisher, D.E. (2006). Malignant melanoma: genetics and therapeutics in the genomic era. Genes Dev. 20(16), 2149-2182., ISSN: 1549-5477

Conway, C., Beswick, S., Elliott, F., Chang, Y.-M., Randerson-Moor, J., Harland, M., Affleck, P., Marsden, J., Sanders, D. S., Boon, A., Knowles, M. A., Bishop, D. T., and Newton-Bishop, J.A. (2010). Deletion at chromosome arm 9p in relation to BRAF/NRAS mutations and prognostic significance for primary melanoma. Genes Chromosomes Cancer. 49(5), 425-438., ISSN: 1098-2264

Conway, K., Edmiston, S.N., Khondker, Z.S., Groben, P.A., Zhou, X., Chu, H., Kuan, P.F., Hao, H., Carson, C., Berwick, M., Olilla, D.W., and Thomas, N.E. (2011). DNA-methylation profiling distinguishes malignant melanomas from benign nevi. Pigment Cell Melanoma Res. 24(2), 352-360., ISSN: 1755-148X

Cronin, J.C., Wunderlich, J., Loftus, S.K., Prickett, T.D., Wei, X., Ridd, K., Vemula, S., Burrell, A.S., Agrawal, N.S., Lin, J.C., Banister, C.E.,Buckhaults ,P., Rosenberg, S.A., Bastian, B.C., Pavan, W.J., and Samuels, Y. (2009). Frequent mutations in the MITF pathway in melanoma. Pigment Cell Melanoma Res. 22(4), 435-444., ISSN: 1755-148X

Dalton, S.R., Gerami, P., Kolaitis, N.A., Charzan, S., Werling, R., LeBoit, P.E., and Bastian, B.C. (2010). Use of fluorescence in situ hybridization (FISH) to distinguish intranodal nevus from metastatic melanoma. Am J Surg Pathol. 34(2), 231-237., ISSN: 0147-5185

Feinberg, A.P., Ohlsson, R., and Henikoff, S. (2006). The epigenetic progenitor origin of human cancer. Nat Rev Genet. 7, 21–33., ISSN: 1471-0064

Furuta, J., Umebayashi, Y., Miyamoto, K., Kikuchi, K., Otsuka, F., Sugimura, T., and Ushijima, T. (2004). Promoter methylation profiling of 30 genes in human malignant melanoma. Cancer Sci. 95, 962-968., ISSN: 1349-7006

Gast, A., Scherer, D., Chen, B., Bloethner, S., Melchert, S., Sucker, A., Hemminki, K., Schadendorf, D., and Kumar, R. (2010). Somatic alterations in the melanoma genome: a high-resolution array-based comparative genomic hybridization study. Genes Chromosomes Cancer. 49(8), 733-745., ISSN: 1098-226

Gerami, P., Jewell, SS, Morrison, LE, Blondin, B, Schulz, J, Ruffalo, T, Matushek, P 4th, Legator, M., Jacobson, K., Dalton, S.R., Charzan, S., Kolaitis, N.A., Guitart J., Lertsbarapa T., Boone S., LeBoit P.E., and Bastian B.C. (2009). Fluorescence in situ hybridization (FISH) as an ancillary diagnostic tool in the diagnosis of melanoma. Am J Surg Pathol. 33(8), 1146-1156., ISSN: 0147-5185

Gerami, P., Beilfuss, B., Haghighat, Z., Fang, Y., Jhanwar, S., and Busam, K.J. (2011). Fluorescence in situ hybridization as an ancillary method for the distinction of desmoplastic melanomas from sclerosing melanocytic nevi.J Cutan Pathol. 38(4), 329-334., ISSN: 1600-0560

Gerami, P., Jewell, S.S., Pouryazdanparast, P., Wayne, J.D., Haghighat, Z., Busam, K.J., Rademaker, A., and Morrison, L. (2011). Copy number gains in 11q13 and 8q34 are highly linked to prognosis in cutaneous malignant melanoma. J Mol Diagn. 13(3), 352-358., ISSN: 1525-1578

Ghosh, P., and Chin, L. (2009). Genetics and genomics of melanoma. Expert Rev Dermatol. 4(2), 131., ISSN: 1746-9872

Hoek, K.S., Schlegel, N.C., Eichhoff, O.M., Widmer, D.S., Praetorius, C., Einarsson, S.O., Valgeirsdottir, S., Bergsteinsdottir, K., Schepsky, A., Dummer, R., and Steingrimsson, E. (2008). Novel MITF targets identified using a two-step DNA microarray strategy. Pigment Cell Melanoma Res. 21, 665–676., ISSN: 1755-148X

Howell, P.M. Jr., Liu, S., Ren, S., Behlen, C., Fodstad, O., and Riker, A.I. (2009). Epigenetics in human melanoma. Cancer Control. 16(3), 200-218., ISSN: 1573-7225

Igbokwe, A., and Lopez-Terrada, D.H. (2011). Molecular testing of solid tumors. Arch Pathol Lab Med. 135(1), 67-82., ISSN: 0003-9985

Jaeger, J., Koczan, D., Thiesen, H.J., Ibrahim, S.M., Gross, G., Spang, R., and Kunz, M. (2007). Gene expression signatures for tumor progression, tumor subtype, and tumor thickness in laser-microdissected melanoma tissues. Clin Cancer Res. 13(3), 806–815., ISSN: 1078-0432

James, S.J, Pogribny, I.P, Pogribna, M., Miller, B.J, Jernigan, S., and Melnyk, S. (2003). Mechanisms of DNA damage. DNA hypomethylation, and tumor progression in the folate/methyl-deficient rat model of hepatocarcinogenesis. J. Nutr. 133, 3740S–3747S, ISSN: 1541-6100

Jeffs, A.R., Glover, A.C., Slobbe, L.J., Wang, L., He, S., Hazlett, J.A., Awasthi, A., Woolley, A.G., Marshall, E.S., Joseph, W.R., Print, C.G., Baguley, B.C., and Eccles, M.R.

(2009). A gene expression signature of invasive potential in metastatic melanoma cells. PLoS One. 4(12), e8461., ISSN: 1932-6203

Jenkins, N.C., Liu, T., Cassidy, P., Leachman, S.A., Boucher, K.M., Goodson, A.G., Samadashwily, G., and Grossman, D. (2011). The p16(INK4A) tumor suppressor regulates cellular oxidative stress. Oncogene. 30(3), 265-274., ISSN: 1476-5594

Ko, J.M., and Fisher, D.E. (2011). A new era: melanoma genetics and therapeutics. J Pathol. 223(2), 241-250., ISSN: 0022-3417

Lahtz, C., Stranzenbach, R., Fiedler, E., Helmbold, P., and Dammann, R.H. (2009). Methylation of PTEN as a Prognostic Factor in Malignant Melanoma of the Skin. J Invest Dermatol. 130, 620-622., ISSN: 1523-1747

Lázár, V., Ecsedi, S., Szöllősi, A.G., Tóth, R., Vízkeleti, L., Rákosy, Z., Bégány, A., Ádány, R., and Balázs, M. (2009). Characterization of candidate gene copy number alterations in the 11q13 region along with BRAF and NRAS mutations in human melanoma Mod Pathol. 22(10), 1367-1378., ISSN: 1530-0285

Levati, L., Alvino, E., Pagani, E., Arcelli, D., Caporaso, P., Bondanza, S., Di Leva, G., Ferracin, M., Volinia, S., Bonmassar, E., Croce, C.M., and D'Atri, S. (2009). Altered expression of selected microRNAs in melanoma: antiproliferative and proapoptotic activity of miRNA-155. Int J Oncol. 35(2), 393-400., ISSN: 1791-2423

Levati, L., Pagani, E., Romani, S., Castiglia, D., Piccinni, E., Covaciu, C., Caporaso, P., Bondanza, S., Antonetti, F.R., Bonmassar, E., Martelli, F., Alvino, E., and D'Atri, S. (2011). MicroRNA-155 Targets the SKI Gene in Human Melanoma Cell Lines. Pigment Cell Melanoma Res. In press, ISSN: 1755-148X

Liu, S., Ren, S., Howell, P., Fodstad, O., Riker, A.I. (2008). Identification of novel epigenetically modified genes in human melanoma via promoter methylation gene profiling. Pigment Cell Melanoma Res. 21, 545-558., ISSN: 1755-148X

Marini, A., Mirmohammadsadegh, A., Nambiar, S., Gustrau, A., Ruzicka, T., and Hengge, U.R. (2006). Epigenetic inactivation of tumor suppressor genes in serum of patients with cutaneous melanoma. J Invest Dermatol. 126, 422-431., ISSN: 1523-1747

Métivier, R., Gallais, R., Tiffoche, C., Le Péron, C., Jurkowska, R.Z., Carmouche, R.P., Ibberson, D., Barath, P., Demay, F., Reid, G., Benes, V., Jeltsch, A., Gannon, F., and Salbert, G. (2008). Cyclical DNA methylation of a transcriptionally active promoter. Nature. 452, 45–50., ISSN: 1476-4687

Meyle, K.D., and Guldberg, P. (2009). Genetic risk factors for melanoma. Hum Genet. 126 (4), 499-510., ISSN: 1432-1203

Mirmohammadsadegh, A., Marini, A., Nambiar, S., Hassan, M., Tannapfel, A., Ruzicka, T., and Hengge, U.R. (2006). Epigenetic silencing of the PTEN gene in melanoma. Cancer Res. 66(13), 6546-6552., ISSN: 1078-0432

Moore, S.R., Persons, D.L., Sosman, J.A., Bobadilla, D., Bedell, V., Smith, D.D., Wolman, S.R., Tuthill, R.J., Moon, J., Sondak, V.K., and Slovak, M.L. (2008). Detection of copy number alterations in metastatic melanoma by a DNA fluorescence in situ hybridization probe panel and array comparative genomic hybridization: a southwest oncology group study (S9431). Clin Cancer Res. 14(10), 2927-2935., ISSN: 1557-3265

Mori, T., Martinez, S.R., O'Day, S.J., Morton, D.L., Umetani, N., Kitago, M., Tanemura, A., Nguyen, S.L., Tran, A.N., Wang, H.J., and Hoon, D.S. (2006). Estrogen receptor-alpha methylation predicts melanoma progression. Cancer Res. 66, 6692-6698., ISSN: 1538-7445

O'Neill, R.J., Eldridge, M.D., and Graves, J.A. (2001). Chromosome heterozygosity and de novo chromosome rearrangements in mammalian interspecies hybrids. Mamm Genome. 12, 256–259., ISSN: 1432-1777

Palmieri, G., Casula, M., Sini, M.C., Ascierto, P.A., and Cossu, A. (2007). Issues affecting molecular staging in the management of patients with melanoma. J Cell Mol Med. 11(5), 1052-1068., ISSN: 1582-4934

Palmieri, G., Capone, M., Ascierto, M.L., Gentilcore, G., Stroncek, D.F., Casula, M., Sini, M.C., Palla, M., Mozzillo, N., and Ascierto, P.A. (2009). Main roads to melanoma. J Transl Med. 7, 86., ISSN: 1479-5876

Poetsch, M., Woenckhaus, C., Dittberner, T., Pambor, M., Lorenz, G., and Herrmann, F.H. (1998). Differences in chromosomal aberrations between nodular and superficial spreading malignant melanoma detected by interphase cytogenetics. Lab Invest. 78(7), 883-888., ISSN: 1530-0307

Poetsch, M., Dittberner, T., and Woenckhaus, C. (2003). Can different genetic changes characterize histogenetic subtypes and biologic behavior in sporadic malignant melanoma of the skin? Cell Mol Life Sci. 60(9), 1923-1932., ISSN: 1420-9071

Rákosy, Z., Vízkeleti, L., Ecsedi, S., Bégány, Á., Emri, G., Ádány, R., and Balázs, M. (2008). Characterization of 9p21 copy number alterations in human melanoma by fluorescence in situ hybridization. Cancer Genet Cytogenet. 182(2), 116-121., ISSN: 0165-4608

Ren, S., Liu, S., Howell, P. Jr., Xi, Y., Enkemann, S., Ju, J., and Riker, A. (2008). The impact of genomics in understanding human melanoma progression and metastasis. Cancer Control. 15(3), 202-215., ISSN: 1573-7225

Rother, J., and Jones, D. (2009). Molecular markers of tumor progression in melanoma. Curr Genomics. 10(4), 231-239., ISSN: 1389-2029

Scolyer, R.A., Murali, R., McCarthy, S.W., and Thompson, J.F. (2010). Histologically ambiguous ("borderline") primary cutaneous melanocytic tumors: approaches to patient management including the roles of molecular testing and sentinel lymph node biopsy. Arch Pathol Lab Med. 134(12), 1770-1777., ISSN: 0003-9985

Sekulic, A., Haluska, P. Jr., Miller, A.J., Genebriera De Lamo, J., Ejadi, S., Pulido, J.S., Salomao, D.R., Thorland, E.C., Vile, R.G., Swanson, D.L., Pockaj, B.A., Laman, S.D., Pittelkow, M.R., and Markovic, S.N. (2008). Malignant melanoma in the 21st century: the emerging molecular landscape. Mayo Clin Proc. 83(7), 825-846., ISSN: 1942-5546

Sigalotti, L., Covre, A., Fratta, E., Parisi, G., Colizzi, F., Rizzo, A., Danielli, R., Nicolay, H.J., Coral, S., and Maio, M. (2010). Epigenetics of human cutaneous melanoma: setting the stage for new therapeutic strategies. J Transl Med. (11)8, 56., ISSN: 1479-5876

Tellez, C.S., Shen, L., Estecio, M.R., Jelinek, J., Gershenwald, J.E., and Issa, J.P. (2009). CpG island methylation profiling in human melanoma cell lines. Melanoma Res. 19, 146-155., ISSN: 1473-5636

Timar, J., Gyorffy, B., and Raso, E. (2010). Gene signature of the metastatic potential of cutaneous melanoma: too much for too little? Clin Exp Metastasis. 27(6), 371-387., ISSN: 1573-7276

Trent, J.M. (1991). Cytogenetics of human malignant melanoma. Cancer Metastasis Rev. 10, 103–113., ISSN: 1573-7233

Treszl, A., Ádány, R., Rákosy, Z., Kardos, L., Bégány, Á., Gilde, K., and Balázs, M. (2004). Extra copies of c-myc are more pronounced in nodular melanomas than in superficial spreading melanomas as revealed by fluorescence in situ hybridisation. Cytometry B Clin Cytom. 60(1), 37-46., ISSN: 1552-4949

Viros, A., Fridlyand, J., Bauer, J., Lasithiotakis, K., Garbe, C., Pinkel, D., and Bastian, B.C. (2008). Improving melanoma classification by integrating genetic and morphologic features. PLoS Med. 5(6), e120., ISSN: 1549-167.

Welch, D.R., and Goldberg, S.F. (1997). Molecular mechanisms controlling human melanoma progression and metastasis. Pathobiology. 65(6), 311–330., ISSN: 1088-7180

Wild, L., and Flanagan, J.M. (2010). Genome-wide hypomethylation in cancer may be a passive consequence of transformation. Biochim Biophys Acta. 1806(1), 50-57., ISSN: 0006-3002

Winnepenninckx, V., Lazar, V., Michiels, S., Dessen, P., Stas, M., Alonso, S.R., Avril, M.F., Ortiz Romero, P.L., Robert, T., Balacescu, O., Eggermont, A.M., Lenoir, G., Sarasin, A., Tursz, T., van den Oord, J.J., and Spatz, A. (2006). Gene expression profiling of primary cutaneous melanoma and clinical outcome. Journal of the National Cancer Institute. 98, 472-482., ISSN: 1460-2105

13

# Melanoma and the Nervous System – Novel Pathways Mediated by Neurotrophins and Their Receptors

Carlo Pincelli, Katiuscia Dallaglio and Francesca Truzzi
*Institute of Dermatology, School of Biosciences and Biotechnologies, University of Modena and Reggio Emilia, Modena*
*Italy*

## 1. Introduction

Human melanoma is the deadliest form of skin cancer in the world, and its incidence is rapidly increasing every year 3-7% on average of the last decades, pointing to melanoma as one of the biggest health problem worldwide (Perlis & Herlyn, 2004). Recent statistics show that melanoma represents 1-3% of all malignant tumors, with Australia and New Zealand having the highest incidence (40 new cases/100 000 inhabitants per year), followed by North European countries and the USA; on the other hand, Japan and central Africa share the lowest incidence. Melanoma is one of the most aggressive tumors. Up to one-fifth of patients progress to metastatic (stage IV) disease, with a median survival of 6 months and a 5-year survival rate of less than 5% (Balch et al., 2001). Melanoma is resistant to conventional therapy such as chemotherapy, radiotherapy and immuno-therapy, as only 5-20% of the patients show a positive response to these treatments. To date, the only FDA-approved chemotherapy for melanoma is the alkylating agent dacarbazine (DTIC), which gives clinical responses in 5–10% of patients and cures in about 1%. The only other approved agents for disseminated melanoma are interleukin (IL)-2 and interferon (IFN)-a, which also have low response rates. During the radial phase, melanoma cells spread horizontally, while during the vertical phase they are able to invade the dermis and become able to generate metastasis (Garbe et al., 2011). Usually, the two phases represent the step-process that leads to aggressive melanomas: once melanoma has spread beyond its original location, it is usually highly resistant to therapies. There are four major types of melanoma: superficial melanoma, the most common type, flat and irregular in shape and colour, nodular melanoma, lentigo maligna melanoma, usually occuring in the elderly, and finally, acral lentiginous melanoma, the least common form of melanoma, which develops at high incidence in African Americans. Melanomas may develop in or near a previously existing precursor lesion or in healthy skin, and they can appear in the mouth, eye, or retina at the back of the eye, vagina, esophagus, anus, urinary tract, and small intestine. Age, sunburns during childhood, close relatives with a history of melanoma, presence of displastyc moles, weak immune-system, long-term exposure to sunlight and exposure to carcinogens are the most common risk factors for melanoma development. Melanoma originates from mutated melanocytes, which share with neurons a common neuroectodermal origin. Among the molecules that act as neurotrophic factors, neurotrophins (NTs) and their receptors constitute an important network.

## 2. Neurotrophins

NTs are a family of structurally and functionally related proteins, initially identified as promoters for neuronal survival. During a search for survival factors, nerve growth factor (NGF) was initially identified (Levi-Montalcini, 1987). Secondly, brain-derived neurotrophic factor (BDNF) was characterized as a survival factor for several neuronal populations not responsive to NGF (Barde et al., 1982). These two proteins revealed conserved features of the sequences, leading to isolation of clones encoding additional members of this family. NT expressed in mammals are four: NGF, BDNF, neurotrophin-3 (NT-3) and NT-4. NTs play a critical role in developmental neurobiology; they are crucial in cellular interactions, in regulating synapse formation and plasticity (Huang et al., 2003), in controlling cell survival and differentiation (Segal, 2003). NTs effects are mediated by two classes of cell-surface receptors, a family of tyrosine kinase receptors called Trks (TrkA, TrkB and TrkC) and the p75 neurotrophin receptor (p75NTR). Trk receptors bind NTs with higher affinity and specificity. In particular, TrkA binds NGF and NT-3, TrkB binds BDNF, NT-3, NT-4/5. TrkC only binds NT-3. On the other hand, p75NTR binds all NTs with low affinity and specificity.

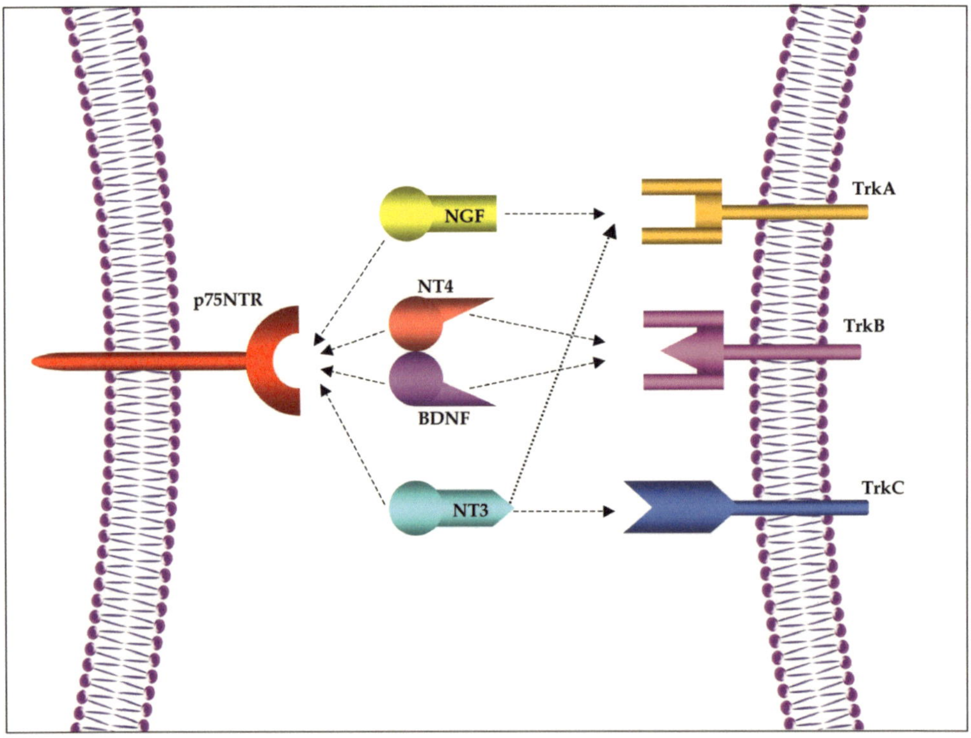


Fig. 1. NTs and their receptors

Trks are tyrosine kinase receptors with similar structure. They are activated by ligand-induced formation of noncovalently associated receptor dimers. In addition to the three full-

length Trk proteins, all three trk genes encode other protein isoforms by alternative splicing in the extracellular and intracellular domains, which include insertions in the extracellular domain (Barker et al., 1993; Tacconelli et al., 2005) and deletions or added residues in the intracytoplasmic domain (Reichardt, 2006). Several different mutation types in the trkA gene have been identified in congenital insensitivity to pain with anhydrosis (CIPA) patients (Indo, 2001). The phenotypes associated with CIPA are believed to result in large part from loss of NGF-dependent neurons, including nociceptive sensory and sympathetic neurons, during embryogenesis. A dominant mutation in TrkB (Y722C) that impairs TrkB kinase signalling has recently been described in a patient with severe hyperphagic obesity and severe impairments in nociception, learning and memory (Yeo et al., 2004).
The biological effects induced by NTs strongly depend on the pattern of NT receptor/co-receptors expression in target cells as well as onset of intracellular adaptor molecules that link NT signaling to different biochemical pathways. The propensity of NTs to produce diametrically opposing effects on cell survival has led to propose a "yin and yang" model of neurotrophin action, where the binary actions of NTs depend on both the form of the neurotrophin (pro- versus mature) and the class of receptor that is activated (Lu et al., 2005). Central to the proposed "yin–yang" model of NTs function is the observation that a mature NT binds preferentially to Trk receptors to enhance cell survival, whereas an unprocessed proNT binds to p75NTR to induce cell death. NTs interaction with Trks require receptor dimerization, autophosphorylation, and the subsequent binding of adaptor molecules that couple Trk receptors to different intracellular signal transduction pathways (Reichardt, 2006). NTs interact with trks receptors at the membrane-proximal immunoglobulin-like domain. The three-dimensional structures of this domain in each of the Trk receptors have been solved (Ultsch et al., 1999). Expression of a specific Trk receptor confers responsiveness to the NT to which it binds. On the other hand the isoform of TrkA including an insert is also activated by NT-3 in addition to NGF (Clary & Reichardt, 1994), while the similar isoform of TrkB is activated by NT-3 and NT-4 in addition to BDNF (Strohmaier, 1996). 36 novel isoforms of TrkB proteins with unique properties have been described recently. This suggests high complexity in the synthesis, regulation and function of this important NTs receptor, emphasizing the need for further study of these novel TrkB variants (Luberg et al., 2010). TrkC has several characteristics of a tumor suppressor: its expression in tumors has often been associated with good prognosis. It was recently demonstrated to be a dependence receptor, transducing different positive signals in the presence of ligand but inducing apoptosis in the absence of ligand. (Tauszig-Delamasure et al., 2007). Differential splicing of trkC mRNA also results in expression of a TrkC isoform with an amino acid insert within the tyrosine kinase domain. This insert appears to modify the substrate specificity of this tyrosine kinase, inhibiting activation of several substrates and interfering with its ability to promote neuronal differentiation (Guiton et al. 1995).
p75NTR was the first NT receptor to be identified as a low-affinity receptor for NGF, but it was subsequently shown to bind each of the neurotrophins with a similar affinity (Rodriguez-Tébar et al., 1990; Frade & Barde, 1998). p75NTR belongs to the tumor necrosis factor receptor superfamily. It has an extra-cellular domain containing four cysteine-rich motifs, a single transmembrane domain and a cytoplasmic domain that includes a 'death' domain, similar to those present in other members of this family (He & Garcia, 2004). This receptor does not contain a catalytic motif, however it interacts with proteins that transmit crucial signals for regulating neuronal survival and differentiation as well as synaptic plasticity. The three-dimensional structure of the extracellular domain of p75NTR in

association with an NGF dimer indicates that each of the four cysteine-rich repeats participates in binding to NGF (He & Garcia, 2004). The binding of NGF to p75NTR may result in dissociation of p75NTR multimers and is compatible with the possibility that Trk and p75NTR monomers simultaneously bind the same NT dimer. A gene related to p75NTR, named NRH-2, has recently been identified. The product of this gene lacks the extracellular cysteine-rich repeats present in p75NTR and fails to bind NGF, but it is able to interact and influence the ligand-binding properties of TrkA (Murray et al., 2004). When p75NTR is expressed alone, mature NTs are capable of inducing apoptosis or promote survival depending on the intracellular adaptor molecules present in target cells by interacting with a mounting number of downstream molecules (Wang et al., 2000). However, signaling through p75NTR may also promote cell survival acting through the NF-κB pathway (Roux & Barker, 2002). The coexpression of Trks and p75NTR increases high affinity NT binding, enhances Trk ability to discriminate a preferred ligand from the other NT, and promotes NT survival effects (Teng & Hempstead, 2004). On the other hand, the proform of NT, proNGF, binds p75NTR in association with its co-receptor sortilin, but not Trk (Nykjaer et al., 2004). More specifically, sortilin, a member of the vps-10 protein family, binds the "pro" region of NGF, whereas p75NTR binds mature NGF. The p75NTR–sortilin complex couples with proNGF to induce apoptosis (Kaplan & Miller, 2004).

## 3. NTs and skin microenviroment

NTs also operate in a number of non-neuronal tissues, including skin where a complex NT network exists with various cells that are either the target or the source of NTs, thus playing autocrine and paracrine functions (Botcharev et al., 2006). Moreover, given the common neuroectodermal origin of the skin with the nervous system, different studies have been carried out on the role of NTs and their receptors in the cutaneous system. First, NGF, which is synthesized in the epidermis, is retrogradelly transported to the ganglia to stimulate the release of neuropeptides in the skin, thus favoring cutaneous neurogenic inflammation (Davis et al., 1997). Moreover, null mutations of genes in the NTs and their receptors lead to loss/reduction of specific neurons in sensory ganglia; conversely, cutaneous overexpression of NTs results in skin hyperinnervation and increase in the number of sensory neurons innervating the skin (Montaño et al., 2010). Not only NGF is neurotrophic at the skin level, but it possesses a number of biological effects also in cutaneous cells. Normal human keratinocytes synthesize and release NGF that can act as a growth factor for these cells (Pincelli et al., 1994). The most common type of skin cells is the keratinocyte. These cells synthesize and secrete all NTs (Di Marco et al., 1991), NGF being secreted at highest levels as compared to the other NT. In human keratinocytes, NT-3 and NGF upregulate each other's secretion. UVB irradiation downregulate NGF, while UVA augment NT-3 release (Marconi et al., 1999; Stefanato et al., 2003). Human keratinocytes release NGF in increasing amounts while proliferating, whereas secretion ends in more differentiated cells (Pincelli et al., 1994). NGF induces human keratinocyte proliferation (Di Marco et al., 1993) and it can either stimulate or inhibit murine epidermal and hair follicle keratinocyte proliferation *in situ (*Paus et.al., 1994). Human keratinocytes express the high affinity receptors TrkA and TrkC, but not the functional form of the TrkB (Marconi et al., 2004). Endogenous NGF autocrinally sustains keratinocyte proliferation. NTs together with their receptors TrkA and TrkB can stimulate proliferation of mouse keratinocyte in *ex-vivo* cultured skin explants (Paus et al., 1994; Botchkarev et al., 1999). Moreover, NTs modulate susceptibility to

apoptosis in the epidermis. Autocrine NGF protects human keratinocytes from UVB-induced apoptosis, while UVB downregulates both NGF and TrkA expression in these cells (Marconi et al., 1999). Because in normal human keratinocytes TrkB lacks functional isoform, NT may exert different functions by binding p75NTR alone. In this context, p75NTR acts as a proapoptotic receptor. This is exemplified by BDNF and NT4, which induce a higher rate of apoptosis in normal human keratinocytes overexpressing p75NTR, as compared to mock-transfected cells. On the other hand, p75NTRsiRNA-transfected keratinocytes fail to undergo cell death after administration of NT4 (Truzzi et al., 2010). Interestingly, stem keratinocytes (KSC) expresses most of the NGF produced by human keratinocytes (Marconi et al., 2004), and inhibition of TrkA reduces the proliferation of this keratinocyte subpopulation (Marconi et al., 2004). This suggests that the presence of a NGF-TrkA autocrine loop, which acts both as mitogenic and as survival factor, contributing to the maintenance of the so-called "stemness" in keratinocytes. Conversely, p75NTR is mostly expressed in the differentiated transit amplifying (TA) cells, and it is barely detected in KSC. TA cells have been shown to be more susceptible than KSC to apoptosis (Tiberio et al., 2002). Therefore, the espression of p75NTR predominantly in TA cells seems to be consistent with the pro-apoptotic role of this receptor in human keratinocytes (Truzzi et al., 2011).
Another important epidermal cell is the melanocyte that localizes in the dermo-epidermal junction and in the hair matrix. NTs are important for melanocyte migration, viability and differentiation together with other paracrine signalling molecules (Pincelli et al., 1997). Normal human melanocytes are a target of the NTs skin network, because they express all the NTs receptors both *in vitro* and *in vivo* (Marconi et al., 2006). Normal human melanocytes also express p75NTR, which is upregulated by different stimuli, like UV irradiation (Peacocke et al., 1988). NTs influence melanocytes in a paracrine fashion. NGF is implicated in melanocyte survival (Zhai et al., 1996), migration and dendricity (Yaar et al., 1991), and its synthesis and secretion are enhanced by UV irradiation (Tron et al., 1990). Moreover, NGF reduces apoptosis when melanocytes are irradiated with UV, through upregulation of the anti-apoptotic Bcl-2 protein *in vivo* (Stefanato et al., 2003). Thus, NTs are important for protection of UV-induced oxidative stress and apoptosis in melanocytes. Melanocytes produce all NTs, while when these factors are added to the cultures, they fail to stimulate cell proliferation (Marconi et al., 2006). When melanocytes are maintained in growth factor-depleted medium, NGF and NT-3 promote melanocyte survival (Yaar et al., 1994). Both NT3 and NT4 secretion promotes the synthesis of tyrosinase and tyrosinase-related peptide (TRP)-1, critical enzyme of melanin biosynthesis (Marconi A et al., 2006). Human melanocytes express Trk receptors (Marconi et al., 2006; Yaar et al., 1994). Interestingly, phorbol 12-tetra decantate 13 acetate (TPA), a strong activator of protein kinase C, induces the expression of TrkA (Yaar et al., 1994) and decreases the expression of TrkC, suggesting that NGF and NT3 mediate different signals through their specific high affinity receptors. Melanocytes express also the NT low affinity receptor p75NTR, which expression is upregulated after TPA treatment (Yaar et al., 1994).
NTs and their receptors are expressed both in dermal fibroblasts and in the more differentiated myofibroblasts. p75NTR and TrkB are expressed at higher levels in myofibroblasts than in fibroblasts, which in contrast express higher levels of TrkA. Dermal fibroblast and myofibroblasts secrete all NTs, modulating dermal fibroblast proliferation. Interestingly, NTs also promote fibroblast differentiation into myofibroblasts, by inducing $\alpha$-SMA expression. This indicates that NTs could have a functional role in the fibro-myofibroblast system (Palazzo et al., 2011). It has been shown that NGF induces fibroblast-

like keratinocyte differentiation into myofibroblasts (Micera et al., 2001), their contraction in 3D collagen matrix (Micera et al., 2001) and the expression of MMP-9 (Metalloprotease-9) in keratoconjunctivitis-derived fibroblasts (Micera et al., 2007b), and different works show the applicative possibility of this NGF function (Landi et al., 2003; Aloe et al., 2008; Sun et al., 2010). All NTs promote fibroblast migration, while NGF and BDNF promote their contractile activity. Therefore, NGF and BDNF, produced by dermal and epidermal cells, could be key regulators of the biomechanical properties in the dermis.

In the skin network, NT and their receptors are also important for other epidermal cells. Skin mast cells express functional TrkA, produce NGF (Marshall et al., 1999), and express p75NTR (Fischer et al., 2008). Merkel cells are sensory cells of neural crest origin. During development, neither NT-3 nor TrkC and p75NTR are expressed by Merkel cells in the murine whisker. However, NT-3 is essential for mice postnatal survival (Szeder et al., 2003). Moreover, both TrkB and p75NTR were shown to be important for Merkel cell development (Perez-Pinera et al., 2008; Kinkelin et al., 1999).

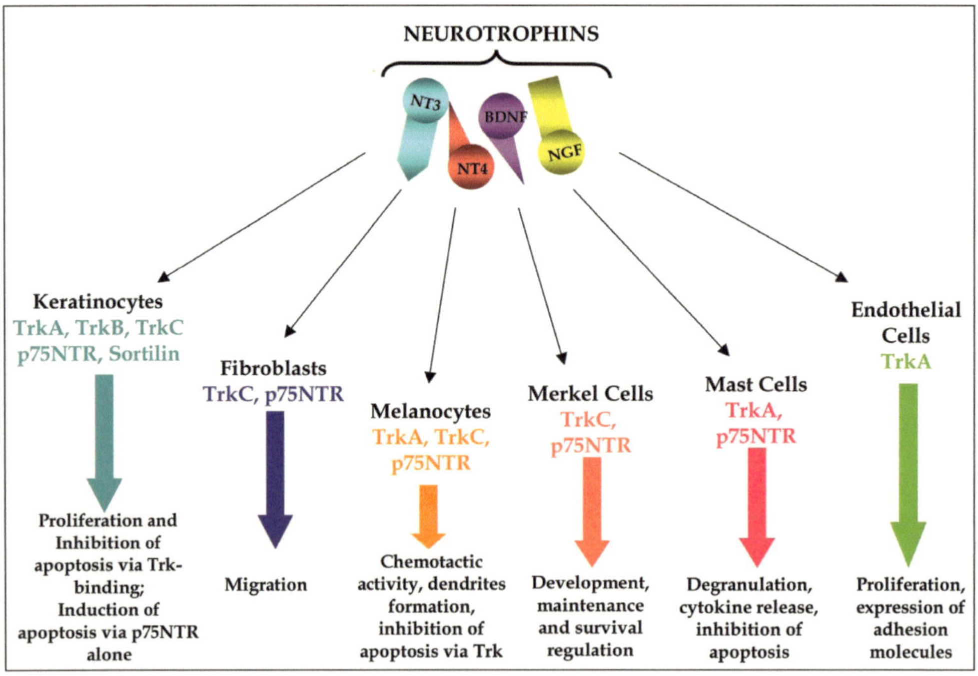


Fig. 2. NTs in the skin network

## 4. NTs and the origin of melanoma

Melanocytes, the cells that originate melanomas, are melanin-producing cells responsible for skin, hair and eye pigmentation. The principal role of melanocytes is to protect human skin from UVB radiation-induced stress. To understand melanoma origin, it is of paramount importance to elucidate the characteristics of the cells that originate the tumor. Indeed, melanocytes have intrinsic properties such as migratory capacity and self-renewal, which are shared with melanoma cells, and that could be partially responsible for the high susceptibility of melanoma to metastasize and recur in patients. Human melanocytes derive from a group of embryonic cells that form, during embryogenesis, the neural crest (NC). Neural crest cells (NCC) are multipotent, giving rise to different cell lineages depending on their anatomic location, and are therefore referred to as NC stem cells (NCSC). Melanocytes appear to derive from both cranial and trunk neural crest, while cells derived from the vagal, sacral, mid/hindbrain regions of the crest originate neurons cartilage, bones, smooth muscle, peripheral and enteric neurons and glia (Anderson et al., 2000). These multipotent cells give rise to a bipotent NCSC that generate both glia and melanoblasts (Dupin et al., 2000). Although the mechanism of lineage restriction towards melanoblasts specification has been deeply studied, it is only partially understood. However, it seems that signals from surrounding cells control this mechanism, both during cell homing and in their final environment. The bipotent progenitor is able to generate a melanocyte-restricted cell, which is referred to as melanoblast. Melanoblasts are unpigmented cells that migrate from the neural crest site along the dorsolateral pathway, throughout the developing epidermis. They colonize both interfollicular epidermis, localizing at the basement membrane, and developing hair follicles. In interfollicular epidermis, melanoblasts differentiate into mature melanocytes, upon stimulation from neighbor keratinocytes. In the hair follicle, melanoblast can then further segregate into a committed melanocyte or an adult melanocyte stem cell (Nishikawa & Osawa, 2007). The committed melanocyte resides in the hair matrix of the follicle and differentiates into a melanin-producing cell, thus being responsible for hair pigmentation. As opposite, melanocyte stem cells, which reside in the bulge area of hair follicles, are amelanotic and conserve characteristics of stem cells such as slow-cell cycle/quiescence and self-renewal capacity (Nishimura et al., 2002). The presence of these cells ensures the pigmentation of hair follicles in subsequent hair cycles. In humans, melanocyte stem cells have not been isolated yet (Sabatino et al., 2009). However, in patients affected by vitiligo, a progressive skin disease with defective pigmentation, the repigmentation process starts from perifollicular areas, thus implying that, during this process, undifferentiated melanocytes in interfollicular epidermis may derive from melanocyte stem cells of the hair follicle bulge area (Falabella & Barona 2009). Consistently, a migration process of bulge melanoblasts towards interfollicular epidermis has been previously observed (Cui et al., 1991). Overall, these observations may suggest that melanoblasts in the hair follicles function as a reservoir population both for the bulb hair follicle and for interfollicular epidermis.

Upon UVB radiations and exogenous stress stimuli, melanocytes can acquire genetic mutations. Although apoptosis usually eliminates highly damaged mutated cells, some of these mutations can confer resistance to apoptosis and proliferative advantage to the cells, thus leading to accumulation of mutations and to the formation of melanocytic lesions. The old carcinogenesis model, namely "the stochastic model", suggests that virtually any cell could be the target of mutations and subsequent transformation. As opposite, different works suggest that only some cells retain the susceptibility to acquire mutations and generate cancer, and that these cells can either be differentiated or have stem cells characteristics. Whether melanoma arises from melanocyte stem cells or a differentiated melanocyte is still matter of debate (Hoek & Godin, 2010). It is possible that differentiated melanocytes undergo a process of de-differentiation, thus acquiring stem cell characteristics. Melanocyte stem cells in the hair follicle generate an amplifying progeny, which is differentiated, still retaining self-renewal capacity. After exiting stem cell niche, transit amplifying melanocytes colonize adjacent vacant spaces and repopulate them, thus functioning as stem cells (Nishimura et al., 2002). In quails, melanocytes removed from their niche and clonally cultured, can generate multipotent cells retaining self-renewal capacity, thus confirming that de-differentiation of melanocytes is indeed possible (Real et al., 2006). It has been proposed that melanoma arises in a stepwise process, starting from nevus and dysplastic nevus stages to in situ melanoma and finally, to metastatic melanoma. Because nevi seems to originate from mutations in a precursor cell, which then activates proliferative pathways, while suppressing apoptosis, it would be more likely that melanoma arises from a mutated cell with stem characteristics. However, this model does not mimic precisely melanoma biology, as melanoma can arise in absence of nevus precursor, and displastyc nevi do not necessarily evolve into melanomas (Beona et al., 2003). In many other systems, stem cells are considered the best candidate for accumulation of mutations, given their long persistence in the tissue and retaining the highest proliferative potential. Although the cell at the origin of melanoma is still unidentified, recent works suggest that melanocyte stem cells located in the hair bulge may not be the right candidate. Indeed, primary melanoma localizes at the junction between dermis and epidermis, suggesting that stem melanocytes should migrate from hair follicles to the epidermis before generating melanomas. Moreover, while epidemiological studies demonstrate a correlation between melanoma formation and UV-radiation-induced sunburn in childhood, hair follicles are only marginally reached by UV, because of their deep localization in the tissue. On the other hand, transgenic mice overexpressing NRAS and β-catenin develop melanocytic lesion in the follicle bulge, thus indicating that melanocyte stem cells in the hair bulge are potentially able to mutate and generate melanocytic lesions (Delmas et al., 2007). Up to now, the exact localization of the melanoma precursor and the differentiation state of this cell are still unclear.

Although NCSC contribution to melanoma formation is still controversial, NCSC migration during embryogenesis and tumor formation are tightly connected. Indeed, extravascular migration process, which guides cells towards their final sites, is shared between melanoma cells and NCSC (Lugassy & Barnhill, 2007). In addition, NCSC behavior is influenced by NTs and their receptors, which in turn are part of melanoma microenvironment. Epidermal-restricted NCSC express all NTs, while NGF and NT-3 support their proliferation as well as survival of daughter cells, in that NGF and NT-3 depletion results in loss of 70% and 60% neurons, respectively (Dasari et al., 2008; Zhang et al., 1997). Moreover, NTs can either support proliferation or induce apoptosis in NCC, depending on their lineage/differentiation stage (Langtimm-Sedlak et al., 1996). Consistently, different expression of trk receptors may identify distinct subpopulations of early NCC. While Trk receptors are not expressed at early stages of embryonic development, p75NTR is the first NT receptor to be expressed in NCC (Rifkin et al., 2000). NCSC have been previously isolated from mouse trunk neural tubes by using a monoclonal antibody against p75NTR. p75NTR-positive cells derived from mouse neural tubes are multipotent and have self renewal capacity, generating multipotent progeny. These cells can differentiate into smooth muscle cells, neurons and glial cells, melanocytes, cartilage and bone. They can also generate clonal subpopulations of cells able to generate only glia and neurons, thus suggesting their ability to generate also committed progenitors (Stemple & Anderson, 1992). p75NTR, also knwon as CD271 (Rogers et al., 2008), was successfully used to isolate multipotent stem cells also from rat sciatic nerves (Morrison et al., 1999). These cells generate neurons and glial cells when injected into chick embryos, and retain self-renewal capacity. Multipotent NCSC can be isolated from hairy skin in humans and mice (Sieber-Blum & Grim, 2004; Sieber-Blum et al., 2004). Consistently, p75NTR-positive cells, isolated from human hair follicle dermal papillae, retain multipotency and contribute to the renewal of neural and non-neural cells, including melanocytes (Yu et al., 2006). Recently, multipotent cells with NCSC characteristics have been extracted by sphere formation from the dermis of human foreskins lacking hair follicles. These cells, not only express stem cells markers such as Oct-4 and nestin, but display also multipotency and the ability to differentiate into multiple lineages, including melanocytes. Moreover, they express p75NTR, thus suggesting that p75NTR can be considered a good marker for NCSC (Li et al., 2010; Paratore et al., 2001).

Melanoma development is considered a stepwise process in which mature melanocytes in the epidermis progressively acquire genetic mutations in oncogenes or tumor-suppressor genes that lead from benign to dysplastic nevi, progressing toward radial growth phase to vertical growth phase, ultimately followed by metastatic melanoma. Melanomas arise within the epidermis and then invade the basement membrane to eventually disseminate to multiple organs. During progression, melanoma moves from the epidermal to the dermal microenvironment by virtue of various mechanisms that involve different cell types, such as keratinocytes, fibroblasts and a number of cytokines and growth factors. While in human epidermis, a functional symbiosis exists between keratinocytes and melanocytes, melanoma cells are refractory to the regulation by keratinocytes and become independent, by autocrinally producing their growth factors (Crowson et al., 2007). The NTs network involves most skin cell types and is responsible for various activities. (Botchkarev et al., 2006). In particular, melanocytes, which share with neurons a common neuroectodermal origin, express all NTs and their receptors.

## 5. NTs and melanoma

As for many other growth factors, dysregulation of NT signal transduction is found in a number of tumors inside and outside the nervous system where they accompany or contribute to malignant transformation (Kruttgen et al., 2006). Yet, the precise role of NTs and their receptors has to be clarified (Thiele et al., 2009; Papatsoris et al., 2009). On the other hand, NTs have been widely investigated in neuroblastoma (NB) and medulloblastoma, tumors derived from the neural crest. Trk-receptors have been identified as important prognostic factors, influencing the heterogeneous clinical behavior of NB (Nakagawara, 1993). TrkA and/or TrkC expression is present in favorable NBs, which tend to show a more differentiated neuronal phenotype and highly correlates with patient survival (Nakagawara, 2001; Brodeur, 2009; Yamashiro, 1996). The tendency of NBs to regress may be related to their dependence on an inadequate amount of NGF supplied from stromal cells and a differentiating rather than a proliferative response to this NT. Therefore, an autocrine or paracrine TrkB/BDNF pathway may contribute to an unfavorable outcome in primary NBs. The different clinical implications of the Trk receptors and their isoforms strongly suggest that the activation of full-length and truncated TrkA and TrkB may exert different influences on the biological behavior of NB cells (Barbacid, 1994). Like NB, medulloblastoma can be subdivided in many subtypes with different prognosis (Johnsen et al., 2009). TrkA or TrkC has been detected in such areas, in parallel with concentrations of apoptotic or differentiating cells (Ohta et al., 2006). TrkC has been correlated to positive prognosis in medulloblastoma (Segal et al., 1994) and to apoptosis *in vitro* in primary medulloblastoma (Kim et al.,1999). Nevertheless, the effect of p75NTR on the cellular response to NT is complex and may depend on the concentration of ligand, the ratio of receptors, the cell type in which it is expressed, and its stage of differentiation (Greene et al., 1995; Chao et al.,

1995). Overexpression of p75NTR increases the number of high- and low-affinity NGF binding sites in TrkA- expressing PC12 cells (Hempstead et al., 1992). Moreover, p75NTR induces apoptosis in the presence of NGF (Bunone et al., 1997), but this apoptotic signaling is inhibited by the presence of TrkA receptors (Eggert et al., 2000). Recently, it has been demonstrated that the effects of necdin, a protein known to interact with NTs receptors, on the susceptibility of NB cells to oxidant stress depend on the p75NTR/TrkA ratio in the cell (Ingraham et al., 2011).

Although melanoma is a tumor derived from the neural crest, and shares with cancers of the same origin embryogenic and oncogenic pathways as well as common transcription factors (Wang et al., 2008; Gershon et al., 2005), it has been given less attention, as far as the role of NT. Melanomas can be morphologically subdivided in several subtypes, such as epithelioid, pleomorphic spindle cell and desmoplastic melanoma. Iwamoto et al. found detectable p75NTR in 13 of 14 benign nevi, primarily in the spindled nevocytic structures within the dermis (Iwamoto et al., 2001). Moreover, p75NTR is weakly expressed in the epithelioid melanomas, while it is highly expressed in desmoplastic and spindle cell melanomas (Iwamoto et al., 1996). This was confirmed by others who showed p75NTR staining to be more diffuse and intense as compared with S100 (Kanik et al., 1996; Lazova et al., 2010). On the contrary, Huttenbach and co-workers detected p75NTR positive cells only in 33% of desmoplastic melanomas (Huttenbach et al., 2002). Marchetti et al, by using melanoma cell lines, observed that NGF/p75NTR signaling promotes the survival of melanoma cells (Marchetti et al., 2003). They also observed the presence of NGF and NT-3 in tumor adjacent tissues at the invasive front of melanoma brain metastases, which might indicate a paracrine activation of p75NTR and TrkC in melanoma cells by NGF and NT-3 produced by nearby glial cells. Besides promoting melanoma cell survival, NTs also induce the expression in melanoma cells of heparanase, an important enzyme for local invasion and metastasis, that cleaves heparan sulfate chains of proteoglycans, thus modifying the extracellular matrix of tumor cells (Walch et al., 1999). Moreover, Shonukan et al showed that NTs are chemotactic for melanoma cells, and that the actin-bundling protein fascin co-immunoprecipitates with p75NTR in an NGF-dependent manner (Shonukan et al., 2003). In addition, TrkA is expressed by primary and metastatic melanomas and is associated with poor clinical outcome (Flørenes et al., 2004). Recently, during a functional characterization of human cancer-derived TrkB mutations, one additional TRKB point mutation proximal to the kinase domain (TRKB(P507L)) in a human melanoma cell line was found, even if it was functionally indistinguishable from wild-type TRKB in both *in-vitro* and *in-vivo* (Geiger et al., 2011). As melanoma could originate from melanocytes and melanocytes seem to benefit from the cutaneous neurotrophic network mainly as paracrine targets, once malignant transformation occurs, melanoma cells acquire self-renewal capabilities mediated also by autocrine NTs loops. Indeed, all NTs, particularly NT-3 and NT-4, have been detected in conditioned medium of different melanoma cell lines (Truzzi et al., 2008). Recent results show that melanoma cells proliferate through autocrine NTs stimulation. K252a significantly reduces melanoma cell proliferation by inhibiting Trks phosphorylation. Proliferation is significantly reduced when endogenous NTs are removed from the culture medium by soluble Trk/Fc receptors. NTs appeared to be important for melanoma cell migration *in vitro*, with special respect for metastatic cell lines. The migratory phenotype is necessarily dependent on the presence of both the high- and low-affinity NTs receptors. Cells treated with p75NTR small interfering RNA (p75NTRsiRNA) fail to respond to NTs stimulation. Similarly, the administration of K252a blocks melanoma cell migration, confirming that NTs stimulate melanoma cell migration and invasion with the cooperation of the low- and high-affinity receptors (Truzzi et al., 2008).

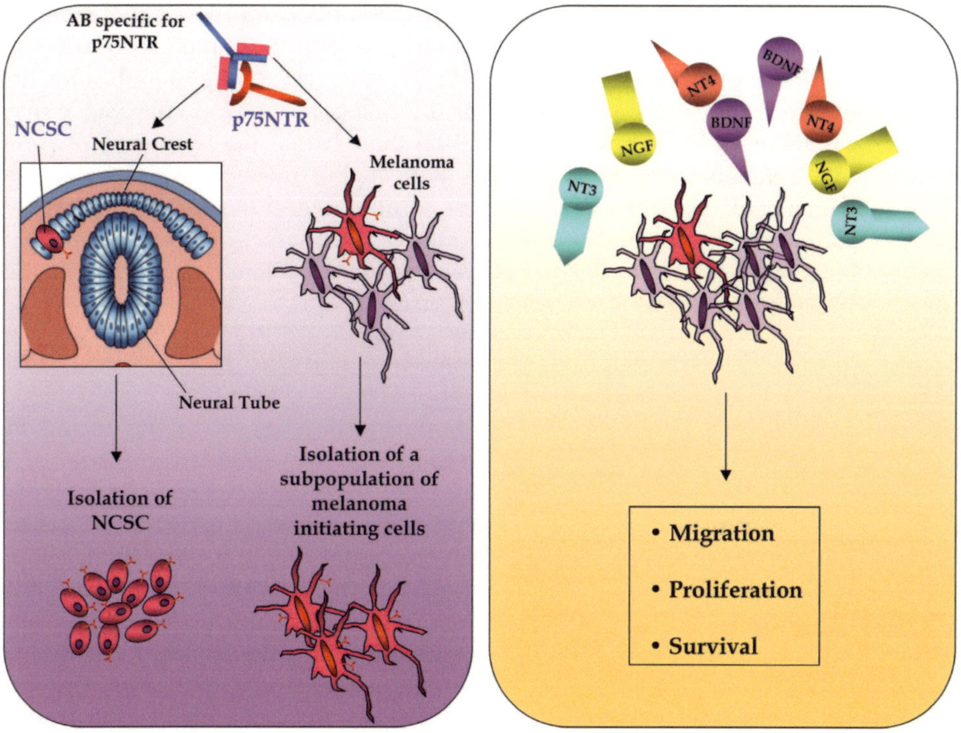


Fig. 3. NTs and their receptors in melanoma biology

Although melanoma may develop in a stepwise manner from a pre-existing lesion, only 26% of melanomas evolve from nevi, while the majority of melanomas arise from normal-appearing skin, suggesting that melanoma development may not follow the classical linear mode of progression (Zabierowsky & Herlyn, 2008). The constant recurrence of melanoma after any therapy is likely due to the survival of a subset of cancer cells that display a resistance to treatment. The "Cancer Stem Cell hypothesis" states that within tumor heterogeneity, only few cells are responsible for tumor initiation and maintenance, sharing with normal stem cells the ability to self renew and to persist in the tissue for years. Although in some tumors, such as leukemia, the CSC model is valid, in melanoma, cells able to initiate tumor formation are not a rare population (Quintana et al., 2010; Held et al., 2010; Roesch et al., 2010). Given the role of NTs and their receptors in melanoma biology, this complex network of growth factors is likely to be involved both in melanoma recurrence and metastasis in the patients. NCSC, that have been proposed as the cells responsible for melanoma origin (see above), have been previously isolated both from neural crest and from adult tissues by using p75NTR (Kruger et al., 2002). Similarly, Boiko and coworkers showed that p75NTR expression characterizes a population of melanoma cells with tumor initiating properties (Boiko et al., 2010). However, the number of cells capable of recapitulating the tumors *in vivo* may vary depending on the assay conditions (Quintana et al., 2008). The use of sensitive mouse models, such as the NOD/SCID IL2R_(null) mice, demonstrated that cell isolation through p75NTR does not enrich melanoma CSC, and melanoma cells are able to metastasize independently from their expression pattern, being able to reverse their phenotype through clonal expansion (Quintana et al., 2010; Civenni et al., 2011). Consistently, in another study CD34-neg/p75NTR-pos cells from mouse melanomas only rarely form tumors, while the p75NTR-negative counterpart frequently forms tumors, depending on CD34 expression (Held et al., 2010). This suggests that although some lines of evidence point at p75NTR as a good marker for the isolation of melanoma CSC, it may not be the right candidate. It is interesting to mention though that the frequency of p75NTR-positive cells in melanoma samples correlates with higher metastasis and worse patient prognosis (Civenni et al., 2011). Altogether, these results suggest that p75NTR-positive cells are not the CSC population in melanoma, but may retain characteristics of aggressiveness and susceptibility to metastasize. Further characterization of these cells and evaluation of the role of p75NTR in melanoma stem cells is still needed.

## 6. Conclusions

A significant progress in understanding NTs signaling in skin has been done during the last fiftheen years. Although more studies are needed to better elucidate the role of these molecules in cutaneous physiology and pathology, there is a large body of evidence indicating that NTs form a complex network with autocrine and paracrine functions. In this context, NTs and their receptors seem to play an important role in the origin, development and invasiveness of malignant melanoma. Given the premise and the common neuroectodermal origin of the skin and the nervous system, future studies will allow a better understanding of the cell of origin of melanoma and of the environment that favors the growth and metastasis of the tumor. Translating these data into clinically oriented research will possibly unravel novel strategies for the treatment of melanoma. In particular, blocking Trks will inhibit melanoma cell migration and survival, thus acting in a less toxic and more specific manner, as compared to chemotherapy. Interestingly, Lestaurtinib (CEP-701), a Trk-selective inhibitor, is effective and well tolerated in patients with refractory neuroblastoma (Minturn JE et al., 2011; Evans AE et al., 2001). In addition, inhibitors of Trk kinase activity, such as K-252a family members, have a significant anti-tumor activity in prostatic and pancreatic carcinomas, in preclinical studies.

## 7. References

Aloe, L.; Tirassa, P. & Lambiase, A. (2008). The topical application of nerve growth factor as a pharmacological tool for human corneal and skin ulcers. *Pharmacol Res*, Vol.57, pp. 253-258.

Anderson, D.J. (2000). Genes, lineages and the neural crest: a speculative review. *Philos Trans R Soc Lond B Biol Sci.* Vol.29; No.355(1399), pp.953-964.

Balch, C.M.; Buzaid, A.C.; Soong, S.J.; Atkins, M.B.; Cascinelli, N.; Coit, D.G.; Fleming, I.D.; Gershenwald, J.E.; Houghton, A. Jr; Kirkwood, J.M.; McMasters, K.M.; Mihm, M.F.; Morton, D.L.; Reintgen, D.S.; Ross, M.I.; Sober, A.; Thompson, J.A. & Thompson, J.F. (2001). Final version of the American Joint Committee on Cancer staging system for cutaneous melanoma. *J Clin Oncol*. Vol. 19, No.16, pp. 3635-3648.

Barbacid, M. (1994). The trk family of neurotrophin receptors. *J.Neurobiol,* Vol.25, pp. 1386–1403.

Barde, Y.A.; Edgar, D. & Thoenen, H. (1982). Purification of a new neurotrophic factor from mammalian brain. *EMBO J*, Vol.1, pp. 549-553.

Barker, P.A.; Lomen-Hoerth, C.; Gensch, E.M.; Meakin, S.O.; Glass, D.J. & Shooter, E.M. (1993). Tissue-specific alternative splicing generates two isoforms of the trkA receptor. *J Biol Chem,* Vol.268, pp. 15150–15157.

Beona, C.; Goggins, W.; Quinn, T.; Fullerton, J. & Tsao, H. (2003). Cutaneous melanomas associated with nevi. *Arch Dermatol,* Vol.139, No.12, pp. 1620-1624.

Boiko, A.D.; Razorenova, O.V.; van de Rijn, M.; Swetter, S.M.; Johnson, D.L.; Ly, D.P.; Butler, P.D.; Yang, G.P.; Joshua, B.; Kaplan, M.J.; Longaker, M.T. & Weissman, I.L. (2011). Human melanoma-initiating cells express neural crest nerve growth factor receptor CD271. *Nature.* Vol.470, No.7334, pp. 424.

Botchkarev, V.A.; Metz, M.; Botchkareva, N.V.; Welker, P.; Lommatzsch, M.; Renz, H. & Paus, R. (1999). Brain-derived neurotrophic factor, neurotrophin-3, and neurotrophin-4 act as "epitheliotrophins" in murine skin. *Lab Invest,* Vol.79, pp. 557-572.

Botchkarev, V.A.; Yaar, M.; Peters, E.M.; Raychaudhuri, S.P.; Botchkareva, N.V.; Marconi, A.; Raychaudhuri, S.K.; Paus, R. & Pincelli, C. (2006). Neurotrophins in skin biology and pathology. *J Invest Dermatol,* Vol.126, No.8, pp.1719-1727.

Brodeur, G.M.; Minturn, J.E.; Ho, R.; Simpson, A.M.; Iyer, R.; Varala, C.R.; Light, J.E.; Kolla, V. & Evans, A.E. (2009). Trk receptor expression and inhibition in neuroblastomas. *Clin Cancer Res,* Vol.15, pp. 3244–3250.

Bunone, G.; Margotti, A.; Compagni, A.; Moranti, E. & Della Valle, G. (1997). Induction of apoptosis by p75 neurotrophin receptor in human neuroblastoma cells. *Oncogene,* Vol.14, pp. 1463–1470.

Chao, M.V. & Hempstead, B.L. (1995). p75 and Trk: a tworeceptor system. *Trends Neurosi,* Vol.18, pp. 321–326.

Civenni, G.; Walter, A.; Kobert, N.; Mihic-Probst, D.; Zipser, M.; Belloni, B.; Seifert, B.; Moch, H.; Dummer, R.; van den Broek, M. & Sommer, L. (2011). Human CD271-Positive Melanoma Stem Cells Associated with Metastasis Establish Tumor Heterogeneity and Long-Term Growth. *Cancer Res.* Epub ahead of print

Clary, D.O. & Reichardt, L.F. (1994). An alternatively spliced form of the nerve growth factor receptor TrkA confers an enhanced response to neurotrophin 3. *Proc Natl Acad Sci U S A,* Vol.91, pp. 11133-11137.

Crowson, A.N.; Magro, C.; Miller, A. & Mihm, M.C. Jr. (2007). The molecular basis of melanomagenesis and the metastatic phenotype. *Semin Oncol.* Vol.34, No.6, pp.476-490.

Cui, J.; Shen, L.Y. & Wang, G.C. (1991). Role of hair follicles in the repigmentation of vitiligo. *J Invest Dermatol.* Vol.97, No.3, pp. 410-416.

Dasari, V.R.; Spomar, D.G.; Li L.; Gujrati, M.; Rao, J.S. & Dinh, D.H. (2008). Umbilical cord blood stem cell mediated downregulation of fas improves functional recovery of rats after spinal cord injury, *Neurochem. Res,* Vol.33, pp. 134–149.

Davis, B.M.; Fundin, B.T.; Albers, K.M.; Goodness, T.P.; Cronk, K.M. & Rice, F.L. (1997). Overexpression of nerve growth factor in skin causes preferential increases among innervation to specific sensory targets. *J Comp Neurol,* Vol.387, pp. 489-506.

Delmas, V.; Beermann, F.; Martinozzi, S.; Carreira, S.; Ackermann, J.; Kumasaka, M.; Denat, L.; Goodall, J.; Luciani, F.; Viros, A.; Demirkan, N.; Bastian, B.C.; Goding, C.R. &

Larue, L. Beta-catenin induces immortalization of melanocytes by suppressing p16INK4a expression and cooperates with N-Ras in melanoma development. *Genes Dev*. Vol.21, No.22, pp. 2923-2935.

Di Marco, E.; Marchisio, P.C.; Bondanza, S.; Franzi, A.T.; Cancedda, R. & De Luca, M. (1991). Growth-regulated synthesis and secretion of biologically active nerve growth factor by human keratinocytes. *J Biol Chem*, Vol.266, pp. 21718-21722.

Di Marco, E.; Mathor, M.; Bondanza, S.; Cutuli, N.; Marchisio, P.C.; Cancedda, R. & De Luca, M. (1993). Nerve growth factor binds to normal human keratinocytes through high and low affinity receptors and stimulates their growth by a novel autocrine loop. *J Biol Chem*, Vol.268, pp. 22838-22846.

Dupin, E.; Glavieux, C.; Vaigot, P. & Le Douarin, N.M. (2000). Endothelin 3 induces the reversion of melanocytes to glia through a neural crest-derived glial-melanocytic progenitor. *Proc Natl Acad Sci USA*, Vol.97, No.14, pp.7882-7887.

Eggert, A.; Sieverts, H.; Ikegaki, N. & Brodeur, G.M. (2000). p75 mediated apoptosis in neuroblastoma cells is inhibited by expression of TrkA. *Med Pediatr Oncol*, Vol.35, pp. 573–576.

Falabella, R., & Barona, M.I. (2009). Update on skin repigmentation therapies in vitiligo. *Pigment Cell Melanoma Res.* Vol.22, No.1, pp.42-65.

Flørenes, V.A.; Maelandsmo, G.M.; Holm, R.; Reich, R.; Lazarovici, P. & Davidson, B. (2004). Expression of activated TrkA protein in melanocytic tumors: relationship to cell proliferation and clinical outcome. *Am J Clin Pathos*, Vol.122, pp. 412–420.

Fischer, T.C.; Lauenstein, H.D.; Serowka, F.; Pilzner, C.; Groneberg, D.A. & Welker, P. (2008). Pan-neurotrophin receptor p75NTR expression is strongly induced in lesional atopic mast cells. *Clin Exp Allergy*, Vol.38, pp. 1168-1173

Frade, J.M & Barde, Y.A. (1998). Nerve growth factor: two receptors, multiple functions. *Bioessays*, Vol. 20, pp. 137-145.

Garbe, C.; Eigentler, T.K.; Keilholz, U.; Hauschild, A. & Kirkwood, J.M. (2011). Systematic review of medical treatment in melanoma: current status and future prospects. *Oncologist*. Vol.16, No.1, pp. 5-24.

Geiger, T.R.; Song, J.Y.; Rosado, A. & Peeper, D.S. (2011). Functional Characterization of Human Cancer-Derived TRKB Mutations. *PLoS One*, Vol.6, No.2, pp. e16871.

Gershon, T.R.; Oppenheimer, O.; Chin, S.S. & Gerald, W.L. (2005). Temporally regulated neural crest transcription factors distinguish neuroectodermal tumors of varying malignancy and differentiation. *Neoplasia*. Vol.7, No.6, pp.575-84.

Greene, L.A. & Kaplan, D.R. (1995). Early events in neurotrophin signalling via Trk and p75 receptors. *Curr Opin Neurobiol*, Vol.5, pp. 579–587.

Guiton, M., Gunn-Moore, F. J., Glass, D. J., Geis, D. R., Yancopoulos, G. D. & Tavare, J. M. (1995). Naturally occurring tyrosine kinase inserts block high affinity binding of phospholipase C gamma and Shc to TrkC and neurotrophin-3 signaling. *J. Biol. Chem*, Vol.270, No.20, pp. 384–390.

He, X.L. & Garcia, K.C. (2004). Structure of nerve growth factor complexed with the shared neurotrophin receptor p75. *Sciente*, Vol.304, pp. 870-875.

Held, M.A.; Curley, D.P.; Dankort, D.; McMahon, M.; Muthusamy, V. & Bosenberg, M.W. (2010). Characterization of melanoma cells capable of propagating tumors from a single cell. *Cancer Res*, Vol.70, No.1, pp. 388-397.

Hempstead, B.L.; Rabin, S.J.; Kaplan, L.; Reid, S.; Parada, L.F. & Kaplan, D.R. (1992). Overexpression of the trk tyrosine kinase rapidly accelerates nerve growth factor-induced differentiation. *Neuron*, Vol.9, pp. 883–896.

Hoek, K.S. & Godine, C.R. (2010). Cancer stem cells versus phenotype-switching in melanoma. *Pigment Cell Melanoma Res.*, Vol.23, No.6, pp.746-759.

Huang, E.J. & Reichardt, L.F. (2003). Trk receptors: roles in neuronal signal transduction. *Annu Rev Biochem*; Vol. 72, pp. 609-642.

Huttenbach, Y.; Prieto, V.G. & Reed, J.A. (2002). Desmoplastic and spindle cell melanomas express protein markers of the neural crest but not of later committed stages of Schwann cell differentiation. *J Cutan Pathos*, Vol.29, pp. 562-568.

Kaplan, D.R. & Miller, F.D. (2004). Neurobiology: a move to sort life from death. *Nature*, Vol.427, pp. 798-799.

Kinkelin, I.; Stucky, C.L. & Koltzenburg, M. (1999). Postnatal loss of Merkel cells, but not of slowly adapting mechanoreceptors in mice lacking the neurotrophin receptor p75. *Eur J Neurosi*, Vol.11, pp. 3963-3969.

Iwamoto, S.; Burrows, R.C.; Agoff, S.N.; Piepkorn, M.; Bothwell, M. & Schmidt, R. (2001). The p75 neurotrophin receptor, relative to other Schwann cell and melanoma markers, is abundantly Expressed in spindled melanomas. *Am J Dermatopathol*, Vol.23, pp. 288-294.

Indo, Y. (2001). Molecular basis of congenital insensitivity to pain with anhidrosis (CIPA): mutations and polymorphisms in TRKA (NTRK1) gene encoding the receptor tyrosine kinase for nerve growth factor. *Hum Mutat*, Vol.18, pp. 462-471.

Ingraham, C.A.; Wertalik, L. & Schor, N.F. (2011). Necdin and neurotrophin receptors: interactors of relevance for neuronal resistance to oxidant stress. *Pediatr Res*, Vol.69, No.4, pp. 279-284.

Johnsen, J.I.; Kogner, P.; Albihn, A. & Henriksson, M.A. (2009). Embryonal neural tumours and cell death. *Apoptosis*, Vol.14, pp. 424–438.

Kanik, A.B.; Yaar, M. & Bhawan, J. (1996). P75 nerve growth factor receptor staining helps identify desmoplastic and neurotropic melanoma. *J Cutan Pathol*, Vol.23, pp. 205-210.

Kim, J.Y.; Sutton, M.E.; Lu, D.J.; Cho, T.A.; Goumnerova, L.C.; Goritchenko, L.; Kaufman, J.R.; Lam, K.K.; Billet, A.L.; Tarbell, N.J.; Wu, J.; Allen, J.C.; Stiles, C.D.; Segal, R.A. & Pomeroy, S.L. (1999). Activation of neurotrophin-3 receptor TrkC induces apoptosis in medulloblastomas. *Cancer Res*, Vol.59, pp. 711–719.

Kruger, G.M.; Mosher, J.T.; Bixby, S.; Joseph, N.; Iwashita, T.; Morrison, S.J. (2002). Neural crest stem cells persist in the adult gut but undergo changes in self-renewal, neuronal subtype potential, and factor responsiveness. *Neuron*, Vol.35, No.4, pp. 657-669.

Krüttgen, A.; Schneider, I. & Weis, J. (2006). The dark side of the NGF family: neurotrophins in neoplasias. *Brain Pathol*, Vol.16, No.4, pp. 304-310.

Landi, F.; Aloe, L.; Russo, A.; Cesari, M.; Onder, G.; Bonini, S.; Carbonin, P.U. & Bernabei, R. (2003). Topical Treatment of Pressure Ulcers with Nerve Growth Factor. A Randomized Clinical Trial. *Ann Int Med*, Vol.139 , No.8, pp. 635-641.

Langtimm-Sedlak, C.J.; Schroeder, B.; Saskowski, J.L.; Carnahan, J.F.; & Sieber-Blum, M. (1996). Multiple actions of stem cell factor in neural crest cell differentiation in vitro. *Dev Biol*, Vol.174, No.2, pp. 345-359.

Lazova, R.; Tantcheva-Poor, I. & Sigal, A.C. (2010). p75 nerve growth factor receptor staining is superior to S100 in identifying spindle cell and desmoplastic melanoma. *J Am Acad Dermatol*, Vol.63, pp. 852-858.

Levi-Montalcini, R. (1987). The nerve growth factor 35 years later. *Sciente*, Vol.237, pp. 1154-1162.

Li, L.; Fukunaga-Kalabis, M.; Yu, H.; Xu, X.; Kong, J.; Lee, J.T. & Herlyn, M. (2010). Human dermal stem cells differentiate into functional epidermal melanocytes. *J Cell Sci*, Vol.123, pp. 853-860.

Lu, B.; Pang, P.T. & Woo, N.H. (2005). The yin and yang of neurotrophin action. *Nat Rev Neurosi*, Vol.6, No8, pp. 603-614.

Luberg, K.; Wong, J.; Weickert, C.S. & Timmusk, T. (2010). Human TrkB gene: novel alternative transcripts, protein isoforms and expression pattern in the prefrontal cerebral cortex during postnatal development. *J Neurochem*, Vol.113, pp. 952-964.

Lugassy, C. & Barnhill, R.L. (2007). Angiotropic melanoma and extravascular migratory metastasis: a review. *Adv Anat Pathol.* Vol.14, No.3, pp. 195-201.

Marconi, A.; Vaschieri, C.; Zanoli, S.; Giannetti, A. & Pincelli, C. (1999). Nerve growth factor protects human keratinocytes from ultraviolet-B-induced apoptosis. *J Invest Dermatol*, Vol.113, pp. 920-927.

Marconi, A.; Terracina, M.; Fila, C.; Franchi, J.; Bonté, F.; Romagnoli, G.; Maurelli, R.; Failla, C.M.; Dumas, M. & Pincelli, C. (2003). Expression and function of neurotrophins and their receptors in cultured human keratinocytes. *J Invest Dermatol*, Vol.121, pp. 1515-21. Erratum in: J Invest Dermatol 2004; 123:803.

Marconi, A.; Panza, M.C.; Bonnet-Duquennoy, M.; Lazou, K.; Kurfurst, R.; Truzzi, F.; Lotti, R.; De Santis, G.; Dumas, M.; Bonté, F. & Pincelli, C. (2006). Espression and function of neurotrophins and their receptors in human melanocytes. *Int.J Cosmet Sci*, Vol.28, pp. 255-261.

Marchetti, D.; Denkins, Y.; Reiland, J.; Greiter-Wilke, A.; Galjour, J.; Murry, B.; Blust, J. & Roy, M. (2003). Brain-metastatic melanoma: a neurotrophic perspective. *Pathol Oncol Res*, Vol.9, pp. 147–158

Marshall, J.S.; Gomi, K.; Blennerhassett, M.G. & Bienenstock, J. (1999). Nerve growth factor modifies the expression of inflammatory cytokines by mast cells via a prostanoid-dependent mechanism. *J Immunol*, Vol.162, pp. 4271-4276.

Micera, A.; Vigneti, E.; Pickholtz, D.; Reich, R.; Pappo, O.; Bonini, S.; Maquart, F.X.; Aloe, L. & Levi-Schaffer, F. (2001). Nerve growth factor displays stimulatory effects on human skin and lung fibroblasts, demonstrating a direct role for this factor in tissue repair. *Proc Natl Acad Sci USA*, Vol.98, pp. 6162-6167.

Micera, A.; Lambiase, A.; Stampachiacchiere, B.; Sgrulletta, R.; Normando, E.M.; Bovini, S. & Bovini, S. (2007b). Nerve growth factor has a modulatory role on human primary fibroblast cultures derived from vernal keratoconjunctivitis-affected conjunctiva. *Mol Vis*, Vol.13, pp. 981-987.

Montaño, J.A.; Pérez-Piñera, P.; García-Suárez, O.; Cobo, J. & Vega, J.A. (2010). Development and neuronal dependence of cutaneous sensory nerve formations: Lessons from neurotrophins. *Microsc Res Tech*, Vol.73, pp. 513-529.

Murray, S.S.; Perez, P.; Lee, R. Hempstead, B.L. & Chao, M.V. (2004). A novel p75 neurotrophin receptor-related protein, NRH2, regulates nerve growth factor binding to the TrkA receptor. *J Neurosi*, Vol.24, pp. 2742-2749.

Nakagawara, A.; Arima-Nakagawara, M.; Scavarla, N.J.;. Azar, C.G.; Cantor, A.B. & Brodeur, G.M. (1993). Association between high levels of expression of the Trk gene and favorable outcome in human neuroblastomas *N. Engl. J. Med.*, Vol.328, pp. 847–854.

Nakagawara, A. (2001). Trk receptor tyrosine kinases: a bridge between cancer and neural development, *Cancer Lett*, Vol.169, pp.107–114.

Nishikawa, S. & Osawa, M. (2007). Generating quiescent stem cells. *Pigment Cell Res*, Vol.20, No.4, pp. 263-270.

Nishimura, E.K.; Jordan, S.A.; Oshima, H.; Yoshida, H.; Osawa, M.; Moriyama, M.; Jackson, I.J.; Barrandon, Y.; Miyachi, Y. & Nishikawa, S. (2002). Dominant role of the niche in melanocyte stem-cell fate determination. *Nature*, Vol.416, No.6883, pp. 854-860.

Nykjaer, A.; Lee, R.; Teng, K.K.; Jansen, P.; Madsen, P.; Nielsen, M.S.; Jacobsen, C.; Kliemannel, M.; Schwarz, E.; Willnow, T.E.; Hempstead, B.L. & Petersen, C.M. (2004). Sortilin is essential for proNGF-induced neuronal cell death. *Nature*, Vol.427, No.6977, pp. 843-848.

Ohta, T.; Watanabe, T.; Katayama, Y.; Kurihara, J.; Yoshino, A.; Nishimoto, H. & Kishimoto, H. (2006). TrkA expression is associated with an elevated level of apoptosis in classic medulloblastomas. *Neuropathology*, Vol.26, pp. 170–177.

Palazzo, E.; Marconi, A.; Truzzi, F.; Dallaglio, K.; Petrachi, T.; Humbert, P.; Schnebert, S.; Perrier, E.; Dumas, M. & Pincelli, C. (2011). Role of neurotrophins on dermal fibroblast survival and differentiation. *J Cell Physiol.*, doi: 10.1002/jcp.22811.

Papatsoris, A.G.; Liolitsa, D. & Deliveliotis, C. (2007). Manipulation of the nerve growth factor network in prostate cancer. *Expert Opin Investig Drugs*, Vol.16, No.3, pp. 303-309.

Paratore, C.; Goerich, D.E.; Suter, U.; Wegner, M. & Sommer, L. (2001). Survival and glial fate acquisition of neural crest cells are regulated by an interplay between the transcription factor Sox10 and extrinsic combinatorial signaling. *Development*, Vol.128, No.20, pp. 3949-3961.

Paus, R.; Lüftl, M. & Czarnetzki, B.M. (1994). Nerve growth factor modulates keratinocyte proliferation in murine skin organ culture. *Br J Dermatol*, Vol.130, pp. 174-180.

Peacocke, M.; Yaar, M.; Mansur, C.P.; Chao, M.V. & Gilchrest, B.A. (1988). Induction of nerve growth factor receptor on cultured human melanocytes. *Proc Natl Acad Sci USA*, Vol.85, pp. 5282-5286.

Perez-Pinera, P.; García-Suarez, O.; Germanà, A.; Díaz-Esnal, B.; de Carlos, F.; Silos-Santiago, I.; del Valle, M.E.; Cobo,J. & Vega, J.A. (2008). Characterization of sensory deficits in TrkB knockout mice. *Neurosci Lett*, Vol.433, pp. 43-47.

Perlis, C. & Herlyn, M. (2004). Recent advances in melanoma biology. *Oncologist*, Vol.9, pp.182–187.

Pincelli, C.; Fantini, F. & Giannetti, A. (1994). Nerve growth factor and the skin. *Int J Fermato*, Vol.33, pp. 308-312.

Pincelli, C.; Haake, A.R.; Benassi, L.; Grassilli, E.; Magnoni, C.; Ottani, D.; Polakowska, R.; Franceschi, C. & Giannetti, A. (1997). Autocrine nerve growth factor protects human keratinocytes from apoptosis through its high affinity receptor (TRK): a role for BCL-2. *J Invest Dermatol*, Vol.109, pp. 757-764.

Quintana, E.; Shackleton, M.; Sabel, M.S.; Fullen, D.R.; Johnson, T.M. & Morrison, S.J. (2008). Efficient tumour formation by single human melanoma cells. *Nature*, Vol.456, No.7222, pp. 593-598.

Quintana, E.; Shackleton, M.; Foster, H.R.; Fullen, D.R.; Sabel, M.S.; Johnson, T.M. & Morrison, S.J. (2010). Phenotypic heterogeneity among tumorigenic melanoma cells from patients that is reversible and not hierarchically organized. *Cancer Cell*, Vol.18, No.5, pp. 510-523.

Real, C.; Glavieux-Pardanaud, C.; Le Douarin, N.M. & Dupin, E. (2006). Clonally cultured differentiated pigment cells can dedifferentiate and generate multipotent progenitors with self-renewing potential. *Dev Biol*, Vol.300, No.2, pp.656-669.

Reichardt, L.F. (2006). Neurotrophin-regulated signalling pathways. *Philos Trans R Soc Lond B Biol Sci*, Vol.361, pp.1545–1564.

Rifkin, J.T.; Todd, V.J.; Anderson, L.W. & Lefcort, F. (2000). Dynamic expression of neurotrophin receptors during sensory neuron genesis and differentiation. *Dev Biol.* Vol.227, No.2, pp. 465-480.

Rodriguez-Tébar, A.; Dechant, G. & Barde, Y.A. (1990). Binding of brain-derived neurotrophic factor to the nerve growth factor receptor. *Neuron*, Vol.4, pp. 487-492.

Roesch, A.; Fukunaga-Kalabis, M.; Schmidt, E.C.; Zabierowski, S.E.; Brafford, P.A.; Vultur, A.; Basu, D.; Gimotty, P.; Vogt, T. & Herlyn, M. (2010). A temporarily distinct subpopulation of slow-cycling melanoma cells is required for continuous tumor growth. *Cell*, Vol.141, pp. 583–594.

Rogers, M.L.; Beare, A.; Zola, H. & Rush, R.A. (2008). CD 271 (P75 neurotrophin receptor). *J Biol Regul Homeost Agents.* Vol.22, No.1, pp. 1-6.

Roux, P.P. & Barker, P.A. (2002). Neurotrohin signaling through the p75 neurotrophin receptor. *Prog Neurobiol*, Vol.67, pp. 203–233.

Sabatino, M.; Stroncek, D.F.; Klein, H.; Marincola, F.M. & Wang, E. (2009). Stem cells in melanoma development. *Cancer Lett.*, Vol.279, No.2, pp. 119-125.

Segal, R.A. (2003). Selectivity in neurotrophin signaling: theme and variations. *Annu Rev Neurosi*, Vol.26, pp. 299-330.

Segal, R.A.; Goumnerova, L.C.; Kwon, Y.K.; Stiles, C.D. & Pomeroy, S.L. (1994). Expression of the neurotrophin receptor TrkC is linked to a favorable outcome in medulloblastoma. *Proc Natl Acad Sci U S A.* Vol.91, No.26, pp. 12867-12871.

Shonukan, O.; Bagayogo, I.; McCrea, P.; Chao, M. & Hempstead, B. (2003). Neurotrophin-induced melanoma cell migration is mediated through the actin-bundling protein fascin. *Oncogene*, Vol.22, pp. 3616-3623.

Sieber-Blum, M. & Grim, M. (2004). The adult hair follicle: cradle for pluripotent neural crest stem cells, *Birth Defects Res. C: Embryo Today*, Vol.72 , No.2, pp. 162–172.

Sieber-Blum, M.; Grim, M.; Hu, Y.F. & Szeder, V. (2004). Pluripotent neural crest stem cells in the adult hair follicle. *Dev. Dyn*, Vol.231, pp. 258–269.

Stefanato, C.M.; Yaar, M.; Bhawan, J.; Philips, T.J.; Kosmadaki, M.G.; Botchkarev, V. & Gilchrest, B.A. (2003). Modulations of nerve growth factor and Bcl-2 in ultraviolet-irradiated human epidermis. *J Cutan Pathos*, Vol.30, pp. 351-357.

Stemple, D.L. & Anderson, D.J. (1992). Isolation of a stem cell for neurons and glia from the mammalian neural crest. *Cell*, Vol.71, No.6, pp. 973-985.

Sun, W.; Lin, H.; Chen, B.; Zhao, W.; Zhao, Y.; Xiao, Z. & Dai, J. (2010). Collagen scaffolds loaded with collagen-binding NGF-beta accelerate ulcer healing. *J Biomed Mater Res A*, Vol.92, pp. 887-895.

Szeder, V.; Grim, M.; Kucera, J. & Sieber-Blum, M. (2003). Neurotrophin-3 signaling in mammalian Merkel cell development. *Dev Dyn*, Vol. 228, pp. 623-629.

Strohmaier, C.; Carter, B.D.; Urfer, R.; Barde, Y.A. & Dechant, G. (1996). A splice variant of the neurotrophin receptor trkB with increased specificity for brain-derived neurotrophic factor. *EMBO J*, Vol.15, pp. 3332-3337.

Tacconelli, A.; Farina, A.R.; Cappabianca, L.; Gulino, A. & Mackay, A.R. (2005). TrkAIII. A novel hypoxia-regulated alternative TrkA splice variant of potential physiological and pathological importance. *Cell Cycle*, Vol.4, pp. 8–9.

Tauszig-Delamasure, S.; Yu, L.Y.; Cabrera, J.R.; Bouzas-Rodriguez, J.; Mermet-Bouvier, C.; Guix, C.; Bordeaux, M.C.; Arumäe, U. & Mehlen, P. (2007). The TrkC receptor induces apoptosis when the dependence receptor notion meets the neurotrophin paradigm. *Proc Natl Acad Sci USA*, Vol.14, No.104, pp.13361-13366.

Teng, K.K. & Hempstead, B.L. (2004). Neurotrophins and their receptors: Signaling trios in complex biological systems. *Cell Mol Life Sci*, Vol.61, pp.35–48.

Thiele, C.J.; Li, Z. & McKee, A.E. (2009). On Trk--the TrkB signal transduction pathway is an increasingly important target in cancer biology. *Clin Cancer Res*, Vol.15, No.19, pp. 5962-5967.

Tiberio, R.; Marconi, A.; Fila, C.; Fumelli, C.; Pignatta, M.; Krajewski, S.; Giannetti, A.; Reed, J.C. & Pincelli, C. (2002). Keratinocytes enriched for stem cells are protected from anoikis via an integrin signaling pathway in a Bcl-2 dependent manner. *FEBS Lett*, Vol.524, pp. 139-144.

Tron, V.A.; Coughlin, M.D.; Jang, D.E.; Stanisz, J. & Sauder, D.N. (1990). Expression and modulation of nerve growth factor in murine keratinocytes (PAM 212). *J Clin Invest*, Vol.85, pp. 1085.

Truzzi, F.; Marconi, A.; Lotti, R.; Dall'aglio, K.; French, L.E. & Hempstead, B.L. & Pincelli, C. (2008). Neurotrophins and their receptors stimulate melanoma cell proliferation and migration. *J Invest Dermatol*, Vol.128, pp. 2031-2040.

Truzzi, F.; Marconi, A.; Atzei, P.; Panza, M.C.; Lotti, R.; Dall'aglio, K.; Tiberio, R.; Palazzo, E.; Vaschieri C. & Pincelli, C. p75 neurotrophin receptor mediates apoptosis in transit-amplifying cells and its overexpression restores cell death in psoriatic keratinocytes. *Cell Death Differ*. (2011) Vol.18, pp. 948-958.

Ultsch, M.H.; Wiesmann, C.; Simmons, L.C.; Henrich, J.; Yang, M.; Reilly, D.; Bass, S.H. & de Vos,A.M. (1999). Crystal structures of the neurotrophin-binding domain of TrkA, TrkB and TrkC. *J Mol Biol*, Vol.290, pp.149-159.

Yeo, G.S.; Conie Hung, C.C.; Rochford, J.; Keogh. J.; Gray, J.; Sivaramakrishnan, S.; O'Rahilly, S. & Faroogi, I.S. (2004). A de novo mutation affecting human TrkB associated with severe obesity and developmental delay. *Nat Neurosi*, Vol.7, pp. 1187-1189.

Walch, E.T.; Albino, A.P. & Marchetti, D. (1999). Correlation of overexpression of the low-affinity p75 neurotrophin receptor with augmented invasion and heparanase production in human malignant melanoma cells. *Int J Cancer*, Vol.82, pp. 112–120.

Wang, J.J.; Tapinat, A.; Ethell, D.W.; Testa, M.P. & Bredesen, D.E. (2000). Phosphorylation of the common neurotrophin receptor p75 by p38beta2 kinase affects NF-kappaB and AP-1 activities. *J Mol Neurosi*, Vol.15, pp. 19-29.

Yaar, M.; Grossman, K.; Eller, M. & Gilchrest, B.A. (1991). Evidente for nerve growth factor-mediated paracrine effects in human epidermis. *J Cell Biol*, Vol.115, pp. 821-828.

Yaar, M., Eller, M.S.; DiBenedetto, P.; Reenstra, W.R.; Zhai, S.; McQuaid, T.; Archambault, M. & Gilchrest, B.A. (1994). The trk family of receptors mediates nerve growth factor and neurotrophin-3 effects in melanocytes. *J Clin Invest.*, Vol.94, pp. 1550-1562.

Yamashiro, D.J.; Nakagawara, A.; Ikegaki, N.; Liu, X.G. & Brodeur, G.M. (1996). Expression of TrkC in favorable human neuroblastomas. *Oncogene*, Vol.12, pp. 37–41.

Yu, H.; Fang, D.; Kumar, S. M.; Li, L.; Nguyen, T. K.; Acs, G.; Herlyn, M. & Xu, X. (2006). Isolation of a novel population of multipotent adult stem cells from human hair follicles. *Am. J. Pathos*, Vol.168, pp. 1879-1888.

Zabierowski, S.E. & Herlyn, M. (2008). Learning the ABCs of melanoma-initiating cells. *Cancer Cell*. Vol.13, No.3, pp.185-187.

Zhai, S.; Yaar, M.; Doyle, S.M. & Gilchrest, B.A. (1996). Nerve growth factor rescues pigment cells from ultraviolet-induced apoptosis by upregulating BCL-2 levels. *Exp Cell Res*, pp. 224-335.

Zhang, J.M.; Hoffmann, R. & Sieber-Blum, M. (1997). Mitogenic and anti-proliferative signals for neural crest cells and the neurogenic action of TGF-beta1. *Dev Dyn*, Vol.208, No.3, pp.375-386.

Wang, Q.; Fang, W.H.; Krupinski, J.; Kumar, S.; Slevin, M. & Kumar, P. (2008). Pax genes in embryogenesis and oncogenesis. *J Cell Mol Med.* Vol.12, No.6A, pp. 2281-2294.

# 14

# The Jak-STAT Signal Transduction Pathway in Melanoma

Courtney Nicholas and Gregory B. Lesinski
*The Ohio State University*
*Department of Internal Medicine*
*Division of Medical Oncology*
*USA*

## 1. Introduction

The Janus-activated kinase (Jak)-signal transducer and activator of transcription (STAT) pathway is thought to play a central role in melanoma cell biology. Membrane-associated Jak proteins can couple with a variety of receptors to transmit signals into the cytoplasm. Immediately downstream, are the STAT family of transcription factors, which can be influenced by a variety of post-translational modifications and localize to the cell nucleus, directly binding DNA. In response to extracellular stimuli or through dysregulated activation of other signaling molecules, STAT proteins are often constitutively phosphorylated or 'activated' in melanoma cells. The balance between the activation of individual STAT proteins influences unique gene expression profiles within melanoma cells. For example, gene expression driven via the STAT1 transcription factor is associated with growth inhibition, resistance to apoptosis and reduced angiogenesis. Conversely, the STAT3 transcription factor mediates a gene expression profile associated with cell growth, anti-apoptosis, angiogenesis, metastasis and immune suppression. Altered activity of STAT proteins has been demonstrated in both melanoma cells, and interestingly, in the immune system of patients with melanoma. Recent data suggest that targeting the aberrant activation of this signal transduction pathway could have therapeutic effects via both modulating tumor cell and host immune function. In this chapter, we aim to summarize the role of the Jak-STAT pathway in melanoma, with a focus on the seemingly divergent effect of the STAT1 and STAT3 transcription factors. We will also highlight recent data suggesting that inhibition of signal transduction via the STAT3 pathway may be of interest as a future therapeutic approach for melanoma.

## 2. Melanoma

Melanoma represents a complex and heterogeneous form of cancer that relies on altered molecular pathways within the tumor cell and cooperation from the host immune system to permit its growth and progression. The incidence of malignant melanoma is rising faster than any other cancer. In the United States alone, more than 68,000 new cases of melanoma were diagnosed in the year 2009 (Jemal, A. et al. 2010). The median survival of patients with metastatic melanoma is approximately 10 months even with aggressive systemic therapy (Atkins, M. B. 1998). Limited treatment options are available to patients with metastatic disease, and standard chemotherapeutic and immunologic agents are ineffective in a majority of patients. Therefore, there remains an urgent need to understand melanoma biology so that novel targets for therapeutic intervention can be identified and evaluated. Over the past several years, an increased understanding of the molecular pathways driving melanoma have allowed for some advances to be made in our ability to treat this disease. Namely, discovery of an activating mutation of the B-Raf protein at the V600 locus has led to the development of small molecule inhibitors of this mutated protein or its downstream pathways, such as MAPK, ERK and MEK (Ball, N. J. et al. 1994; Davies, H. et al. 2002; Pollock, P. M. et al. 2003; Smalley, K. S. et al. 2008). The agents targeting mutated B-Raf have produced impressive regression of established melanoma lesions, leading to their FDA-approval. However, these dramatic responses do not typically persist for more than several months before new melanoma lesions arise and many patients progress (Aplin, A. E. et al. 2011) . Clearly there remains a need for identifying novel pathways in melanoma that could serve as therapeutic targets and be utilized to improve both single-agent or combination treatment options for this disease.

In addition to aberrant molecular pathways within malignant cells, there is strong evidence that the immune system plays a role in regulating the development and progression of melanoma. For example, melanoma incidence is increased in patients who are immunosuppressed (Vajdic, C. M. et al. 2009) and circulating, tumor-antigen specific T cells are present in patients with melanoma (Kawakami, Y. et al. 1994). Melanoma is also considered a tumor in which immune-based therapies can elicit dramatic clinical responses in a subset of patients. Recombinant cytokines such as interleukin-2 (IL-2), interferon-alpha (IFN-α) and granulocyte macrophage colony stimulating factor (GM-CSF) have been clinically utilized for treatment for melanoma patients at various disease stages ranging from metastatic disease to adjuvant therapy. In addition, the use of Ipilimumab, an antibody targeting the negative regulatory CTLA-4 receptor on T cells has recently gained FDA-approval for the treatment of metastatic melanoma (Traynor, K. 2011). In those melanoma patients who respond to immune-based therapies, vitiligo and autoimmune phenomena are often observed, further supporting a role for the immune system in regulating this malignancy (Bouwhuis, M. G. et al. 2010; Gogas, H. et al. 2006). As we gain experience with using new molecular-targeted agents for melanoma therapy, it will also be important to assess how these compounds modulate immune function of patients, as it relates to cancer progression or anti-tumor immune responses.

## 3. The Jak-STAT signal transduction pathway

The Janus-activated kinase (Jak)-signal transducer and activator of transcription (STAT) pathway is a signal transduction pathway that has been well-characterized in basic biologic study (Darnell, J. E., Jr. et al. 1994; Haque, S. J. et al. 1998). This pathway is thought to play a major role in regulating both the development and elimination of cancer. The various protein components of the Jak-STAT pathway are expressed ubiquitously within a majority of somatic cells. Four individual members of the Jak family of proteins (Jak1, Jak2, Jak3, Tyk2) and seven unique STAT proteins (STAT1-STAT7) have been identified. The structural features of these proteins are presented in Figures 1 and 2 in this section.

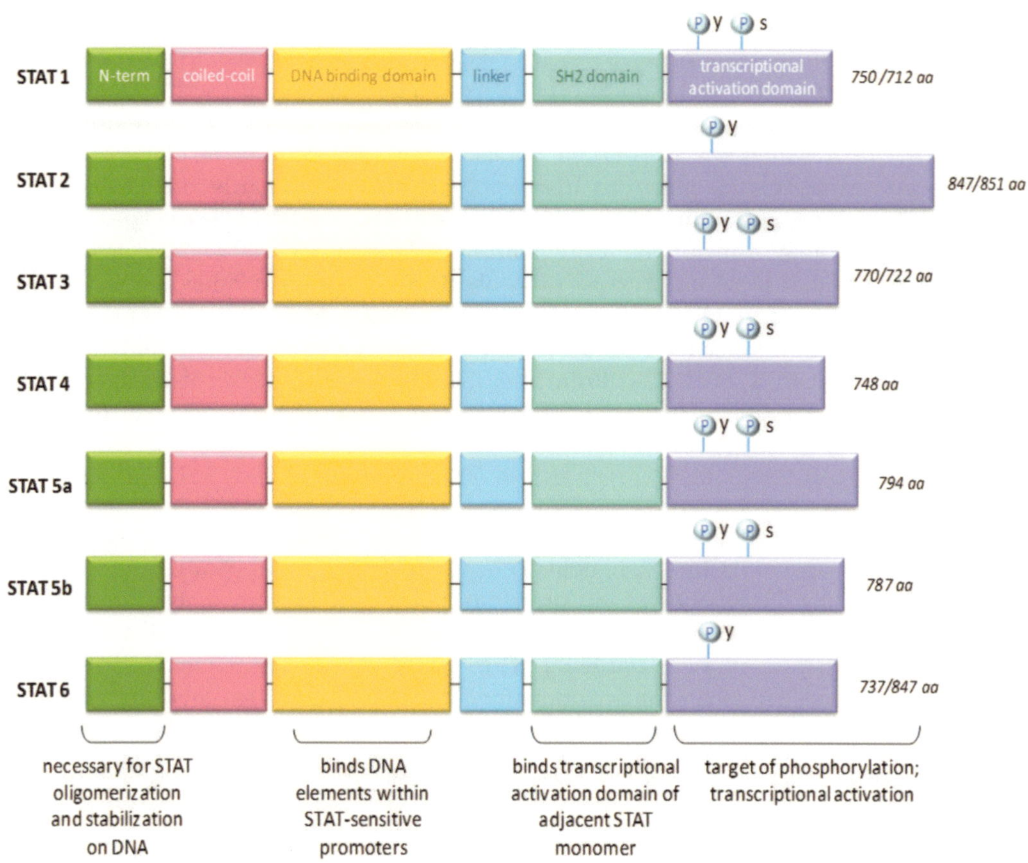


Fig. 1. Structural homology of the STAT family of transcription factors. P = phosphorylation, y = tyrosine, s = serine; isoforms are indicated by number of amino acids (aa). Adapted from (Jatiani, S. S. et al. 2010; Yue, P. et al. 2009)

A number of extracellular receptors can directly associate with Jak proteins residing in the cell membrane. The Jak proteins are typically activated upon binding of a ligand (typically a cytokine) to the receptor in normal cells, although they can be constitutively activated in malignant cells. Activation of Jak proteins leads to post-translational modifications of cytoplasmic STAT proteins that influence their subsequent cellular actions. Phosphorylation of STAT proteins is the most well-characterized of these modifications, an action which typically allows for STAT proteins to dimerize and translocate to the nucleus.

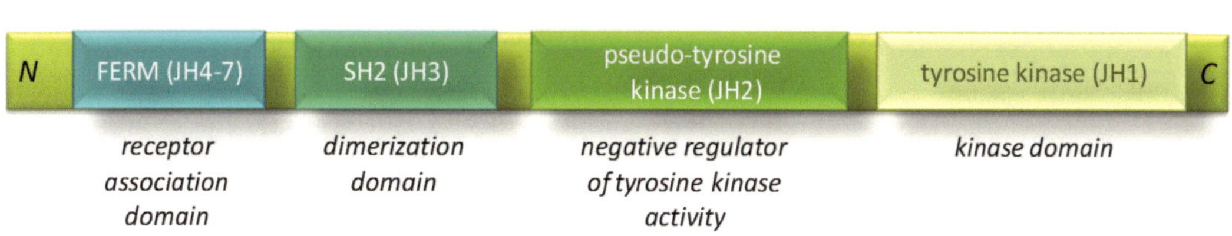


Fig. 2. Basic structure of Jak/Tyk kinases involved in STAT pathways. Adapted from (Jatiani, S. S. et al. 2010)

Other kinases such as Src or Abelson (Abl) kinases can also lead to STAT protein phosphorylation (Al Zaid Siddiquee, K. et al. 2008). Once in the nucleus, STAT proteins can cooperate with other co-factors, bind to promoters and activate the transcription of specific genes involved in a diverse array of cellular processes. The profile of individual STAT proteins that are activated has a profound influence upon the biologic response of the cell. For the purposes of this chapter, our discussion will focus primarily on the difference between biologic responses induced by STAT1 as compared to STAT3. These specific STAT proteins appear to play a major role in regulating melanoma biology and the response of this cancer to various types of therapy (Ransohoff, R. M. 1998). Under normal biologic conditions, activation of STAT proteins is rapid and transient. However, aberrant activation of the STAT proteins is associated with a variety of human malignancies (Al Zaid Siddiquee, K. et al. 2008) (Bowman, T. et al. 2000; Bromberg, J. F. 2001; Buettner, R. et al. 2002; Darnell, J. E., Jr. 2002; Darnell, J. E. 2005; Turkson, J. 2004; Turkson, J. et al. 2000; Yu, H. et al. 2004).

## 4. STAT1

The STAT1 transcription factor has been traditionally viewed as a 'tumor suppressor' (Bromberg, J. F. et al. 1996; Chin, Y. E. et al. 1997; Kaplan, D. H. et al. 1998). A great deal of knowledge regarding the function of this protein has been gained from analysis of its role in mediating signal transduction in response to cytokines such as the Type I and Type II interferons (Darnell, J. E., Jr. 1998; Darnell, J. E., Jr. et al. 1994; Haque, S. J. et al. 1998). These studies have established that transcriptionally active STAT1 is required for the anti-proliferative effects of interferons (Bromberg, J. F. et al. 1996). This is particularly relevant in the setting of melanoma, where aside from their immunostimulatory effects, interferons can bind their receptors and exert direct anti-proliferative effects against the tumor cell.

It has also been observed that some interferon-resistant human melanoma cell lines exhibited defects in specific Jak-STAT intermediates, which when reversed led to the recovery of in vitro sensitivity to interferons (Kaplan, D. H. et al. 1998; Pansky, A. et al. 2000; Huang, M. et al. 2002; Wong, L. H. et al. 1998). Interestingly, the most common defect appeared to be the loss of STAT1. These data support a role for STAT1 as a negative regulator of melanoma cell proliferation. In other cell types, STAT1 has been shown to negatively regulate the cell cycle by down-regulating the expression of cyclins, c-myc and by inducing the CDK inhibitors p21 and p27 (Regis, G. et al. 2008). A brief overview of STAT1 transcriptional targets can be found in Figure 3.

The STAT1 transcription factor is also important for mediating melanoma cell sensitivity to various pro-apoptotic stimuli. In a sentinel study by Kumar et al., it was shown that STAT1-deficient human fibrosarcoma cells were less susceptible to tumor necrosis factor alpha (TNF-α) induced cell death as compared to parental cells containing STAT1 (Kumar, A. et al. 1997). This STAT1 dependent regulation of cell death is largely dependent on a transcriptional mechanism such as the activation of death-promoting genes, or induction of the Interferon Regulatory Factor 1 (IRF1) (Bernabei, P. et al. 2001; Sato, T. et al. 1997; Regis, G. et al. 2005; Kim, H. S. et al. 2007). For example, STAT1 can regulate the expression of death-receptor-4 (DR4) expression on melanoma cells, which could affect TRAIL sensitivity (Meng, R. D. et al. 2001). Similarly, STAT1 has also been shown to upregulate the expression of caspases, Fas, and FasL, (Kumar, A. et al. 1997; Chin, Y. E. et al. 1996; Lee, C. K. et al. 2000; Ouchi, T. et al. 2000; Stephanou, A. et al. 2005). Non-transcriptional mechanisms such as the ability of STAT1 to interact with TRADD, p53 or HDAC have also been implicated in the regulation of cell death by STAT1 (Kim, H. S. et al. 2007). The precise role for these STAT1-mediated factors in regulating apoptosis specifically in melanoma cells is an area of interest that could be exploited for further therapeutic benefit.

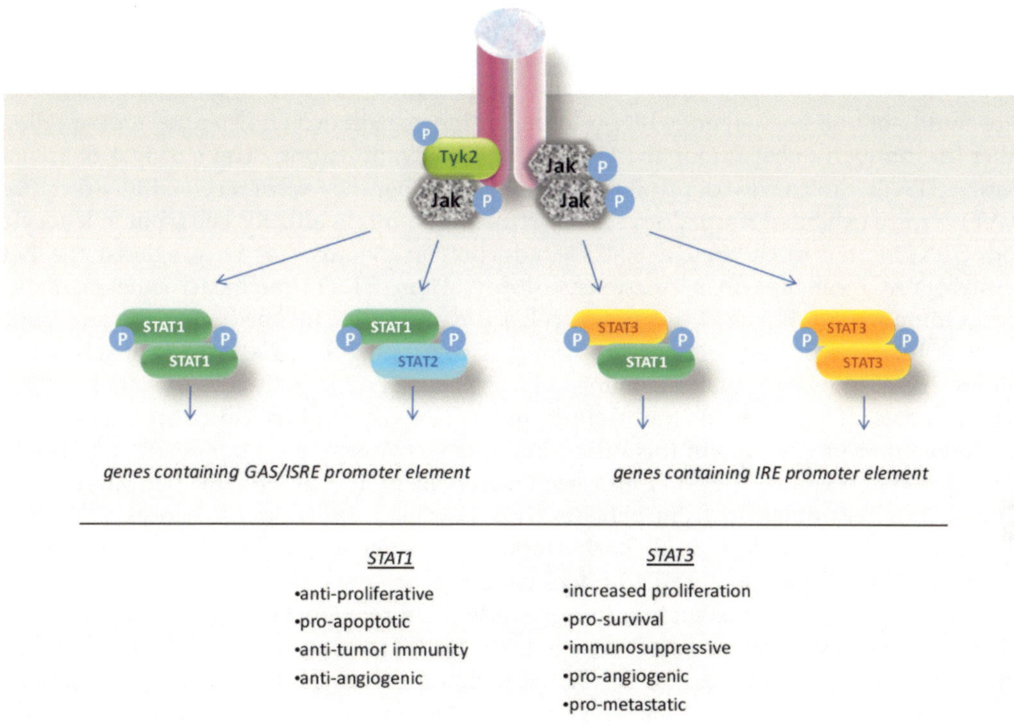


Fig. 3. Comparison of STAT1 and STAT3 signaling and their effects in cancer. Adapted from (Yu, H. et al. 2009)

Other evidence that supports a role for STAT1 as a tumor suppressor gene has come from STAT1-deficient mice. These animals were initially described by Durbin *et al.*, and found to be more susceptible to infection with microbial pathogens. It was discovered that these animals had defective immune responses, and more specifically in their lack of interferon-responsiveness (Durbin, J. E. et al. 1996). Later studies showed that these animals were also more susceptible to tumorigenesis induced by exposure to chemical carcinogens as compared to their wild-type counterparts (Kaplan, D. H. et al. 1998). Finally, when crossed on to a p53-deficient background, STAT1-deficient mice demonstrated a greater propensity for tumor development as compared to mice lacking either p53 or STAT1 alone (Kaplan, D. H. et al. 1998). Together these data support a role for STAT1 as a negative regulator of tumor development (Bromberg, J. F. 2001).

In addition to its putative role as a tumor suppressor, STAT1 signal transduction within non-malignant cells can also regulate the outgrowth of tumors and the response to therapy with exogenous IFN-α. Since STAT1 deficient (STAT1$^{-/-}$) mice manifested deficiencies in IFN-mediated anti-viral immunity, we postulated that the anti-tumor effects of IFN-α might proceed primarily via immunologic mechanisms (Durbin, J. E. et al. 1996). To explore the contribution of STAT1-mediated gene regulation within the tumor, our group generated a

STAT1-deficient murine melanoma cell line, AGS-1 (Badgwell, B. et al. 2004; Lesinski, G. B. et al. 2003). STAT1 was reconstituted within AGS-1 cells by retroviral gene transfer. The resulting cell line (AGS-1$^{STAT1}$) showed normal regulation of IFN-α-stimulated genes (H2k, ISG-54) as compared to AGS-1 cells infected with the empty vector (AGS-1$^{MSCV}$). However, mice challenged with the AGS-1, AGS-1$^{STAT1}$, and AGS-1$^{MSCV}$ cell lines exhibited nearly identical survival in response to IFN-α treatment, indicating that restored STAT1 signaling within the tumor did not augment the anti-tumor activity of IFN-α. In contrast, STAT1$^{-/-}$ mice could not utilize exogenous IFN-α to inhibit the growth of STAT1$^{+/+}$ melanoma cells in either an intraperitoneal tumor model or in the adjuvant setting. The survival of tumor-bearing STAT1$^{-/-}$ mice was identical regardless of whether they were received IFN-α or PBS. STAT1$^{-/-}$ mice exhibited normal levels of circulating immune effector cells, but splenocytes from STAT1$^{-/-}$ mice exhibited a 90-95% reduction in cytotoxic activity against the NK-sensitive YAC1 cell line in a $^{51}$Cr-release assay. Thus, STAT1-mediated gene regulation within immune effectors (but not tumor cells) was necessary for mediating the anti-tumor effects of IFN-α in this experimental system (Lesinski, G. B. et al. 2003). Several subsequent studies have indicated that signaling via the Jak-STAT1 pathway in other cellular compartments is altered in the setting of melanoma, and could contribute to the development or progression of this tumor in humans. For example, significant impairments in the phosphorylation of STAT1 has been observed in T cells or bulk peripheral blood mononuclear cells obtained from patients with metastatic melanoma (Lesinski, G. B. et al. 2004; Critchley-Thorne, R. J. et al. 2009; Mortarini, R. et al. 2009). Other evidence suggests that intratumoral expression of STAT1 does not correlate with effectiveness of IFN-α used as an adjuvant therapy for melanoma. In one study, a large cohort of high-risk patients that exhibited prolonged survival in response to adjuvant IFN-α was identified. In some of these patients, loss of STAT1 expression was noted within their tumor. In contrast, other patients, who had normal expression of Jak-STAT proteins, recurred after just a few months of IFN therapy (Lesinski, G. B. et al. 2005). These results have been confirmed by a second group, who showed that while phosphorylation of STAT1 at Tyr$^{701}$ and Ser$^{727}$ was not inducible in 63% of patient tumors, STAT1 activation defects showed no correlation with disease outcome or response to IFN-α-2b immunotherapy as indicated by progression-free survival (Boudny, V. et al. 2003). Recent studies have further shown that patient melanoma cells exhibit negligible levels of STAT1 activation following IFN-α stimulation (as compared to immune cells from the same patient), even when all major components of the Jak-STAT signaling pathway were present (Lesinski, G. B. et al. 2007). These experiments provide compelling evidence that STAT1 signal transduction within non-transformed cellular compartments may be altered in patients with melanoma and required for effective anti-tumor immune responses.

Although STAT1 has traditionally been associated with anti-tumor effects mentioned above, more recent studies have suggested that in certain situations, STAT1 may play a paradoxical role in promoting melanoma progression. In murine tumor models, it has been shown that stable knockdown of STAT1 from B16F1 melanoma cells constitutively over-expressing STAT1 led to a less aggressive tumor phenotype and decreased colonization of tumor cells into the lung (Khodarev, N. N. et al. 2009). In another study, a large-scale gene expression analysis of melanoma metastases was conducted to identify genes involved in late-stage tumor progression. A comparison of differential gene expression between peripheral areas of the tumor (around the 'invasion front') with that of central tumor areas revealed that

STAT1 was highly expressed within peripheral, compared with central tumor areas. Furthermore, STAT1 knockdown reduced the metastatic behavior of melanoma cells in a murine model (Schultz, J. et al. 2010). These studies suggest that STAT1 might play a role in promoting the progression of certain late stage melanomas. These seemingly pro-tumor properties of activated STAT1 within a subset of melanoma cells could be due to the ability of STAT1 to serve as a central mediator of inflammation. Indeed, STAT1 is activated following stimulation with pro-inflammatory cytokines in other tumor such as tumor-associated macrophages. For example, STAT1 can regulate the expression of arginase and nitric oxide (NO), which in turn suppress tumor-specific T cells (Kusmartsev, S. et al. 2005). In addition, STAT1 can induce the expression of indoleamine 2,3-dioxygenase, an enzyme that is expressed in cancer that can block T cell activation (Uyttenhove, C. et al. 2003). However, the approach of STAT1 inhibition as a potential therapeutic strategy should be approached with caution. Prior studies have shown that in the absence of STAT1, IFN-γ stimulation leads to a strong and prolonged activation of STAT3, which could exacerbate tumorigenesis or metastasis (Qing, Y. et al. 2004).

## 5. STAT3

The STAT3 transcription factor plays a key role in the setting of melanoma and numerous other cancers. This protein induces unique transcriptional profiles in response to a variety of growth factors, cytokines, hormones and oncogenes (e.g. IL-6, leptin, IL-12, IFNs, IL-10, G-CSF, prolactin, growth hormone, EGF, HGF, bFGF, v-Src, v-Fps, v-Sis) (Dewilde, S. et al. 2008). A brief overview of STAT3 transcriptional targets can be found in Figure 3. STAT3 is considered an oncogene due to prior studies showing that over-expression of its constitutively active form could transform cultured cells or form tumors in nude mice (Bromberg, J. F. et al. 1999; Dechow, T. N. et al. 2004; Azare, J. et al. 2007). In the malignant cell, this protein is a key mediator which promotes cell proliferation and angiogenesis, inhibits apoptosis, and promotes the transcription of genes important for invasion and metastasis. Phosphorylation of STAT3 on specific tyrosine residues can modulate its propensity to dimerize with other STAT proteins (STAT1, STAT3, or STAT5), or to increase its affinity for DNA once it has dimerized and translocated to the nucleus. In contrast to other STAT proteins, loss of STAT3 in a whole organism is embryonic lethal (Takeda, K. et al. 1997). However, tissue specific knockout of STAT3 has been possible, and has led to a great appreciation as to the complexity of STAT3 in regulating various inflammatory, growth or physiologic processes (Dewilde, S. et al. 2008). In contrast to normal cells, where STAT3 activation is rapid and transient, neoplastic cells often display constitutive STAT3 activation (Fletcher, S. et al. 2008). Like other STAT proteins, STAT3 exists in two isoforms generated by alternative splicing, the full length STAT3α and the truncated STAT3β. These distinct isoforms add further to the complexity of this protein, as the STAT3β isoform is thought to act as a dominant negative factor, and to be transcriptionally active (Dewilde, S. et al. 2008). Two additional STAT3 isoforms, gamma and delta are generated proteolytically in myeloid cells, however their role in these or other cells remains unclear (Hevehan, D. L. et al. 2002; Chakraborty, A. et al. 1996). STAT3 was initially identified as Acute Phase Response Factor (APRF), which was shown to activate promoters of acute phase genes following IL-6 (Wegenka, U. M. et al. 1993).

Constitutive activation of STAT3 is a common characteristic of multiple tumor types. This observation was first noted associated with oncogenic transformation by the viral Src oncoprotein (Al Zaid Siddiquee, K. et al. 2008; Yu, C. L. et al. 1995). In a majority of melanoma cell lines and clinical specimens, constitutive phosphorylation of STAT3 at the Tyr705 residue has also been observed (Alas, S. et al. 2003; Buettner, R. et al. 2002; Duan, Z. et al. 2007; Real, P. J. et al. 2002; Shen, Y. et al. 2001; Wang, T. et al. 2004; Yu, H. et al. 2004). This post-translational modification can occur in response to receptor-ligand interactions such as cytokines (interleukin-6), growth factors (vascular endothelial growth factor) or other soluble mediators (oncostatin M) that may be secreted in an autocrine fashion by melanoma cells or in a paracrine manner by other cells present in the microenvironment. In addition to soluble mediators, constitutive activation of other intracellular proteins such as Src within melanoma cells can also promote STAT3 phosphorylation and its downstream effects. Recent studies have led to further insight as to the mechanism by which STAT3 is persistently activated in tumors. In a study by Lee *et al.*, it was shown that expression of the sphingosine-1-phosphate receptor-1 (S1PR1), a G protein-coupled receptor for the lysophospholipid sphingosine-1-phosphate (S1P), is elevated in STAT3 positive tumors, including melanoma (Lee, H. et al. 2010). In this report, the authors further showed that STAT3 was a transcription factor for the S1pr1 gene, and that enhanced S1pr1 expression led to STAT3 activation and upregulated IL-6 expression. This reciprocal relationship led to accelerated tumor growth and metastasis in a STAT3 dependent manner. Together these data identify that STAT3 and S1PR1 participate in a positive feedback loop to sustain STAT3 activation in cancer cells (Lee, H. et al. 2010).

Constitutive activation of STAT3 in melanoma tumors is associated with a poor prognosis (Kortylewski, M. et al. 2005; Xie, T. X. et al. 2006; Niu, G. et al. 2002). Besides melanoma, STAT3 is thought to play a critical role in promoting an oncogenic, metastatic and drug-resistant phenotype in several types of cancer including breast, lung, and pancreatic among others (Alas, S. et al. 2003; Buettner, R. et al. 2002; Duan, Z. et al. 2007; Real, P. J. et al. 2002; Shen, Y. et al. 2001; Wang, T. et al. 2004; Yu, H. et al. 2004). The transcriptional signature mediated by STAT3 activation consists of numerous genes that contribute to retaining a malignant phenotype. For example, the oncogenic role of STAT3 is highlighted through its ability to regulate the expression of genes which mediate proliferation (c-myc, cyclin D1), inhibit apoptosis (Bcl-xL, survivin), and promote metastasis (e.g. matrix metalloproteinases) (Bromberg, J. 2002; Bromberg, J. F. et al. 1996; Fletcher, S. et al. 2008). STAT3 is also associated with regulating apoptosis by the noncanonical nuclear factor-κB (NF-κB) (Barre, B. et al. 2007) and induces VEGF or HIF1-α expression to promote angiogenesis (Barre, B. et al. 2007; Chauhan, D. et al. 2001; Xi, S. et al. 2005; Niu, G. et al. 2002; Xu, Q. et al. 2005; Xie, T. X. et al. 2006). STAT3 can also indirectly repress pro-apoptotic factors via its ability to repress the expression of the p53 tumor suppressor gene. Finally, studies in preclinical models of melanoma have also shown that STAT3 stimulates invasion and metastasis by inducing matrix metalloproteinase-2 (MMP-2) *in vitro* and *in vivo* (Xie, T. X. et al. 2006).

Unphosphorylated STAT3 has also been shown to regulate a specific subset of genes in fibroblast cell lines. Some of the genes present in the transcriptional profile induced by unphosphorylated STAT3 included well-known oncoproteins (e.g. MRas, MET, CDC2, Cyclin B1, E2F1) (Yang, J. et al. 2005). High levels of unphosphorylated STAT3 typically occur via a transcriptional mechanism following IL-6 stimulation. However to the best of our knowledge, the role of this mechanism has not been investigated specifically in melanoma.

## 6. Balance between STAT1 and STAT3 in Melanoma

The balance between phosphorylated STAT1 and STAT3 may be important in melanoma cell biology. Since IFN-α is a clinically-relevant therapy for melanoma, much investigation has occurred into differential regulation of STAT1 and STAT3 by this cytokine. Studies have shown that the differential phosphorylation of STAT1 and STAT3 regulates the cellular response to IFNs, and influences their anti-tumor activity (Ho, H. H. et al. 2006; Lesinski, G. B. et al. 2007; Wang, W. et al. 2007). STAT3 may act as a molecular "sink" for phosphorylation events upon ligand binding to a receptor. This functional property of STAT3 can negatively regulate the transcriptional response mediated via other STAT proteins.

The concept that the ratio of phosphorylated STAT1 to STAT3 could serve as a biomarker for melanoma progression has recently gained attention. For example, in a study by Wang et al., the level of pSTAT1 and pSTAT3 was evaluated in biopsies of atypical nevi from patients receiving IFN-α (Wang, W. et al. 2008). Results from these studies showed that the percentage of pSTAT3-positive melanocytes was positively associated with the atypical degree of nevi. These data showed that the relative balance of pSTAT1/pSTAT3 may be associated with melanocyte differentiation *in vivo*. Studies from our group have also shown that the level of pSTAT3 present in melanoma cell lines was inversely correlated with IFN-α induced STAT1 phosphorylation (Lesinski, G.B. et al. 2007). The therapeutic utility of this inverse relationship between STAT1 and STAT3 is currently being evaluated in pre-clinical studies of melanoma utilizing combinations of STAT3 pathway inhibitors with cytokines that activate STAT1 (Kong, L. Y. et al. 2010). These studies are described in detail below in section 9.

## 7. Rationale for STAT3 as a molecular target for therapy

In melanoma and numerous other cancers, constitutively active STAT3 is a poor prognostic indicator and potential therapeutic target. Indeed constitutive phosphorylation of STAT3 can afford melanoma cells a survival advantage and promote an aggressive phenotype. Constitutive STAT3 phosphorylation is mediated by several kinases including Jak2, members of the Src family (hck, src), Erb B1, Erb B2, anaplastic lymphoma kinase, protein kinase C (PKC)-d, c-fos, gp130, and epithelial growth factor (EGF) receptor (Jain, N. et al. 1999; Nelson, K. L. et al. 1998; Ren, Z. et al. 2002; Sellers, L. A. et al. 1999; Smithgall, T. E. et al. 2000; Zhang, Y. et al. 2000). Interestingly, despite its necessity in early embryogenesis, STAT3 appears to be largely dispensable in most normal adult cell and tissue types (Akira, S. 2000; Takeda, K. et al. 1997). In addition to the role of STAT3 in tumor cells, recent studies have demonstrated that STAT3 also promotes immune tolerance in the setting of cancer (reviewed in (Yu, H. et al. 2007)). Together these data suggest that inhibition of STAT3 represents a rational approach to cancer therapy as it could have both an effect directly on the tumor cell while also promoting the ability of immune cells to recognize and eliminate cancer. Interestingly, recent studies from our group and others have demonstrated that the presence of constitutively active STAT3 can inhibit the response to cytokines which act via STAT1 signal transduction (Lesinski, G. B. et al. 2007). These data suggest that the balance between pSTAT1 and pSTAT3 may influence the responsiveness of cells to immunostimulatory cytokines and ultimately immune-mediated tumor regression (Lesinski, G. B. et al. 2007; Wang, W. et al. 2007). Based on these data, it is rational to suggest that inhibition of STAT3 could augment responsiveness to standard or experimental immune-based therapies that act via the STAT1 transcription factor.

Notably, administration of IFN-α2b is currently the standard of care and only FDA-approved agent for use as an adjuvant therapy in melanoma patients after surgical resection of high-risk cutaneous lesions (Balch, C. M. 1998). Therefore, STAT3 inhibition could enhance the anti-tumor properties of these existing therapies for melanoma patients.

## 8. Relevant structural features of STAT3 for inhibitor development

The structure of STAT3 includes a STAT dimerization domain at the amino-terminus, a coiled-coil domain important in protein interactions, a DNA binding domain, a SH2 domain, and a carboxy terminus that controls transcriptional activation (Frank, D. A. 2007; Levy, D. E. et al. 2002; Turkson, J. et al. 2000). Disrupting SH2 homodimerization of STAT3 can be achieved through inhibitor competition with the phosphoryl tyrosine 705 (Y705) binding site. These two SH2 domains are hinged together by a loop segment from each monomer. The pY705 critical for the biological function of STAT3 locates right on this loop segment, and binds, together with several adjacent amino acid residues (leucine 706, threonine 708, and phenyalanine 710), to a cavity on the SH2 domain of the other monomer.

## 9. Experimental strategies for STAT3 inhibition

Several strategies have been used to inhibit the STAT3 pathway as a therapeutic approach for treating various types of cancer including malignant melanoma. Direct STAT3 inhibitors can be categorized into different classes of compounds: peptides, peptidomimetics, small molecules, platinum complexes, siRNA and plant polyphenols (Fletcher, S. et al. 2008). Indeed, a number of peptides, peptidomimetics and peptide aptamers have been reported to inhibit STAT3 via their interaction with the DNA binding domain or the dimerization domain of the protein (Alas, S. et al. 2003; Yu, H. et al. 2007). These various strategies of STAT3 inhibition are outlined briefly in Figure 4. Each of these strategies for STAT3 inhibition have their strengths and weaknesses. For example, although there is a high degree of specificity using peptide-based approaches, these agents traditionally suffer from limited cell permeability and *in vivo* stability. Unfortunately, these properties have restricted their practical application *in vivo* (Fletcher, S. et al. 2008). More recently, however, advances have been made in designing cell-permeable, STAT3 SH2 domain mimetics. These mimetics have shown promising anti-tumor effects *in vitro* against a variety of solid tumor types (Zhao, W. et al. 2010). Moreover, siRNA specific for the SH2 coding region of STAT3 could induce apoptosis in prostate cancer cells *in vitro* and in nude mice bearing human xenograft tumors (Bromberg, J. F. et al. 1996). Recent studies have also shown that platinum complexes promote anti-tumor activity by their ability to inhibit STAT3 (Turkson, J. et al. 2004). A variety of plant polyphenols (e.g. resveratrol, flavopiridol, indirubin, magnolol, picetannol, parthenolide, EGCG, curcubitacin Q and curcumin) have also been shown to down-regulate the activity of STAT3 and other targets in malignant cells (Bharti, A. C. et al. 2003; Blaskovich, M. A. et al. 2003; Chakravarti, N. et al. 2006; Chen, S. C. et al. 2006; Lee, Y. K. et al. 2006; Masuda, M. et al. 2001; Nam, S. et al. 2005; Sobota, R. et al. 2000; Su, L. et al. 2000; Wung, B. S. et al. 2005). Collectively, these studies provide precedent for targeting STAT3 as a means of inducing apoptosis of tumor cells. However, the specificity of many existing inhibitory strategies for STAT3 and not other STAT proteins (e.g. STAT1) or oncogenic pathways is still being validated in biological systems. Arguably, numerous early generation small molecule STAT3 inhibitors (e.g. Stattic, STA-21, S32-M2001, S3I-201) have shown particular promise, due to their ability induce apoptosis (Fletcher, S. et al. 2008). In the past, our ability to identify novel small molecule inhibitors that disrupt SH2 domain phosphotyrosine interactions has been limited due to the very high degree of hydrophobic interactions present within this portion of the molecule. However, recent advances from a number of groups have shown that this is indeed possible. For example, Zhang *et al.* have recently described a novel small molecule S3I-201.1066, a structural derivative of S3I-201 that can disrupt phosphotyrosine interactions at the STAT3 SH2 domain (Zhang, X. et al. 2010). Similarly, other derivatives of the early generation STAT3 inhibitor LLL-3 (designated LLL-12) (Ball, S. et al. 2011; Lin, L. et al. 2011; Onimoe, G. I. et al. 2011; Wei, C. C. et al. 2011; Lin, L. et al. 2010) or purine scaffolds (Shahani, V. M. et al. 2011) show similar activity in a variety of tumor models. Finally, recent studies have described that FLLL32, a structural analog of curcumin, can preferentially target STAT3 while retaining STAT1 mediated signal transduction within melanoma and immune effector cells. Treatment of human melanoma cell lines, and early passage primary melanoma tumors with FLLL32 led to caspase-dependent apoptosis via its inhibition of STAT3 (Bill, M. A. et al. 2010).

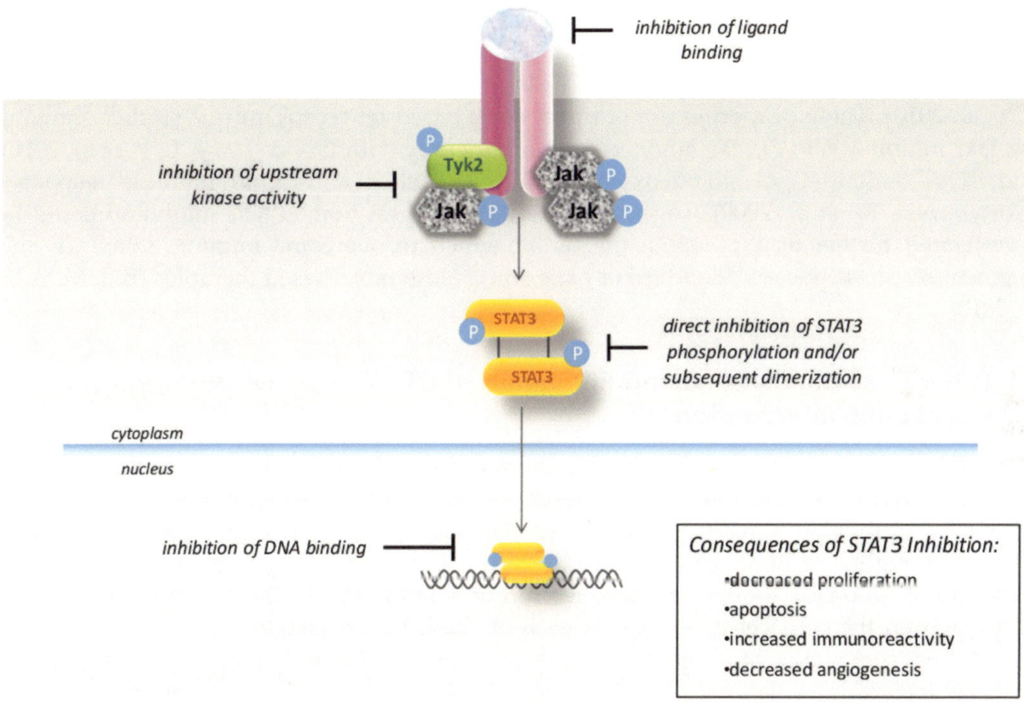


Fig. 4. Strategies of STAT3 pathway inhibition

Because STAT3 can promote immune tolerance in the setting of cancer, this pathway represents an attractive target to enhance immunotherapy (Reviewed in (Yu, H. et al. 2007)). Recent studies have demonstrated that the presence of constitutively phosphorylated STAT3 in melanoma cells is correlated with reduced responsiveness to cytokines which act via STAT1 signal transduction (Lesinski, G. B. et al. 2007). These data suggest that the balance between pSTAT1 and pSTAT3 may influence cellular responsiveness to immunostimulatory cytokines and ultimately immune-mediated tumor regression (Lesinski, G. B. et al. 2007; Wang, W. et al. 2007).

It is apparent that STAT3 inhibition may serve as a means to sensitize melanoma cells, or the immune system of a tumor bearing host to interferon-alpha, a cytokine that exerts its anti-tumor effects in a manner dependent upon STAT1 signaling. For example, Kong *et al.* demonstrated that combined therapy with the Jak2/STAT3 pathway inhibitor WP1193 (a third generation AG490 analog) and IFN-$\alpha$ could enhance innate and adaptive cytotoxic T cell activity and elicit impressive anti-tumor activity in an intracerebral murine tumor model of melanoma (Kong, L. Y. et al. 2010). Further supporting the concept that STAT3 inhibition may augment immunotherapy with IFN-$\alpha$ was a study by Ito *et al* performed in patients with renal cell carcinoma. In this report, linkage disequilibrium mapping revealed that a SNP in the 5′ region of STAT3, rs4796793, leads to reduced STAT3 protein expression. Importantly this SNP was a significant predictor of clinical response to IFN-$\alpha$. The authors of this study concluded that patients with a minor rs4796793 allele had better intrinsic immunosurveillance. Although immunomodulation was the focus of these prior studies, it remains possible that this strategy could also enhance the direct anti-proliferative or pro-apoptotic effects of IFN-$\alpha$ on melanoma cells (Ito, N. et al. 2007).

With these studies in mind, recent data indicate that inhibition of STAT3 with the FLLL32 small molecule does not alter production of granzyme b or IFN-$\gamma$ by NK cells from normal donors when cultured with K562 targets, or their viability when cultured with IL-2 (Bill, M. A. et al. 2010). These properties are of importance based on recent murine studies showing the Jak2 inhibitor WP1193 can augment immunotherapy with IFN-$\alpha$ (Kong, L. Y. et al. 2010), and STAT3 siRNA-CpG oligodeoxynucleotides can elicit anti-tumor immune responses (Kortylewski, M. et al. 2009). Together these data suggest that STAT3 inhibition could be investigated further as a potential means by which to overcome immune tolerance and augment responsiveness to standard or experimental immune-based therapies (Bill, M. A. et al. 2010).

## 10. Other post-translational modifications of STAT proteins: An opportunity for therapeutic intervention

In addition to phosphorylation, other post-translational modifications can regulate the activity of STAT proteins and deserve mention in this chapter. Among these modifications are methylation, ubiquitination, sumoylation, isgylation and acetylation (O'Shea, J. J. et al. 2005). Although we will not provide an exhaustive review of these processes, the balance of these modifications is thought to have a profound influence on the gene expression that occurs within the cell. The relevance of each of these post-translational modifications is a rapidly emerging area of research, and is not completely understood in most cellular systems including melanoma. These various post-translational modifications of STAT proteins are a clear opportunity for further study. Below we will highlight a few brief examples that provide great insight into how these events might regulate cellular function.

First, in an eloquent study by Yuan *et al.*, it was demonstrated that STAT proteins undergo acetylation of a single amino acid residue, lysine 685, in response to cytokine stimulation. The authors were able to conclude that this modification was essential for STAT proteins to dimerize and initiate gene transcription (O'Shea, J. J. et al. 2005; Yuan, Z. L. et al. 2005). These initial data were instrumental in demonstrating that acetylation of STAT proteins is a cytokine-induced post-translational modification that is critical for initiating the downstream gene expression characteristic of these transcription factors.

Acetylation has also been shown to be critical for crosstalk between STAT proteins and other signal transduction pathways. For example, a study by Kramer *et al.* demonstrated that only acetylated STAT1 was able to interact with NF-κB p65. As a consequence, p65 DNA binding, nuclear localization, and expression of anti-apoptotic NF-κB target genes decreased (Kramer, O. H. et al. 2006). In addition, STAT1 protein acetylation is a process that is tightly controlled by histone deacetylases (HDAC) and may play a negative regulatory role by counteracting interferon-stimulated gene expression (Kramer, O. H. et al. 2010).

The importance of these post-translational modifications to melanoma cell biology represents an area of great interest and importance. A greater understanding of their role in melanoma could be utilized to develop novel therapeutic agents that alter cell survival and response to therapy.

## 11. Negative regulation of Jak-STAT signal transduction

Negative regulation of cytokine-induced STAT protein phosphorylation can be mediated by a variety of mechanisms. Proteins involved in the negative regulation of this pathway are cytokine receptors, kinases, phosphatases (PTPs), suppressors of cytokine signaling (SOCS), and protein inhibitors of activated STAT (PIAS). Accurate 'tuning' of the Jak-STAT pathway is instrumental in regulating the cellular response to various cytokines or growth factors to maintain physiological processes in normal and malignant cells. Thus, altering negative regulatory mediators involved in Jak-STAT signal transduction can have dramatic consequences on cellular function and survival. Because many STAT proteins are constitutively active in melanoma cells, these various negative regulatory proteins are currently under investigation as novel therapeutic targets, primarily in pre-clinical models.

The negative regulatory SOCS proteins (briefly illustrated in Figure 5) are a particularly promising target for melanoma (Alexander, W. S. 2002). The SOCS family of proteins has eight members, all of which have a central SH2 domain, an amino terminal domain, and a 40-amino acid motif at the carboxy terminus that is known as the SOCS box. In unstimulated cells, signaling molecules (such as the Jaks and STATs) are typically inactive, and SOCS genes are generally not expressed. The induction of SOCS proteins following cytokine stimulation defines a negative feedback loop, and serves to regulate cytokine-induced signal transduction. SOCS1 possesses a kinase inhibitory region (KIR) that binds to the catalytic groove of Jak2 and inhibits its activity (Nicholson, S. E. et al. 1999; Yasukawa, H. et al. 1999). SOCS3 has significant sequence homology to SOCS1 and appears to inhibit Jak catalytic activity via its KIR region. SOCS3 does not bind directly to Jaks but instead utilizes direct receptor binding to access to the Jak activation loop (Belardelli, F. et al. 2002).

Since melanoma is traditionally viewed as an immune-reactive tumor, targeting SOCS proteins in immune effector cells is attracting interest as a potential therapeutic approach. This concept is founded on the fact that SOCS proteins are important for regulating multiple cytokine-induced processes in immune cells. Several lines of evidence point to SOCS proteins as important regulators of T cell development and function. For example, previous studies have demonstrated that over-expression of SOCS3 inhibits the proliferation of T cells following TCR ligation and exposure to cytokines. Mice with a targeted deficiency of SOCS1 within the T cell compartment exhibit an increased ratio of CD8/CD4 mature thymic cells and a significant increase in the prevalence of $CD44^{hi}$ $CD8^{+}$ memory T cells within the periphery (Davey, G. M. et al. 2005). SOCS1-deficiency has also been shown to promote the processing of tumor antigens by DC and their recognition by effector T cells (Hanada, T. et al. 2005; Shen, L. et al. 2004). One recent study has also demonstrated that vaccination of mice with melanoma antigen-primed, SOCS1-deficient DC elicited protection against lethal melanoma tumors (Shen, L. et al. 2004). Other studies have demonstrated that mice lacking both SOCS1 and IFN-γ can be cured of otherwise lethal melanoma tumors through exogenous administration of IFN-α (Zimmerer, J. M. et al. 2007; Guenterberg, K. D. et al. 2011). Finally, studies from Hashimoto *et al.* have demonstrated that silencing SOCS1 in macrophages enhances the survival of mice bearing B16 melanoma tumors (Hashimoto, K. et al. 2009). Together these data suggest that SOCS proteins within the adaptive immune system play an instrumental role in regulating the anti-tumor response against melanoma.

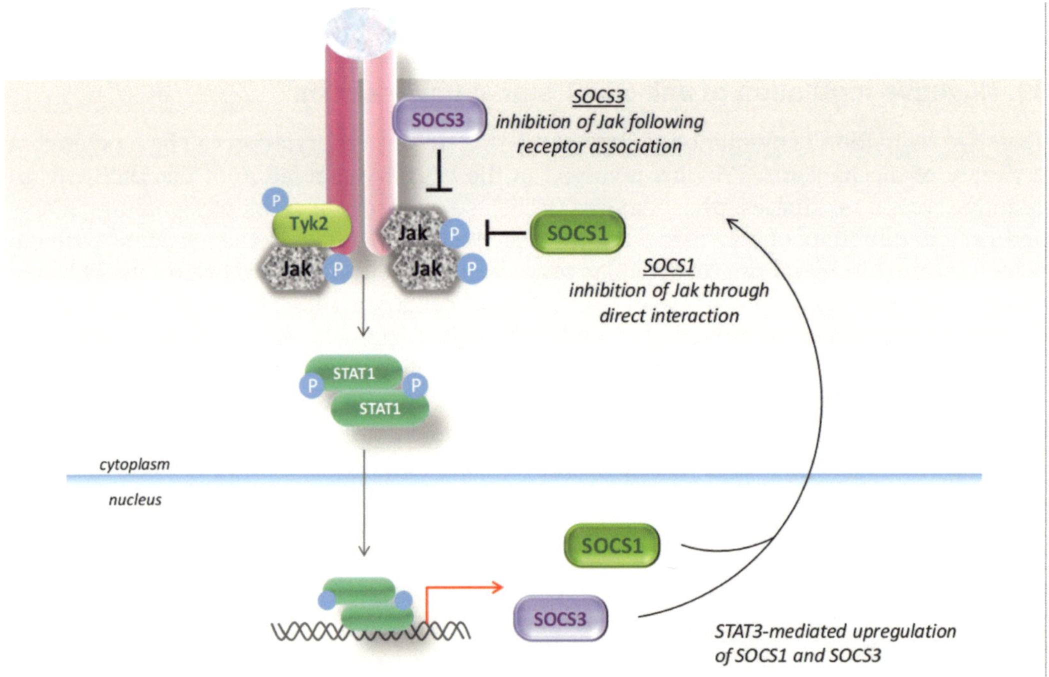


Fig. 5. Negative feedback inhibition of the STAT pathway through SOCS1 and SOCS3 (Alexander, W. S. 2002)

Jak-STAT activation is also negatively regulated by other mechanisms including protein inhibitors of activated STATs (PIAS), SHP-1 and SHP-2 (which de-phosphorylate activated receptors), truncated STAT isoforms (Brassard, D. L. et al. 2002; Liu, B. et al. 1998; Sakai, I. et al. 2002; You, M. et al. 1999) and acetylation, as mentioned previously in this chapter (Kramer, O. H. et al. 2010; O'Shea, J. J. et al. 2005). Moreover, other post-translational modifications such as sumoylation of STAT1 can influence IFN-induced signal transduction (Liu, B. et al. 2008; Lim, C. P. et al. 2006; Kim, H. S. et al. 2007). These data highlight the diversity of intracellular mechanisms available to limit Jak-STAT signal transduction and suggest numerous potential molecular targets for future study in melanoma. Despite the various data demonstrating upregulated negative regulatory proteins such as SOCS1 and SOCS3 in melanoma, it remains somewhat unclear as to how constitutive STAT protein phosphorylation can occur in a highly prevalent manner along with consistent upregulation of the negative regulatory factors.

## 12. Conclusions

The Jak-STAT pathway plays an instrumental role in mediating the biology of malignant melanoma cells. This signal transduction pathway also holds great opportunity for therapeutic targeting of melanoma. In particular, the STAT3 transcription factor represents an area of increasing interest for development of small molecule inhibitors or other approaches for therapeutic use. Finally, there lies a tremendous opportunity to better understand melanoma biology through our investigation into novel post-translational modifications and negative regulation of signal transduction via the Jak-STAT pathway.

## 13. References

Akira, S. (2000). Roles of STAT3 defined by tissue-specific gene targeting. *Oncogene,* 19, 21, 2607-2611.

Al Zaid Siddiquee, K. and J. Turkson. (2008). STAT3 as a target for inducing apoptosis in solid and hematological tumors. *Cell Res,* 18, 2, 254-267.

Alas, S. and B. Bonavida. (2003). Inhibition of constitutive STAT3 activity sensitizes resistant non-Hodgkin's lymphoma and multiple myeloma to chemotherapeutic drug-mediated apoptosis. *Clin Cancer Res,* 9, 1, 316-326.

Alexander, W. S. (2002). Suppressors of cytokine signalling (SOCS) in the immune system. *Nat Rev Immunol,* 2, 6, 410-416.

Aplin, A. E., F. M. Kaplan and Y. Shao. (2011). Mechanisms of Resistance to RAF Inhibitors in Melanoma. *J Invest Dermatol,*

Atkins, M. B. (1998). Immunotherapy and experimental approaches for metastatic melanoma. *Hematol Oncol Clin North Am,* 12, 4, 877-902, viii.

Azare, J., K. Leslie, H. Al-Ahmadie, W. Gerald, P. H. Weinreb, S. M. Violette and J. Bromberg. (2007). Constitutively activated Stat3 induces tumorigenesis and enhances cell motility of prostate epithelial cells through integrin beta 6. *Mol Cell Biol,* 27, 12, 4444-4453.

Badgwell, B., G. B. Lesinski, C. Magro, G. Abood, A. Skaf and W. Carson, 3rd. (2004). The antitumor effects of interferon-alpha are maintained in mice challenged with a STAT1-deficient murine melanoma cell line. *J Surg Res,* 116, 1, 129-136.

Balch, C. M. (1998). Cutaneous melanoma. St. Louis, Mo., Quality Medical Pub.

Ball, N. J., J. J. Yohn, J. G. Morelli, D. A. Norris, L. E. Golitz and J. P. Hoeffler. (1994). Ras mutations in human melanoma: a marker of malignant progression. *J Invest Dermatol,* 102, 3, 285-290.

Ball, S., C. Li, P. K. Li and J. Lin. (2011). The Small Molecule, LLL12, Inhibits STAT3 Phosphorylation and Induces Apoptosis in Medulloblastoma and Glioblastoma Cells. *PLoS One,* 6, 4, e18820.

Barre, B., A. Vigneron, N. Perkins, I. B. Roninson, E. Gamelin and O. Coqueret. (2007). The STAT3 oncogene as a predictive marker of drug resistance. *Trends Mol Med,* 13, 1, 4-11.

Belardelli, F., M. Ferrantini, E. Proietti and J. M. Kirkwood. (2002). Interferon-alpha in tumor immunity and immunotherapy. *Cytokine Growth Factor Rev,* 13, 2, 119-134.

Bernabei, P., E. M. Coccia, L. Rigamonti, M. Bosticardo, G. Forni, S. Pestka, C. D. Krause, A. Battistini and F. Novelli. (2001). Interferon-gamma receptor 2 expression as the deciding factor in human T, B, and myeloid cell proliferation or death. *J Leukoc Biol,* 70, 6, 950-960.

Bharti, A. C., N. Donato and B. B. Aggarwal. (2003). Curcumin (diferuloylmethane) inhibits constitutive and IL-6-inducible STAT3 phosphorylation in human multiple myeloma cells. *J Immunol,* 171, 7, 3863-3871.

Bill, M. A., J. R. Fuchs, C. Li, J. Yui, C. Bakan, D. M. Benson, Jr., E. B. Schwartz, D. Abdelhamid, J. Lin, D. G. Hoyt, S. L. Fossey, G. S. Young, W. E. Carson, 3rd, P. K. Li and G. B. Lesinski. (2010). The small molecule curcumin analog FLLL32 induces apoptosis in melanoma cells via STAT3 inhibition and retains the cellular response to cytokines with anti-tumor activity. *Mol Cancer,* 9, 165.

Blaskovich, M. A., J. Sun, A. Cantor, J. Turkson, R. Jove and S. M. Sebti. (2003). Discovery of JSI-124 (cucurbitacin I), a selective Janus kinase/signal transducer and activator of transcription 3 signaling pathway inhibitor with potent antitumor activity against human and murine cancer cells in mice. *Cancer Res,* 63, 6, 1270-1279.

Boudny, V., I. Kocak, L. Lauerova and J. Kovarik. (2003). Interferon inducibility of STAT 1 activation and its prognostic significance in melanoma patients. *Folia Biol (Praha),* 49, 4, 142-146.

Bouwhuis, M. G., T. L. Ten Hagen, S. Suciu and A. M. Eggermont. (2010). Autoimmunity and treatment outcome in melanoma. *Curr Opin Oncol,*

Bowman, T., R. Garcia, J. Turkson and R. Jove. (2000). STATs in oncogenesis. *Oncogene,* 19, 21, 2474-2488.

Brassard, D. L., M. J. Grace and R. W. Bordens. (2002). Interferon-alpha as an immunotherapeutic protein. *J Leukoc Biol,* 71, 4, 565-581.

Bromberg, J. (2002). Stat proteins and oncogenesis. *J Clin Invest,* 109, 9, 1139-1142.

Bromberg, J. F. (2001). Activation of STAT proteins and growth control. *Bioessays,* 23, 2, 161-169.

Bromberg, J. F., C. M. Horvath, Z. Wen, R. D. Schreiber and J. E. Darnell, Jr. (1996). Transcriptionally active Stat1 is required for the antiproliferative effects of both interferon alpha and interferon gamma. *Proc Natl Acad Sci U S A,* 93, 15, 7673-7678.

Bromberg, J. F., M. H. Wrzeszczynska, G. Devgan, Y. Zhao, R. G. Pestell, C. Albanese and J. E. Darnell, Jr. (1999). Stat3 as an oncogene. *Cell,* 98, 3, 295-303.

Buettner, R., L. B. Mora and R. Jove. (2002). Activated STAT signaling in human tumors provides novel molecular targets for therapeutic intervention. *Clin Cancer Res,* 8, 4, 945-954.

Chakraborty, A., S. M. White, T. S. Schaefer, E. D. Ball, K. F. Dyer and D. J. Tweardy. (1996). Granulocyte colony-stimulating factor activation of Stat3 alpha and Stat3 beta in immature normal and leukemic human myeloid cells. *Blood,* 88, 7, 2442-2449.

Chakravarti, N., J. N. Myers and B. B. Aggarwal. (2006). Targeting constitutive and interleukin-6-inducible signal transducers and activators of transcription 3 pathway in head and neck squamous cell carcinoma cells by curcumin (diferuloylmethane). *Int J Cancer,* 119, 6, 1268-1275.

Chauhan, D. and K. C. Anderson. (2001). Apoptosis in multiple myeloma: therapeutic implications. *Apoptosis,* 6, 1-2, 47-55.

Chen, S. C., Y. L. Chang, D. L. Wang and J. J. Cheng. (2006). Herbal remedy magnolol suppresses IL-6-induced STAT3 activation and gene expression in endothelial cells. *Br J Pharmacol,* 148, 2, 226-232.

Chin, Y. E., M. Kitagawa, K. Kuida, R. A. Flavell and X. Y. Fu. (1997). Activation of the STAT signaling pathway can cause expression of caspase 1 and apoptosis. *Mol Cell Biol,* 17, 9, 5328-5337.

Chin, Y. E., M. Kitagawa, W. C. Su, Z. H. You, Y. Iwamoto and X. Y. Fu. (1996). Cell growth arrest and induction of cyclin-dependent kinase inhibitor p21 WAF1/CIP1 mediated by STAT1. *Science,* 272, 5262, 719-722.

Critchley-Thorne, R. J., D. L. Simons, N. Yan, A. K. Miyahira, F. M. Dirbas, D. L. Johnson, S. M. Swetter, R. W. Carlson, G. A. Fisher, A. Koong, S. Holmes and P. P. Lee. (2009). Impaired interferon signaling is a common immune defect in human cancer. *Proc Natl Acad Sci U S A,* 106, 22, 9010-9015.

Darnell, J. E. (2005). Validating Stat3 in cancer therapy. *Nat Med,* 11, 6, 595-596.

Darnell, J. E., Jr. (1998). Studies of IFN-induced transcriptional activation uncover the Jak-Stat pathway. *J Interferon Cytokine Res,* 18, 8, 549-554.

Darnell, J. E., Jr. (2002). Transcription factors as targets for cancer therapy. *Nat Rev Cancer,* 2, 10, 740-749.

Darnell, J. E., Jr., I. M. Kerr and G. R. Stark. (1994). Jak-STAT pathways and transcriptional activation in response to IFNs and other extracellular signaling proteins. *Science,* 264, 5164, 1415-1421.

Davey, G. M., R. Starr, A. L. Cornish, J. T. Burghardt, W. S. Alexander, F. R. Carbone, C. D. Surh and W. R. Heath. (2005). SOCS-1 regulates IL-15-driven homeostatic proliferation of antigen-naive CD8 T cells, limiting their autoimmune potential. *J Exp Med,* 202, 8, 1099-1108.

Davies, H., G. R. Bignell, C. Cox, P. Stephens, S. Edkins, S. Clegg, J. Teague, H. Woffendin, M. J. Garnett, W. Bottomley, N. Davis, E. Dicks, R. Ewing, Y. Floyd, K. Gray, S. Hall, R. Hawes, J. Hughes, V. Kosmidou, A. Menzies, C. Mould, A. Parker, C. Stevens, S. Watt, S. Hooper, R. Wilson, H. Jayatilake, B. A. Gusterson, C. Cooper, J. Shipley, D. Hargrave, K. Pritchard-Jones, N. Maitland, G. Chenevix-Trench, G. J. Riggins, D. D. Bigner, G. Palmieri, A. Cossu, A. Flanagan, A. Nicholson, J. W. Ho, S. Y. Leung, S. T. Yuen, B. L. Weber, H. F. Seigler, T. L. Darrow, H. Paterson, R. Marais, C. J. Marshall, R. Wooster, M. R. Stratton and P. A. Futreal. (2002). Mutations of the BRAF gene in human cancer. *Nature,* 417, 6892, 949-954.

Dechow, T. N., L. Pedranzini, A. Leitch, K. Leslie, W. L. Gerald, I. Linkov and J. F. Bromberg. (2004). Requirement of matrix metalloproteinase-9 for the transformation of human mammary epithelial cells by Stat3-C. *Proc Natl Acad Sci U S A,* 101, 29, 10602-10607.

Dewilde, S., A. Vercelli, R. Chiarle and V. Poli. (2008). Of alphas and betas: distinct and overlapping functions of STAT3 isoforms. *Front Biosci,* 13, 6501-6514.

Duan, Z., J. Bradner, E. Greenberg, R. Mazitschek, R. Foster, J. Mahoney and M. V. Seiden. (2007). 8-benzyl-4-oxo-8-azabicyclo[3.2.1]oct-2-ene-6,7-dicarboxylic acid (SD-1008), a novel janus kinase 2 inhibitor, increases chemotherapy sensitivity in human ovarian cancer cells. *Mol Pharmacol,* 72, 5, 1137-1145.

Durbin, J. E., R. Hackenmiller, M. C. Simon and D. E. Levy. (1996). Targeted disruption of the mouse Stat1 gene results in compromised innate immunity to viral disease. *Cell,* 84, 3, 443-450.

Fletcher, S., J. Turkson and P. T. Gunning. (2008). Molecular approaches towards the inhibition of the signal transducer and activator of transcription 3 (Stat3) protein. *ChemMedChem,* 3, 8, 1159-1168.

Frank, D. A. (2007). STAT3 as a central mediator of neoplastic cellular transformation. *Cancer Lett,* 251, 2, 199-210.

Gogas, H., J. Ioannovich, U. Dafni, C. Stavropoulou-Giokas, K. Frangia, D. Tsoutsos, P. Panagiotou, A. Polyzos, O. Papadopoulos, A. Stratigos, C. Markopoulos, D. Bafaloukos, D. Pectasides, G. Fountzilas and J. M. Kirkwood. (2006). Prognostic significance of autoimmunity during treatment of melanoma with interferon. *N Engl J Med,* 354, 7, 709-718.

Guenterberg, K. D., G. B. Lesinski, B. L. Mundy-Bosse, V. I. Karpa, A. C. Jaime-Ramirez, L. Wei and W. E. Carson, 3rd. (2011). Enhanced anti-tumor activity of interferon-alpha in SOCS1-deficient mice is mediated by CD4(+) and CD8 (+) T cells. *Cancer Immunol Immunother,*

Hanada, T., K. Tanaka, Y. Matsumura, M. Yamauchi, H. Nishinakamura, H. Aburatani, R. Mashima, M. Kubo, T. Kobayashi and A. Yoshimura. (2005). Induction of hyper Th1 cell-type immune responses by dendritic cells lacking the suppressor of cytokine signaling-1 gene. *J Immunol,* 174, 7, 4325-4332.

Haque, S. J. and B. R. Williams. (1998). Signal transduction in the interferon system. *Semin Oncol,* 25, 1 Suppl 1, 14-22.

Hashimoto, K., K. Ishibashi, K. Ishioka, D. Zhao, M. Sato, S. Ohara, Y. Abe, Y. Kawasaki, Y. Sato, S. Yokota, N. Fujii, R. S. Peebles, Jr., M. Hosoya and T. Suzutani. (2009). RSV replication is attenuated by counteracting expression of the suppressor of cytokine signaling (SOCS) molecules. *Virology,* 391, 2, 162-170.

Hevehan, D. L., W. M. Miller and E. T. Papoutsakis. (2002). Differential expression and phosphorylation of distinct STAT3 proteins during granulocytic differentiation. *Blood,* 99, 5, 1627-1637.

Ho, H. H. and L. B. Ivashkiv. (2006). Role of STAT3 in type I interferon responses. Negative regulation of STAT1-dependent inflammatory gene activation. *J Biol Chem,* 281, 20, 14111-14118.

Huang, M., J. F. Dorsey, P. K. Epling-Burnette, R. Nimmanapalli, T. H. Landowski, L. B. Mora, G. Niu, D. Sinibaldi, F. Bai, A. Kraker, H. Yu, L. Moscinski, S. Wei, J. Djeu, W. S. Dalton, K. Bhalla, T. P. Loughran, J. Wu and R. Jove. (2002). Inhibition of Bcr-Abl kinase activity by PD180970 blocks constitutive activation of Stat5 and growth of CML cells. *Oncogene,* 21, 57, 8804-8816.

Ito, N., M. Eto, E. Nakamura, A. Takahashi, T. Tsukamoto, H. Toma, H. Nakazawa, Y. Hirao, H. Uemura, S. Kagawa, H. Kanayama, Y. Nose, N. Kinukawa, T. Nakamura, N. Jinnai, T. Seki, M. Takamatsu, Y. Masui, S. Naito and O. Ogawa. (2007). STAT3 polymorphism predicts interferon-alfa response in patients with metastatic renal cell carcinoma. *J Clin Oncol,* 25, 19, 2785-2791.

Jain, N., T. Zhang, W. H. Kee, W. Li and X. Cao. (1999). Protein kinase C delta associates with and phosphorylates Stat3 in an interleukin-6-dependent manner. *J Biol Chem,* 274, 34, 24392-24400.

Jatiani, S. S., S. J. Baker, L. R. Silverman and E. P. Reddy. (2010). JAK/STAT Pathways in Cytokine Signaling and Myeloproliferative Disorders: Approaches for Targeted Therapies. *Genes Cancer,* 1, 10, 979-993.

Jemal, A., R. Siegel, J. Xu and E. Ward. (2010). Cancer statistics, 2010. *CA Cancer J Clin,* 60, 5, 277-300.

Kaplan, D. H., V. Shankaran, A. S. Dighe, E. Stockert, M. Aguet, L. J. Old and R. D. Schreiber. (1998). Demonstration of an interferon gamma-dependent tumor surveillance system in immunocompetent mice. *Proc Natl Acad Sci U S A,* 95, 13, 7556-7561.

Kawakami, Y., S. Eliyahu, C. H. Delgado, P. F. Robbins, K. Sakaguchi, E. Appella, J. R. Yannelli, G. J. Adema, T. Miki and S. A. Rosenberg. (1994). Identification of a human melanoma antigen recognized by tumor-infiltrating lymphocytes associated with in vivo tumor rejection. *Proc Natl Acad Sci U S A,* 91, 14, 6458-6462.

Khodarev, N. N., P. Roach, S. P. Pitroda, D. W. Golden, M. Bhayani, M. Y. Shao, T. E. Darga, M. G. Beveridge, R. F. Sood, H. G. Sutton, M. A. Beckett, H. J. Mauceri, M. C. Posner and R. R. Weichselbaum. (2009). STAT1 pathway mediates amplification of metastatic potential and resistance to therapy. *PLoS One,* 4, 6, e5821.

Kim, H. S. and M. S. Lee. (2007). STAT1 as a key modulator of cell death. *Cell Signal,* 19, 3, 454-465.

Kong, L. Y., A. Gelbard, J. Wei, C. Reina-Ortiz, Y. Wang, E. C. Yang, Y. Hailemichael, I. Fokt, A. Jayakumar, W. Qiao, G. N. Fuller, W. W. Overwijk, W. Priebe and A. B. Heimberger. (2010). Inhibition of p-STAT3 enhances IFN-alpha efficacy against metastatic melanoma in a murine model. *Clin Cancer Res,* 16, 9, 2550-2561.

Kortylewski, M., R. Jove and H. Yu. (2005). Targeting STAT3 affects melanoma on multiple fronts. *Cancer Metastasis Rev,* 24, 2, 315-327.

Kortylewski, M., M. Kujawski, A. Herrmann, C. Yang, L. Wang, Y. Liu, R. Salcedo and H. Yu. (2009). Toll-like receptor 9 activation of signal transducer and activator of transcription 3 constrains its agonist-based immunotherapy. *Cancer Res,* 69, 6, 2497-2505.

Kramer, O. H., D. Baus, S. K. Knauer, S. Stein, E. Jager, R. H. Stauber, M. Grez, E. Pfitzner and T. Heinzel. (2006). Acetylation of Stat1 modulates NF-kappaB activity. *Genes Dev,* 20, 4, 473-485.

Kramer, O. H. and T. Heinzel. (2010). Phosphorylation-acetylation switch in the regulation of STAT1 signaling. *Mol Cell Endocrinol,* 315, 1-2, 40-48.

Kumar, A., M. Commane, T. W. Flickinger, C. M. Horvath and G. R. Stark. (1997). Defective TNF-alpha-induced apoptosis in STAT1-null cells due to low constitutive levels of caspases. *Science,* 278, 5343, 1630-1632.

Kusmartsev, S. and D. I. Gabrilovich. (2005). STAT1 signaling regulates tumor-associated macrophage-mediated T cell deletion. *J Immunol,* 174, 8, 4880-4891.

Lee, C. K., E. Smith, R. Gimeno, R. Gertner and D. E. Levy. (2000). STAT1 affects lymphocyte survival and proliferation partially independent of its role downstream of IFN-gamma. *J Immunol,* 164, 3, 1286-1292.

Lee, H., J. Deng, M. Kujawski, C. Yang, Y. Liu, A. Herrmann, M. Kortylewski, D. Horne, G. Somlo, S. Forman, R. Jove and H. Yu. (2010). STAT3-induced S1PR1 expression is crucial for persistent STAT3 activation in tumors. *Nat Med,* 16, 12, 1421-1428.

Lee, Y. K., C. R. Isham, S. H. Kaufman and K. C. Bible. (2006). Flavopiridol disrupts STAT3/DNA interactions, attenuates STAT3-directed transcription, and combines with the Jak kinase inhibitor AG490 to achieve cytotoxic synergy. *Mol Cancer Ther,* 5, 1, 138-148.

Lesinski, G. B., M. Anghelina, J. Zimmerer, T. Bakalakos, B. Badgwell, R. Parihar, Y. Hu, B. Becknell, G. Abood, A. R. Chaudhury, C. Magro, J. Durbin and W. E. Carson, 3rd. (2003). The antitumor effects of IFN-alpha are abrogated in a STAT1-deficient mouse. *J Clin Invest,* 112, 2, 170-180.

Lesinski, G. B., S. V. Kondadasula, T. Crespin, L. Shen, K. Kendra, M. Walker and W. E. Carson, 3rd. (2004). Multiparametric flow cytometric analysis of inter-patient variation in STAT1 phosphorylation following interferon Alfa immunotherapy. *J Natl Cancer Inst,* 96, 17, 1331-1342.

Lesinski, G. B., J. Trefry, M. Brasdovich, S. V. Kondadasula, K. Sackey, J. M. Zimmerer, A. R. Chaudhury, L. Yu, X. Zhang, T. R. Crespin, M. J. Walker and W. E. Carson, 3rd. (2007). Melanoma cells exhibit variable signal transducer and activator of transcription 1 phosphorylation and a reduced response to IFN-alpha compared with immune effector cells. *Clin Cancer Res,* 13, 17, 5010-5019.

Lesinski, G. B., D. Valentino, E. M. Hade, S. Jones, C. Magro, A. R. Chaudhury, M. J. Walker and W. E. Carson, 3rd. (2005). Expression of STAT1 and STAT2 in malignant melanoma does not correlate with response to interferon-alpha adjuvant therapy. *Cancer Immunol Immunother,* 54, 9, 815-825.

Levy, D. E. and C. K. Lee. (2002). What does Stat3 do? *J Clin Invest,* 109, 9, 1143-1148.

Lim, C. P. and X. Cao. (2006). Structure, function, and regulation of STAT proteins. *Mol Biosyst,* 2, 11, 536-550.

Lin, L., D. M. Benson, Jr., S. Deangelis, C. E. Bakan, P. K. Li, C. Li and J. Lin. (2011). A small molecule, LLL12 inhibits constitutive STAT3 and IL-6-induced STAT3 signaling and exhibits potent growth suppressive activity in human multiple myeloma cells. *Int J Cancer,*

Lin, L., B. Hutzen, P. K. Li, S. Ball, M. Zuo, S. DeAngelis, E. Foust, M. Sobo, L. Friedman, D. Bhasin, L. Cen, C. Li and J. Lin. (2010). A novel small molecule, LLL12, inhibits STAT3 phosphorylation and activities and exhibits potent growth-suppressive activity in human cancer cells. *Neoplasia,* 12, 1, 39-50.

Liu, B., J. Liao, X. Rao, S. A. Kushner, C. D. Chung, D. D. Chang and K. Shuai. (1998). Inhibition of Stat1-mediated gene activation by PIAS1. *Proc Natl Acad Sci U S A,* 95, 18, 10626-10631.

Liu, B. and K. Shuai. (2008). Targeting the PIAS1 SUMO ligase pathway to control inflammation. *Trends Pharmacol Sci,* 29, 10, 505-509.

Masuda, M., M. Suzui and I. B. Weinstein. (2001). Effects of epigallocatechin-3-gallate on growth, epidermal growth factor receptor signaling pathways, gene expression, and chemosensitivity in human head and neck squamous cell carcinoma cell lines. *Clin Cancer Res,* 7, 12, 4220-4229.

Meng, R. D. and W. S. El-Deiry. (2001). p53-independent upregulation of KILLER/DR5 TRAIL receptor expression by glucocorticoids and interferon-gamma. *Exp Cell Res,* 262, 2, 154-169.

Mortarini, R., C. Vegetti, A. Molla, F. Arienti, F. Ravagnani, A. Maurichi, R. Patuzzo, M. Santinami and A. Anichini. (2009). Impaired STAT phosphorylation in T cells from melanoma patients in response to IL-2: association with clinical stage. *Clin Cancer Res,* 15, 12, 4085-4094.

Nam, S., R. Buettner, J. Turkson, D. Kim, J. Q. Cheng, S. Muehlbeyer, F. Hippe, S. Vatter, K. H. Merz, G. Eisenbrand and R. Jove. (2005). Indirubin derivatives inhibit Stat3 signaling and induce apoptosis in human cancer cells. *Proc Natl Acad Sci U S A*, 102, 17, 5998-6003.

Nelson, K. L., J. A. Rogers, T. L. Bowman, R. Jove and T. E. Smithgall. (1998). Activation of STAT3 by the c-Fes protein-tyrosine kinase. *J Biol Chem*, 273, 12, 7072-7077.

Nicholson, S. E., T. A. Willson, A. Farley, R. Starr, J. G. Zhang, M. Baca, W. S. Alexander, D. Metcalf, D. J. Hilton and N. A. Nicola. (1999). Mutational analyses of the SOCS proteins suggest a dual domain requirement but distinct mechanisms for inhibition of LIF and IL-6 signal transduction. *EMBO J*, 18, 2, 375-385.

Niu, G., T. Bowman, M. Huang, S. Shivers, D. Reintgen, A. Daud, A. Chang, A. Kraker, R. Jove and H. Yu. (2002). Roles of activated Src and Stat3 signaling in melanoma tumor cell growth. *Oncogene*, 21, 46, 7001-7010.

Niu, G., K. L. Wright, M. Huang, L. Song, E. Haura, J. Turkson, S. Zhang, T. Wang, D. Sinibaldi, D. Coppola, R. Heller, L. M. Ellis, J. Karras, J. Bromberg, D. Pardoll, R. Jove and H. Yu. (2002). Constitutive Stat3 activity up-regulates VEGF expression and tumor angiogenesis. *Oncogene*, 21, 13, 2000-2008.

O'Shea, J. J., Y. Kanno, X. Chen and D. E. Levy. (2005). Cell signaling. Stat acetylation--a key facet of cytokine signaling? *Science*, 307, 5707, 217-218.

Onimoe, G. I., A. Liu, L. Lin, C. C. Wei, E. B. Schwartz, D. Bhasin, C. Li, J. R. Fuchs, P. K. Li, P. Houghton, A. Termuhlen, T. Gross and J. Lin. (2011). Small molecules, LLL12 and FLLL32, inhibit STAT3 and exhibit potent growth suppressive activity in osteosarcoma cells and tumor growth in mice. *Invest New Drugs*,

Ouchi, T., S. W. Lee, M. Ouchi, S. A. Aaronson and C. M. Horvath. (2000). Collaboration of signal transducer and activator of transcription 1 (STAT1) and BRCA1 in differential regulation of IFN-gamma target genes. *Proc Natl Acad Sci U S A*, 97, 10, 5208-5213.

Pansky, A., P. Hildebrand, E. Fasler-Kan, L. Baselgia, S. Ketterer, C. Beglinger and M. H. Heim. (2000). Defective Jak-STAT signal transduction pathway in melanoma cells resistant to growth inhibition by interferon-alpha. *Int J Cancer*, 85, 5, 720-725.

Pollock, P. M., U. L. Harper, K. S. Hansen, L. M. Yudt, M. Stark, C. M. Robbins, T. Y. Moses, G. Hostetter, U. Wagner, J. Kakareka, G. Salem, T. Pohida, P. Heenan, P. Duray, O. Kallioniemi, N. K. Hayward, J. M. Trent and P. S. Meltzer. (2003). High frequency of BRAF mutations in nevi. *Nat Genet*, 33, 1, 19-20.

Qing, Y. and G. R. Stark. (2004). Alternative activation of STAT1 and STAT3 in response to interferon-gamma. *J Biol Chem*, 279, 40, 41679-41685.

Ransohoff, R. M. (1998). Cellular responses to interferons and other cytokines: the JAK-STAT paradigm. *N Engl J Med*, 338, 9, 616-618.

Real, P. J., A. Sierra, A. De Juan, J. C. Segovia, J. M. Lopez-Vega and J. L. Fernandez-Luna. (2002). Resistance to chemotherapy via Stat3-dependent overexpression of Bcl-2 in metastatic breast cancer cells. *Oncogene*, 21, 50, 7611-7618.

Regis, G., M. Bosticardo, L. Conti, S. De Angelis, D. Boselli, B. Tomaino, P. Bernabei, M. Giovarelli and F. Novelli. (2005). Iron regulates T-lymphocyte sensitivity to the IFN-gamma/STAT1 signaling pathway in vitro and in vivo. *Blood*, 105, 8, 3214-3221.

Regis, G., S. Pensa, D. Boselli, F. Novelli and V. Poli. (2008). Ups and downs: the STAT1:STAT3 seesaw of Interferon and gp130 receptor signalling. *Semin Cell Dev Biol*, 19, 4, 351-359.

Ren, Z. and T. S. Schaefer. (2002). ErbB-2 activates Stat3 alpha in a Src- and JAK2-dependent manner. *J Biol Chem,* 277, 41, 38486-38493.

Sakai, I., K. Takeuchi, H. Yamauchi, H. Narumi and S. Fujita. (2002). Constitutive expression of SOCS3 confers resistance to IFN-alpha in chronic myelogenous leukemia cells. *Blood,* 100, 8, 2926-2931.

Sato, T., C. Selleri, N. S. Young and J. P. Maciejewski. (1997). Inhibition of interferon regulatory factor-1 expression results in predominance of cell growth stimulatory effects of interferon-gamma due to phosphorylation of Stat1 and Stat3. *Blood,* 90, 12, 4749-4758.

Schultz, J., D. Koczan, U. Schmitz, S. M. Ibrahim, D. Pilch, J. Landsberg and M. Kunz. (2010). Tumor-promoting role of signal transducer and activator of transcription (Stat)1 in late-stage melanoma growth. *Clin Exp Metastasis,* 27, 3, 133-140.

Sellers, L. A., W. Feniuk, P. P. Humphrey and H. Lauder. (1999). Activated G protein-coupled receptor induces tyrosine phosphorylation of STAT3 and agonist-selective serine phosphorylation via sustained stimulation of mitogen-activated protein kinase. Resultant effects on cell proliferation. *J Biol Chem,* 274, 23, 16423-16430.

Shahani, V. M., P. Yue, S. Haftchenary, W. Zhao, J. L. Lukkarila, X. Zhang, D. Ball, C. Nona, P. T. Gunning and J. Turkson. (2011). Identification of Purine-Scaffold Small-Molecule Inhibitors of Stat3 Activation by QSAR Studies. *ACS Med Chem Lett,* 2, 1, 79-84.

Shen, L., K. Evel-Kabler, R. Strube and S. Y. Chen. (2004). Silencing of SOCS1 enhances antigen presentation by dendritic cells and antigen-specific anti-tumor immunity. *Nat Biotechnol,* 22, 12, 1546-1553.

Shen, Y., G. Devgan, J. E. Darnell, Jr. and J. F. Bromberg. (2001). Constitutively activated Stat3 protects fibroblasts from serum withdrawal and UV-induced apoptosis and antagonizes the proapoptotic effects of activated Stat1. *Proc Natl Acad Sci U S A,* 98, 4, 1543-1548.

Smalley, K. S., R. Contractor, T. K. Nguyen, M. Xiao, R. Edwards, V. Muthusamy, A. J. King, K. T. Flaherty, M. Bosenberg, M. Herlyn and K. L. Nathanson. (2008). Identification of a novel subgroup of melanomas with KIT/cyclin-dependent kinase-4 overexpression. *Cancer Res,* 68, 14, 5743-5752.

Smithgall, T. E., S. D. Briggs, S. Schreiner, E. C. Lerner, H. Cheng and M. B. Wilson. (2000). Control of myeloid differentiation and survival by Stats. *Oncogene,* 19, 21, 2612-2618.

Sobota, R., M. Szwed, A. Kasza, M. Bugno and T. Kordula. (2000). Parthenolide inhibits activation of signal transducers and activators of transcription (STATs) induced by cytokines of the IL-6 family. *Biochem Biophys Res Commun,* 267, 1, 329-333.

Stephanou, A. and D. S. Latchman. (2005). Opposing actions of STAT-1 and STAT-3. *Growth Factors,* 23, 3, 177-182.

Su, L. and M. David. (2000). Distinct mechanisms of STAT phosphorylation via the interferon-alpha/beta receptor. Selective inhibition of STAT3 and STAT5 by piceatannol. *J Biol Chem,* 275, 17, 12661-12666.

Takeda, K., K. Noguchi, W. Shi, T. Tanaka, M. Matsumoto, N. Yoshida, T. Kishimoto and S. Akira. (1997). Targeted disruption of the mouse Stat3 gene leads to early embryonic lethality. *Proc Natl Acad Sci U S A,* 94, 8, 3801-3804.

Traynor, K. (2011). Ipilimumab approved for metastatic melanoma. *Am J Health Syst Pharm,* 68, 9, 768.

Turkson, J. (2004). STAT proteins as novel targets for cancer drug discovery. *Expert Opin Ther Targets,* 8, 5, 409-422.

Turkson, J. and R. Jove. (2000). STAT proteins: novel molecular targets for cancer drug discovery. *Oncogene,* 19, 56, 6613-6626.

Turkson, J., S. Zhang, J. Palmer, H. Kay, J. Stanko, L. B. Mora, S. Sebti, H. Yu and R. Jove. (2004). Inhibition of constitutive signal transducer and activator of transcription 3 activation by novel platinum complexes with potent antitumor activity. *Mol Cancer Ther,* 3, 12, 1533-1542.

Uyttenhove, C., L. Pilotte, I. Theate, V. Stroobant, D. Colau, N. Parmentier, T. Boon and B. J. Van den Eynde. (2003). Evidence for a tumoral immune resistance mechanism based on tryptophan degradation by indoleamine 2,3-dioxygenase. *Nat Med,* 9, 10, 1269-1274.

Vajdic, C. M., M. T. van Leeuwen, A. C. Webster, M. R. McCredie, J. H. Stewart, J. R. Chapman, J. Amin, S. P. McDonald and A. E. Grulich. (2009). Cutaneous melanoma is related to immune suppression in kidney transplant recipients. *Cancer Epidemiol Biomarkers Prev,* 18, 8, 2297-2303.

Wang, T., G. Niu, M. Kortylewski, L. Burdelya, K. Shain, S. Zhang, R. Bhattacharya, D. Gabrilovich, R. Heller, D. Coppola, W. Dalton, R. Jove, D. Pardoll and H. Yu. (2004). Regulation of the innate and adaptive immune responses by Stat-3 signaling in tumor cells. *Nat Med,* 10, 1, 48-54.

Wang, W., H. D. Edington, U. N. Rao, D. M. Jukic, S. R. Land, S. Ferrone and J. M. Kirkwood. (2007). Modulation of signal transducers and activators of transcription 1 and 3 signaling in melanoma by high-dose IFNalpha2b. *Clin Cancer Res,* 13, 5, 1523-1531.

Wang, W., H. D. Edington, U. N. Rao, D. M. Jukic, H. Wang, J. M. Shipe-Spotloe and J. M. Kirkwood. (2008). STAT3 as a biomarker of progression in atypical nevi of patients with melanoma: dose-response effects of systemic IFNalpha therapy. *J Invest Dermatol,* 128, 8, 1997-2002.

Wegenka, U. M., J. Buschmann, C. Lutticken, P. C. Heinrich and F. Horn. (1993). Acute-phase response factor, a nuclear factor binding to acute-phase response elements, is rapidly activated by interleukin-6 at the posttranslational level. *Mol Cell Biol,* 13, 1, 276-288.

Wei, C. C., S. Ball, L. Lin, A. Liu, J. R. Fuchs, P. K. Li, C. Li and J. Lin. (2011). Two small molecule compounds, LLL12 and FLLL32, exhibit potent inhibitory activity on STAT3 in human rhabdomyosarcoma cells. *Int J Oncol,* 38, 1, 279-285.

Wong, L. H., I. Hatzinisiriou, R. J. Devenish and S. J. Ralph. (1998). IFN-gamma priming up-regulates IFN-stimulated gene factor 3 (ISGF3) components, augmenting responsiveness of IFN-resistant melanoma cells to type I IFNs. *J Immunol,* 160, 11, 5475-5484.

Wung, B. S., M. C. Hsu, C. C. Wu and C. W. Hsieh. (2005). Resveratrol suppresses IL-6-induced ICAM-1 gene expression in endothelial cells: effects on the inhibition of STAT3 phosphorylation. *Life Sci,* 78, 4, 389-397.

Xi, S., W. E. Gooding and J. R. Grandis. (2005). In vivo antitumor efficacy of STAT3 blockade using a transcription factor decoy approach: implications for cancer therapy. *Oncogene,* 24, 6, 970-979.

Xie, T. X., F. J. Huang, K. D. Aldape, S. H. Kang, M. Liu, J. E. Gershenwald, K. Xie, R. Sawaya and S. Huang. (2006). Activation of stat3 in human melanoma promotes brain metastasis. *Cancer Res,* 66, 6, 3188-3196.

Xu, Q., J. Briggs, S. Park, G. Niu, M. Kortylewski, S. Zhang, T. Gritsko, J. Turkson, H. Kay, G. L. Semenza, J. Q. Cheng, R. Jove and H. Yu. (2005). Targeting Stat3 blocks both HIF-1 and VEGF expression induced by multiple oncogenic growth signaling pathways. *Oncogene,* 24, 36, 5552-5560.

Yang, J., M. Chatterjee-Kishore, S. M. Staugaitis, H. Nguyen, K. Schlessinger, D. E. Levy and G. R. Stark. (2005). Novel roles of unphosphorylated STAT3 in oncogenesis and transcriptional regulation. *Cancer Res,* 65, 3, 939-947.

Yasukawa, H., H. Misawa, H. Sakamoto, M. Masuhara, A. Sasaki, T. Wakioka, S. Ohtsuka, T. Imaizumi, T. Matsuda, J. N. Ihle and A. Yoshimura. (1999). The JAK-binding protein JAB inhibits Janus tyrosine kinase activity through binding in the activation loop. *EMBO J,* 18, 5, 1309-1320.

You, M., D. H. Yu and G. S. Feng. (1999). Shp-2 tyrosine phosphatase functions as a negative regulator of the interferon-stimulated Jak/STAT pathway. *Mol Cell Biol,* 19, 3, 2416-2424.

Yu, C. L., D. J. Meyer, G. S. Campbell, A. C. Larner, C. Carter-Su, J. Schwartz and R. Jove. (1995). Enhanced DNA-binding activity of a Stat3-related protein in cells transformed by the Src oncoprotein. *Science,* 269, 5220, 81-83.

Yu, H. and R. Jove. (2004). The STATs of cancer--new molecular targets come of age. *Nat Rev Cancer,* 4, 2, 97-105.

Yu, H., M. Kortylewski and D. Pardoll. (2007). Crosstalk between cancer and immune cells: role of STAT3 in the tumour microenvironment. *Nat Rev Immunol,* 7, 1, 41-51.

Yu, H., D. Pardoll and R. Jove. (2009). STATs in cancer inflammation and immunity: a leading role for STAT3. *Nat Rev Cancer,* 9, 11, 798-809.

Yuan, Z. L., Y. J. Guan, D. Chatterjee and Y. E. Chin. (2005). Stat3 dimerization regulated by reversible acetylation of a single lysine residue. *Science,* 307, 5707, 269-273.

Yue, P. and J. Turkson. (2009). Targeting STAT3 in cancer: how successful are we? *Expert Opin Investig Drugs,* 18, 1, 45-56.

Zhang, X., P. Yue, S. Fletcher, W. Zhao, P. T. Gunning and J. Turkson. (2010). A novel small-molecule disrupts Stat3 SH2 domain-phosphotyrosine interactions and Stat3-dependent tumor processes. *Biochem Pharmacol,* 79, 10, 1398-1409.

Zhang, Y., J. Turkson, C. Carter-Su, T. Smithgall, A. Levitzki, A. Kraker, J. J. Krolewski, P. Medveczky and R. Jove. (2000). Activation of Stat3 in v-Src-transformed fibroblasts requires cooperation of Jak1 kinase activity. *J Biol Chem,* 275, 32, 24935-24944.

Zhao, W., S. Jaganathan and J. Turkson. (2010). A cell-permeable Stat3 SH2 domain mimetic inhibits Stat3 activation and induces antitumor cell effects in vitro. *J Biol Chem,* 285, 46, 35855-35865.

Zimmerer, J. M., G. B. Lesinski, S. V. Kondadasula, V. I. Karpa, A. Lehman, A. Raychaudhury, B. Becknell and W. E. Carson, 3rd. (2007). IFN-alpha-induced signal transduction, gene expression, and antitumor activity of immune effector cells are negatively regulated by suppressor of cytokine signaling proteins. *J Immunol,* 178, 8, 4832-4845.

# Part 4

## Receptor

# 15

# Targeting Adenosine Receptors for the Treatment of Melanoma

Sarvesh Jajoo, Sandeep Sheth,
Debashree Mukherjea, Leonard P. Rybak and Vickram Ramkumar
*Southern Illinois University School of Medicine, Springfield, IL*
*USA*

## 1. Introduction

Melanoma is the malignant tumor of melanocytes, skin cells which produce the pigment melanin. According to the 2010 statistics from American Cancer Society, around 68,130 new cases will be diagnosed with melanoma, of which 8,700 individuals will die (http://www.cancer.gov/cancertopics/types/melanoma). Melanoma is one of the most fatal forms of skin cancer, accounting for almost 65% of all the skin cancer related deaths. Despite a decrease in the mortality rate in the population under the age of 65 years, the incidence of melanoma has increased annually in both Caucasian men and women. It is ranked as the 5$^{th}$ most common cancer in men and the 6$^{th}$ most common cancer in women (Sober et al., 2008). Additionally, the 5-year survival for the metastatic melanoma is still significantly high, when compared to the non-metastatic type (O'Day et al., 2002). This is due, in part, to the relative resistance of metastatic melanoma to chemotherapeutic agents (O'Day et al., 2002). Thus, it is essential to develop new therapeutic agents targeting unique molecular signaling pathways important for the development of the malignant and invasive neoplasm.

Factors which predispose individual to developing melanomas include, among others, exposure to sunlight (UVB irradiation) (Lee, 1982). UVB radiation is linked to DNA damage and depressed immune function. This is supported by demographic data which show high prevalence of melanomas in white skin individuals living in the equatorial zone (compared to those living in northern latitudes) (Lee and Scotto, 1993), the prevalence of melanomas to sun exposed areas of the body, early exposures and sunburns, and increased outdoor recreational sports (Balch et al., 1997). However, sunlight may not be the only cause, but one of several causes. For example, the incidence of melanomas is higher in white collar workers (mostly likely to work inside) than in blue collar workers (more likely to work outside). Susceptibility to sunburns, light skin color and freckling are associated with increased incidence of melanomas (Balch et al., 1997). Measures which could be taken to decrease the incidence of melanomas include the use of UV-A/UV-B sunblock with sun protection factor ≥15, avoiding mid-day sunlight, restriction of activity in a shaded area, and the use of umbrellas and protective clothing. In addition, it is also recommended that individuals avoid tanning in a UV tanning salon (Balch et al., 1997).

Several genes have been identified which increases susceptibility to melanomas. These include p16, the product of which regulates the cell cycle by inhibiting cyclin-dependent kinase 4 (cdk4) (Serrano et al., 1993). Mutation of this gene would allow for uncontrolled cell proliferation. Screening could identify patients who are likely to develop melanoma and help them to institute life-style changes to limit UV exposure.

Melanoma progresses from a common acquired nevus to a primary dysplastic nevus. This can then develop into a primary melanoma and subsequently to metastatic melanoma. Early detection of melanoma is essential for initiation of its management. This is aided by evaluation of antigenic markers linked to differentiation and pathogenesis. One such protein, S-100 protein, is expressed in all melanomas and could serve as a marker for melanoma (Harpio and Einarsson, 2004). However, it is also expressed in sarcomas and other cancers. Another protein, HMB-45, is more specific for melanoma but is not always accurate for metastatic melanoma (Wick et al., 1988). Various other markers include cytokeratins and leukocyte common antigen.

Management of melanoma includes surgical excision of the superficial skin lesions and local metastases which are accessible. In addition, radiation of cutaneous and lymph node metastases could be performed. Chemotherapy is also useful for the management of melanoma. The infusion of the alkylating agent, decarbazine, is a standard treatment. Other agents include melphalan, nitrosureas, platinum compounds, vincristine and others. However, the response rates of chemotherapy are low, ranging from 10-23%. In some cases, limb perfusion with melphalan alone or in combination with immune modulators, such as tumor necrosis factor-$\alpha$ (TNF-$\alpha$) and interferons (IFNs) have been shown to be effective. However, the prolonged use of IFNs is limited by the development of flu-like symptoms and hepatotoxicity (Atallah and Flaherty, 2005). Other forms of immunotherapy, such as the use of tumor vaccines and monoclonal antibodies, are under investigation (Weber, 2011). Melanomas are associated with specific antigens on their cell surfaces, which serve as homing targets of cytotoxic T cells (CTLs). These include MAGE-1 (Van der Bruggen et al., 1991; De Plaen et al., 1994), which could be a suitable target for immune-based therapies (Marchand et al., 1993). Other targets include tyrosinase and MART-1 melanoma antigens (Kawakami and Rosenberg, 1996). CTLs generated against these proteins could serve as novel targets for immunotherapy.

This chapter provides a review of studies on the types of adenosine receptors present on melanoma cells and discusses how these receptors mediate the progression or inhibit the growth and metastasis of melanoma. These receptors present on melanoma cells or immune cells mediate a direct or indirect effect on the growth and metastasis of melanoma. Selective agonists or antagonists of these receptor types could serve as novel treatments for melanoma.

## 2. Adenosine and its receptors

Adenosine is a purine nucleoside composed of adenine attached to a ribose molecule via glycosidic linkage. It is a ubiquitously produced by stepwise dephosphorylation of ATP. Extracellular adenosine acts as a signaling molecule which mediates a number of physiological and metabolic effects (Gorlach, 2005). Adenosine accumulation during ischemia and inflammation protects tissue from injury (Linden, 2001). Some effects of adenosine which are considered tissue or cytoprotective are mediated by a variety of cellular mechanisms. These include stimulation of glycogen breakdown to provide glucose for ATP production via anaerobic glycolysis, reduction in neuronal excitability as well as neurotransmitter release to reduce neuronal energy demands (Gorlach, 2005), increasing the

ratio of oxygen supply to demand by causing vasodilation, reducing inflammation and promoting angiogenesis (Adair, 2005; Jacobson and Gao, 2006).
The idea that adenosine has an important role in cardiovascular function was first introduced more than 80 years ago when Drury and Szent-Gyorgyi (1929) found that extracts from heart and other tissues produced vasodilation, hypotension, bradycardia, and a decrease in atrioventricular conduction velocity. It was later shown by Berne et al (1983) that adenosine acts as a retaliatory metabolite which tend to counter the processes which led to increased oxygen demand. This action helps to maintain tissue oxygenation within a normal range in hypoxia. Such a retaliatory action could be demonstrated in the heart, brain, and skeletal muscle, where adenosine increases oxygen supply by promoting vasodilation and increased blood flow to these tissues (Berne et al., 1983). Adenosine also mediates an anti-adrenergic effect which decreases oxygen demand in the heart (Adair, 2005). While these actions of adenosine are relatively short-term, the nucleoside can also promote long-term changes to enhance survival. For example, adenosine promotes angiogenesis, a process of new blood vessel growth (Adair, 2005). Angiogenesis may be important in coronary artery disease, ischemia, stroke and in delayed wound healing for the repair and regeneration of tissue (Gupta and Zhang, 2005). Such an action may also provide oxygen and nutrient to tumors as they grow away from their primary blood vessel supplies.

### 2.1 Adenosine: Formation and metabolism

Adenosine accumulates in tissues when oxygen demand exceeds oxygen supply, as would be encountered during vigorous exercise or during an ischemic attack (Adair, 2005) or in the microenvironment of tumors. It is generated and metabolized through stepwise dephosphorylation of ATP (Figure 1). ATP and ADP are converted by CD39 (ecto-ATP apyrase) to AMP through a process activated by hypoxia (Gorlach, 2005). Dephosphorylation of AMP is mediated intracellularly by cytosolic-5′-nucleotidase and extracellularly by membrane-bound ecto-5′-nucleotidase (CD73), respectively. Intracellularly, adenosine is also produced from the hydrolysis of S-adenosylhomocysteine (SAH). However, hydrolysis of SAH to adenosine contributes marginally to its production (Adair, 2005). Adenosine deaminase is widely distributed in many cells and tissues where it metabolizes adenosine to form inosine and hypoxanthine. Adenosine kinase catalyses the formation of AMP from adenosine in order to replenish the stores of cellular ATP (Adair, 2005; Gorlach, 2005).
The cellular uptake and release of adenosine is accomplished by two main groups of membrane nucleoside transporters. Concentrative nucleoside transporter family (SLC28) is found in specialized epithelial tissue and it mediates active $Na^+$-dependent nucleoside transport. Passive nucleoside transport processes are ubiquitous and are mediated by members of the equilibrative nucleoside transporter (ENT) family (SLC29) (Baldwin et al., 2004). ENTs are bidirectional and four ENT isoforms are identified in human and rodent genome. Inhibition of ENTs by dipyridamole, a coronary vasodilatory and cardio-protective agent, prevents the reuptake of adenosine into the endothelial cells, increases its extracellular concentration and thus enhances AR activation (Adair, 2005; Gorlach, 2005). Thus, extracellular adenosine concentrations can increase by increasing the activities of nucleotidases (major pathway) and adenosine kinases (minor pathway) along with their substrates (such as AMP). In addition, inhibition of ENTs would also lead to increased extracellular adenosine (Adair, 2005). Exposing cells to a hypoxic environment can increase

the activities of nucleotidases and decrease the activities of adenosine kinases, leading to a net increase in the production of adenosine (Linden, 2001). The induction of ecto-5′-nucleotidase (CD73) activity in hypoxic condition has been shown in the ischemic heart (Minamino et al., 1996) and brain (Braun et al., 1997) of intact animal, possibly by hypoxia inducible factor (HIF-1- dependent pathway (Synnestvedt et al., 2002). Hypoxia also down-regulates ENT1 expression in different mouse tissues (Chaudry et al., 2004; Eltzschig et al., 2005), thereby increasing extracellular concentrations of adenosine.

Higher adenosine concentrations in the extracellular fluids are important to activate the ARs present on a variety of cells. Studies have estimated the physiological extracellular adenosine concentrations in normal brain to be approximately 30-300 nM (Fredholm et al., 2001). *In vivo* studies by Blay et al. (1997) revealed that the adenosine concentrations in the extracellular fluids of solid tumor in mice range from 0.2-2.4 μM, which is 10- to 20-fold higher compared to concentrations in adjacent subcutaneous tissue. Furthermore, treatment with inhibitors of adenosine deaminase and adenosine kinase can increase adenosine levels in tumors to as high as 13 μM (Blay et al., 1997).

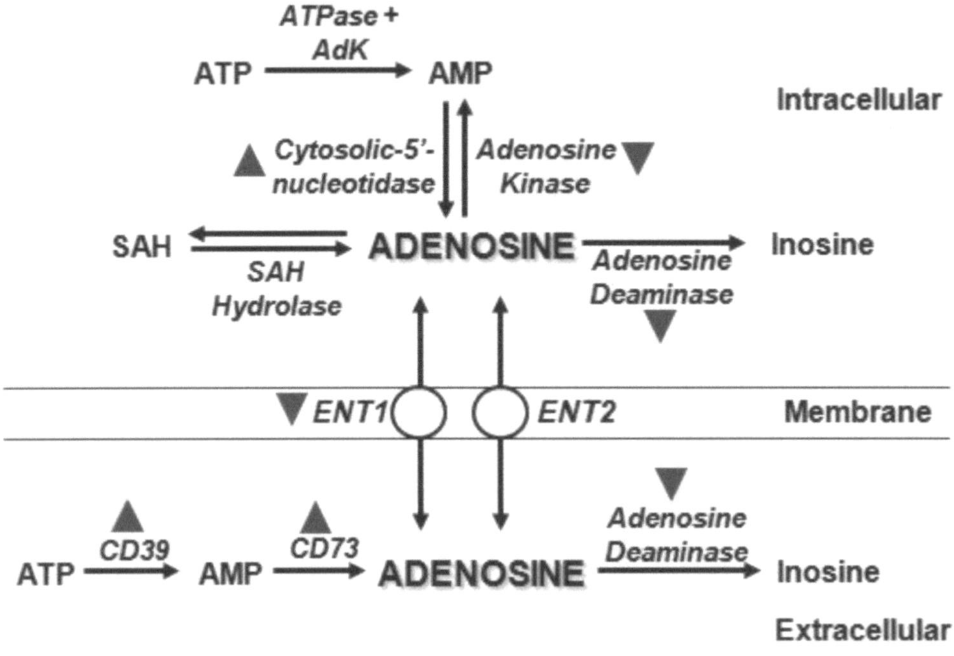


Fig. 1. Metabolic pathways for adenosine production and consumption. Adenosine is produced by the dephosphorylation of ATP and ADP by ATPases and the action of 5′-nucleotidase. Additionally, the nucleoside is produced from SAH by SAH hydrolase. Once produced, adenosine could be transported in or out of the cell by bidirectional transporters , ENT1 and 2. Adenosine is rapidly degraded by adenosine deaminase. Abbreviations: ATPase, ATP hydrolyzing enzymes; AdK, adenylate kinase; SAH, S-adenosylhomocysteine; ENT: Equilibrative nucleoside transporter. The arrow heads ▲ and ▼ indicate up-regulation or down-regulation of enzymes and the transporter during hypoxia. [Modified from (Adair, 2005; Gorlach, 2005)]

### 2.2 Adenosine receptors

Studies have shown that adenosine levels are highest in the tumor microenvironment which is severely hypoxic. The physiological concentrations of adenosine produced under such conditions are sufficient enough to activate ARs present on the tumor cells (Ohta et al., 2006). The effects of extracellular adenosine are mediated by four known ARs subtypes, namely the $A_1$, $A_{2A}$, $A_{2B}$ and $A_3AR$. All of these ARs are cell surface G protein-coupled receptor which have distinct tissue-specific distributions (Fredholm et al., 2001). These ARs were classified on the basis of their inhibiting ($A_1$ and $A_3AR$) or stimulating ($A_{2A}$ and $A_{2B}AR$) adenylyl cyclase by coupling to either $G_i$ or $G_s$ types of guanine nucleotide regulatory (G) proteins, respectively (Fredholm et al., 2006). Inhibition or activation of adenylyl cyclase reduces or increases intracellular cyclic AMP, respectively. This second messenger mediates a number of cellular functions, which could be altered depending on the presence of extracellular adenosine and the AR profile expressed on the cell surface. In addition, there is some evidence that the ARs may signal via other G-proteins (Fredholm et al., 2001), which activate other pathways such as phospholipase C (PLC), $Ca^{2+}$ and mitogen-activated protein kinases (MAPKs) (Jacobson and Gao, 2006). Activation of $A_1AR$ inhibits adenylyl cyclase by stimulating pertussis toxin-sensitive $G_i$ proteins, leading to increased activity of PLC. The $A_1AR$ is also coupled to the activation of $K^+$ channels and inhibition of N-, P- and Q-type $Ca^{2+}$ channels (Fredholm et al., 2001; Jacobson and Gao, 2006). The same appears to be true for $A_3AR$, which also binds to $G_q$ G-proteins and activates PLC (Fredholm et al., 2001). In contrast, the $A_{2A}AR$ interacts with the stimulatory $G_s$ and $G_{olf}$ G-proteins to activate adenylyl cyclase and increase cyclic AMP concentrations (Fredholm et al., 2001). Activation of $A_{2A}AR$ also induces the formation of inositol 1,4,5-trisphosphate ($IP_3$) to raise intracellular $Ca^{2+}$ and activate PKC in COS-7 cells via pertussis toxin-insensitive $G_{\alpha 15}$ and $G_{\alpha 16}$ proteins (Fredholm et al., 2001). Like the $A_{2A}AR$, the $A_{2B}AR$ is positively coupled to both $G_s$ and $G_q$ proteins and therefore can modulate both intracellular cyclic AMP and $IP_3$ concentrations (Fredholm et al., 2001). $A_{2B}AR$ has lower affinity for adenosine as compared to $A_{2A}AR$ (Feoktistov and Biaggioni, 1997). $A_{2A}AR$ expression could be induced by inflammatory cytokines, such as interleukin (IL)-1 and tumor necrosis factor (TNF)-α (Khoa et al., 2001). $A_{2B}AR$ expression is induced by hypoxia inducible factor (HIF)-1α in hypoxia (Kong et al., 2006), TNF-α and interferon (IFN)-γ (St Hilaire et al., 2008; Xaus et al., 1999). Such regulations could be important in a tumor microenvironment associated with significant hypoxia and/or inflammation.

Several studies have shown that the adenosine-induced activation of MAPK is essential for mediating cell differentiation, survival, proliferation, and death (Fredholm et al., 2001). Extracellular regulated kinases (ERK1/2) are members of the MAPK family linked to cellular proliferation. $A_1AR$ transiently expressed in COS-7 cells activated ERK1/2 via β,γ-subunits released from $G_{i/o}$ G-proteins (Faure et al., 1994). Studies on stably expressed $A_1AR$ in CHO cells demonstrated that the $A_1AR$ can also induce ERK1/2 activation (Dickenson et al., 1998; Schulte and Fredholm, 2000). $A_{2A}AR$ activation stimulates ERK1/2 via a cyclic AMP/Ras/MAPK kinase pathway in endothelial cells (Sexl et al., 1997). $A_{2B}AR$-mediated activation of MAPK is important for interleukin (IL)-8 secretion, a pro-angiogenic growth factor, and consequently for mast cell activation (Fredholm et al., 2001). Another pathway has been demonstrated in human umbilical vascular endothelial cell (HUVEC) which involves cyclic AMP-dependent but protein kinase A (PKA)-independent activation of ERK1/2, associated with cell proliferation (Fang and Olah, 2007). The cyclic AMP activation of exchange protein activated by cyclic AMP-1 (Epac1) stimulates ERK1/2 activity. This provides an alternate pathway for ERK1/2 activation by the $A_{2B}AR$. (Fang and Olah, 2007).

### 2.3 Adenosine receptors in cancer

ARs are differentially expressed on tumor cell lines and tumor samples. High levels of $A_1AR$ are expressed in breast cancer tissues, compared to normal breast tissues (Mirza et al., 2005). Activation of the $A_1AR$ was shown to reduce the proliferation of these cells by inhibiting the $G_1$ checkpoint in the cell cycle (Mirza et al., 2005). Increased $A_1AR$ was also observed in the peritumoral regions of experimental F98 glioma cells. The sources of the increased $A_1AR$ expression were activated astrocytes and microglia which suppress glioblastoma (Synowitz et al., 2006). In addition, activation of $A_1AR$ on colon cancer cells increased apoptosis by activating caspases (Saito et al., 2010). Studies have also shown an anti-tumor action of $A_{2A}AR$ in A375 melanoma (Merighi et al., 2002) and human colon cancer cells (Yasuda et al., 2009), the latter mediated by activation of caspases. In contrast, the $A_{2A}AR$ promotes growth of breast cancer MCF-7 breast cancer cells (Etique et al., 2009) and increases angiogenesis by inducing VEGF expression (Montesinos et al., 2002). These studies suggest that $A_{2A}AR$ antagonists could be useful in cancer by blocking angiogenesis. Activation of the $A_{2B}AR$ is also linked to angiogenesis and promotes growth and tumor metastasis (Grant et al., 1999). In support of this, $A_{2B}AR$ knockout mice, administered Lewis lung carcinoma, demonstrated reduced tumor growth and survival times (Ryzhov et al., 2008). Studies performed on U87 MG human glioblastoma cells only detected transcripts for $A_1$, $A_{2A}$ and $A_{2B}ARs$, but no transcript for $A_3AR$ (Zeng et al., 2003). However, Merighi et al. (2006) were able to detect $A_3AR$ in these cells. $A_3AR$ is also highly expressed in tumors like colon and breast carcinoma tissues as compared to non-neoplastic or normal tisues (Madi et al., 2004). A role of the $A_3AR$ in mediating anti-tumor actions *in vitro* and *in vivo* has been demonstrated. For example, $A_3AR$ agonists inhibit the growth of melanoma (Madi et al., 2003), colon (Ohana et al., 2003) and prostate cancers (Fishman et al., 2004) in animal models. Induction of the $A_3AR$ occurs in several types of cancers (Madi et al., 2004), when compared to normal adjacent tissue, suggesting that these receptors could serve as potential molecular markers of these cancers. One study demonstrated inhibition of liver metastasis in mice inoculated with human HCT-116 or murine CT-26 colon carcinoma cells by $A_3AR$ agonists (Ohana et al., 2003). The anti-tumor action of $A_3AR$ agonists could be explained by an increase in natural killer (NK) cell activity, which promotes killing of tumor cells (Harish et al., 2003).

## 3. Adenosine receptors in melanoma

Studies have demonstrated both pro- and anti-tumorigenic effects of AR activation in melanoma. Early studies showed that topical application of an $A_{2A}AR$ agonist to the skin enhanced wound closure in animals as well as in the animals (Montesinos et al., 1997). Adenosine suppressed the proliferation of transformed keratinocytes in both $G_1$ and S phases of the cell cycle (Brown et al., 2000). Furthermore, activation of $A_3AR$ protected skin mast cells from UV light-induced cell death (Gao et al., 2001). This suggests that $A_3AR$ agonists can also mediate similar protection in different skin cell types. Studies described below demonstrate the actions of different AR subtypes on melanoma and support the utility of these receptor for treating melanoma. These receptors are described in order of their importance in melanoma treatment.

### 3.1 $A_3$ adenosine receptors and melanoma

The actions of this AR subtype has been best studied in melanoma. This receptor is highly expressed in melanoma cell lines and tissues, compared to normal tissues. Measurements of the mRNA levels of $A_3$AR in paraffin-embedded melanoma tissue slides showed almost 2-fold increased expression of $A_3$AR in cancerous tissues, as compared to the normal tissues (Madi et al., 2004). Human malignant melanoma A375 cells expressed high levels of $A_3$AR, as determined by radioligand binding assays. Activation of these receptors did not decrease forskolin-stimulated adenylyl cyclase activity (Merighi et al., 2001), suggesting coupling of these receptors to an alternate signaling system. In fact, $A_3$AR activation increased intracellular calcium release which was suppressed by an $A_3$AR antagonist. This finding suggests that $A_3$AR preferentially couples to a $G_q$-PLC pathway in A375 melanoma cells. Activation of $A_3$ARs in these cells improved survival and reduced $A_{2A}$AR-induced cell death. However, $A_3$AR agonist decreased melanoma cell proliferation in a PKC- and MAPK-dependent manner. Furthermore, $A_3$AR activation arrested cells in the $G_1$ phase, leading to decreased cell number in the $G_2$/M phase (Merighi et al., 2002). The reason for the apparent discrepancy between improving survival and decreasing cell proliferation following $A_3$AR activation in A375 melanoma cells is unclear.

In an earlier study, Bar-Yehuda et al. (2001) showed that the $A_3$AR agonist, 1-deoxy-1-[6-[((3-iodophenyl)methyl)amino]-9H-purin-9-yl]-N-methyl-β-D-ribofuranuronamide, N6-(3-iodobenzyl)adenosine-5'-N-methyluronamide (IB-MECA), inhibited the growth of murine melanoma (B16-F10) cells in culture and suppressed the tumor growth in mice injected with these cells. B16-F10 melanoma cells express high levels of $A_3$AR, as detected by western blotting, immunocytochemistry and RT-PCR (Madi et al., 2003). The authors showed that the $A_3$AR in these cells were negatively coupled to adenylyl cyclase and reduced PKA activity. In addition to the primary melanoma growth, the $A_3$AR agonist reduced the number of metastatic lung foci, suggesting that $A_3$AR activation also suppresses metastasis of these cells. There was also an additive effect of $A_3$AR agonist and cyclophosphamide, a chemotherapeutic drug (Fishman et al., 2001). $A_3$AR expression has also been studied in another murine melanoma cell line (B16-BL6). Cordycepin, a product of the parasitic fungus, *Cordyceps sinensis*, inhibited the growth of these melanoma cells, both *in vivo* and *in vitro* by activating the $A_3$AR (Yoshikawa et al., 2008).

In addition to melanoma cells, $A_3$ARs are also expressed by the anti-tumor T-cells and possibly by NK cells (Gessi et al., 2004; Hoskin et al., 2008). $A_3$AR agonist activates NK cells in the mouse melanoma model, leading to the suppression of tumor growth and lung metastases (Harish et al., 2003). In a recent study, Morello et al. (2011) showed that $A_3$AR agonist recruits NK cells to the tumor region to increase the killing of the tumor cells and reduce tumor growth.

The studies described in this section suggest an important anti-tumor action of $A_3$AR agonists mediated via inhibition of the cyclic AMP-PKA pathway, which appears important for tumor growth. Additionally, due to the additive effects seen with other chemotherapeutic drugs, such as cyclophosphamide, the $A_3$AR agonists can also be used as part of a combination therapy against melanoma. Importantly, these studies support an indirect role of $A_3$AR in mediating its anti-tumor action, primarily via T lymphocytes and NK cells.

### 3.2 $A_{2A}$ adenosine receptors and melanoma

The $A_{2A}$ARs mediate anti-tumor action via a direct and an indirect pathway, the latter pathway involving immune cells. Expression of $A_{2A}$ARs in melanoma cell line A375 was first reported by Merighi et al (2001). These cells express $A_{2A}$AR, as determined by RT-PCR and radioligand binding assays. Activation of $A_{2A}$AR on these melanoma cells increased cyclic AMP levels and led to death of melanoma cells (Merighi et al., 2002).

The $A_{2A}$AR could mount a significant anti-tumor action against melanoma through an indirect mechanism. $A_{2A}$ARs are expressed on $CD4^+$ and $CD8^+$ T-lymphocytes (Koshiba et al., 1999), the immune cells that infiltrate the tumor microenvironment as part of the anti-tumor defense mechanism (Shankaran et al., 2001). The importance of specific anti-melanoma T-cells lies in the fact that the adoptive transfer of such cells in patients with metastatic melanoma resulted in the regression of the tumor at metastatic sites along with the mounting of an immune response against the melanoma cells (Dudley et al., 2002). Functionally, adenosine and $A_{2A}$AR specific agonists suppressed the activity of the anti-tumor T-cells (Butler et al., 2003; Zhang et al., 2004), leading to enhanced tumor growth. In fact, mice deficient in $A_{2A}$AR developed an autoimmune response against the immunogenic melanoma cells and complete tumor rejection in ~60% of the mice (Ohta et al., 2006).

$A_{2A}$ARs have also been studied in lymphokine-activated killer (LAK) cells (Raskovalova et al., 2005). LAK cells are the NK cells that become activated by cytokines and demonstrate enhanced anti-tumor activity against cancer cells (Zamai et al., 2007). Although expression of $A_{2A}$ARs have not been well established in these cells, it has been shown that the LAK cells generated from $A_1$AR- and $A_3$AR-deficient mice failed to show any inhibitory effects of adenosine. In contrast, LAK cells from $A_{2A}$AR-deficient mice were resistant to adenosine response (Raskovalova et al., 2005).

The preceding discussion does not provide a clear outcome of the responses of adenosine via a direct and indirect pathway *in vivo* or in the clinical settings. However, the indirect pathway of $A_{2A}$AR action appears to be dominant since inhibition or knockout of these receptors enhanced tumor regression *in vivo* (Ohta et al., 2006, Raskovalova et al., 2007).

### 3.3 $A_{2B}$ adenosine receptors and melanoma

$A_{2B}$ARs are the low affinity adenosine receptors (Fredholm et al., 2001) which are over-expressed in various tumors (Panjehpour et al., 2005, Li et al., 2005, Phelps et al., 2006). These receptors are involved in promotion of the tumor growth (Ryzhov et al., 2008). $A_{2B}$AR has been characterized in A375 human malignant melanoma cells where its activation led to increases in cyclic AMP levels (Merighi et al., 2001).

As with the $A_{2A}$ARs, $A_{2B}$ARs are also expressed by the normal as well as activated T-lymphocytes (Mirabet et al., 1999). As mentioned above, these activated T-lymphocytes provide host defense response against the tumor cells. Similar to the $A_{2A}$AR, the $A_{2B}$AR inhibits T-lymphocytes function and promotes tumor growth (Ohta et al., 2006). These investigators demonstrated that mice in which $A_{2A}$AR was deleted showed a 60% tumor regression, suggesting a tumor enhancing action of the $A_{2B}$AR (Ohta et al. (2006).

### 3.4 $A_1$ adenosine receptors and melanoma

One of the first studies of ARs in melanoma examined the role of $A_1$AR on the motility of A2058 melanoma cells *in vitro* (Woodhouse et al., 1998). In this study, the authors showed that adenosine- and AMP-dependent chemotactic responses of melanoma cells were mediated via $A_1$AR stimulation. This response was prevented by $A_1$AR specific antagonist and also by pre-treatment with pertussis toxin, to uncouple the $A_1$AR from its G proteins. These data implicate the $A_1$AR in chemotaxis of melanoma cells. The normal physiological extracellular concentrations of adenosine are low, ranging between 30-200 nM (Ballarín et al., 1991). However, there is a drastic increase in extracellular adenosine levels to micromolar levels under conditions of oxidative stress, such as hypoxia and ischemia (Rudolphi et al., 1992), as would be expected in the core of the solid tumors. Therefore, is highly likely that adenosine produced in the microenvironment of the melanoma could facilitate motility and metastasis. One potential target of $A_1$AR-mediated chemotaxis of melanoma cells is the central nervous system (Woodhouse et al., 1998). The melanoma cells have a high propensity for metastasizing to the brain. Malignant melanoma ranks as the fourth most common primary malignancy to metastasize to the brain (Wen et al., 2001), with almost 75% prevalence rate determined at autopsies (Patel et al., 1978). One of the possible explanations for the increased brain metastases in melanoma could be increased adenosine levels in the brain produced by high rates of ATP consumption following neuronal activity (Woodhouse et al., 1998).

$A_1$AR expression along with its biochemical and functional characterization has also been described in A375 human malignant melanoma cells (Merighi et al., 2001). It was shown that these cells express relatively low levels of $A_1$ARs both at the transcript (as determine by low mRNA expression), and at the protein levels (as suggested by the low radioligand binding). These investigators observed no significant functional response of $A_1$AR agonist on cyclic AMP levels in these cells (Merighi et al., 2001). Furthermore, $A_1$AR antagonist failed to suppress the increased levels of IL-8 and VEGF induced by two chemotherapeutic drugs (Merighi et al., 2009). These studies suggest that the $A_1$AR are expressed in melanoma cell lines used *in vitro*, which could account for the response to $A_1$AR agonists. Whether the $A_1$AR are expressed in melanoma tissues is not yet clear.

## 4. Adenosine receptors signaling in melanoma

The signaling mechanisms involved in the suppression or promotion of melanoma growth by adenosine receptors can be further sub-divided into direct (by acting on the melanoma cells), or indirect (by regulating the melanoma cell growth via immune cells).

### 4.1 Direct signaling mechanisms

Activation of the $A_3$AR in melanoma has been shown to couple to activation of PLC leading (via $G_q$) to enhanced survival of A375 melanoma cells (Merighi et al., 2001). In contrast, activation of the $A_3$AR negatively couples to adenylyl cyclase in melanoma cells which suppresses the Wnt signaling pathway. In these cells cyclic AMP, via PKA, increases glycogen synthase kinase (GSK)-β and increased phosphorylation of β-catenin. This allow for enhanced transcription of genes, such as c-myc and cyclin D, which enhance tumor growth. As such, the $A_3$AR suppress tumor growth by inhibiting adenylyl cyclase activity. Activation of the $A_3$AR inhibits nuclear factor (NF)-κB, which also negatively regulates tumor growth (Fishman et al., 2002; Fishman et al., 2004).

### 4.2 Indirect signaling mechanisms

As discussed above, the $A_{2A}$AR plays a critical role in tumor progression through their inhibitory action on anti-tumor immune cells, such as T-lymphocytes and LAK cells. This inhibition is exerted mainly by increasing the levels of cyclic AMP in these cells and activating PKA-dependent pathways. In a recently published study, anti-melanoma specific $CD8^+$ and $CD4^+$ T-cells activity was suppressed by adenosine and 2-chloroadenosine

(Raskovalova et al., 2007). Furthermore, this inhibition was mimicked by $A_{2A}AR$ specific agonist 2-p-(2-Carboxyethyl)phenethylamino-5'-N-ethylcarboxamidoadenosine hydrochloride hydrate (CGS21680), and was blocked by $A_{2A}AR$ specific antagonist, 4-(-2-[7-amino-2-{2-furyl}{1,2,4}triazolo{2,3-a} {1,3,5}triazin-5-yl-amino]ethyl)phenol (ZM241385). The $A_{2A}AR$-dependent effect was mediated by the cyclic AMP/PKA pathway. $A_{2A}AR$ activation increased cyclic AMP levels, which activate PKA and regulate different cellular function by phosphorylation of cellular targets. PKA consists of two regulatory and two catalytic subunits (Francis & Corbin, 1999). Furthermore, two isoforms of PKA are known, PKA-I and PKA-II (Chin et al., 2002). In particular, activation of the PKA-I regulatory subunit was responsible for the T-cell suppressive effects of adenosine, as blockade of catalytic subunits of PKA was not able to reduce the adenosine effects while the PKA-I blocker efficiently suppressed the adenosine response (Raskovalova et al., 2007). The inhibitory effects of adenosine and its analogues reduced cytotoxicity of anti-melanoma specific T-cells and reduced production of cytokines, such as IFN-γ, IL-2 and TNF-α (Raskovalova et al., 2007). IFN-γ is one of the critical cytokines involved in the anti-tumor action of the T-cells, as it inhibits the process of angiogenesis (Qin and Blankenstein, 2000). Thus, $A_{2A}AR$ inhibition could be used in combination with the anti-angiogenic therapy. In this situation, $A_{2A}AR$ inhibitors will enhance the immune response against the tumor cells and increase IFN-γ secretion, leading to tumor cell killing and decreased angiogenesis.

Similar to the anti-tumor T-cell inhibition, adenosine and $A_{2A}AR$-specific agonists also reduce the LAK cells-mediated anti-tumor response via cyclic AMP-PKA signaling (Lokshin et al., 2006). In addition to the involvement of the regulatory subunit of the PKA, PKA-I, the $A_{2A}AR$-dependent response also exhibits complimentary inhibitory effect on LAK cells along with prostaglandin E2 (PGE2) (Lokshin et al., 2006; Su et al., 2008). The co-operative response of adenosine and PGE2 involves amplification of the cyclic AMP-PKA signaling, in addition to the increased CREB phosphorylation and inhibition of Akt (Su et al., 2008). This co-operative response of adenosine and PGE2 also leads to the activation of Csk, an inhibitor of the T-cell receptor (TCR) signaling (Su et al., 2011). Activated Csk in turn inhibits Lck, ZAP-70 and phosphorylated Akt. The interesting aspect of this co-operative action of adenosine and PGE2 is that pre-treatment with sub-suppressive doses of adenosine or PGE2 results in lack of inhibition of the tumor infiltrating lymphocytes (TILs). This effect is explained due to cross desensitization of the PGE2 and ARs. This process gives a new direction for the use of adoptive immunotherapy against the tumor cells. It is possible to improve the effectiveness of the anti-tumor immune cells by pre-treating them with low doses of PGE2 or $A_{2A}AR$ agonist before their adoptive transfer (Su et al., 2011).

In contrast to the above mentioned mechanisms of $A_{2A}AR$ in regulating the immune cells in the tumor microenvironment, an additional concept has been put forward that describes the role of $A_{2A}ARs$ in suppressing the activation-induced cell death (AICD) of the $CD4^+$ T cells (Himer et al., 2010). AICD is a phenomenon that results from TCR-mediated stimulation of the already activated T-cells, resulting in apoptosis. This action involves the interaction of Fas and Fas ligand (Green et al., 2003). Activation of $A_{2A}AR$ by specific agonist reduced the expression of Fas and Fas ligand and prevented the killing of CD4+ cells by AICD. This process was PKA-dependent and it also involved the suppression of various transcription factors, such as NF-κB, nuclear factor of activated T cells (NF-AT) and early growth response (Egr)-1 and Egr-3 proteins (Himer et al., 2010). This anti-apoptotic response of $A_{2A}AR$ on $CD4^+$ T cells could promote a prolonged immune response by these cells. This action contrasts the inhibitory actions of $A_{2A}AR$ on T-lymphocytes and LAK cells, which reduces their anti-tumor immune response. Although, this anti-AICD process has not been described in connection to the tumor cells, it will be interesting to determine if this is also true in the anti-tumor immune cells.

Although, $A_{2A}$ and $A_{2B}$ ARs have been primarily studied in context to anti-tumor immune cells functions, immune cells also express $A_3$ARs (Hoskin et al., 2008). However, in contrast to the $A_{2A}$ and $A_{2B}$AR, activation of $A_3$AR boost the anti-tumor immune response (Harish et al., 2003; Morello et al., 2011). Treatment with $A_3$AR agonist in the murine B16-F10 melanoma model resulted in an increased infiltration and activation of the NK and $CD8^+$ T cells in the melanoma tissues which was associated with increased levels of IL-12. Furthermore, transfer of splenocytes from the $A_3$AR agonist-treated mice suppressed metastasis to the lungs of recipient mice (Harish et al., 2003). In contrast, treatment of nude mice with $A_3$AR agonist failed to have any effect on the melanoma growth (Morello et al., 2011). This effect of $A_3$AR agonist on NK and T-cells was associated with increased TNF-α and IFN-γ levels in the melanoma tissues, suggestive of heightened immune response against the tumor cells (Morello et al., 2011). Thus, the use of $A_3$AR agonists can provide strong anti-tumor actions on melanoma cells by a direct inhibitory effects on the tumor cells and indirectly via activation of the immune system.

## 5. Reactive oxygen species and melanoma

A number of studies support a role of reactive oxygen species (ROS) in the proliferation and metastasis of melanoma cells. For example, ROS can select for chemoresistance by increasing the expression of glutathione, an antioxidant. ROS can promote cell survival through activation of NF-κB and MAPK pathways and inhibition of p53. ROS can also promote melanoma metastasis. High ROS levels in the tumor microenvironment is important for killing melanoma cells that are susceptible to ROS and for "selecting" those cells which are resistant. These resistant cells are endowed with higher levels of glutathione. High ROS levels can induce DNA mitochondrial damage in melanoma cells which can facilitate the invasive and metastatic process (Poetsch et al., 2004). In addition high levels of ROS can induce epigenetic changes through stimulating DNA methylation (Campos et al., 2007), which also can promote invasiveness (Seftor et al., 2005). ROS can also contribute to increased melanoma cell proliferation by activating redox-sensitive transcription factors, such as NF-κB, activator protein-1 (AP-1) and c-myc (Karin et al., 2001). High ROS levels could also increase killing of normal cells in the tumor microenvironment (such as vascular endothelial cells) and promote extravasation and metastasis (Offner et al., 1992, 1996). ROS could also induce expression of cell adhesion molecules on the primary tumor cells and endothelial cells which could promote the metastatic process. In support of these findings, a number of *in vivo* studies in experimental animals demonstrated that antioxidants/antioxidant enzymes were effective in lowering the metastatic potential of melanoma cells (for review, see Joosse et al., 2010). However, all antioxidants/antioxidant enzymes were not effective. While catalase and superoxide dismutase clearly demonstrated antitumor actions, glutathione appeared to increase metastasis (Joosse et al., 2010).

However, ROS has also been linked to the antitumor action of drugs against metastatic melanoma. The effectiveness of the agent elesclomol against melanoma has been attributed to its ability to promote intracellular ROS generation. When used in association with paclitaxel in a Phase 2 clinical trial, elesclomol increased the progression-free survival of patients to 3.7 months versus 1.8 months for the second group of patients treated with paclitaxel alone (Fruehauf and Trapp, 2008).

### 5.1 NADPH oxidase: source of ROS in melanoma

The nicotinamide adenine dinucleotide phosphate (NADPH) oxidase system is a superoxide producing enzyme complex that has historically been studied in the phagocytes as the source of respiratory burst against the ingested microbes. However, this enzyme system is also found in other tissues including many cancer tissues and cells. NADPH oxidase complex consists of different subunits of which $gp91^{phox}$, $p47^{phox}$, $p67^{phox}$ and $p22^{phox}$ are required for the activity of the enzyme system. The $p40^{phox}$ and small GTP-binding proteins, Rac1 and Rap1A, form the holoenzyme component that promote enzyme activity and ROS generation (Lassègue & Clempus, 2003).

Melanoma cell lines express high levels of $p22^{phox}$, $gp91^{phox}$, NOX4 (a homolog of $gp91^{phox}$) and $p67^{phox}$ subunits, with relatively lower expression of $p47^{phox}$ subunit (Brar et al., 2002). Over expression of these subunits in M1619 melanoma cells is associated with increased activity of NADPH oxidase and high ROS generation, which in turn leads to high rates of cell proliferation. This process is dependent on the cyclic AMP responsive element (CRE), as inhibition of NADPH oxidase suppressed the cell growth as well as CRE-binding activity (Brar et al., 2002).

Both $gp91^{phox}$ and its homolog NOX4 are expressed in melanoma cells and appear to mediate differential effects on these cells. NOX4 appears to be critical for the melanoma growth. This observation is supported by the following observations. First, increased NOX4 expression is observed in human melanoma tissues and cell lines. Second, suppression of melanoma tumor growth in nude mice could be produced by silencing the NOX4 expression. Third, inhibition of melanoma cell proliferation and $G_2$-M cell cycle transition in cultures is produced by small interfering (si) RNA against NOX4 (Yamaura et al., 2009). However, $gp91^{phox}$ subunit might play an important role in the invasiveness and metastasis of melanoma cells. The primary melanoma tumors were not different in the gp91 knockout mice, compared to wild type, but they showed reduced invasion and lung metastases. Additionally, when $gp91^{phox}$ knockout mice were injected with the phagocytes from wild type mice, they showed increased in metastatic ability (Okada et al., 2006).

In addition to the role of NOX isoforms discussed in the previous paragraph, two other subunits of NADPH oxidase, Rac1 and $p47^{phox}$, also play important roles in ROS generation, proliferation and motility of the melanoma cells. Rac1 is a small GTP-binding protein that is involved in cell motility and ROS generation as a component of the NADPH oxidase system (Hall, 1992; Lassègue & Clempus, 2003 ). In B16F10 melanoma cells, hyaluronidase increased ROS generation and cell motility in Rac1-dependent fashion. Furthermore, Rac1 is also involved in the membrane translocation and activation of $p47^{phox}$ subunit. Inhibition of Rac1 activity by a dominant-negative Rac1 (Rac1N17) and by siRNA again $p47^{phox}$ reduced the ROS generation by hyaluronidase and the cell migration ability of these cells (Kim et al., 2008). In addition to stimulating proliferation and motility, both Rac1 and $p47^{phox}$ can also regulate differentiation of the melanoma cells. The NADPH oxidase inhibitor, diphenylene iodonium, changed the morphology of the melanoma cells, increased the production of melanin pigment and also increased the expression of a pro-melanocyte differentiation factor microphthalmia–associated transcription factor (MITF). Expression of MITF was also increased by suppressing the expression of Rac1 and $p47^{phox}$ by their respective siRNAs (Zhao et al., 2008). Hence, targeting the NADPH oxidase system to reduce the high ROS levels in melanoma cells could provide an effective therapeutic strategy to suppress the growth, migration and metastasis of the melanoma cells.

### 5.2 $A_3$AR inhibits NADPH oxidase

As discussed above, the $A_3$AR mediates both direct and indirect inhibition of melanoma cell growth (see section 4.1 and 4.2). In a recently published study, we showed that one of the potential targets for $A_3$AR is the NADPH oxidase ROS generating system (Jajoo et al., 2009). In this study $A_3$AR agonist decreased the NADPH oxidase-dependent high ROS generation in prostate cancer cells, resulting in inhibition of tumor growth and metastasis (Jajoo et al., 2009). Although this study was performed in androgen-resistant prostate cancer cells, these findings could be applied to the melanoma cells due to inherent similarities with the prostate cancer cells at the biochemical and molecular level. First, melanoma cells generate high ROS mediated by the NADPH oxidase system. Further, high ROS levels are responsible for the tumor cell growth, migration and invasiveness (Brar et al, 2002; Kim et al., 2008; Yamaura et al., 2009). Second, $A_3$AR expression is well characterized in melanoma cells along with the anti-tumor effects of the $A_3$AR agonists (Merighi et al., 2001; Fishman et al., 2002). Third, similar to our findings in prostate cancer cells, melanoma cells also exhibit higher levels of cyclic AMP resulting in increased activation of PKA and its downstream signaling pathways. Furthermore, $A_3$AR activation in both types of tumor cells exerted its effect by regulating the Wnt signaling pathways (Fishman et al., 2002; 2003). Fourth, we found increased ERK1/2-MAP kinase activation in the prostate cancer cells, which was reduced by $A_3$AR agonist (Jajoo et al., 2009). In melanoma, $A_3$AR activation reduced the p-ERK1/2 levels and the ERK1/2-MAP kinase pathway (Merighi et al., 2005). As such, we propose that inhibition of NADPH oxidase system resulting in reduced levels of ROS generation can also account for $A_3$AR mediated anti-melanoma effects.

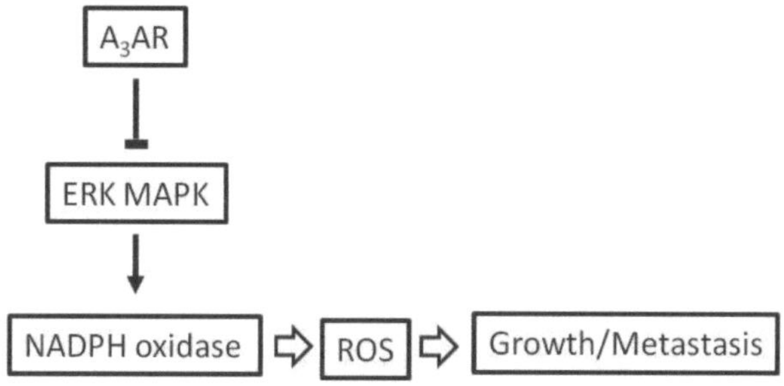


Fig. 2. Proposed mechanism of inhibition of the growth and metastasis of melanoma cells by $A_3$AR agonists. Activation of the $A_3$AR is expected to inhibit ERK MAPK activity by inhibiting an upstream cyclic AMP-PKA pathway. Inhibition of ERK reduces activation of NADPH oxidase, thereby reducing ROS production. ROS contributes significantly to the growth and metastasis of melanoma cells

## 6. Conclusion

Adenosine plays an important role in modulating the progression of melanoma. Several AR types present on these cells would determine whether endogenously released adenosine promote or inhibit tumor growth and metastasis. In general, agonists of the $A_{2A}$ and $A_{2B}$ARs are expected to promote the growth and metastasis of melanoma by inhibiting an indirect pathway which involves T-lymphocytes and NK cells-promoted killing of melanoma cells. As such, antagonists of these receptors should increase activity of these immune cells and promote anti-tumor actions. On the other hand, agonists of the $A_3$AR are expected to provide anti-tumor action by activating these receptors directly on melanoma cells to reduce proliferation and metastasis. In addition, activation of the $A_3AR$ is expected to provide anti-tumor actions indirectly by activating T-lymphocytes and NK cells to promote tumor cell destruction. Therefore, antagonists of the $A_{2A}$ and $A_{2B}AR$ and agonists of the $A_3AR$ should be considered as potential treatments for melanoma. These drugs could be combined with standard treatment regimen to enhance treatment efficacy.

## 7. Acknowledgement

The authors are funded by grants R15-CA135494, RO1-DC 002396 and F32DC009950 from the National Institute of Health and an Excellence in Academic Medicine Award from SIU School of Medicine.

## 8. References

Adair, T.H. (2005). Growth regulation of the vascular system: an emerging role for adenosine. *Am J Physiol Regul Integr Comp Physiol,* Vol. 289, No. 2, pp. R283-R296.

Arslan, G. & Fredholm, B.B. (2000). Stimulatory and inhibitory effects of adenosine A(2A) receptors on nerve growth factor-induced phosphorylation of extracellular regulated kinases 1/2 in PC12 cells. *Neurosci Lett,* Vol. 292, No. 3, pp. 183-186.

Atallah, E. & Flaherty, L. (2005). Treatment of metastatic malignant melanoma. *Curr Treat Options Oncol,* Vol. 6, No. 3, pp. 185-193.

Balch, C.M.; Reintgen, D.S.; Kirkwood, J.M.; Houghton, A.; Peters, L. & Ang, K.K. (1997). Cutaneous Melanoma. *Cancer: Principles and Practice of Oncology* (5th Ed.), Lippincott-Raven, Philadelphia.

Baldwin, S.A.; Beal, P.R.; Yao, S.Y.; King, A.E.; Cass, C.E. & Young, J.D. (2004). The equilibrative nucleoside transporter family, SLC29. *Pflugers Arch,* Vol. 447, No. 5, pp. 735-743.

Ballarín, M.; Fredholm, B.B.; Ambrosio, S. & Mahy, N. (1991). Extracellular levels of adenosine and its metabolites in the striatum of awake rats: inhibition of uptake and metabolism. *Acta Physiol Scand,* Vol. 142, No. 1, pp. 97–103.

Bar-Yehuda, S.; Barer, F.; Volfsson, L. & Fishman, P. (2001). Resistance of muscle to tumor metastases: a role for a3 adenosine receptor agonists. *Neoplasia,* Vol. 3, No. 2, pp. 125-131.

Berne, R.M.; Knabb, R.M.; Ely, S.W. & Rubio, R. (1983). Adenosine in the local regulation of blood flow: a brief overview. *Fed Proc,* Vol. 42, No. 15, pp. 3136-3142.

Blay, J.; White, T.D. & Hoskin, D.W. (1997). The extracellular fluid of solid carcinomas contains immunosuppressive concentrations of adenosine. *Cancer Res,* Vol. 57, No. 13, pp. 2602-2605.

Braun, N.; Lenz, C.; Gillardon, F.; Zimmermann, M. & Zimmermann, H. (1997). Focal cerebral ischemia enhances glial expression of ecto-5'-nucleotidase. *Brain Res,* Vol. 766, No. 1-2, pp. 213-226.

Brar, S.S.; Kennedy, T.P.; Sturrock, A.B.; Huecksteadt, T.P.; Quinn, M.T.; Whorton, A.R. & Hoidal, J.R. (2002). An NAD(P)H oxidase regulates growth and transcription in melanoma cells. *Am J Physiol Cell Physiol,* Vol. 282, No. 6, pp. C1212-C1224.

Brown, J.R.; Cornell, K. & Cook, P.W. (2000). Adenosine- and adenine-nucleotide-mediated inhibition of normal and transformed keratinocyte proliferation is dependent upon dipyridamole-sensitive adenosine transport. *J Invest Dermatol*, Vol. 115, No. 5, pp. 849-859.

Butler, J.J.; Mader, J.S.; Watson, C.L.; Zhang, H.; Blay, J. & Hoskin, D.W. (2003). Adenosine inhibits activation-induced T cell expression of CD2 and CD28 co-stimulatory molecules: role of interleukin-2 and cyclic AMP signaling pathways. *J Cell Biochem*, Vol. 89, No. 5, pp. 975-991.

Campos, A.C.; Molognoni, F.; Melo, F.H.; Galdieri, L.C.; Carneiro, C.R.; D'Almeida, V.; Correa, M. & Jasiulionis, M.G. (2007). Oxidative stress modulates DNA methylation during melanocyte anchorage blockade associated with malignant transformation. *Neoplasia*, Vol. 9, No. 12, pp. 1111-1121.

Chaudary, N.; Naydenova, Z.; Shuralyova, I. & Coe, I.R. (2004). Hypoxia regulates the adenosine transporter, mENT1, in the murine cardiomyocyte cell line, HL-1. *Cardiovasc Res*, Vol. 61, No. 4, pp. 780-788.

Chin, K.V.; Yang, W.L.; Ravatn, R.; Kita, T.; Reitman, E.; Vettori, D.; Cvijic, M.E.; Shin, M. & Iacono, L. (2002). Reinventing the wheel of cyclic AMP: novel mechanisms of cAMP signaling. *Ann N Y Acad Sci*, Vol. 968, pp. 49-64.

De Plaen, E.; Arden, K.; Traversari, C.; Gaforio, J.J.; Szikora, J.P.; De Smet, C.; Brasseur, F.; van der Bruggen, P.; Lethé, B.; Lurquin, C.; et al. (1994). Structure, chromosomal localization, and expression of 12 genes of the MAGE family. *Immunogenetics*, Vol. 40, No. 5, pp. 360-369.

Dickenson, J.M.; Blank, J.L. & Hill, S.J. (1998). Human adenosine A1 receptor and P2Y2-purinoceptor-mediated activation of the mitogen-activated protein kinase cascade in transfected CHO cells. *Br J Pharmacol*, Vol. 124, No. 7, pp. 1491-1499.

Drury, A.N. & Szent-Gyorgyi, A. (1929). The physiological activity of adenine compounds with especial reference to their action upon the mammalian heart. *J Physiol*, Vol. 68, No. 3, pp. 213-237.

Dudley, M.E.; Wunderlich, J.R.; Robbins, P.F.; Yang, J.C.; Hwu, P.; Schwartzentruber, D.J.; Topalian, S.L.; Sherry, R.; Restifo, N.P.; Hubicki, A.M.; Robinson, M.R.; Raffeld M.; Duray, P.; Seipp, C.A.; Rogers-Freezer, L.; Morton, K.E.; Mavroukakis, S.A.; White, D.E. & Rosenberg, S.A. (2002). Cancer regression and autoimmunity in patients after clonal re-population with antitumor lymphocytes. *Science*, Vol. 298, No. 5594, pp. 850-854.

Eltzschig, H.K.; Abdulla. P.; Hoffman, E.; Hamilton, K.E.; Daniels, D.; Schonfeld, C.; Löffler, M.; Reyes, G.; Duszenko, M.; Karhausen, J.; Robinson, A.; Westerman, K.A.; Coe, I.R. & Colgan, S.P. (2005). HIF-1-dependent repression of equilibrative nucleoside transporter (ENT) in hypoxia. *J Exp Med*, Vol. 202, No. 11, pp. 1493-1505.

Etique, N., Grillier-Vuissoz, I., Lecomte, J., & Flament, S. (2009) Crosstalk between adenosine receptor ($A_{2A}$ isoform) and ERalpha mediates ethanol action in MCF-7 breast cancer cells. *Oncol Rep*, Vol. 21, No. 4, pp. 977-981.

Fang,Y. & Olah, M.E. (2007). Cyclic AMP-dependent, protein kinase A-independent activation of extracellular signal-regulated kinase 1/2 following adenosine receptor stimulation in human umbilical vein endothelial cells: role of exchange protein activated by cAMP 1 (Epac1). *J Pharmacol Exp Ther*, Vol. 322, No. 3, pp. 1189-2000.

Faure, M.; Voyno-Yasenetskaya, T.A. & Bourne, H.R. (1994). cAMP and beta gamma subunits of heterotrimeric G proteins stimulate the mitogen-activated protein kinase pathway in COS-7 cells. *J Biol Chem*, Vol. 269, No. 11, pp. 7851-7854.

Feoktistov, I. & Biaggioni, I. (1997). Adenosine A2B receptors. *Pharmacol Rev,* Vol. 49, No. 4, pp. 381-402.

Fishman, P.; Bar-Yehuda, S.; Barer, F.; Madi, L.; Multani, A.S. & Pathak, S. (2001). The A3 adenosine receptor as a new target for cancer therapy and chemoprotection. *Exp Cell Res,* Vol. 269, No. 2, pp. 230-236.

Fishman, P.; Madi, L.; Bar-Yehuda, S.; Barer, F.; Del Valle, L. & Khalili, K. (2002). Evidence for involvement of Wnt signaling pathway in IB-MECA mediated suppression of melanoma cells. *Oncogene,* Vol. 21, No. 25, pp. 4060-4064.

Fishman, P.; Bar-Yehuda, S.; Ohana, G.; Barer, F.; Ochaion, A.; Erlanger, A. & Madi, L. (2004) An agonist to the A3 adenosine receptor inhibits colon carcinoma growth in mice via modulation of GSK-3 β and NF-κB. *Oncogene,* Vol. 23, No. 14, pp. 2465-2471.

Fishman, P.; Bar-Yehuda, S.; Ardon, E.; Rath-Wolfson, L.; Barrer, F.; Ochaion, A. & Madi, L. (2003). Targeting the $A_3$ adenosine receptor for cancer therapy: inhibition of prostate carcinoma cell growth by $A_3$AR agonist. *Anticancer Res,* Vol. 23, No. 3A, pp. 2077-2083.

Francis, S.H. & Corbin, J.D. (1999). Cyclic nucleotide-dependent protein kinases: intracellular receptors for cAMP and cGMP action. *Crit Rev Clin Lab Sci,* Vol. 36, No. 4, pp. 275-328.

Fredholm, B.B.; AP, I.J.; Jacobson, K.A.; Klotz, K.N. & Linden, J. (2001). International Union of Pharmacology. XXV. Nomenclature and classification of adenosine receptors. *Pharmacol Rev,* Vol. 53, No. 4, pp. 527-552.

Fredholm, B.B.; IJzerman, A.P.; Jacobson, K.A.; Klotz, K.N. & Linden, J. (2001). International Union of Pharmacology. XXV. Nomenclature and classification of adenosine receptors. *Pharmacol Rev,* Vol. 53, No. 4, pp. 527-552.

Fruehauf, J.P. & Trapp, V. (2008). Reactive oxygen species: an Achilles' heel of melanoma? *Expert Rev Anticancer Ther,* Vol. 8, No. 11, pp. 1751-1757.

Gao, Z.; Li, B.S.; Day, Y.J. & Linden, J. (2001). $A_3$ adenosine receptor activation triggers phosphorylation of protein kinase B and protects rat basophilic leukemia 2H3 mast cells from apoptosis. *Mol Pharmacol,* Vol. 59, No. 1, pp. 76-82.

Gessi, S.; Varani, K.; Merighi, S.; Cattabriga, E.; Avitabile, A.; Gavioli, R.; Fortini, C.; Leung, E.; Mac Lennan, S. & Borea, P.A. (2004). Expression of A3 adenosine receptors in human lymphocytes: up-regulation in T cell activation. *Mol Pharmacol,* Vol. 65, No. 3, pp. 711-719.

Grant, M.B.; Tarnuzzer, R.W.; Caballero, S.; Ozeck, M.J.; Davis, M.I.; Spoerri, P.E.; Feoktistov, I.; Biaggioni, I.; Shryock, J.C. & Belardinelli L. (1999) Adenosine receptor activation induces vascular endothelial growth factor in human retinal endothelial cells. *Circ Res,* Vol. 85, No. 8, pp. 699-706.

Green, D.R.; Droin, N. & Pinkoski, M. (2003). Activation-induced cell death in T cells. *Immunol Rev,* Vol. 193, pp. 70-81.

Gorlach, A. (2005). Control of adenosine transport by hypoxia. *Circ Res,* Vol. 97, No. 1, pp. 1-3.

Gupta, K. & Zhang, J. (2005). Angiogenesis: a curse or cure? *Postgrad Med J,* Vol. 81, No. 954, pp. 236-242.

Hall, A. (1992). Ras-related GTPases and the cytoskeleton. *Mol Biol Cell,* Vol. 3, No. 5, pp. 475-479.

Harish, A.; Hohana, G.; Fishman, P.; Arnon, O. & Bar-Yehuda, S. (2003). $A_3$ adenosine receptor agonist potentiates natural killer cell activity. *Int J Oncol,* Vol. 23, No. 4, pp. 1245-1249.

Harpio, R. & Einarsson, R. (2004). S100 proteins as cancer biomarkers with focus on S100B in malignant melanoma. *Clin Biochem,* Vol. 37, No. 7, pp. 512-518.

Hart, M.L.; Grenz, A.; Gorzolla, I.C.; Schittenhelm, J.; Dalton, J.H., & Eltzschig, H.K. (2011) Hypoxia-inducible factor-1α-dependent protection from intestinal ischemia/reperfusion injury involves ecto-5'-nucleotidase (CD73) and the $A_{2B}$ adenosine receptor. *J Immunol,* Vol. 186, No.7, pp. 4367-4374.

St Hilaire, C.; Koupenova, M.; Carroll, S.H.; Smith, B.D., & Ravid, K. (2008)TNF-α upregulates the $A_{2B}$ adenosine receptor gene: The role of NAD(P)H oxidase 4. *Biochem Biophys Res Commun,* Vol. 375, No. 3, pp. 292-296.

Himer, L.; Csóka, B.; Selmeczy, Z.; Koscsó, B.; Pócza, T.; Pacher, P.; Németh, Z.H.; Deitch, E.A.; Vizi, E.S.; Cronstein, B.N. & Haskó, G. (2010). Adenosine A2A receptor activation protects CD4+ T lymphocytes against activation-induced cell death. *FASEB J,* Vol. 24, No. 8, pp. 2631-2640.

Hoskin, D.W.; Mader, J.S.; Furlong, S.J.; Conrad, D.M. & Blay, J. (2008) Inhibition of T cell and natural killer cell function by adenosine and its contribution to immune evasion by tumor cells (Review). *Int J Oncol,* Vol. 32, No. 3, pp. 527-535.

Jacobson, K.A. Gao, Z.G. (2006). Adenosine receptors as therapeutic targets. *Nat Rev Drug Discov,* Vol. 5, No. 3, pp. 247-264.

Jajoo, S.; Mukherjea, D.; Watabe, K. & Ramkumar, V. (2009). Adenosine $A_3$ receptor suppresses prostate cancer metastasis by inhibiting NADPH oxidase activity. *Neoplasia,* Vol. 11 No. 11, pp. 1132-1145.

Joosse, A.; De Vries, E.; van Eijck, C.H.; Eggermont, A.M.; Nijsten, T. & Coebergh, J.W. (2010). Reactive oxygen species and melanoma: an explanation for gender differences in survival? *Pigment Cell Melanoma Res,* Vol. 23, No. 3, pp. 352-364.

Karin, M.; Takahashi, T.; Kapahi, P.; Delhase, M.; Chen, Y.; Makris, C.; Rothwarf, D.; Baud, V.; Natoli, G.; Guido, F. & Li, N. (2001). Oxidative stress and gene expression: the AP-1 and NF-kappaB connections. *Biofactors,* Vol. 15, Vol. 2-4, pp. 87-89.

Kawakami, Y. & Rosenberg, S.A. (1996). T-cell recognition of self peptides as tumor rejection antigens. *Immunol Res,* Vol. 15, No. 3, pp. 179-180.

Kim, Y.; Lee, Y.S.; Choe, J.; Lee, H.; Kim, Y.M. & Jeoung D. (2008). CD44-epidermal growth factor receptor interaction mediates hyaluronic acid-promoted cell motility by activating protein kinase C signaling involving Akt, Rac1, Phox, reactive oxygen species, focal adhesion kinase, and MMP-2. *J Biol Chem,* Vol. 283, No. 33, pp. 22513-22528.

Khoa, N.D.; Montesinos, M.C.; Reiss, A.B.; Delano, D.; Awadallah, N. & Cronstein, B.N. (2001) Inflammatory cytokines regulate function and expression of adenosine A(2A) receptors in human monocytic THP-1 cells. *J Immunol,* Vol. 167, No. 7, pp. 4026-4032.

Koshiba, M.; Rosin, D.L.; Hayashi, N.; Linden, J. & Sitkovsky, M.V. (1999). Patterns of A2A extracellular adenosine receptor expression in different functional subsets of human peripheral T cells: flow cytometry studies with anti-A2A receptor monoclonal antibodies. *Mol Pharmacol,* Vol. 55, No. 3, pp. 614-624.

Lassègue, B. & Clempus, R.E. (2003). Vascular NAD(P)H oxidases: specific features, expression, and regulation. *Am J Physiol Regul Integr Comp Physiol,* Vol. 285, No. 2, pp. R277-R297.

Lee, J.A. (1982). Melanoma and exposure to sunlight. *Epidemol Rev,* Vol. 4, pp. 110-106.

Lee, J.A. & Scotto, J. (1993). Melanoma: linked temporal and latitude changes in the United States. *Cancer Causes Control,* Vol. 4, No. 5, pp. 413-418.

Li, S.; Huang, S. & Peng, S.B. (2005). Overexpression of G protein-coupled receptors in cancer cells: involvement in tumor progression. *Int J Oncol,* Vol. 27, No. 5, pp. 1329-1339.

Linden, J. (1991) Structure and function of A1 adenosine receptor. *FASEB J,* Vol. 5, No. 12, pp. 2668-2676.

Lokshin, A.; Raskovalova, T.; Huang, X.; Zacharia, L.C.; Jackson, E.K. & Gorelik, E. (2006). Adenosine-mediated inhibition of the cytotoxic activity and cytokine production by activated natural killer cells. *Cancer Res,* Vol. 66, No. 15, pp. 7758-7765.

Madi, L.; Bar-Yehuda, S.; Barer, F.; Ardon, E.; Ochaion, A. & Fishman, P. (2003). $A_3$ adenosine receptor activation in melanoma cells: association between receptor fate and tumor growth inhibition. *J Biol Chem,* Vol. 278, No. 43, pp. 42121-42130.

Madi, L.; Ochaion, A.; Rath-Wolfson, L.; Bar-Yehuda, S.; Erlanger, A.; Ohana, G.; Harish, A.; Merimski, O.; Barer, F. & Fishman, P. (2004). The $A_3$ adenosine receptor is highly expressed in tumor versus normal cells: potential target for tumor growth inhibition. *Clin Cancer Res,* Vol. 10, No. 13, pp. 4472-4479.

Marchand, M.; Brasseur, F.; van der Bruggen, P.; Coulie, P. & Boon, T. (1993). A gene encoding an antigen recognized by cytolytic T lymphocytes on a human melanoma. *Dermatology,* Vol. 186, No. 4, pp. 278-280.

Merighi, S.; Varani, K.; Gessi, S.; Cattabriga, E.; Iannotta, V.; Ulouglu, C.; Leung, E. & Borea, P.A. (2001). Pharmacological and biochemical characterization of adenosine receptors in the human malignant melanoma A375 cell line. *Br J Pharmacol,* Vol. 134, No. 6, pp. 1215-1226.

Merighi, S.; Mirandola, P.; Milani, D.; Varani, K.; Gessi, S.; Klotz, K.N.; Leung, E.; Baraldi, P.G. & Borea, P.A. (2002). Adenosine receptors as mediators of both cell proliferation and cell death of cultured human melanoma cells. *J Invest Dermatol,* Vol. 119, No. 4, pp. 923-933.

Merighi, S.; Benini, A.; Mirandola, P.; Gessi, S.; Varani, K.; Leung, E.; Maclennan, S. & Borea, P.A. (2005). A3 adenosine receptor activation inhibits cell proliferation via phosphatidylinositol 3-kinase/Akt-dependent inhibition of the extracellular signal-regulated kinase 1/2 phosphorylation in A375 human melanoma cells. *J Biol Chem,* Vol. 280, No. 20, pp. 19516-19526.

Merighi, S.; Benini, A.; Mirandola, P.; Gessi, S.; Varani, K.; Leung, E.; Maclennan, S. & Borea, P.A. (2006). Adenosine modulates vascular endothelial growth factor expression via hypoxia-inducible factor-1 in human glioblastoma cells. *Biochem Pharmacol,* Vol. 72, No. 1, pp. (19-31).

Merighi, S.; Simioni, C.; Gessi, S.; Varani, K.; Mirandola, P.; Tabrizi, M.A.; Baraldi, P.G. & Borea, P.A. (2009). A(2B) and A(3) adenosine receptors modulate vascular endothelial growth factor and interleukin-8 expression in human melanoma cells treated with etoposide and doxorubicin. *Neoplasia,* Vol. 10, No. 10, pp. 1064-1073.

Mirabet, M.; Herrera, C.; Cordero, O.J.; Mallol, J.; Lluis, C. & Franco, R. (1999). Expression of A2B adenosine receptors in human lymphocytes. Their role in T cell activation. *J Cell Sci*, Vol. 112, Pt. 4, pp. 491-502.

Mirza, A.; Basso, A.; Black, S.; Malkowski, M.; Kwee, L.; Pachter, J.A.; Lachowicz, J.E.; Wang, Y. and Liu, S. (2005). RNA interference targeting of A1 receptor-overexpressing breast carcinoma cells leads to diminished rates of cell proliferation and induction of apoptosis. *Cancer Biol Ther*, Vol. 4, No. 12, pp. 1355-1360.

Montesinos, M.C.; Gadangi, P.; Longaker, M.; Sung, J.; Levine, J.; Nilsen, D.; Reibman, J.; Li, M.; Jiang, C.K.; Hirschhorn, R.; Recht, P.A.; Ostad, E.; Levin, R.I. & Cronstein, B.N. (1997). Wound healing is accelerated by agonists of adenosine $A_2$ (G alpha s-linked) receptors. *J Exp Med*, Vol. 186, No. 9, pp. 1615-1620.

Montesinos, M.C.; Desai, A.; Chen, J.F.; Yee, H.; Schwarzschild, M.A.; Fink, J.S. and Cronstein B.N. (2002). Adenosine promotes wound healing and mediates angiogenesis in response to tissue injury via occupancy of A2A receptors. *Am J Pathol* Vol. 160, No. 6, pp. 2009-2018.

Morello, S.; Sorrentino, R.; Montinaro, A.; Luciano, A.; Maiolino, P.; Ngkelo, A.; Arra, C.; Adcock, I.M. & Pinto, A. (2011). NK1.1+ cells and CD8+T cells mediate the anti-tumour activity of Cl-IB-MECA in a mouse melanoma model. *Neoplasia*, Vol. 13, No. 4, pp. 365-373.

O'Day, S.J.; Kim, C.J. & Reintgen, D.S. (2002). Metastatic melanoma: chemotherapy to biochemotherapy. *Cancer Control*, Vol. 9, No. 1, pp. 31-38.

Offner, F.A.; Wirtz, H.C.; Schiefer, J.; Bigalke, I.; Klosterhalfen, B.; Bittinger, F.; Mittermayer, C. & Kirkpatrick, C.J. (1992). Interaction of human malignant melanoma (ST-ML-12) tumor spheroids with endothelial cell monolayers. Damage to endothelium by oxygen-derived free radicals. *Am J Pathol*, Vol. 141, No. 3, pp. 601-610.

Offner, F.A.; Schiefer, J.; Wirtz, H.C.; Bigalke, I.; Pavelka, M.; Hollweg, G.; Ensinger, C.; Klosterhalfen, B.; Mittermayer, C. & Kirkpatrick, C.J. (1996). Tumour-cell-endothelial interactions: free radicals are mediators of melanoma-induced endothelial cell damage. *Virchows Arch*, Vol. 428, No. 2, pp. 99-106.

Ohana, G.; Bar-Yehuda, S.; Arich, A.; Madi, L.; Dreznick, Z.; Rath-Wolfson, L.; Silberman, D.; Slosman, G., & Fishman, P. (2003) Inhibition of primary colon carcinoma growth and liver metastasis by the $A_3$ adenosine receptor agonist CF101. *Br J Cancer*, Vol. 89, No. 8, pp. 1552-1558.

Ohta, A.; Gorelik, E.; Prasad, S.J.; Ronchese, F.; Lukashev, D.; Wong, M.K.; Huang, X.; Caldwell, S.; Liu, K.; Smith, P.; Chen, J.F.; Jackson, E.K.; Apasov, S.; Abrams, S. & Sitkovsky, M. (2006). A2A adenosine receptor protects tumors from antitumor T cells. *Proc Natl Acad Sci USA*, Vol. 103, No. 35, pp. 13132-13137.

Okada, F.; Kobayashi, M.; Tanaka, H.; Kobayashi, T.; Tazawa, H.; Iuchi, Y.; Onuma, K.; Hosokawa, M.; Dinauer, M.C. & Hunt, N.H. (2006). The role of nicotinamide adenine dinucleotide phosphate oxidase-derived reactive oxygen species in the acquisition of metastatic ability of tumor cells. *Am J Pathol*, Vol. 169, No. 1, pp. 294-302.

Panjehpour, M.; Castro, M. & Klotz, K.N. (2005). Human breast cancer cell line MDA-MB-231 expresses endogenous $A_{2B}$ adenosine receptors mediating a $Ca^{2+}$ signal. *Br J Pharmacol*, Vol. 145, No. 2, pp. 211–218.

Patel, J.K.; Didolkar, M.S.; Pickren, J.W. & Moore, R.H. (1978). Metastatic pattern of malignant melanoma. A study of 216 autopsy cases. *American Journal of Surgery,* Vol. 135, No. 6, pp. 807–810.

Phelps, P.T.; Anthes, J.C. & Correll, C.C. (2006). Characterization of adenosine receptors in the human bladder carcinoma T24 cell line. *Eur J Pharmacol,* Vol. 536, No. 1-2, pp. 28–37.

Poetsch, M.; Dittberner, T.; Petersmann, A. & Woenckhaus, C. (2004). Mitochondrial DNA instability in malignant melanoma of the skin is mostly restricted to nodular and metastatic stages. *Melanoma Res,* Vol. 14, No. 6, pp. 501-508.

Qin, Z. & Blankenstein, T. (2000). CD4+ T cell--mediated tumor rejection involves inhibition of angiogenesis that is dependent on IFN gamma receptor expression by nonhematopoietic cells. *Immunity,* Vol. 12, No. 6, pp. 677-686.

Raskovalova, T.; Huang, X.; Sitkovsky, M.; Zacharia, L.C.; Jackson, E.K. & Gorelik, E. (2005). Gs protein-coupled adenosine receptor signaling and lytic function of activated NK cells. *J Immunol,* Vol. 175, No. 7, pp. 4383-4391.

Raskovalova, T.; Lokshin, A.; Huang, X.; Su, Y.; Mandic, M.; Zarour, H.M.; Jackson, E.K. & Gorelik, E. (2007). Inhibition of cytokine production and cytotoxic activity of human antimelanoma specific CD8+ and CD4+ T lymphocytes by adenosine-protein kinase A type I signaling. *Cancer Res,* Vol. 67, No. 12, pp. 5949-5956.

Rudolphi, K.A.; Schubert, P.; Parkinson, F.E. & Fredholm, B.B. (1992). Adenosine and brain ischemia. *Cerebrovasc Brain Metab Rev,* Vol. 4, No. 4, pp. 346-369.

Ryzhov, S.; Novitskiy, S.V.; Zaynagetdinov, R.; Goldstein, A.E.; Carbone, D.P.; Biaggioni, I.; Dikov, M.M. & Feoktistov, I. (2008). Host A(2B) adenosine receptors promote carcinoma growth. *Neoplasia,* Vol. 10, No. 9, pp. 987-995.

Saito, M.; Yaguchi, T.; Yasuda, Y.; Nakano, T. & Nishizaki, T. (2010). Adenosine suppresses CW2 human colonic cancer growth by inducing apoptosis via $A_1$ adenosine receptors. *Cancer Lett,* Vol. 290, No. 2, pp. 211-215.

Schulte, G. & Fredholm, B.B. (2000). Human adenosine $A_1$, $A_{2A}$, $A_{2B}$, and $A_3$ receptors expressed in Chinese hamster ovary cells all mediate the phosphorylation of extracellular-regulated kinase 1/2. *Mol Pharmacol,* Vol. 58, No. 3, pp. 477-82.

Seftor, E.A.; Brown, K.M.; Chin, L.; Kirschmann, D.A.; Wheaton, W.W.; Protopopov, A.; Feng, B.; Balagurunathan, Y.; Trent, J.M.; Nickoloff, B.J.; Seftor, R.E. & Hendrix, M.J. (2005). Epigenetic transdifferentiation of normal melanocytes by a metastatic melanoma microenvironment. *Cancer Res,* Vol. 65, No. 22, pp. 10164-10169.

Serrano, M.; Hannon, G.J. & Beach, D. (1993). A new regulatory motif in cell-cycle control causing specific inhibition of cyclin D/CDK4. *Nature,* Vol. 366, No. 6456, pp. 704-707.

Sexl, V.; Mancusi, G.; Höller, C.; Gloria-Maercker, E.; Schütz, W., & Freissmuth, M. (1997) Stimulation of the mitogen-activated protein kinase via the A2A-adenosine receptor in primary human endothelial cells. *J Biol Chem,* Vol. 272, No. 9, pp. 5792-5799.

Shankaran, V.; Ikeda, H.; Bruce, A.T.; White, J.M.; Swanson, P.E.; Old, L.J. & Schreiber, R.D. (2001). IFNgamma and lymphocytes prevent primary tumour development and shape tumour immunogenicity. *Nature,* Vol. 410, No. 6832, pp. 1107-1111.

Sober, A.J.; Tsao, H. & Washington, C.V. (2008). Cancer of the Skin. *Harrison's: Principles of Internal Medicine* (17th Ed.), McGraw Hill Medical, New York.

Su, Y.; Huang, X.; Raskovalova, T.; Zacharia, L.; Lokshin, A.; Jackson, E. & Gorelik, E. (2008). Cooperation of adenosine and prostaglandin E2 (PGE2) in amplification of cAMP-PKA signaling and immunosuppression. *Cancer Immunol Immunother,* Vol. 57, No. 11, pp. 1611-1623.

Su, Y.; Jackson, E.K. & Gorelik, E. (2011). Receptor desensitization and blockade of the suppressive effects of prostaglandin E(2) and adenosine on the cytotoxic activity of human melanoma-infiltrating T lymphocytes. *Cancer Immunol Immunother,* Vol. 60, No. 1, pp. 111-122.

Synnestvedt, K.; Furuta, G.T.; Comerford, K.M.; Louis, N.; Karhausen, J.; Eltzschig, H.K.; Hansen, K.R.; Thompson, L.F., & Colgan, S.P. (2002) Ecto-5'-nucleotidase (CD73) regulation by hypoxia-inducible factor-1 mediates permeability changes in intestinal epithelia. *J Clin Invest*, Vol. 110, No. 7, pp. 993-1002.

Synowitz, M.; Glass, R.; Färber, K.; Markovic, D.; Kronenberg, G.; Herrmann, K.; Schnermann, J.; Nolte, C.; van Rooijen, N.; Kiwit, J. & Kettenmann, H. (2006). A1 adenosine receptors in microglia control glioblastoma-host interaction. *Cancer Res,* Vol. 66, No.17, pp. 8550-8557.

van der Bruggen, P.; Traversari, C.; Chomez, P.; Lurquin, C.; De Plaen, E.; Van den Eynde, B.; Knuth, A. & Boon, T. (1991). A gene encoding an antigen recognized by cytolytic T lymphocytes on a human melanoma. *Science,* Vol. 254, No. 5038, pp. 1643-1647.

Weber, J. (2011). Immunotherapy for melanoma. *Curr Opin Oncol,* Vol. 23, No. 2, pp. 163-169.

Wen, P.Y.; Black, P.M. & Joeffler, S.L. (2001). Treatment of metastatic cancer. *Cancer: principles and practice of oncology (6),* Lippincott, Williams & Wilkins, Philadelphia, pp. 2655–2670.

Wick, M.R.; Swanson, P.E. & Rocamora, A. (1988). Recognition of malignant melanoma by monoclonal antibody HMB-45. An immunohistochemical study of 200 paraffin-embedded cutaneous tumors. *J Cutan Pathol,* Vol. 15, No. 4, pp. 201-207.

Woodhouse, E.C.; Amanatullah, D.F.; Schetz, J.A.; Liotta, L.A.; Stracke, M.L. & Clair, T. (1998). Adenosine receptor mediates motility in human melanoma cells. *Biochem Biophys Res Commun,* Vol. 246, No. 3, pp. 888-894.

Xaus, J.; Mirabet, M.; Lloberas, J.; Soler, C.; Lluis, C.; Franco, R., & Celada, A. (1999) IFN-gamma up-regulates the $A_{2B}$ adenosine receptor expression in macrophages: a mechanism of macrophage deactivation. *J Immunol,* Vol. 162, No. 6, pp. 3607-3614.

Yamaura, M.; Mitsushita, J.; Furuta, S.; Kiniwa, Y.; Ashida, A.; Goto, Y.; Shang, W.H.; Kubodera, M.; Kato, M.; Takata, M.; Saida, T. & Kamata, T. (2009). NADPH oxidase 4 contributes to transformation phenotype of melanoma cells by regulating G2-M cell cycle progression. *Cancer Res,* Vol. 69, No. 6, pp. 2647-2654.

Yasuda, Y.; Saito, M.; Yamamura, T.; Yaguchi, T. & Nishizaki, T. (2009) Extracellular adenosine induces apoptosis in Caco-2 human colonic cancer cells by activating caspase-9/-3 via A(2a) adenosine receptors. *J Gastroenterol,* Vol. 44, No. 1, pp 56-65.

Yoshikawa, N.; Yamada, S.; Takeuchi, C.; Kagota, S.; Shinozuka, K.; Kunitomo, M. & Nakamura, K. (2008). Cordycepin (3'-deoxyadenosine) inhibits the growth of B16-BL6 mouse melanoma cells through the stimulation of adenosine A3 receptor followed by glycogen synthase kinase-3beta activation and cyclin D1 suppression. *Naunyn Schmiedebergs Arch Pharmacol,* Vol. 377, No. 4-6, pp. 591-595.

Zamai, L.; Ponti, C.; Mirandola, P.; Gobbi, G.; Papa, S.; Galeotti, L.; Cocco, L. & Vitale, M. (2007). NK cells and cancer. *J Immunol,* Vol. 178, No. 7, pp. 4011-4016.

Zhang, H.; Conrad, D.M.; Butler, J.J.; Zhao, C.; Blay, J. & Hoskin, D.W. (2004). Adenosine acts through A2 receptors to inhibit IL-2-induced tyrosine phosphorylation of STAT5 in T lymphocytes: role of cyclic adenosine 3',5'-monophosphate and phosphatases. *J Immunol,* Vol. 173, No. 2, pp. 932-944.

Zhao, Y.; Liu, J. & McMartin, K.E. (2008). Inhibition of NADPH oxidase activity promotes differentiation of B16 melanoma cells. *Oncol Rep,* Vol. 19, No. 5, pp. 1225-1230.

Zeng, D.; Maa, T.; Wang, U.; Feoktistov, I. Biaggioni, I. & Belardinelli, L. (2003). Expression and function of $A_{2B}$ adenosine receptors in the U87MG tumor cells. *Drug Development Research,* Vol. 58, No. 4, pp. 405-411.

# 16

# The Roles of S100 Proteins and RAGE in Melanoma

Estelle Leclerc
*North Dakota State University/Department of Pharmaceutical Sciences*
*U.S.A*

## 1. Introduction

The incidence of melanoma continues to rise worldwide and increases annually by 4% to 6% in the United States (Darrell and Rigel 2010). Once metastatic, invasive melanoma offers poor prognosis to patients (Bhatia, Tykodi and Thompson, 2009). The classic prognostic factors in melanoma include primary tumor thickness, patient gender, primary melanoma ulceration, mitotic activity and the presence of tumor infiltrating lymphocytes (Spatz et al. 2010). Besides these established prognostic markers, the S100 protein family member S100B has emerged in recent years as a new prognostic marker and is now incorporated into the American Joint Committee on Cancer (AJCC) melanoma staging system for stage IV melanoma patients (Balch et al. 2009; Chun et al. 2008; Gogas et al. 2009). High S100B serum concentration correlates with poor survival rate (Hauschild et al. 1999). Current studies are also analyzing the prognostic value of S100B in earlier melanoma stages (IIB-III) (Bouwhuis et al. 2010).

The role of S100B in the progression of melanoma is not clearly understood. For instance, although it is established that S100B is released from melanoma tumor cells, its role in tumor development, invasion and metastasis is currently under investigation. This chapter will discuss the role of S100B and other members of the S100 protein family in the biology of melanoma. We will focus on the relation between the S100 proteins and their common receptor, the receptor for advanced glycation endproducts (RAGE), in the context of melanoma.

## 2. Generalities about RAGE

RAGE is a multiligand receptor of the immunoglobulin superfamily and is involved in a large number of pathologies such as complications of diabetes, cardiovascular diseases, Alzheimer's disease, and cancer (Schmidt et al. 2000; Deane et al. 2003; Lue et al. 2009; Fang et al. 2010; Yan, Bierhaus et al. 2009; Bierhaus and Nawroth 2009; Sparvero et al. 2009).

RAGE is often described as a pattern recognition receptor and it is activated by structurally unrelated ligands. RAGE ligands include the advanced glycation endproducts (AGE) (Schmidt et al. 1992), the high mobility group box 1 protein (HMGB1 = amphoterin), amyloid forming peptides and proteins (amyloid β-peptide) and members of the S100 protein family (Heizmann, Ackermann, and Galichet 2007; Leclerc et al. 2009; Schmidt et al. 2000).

AGEs are the result of non-enzymatic modification of proteins or lipids by reducing carbohydrates and are therefore very heterogeneous in nature (reviewed in (Ahmed et al. 2005)). Due to poorly regulation of glucose concentration, AGEs are found elevated in patients suffering for diabetes but are also present at high concentration at sites of active inflammation (Yan et al. 2003). In addition, elevated concentration of AGEs have been found in melanoma tissue samples (Sander et al. 2003; Wondrak, Jacobson, and Jacobson 2006; Abe et al. 2004). Other ligands of RAGE include amyloid forming proteins or peptides such as Aβ peptide, responsible for Alzheimer's disease (Yan et al. 1996; Sturchler et al. 2008) or transthyretin, responsible for familial amyloid polyneuropathy or cardiomyopathy (Sousa et al. 2000).

The DNA binding protein HMGB1 is another RAGE ligand that plays important functions in neuronal development, inflammation, and cancer (Hori et al. 1995)(reviewed in (Sims et al. 2010; Rauvala and Rouhiainen 2010)). Interestingly, HMGB1 was shown to be secreted from melanoma cells following treatment with cytolytic lymphoid cells (Ito et al. 2007). Secreted HMGB1 could contribute to enhanced RAGE signaling in the tumor environment.

The S100 proteins constitute a large group of RAGE ligands with more than 20 members. S100 proteins are small calcium binding proteins that play diverse intra- and extracellular functions. These functions will be described in more details in the next chapter. S100A12 was the first member of the family to be identified as a RAGE ligand (Hofmann et al. 1999). Many other members of the family have since been identified as ligand (Donato 2007; Leclerc et al. 2009).

The physiological function of RAGE is not yet fully understood. Among human tissues, RAGE is expressed at the highest level in the lung where it is believed to exert a protective effect (Brett et al. 1993; Queisser et al. 2008; Ramsgaard et al. 2010; Buckley and Ehrhardt 2010). RAGE has also been suggested to have a beneficial function in peripheral nerve regeneration (Rong, Trojaborg et al. 2004; Rong, Yan et al. 2004), and in auditory stimuli in mice (Sakatani et al. 2009).

RAGE is expressed in different isoforms. The main two isoforms are the membrane bound and the soluble forms. The membrane bound full-length form of RAGE, is composed of an extracellular part (314 amino-acids), followed by a single transmembrane spanning helix (27 aa) and a short cytosolic domain (41 aa) (Figure 1) (Neeper et al. 1992). The extracellular part itself is composed of three Ig-like domains: a variable and two constant C1 and C2 domains. The structures of the V and VC1 domains of RAGE have been solved recently and showed similarities with other immunoglobulins (Matsumoto et al. 2008; Koch et al. 2010). RAGE is glycosylated *in vivo* and RAGE glycosylation has been shown to modulate the interaction of RAGE with AGEs, amphoterin and several S100 proteins (S100A8/A9, S100A12) (Neeper et al. 1992; Wilton et al. 2006; Osawa et al. 2007; Srikrishna et al. 2010).

The second important isoform of RAGE is soluble RAGE (sRAGE). sRAGE can be generated from splicing (RAGE_v1) or shedding by ADAM10 (Ohe et al. 2010; Hudson et al. 2008; Galichet, Weibel, and Heizmann 2008; Raucci et al. 2008; Zhang et al. 2008; Ding and Keller 2005; Yonekura et al. 2003). sRAGE is composed only of the extracellular part of receptor and is released in the extracellular space. sRAGE was suggested to play the role of decoy and to prevent RAGE activation by its ligands (Santilli et al. 2009). However, this role has been questioned due to the low concentration of sRAGE present in serum (Bierhaus and Nawroth 2009). Indeed, this concentration varies between 10pM and 50pM in normal conditions and might not be sufficient to conteract the effect of circulating RAGE ligands whose affinity towards RAGE are in the nanomolar RAGE (Tesarova et al. 2007; Nakamura et al. 2008; Bierhaus and Nawroth 2009; Kislinger et al. 1999; Dattilo et al. 2007).

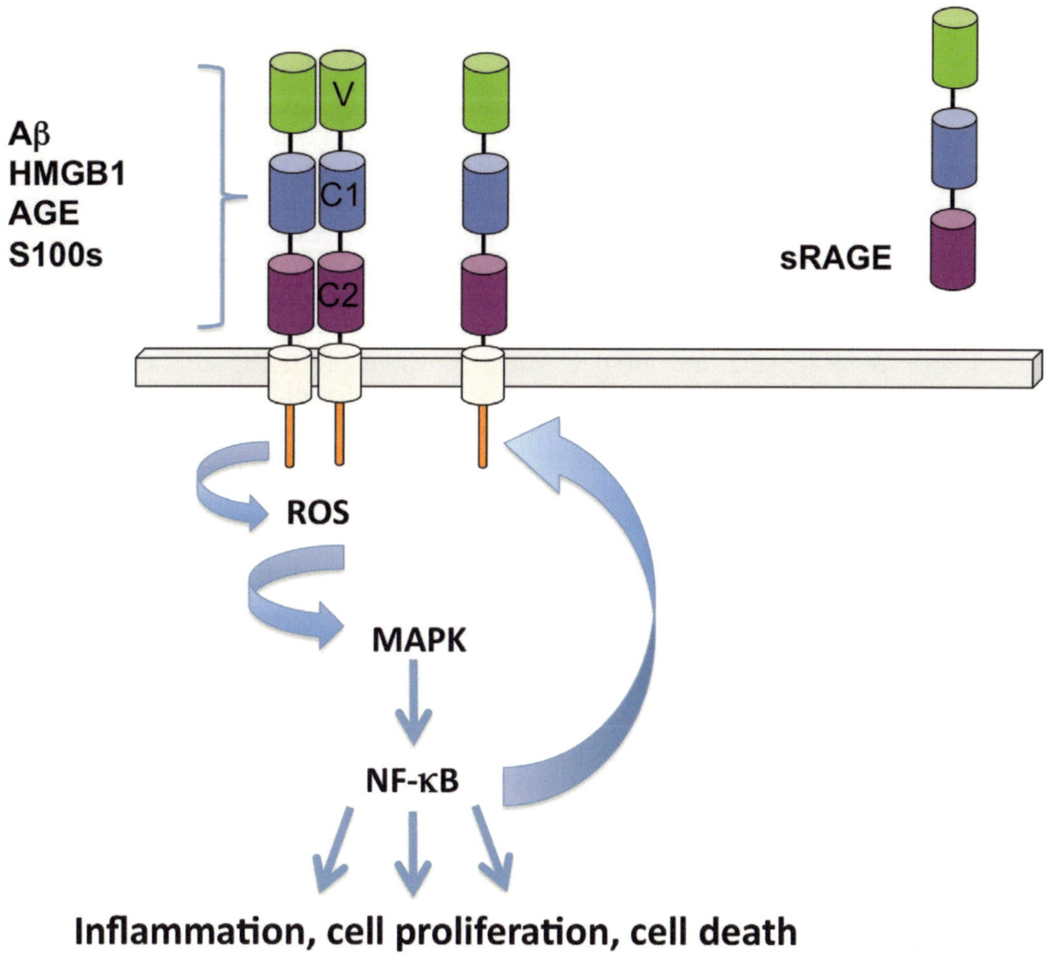


Fig. 1. RAGE and its ligands. RAGE is activated by structurally unrelated ligands. These ligands include the advanced glycation endproducts (AGE), amyloid β peptides, high mobility group box 1 protein and members of the S100 protein family. Recent evidences suggest that RAGE dimerize on the cell surface. Engagement of RAGE by its ligands triggers the formation of reactive oxygen species (ROS), the activation of members of the MAP kinase family (MAPK) and often leads to activation of NF-κB. Since RAGE expression is under the control of NF-κB, initial activation of RAGE leads to up-regulation of RAGE expression and sustained RAGE activation and inflammation. RAGE activation can also result in cell proliferation or cell death depending of the ligand and cell type. Soluble RAGE or sRAGE can also be generated by splicing or proteolytic shedding. sRAGE can counteract the activation of RAGE by its circulating ligands and serves as a decoy receptor

sRAGE has also been suggested to be a biomarker in certain pathologies such as Alzheimer's disease and diabetes (Emanuele et al. 2005; Nozaki et al. 2007; Nakamura et al. 2008; Yan, Ramasamy, and Schmidt 2010). However, many studies are contradictory and show either positive or negative correlation between the concentration of sRAGE and the stage of the disease (Bierhaus and Nawroth 2009; Humpert et al. 2007; Koyama, Yamamoto, and Nishizawa 2007). We recently evaluated the change of transcript levels of the spliced form of RAGE (RAGE_v1) in 40 melanoma stage III and stage IV tissue samples. We showed that 90 % of those samples showed a significant reduction in the transcript level of RAGE_v1 (Leclerc, Heizmann, and Vetter 2009). However, further studies are necessary to demonstrate that the protein level of RAGE_v1 can be associated with distinct stages of melanoma.

The activation of RAGE by its ligands triggers the activation of multiple signaling pathways resulting in the production of reactive oxygen species, the activation of the extracellular signal regulated kinase (ERK1/2) and NF-κB, leading to the initiation of inflammation (Bierhaus et al. 2005; Yan, Du Yan et al. 2009; Coughlan et al. 2009). Since the transcription of RAGE is under the control of NF-kB itself and of other pro-inflammatory transcription factors such as SP-1, AP-2 and NF-IL6, RAGE activation by its ligands also result in sustained inflammation through a positive feedback loop (Schmidt et al. 2001; Bierhaus and Nawroth 2009). Other signaling pathways have been described and include RAC-1, NADPH-oxidase, p38, PI3K, JNK or JAK/STAT (Leclerc et al. 2007; Lin, Park, and Lakatta 2009; Bierhaus and Nawroth 2009; Donato 2007).

## 3. Generalities about S100 proteins

S100 proteins are small EF-hand calcium binding proteins that show tissue and cell specific expression (Donato 2003; Heizmann 2002). The cell expression specificity of some of the S100s has been suggested to be regulated by DNA methylation (reviewed in (Lesniak 2011)). 21 members have been described so far. Many of the genes coding for the S100 proteins identified as S100A1 to S100A16, are clustered onto one region of chromosome 1 (1q21), which is often prone to deletion and rearrangements, linking S100 proteins to cancer (Marenholz, Lovering, and Heizmann 2006). Binding of calcium to the S100 proteins occurs in the EF-hands (Fritz and Heizmann 2004). Most S100 proteins form dimers. Each S100 monomer contains two EF-hands: the C terminal EF-hand is present in all S100 proteins and is described as canonical. The N-terminal EF-hand is specific for each S100 protein. Binding of calcium to the C-terminal EF-hand is in average 100 times stronger than binding to the N-terminal site. Although most S100 proteins contain two functional EF-hands, some S100 protein present only one functional EF-hand (example). S100 proteins display a large range of calcium binding affinity ($K_D$ = 20-500 μM) (Heizmann, Ackermann, and Galichet 2007; Zimmer and Weber 2010). Certain S100 proteins possess additional metal binding sites for zinc and copper (Moroz, Wilson, and Bronstein 2010).

S100 proteins form a family of proteins with high similarities in amino-acid sequence and tri-dimensional structure (Fritz and Heizmann 2004; Heizmann, Fritz, and Schäfer 2002). For this reason, S100 proteins can share the same target proteins. For instance, fructose-1,6-biphosphate aldolase can be activated by both S100B and S100A1 (Zimmer and Van Eldik 1986). However, the slight differences in sequence and structure also explain that two S100 proteins can modulate the activity of the same target protein with different or opposite results. Indeed, whereas S100A1 activates phosphoglucomutase, S100B inhibits this enzyme (Landar et al. 1996). Similarly many members of the S100 protein family that include S100B, S100A1, S100A2, S100A4, S100A6 and S100A10 have been shown to interact in different manners to the tumor suppressor p53 protein (Baudier et al. 1992; Wilder et al. 2006; Mueller et al. 2005; Fernandez-Fernandez, Rutherford, and Fersht 2008; van Dieck, Teufel et al. 2009; van Dieck, Fernandez-Fernandez et al. 2009).

S100 proteins can exert both intra- and extracellular functions through the activation of their target proteins (Heizmann, Fritz, and Schäfer 2002; Donato 2003; Santamaria-Kisiel, Rintala-Dempsey, and Shaw 2006). Most of the S100 proteins exert their functions principally as dimers, but higher orders of oligomerisation have been observed. For example, functional tetramers of S100B and S100A8/A9, hexamers of S100A12 and oligomers of S100A4 have been described (Ostendorp et al. 2007; Vogl et al. 2006; Moroz et al. 2002; Kiryushko et al. 2006).

S100 proteins are found in many cell types constituting the epidermis (Eckert et al. 2004). S100B and S100A6 have been described in both melanocytes and Langerhan's cells (Ito and Kizawa 2001; Boni, Burg et al. 1997; Ribe and McNutt 2003). S100A2, A7, A10, A11, A12 and S100A15 have been identified in basal keratinocytes (Ribe and McNutt 2003; Ito and Kizawa 2001; Boni, Burg et al. 1997; Zhang, Woods, and Elder 2002; Deshpande et al. 2000; Broome, Ryan, and Eckert 2003; Robinson et al. 2002; Mirmohammadsadegh et al. 2000). The role of these S100 proteins in normal skin is not fully understood. However, up-regulation of many S100 proteins has been described in inflamed keratinocytes and in melanoma (Broome, Ryan, and Eckert 2003; Eckert et al. 2004).

In this chapter we will discuss about the role of certain members of the S100 protein family that have been found to play a role in melanoma. These S100 proteins include S100B, S100A2, A4, A6 and S100A11 (Table 1).

| S100 name | Expression | References |
|---|---|---|
| S100B | Melanoma | (Boni, Heizmann et al. 1997)<br>(Harpio and Einarsson 2004)<br>(Donato 2009)<br>(Lin et al. 2010)<br>(Hsieh et al. 2003)<br>(Leclerc, Heizmann, and Vetter 2009) |
| S100A2 | Keratinocytes<br>Melanoma | (Ribe and McNutt 2003)<br>(Boni, Burg et al. 1997)<br>(Shrestha et al. 1998)<br>(Leclerc, Heizmann, and Vetter 2009) |
| S100A4 | Melanoma | (Hsieh et al. 2003)<br>(Maelandsmo et al. 1997)<br>(Andersen et al. 2004)<br>(Leclerc, Heizmann, and Vetter 2009) |
| S100A6 | Melanoma<br>Keratinocytes<br>Langerhans' cells | (Ribe and McNutt 2003)<br>(Maelandsmo et al. 1997)<br>(Weterman et al. 1992)<br>(Boni, Heizmann et al. 1997)<br>(Hsieh et al. 2003)<br>(Leclerc, Heizmann, and Vetter 2009) |
| S100A11 | Keratinocytes<br>Uveal melanoma | (Sakaguchi et al. 2008)<br>(Van Ginkel et al. 1998) |

Table 1. S100 proteins involved in melanoma

## 4. S100 proteins in melanoma

### 4.1 S100B

S100B is predominantly expressed in the brain (Moore 1965). It is mainly secreted by astrocytes and triggers neurotrophic or neurotoxic effects dependent of its concentration (reviewed in (Donato 2009)). S100B is also secreted by melanoma cells and is a biomarker for stage IV malignant melanoma: a high concentration of serum S100B correlates with poor prognosis (Balch et al. 2009; Ghanem et al. 2001; Harpio and Einarsson 2004). S100B binds two calcium ions with micromolar affinity (2-20 μM) (Baudier and Gerard 1986). Binding to calcium triggers large conformational changes in the C-terminal EF-hand leading to interaction with target proteins (Heizmann, Fritz, and Schäfer 2002). S100B also binds zinc and copper ions. It is important to note that binding of zinc to S100B is tighter ($K_D$ = 0.1-1 μM) that binding of calcium. Binding of zinc to histidine and glutamic acid residues present at the dimer interface leads to major conformational changes within S100B resulting in modulation of the interaction with the target proteins (Wilder et al. 2005; Ostendorp et al. 2010).

S100B interacts with more than a dozen intracellular targets *in vitro* (Donato et al. 2009). Many of these targets have important functions in cancer and cell proliferation. For instance, S100B activates the glycolytic enzyme fructose-1,6-biphosphate aldolase, (Zimmer and Van Eldik 1986). S100B secreted by melanoma may therefore contribute to higher glycolysis of cancer cells. Cancer cells are known to have increased metabolism and glycolysis activity and inhibition of metabolism is currently a therapeutic approach to treat melanoma (Hersey et al. 2009; Xu et al. 2005). S100B may also contribute to cellular proliferation by interacting with many proteins of the cytoskeleton. As an example, S100B activates microtubule depolymerization in a calcium dependent manner (Donato 1988). S100B has been shown to directly interact with other constituents of the microtubules such as tubulin (Donato 1988), the microtubule associated tau protein (Baudier and Cole 1988), the actin binding protein caldesmon (Skripnikova and Gusev 1989) or the small GTPase Rac1 and cdc42 effector IQGAP1 (Mbele et al. 2002). S100B may also play a role in cellular division and proliferation through the activation of Nuclear Dbf2 related (ndr) kinase (Millward et al. 1998). S100B also binds to the giant phosphoprotein AHNAK/desmoyokin in a calcium dependent manner, resulting in the regulation of calcium homeostasis (Gentil et al. 2001). AHNAK is a protein of neuroectodermal origin and is present in melanoma cells (Shtivelman and Bishop 1993). Since changes in calcium homeostasis have been shown to play important roles in melanoma through the activation of protein kinase B/Akt, the interaction of S100B with AHNAK might be of high relevance in the disease (Fedida-Metula et al. 2008).

Among the intracellular proteins, the transcriptional factors p53 and its related factors p63 and p73 are also target proteins. Binding of S100B inhibits p53 phosphorylation and oligomerization resulting in inhibition of p53 apoptotic function (Lin et al. 2010).

As mentioned earlier, S100B is secreted from melanoma cells. The mechanisms of S100B secretion are still poorly understood but recent studies have suggested that RAGE may participate in the translocation of several S100s including S100B (Hsieh et al. 2004; Perrone, Peluso, and Melone 2008). The role of S100B, ounce secreted in the extracellular medium is currently unknown. Secreted S100B could act in an autocrine or paracrine manner through the activation of cell surface receptors. RAGE is among the potential candidates that could play the role of receptor.

### 4.2 S100A2

Although S100B is an established biomarker in melanoma, the role of S100A2 is not yet completely understood. S100A2 is expressed in many cells of the normal epidermis (Table 1) (Boni, Burg et al. 1997; Eckert et al. 2004; Maelandsmo et al. 1997). S100A2 is dimeric and binds both zinc ($K_D$ = 25 nM) and calcium ($K_D$= 470 μM) and binding to zinc reduces significantly the affinity for calcium (Franz et al. 1998; Koch et al. 2007).

S100A2 is mainly localized in the cell nucleus where it is believed to play the role of tumor suppressor (Glenney, Kindy, and Zokas 1989). In line with this hypothesis, S100A2 is found down-regulated in melanoma and other cancers that include prostate, oral, lung and breast cancers (Maelandsmo et al. 1997; Leclerc, Heizmann, and Vetter 2009; Gupta et al. 2003; Suzuki et al. 2005; Feng et al. 2001; Lee et al. 1992). However, recent studies also showed that S100A2 could be up-regulated in other cancers such as esophageal squamous carcinoma, gastric, and ovarian cancer (Imazawa et al. 2005; El-Rifai et al. 2002; Hough et al. 2001). Both down- and up-regulation of S100A2 have been found in different tumors of non-small cell lung cancer (NSCLC) (Smith et al. 2004; Strazisar, Mlakar, and Glavac 2009). In a mouse model of NSCLC over-expression of S100A2 correlated with strong metastasis (Bulk et al. 2009).

The expression pattern of S100A2 in melanoma is opposite to that of S100B. An earlier study showed that although most of benign nevi showed the presence of S100A2 mRNA, none of the metastatic tissue sample showed detectable levels of S100A2 mRNA (Maelandsmo et al. 1997). We recently confirmed this observation using a panel of 40 stage III and stage IV melanoma tissue samples and we showed a significant reduction in S100A2 mRNA level in both stage III and stage IV compared to the control samples (Leclerc, Heizmann, and Vetter 2009).

A role of S100A2 in uveal melanoma was also suggested by a recent study where co-treatment of uveal melanoma cells with decitabine and cell death inducing interferon-γ resulted in a dose-dependent increase in S100A2 expression, both at the transcription and protein level (Gollob and Sciambi 2007).

As mentioned earlier, S100A2 locates in the nucleus where its most evident target appears to be p53. Numerous studies have shown and characterized *in vitro* the interaction of S100A2 and p53. Binding of S100A2 with p53 results in increase of the transcriptional activity of the nuclear factor (Mueller et al. 2005; Fernandez-Fernandez, Rutherford, and Fersht 2008; van Dieck, Teufel et al. 2009). Binding of S100A2 to p53 is increased when p53 is phosphorylated (van Dieck, Teufel et al. 2009). A recent study shows that over-expression of S100A2 in nude mice resulted in the induction of metastatic melanoma (Bulk et al. 2009). The presence of S100A2 was also found to correlate with a favorable outcome in patients carrying p53 negative tumors (Matsubara et al. 2005).

The transcription of S100A2 itself has been shown to be under the control of p53 and of the p53 related factors p63 and p73 suggesting complex mechanisms of regulation of S100A2 and p53 (Tan et al. 1999; Kirschner et al. 2008).

S100A2 could also play a role in tumor suppression though the interaction with cyclophilin CyP40. Indeed S100A2 has been shown to interact with CyP40, resulting in inhibition of the complex formation between CyP40 and HsP90 and therefore resulting in alteration of protein folding (Shimamoto et al. 2010).

Although some mutations and polymorphisms within S100A2 have been reported in NSCLC, none have been reported in melanoma so far (Strazisar, Rott, and Glavac 2009).

We recently showed that S100A2 could interact with RAGE *in vitro* (Leclerc et al. 2009). However, the role of this interaction in melanoma or others pathologies has not yet been demonstrated.

### 4.3 S100A4

S100A4 is characterized by its involvement in cancer progression and metastasis (Boye and Maelandsmo 2010). S100A4 forms dimers, binds calcium and zinc and similarly to other S100 proteins, shows cell- and tissue-specific expression (Helfman et al. 2005; Garrett et al. 2006; Chen et al. 2009). In normal conditions, S100A4 is found in a large variety of cells that include fibroblasts, leukocytes, smooth muscle cells, and endothelial cells (Gibbs et al. 1995). It is also found in the brain where it is believed to play a role in neuronal plasticity (Kozlova and Lukanidin 2002).

The role of S100A4 in cancer was first suggested in mouse adenocarcinoma and later confirmed in many animal studies (Grum-Schwensen et al. 2005; Ambartsumian, Grigorian, and Lukanidin 2005). In one study, the injection of highly metastatic mouse mammary carcinoma did not generate metastasis in S100A4 knock-out mice whereas many metastases were found in the control animals (Grum-Schwensen et al. 2005).

The role of S100A4 in melanoma has not yet been clearly established. An earlier study aiming at measuring the mRNA levels of S100A4 in melanoma samples did not showed any significant difference in S100A4 mRNAs between melanoma samples and benign nevi (Maelandsmo et al. 1997). Our recent analysis of 40 samples of stage III and stage IV melanoma tissues showed a significantly reduction of S100A4 mRNA in stage IV tissue samples compared to control samples.

Although S100A4 might not possess the properties of prognostic marker for stage III and IV melanoma, it might predict the outcome of patients at earlier stages of the disease. Indeed, a study by Andersen et al. showed a positive correlation between the level of S100A4 and the depth of the primary nodular melanoma tumor, with a higher expression of S100A4 correlating with a decreased disease free survival rate (Andersen et al. 2004). Accordingly, loss of S100A4 expression was found in the metastatic tumors deriving from the nodular tumors (Andersen et al. 2004).

At the molecular level, S100A4 has been shown to interact with both intracellular (non-muscle myosin, tropomyosin) and extracellular targets (annexin II, plasminogen, EGFR ligands) (Kim and Helfman 2003; Takenaga et al. 1994; Ford et al. 1995; Li et al. 2003; Semov et al. 2005; Klingelhofer et al. 2009). The control of the interaction of S100A4 with its target proteins might involve S100A4 oligomerization, as suggested by recent studies with myosin-IIA (Malashkevich et al. 2010). In another study, self-association of S100A4 has been shown to be essential for S100A4 induced metastasis formation (Ismail et al. 2010). Importantly, as described for S100B and S100A2, S100A4 interacts with the tumor suppressor p53 protein, resulting in the inhibition of p53 oligomerization and its interaction with its target DNA (Grigorian et al. 2001; Fernandez-Fernandez, Rutherford, and Fersht 2008; van Dieck, Teufel et al. 2009; Berge and Maelandsmo 2010).

Both S100A4 dimers and oligomers have been found to interact with RAGE *in vitro* as demonstrated by biophysical studies (Kiryushko et al. 2006). *In vivo* the activation of RAGE by S100A4 appears to depend of the cell type. S100A4 has been shown to trigger RAGE dependent signaling in osteoarthritic cartilage and pulmonary artery smooth muscle cells but not in neurons (Yammani et al. 2006; Spiekerkoetter et al. 2009; Kiryushko et al. 2006).

### 4.4 S100A6

The gene of S1000A6 was identified and cloned from human melanoma cells (Weterman et al. 1993). S100A6 is structurally very similar to S100B (Sastry et al. 1998; Otterbein et al. 2002) but is present in a larger number of tissues and cells than S100B. It is found in muscle tissues, lung, kidney, spleen, and brain (Kuznicki et al. 1989). S100A6 binds both calcium and zinc (Filipek, Heizmann, and Kuznicki 1990). S100A6 has been found in high levels in several cancers including colorectal cancer, pancreatic, hepato-cellular carcinoma, melanoma, lung cancer or gastric cancer and has been suggested to play a role in proliferation and tumorigenesis (Komatsu et al. 2000; Maelandsmo et al. 1997; Nedjadi et al. 2009; De Petris et al. 2009; Ohuchida et al. 2007; Yang et al. 2007; Lesniak, Slomnicki, and Filipek 2009; Vimalachandran et al. 2005).

S100A6 was identified by comparing metastatic melanoma samples with normal nevi (Weterman et al. 1993). An increase in S100A6 staining intensity correlated with the stage of the melanoma sample (Weterman et al. 1993). In a later study, Maelandsmo et al. confirmed that S100A6 mRNA expression was significantly higher in samples from patients with thick primary lesions and short survival time than in samples from patients with thin primary lesions and longer survival time (Maelandsmo et al. 1997). S100A6 over-expression has been described in occular and non-occular melanoma tissue samples (Van Ginkel et al. 1998; Hsieh et al. 2003). We recently examined by quantitative PCR a panel of 40 stage III and stage IV melanoma samples. Our study showed that 43% of stage III melanoma tissue samples presented significant over-expression of S100A6 mRNA (Leclerc, Heizmann, and Vetter 2009). Our results were in agreement with those of Ribe et al. where 33% of melanoma samples showed the expression of S100A6 at the protein level (Ribe and McNutt 2003).

At the molecular level, S100A6 interacts with the tumor suppressor p53. However, contrarily to the interaction of S100B or S100A2 with p53, binding of S100A6 to p53 does not affect p53 interaction with its target proteins (Fernandez-Fernandez, Rutherford, and Fersht 2008; Slomnicki, Nawrot, and Lesniak 2009). S100A6 also interacts with RAGE and triggers RAGE dependent intracellular signaling (Leclerc et al. 2007). We showed that S100A6 triggered cell death through the C2 domain of RAGE whereas on the same cells, S100B triggered cell proliferation through the V domain of the receptor (Leclerc et al. 2007).

### 4.5 S100A11

S100A11 shows 50% amino-acid homology with S100A2 (Kondo et al. 2002). It has a large tissue and cell distribution (Allen et al. 1996). S100A11 plays dual roles in cancer (reviewed in (He et al. 2009)). S100A11 was shown to promote tumor formation in prostate, breast, and pancreatic cancer (Rehman et al. 2004; Cross et al. 2005; Ohuchida et al. 2006). Surprisingly, it was also shown to play the role of tumor suppressor in bladder and renal carcinoma (Memon et al. 2005; Kondo et al. 2002). S100A11 has been found over-expressed in malignant melanoma of the uvea suggesting a role in this type of cancer as well (Van Ginkel et al. 1998).

At the molecular level, S100A11 interacts with a number of targets that have key functions in cell proliferation and repair mechanisms. For instance, S100A11 translocates from the cytoplasm to the nucleus where it regulates cell proliferation in response to DNA damage (Gorsler et al. 2010). S100A11 also interacts with annexin II which has been associated with many cancer (Diaz et al. 2004; Emoto et al. 2001; Esposito et al. 2006; Rintala-Dempsey et al. 2006). S100A11 binds to p53 and to the DNA repair protein Rad54B as well (Fernandez-Fernandez, Rutherford, and Fersht 2008; Murzik et al. 2008).

S100A11 has also been found to interact with RAGE and to trigger RAGE dependent intracellular signaling in osteoarthritis (OA) and in human keratinocytes (Cecil et al. 2005; Sakaguchi et al. 2008).

### 4.6 Other S100 proteins

The S100 proteins described above have been found in melanoma cells or tumor samples. However, melanoma tumors, like many solid tumors, are in constant communication with the tumor micro-environment through the activation of various signal transduction pathways. For instance, although S100A8/A9 are not over-expressed in melanoma tissue samples, the heterodimer was suggested to be released from the tumor environment and to participate in melanoma tumor growth through RAGE (Figure 2A, B) (Saha et al. 2010). S100A8 and S100A9 form heterodimers that are mainly expressed and secreted by monocytes and macrophages and were initially described as pro-inflammatory cytokines (Hsu et al. 2009). However, in recent years many studies have demonstrated that S100A8/A9 also play an increasing role in cancer (Ehrchen et al. 2009; Ghavami et al. 2009; Ang et al. 2010). Interestingly several studies have shown that S10A8/A9 may play a role in cancer through RAGE and the activation of MAPK and NF-κB (Ghavami et al. 2008; Ang et al. 2010; Ichikawa et al. 2011).

S100A10 has also been suggested to play a role in melanoma and was found expressed at various levels in melanoma tumor samples and melanocytes (Petersson et al. 2009; Leclerc, Heizmann, and Vetter 2009).

## 5. Role of RAGE in melanoma and therapeutic approach

The role of RAGE in melanoma tumor growth and metastasis has been suggested by studies in mice (Huttunen et al. 2002; Abe et al. 2004). In the study by Huttunen et al., the metastatic activity of melanoma B16-F1 cells overexpressing either full-length RAGE (B16-F1 RAGE) or a truncated form of the receptor lacking the intracellular part (B16-F1 RAGEΔcyto), were compared. The study showed that mice that received the B16-F1 RAGEΔcyto cells developed about 70% less lung metastasis than the mice that were injected with B16-F1 RAGE cells (Huttunen et al. 2002). In a study by Abe et al., blockade of RAGE using anti-RAGE antibodies suppressed growth of melanoma tumors implanted in mice and originating from G361 melanoma cells (Abe et al. 2004). The presence of RAGE in melanoma tissue samples from human patients was demonstrated by Hsieh et al. (Hsieh et al. 2003) using tumor tissue microarrays. We have recently shown that the transcript levels of RAGE in melanoma patient tissue samples were significantly higher in stage IV than in stage III melanoma and that large variations were present between samples (>100 fold) (Leclerc, Heizmann, and Vetter 2009). A recent study also showed that the inhibition of proliferation of the melanoma cell line SK-MEL-28 following the treatment with the MK615 compound was accompanied with a decrease in the protein expression level of RAGE (Matsushita et al. 2010). In addition, Saha et al. demonstrated that in the uteroglobin-KO mouse model of pulmonary inflammation, RAGE expressing B16F10 melanoma cells were more prone to pulmonary metastatic colonization than in the control mice (Saha et al. 2010). More importantly, these authors demonstrated that metastatic melanoma cells were chemoattracted by S100A8 and S100A9 overproduced by the uteroglobin-KO mouse and that blocking RAGE with a specific antibody resulted in the inhibition of the chemotactic migration (Saha et al. 2010).

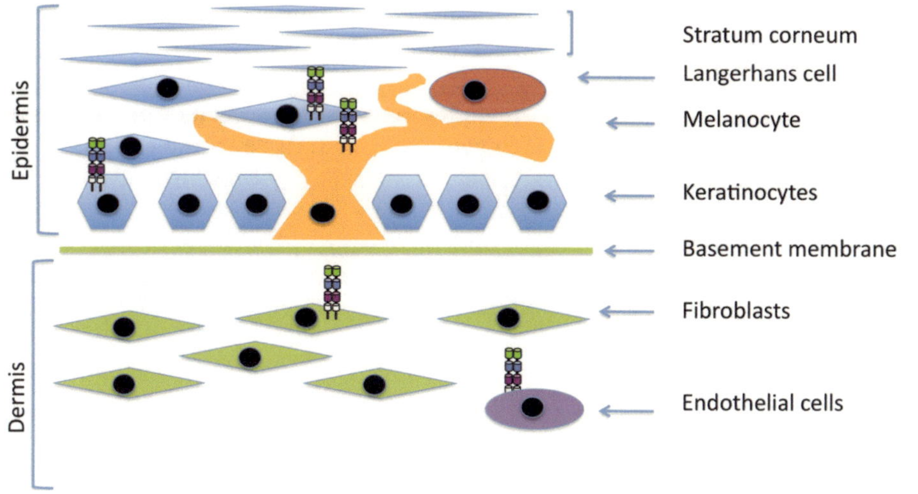


(a)

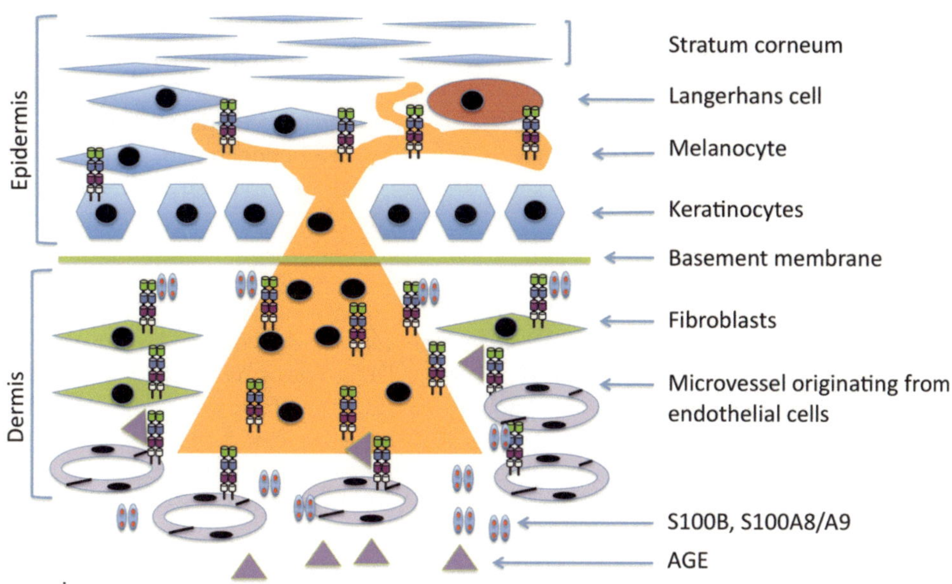


(b)

Fig. 2. a) Cells of the epidermis and dermis. In the epidermis, RAGE is expressed in skin fibroblasts, keratinocytes, endothelial cells and melanocytes (Lohwasser et al. 2006). In the dermis, RAGE is expressed on the surface of fibroblasts and endothelial cells. b) Invasion of melanocytes through the dermis. Melanocytes have invaded the dermis and have multiplied. Melanoma cells express RAGE and secrete S100B. Secreted S100B may activate other melanoma cells, fibroblasts or endothelial cells present in the environment through the interaction with RAGE, resulting in tumor growth. Other cells within the tumor environment produce S100A8/A9 and AGEs. Endothelial cells start forming new blood vessels. Activation of RAGE by its ligands results in up-regulation of RAGE and amplification of RAGE dependent signaling

There is currently no treatment that efficiently cures metastatic melanoma. For primary melanoma tumors, the therapeutic approach consists in the surgical removal of the lesion and the survival rate is very high (>90%). For metastatic melanoma, the FDA approved therapies include chemotherapy with alkylating agents (Dacarbazine) or immunotherapy with interleukin-2 (Atkins et al. 1999). However, even with these therapies, the survival rate of patients with advanced melanoma (stage III and IV) is only around 10%. There is therefore a need for new therapeutic targets.

RAGE appears to be a promising target and in two independent animal models, RAGE blockade resulted in decreased cell proliferation and tumor growth rate (Abe et al. 2004) as well as in the reduction of the number of metastasis (Huttunen et al. 2002). Due to the broad variety of its ligands, RAGE is at the crossroad of several pathways. The increased metabolic activity (glycolysis, mitochondrial oxidative stress) of tumor cells leads to the formation of reactive carbonyl species (RCS) that react with tumor proteins to form AGEs (Sander et al. 2003; Abe et al. 2004; Wondrak, Jacobson, and Jacobson 2006). AGEs react with RAGE and trigger proliferative signaling pathways. Blocking AGE formation through carbonyl scavengers have been tested in melanoma cell lines and showed encouraging results (Wondrak, Jacobson, and Jacobson 2006). Blocking RAGE activation by AGEs is another option. Blockade of RAGE/HMGB1 with an HMGB1 derived peptide was also shown to efficiently reduce the number of metastatic tumors generated by the melanoma cell line B16-F1 (Huttunen et al. 2002).

Blockage of RAGE/ligand might not be successful in each melanoma patient. As we recently showed, large variation in the transcript levels of RAGE exist between patients and blockade of RAGE might be efficient only in patients showing high expression of RAGE (Leclerc, Heizmann, and Vetter 2009).

## 6. Conclusion

The prevalence of metastatic melanoma is on the rise worldwide and new targets are urgently needed to treat this cancer. In recent years, S100 proteins have evolved from simple calcium binding proteins into proteins that participate actively in many diseases such as cancer. We have discussed in this chapter how S100 proteins could play important role in melanoma proliferation and metastasis through their interaction with key target proteins such as p53, tubulin associated protein, CyP40 or RAGE. In particular, RAGE appears to be a promising therapeutic target and efforts should be devoted to develop inhibitors of RAGE/S100 protein interaction.

## 7. Acknowledgements

The author thanks ND-EPSCoR (FAR0016296) and the College of Pharmacy, Nursing and Allied Sciences at North Dakota State University for financial support.

## 8. References

Abe, R., T. Shimizu, H. Sugawara, H. Watanabe, H. Nakamura, H. Choei, N. Sasaki, S. Yamagishi, M. Takeuchi, and H. Shimizu. 2004. Regulation of human melanoma growth and metastasis by AGE-AGE receptor interactions. *J Invest Dermatol* 122 (2):461-7.

Ahmed, N., U. Ahmed, P. J. Thornalley, K. Hager, G. Fleischer, and G. Munch. 2005. Protein glycation, oxidation and nitration adduct residues and free adducts of cerebrospinal fluid in Alzheimer's disease and link to cognitive impairment. *J Neurochem* 92 (2):255-63.

Allen, B. G., I. Durussel, M. P. Walsh, and J. A. Cox. 1996. Characterization of the $Ca^{2+}$-binding properties of calgizzarin (S100C) isolated from chicken gizzard smooth muscle. *Biochem Cell Biol* 74 (5):687-94.

Ambartsumian, N., M. Grigorian, and E. Lukanidin. 2005. Genetically modified mouse models to study the role of metastasis-promoting S100A4(mts1) protein in metastatic mammary cancer. *J Dairy Res* 72 Spec No:27-33.

Andersen, K., J. M. Nesland, R. Holm, V. A. Florenes, O. Fodstad, and G. M. Maelandsmo. 2004. Expression of S100A4 combined with reduced E-cadherin expression predicts patient outcome in malignant melanoma. *Mod Pathol* 17 (8):990-7.

Ang, C. W., T. Nedjadi, A. A. Sheikh, E. M. Tweedle, S. Tonack, S. Honap, R. E. Jenkins, B. K. Park, I. Schwarte-Waldhoff, I. Khattak, B. Azadeh, A. Dodson, H. Kalirai, J. P. Neoptolemos, P. S. Rooney, and E. Costello. 2010. Smad4 loss is associated with fewer S100A8-positive monocytes in colorectal tumors and attenuated response to S100A8 in colorectal and pancreatic cancer cells. *Carcinogenesis* 31 (9):1541-51.

Atkins, M. B., M. T. Lotze, J. P. Dutcher, R. I. Fisher, G. Weiss, K. Margolin, J. Abrams, M. Sznol, D. Parkinson, M. Hawkins, C. Paradise, L. Kunkel, and S. A. Rosenberg. 1999. High-dose recombinant interleukin 2 therapy for patients with metastatic melanoma: analysis of 270 patients treated between 1985 and 1993. *J Clin Oncol* 17 (7):2105-16.

Balch, C. M., J. E. Gershenwald, S. J. Soong, J. F. Thompson, M. B. Atkins, D. R. Byrd, A. C. Buzaid, A. J. Cochran, D. G. Coit, S. Ding, A. M. Eggermont, K. T. Flaherty, P. A. Gimotty, J. M. Kirkwood, K. M. McMasters, M. C. Mihm, Jr., D. L. Morton, M. I. Ross, A. J. Sober, and V. K. Sondak. 2009. Final version of 2009 AJCC melanoma staging and classification. *J Clin Oncol* 27 (36):6199-206.

Baudier, J., and R. D. Cole. 1988. Interactions between the microtubule-associated tau proteins and S100B regulate tau phosphorylation by the $Ca^{2+}$/calmodulin-dependent protein kinase II. *J Biol Chem* 263 (12):5876-83.

Baudier, J., C. Delphin, D. Grunwald, S. Khochbin, and J. J. Lawrence. 1992. Characterization of the tumor suppressor protein p53 as a protein kinase C substrate and a S100b-binding protein. *Proc Natl Acad Sci U S A* 89 (23):11627-31.

Baudier, J., and D. Gerard. 1986. Ions binding to S100 proteins. II. Conformational studies and calcium-induced conformational changes in S100 alpha alpha protein: the effect of acidic pH and calcium incubation on subunit exchange in S100a (alpha beta) protein. *J Biol Chem* 261 (18):8204-12.

Berge, G., and G. M. Maelandsmo. 2010. Evaluation of potential interactions between the metastasis-associated protein S100A4 and the tumor suppressor protein p53. *Amino Acids*: [Epub ahead of print].

Bhatia, S., S. S. Tykodi, and J. A. Thompson. 2009. Treatment of metastatic melanoma: an overview. *Oncology (Williston Park)* 23 (6):488-96.

Bierhaus, A., P. M. Humpert, M. Morcos, T. Wendt, T. Chavakis, B. Arnold, D. M. Stern, and P. P. Nawroth. 2005. Understanding RAGE, the receptor for advanced glycation end products. *J Mol Med* 83 (11):876-86.

Bierhaus, A., and P. P. Nawroth. 2009. Multiple levels of regulation determine the role of the receptor for AGE (RAGE) as common soil in inflammation, immune responses and diabetes mellitus and its complications. *Diabetologia* 52 (11):2251-63.

Boni, R., G. Burg, A. Doguoglu, E. C. Ilg, B. W. Schafer, B. Muller, and C. W. Heizmann. 1997. Immunohistochemical localization of the Ca2+ binding S100 proteins in normal human skin and melanocytic lesions. *Br J Dermatol* 137 (1):39-43.

Boni, R., C. W. Heizmann, A. Doguoglu, E. C. Ilg, B. W. Schafer, R. Dummer, and G. Burg. 1997. Ca(2+)-binding proteins S100A6 and S100B in primary cutaneous melanoma. *J Cutan Pathol* 24 (2):76-80.

Bouwhuis, M. G., S. Suciu, W. Kruit, F. Sales, K. Stoitchkov, P. Patel, V. Cocquyt, J. Thomas, D. Lienard, A. M. Eggermont, and G. Ghanem. 2010. Prognostic value of serial blood S100B determinations in stage IIB-III melanoma patients: A corollary study to EORTC trial 18952. *Eur J Cancer* 47 (3):361-368

Boye, K., and G. M. Maelandsmo. 2010. S100A4 and metastasis: a small actor playing many roles. *Am J Pathol* 176 (2):528-35.

Brett, J., A. M. Schmidt, S. D. Yan, Y. S. Zou, E. Weidman, D. Pinsky, R. Nowygrod, M. Neeper, C. Przysiecki, A. Shaw, and et al. 1993. Survey of the distribution of a newly characterized receptor for advanced glycation end products in tissues. *Am J Pathol* 143 (6):1699-712.

Broome, A. M., D. Ryan, and R. L. Eckert. 2003. S100 protein subcellular localization during epidermal differentiation and psoriasis. *Journal of Histochemistry & Cytochemistry* 51 (5):675-685.

Buckley, S. T., and C. Ehrhardt. 2010. The receptor for advanced glycation end products (RAGE) and the lung. *J Biomed Biotechnol*:in press.

Bulk, E., B. Sargin, U. Krug, A. Hascher, Y. Jun, M. Knop, C. Kerkhoff, V. Gerke, R. Liersch, R. M. Mesters, M. Hotfilder, A. Marra, S. Koschmieder, M. Dugas, W. E. Berdel, H. Serve, and C. Muller-Tidow. 2009. S100A2 induces metastasis in non-small cell lung cancer. *Clin Cancer Res* 15 (1):22-9.

Cecil, D. L., K. Johnson, J. Rediske, M. Lotz, A. M. Schmidt, and R. Terkeltaub. 2005. Inflammation-induced chondrocyte hypertrophy is driven by receptor for advanced glycation end products. *J Immunol* 175 (12):8296-302.

Chen, M., M. Sinha, B. A. Luxon, A. R. Bresnick, and K. L. O'Connor. 2009. Integrin alpha6beta4 controls the expression of genes associated with cell motility, invasion, and metastasis, including S100A4/metastasin. *J Biol Chem* 284 (3):1484-94.

Chun, Y.S., Y. Wang, D.Y. Wang, D.M. McClain, A. Lucci, P.F. Mansfield, J.N. Cormier, M.I. Ross, J.E. Gershenwald, and J.E. Lee. 2008. Prognostic value of s100B levels and LDH levels in melanoma patients. *J Clin Oncol* 26:abstract 9002.

Coughlan, M. T., D. R. Thorburn, S. A. Penfold, A. Laskowski, B. E. Harcourt, K. C. Sourris, A. L. Tan, K. Fukami, V. Thallas-Bonke, P. P. Nawroth, M. Brownlee, A. Bierhaus, M. E. Cooper, and J. M. Forbes. 2009. RAGE-induced cytosolic ROS promote mitochondrial superoxide generation in diabetes. *J Am Soc Nephrol* 20 (4):742-52.

Cross, S. S., F. C. Hamdy, J. C. Deloulme, and I. Rehman. 2005. Expression of S100 proteins in normal human tissues and common cancers using tissue microarrays: S100A6, S100A8, S100A9 and S100A11 are all overexpressed in common cancers. *Histopathology* 46 (3):256-69.

Darrell, S., and M.D. Rigel. 2010. Trends in Dermatology: Melanoma Incidence. *Archives in Dermatology* 146:318.

Dattilo, B. M., G. Fritz, E. Leclerc, C. W. Kooi, C. W. Heizmann, and W. J. Chazin. 2007. The extracellular region of the receptor for advanced glycation end products is composed of two independent structural units. *Biochemistry* 46 (23):6957-70.

De Petris, L., L. M. Orre, L. Kanter, M. Pernemalm, H. Koyi, R. Lewensohn, and J. Lehtio. 2009. Tumor expression of S100A6 correlates with survival of patients with stage I non-small-cell lung cancer. *Lung Cancer* 63:410-417.

Deane, R., S. Du Yan, R. K. Submamaryan, B. LaRue, S. Jovanovic, E. Hogg, D. Welch, L. Manness, C. Lin, J. Yu, H. Zhu, J. Ghiso, B. Frangione, A. Stern, A. M. Schmidt, D. L. Armstrong, B. Arnold, B. Liliensiek, P. Nawroth, F. Hofman, M. Kindy, D. Stern, and B. Zlokovic. 2003. RAGE mediates amyloid-beta peptide transport across the blood-brain barrier and accumulation in brain. *Nat Med* 9 (7):907-13.

Deshpande, R., T. L. Woods, J. Fu, T. Zhang, S. W. Stoll, and J. T. Elder. 2000. Biochemical characterization of S100A2 in human keratinocytes: subcellular localization, dimerization, and oxidative cross-linking. *J Invest Dermatol* 115 (3):477-85.

Diaz, V. M., M. Hurtado, T. M. Thomson, J. Reventos, and R. Paciucci. 2004. Specific interaction of tissue-type plasminogen activator (t-PA) with annexin II on the membrane of pancreatic cancer cells activates plasminogen and promotes invasion in vitro. *Gut* 53 (7):993-1000.

Ding, Q., and J. N. Keller. 2005. Splice variants of the receptor for advanced glycosylation end products (RAGE) in human brain. *Neurosci Lett* 373 (1):67-72.

Donato, R. 1988. Calcium-independent, pH-regulated effects of S-100 proteins on assembly-disassembly of brain microtubule protein in vitro. *J Biol Chem* 263 (1):106-10.

2003. Intracellular and extracellular roles of S100 proteins. *Microsc Res Tech* 60 (6):540-51.

2007. RAGE: a single receptor for several ligands and different cellular responses: the case of certain S100 proteins. *Curr Mol Med* 7 (8):711-24.

2009. S100B's double life: intracellular and extracellular signal. *Biochemica Biophysica Acta: Molecular Cell Research* 1793 (6):1008-1022..

Donato, R., G. Sorci, F. Riuzzi, C. Arcuri, R. Bianchi, F. Brozzi, C. Tubaro, and I. Giambanco. 2009. S100B's double life: intracellular regulator and extracellular signal. *Biochim Biophys Acta* 1793 (6):1008-22.

Eckert, R. L., A. M. Broome, M. Ruse, N. Robinson, D. Ryan, and K. Lee. 2004. S100 proteins in the epidermis. *Journal of Investigative Dermatology* 123 (1):23-33.

Ehrchen, J. M., C. Sunderkotter, D. Foell, T. Vogl, and J. Roth. 2009. The endogenous Toll-like receptor 4 agonist S100A8/S100A9 (calprotectin) as innate amplifier of infection, autoimmunity, and cancer. *J Leukoc Biol* 86 (3):557-66.

El-Rifai, W., C. A. Moskaluk, M. K. Abdrabbo, J. Harper, C. Yoshida, G. J. Riggins, H. F. Frierson, Jr., and S. M. Powell. 2002. Gastric cancers overexpress S100A calcium-binding proteins. *Cancer Res* 62 (23):6823-6.

Emanuele, E., A. D'Angelo, C. Tomaino, G. Binetti, R. Ghidoni, P. Politi, L. Bernardi, R. Maletta, A. C. Bruni, and D. Geroldi. 2005. Circulating levels of soluble receptor for advanced glycation end products in Alzheimer disease and vascular dementia. *Arch Neurol* 62 (11):1734-6.

Emoto, K., H. Sawada, Y. Yamada, H. Fujimoto, Y. Takahama, M. Ueno, T. Takayama, H. Uchida, K. Kamada, A. Naito, S. Hirao, and Y. Nakajima. 2001. Annexin II overexpression is correlated with poor prognosis in human gastric carcinoma. *Anticancer Res* 21 (2B):1339-45.

Esposito, I., R. Penzel, M. Chaib-Harrireche, U. Barcena, F. Bergmann, S. Riedl, H. Kayed, N. Giese, J. Kleeff, H. Friess, and P. Schirmacher. 2006. Tenascin C and annexin II expression in the process of pancreatic carcinogenesis. *J Pathol* 208 (5):673-85.

Fang, F., L. F. Lue, S. Yan, H. Xu, J. S. Luddy, D. Chen, D. G. Walker, D. M. Stern, A. M. Schmidt, J. X. Chen, and S. S. Yan. 2010. RAGE-dependent signaling in microglia contributes to neuroinflammation, Abeta accumulation, and impaired learning/memory in a mouse model of Alzheimer's disease. *FASEB J* 24 (4):1043-55.

Fedida-Metula, S., S. Elhyany, S. Tsory, S. Segal, M. Hershfinkel, I. Sekler, and D. Fishman. 2008. Targeting lipid rafts inhibits protein kinase B by disrupting calcium homeostasis and attenuates malignant properties of melanoma cells. *Carcinogenesis* 29 (8):1546-54.

Feng, G., X. Xu, E. M. Youssef, and R. Lotan. 2001. Diminished expression of S100A2, a putative tumor suppressor, at early stage of human lung carcinogenesis. *Cancer Res* 61 (21):7999-8004.

Fernandez-Fernandez, M. R., T. J. Rutherford, and A. R. Fersht. 2008. Members of the S100 family bind p53 in two distinct ways. *Protein Sci* 17 (10):1663-70.

Filipek, A., C. W. Heizmann, and J. Kuznicki. 1990. Calcyclin is a calcium and zinc binding protein. *FEBS Lett* 264 (2):263-6.

Ford, H. L., M. M. Salim, R. Chakravarty, V. Aluiddin, and S. B. Zain. 1995. Expression of Mts1, a metastasis-associated gene, increases motility but not invasion of a nonmetastatic mouse mammary adenocarcinoma cell line. *Oncogene* 11 (10):2067-75.

Franz, C., I. Durussel, J. A. Cox, B. W. Schafer, and C. W. Heizmann. 1998. Binding of Ca2+ and Zn2+ to human nuclear S100A2 and mutant proteins. *J Biol Chem* 273 (30):18826-34.

Fritz, G., and C. W. Heizmann. 2004. 3D structures of the calcium and zinc binding S100 proteins. In *Handbook of Metalloproteins Vol. 3*, edited by A. Messerschmidt, W. Bode and M. Cygler. Chichester: Wiley.

Galichet, A., M. Weibel, and C. W. Heizmann. 2008. Calcium-regulated intramembrane proteolysis of the RAGE receptor. *Biochem Biophys Res Commun* 370 (1):1-5.

Garrett, S. C., K. M. Varney, D. J. Weber, and A. R. Bresnick. 2006. S100A4, a mediator of metastasis. *J Biol Chem* 281 (2):677-80.

Gentil, B. J., C. Delphin, G. O. Mbele, J. C. Deloulme, M. Ferro, J. Garin, and J. Baudier. 2001. The giant protein AHNAK is a specific target for the calcium- and zinc-binding S100B protein: potential implications for Ca2+ homeostasis regulation by S100B. *J Biol Chem* 276 (26):23253-61.

Ghanem, G., B. Loir, R. Morandini, F. Sales, D. Lienard, A. Eggermont, and F. Lejeune. 2001. On the release and half-life of S100B protein in the peripheral blood of melanoma patients. *Int J Cancer* 94 (4):586-90.

Ghavami, S., S. Chitayat, M. Hashemi, M. Eshraghi, W. J. Chazin, A. J. Halayko, and C. Kerkhoff. 2009. S100A8/A9: a Janus-faced molecule in cancer therapy and tumorgenesis. *Eur J Pharmacol* 625 (1-3):73-83.

Ghavami, S., I. Rashedi, B. M. Dattilo, M. Eshraghi, W. J. Chazin, M. Hashemi, S. Wesselborg, C. Kerkhoff, and M. Los. 2008. S100A8/A9 at low concentration promotes tumor cell growth via RAGE ligation and MAP kinase-dependent pathway. *J Leukoc Biol* 83 (6):1484-92.

Gibbs, F. E., R. Barraclough, A. Platt-Higgins, P. S. Rudland, M. C. Wilkinson, and E. W. Parry. 1995. Immunocytochemical distribution of the calcium-binding protein p9Ka

in normal rat tissues: variation in the cellular location in different tissues. *J Histochem Cytochem* 43 (2):169-80.
Glenney, J. R., Jr., M. S. Kindy, and L. Zokas. 1989. Isolation of a new member of the S100 protein family: amino acid sequence, tissue, and subcellular distribution. *J Cell Biol* 108 (2):569-78.
Gogas, H., A. M. Eggermont, A. Hauschild, P. Hersey, P. Mohr, D. Schadendorf, A. Spatz, and R. Dummer. 2009. Biomarkers in melanoma. *Ann Oncol* 20 8-13.
Gollob, J. A., and C. J. Sciambi. 2007. Decitabine up-regulates S100A2 expression and synergizes with IFN-gamma to kill uveal melanoma cells. *Clin Cancer Res* 13 (17):5219-25.
Gorsler, T., U. Murzik, T. Ulbricht, J. Hentschel, P. Hemmerich, and C. Melle. 2010. DNA damage-induced translocation of S100A11 into the nucleus regulates cell proliferation. *BMC Cell Biol* 11:100.
Grigorian, M., S. Andresen, E. Tulchinsky, M. Kriajevska, C. Carlberg, C. Kruse, M. Cohn, N. Ambartsumian, A. Christensen, G. Selivanova, and E. Lukanidin. 2001. Tumor suppressor p53 protein is a new target for the metastasis-associated Mts1/S100A4 protein: functional consequences of their interaction. *J Biol Chem* 276 (25):22699-708.
Grum-Schwensen, B., J. Klingelhofer, C. H. Berg, C. El-Naaman, M. Grigorian, E. Lukanidin, and N. Ambartsumian. 2005. Suppression of tumor development and metastasis formation in mice lacking the S100A4(mts1) gene. *Cancer Res* 65 (9):3772-80.
Gupta, S., T. Hussain, G. T. MacLennan, P. Fu, J. Patel, and H. Mukhtar. 2003. Differential expression of S100A2 and S100A4 during progression of human prostate adenocarcinoma. *J Clin Oncol* 21 (1):106-12.
Harpio, R., and R. Einarsson. 2004. S100 proteins as cancer biomarkers with focus on S100B in malignant melanoma. *Clin Biochem* 37 (7):512-8.
Hauschild, A., G. Engel, W. Brenner, R. Glaser, H. Monig, E. Henze, and E. Christophers. 1999. S100B protein detection in serum is a significant prognostic factor in metastatic melanoma. *Oncology* 56 (4):338-44.
He, H., J. Li, S. Weng, M. Li, and Y. Yu. 2009. S100A11: diverse function and pathology corresponding to different target proteins. *Cell Biochem Biophys* 55 (3):117-26.
Heizmann, C. W. 2002. The multifunctional S100 protein family. *Methods Mol Biol* 172:69-80.
Heizmann, C. W., G. E. Ackermann, and A. Galichet. 2007. Pathologies involving the S100 proteins and RAGE. *Subcell Biochem* 45:93-138.
Heizmann, C. W., G. Fritz, and B. W. Schäfer. 2002. S100 proteins: structure, functions and pathology. *Front Biosci* 7:d1356-68.
Helfman, D.M., E.J. Kim, E. Lukanidin, and M. Grigorian. 2005. The metastasis associated protein S100A4: role in tumour progression and metastasis. *Br J Cancer* 92:1955-1958.
Hersey, P., R. N. Watts, X. D. Zhang, and J. Hackett. 2009. Metabolic approaches to treatment of melanoma. *Clin Cancer Res* 15 (21):6490-4.
Hofmann, M. A., S. Drury, C. Fu, W. Qu, A. Taguchi, Y. Lu, C. Avila, N. Kambham, A. Bierhaus, P. Nawroth, M. F. Neurath, T. Slattery, D. Beach, J. McClary, M. Nagashima, J. Morser, D. Stern, and A. M. Schmidt. 1999. RAGE mediates a novel proinflammatory axis: a central cell surface receptor for S100/calgranulin polypeptides. *Cell* 97 (7):889-901.
Hori, O., J. Brett, T. Slattery, R. Cao, J. Zhang, J. X. Chen, M. Nagashima, E. R. Lundh, S. Vijay, D. Nitecki, and et al. 1995. The receptor for advanced glycation end products

(RAGE) is a cellular binding site for amphoterin. Mediation of neurite outgrowth and co-expression of rage and amphoterin in the developing nervous system. *J Biol Chem* 270 (43):25752-61.

Hough, C. D., K. R. Cho, A. B. Zonderman, D. R. Schwartz, and P. J. Morin. 2001. Coordinately up-regulated genes in ovarian cancer. *Cancer Res* 61 (10):3869-76.

Hsieh, H. L., B. W. Schafer, N. Sasaki, and C. W. Heizmann. 2003. Expression analysis of S100 proteins and RAGE in human tumors using tissue microarrays. *Biochem Biophys Res Commun* 307 (2):375-81.

Hsieh, H. L., B. W. Schäfer, B. Weigle, and C. W. Heizmann. 2004. S100 protein translocation in response to extracellular S100 is mediated by receptor for advanced glycation endproducts in human endothelial cells. *Biochem Biophys Res Commun* 316 (3):949-59.

Hsu, K., C. Champaiboon, B. D. Guenther, B. S. Sorenson, A. Khammanivong, K. F. Ross, C. L. Geczy, and M. C. Herzberg. 2009. Anti-Infective Protective Properties of S100 Calgranulins. *Antiinflamm Antiallergy Agents Med Chem* 8 (4):290-305.

Hudson, B. I., A. M. Carter, E. Harja, A. Z. Kalea, M. Arriero, H. Yang, P. J. Grant, and A. M. Schmidt. 2008. Identification, classification, and expression of RAGE gene splice variants. *Faseb J* 22 (5):1572-80.

Humpert, P. M., Z. Djuric, S. Kopf, G. Rudofsky, M. Morcos, P. P. Nawroth, and A. Bierhaus. 2007. Soluble RAGE but not endogenous secretory RAGE is associated with albuminuria in patients with type 2 diabetes. *Cardiovasc Diabetol* 6:9.

Huttunen, H. J., C. Fages, J. Kuja-Panula, A. J. Ridley, and H. Rauvala. 2002. Receptor for advanced glycation end products-binding COOH-terminal motif of amphoterin inhibits invasive migration and metastasis. *Cancer Res* 62 (16):4805-11.

Ichikawa, M., R. Williams, L. Wang, T. Vogl, and G. Srikrishna. 2011. S100A8/A9 activate key genes and pathways in colon tumor progression. *Mol Cancer Res* 9 (2):133-48.

Imazawa, M., K. Hibi, S. Fujitake, Y. Kodera, K. Ito, S. Akiyama, and A. Nakao. 2005. S100A2 overexpression is frequently observed in esophageal squamous cell carcinoma. *Anticancer Res.* 25:1247-1250.

Ismail, T. M., S. Zhang, D. G. Fernig, S. Gross, M. L. Martin-Fernandez, V. See, K. Tozawa, C. J. Tynan, G. Wang, M. C. Wilkinson, P. S. Rudland, and R. Barraclough. 2010. Self-association of calcium-binding protein S100A4 and metastasis. *J Biol Chem* 285 (2):914-22.

Ito, M., and K. Kizawa. 2001. Expression of calcium-binding S100 proteins A4 and A6 in regions of the epithelial sac associated with the onset of hair follicle regeneration. *J Invest Dermatol* 116 (6):956-63.

Ito, N., R. A. DeMarco, R. B. Mailliard, J. Han, H. Rabinowich, P. Kalinski, D. B. Stolz, H. J. Zeh, 3rd, and M. T. Lotze. 2007. Cytolytic cells induce HMGB1 release from melanoma cell lines. *J Leukoc Biol* 81 (1):75-83.

Kim, E. J., and D. M. Helfman. 2003. Characterization of the metastasis-associated protein, S100A4. Roles of calcium binding and dimerization in cellular localization and interaction with myosin. *J Biol Chem* 278 (32):30063-73.

Kirschner, R. D., K. Sanger, G. A. Muller, and K. Engeland. 2008. Transcriptional activation of the tumor suppressor and differentiation gene S100A2 by a novel p63-binding site. *Nucleic Acids Res* 36 (9):2969-80.

Kiryushko, D., V. Novitskaya, V. Soroka, J. Klingelhofer, E. Lukanidin, V. Berezin, and E. Bock. 2006. Molecular mechanisms of $Ca^{2+}$ signaling in neurons induced by the S100A4 protein. *Mol Cell Biol* 26 (9):3625-38.

Kislinger, T., C. Fu, B. Huber, W. Qu, A. Taguchi, S. Du Yan, M. Hofmann, S. F. Yan, M. Pischetsrieder, D. Stern, and A. M. Schmidt. 1999. N(epsilon)-(carboxymethyl)lysine adducts of proteins are ligands for receptor for advanced glycation end products that activate cell signaling pathways and modulate gene expression. *J Biol Chem* 274 (44):31740-9.

Klingelhofer, J., H. D. Moller, E. U. Sumer, C. H. Berg, M. Poulsen, D. Kiryushko, V. Soroka, N. Ambartsumian, M. Grigorian, and E. M. Lukanidin. 2009. Epidermal growth factor receptor ligands as new extracellular targets for the metastasis-promoting S100A4 protein. *FEBS J* 276 (20):5936-48.

Koch, M., S. Bhattacharya, T. Kehl, M. Gimona, M. Vasak, W. Chazin, C. W. Heizmann, P. M. Kroneck, and G. Fritz. 2007. Implications on zinc binding to S100A2. *Biochim Biophys Acta* 1773 (3):457-70.

Koch, M., S. Chitayat, B. M. Dattilo, A. Schiefner, J. Diez, W. J. Chazin, and G. Fritz. 2010. Structural Basis for Ligand Recognition and Activation of RAGE. *Structure* 18 (10):1342-52.

Komatsu, K., A. Andoh, S. Ishiguro, N. Suzuki, H. Hunai, Y. Kobune-Fujiwara, M. Kameyama, J. Miyoshi, H. Akedo, and H. Nakamura. 2000. Increased expression of S100A6 (Calcyclin), a calcium-binding protein of the S100 family, in human colorectal adenocarcinomas. *Clin Cancer Res* 6 (1):172-7.

Kondo, A., M. Sakaguchi, E. Makino, M. Namba, S. Okada, and N. H. Huh. 2002. Localization of S100C immunoreactivity in various human tissues. *Acta Med Okayama* 56 (1):31-4.

Koyama, H., H. Yamamoto, and Y. Nishizawa. 2007. RAGE and soluble RAGE: potential therapeutic targets for cardiovascular diseases. *Mol Med* 13 (11-12):625-35.

Kozlova, E. N., and E. Lukanidin. 2002. Mts1 protein expression in the central nervous system after injury. *Glia* 37 (4):337-48.

Kuznicki, J., A. Filipek, P. Heimann, L. Kaczmarek, and B. Kaminska. 1989. Tissue specific distribution of calcyclin--10.5 kDa Ca2+-binding protein. *FEBS Lett* 254 (1-2):141-4.

Landar, A., G. Caddell, J. Chessher, and D. B. Zimmer. 1996. Identification of an S100A1/S100B target protein: phosphoglucomutase. *Cell Calcium* 20 (3):279-85.

Leclerc, E., G. Fritz, S. W. Vetter, and C. W. Heizmann. 2009. Binding of S100 proteins to RAGE: an update. *Biochim Biophys Acta* 1793 (6):993-1007.

Leclerc, E., G. Fritz, M. Weibel, C. W. Heizmann, and A. Galichet. 2007. S100B and S100A6 differentially modulate cell survival by interacting with distinct RAGE (receptor for advanced glycation end products) immunoglobulin domains. *J Biol Chem* 282 (43):31317-31.

Leclerc, E., C. W. Heizmann, and S.W. Vetter. 2009. RAGE and S100 protein transcription levels are highly variable in human melanoma tumors and cells. *General Physiology and Biophysics* 28 (Focus Issue):F65-F75.

Lee, S. W., C. Tomasetto, K. Swisshelm, K. Keyomarsi, and R. Sager. 1992. Down-regulation of a member of the S100 gene family in mammary carcinoma cells and reexpression by azadeoxycytidine treatment. *Proc Natl Acad Sci U S A* 89 (6):2504-8.

Lesniak, W. 2011. Epigenetic regulation of S100 protein expression. *Clinical Epigenetic*:DOI 10.1007/s13148-011-0023-9.

Lesniak, W., L. P. Slomnicki, and A. Filipek. 2009. S100A6 - new facts and features. *Biochem Biophys Res Commun* 390 (4):1087-92.

Li, Z. H., A. Spektor, O. Varlamova, and A. R. Bresnick. 2003. Mts1 regulates the assembly of nonmuscle myosin-IIA. *Biochemistry* 42 (48):14258-66.

Lin, J., Q. Yang, P. T. Wilder, F. Carrier, and D. J. Weber. 2010. The calcium-binding protein S100B down-regulates p53 and apoptosis in malignant melanoma. *J Biol Chem* 285 (35):27487-98.

Lin, L., S. Park, and E. G. Lakatta. 2009. RAGE signaling in inflammation and arterial aging. *Front Biosci* 14:1403-13.

Lohwasser, C., D. Neureiter, B. Weigle, T. Kirchner, and D. Schuppan. 2006. The receptor for advanced glycation end products is highly expressed in the skin and upregulated by advanced glycation end products and tumor necrosis factor-alpha. *J Invest Dermatol* 126 (2):291-9.

Lue, L. F., D. G. Walker, S. Jacobson, and M. Sabbagh. 2009. Receptor for advanced glycation end products: its role in Alzheimer's disease and other neurological diseases. *Future Neurol* 4 (2):167-177.

Maelandsmo, G. M., V. A. Florenes, T. Mellingsaeter, E. Hovig, R. S. Kerbel, and O. Fodstad. 1997. Differential expression patterns of S100A2, S100A4 and S100A6 during progression of human malignant melanoma. *Int J Cancer* 74 (4):464-9.

Malashkevich, V. N., N. G. Dulyaninova, U. A. Ramagopal, M. A. Liriano, K. M. Varney, D. Knight, M. Brenowitz, D. J. Weber, S. C. Almo, and A. R. Bresnick. 2010. Phenothiazines inhibit S100A4 function by inducing protein oligomerization. *Proc Natl Acad Sci U S A* 107 (19):8605-10.

Marenholz, I., R. C. Lovering, and C. W. Heizmann. 2006. An update of the S100 nomenclature. *Biochim Biophys Acta* 1763 (11):1282-3.

Matsubara, D., T. Niki, S. Ishikawa, A. Goto, E. Ohara, T. Yokomizo, C. W. Heizmann, H. Aburatani, S. Moriyama, H. Moriyama, Y. Nishimura, N. Funata, and M. Fukayama. 2005. Differential expression of S100A2 and S100A4 in lung adenocarcinomas: clinicopathological significance, relationship to p53 and identification of their target genes. *Cancer Sci* 96 (12):844-57.

Matsumoto, S., T. Yoshida, H. Murata, S. Harada, S. Nakamura, Y. Yamamoto, T. Watanabe, H. Yonekura, H. Yamamoto, T. Ohkubo, and Y. Kobayashi. 2008. Solution Structure of the Variable-Type Domain of the Receptor for Advanced Glycation End Products: New Insight into AGE-RAGE Interaction(,). *Biochemistry* 47:12299-12311.

Matsushita, S., K-I Tada, K-I Kawahara, K. Kawai, T. Hashiguchi, I. Maruyama, and T. Kanekura. 2010. Advanced malignant melanoma responds to Prunus mume Sieb. Et Zucc (Ume) extract: Case report and in vitro study. *Experimental and Therapeutic medicine* 1:569-574.

Mbele, G. O., J. C. Deloulme, B. J. Gentil, C. Delphin, M. Ferro, J. Garin, M. Takahashi, and J. Baudier. 2002. The zinc- and calcium-binding S100B interacts and co-localizes with IQGAP1 during dynamic rearrangement of cell membranes. *J Biol Chem* 277 (51):49998-50007.

Memon, A. A., B. S. Sorensen, P. Meldgaard, L. Fokdal, T. Thykjaer, and E. Nexo. 2005. Down-regulation of S100C is associated with bladder cancer progression and poor survival. *Clin Cancer Res* 11 (2 Pt 1):606-11.

Millward, T. A., C. W. Heizmann, B. W. Schafer, and B. A. Hemmings. 1998. Calcium regulation of Ndr protein kinase mediated by S100 calcium-binding proteins. *Embo J* 17 (20):5913-22.

Mirmohammadsadegh, A., E. Tschakarjan, A. Ljoljic, K. Bohner, G. Michel, T. Ruzicka, M. Goos, and U. R. Hengge. 2000. Calgranulin C is overexpressed in lesional psoriasis. *Journal of Investigative Dermatology* 114 (6):1207-1208.

Moore, B. W. 1965. A soluble protein characteristic of the nervous system. *Biochem Biophys Res Commun* 19 (6):739-44.

Moroz, O. V., A. A. Antson, E. J. Dodson, H. J. Burrell, S. J. Grist, R. M. Lloyd, N. J. Maitland, G. G. Dodson, K. S. Wilson, E. Lukanidin, and I. B. Bronstein. 2002. The structure of S100A12 in a hexameric form and its proposed role in receptor signalling. *Acta Crystallogr D Biol Crystallogr* 58 (Pt 3):407-13.

Moroz, O. V., K. S. Wilson, and I. B. Bronstein. 2010. The role of zinc in the S100 proteins: insights from the X-ray structures. *Amino Acids* in press.

Mueller, A., B. W. Schäfer, S. Ferrari, M. Weibel, M. Makek, M. Hochli, and C. W. Heizmann. 2005. The calcium-binding protein S100A2 interacts with p53 and modulates its transcriptional activity. *J Biol Chem* 280 (32):29186-93.

Murzik, U., P. Hemmerich, S. Weidtkamp-Peters, T. Ulbricht, W. Bussen, J. Hentschel, F. von Eggeling, and C. Melle. 2008. Rad54B targeting to DNA double-strand break repair sites requires complex formation with S100A11. *Mol Biol Cell* 19 (7):2926-35.

Nakamura, K., S. Yamagishi, H. Adachi, T. Matsui, Y. Kurita-Nakamura, M. Takeuchi, H. Inoue, and T. Imaizumi. 2008. Serum levels of soluble form of receptor for advanced glycation end products (sRAGE) are positively associated with circulating AGEs and soluble form of VCAM-1 in patients with type 2 diabetes. *Microvasc Res* 76 (1):52-6.

Nedjadi, T., N. Kitteringham, F. Campbell, R. E. Jenkins, B. K. Park, P. Navarro, F. Ashcroft, A. Tepikin, J. P. Neoptolemos, and E. Costello. 2009. S100A6 binds to annexin 2 in pancreatic cancer cells and promotes pancreatic cancer cell motility. *Br J Cancer* 101 (7):1145-54.

Neeper, M., A. M. Schmidt, J. Brett, S. D. Yan, F. Wang, Y. C. Pan, K. Elliston, D. Stern, and A. Shaw. 1992. Cloning and expression of a cell surface receptor for advanced glycosylation end products of proteins. *J Biol Chem* 267 (21):14998-5004.

Nozaki, I., T. Watanabe, M. Kawaguchi, H. Akatsu, K. Tsuneyama, Y. Yamamoto, K. Ohe, H. Yonekura, M. Yamada, and H. Yamamoto. 2007. Reduced expression of endogenous secretory receptor for advanced glycation endproducts in hippocampal neurons of Alzheimer's disease brains. *Arch Histol Cytol* 70 (5):279-90.

Ohe, K., T. Watanabe, S. Harada, S. Munesue, Y. Yamamoto, H. Yonekura, and H. Yamamoto. 2010. Regulation of alternative splicing of the receptor for advanced glycation endproducts (RAGE) through G-rich cis-elements and heterogenous nuclear ribonucleoprotein H. *J Biochem* 147 (5):651-9.

Ohuchida, K., K. Mizumoto, S. Ohhashi, H. Yamaguchi, H. Konomi, E. Nagai, K. Yamaguchi, M. Tsuneyoshi, and M. Tanaka. 2006. S100A11, a putative tumor suppressor gene, is overexpressed in pancreatic carcinogenesis. *Clin Cancer Res* 12 (18):5417-22.

Ohuchida, K., K. Mizumoto, J. Yu, H. Yamaguchi, H. Konomi, E. Nagai, K. Yamaguchi, M. Tsuneyoshi, and M. Tanaka. 2007. S100A6 is increased in a stepwise manner during pancreatic carcinogenesis: clinical value of expression analysis in 98 pancreatic juice samples. *Cancer Epidemiol Biomarkers Prev* 16 (4):649-54.

Osawa, M., Y. Yamamoto, S. Munesue, N. Murakami, S. Sakurai, T. Watanabe, H. Yonekura, Y. Uchigata, Y. Iwamoto, and H. Yamamoto. 2007. De-N-glycosylation or G82S mutation of RAGE sensitizes its interaction with advanced glycation endproducts. *Biochim Biophys Acta* 1770 (10):1468-74.

Ostendorp, T., J. Diez, C. W. Heizmann, and G. Fritz. 2010. The crystal structures of human S100B in the zinc- and calcium-loaded state at three pH values reveal zinc ligand swapping. *Biochim Biophys Acta*. in press

Ostendorp, T., E. Leclerc, A. Galichet, M. Koch, N. Demling, B. Weigle, C. W. Heizmann, P. M. Kroneck, and G. Fritz. 2007. Structural and functional insights into RAGE activation by multimeric S100B. *Embo J* 26 (16):3868-78.

Otterbein, L. R., J. Kordowska, C. Witte-Hoffmann, C. L. Wang, and R. Dominguez. 2002. Crystal structures of S100A6 in the Ca(2+)-free and Ca(2+)-bound states: the calcium sensor mechanism of S100 proteins revealed at atomic resolution. *Structure* 10 (4):557-67.

Perrone, L., G. Peluso, and M. A. Melone. 2008. RAGE recycles at the plasma membrane in S100B secretory vesicles and promotes Schwann cells morphological changes. *J Cell Physiol* 217 (1):60-71.

Petersson, S., E. Shubbar, L. Enerback, and C. Enerback. 2009. Expression patterns of S100 proteins in melanocytes and melanocytic lesions. *Melanoma Res* 19 (4):215-25.

Queisser, M. A., F. M. Kouri, M. Konigshoff, M. Wygrecka, U. Schubert, O. Eickelberg, and K. T. Preissner. 2008. Loss of RAGE in pulmonary fibrosis: molecular relations to functional changes in pulmonary cell types. *Am J Respir Cell Mol Biol* 39 (3):337-45.

Ramsgaard, L., J. M. Englert, J. Tobolewski, L. Tomai, C. L. Fattman, A. S. Leme, A. M. Kaynar, S. D. Shapiro, J. J. Enghild, and T. D. Oury. 2010. The role of the receptor for advanced glycation end-products in a murine model of silicosis. *PLoS One* 5 (3):e9604.

Raucci, A., S. Cugusi, A. Antonelli, S. M. Barabino, L. Monti, A. Bierhaus, K. Reiss, P. Saftig, and M. E. Bianchi. 2008. A soluble form of the receptor for advanced glycation endproducts (RAGE) is produced by proteolytic cleavage of the membrane-bound form by the sheddase a disintegrin and metalloprotease 10 (ADAM10). *Faseb J* 22 (10):3716-27.

Rauvala, H., and A. Rouhiainen. 2010. Physiological and pathophysiological outcomes of the interactions of HMGB1 with cell surface receptors. *Biochim Biophys Acta* 1799 (1-2):164-70.

Rehman, I., A. R. Azzouzi, S. S. Cross, J. C. Deloulme, J. W. Catto, N. Wylde, S. Larre, J. Champigneuille, and F. C. Hamdy. 2004. Dysregulated expression of S100A11 (calgizzarin) in prostate cancer and precursor lesions. *Hum Pathol* 35 (11):1385-91.

Ribe, A., and N. S. McNutt. 2003. S100A6 protein expression is different in Spitz nevi and melanomas. *Mod Pathol* 16 (5):505-11.

2003. S100A protein expression in the distinction between lentigo maligna and pigmented actinic keratosis. *Am J Dermatopathol* 25 (2):93-9.

Rintala-Dempsey, A. C., L. Santamaria-Kisiel, Y. Liao, G. Lajoie, and G. S. Shaw. 2006. Insights into S100 target specificity examined by a new interaction between S100A11 and annexin A2. *Biochemistry* 45 (49):14695-705.

Robinson, M. J., P. Tessier, R. Poulsom, and N. Hogg. 2002. The S100 family heterodimer, MRP-8/14, binds with high affinity to heparin and heparan sulfate glycosaminoglycans on endothelial cells. *J Biol Chem* 277 (5):3658-65.

Rong, L. L., W. Trojaborg, W. Qu, K. Kostov, S. D. Yan, C. Gooch, M. Szabolcs, A. P. Hays, and A. M. Schmidt. 2004. Antagonism of RAGE suppresses peripheral nerve regeneration. *Faseb J* 18 (15):1812-7.

Rong, L. L., S. F. Yan, T. Wendt, D. Hans, S. Pachydaki, L. G. Bucciarelli, A. Adebayo, W. Qu, Y. Lu, K. Kostov, E. Lalla, S. D. Yan, C. Gooch, M. Szabolcs, W. Trojaborg, A. P. Hays, and A. M. Schmidt. 2004. RAGE modulates peripheral nerve regeneration via recruitment of both inflammatory and axonal outgrowth pathways. *Faseb J* 18 (15):1818-25.

Saha, A., Y. C. Lee, Z. J. Zhang, G. Chandra, S. B. Su, and A. B. Mukherjee. 2010. Lack of an Endogenous Anti-inflammatory Protein in Mice Enhances Colonization of B16F10 Melanoma Cells in the Lungs. *Journal of Biological Chemistry* 285 (14):10822-10831.

Sakaguchi, M., H. Sonegawa, H. Murata, M. Kitazoe, J. Futami, K. Kataoka, H. Yamada, and N. H. Huh. 2008. S100A11, an Dual Mediator for Growth Regulation of Human Keratinocytes. *Mol Biol Cell* 19 (1):78-85.

Sakatani, S., K. Yamada, C. Homma, S. Munesue, Y. Yamamoto, H. Yamamoto, and H. Hirase. 2009. Deletion of RAGE causes hyperactivity and increased sensitivity to auditory stimuli in mice. *PLoS One* 4 (12):e8309.

Sander, C. S., F. Hamm, P. Elsner, and J. J. Thiele. 2003. Oxidative stress in malignant melanoma and non-melanoma skin cancer. *Br J Dermatol* 148 (5):913-22.

Santamaria-Kisiel, L., A. C. Rintala-Dempsey, and G. S. Shaw. 2006. Calcium-dependent and -independent interactions of the S100 protein family. *Biochem J* 396 (2):201-14.

Santilli, F., N. Vazzana, L. G. Bucciarelli, and G. Davi. 2009. Soluble forms of RAGE in human diseases: clinical and therapeutical implications. *Curr Med Chem* 16 (8):940-52.

Sastry, M., R. R. Ketchem, O. Crescenzi, C. Weber, M. J. Lubienski, H. Hidaka, and W. J. Chazin. 1998. The three-dimensional structure of Ca(2+)-bound calcyclin: implications for Ca(2+)-signal transduction by S100 proteins. *Structure* 6 (2):223-31.

Schmidt, A. M., M. Vianna, M. Gerlach, J. Brett, J. Ryan, J. Kao, C. Esposito, H. Hegarty, W. Hurley, M. Clauss, and et al. 1992. Isolation and characterization of two binding proteins for advanced glycosylation end products from bovine lung which are present on the endothelial cell surface. *J Biol Chem* 267 (21):14987-97.

Schmidt, A. M., S. D. Yan, S. F. Yan, and D. M. Stern. 2000. The biology of the receptor for advanced glycation end products and its ligands. *Biochim Biophys Acta* 1498 (2-3):99-111.

2001. The multiligand receptor RAGE as a progression factor amplifying immune and inflammatory responses. *J Clin Invest* 108 (7):949-55.

Semov, A., M. J. Moreno, A. Onichtchenko, A. Abulrob, M. Ball, I. Ekiel, G. Pietrzynski, D. Stanimirovic, and V. Alakhov. 2005. Metastasis-associated protein S100A4 induces angiogenesis through interaction with Annexin II and accelerated plasmin formation. *J Biol Chem* 280 (21):20833-41.

Shimamoto, S., Y. Kubota, H. Tokumitsu, and R. Kobayashi. 2010. S100 proteins regulate the interaction of Hsp90 with Cyclophilin 40 and FKBP52 through their tetratricopeptide repeats. *FEBS Lett* 584 (6):1119-25.

Shrestha, P., Y. Muramatsu, W. Kudeken, M. Mori, Y. Takai, E. C. Ilg, B. W. Schafer, and C. W. Heizmann. 1998. Localization of Ca(2+)-binding S100 proteins in epithelial tumours of the skin. *Virchows Arch* 432 (1):53-9.

Shtivelman, E., and J. M. Bishop. 1993. The human gene AHNAK encodes a large phosphoprotein located primarily in the nucleus. *J Cell Biol* 120 (3):625-30.

Sims, G.P., D.C. Rowe, S.T. Rietdijk, R. Herbst, and A.J. Coyle. 2010. HMGB1 and RAGE in Inflammation and Cancer. *Annual Review of Immunology* 28:367-388.

Skripnikova, E. V., and N. B. Gusev. 1989. Interaction of smooth muscle caldesmon with S-100 protein. *FEBS Lett* 257 (2):380-2.

Slomnicki, L. P., B. Nawrot, and W. Lesniak. 2009. S100A6 binds p53 and affects its activity. *Int J Biochem Cell Biol* 41 (4):784-90.

Smith, S. L., M. Gugger, P. Hoban, D. Ratschiller, S. G. Watson, J. K. Field, D. C. Betticher, and J. Heighway. 2004. S100A2 is strongly expressed in airway basal cells, preneoplastic bronchial lesions and primary non-small cell lung carcinomas. *Br J Cancer* 91 (8):1515-24.

Sousa, M. M., S. D. Yan, D. Stern, and M. J. Saraiva. 2000. Interaction of the receptor for advanced glycation end products (RAGE) with transthyretin triggers nuclear transcription factor kB (NF-kB) activation. *Lab Invest* 80 (7):1101-10.

Sparvero, L. J., D. Asafu-Adjei, R. Kang, D. Tang, N. Amin, J. Im, R. Rutledge, B. Lin, A. A. Amoscato, H. J. Zeh, and M. T. Lotze. 2009. RAGE (Receptor for Advanced Glycation Endproducts), RAGE ligands, and their role in cancer and inflammation. *J Transl Med* 7:17.

Spatz, A., N. Stock, G. Batist, and L. C. van Kempen. 2010. The biology of melanoma prognostic factors. *Discov Med* 10 (50):87-93.

Spiekerkoetter, E., C. Guignabert, V. de Jesus Perez, T. P. Alastalo, J. M. Powers, L. Wang, A. Lawrie, N. Ambartsumian, A. M. Schmidt, M. Berryman, R. H. Ashley, and M. Rabinovitch. 2009. S100A4 and bone morphogenetic protein-2 codependently induce vascular smooth muscle cell migration via phospho-extracellular signal-regulated kinase and chloride intracellular channel 4. *Circ Res* 105 (7):639-47.

Srikrishna, G., J. Nayak, B. Weigle, A. Temme, D. Foell, L. Hazelwood, A. Olsson, N. Volkmann, D. Hanein, and H. H. Freeze. 2010. Carboxylated N-glycans on RAGE promote S100A12 binding and signaling. *J Cell Biochem* 110 (3):645-59.

Strazisar, M., V. Mlakar, and D. Glavac. 2009. The expression of COX-2, hTERT, MDM2, LATS2 and S100A2 in different types of non-small cell lung cancer (NSCLC). *Cell Mol Biol Lett* 14 (3):442-56.

Strazisar, M., T. Rott, and D. Glavac. 2009. Frequent polymorphic variations but rare tumour specific mutations of the S100A2 on 1q21 in non-small cell lung cancer. *Lung Cancer* 63 (3):354-9.

Sturchler, E., A. Galichet, M. Weibel, E. Leclerc, and C. W. Heizmann. 2008. Site-specific blockade of RAGE-Vd prevents amyloid-beta oligomer neurotoxicity. *J Neurosci* 28 (20):5149-58.

Suzuki, F., N. Oridate, A. Homma, Y. Nakamaru, T. Nagahashi, K. Yagi, S. Yamaguchi, Y. Furuta, and S. Fukuda. 2005. S100A2 expression as a predictive marker for late cervical metastasis in stage I and II invasive squamous cell carcinoma of the oral cavity. *Oncol Rep* 14 (6):1493-8.

Takenaga, K., Y. Nakamura, S. Sakiyama, Y. Hasegawa, K. Sato, and H. Endo. 1994. Binding of pEL98 protein, an S100-related calcium-binding protein, to nonmuscle tropomyosin. *J Cell Biol* 124 (5):757-68.

Tan, M., C. W. Heizmann, K. Guan, B. W. Schafer, and Y. Sun. 1999. Transcriptional activation of the human S100A2 promoter by wild-type p53. *FEBS Lett* 445 (2-3):265-8.

Tesarova, P., M. Kalousova, M. Jachymova, O. Mestek, L. Petruzelka, and T. Zima. 2007. Receptor for advanced glycation end products (RAGE)--soluble form (sRAGE) and gene polymorphisms in patients with breast cancer. *Cancer Invest* 25 (8):720-5.

van Dieck, J., M. R. Fernandez-Fernandez, D. B. Veprintsev, and A. R. Fersht. 2009. Modulation of the oligomerization state of p53 by differential binding of proteins of the S100 family to p53 monomers and tetramers. *J Biol Chem* 284 (20):13804-11.

van Dieck, J., D. P. Teufel, A. M. Jaulent, M. R. Fernandez-Fernandez, T. J. Rutherford, A. Wyslouch-Cieszynska, and A. R. Fersht. 2009. Posttranslational modifications affect the interaction of S100 proteins with tumor suppressor p53. *J Mol Biol* 394 (5):922-30.

Van Ginkel, P. R., R. L. Gee, T. M. Walker, D. N. Hu, C. W. Heizmann, and A. S. Polans. 1998. The identification and differential expression of calcium-binding proteins associated with ocular melanoma. *Biochim Biophys Acta* 1448 (2):290-7.

Vimalachandran, D., W. Greenhalf, C. Thompson, J. Luttges, W. Prime, F. Campbell, A. Dodson, R. Watson, T. Crnogorac-Jurcevic, N. Lemoine, J. Neoptolemos, and E. Costello. 2005. High nuclear S100A6 (Calcyclin) is significantly associated with poor survival in pancreatic cancer patients. *Cancer Res* 65 (8):3218-25.

Vogl, T., N. Leukert, K. Barczyk, K. Strupat, and J. Roth. 2006. Biophysical characterization of S100A8 and S100A9 in the absence and presence of bivalent cations. *Biochim Biophys Acta* 1763 (11):1298-306.

Weterman, M. A., G. M. Stoopen, G. N. van Muijen, J. Kuznicki, D. J. Ruiter, and H. P. Bloemers. 1992. Expression of calcyclin in human melanoma cell lines correlates with metastatic behavior in nude mice. *Cancer Res* 52 (5):1291-6.

Weterman, M. A., G. N. van Muijen, H. P. Bloemers, and D. J. Ruiter. 1993. Expression of calcyclin in human melanocytic lesions. *Cancer Res* 53 (24):6061-6.

Wilder, P. T., J. Lin, C. L. Bair, T. H. Charpentier, D. Yang, M. Liriano, K. M. Varney, A. Lee, A. B. Oppenheim, S. Adhya, F. Carrier, and D. J. Weber. 2006. Recognition of the tumor suppressor protein p53 and other protein targets by the calcium-binding protein S100B. *Biochim Biophys Acta* 1763 (11):1284-97.

Wilder, P. T., K. M. Varney, M. B. Weiss, R. K. Gitti, and D. J. Weber. 2005. Solution structure of zinc- and calcium-bound rat S100B as determined by nuclear magnetic resonance spectroscopy. *Biochemistry* 44 (15):5690-702.

Wilton, R., M. A. Yousef, P. Saxena, M. Szpunar, and F. J. Stevens. 2006. Expression and purification of recombinant human receptor for advanced glycation endproducts in Escherichia coli. *Protein Expr Purif* 47 (1):25-35.

Wondrak, G. T., M. K. Jacobson, and E. L. Jacobson. 2006. Antimelanoma activity of apoptogenic carbonyl scavengers. *J Pharmacol Exp Ther* 316 (2):805-14.

Xu, R. H., H. Pelicano, Y. Zhou, J. S. Carew, L. Feng, K. N. Bhalla, M. J. Keating, and P. Huang. 2005. Inhibition of glycolysis in cancer cells: a novel strategy to overcome drug resistance associated with mitochondrial respiratory defect and hypoxia. *Cancer Res* 65 (2):613-21.

Yammani, R. R., C. S. Carlson, A. R. Bresnick, and R. F. Loeser. 2006. Increase in production of matrix metalloproteinase 13 by human articular chondrocytes due to stimulation with S100A4: Role of the receptor for advanced glycation end products. *Arthritis Rheum* 54 (9):2901-11.

Yan, S. D., A. Bierhaus, P. P. Nawroth, and D. M. Stern. 2009. RAGE and Alzheimer's disease: a progression factor for amyloid-beta-induced cellular perturbation? *J Alzheimers Dis* 16 (4):833-43.

Yan, S. D., X. Chen, J. Fu, M. Chen, H. Zhu, A. Roher, T. Slattery, L. Zhao, M. Nagashima, J. Morser, A. Migheli, P. Nawroth, D. Stern, and A. M. Schmidt. 1996. RAGE and amyloid-beta peptide neurotoxicity in Alzheimer's disease. *Nature* 382 (6593):685-91.

Yan, S. F., S. Du Yan, R. Ramasamy, and A. M. Schmidt. 2009. Tempering the wrath of RAGE: An emerging therapeutic strategy against diabetic complications, neurodegeneration, and inflammation. *Ann Med*:1-15.

Yan, S. F., R. Ramasamy, Y. Naka, and A. M. Schmidt. 2003. Glycation, inflammation, and RAGE: a scaffold for the macrovascular complications of diabetes and beyond. *Circ Res* 93 (12):1159-69.

Yan, S. F., R. Ramasamy, and A. M. Schmidt. 2010. Soluble RAGE: therapy and biomarker in unraveling the RAGE axis in chronic disease and aging. *Biochem Pharmacol* 79 (10):1379-86.

Yang, Y. Q., L. J. Zhang, H. Dong, C. L. Jiang, Z. G. Zhu, J. X. Wu, Y. L. Wu, J. S. Han, H. S. Xiao, H. J. Gao, and Q. H. Zhang. 2007. Upregulated expression of S100A6 in human gastric cancer. *J Dig Dis* 8 (4):186-93.

Yonekura, H., Y. Yamamoto, S. Sakurai, R. G. Petrova, M. J. Abedin, H. Li, K. Yasui, M. Takeuchi, Z. Makita, S. Takasawa, H. Okamoto, T. Watanabe, and H. Yamamoto. 2003. Novel splice variants of the receptor for advanced glycation end-products expressed in human vascular endothelial cells and pericytes, and their putative roles in diabetes-induced vascular injury. *Biochem J* 370 (Pt 3):1097-109.

Zhang, L., M. Bukulin, E. Kojro, A. Roth, V. V. Metz, F. Fahrenholz, P. P. Nawroth, A. Bierhaus, and R. Postina. 2008. Receptor for advanced glycation end products is subjected to protein ectodomain shedding by metalloproteinases. *J Biol Chem* 283 (51):35507-16.

Zhang, T., T. L. Woods, and J. T. Elder. 2002. Differential responses of S100A2 to oxidative stress and increased intracellular calcium in normal, immortalized, and malignant human keratinocytes. *J Invest Dermatol* 119 (5):1196-201.

Zimmer, D. B., and L. J. Van Eldik. 1986. Identification of a molecular target for the calcium-modulated protein S100. Fructose-1,6-bisphosphate aldolase. *J Biol Chem* 261 (24):11424-8.

Zimmer, D. B., and D. J. Weber. 2010. The Calcium-Dependent Interaction of S100B with Its Protein Targets. *Cardiovasc Psychiatry Neurol* in press.

17

# Understanding Melanocyte Transformation – A Work in Progress

Janet Wangari-Talbot[1,2], James Goydos[1,3] and Suzie Chen[2]
*[1]Graduate School of Biomedical Sciences at Robert Wood Johnson Medical School, Piscataway, New Jersey;*
*[2]Susan Lehman Cullman Laboratory for Cancer Research, Ernest Mario School of Pharmacy, Rutgers, The State University of New Jersey, Piscataway, NJ*
*[3]Cancer Institute of New Jersey, New Brunswick, New Jersey;*
*United States of America*

## 1. Introduction

Malignant melanoma, the most deadly form of skin cancer poses a substantial clinical burden with ~68,000 Americans diagnosed in 2010 and ~8,700 succumbing to the disease (American Cancer Society. 2010). Melanoma is also the fifth most common cancer in men and the sixth most common cancer in women (American Cancer Society. 2010). The incidence of melanoma has been increasing annually at an alarming rate worldwide. In the United States of America, the incidence of melanoma increased by 270% between 1973 and 2002 (Ries, Wingo et al. 2000). In parallel to the increase in melanoma incidence, the mortality rate increased annually by 1.4% between 1970 and 1990 with a slight decrease of 0.3% between 1990 and 2002 (Ries, Wingo et al. 2000). Despite aggressive research towards finding treatments, the prognosis for patients with late stage melanoma remains poor with median survival rates of 9 months with less than 5% probability of surviving 5 years after a diagnosis with disseminated melanoma (Balch, Sober et al. 2003; Balch, Soong et al. 2004). Treatment of the disease is still mainly defined by primary surgical intervention in patients with localized disease or early regional spread (Markovic, Erickson et al. 2007). Surgical resection is only partially effective in extending disease free survival in patients with regional metastases and therefore adjuvant therapies have been used in an attempt to improve patient outcomes. However, only high-dose therapy is applied either by radio-therapy (Geara and Ang 1996; Ballo, Strom et al. 2002) or with interferon α-2b, a FDA approved regiment, has been shown to increase disease free progression and only by 8 months (Kirkwood, Ibrahim et al. 2001). Adjuvant radio-therapy has been shown to control local disease in selected patients but has not had a significant impact on survival in patient with locally or regionally advanced melanoma (Geara and Ang 1996; Ballo, Strom et al. 2002). In patients who develop distant metastatic disease, systemic therapy with dacarbazine provides a modest 22% response rate but no meaningful increase in overall survival (Bellett, Mastrangelo et al. 1976) while immunotherapy with interleukin 2 (IL-2) has proven toxic and only offers a modest survival advantage (White, Schwartzentruber et al. 1994). The, prompting the need for compounds with greater anti-melanoma activity is obvious and has spurred new research into the genetics and pathogenesis of this disease.

The emergence of targeted molecular therapies has changed our view of melanoma as a homogeneous disease to a heterogeneous one where the genetic and epi-genetic makeup of the tumor(s) dictates the type of therapy to be used. Vemurafenib (PLX4032/RG7204) a small tyrosine kinase inhibitor with a higher affinity for mutant $BRAF^{V600E}$, which is found in over 60% of melanomas (Davies, Bignell et al. 2002), has been shown to promote complete or partial tumor regression with a median progression free survival of 7 months, outstanding results that are but which is marred by high rates of recurrence in responding patients (Bollag, Hirth et al.; Flaherty, Puzanov et al.). Ipilimumab, a monoclonal antibody directed against the cytotoxic T-lymphocyte antigen-4 (CTLA-4) expressed by T regulatory cells (Tregs), key negative regulators of T-cell activation (Korman, Peggs et al. 2006; Peggs, Quezada et al. 2006; O'Day, Hamid et al. 2007 ), has been demonstrated to increase overall survival in patients with advanced melanoma by 2 years (Weber, Thompson et al. 2009). Because constitutively high levels of activated ERK seen in melanomas harboring the BRAFV600E mutation appear to suppress immune responses (Sumimoto, Imabayashi et al. 2006). Future trials are expected to combine Vemurafenib and Ipilimumab to investigate whether increased clinical efficacy can be achieved.

Understanding how normal cells develop into malignant cells by overriding essential mechanisms that control cell proliferation is one of the keys to developing effective therapies. Melanoma occurs as a result of neoplastic transformation of melanocytes and can affect any melanocyte containing tissue including the skin, oral mucosa, nasopharynx, uveal tissues, and the urinary tract (Chang, Karnell et al. 1998). The skin, the site affected by cutaneous melanoma, is the largest organ in the body and serves a protective role from constant exposure to toxins in the environment and through the production of melanin, adds a layer of protection from ultraviolet (UV) rays that can result in DNA damage (Chedekel and Zeise 1988). Early studies in the transformation of cells from a normal state to a transformed state evolved from observations of spontaneous neoplastic transformation *in-vitro* in fibroblasts cultured from normal tissue in rats (Gey 1941) or those treated with carcinogens (Earle 1943). This was followed by observations that infection with the polyomavirus could lead to induction of a variety of tumor types in mice (Stewart, Eddy et al. 1957), hamsters (Eddy, Stewart et al. 1958), rats (Eddy, Stewart et al. 1959) and ferrets (Harris, Chesterman et al. 1961). These animal experiments led to epidemiological and genetic studies in humans that also showed a link between herpes virus type-2 infection and development of uterine and cervical carcinomas (Naib, Nahmias et al. 1969; Rawls, Tompkins et al. 1969). Since these discoveries, many laboratories have developed models of cancer through the manipulation of cells in culture or through genetic manipulation of whole organisms. These models have been extremely useful in deriving information about the interaction between genetics and the environment and their roles in the initiation, progression, and maintenance of transformed states validated by tumorigenic phenotypes.

## 2. Immortalization and transformation

Rodent and human cells have been vital in the study of neoplastic transformation *in-vitro*. However, these cells have diferent growth properties with most rodent cells having the ability to immortalize spontaneously and human cells lacking the ability to grow indefinitely under culture conditions. Furthermore, rodent and human cells have differing transformative abilities with human cells being more resistant to transformation. Rodent cells have been shown to be rendered tumorigenic by the expression of two cooperating oncogenes (Land, Parada et al. 1983; Ruley 1983). This process of oncogene assisted transformation however fails to transform normal human cells (Stevenson and Volsky 1986) due to the activation of replicative senescence, a tumor suppressive mechanism (Hayflick 1961; O'Brien, Stenman et al. 1986). Nevertheless, success in deriving human tumor cells in the laboratory was accomplished with the use of chemicals or physical mutagens to select for rare spontaneously immortalized cells (Kang, Sun et al. 1998), or by the use of an entire viral genome (Flore, Rafii et al. 1998). Further studies have shown that alterations in various signaling pathways are required to convert normal cells to neoplastic transformed cells (Hahn, Counter et al. 1999; Elenbaas, Spirio et al. 2001). Ectopic expression of the telomerase catalytic subunit (hTERT), co-expressed with the oncogenic simian virus 40 (SV40) large-T oncoprotein and an oncogenic allele of *H-Ras* resulted in the derivation of tumorigenic cells from normal human epithelial and fibroblast cells (Hahn, Counter et al. 1999). The ectopic expression of hTERT was necessary to allow these cells to proliferate indefinitely in culture as loss of telomerase activity occurs with continuous passage and has been shown to limit proliferation of human cancer cells (Hahn, Stewart et al. 1999). Immortalization has since been identified as a necessary step in achieving malignant transformation with oncogenes (Lundberg, Randell et al. 2002). Also necessary is the disruption of the p53 and Rb tumor suppressor pathways which have also been shown to be necessary for uncontrolled proliferation *in-vitro* and in a variety of human cancers (Hanahan 2000; Sherr and DePinho 2000; Hahn and Weinberg 2002; Hanahan and Weinberg 2011). Following these steps to achieve cell immortalization, the subsequent expression of an oncoprotein has been found to be sufficient to transform cells, rendering them tumorigenic *in-vivo* (Hahn, Counter et al. 1999).

### 2.1 Melanocyte transformation

Attempts had been made to develop animal models of melanoma that recapitulate the human disease to facilitate in delineating molecular mechanisms that result in malignancy. Commonly, the carcinogen, 7,12-dimethylbenz(a)anthracene (DMBA) was applied to induce melanoma initiation followed by application of TPA (Phorbol myristate acetate), to promote tumor growth in mice (Goerttler and Loehrke 1976), hamsters (Goerttler, Loehrke et al. 1980) and guinea pigs (Pawlowski, Haberman et al. 1980). These tumors were sometimes transplanted to normal hosts during which they developed to malignant melanomas that also metastasized to several organs (Goerttler, Loehrke et al. 1980). These models though successful in generating malignant tumors did not mimic the human disease. The culturing of melanocytes *in-vitro* to facilitate pigmentation studies as well as understanding of melanoma development was hampered by the contamination of the cultures with keratinocytes and fibroblasts and by the lack of knowledge on how to sustain long term melanocyte growth in culture. Eisinger et al. (Eisinger, Flores et al. 1982) described the initial culture conditions required to facilitate the maintenance of normal human melanocytes *in-vitro*. They described the requirement for fetal calf serum, TPA - a phorbol ester that up-regulates protein kinase C, and cholera toxin to prevent the growth of keratinocytes and stimulate the proliferation of pure melanocytes *in-vitro*. Modifications to these original culture conditions and the identification of other mitogens have been invaluable in generating various melanocytic lines. Towards the study of malignant transformation of normal melanocytes, Sato et al generated the first immortalized melanoma cells line, TM10, from C57BL/6J mice in the presence of TPA and cholera toxin. These cells were found to have chromosomal aneuploidy but were nevertheless not tumorigenic (Sato, Ito et al. 1985). Shortly after, Bennett et al (Bennett, Cooper et al. 1987) described the generation of a second spontaneously immortalized mouse cell line, Melan-a. These cells which were generated with TPA but without cholera toxin retained a diploid chromosome number but lacked tumorigenicity in both nude and syngenic mice. These immortal cell lines have nevertheless proven to be acquiescent to transformation with exogenous genes and have been used in the construction of numerous transformed lines.

Spontaneous immortalization of human melanocytes has not been described but immortalized lines have been generated with viral oncogenes such as *H-Ras*, *K-Ras* (Albino, Houghton et al. 1986), and SV40 large T antigen (Jambrosic, Mancianti et al. 1989; Melber, Zhu et al. 1989; Zepter, Haffner et al. 1995). *Ras* immortalized melanocytes exhibited characteristics of transformed cells such as the expression of class II histo-compatibility antigens not expressed by normal melanocytes, ability to grow in soft agar and increased expression of the cell surface ganglioside, GD3, but lacked growth factor independence exhibited by melanoma cells (Albino, Houghton et al. 1986). These *Ras* immortalized cells senesced but eventually, some of them were able to escape and became more transformed by acquiring melanoma specific markers and becoming tumorigenic *in-vivo* (Albino 1992). The SV40 immortalized melanocytes also exhibited markers of transformation such as loss of TPA requirement and expression of melanocytic markers but were otherwise non-tumorigenic (Jambrosic, Mancianti et al. 1989; Melber, Zhu et al. 1989). Generation of tumorigenic mouse lines was also achieved with oncogene assisted immortalization and transformation. Several transgenic mouse lines were generated using a tyrosinase promoter-regulated SV40 large T-viral oncogene with the mice developing ocular and cutaneous melanomas (Bradl, Klein-Szanto et al. 1991; Klein-Szanto, Bradl et al. 1991). These melanomas which were histopathologically similar to human melanomas provided an opportunity to study the etiology and progression of melanoma. These transgenic mouse lines were also invaluable to studies examining the role of epigenetic factors such as UV rays on melanoma formation (Larue, Dougherty et al. 1993). Transgenic cells generated from these mice were exposed to levels of UVB determined to be harmless to normal cells, however, these cells became tumorigenic after exposure to low UVB levels and illustrated the multi-step process involved in malignant transformation. The success of these initial models and the discovery that genetic factors are indispensable in melanoma initiation, progression and metastasis has led to the development of numerous malignant melanoma models. In this review, we will address a subset of melanoma models derived from defects in tumor suppressors, aberrant activation of receptor tyrosine kinases, mitogen activated protein kinases as well as variations and mis-expression of G-protein coupled receptors.

## 3. Tumor suppressors

### 3.1 CDKN2A/p16$^{INK4A}$/ARF

Approximately 8-12% of melanomas are thought to be as a result of familial pre-disposition (Greene 1979; Fountain, Karayiorgou et al. 1992). Deletions and rearrangements in the *p16* gene which is located on human chromosome 9p21 have been identified in dysplastic nevi and in patients with sporadic cutaneous melanoma (Cannon-Albright, Goldgar et al. 1992; Goldstein, Dracopoli et al. 1994). In addition, ~75% of human melanoma cell lines analyzed showed homozygous deletions and mutations in *p16* suggesting that this region likely harbored a melanoma tumor suppressor (Fountain, Karayiorgou et al. 1992). Genetic studies in large melanoma-prone families further demonstrated that loss of heterozygosity or mutations at this locus co-segregated with melanoma susceptibility in familial melanoma kindred (Hussussian, Struewing et al. 1994; Kamb, Shattuck-Eidens et al. 1994). The 9p21 locus is complex in that it encodes two distinct proteins; p16INK4A and p19ARF (Kamb, Shattuck-Eidens et al. 1994; Quelle, Zindy et al. 1995). Exon 1α and 1β of the *CDKN2A* gene are driven by two different promoters which results in two alternate transcripts that share exon 2 and 3. The 1α transcript encodes the p16INK4A protein while the 1β transcript encodes the p19ARF protein (Serrano, Hannon et al. 1993; Quelle, Zindy et al. 1995). P16INK4A controls the RB-regulated G1–S transition by inhibiting CDK4/6–cyclin-D-mediated hyper-phosphorylation of RB. P16INK4A maintains the complex of RB with the E2F transcription factor which results in the recruitment of histone deacetylases that promote and repress genes which regulate G1 arrest (DePinho 1998; Sherr and Roberts 1999). The absence of p16INK4A abolishes the RB-E2F complex formation through the phosphorylation of RB by the cyclin dependent kinases CDK4 and CDK6, which leads to the release of the E2F transcription factor and activation of genes that allow S phase progression (Sherr and Roberts 1999). On the other hand, p19ARF blocks oncogenic transformation and acts as a tumor suppressor by stabilizing and enhancing p53 levels through the blockade of MDM2-mediated p53 ubiquitylation and degradation (Chen, Agrawal et al. 1998; Kamijo, Weber et al. 1998; Pomerantz, Schreiber-Agus et al. 1998; Zhang, Xiong et al. 1998).

In addition to the germline mutations reported in *INK4,* (Hussussian, Struewing et al. 1994; Kamb, Shattuck-Eidens et al. 1994), polymorphisms in the 5′ and 3′ untranslated regions (UTRs) which alter translation or regulate messenger RNA stability of p16*INK4A* and promoter mutations of *p16INK4A* have also been identified in association with 9p21-linked familial melanoma (Liu, Dilworth et al. 1999; Kumar, Smeds et al. 2001). This was recapitulated in mouse studies where the inactivation of *p16Ink4a* showed increased susceptibility to both spontaneous melanoma and carcinogen induced melanoma (Krimpenfort, Quon et al. 2001; Sharpless, Bardeesy et al. 2001). Further, rare mutations in the *CDK4* gene whose activity is controlled by p16INK4A have also been identified in melanoma families (Wolfel, Hauer et al. 1995; Soufir, Avril et al. 1998; Molven, Grimstvedt et al. 2005). In this case, the protein becomes insensitive to p16INK4A inhibition even though these patients have been found to have normal *p16INK4A* suggesting that these two mutations are mutually exclusive. A knock-in mouse model created with this CDK4 mutant, *Cdk4* Arg24Cys (R24C), and lacking somatic inactivation of *p16Inka* or *p19Arf* showed increased melanoma susceptibility after carcinogen exposure (Sotillo, Garcia et al. 2001). Cooperation of *p16INK4A* with other oncogenes has also been reported. The combination of *p16INK4a* deficiency with activated *H-Ras* (Serrano, Hannon et al. 1993; Chin, Pomerantz et al. 1997), *N-Ras* (Ackermann, Frutschi et al. 2005) and *K-Ras* (Monahan, Rozenberg et al. 2010) in mouse models have been shown to promote highly penetrant melanomas with short latency.

Inactivation of the tumor suppressor p53 whose stability is controlled by ARF is common in many tumors (Greenblatt, Bennett et al. 1994). In melanoma, the pathological role of *p53* is highly controversial as primary and metastatic melanoma have been found to have low incidences of *p53* point mutations or allelic loss of *p53* (Yang, Merlino et al. 2001). This is in contrast to the role of *p53* inactivation in melanoma development illustrated by Mintz et al., where expression of the SV40 large T antigen inactivates both the RB and p53 pathways leading to highly penetrant and aggressive melanomas (Bradl, Klein-Szanto et al. 1991). The importance of *p53* is also supported by a transgenic mouse model, *Tyr-RAS/Trp53*$^{+/-}$, characterized by the loss of a *p53* allele but with retention of *p19Arf* that also develops melanoma (Bardeesy, Bastian et al. 2001). *p19Arf* deficiency has also been shown to result in melanoma development in a mouse model with *Tyr-RAS+; Ink4a/Arf–/–* and functional *p53* (Chin, Pomerantz et al. 1997). This illustrate a reciprocal role of *p53* inactivation and loss of *Arf* suggesting that they have related functions which have been confirmed with the studies showing that Arf does indeed serve as a regulator of p53 (Sharpless and Chin 2003).

### 3.2 PTEN

The tumor suppressor on chromosome 10, PTEN (phosphatase with tensin homology) acts as a negative regulator of the phosphatidylinositol 3-kinase (PI3K) signalling pathway and has been implicated in a multitude of cancers. Deletion, mutation or inactivation of *PTEN* results in aberrant activation of the PI3K pathway effectors such as Protein Kinase B/AKT which drives cell proliferation and cell survival (Stambolic, Suzuki et al. 1998; Suzuki, de la Pompa et al. 1998). Allelic loss of *PTEN* has been identified in 20% of melanomas while altered expression has been detected in 40% of melanoma tumors while hemizygous deletions and inactivation of PTEN by homozygous deletions or mutations have been noted in 57% - 60% of melanoma cell lines (Pollock, Walker et al. 2002; Goel, Lazar et al. 2006; Li and Ross 2007; Yin and Shen 2008). The relevance of *PTEN* in melanoma has been demonstrated with ectopic expression of *PTEN* in melanoma cells lacking functional PTEN protein resulting in inhibition of Akt phosphorylation, increased apoptosis and decreased cell proliferation (Stewart, Mhashilkar et al. 2002). In addition, siRNA-mediated inhibition in a cell line harboring wild-type *PTEN* led to increased phosphorylation of Akt3 and radial growth reinforcing its involvement in melanoma development and its preferential regulation of Akt3 (Stahl, Sharma et al. 2004). Cells lacking functional PTEN also appear to have an added advantage in sustaining their survival by exhibiting increased Bcl2 expression, resistance to growth factors, altered cell cycle progression, impaired migration and insensitivity to chemotherapeutic agents compared to cells with functional PTEN (Wu, Goel et al. 2003; Stahl, Sharma et al. 2004; Madhunapantula, Sharma et al. 2007). *PTEN* is thought to be lost early in melanoma development as shown by early melanocytic lesions harboring loss of one allele of *PTEN*, or *PTEN* haplo-insufficiency due to the loss of the entire chromosome 10 resulting in increased AKT phosphorylation (Parmiter and Nowell 1988; Bastian, LeBoit et al. 1998; Wu, Goel et al. 2003). In addition, loss of *PTEN* has recently been shown to cooperate with *BRAF*$^{V600E}$, a commonly mutated genetic component of the MAPK pathway found in nevi and in melanoma, in promoting melanoma development (Tsao, Zhang et al. 2000; Dankort, Curley et al. 2009). Here, the phosphorylation of Akt3 was shown to promote a transformed phenotype and anchorage independent growth. It was also postulated that since nevi that contain BRAF$^{V600E}$ rarely developed into melanoma, further oncogenic events are necessary for them to become melanoma. It thus appears that aberrant Akt3 phosphorylation reduces the levels and activities of BRAF$^{V600E}$ which in this case appears to promote rather than inhibit melanomagenesis (Cheung, Sharma et al. 2008). Further interaction of the PI3K pathway and MAPK pathway is also demonstrated by the activation of the p110 catalytic subunit of PI3K through interaction with Ras (Kodaki, Woscholski et al. 1994; Rodriguez-Viciana, Warne et al. 1994). It has been reported that in melanoma and endometrial cancer derived cell lines, RAS and PI3K are mutually exclusive due to functional and genetic redundancy given that the *PTEN* inactivation and *RAS* activating mutations can drive constitutive AKT activation (Ikeda, Yoshinaga et al. 2000; Tsao, Zhang et al. 2000). This was supported by mouse models of DMBA induced tumorigenesis where *Ras* mutations arose in *Pten+/+* mice while *Pten+/–* mice showed a decreased incidence of *Ras* mutations (Mao, To et al. 2004). Furthermore, tumors that lacked

*Ras* mutations also had complete loss of Pten as a result of deletion of the wild-type allele. However, this has recently been contradicted by a study that found that ~14% of human melanomas that had an *N-RAS* mutation also harbored *PTEN* loss (Nogueira, Kim et al. 2010). A subsequent mouse model of *Tyr-HRAS*$^{V21G}$*ink4a/Arf-/-* in a *Pten+/+* or *Pten+/-* background showed that inactivation of one copy of *Pten* led to earlier onset of melanoma whereas mice lacking expression of activated *Ras* in the *Pten+/-Ink4aArf-/-* did not develop melanoma establishing that activation of *Ras* and loss of *Pten* cooperates in a subset of melanomas (Nogueira, Kim et al. 2010).

In agreement with the notion that the lack of *PTEN* leads to aberrant activation of AKT, constitutive expression of AKT has been implicated in melanocyte transformation and poor prognosis in a variety of human cancers (Dai, Martinka et al. 2005). Amplification of *AKT1* and *AKT2* have been reported in stomach, breast, pancreatic and ovarian adeno-carcinoma (Staal 1987; Cheng, Godwin et al. 1992; Bellacosa, de Feo et al. 1995; Cheng, Ruggeri et al. 1996). In melanoma, AKT3 has been found to be activated in 43-60% of sporadic metastatic melanoma cases which has been attributed to increased copy number of the *AKT3* gene as well as loss of *PTEN* (Stahl, Sharma et al. 2004). Additionally, *AKT3* has been shown to cooperate with *BRAF*$^{V600E}$ in promoting a transformed phenotype in melanocytes (Cheung, Sharma et al. 2008; Tran, Gowda et al. 2008). In validating AKT3 as a potential therapeutic target, siRNA mediated down-regulation results in reduced cell survival and inhibition of tumor growth (Stahl, Sharma et al. 2004; Tran, Gowda et al. 2008). AKT2 over-activation has also been identified in melanoma and ovarian cancer (Yuan, Feldman et al. 2003; Nogueira, Kim et al. 2010; Shin, Wall et al. 2010). Examination of primary melanomas, nodal and in-transit metastasis found to express *GRM1*, a metabotropic glutamate receptor implicated in melanoma development, (Pollock, Cohen-Solal et al. 2003) indicated predominant expression of the AKT2 isoform but not AKT3. Furthermore, in an animal model of *Grm1* expression in melanoma, Akt2 but not Akt3 was the isoform of Akt found to be highly activated. In this model, siRNA against Akt2 lead to growth suppression *in-vitro* and *in-vivo* (Shin, Wall et al. 2010). This has been recapitulated with dominant negative inhibition of AKT2 expression in the invasive melanoma cell line, CN44, where invasion was inhibited indicating a pro-invasive role of AKT2 in melanoma (Nogueira, Kim et al. 2010). Regardless of the discrepancies in the activation of various AKT isoforms, one or more isoforms of AKT remain excellent therapeutic targets due to their involvement in mediating melanoma invasion and chemoresistance.

## 4. Receptor tyrosine kinases

Receptor tyrosine kinases (RTKs) are integral components in signal transduction where they mediate normal cell growth, survival, differentiation and oncogenesis among other processes (Barnhill, Xiao et al. 1996; Hanahan and Weinberg 2000; Eckstein, Servan et al. 2008; Hunter 2009). RTKs are transmembrane proteins with conserved intracellular catalytic domains and extracellular ligand-binding domains. Following binding of a ligand such as a growth factor or cytokines, the receptor forms dimers or oligomers allowing auto-phosphorylation and substrate phosphorylation on tyrosine residues (Ullrich and Schlessinger 1990; Lemmon and Schlessinger 2010). Signalling cascades requires the recruitment of adaptor proteins and intracellular kinases, which physically bind tyrosine phosphates on the activated RTK via either SRC (sarcoma) homology domains or phosphotyrosine binding (PTB) domains (Ullrich and Schlessinger 1990; Cadena and Gill 1992; Seger, Rodeck et al.

2008). Activation of the RTKs leads to activation of cell specific signaling cascades such as the RAS/RAF/MEK/ERK pathway or the PI3K pathway which are essential in mediating growth, survival and differentiation signals (Hunter 2009). In melanoma, aberrant RTK signaling has been implicated in development and progression due to mutations and overexpression of these receptors.

### 4.1 Epidermal growth factor receptor (EGFR/ ErbB1/HER1)

The epidermal growth factor receptor belongs to the ErbB family of RTKs activated by the EGF family of growth factors. *EGFR* and EGF-like peptides are often over-expressed in human carcinomas and have been shown to induce cell transformation *in-vivo* and *in-vitro* (Normanno, Kim et al. 1995; Salomon, Brandt et al. 1995; Yarden 2001; Normanno, Bianco et al. 2003). Gene amplification of *EGFR* has been described in different tumor types and is usually associated with overexpression of *EGFR* even though overexpression without gene amplification has also been reported (Salomon, Brandt et al. 1995; Normanno, Bianco et al. 2003; Bhargava, Gerald et al. 2005; Suzuki, Dobashi et al. 2005). Expression of *EGFR* in melanoma cells has been shown to be as a result of increased copies of chromosome 7 and is associated with late stage melanoma (Koprowski, Herlyn et al. 1985; Bastian, LeBoit et al. 1998). In metastatic melanoma, the incidence of the overexpression of EGFR or its ligand, EGF has been reported in about 90% of melanoma cases making it a likely therapeutic target (de Wit, Moretti et al. 1992; Mattei, Colombo et al. 1994; Salomon, Brandt et al. 1995). Gefitinib and Erlotinib are two orally available specific small molecule inhibitors of the *EGFR* kinase approved for the treatment of non-small-cell-lung carcinoma that compete with ATP for binding to the intracellular catalytic domain of the receptor kinase, thereby inhibiting autophosphorylation of the receptor which is critical for binding to downstream signaling proteins (Moyer, Barbacci et al. 1997; Arora and Scholar 2005; Hirsch and Bunn 2005). The efficacies of these inhibitors seem to be dependent on increased *EGFR* copy number and/or increased *EGFR* mRNA expression levels (Cappuzzo, Varella-Garcia et al. 2005). Patients with an amplified *EGFR* gene and/or elevated *EGFR* mRNA expression have higher response rates and improved survival than those with low *EGFR* copy number and/or mRNA expression level upon treatment with the Gefitinib (Hirsch, Varella-Garcia et al. 2005; Dziadziuszko, Witta et al. 2006). *In-vivo,* melanoma cells treated with Erlotinib exhibited decreased invasiveness, increased apoptosis and a decrease in phosphorylated ERK and AKT (Schicher, Paulitschke et al. 2009). Clinical results of Erlotinib in melanoma patients have been disappointing with minimal objective responses obtained (Wyman 2006). Combination of Erlotibin with Bevacizumab, an inhibitor of VEGF (vascular endothelial growth factor), a potent contributor to angiogenesis, tumor proliferation, and lymphangiogenesis in malignant melanoma has shown synergistic efficacy *in-vivo* (Schicher, Paulitschke et al. 2009) and is currently being tested clinically. In addition, the combination of Erlotinib with the cytokine interleukin-24 (IL-24) has shown that IL-24 sensitizes melanoma cells to the EGFR inhibitor through modulation of Akt and induction of Apaf-1 dependent apoptosis (Deng, Kwon et al. 2010).

### 4.2 c-MET (Hepatocyte growth factor/ scatter factor receptor)

c-MET is a RTK normally expressed on the surface of melanocytes and epithelial cells and is activated by the cytokine hepatocyte growth factor/scatter factor (HGF-SF) (Bottaro, Rubin et al. 1991). It has been identified as a part of the oncogenic fusion protein TRP-MET with mutations identified in multiple tumor types including renal papillary carcinoma, lung cancer, thyroid cancer, lymphoma and melanoma (Dean, Park et al. 1987; Park, Dean et al. 1987; Natali, Nicotra et al. 1993; Schmidt, Junker et al. 1998; Ma, Jagadeeswaran et al. 2005; Wasenius, Hemmer et al. 2005; Tjin, Groen et al. 2006). In melanoma, c-Met expression was undetectable in benign nevi, detectable in a small fraction of primary melanomas and significantly expressed in metastatic melanoma lesions (Natali, Nicotra et al. 1993). In normal melanocytes, HGF-SF is a potent mitogen and promotes motility and expression of high levels of tyrosinase activity and melanin content (Halaban, Rubin et al. 1993). Stimulation of c-MET in normal melanocytes is via a paracrine loop which is subverted by autocrine signaling in melanoma where it is associated with metastatic progression (Otsuka, Takayama et al. 1998). c-MET expression in metastatic melanoma is associated with gains in copy number of the *c-MET* locus at 7q33 and not due to focal *MET* amplifications or activating *MET* point mutations which have been observed in other cancers but not in melanoma (Wiltshire, Duray et al. 1995; Bastian, LeBoit et al. 1998; Schmidt, Junker et al. 1998; Smolen, Muir et al. 2006). Additionally, c-Met activation and HGF autocrine signaling have been shown to cooperate with other factors such as UVB exposure (Noonan, Dudek et al. 2003) and *Ink4a/Arf* deficiency (Recio, Noonan et al. 2002) in promoting melanoma progression. Given the role of c-MET in melanoma, inhibitors of this RTK might play a role in suppressing metastasis. Several inhibitors of c-MET, PHA-665752 (Christensen, Schreck et al. 2003) and SU11274 (Sattler, Pride et al. 2003) have been shown to have inhibitory activity in *in-vitro* and *in-vivo* assays but lack clinical viability due to poor pharmaceutical properties and oral bioavailability. Nevertheless, further studies on inhibitors of c-Met have recently identified another small molecule inhibitor that is orally bio-available, with which a dose-dependent suppression of c-Met, induction of apoptosis and inhibition of angiogenesis has been reported (Zou, Li et al. 2007)

### 4.3 c-KIT (CD117/K14/stem cell factor receptor)

The *c-Kit* gene encodes a RTK that serves as the receptor for stem cell factor (SCF) ligand and has been identified as a growth factor involved in melanocyte migration and proliferation (Luo, Gao et al. 2003; Wehrle-Haller 2003). Oncogenic mutations and increases in copy number in *c-KIT* have been identified in melanomas, particularly in mucosal and acral melanomas than in cutaneous melanomas (Curtin, Busam et al. 2006; Antonescu, Busam et al. 2007). Contrary to this, other reports have indicated that progressive loss of c-KIT protein expression is associated with progression from benign nevi to primary and metastatic melanoma (Montone, van Belle et al. 1997; Isabel Zhu and Fitzpatrick 2006). Despite these inconsistencies, c-KIT remains of interest given the identification of a recurrent mutation in melanoma (Willmore-Payne, Holden et al. 2005). The L576P mutation has been identified in metastatic melanomas with increased c-KIT expression (Antonescu, Busam et al. 2007). This mutation is also common in gastro-intestinal stromal tumors where it acts as a marker for neoplastic growth (Willmore-Payne, Holden et al. 2005; Willmore-Payne, Layfield et al. 2005). Success in the inhibition of *c-KIT* activating mutations in gastro-intestinal stromal tumors with imatinib (Gleevec) lead to speculation that this might be a successful approach in melanoma (Hodi, Friedlander et al. 2008). Unfortunately, clinical testing has been largely unsuccessful in melanoma patients with imatinib (Alexis, Martinez et al. 2005; Ugurel, Hildenbrand et al. 2005; Wyman, Atkins et al. 2006) or with another c-KIT inhibitor, PKC412 (Millward, House et al. 2006). To enhance response to these inhibitors, effective screening might be necessary given that only a subset of melanoma show c-KIT expression. In examining melanoma samples with increased c-KIT expression, it was also noted that mutations in *KIT*, *BRAF* and *N-RAS* tend to be mutually exclusive (Cohen, Rosenbaum et al. 2004; Curtin, Busam et al. 2006; Beadling, Jacobson-Dunlop et al. 2008). This might have an implication in response to therapy as each genotype may represent a distinct melanoma sub-population.

## 5. Mitogen activated protein kinase (MAPK) pathway

The MAPK pathway is a highly conserved phosphorylation signaling cascade that is involved in various cellular functions, including cell proliferation, differentiation and migration. The kinase activated pathway consists of ubiquitous proline-directed, protein kinases which phosphorylate hydroxyl side chains of serine/threonine and tyrosine residues in their MAP kinase substrates. Mammals have conserved MAPK pathways that are mediated through phosphorylation of the kinases ERK1/2 (Boulton, Nye et al. 1991; Cobb, Robbins et al. 1991), JNK/SAPK (Hibi, Lin et al. 1993) and p38 (Rouse, Cohen et al. 1994). The activation module consists of a receptor that acts in response to stimuli and leads to the activation of three kinases: a MAPK kinase kinase (MAPKKK) that phosphorylates and activates a MAPK kinase (MAPKK), which in turn activates MAPK (Pearson, Robinson et al. 2001). The activation of the classical MAPK pathway with ERK as the terminal kinase is a frequent event in human cancer and is often the result of activating mutations in the oncogenes *BRAF* (7%) (Davies, Bignell et al. 2002) and *RAS* (15-30%) (Bos 1989) in overall cancer cases.

### 5.1 *Ras* oncogenes

Ras proteins are usually associated with the cell membrane and require stimuli to convert to an active conformation by inducing the exchange of GDP with GTP which is facilitated by the recruitment of GDP-GTP exchange factors such as SOS to the cell membrane (Boguski and McCormick 1993; McCormick 1993). The active GTP-bound form of Ras is then unconstrained and can interact with diverse effectors including Raf, phosphatidylinositol 3-kinase (PI3K), Ral-GDS, and other molecules to transmit downstream signals (Boguski and McCormick 1993; McCormick 1993). *N-RAS* is the most common of the RAS isoforms found mutated and activated in human melanoma and in melanocytic nevi. Mutational analysis have shown that ~56% of congenital nevi exhibit *RAS* mutations in comparison to 33% of primary and 26% of metastatic melanoma implying that this activation might be a risk factor in melanoma formation even though they are rare in dysplastic nevi (Albino, Nanus et al. 1989; Jafari, Papp et al. 1995; Demunter, Ahmadian et al. 2001). In line with this, activating *RAS* mutations are associated with sun and UV exposure (van 't Veer, Burgering et al. 1989; Jafari, Papp et al. 1995; van Elsas, Zerp et al. 1996; Papp, Pemsel et al. 1999). Codons 12, 13 and 61 have been identified as the most mutated hot spots in *RAS* mutations (Der, Finkel et al. 1986; Trahey and McCormick 1987; Trahey, Milley et al. 1987). An alteration in these codons reduces intrinsic GTPase activity of the Ras proteins and makes them insensitive to GTPase-activating proteins. N-*RAS* codon 61 mutations are the most common *RAS* alterations in malignant melanoma and appear to be preserved throughout melanoma progression. Interestingly, the presence of an *N-Ras* mutation in patients was found to have no effect on metastasis as primary tumors that were wild-type for *N-RAS* codon 61 were found to lack the mutation in their metastatic tumors (Albino, Nanus et al. 1989; Omholt, Karsberg et al. 2002). This lack of activity in enhancing metastasis should however not be ignored as Ras has been shown to cross talk with the PI3K/Akt which promotes cell

survival and suppresses apoptotic responses (Kodaki, Woscholski et al. 1994; Rodriguez-Viciana, Warne et al. 1994).
The activation of *K-RAS* in melanoma appears to be an extremely rare event described in a singular study (Shukla, Hughes et al. 1989). *H-Ras* activation has been reported in a rare population of sporadic melanomas and in Spitz nevi based on amplification of its genomic locus on 11p and oncogenic point mutations (Bastian, LeBoit et al. 2000). Animal models that utilize activated *H-Ras* in *Ink4a*, *Arf* and *p53* null backgrounds support the notion of *H-Ras* being a weak oncogene in human melanomas as these mice develop non-metastatic melanomas (Chin, Pomerantz et al. 1997; Bardeesy, Bastian et al. 2001; Sharpless, Kannan et al. 2003).

### 5.2 BRAF

BRAF is a serine/threonine kinase that is activated by RAS and triggers its down-stream substrate MEK in the MAPK signaling pathway. *BRAF* mutations are prevalent in 7% of human cancers. The highest incidence of *BRAF* mutations is in malignant melanoma (27%-70%), papillary thyroid cancer (36%-53%), colorectal cancer (5%-22%) and serous ovarian cancer (30%) (Davies, Bignell et al. 2002; Kumar, Angelini et al. 2003; Pollock, Harper et al. 2003b; Young, Barker et al. 2005). Over 40 *BRAF* activating mutations have been identified with the $BRAF^{V600E}$ being the most common and accounting for 92% of *BRAF* mutations in melanoma (Davies, Bignell et al. 2002; Kumar, Angelini et al. 2003). This mutation is not found in familial melanomas and occurs as a result of a single-base mis-sense substitution (T to A at nucleotide 1,799) that changes the valine to glutamic acid at codon 600 (V600E) in exon 15 (Davies, Bignell et al. 2002). The insertion of the glutamic acid between Thr 598 and Ser 601 mimics the phosphorylation in the BRAF activation sequence and alters the protein structure to a constitutively activated conformation (Davies, Bignell et al. 2002; Garnett and Marais 2004; Wan, Garnett et al. 2004). This constitutive activation of BRAF has been shown to not only have 500-fold greater basal activity than wild-type BRAF but is also capable of inducing focus formation in NIH3T3 cells and mouse melanocytes, stimulate ERK phosphorylation and promote proliferation and transformation *in-vivo* (Houben, Becker et al. 2004; Ikenoue, Hikiba et al. 2004; Wan, Garnett et al. 2004; Wellbrock, Karasarides et al. 2004). This $BRAF^{V600E}$ mutation has been identified in pre-malignant colon polyps, early stage colorectal cancer (Rajagopalan, Bardelli et al. 2002; Yuen, Davies et al. 2002) and in ~82% of benign nevi implying that it might be involved in the progression from a benign to a cancerous state (Yazdi, Palmedo et al. 2003; Pollock, Harper et al. 2003b). This suggests that *BRAF* mutations might occur early on in cancer initiation but other mutations are required to further drive tumor development. Benign melanocytic nevi with *BRAF* mutations exhibit growth arrest characteristics including the expression of the senescence marker, β-galactosidase, which may support this theory (Michaloglou, Vredeveld et al. 2005). Additionally, normal murine and human melanocytes with enforced expression of $BRAF^{V600E}$ exhibit oncogene induced senescence in the absence of additional cancer driving mechanisms such as loss of *Ink4a* (Gray-Schopfer, Cheong et al. 2006; Dhomen, Reis-Filho et al. 2009). Furthermore, the generation of nevi in normal mouse and human melanocytes is in contrast to observations in immortalized melanocytes transformed with activating mutations in NRAS or PI3K which were found to result in the development of invasive melanomas (Chudnovsky, Adams et al. 2005). This was also recapitulated in a zebra fish model of melanoma development where BRAF activation was shown to result in the development of benign nevi, with melanoma progression requiring additional loss of p53

(Patton, Widlund et al. 2005). Some $BRAF^{V600E}$ cells are however able to escape senescence and develop into melanoma (Dhomen, Reis-Filho et al. 2009) which might explain the high percentage of this mutation in sporadic melanoma. Even though a lot of studies show that *$BRAF^{V600E}$* results in senescence and the formation of benign nevi, others have successfully shown that it can serve as an oncogene in transforming immortalized melanocytes (Wellbrock, Ogilvie et al. 2004; Dhomen, Reis-Filho et al. 2009). Importantly, they showed that low levels of *$BRAF^{V600E}$* were sufficient to drive transformation and result in melanomas while high levels of $BRAFV^{600E}$ resulted in higher levels of ERK that were intolerable to the cells (Dhomen, Reis-Filho et al. 2009).

Therapeutically, small kinase inhibitors have been developed to target $BRAF^{V600E}$ activation. A multi-kinase inhibitor, Sorafenib (Nexavar, Bay 43-9006) was produced as a specific inhibitor of CRAF but was found to have inhibitory activity towards BRAF (Lyons, Wilhelm et al. 2001; Wilhelm, Carter et al. 2004). Sorafenib was shown to potently inhibit not only the wild type and oncogenic BRAF signaling through the MAPK pathway, but also other kinases including the pro-angiogenic vascular endothelial growth factor receptors (VEGFRs) 1/2/3, platelet derived growth factor receptors β (PDGFR-β), fibroblast growth factor receptor 1 (FGFR-1) and other tumorigenic RTKs including c-kit, Flt-3 and RET (Wilhelm, Carter et al. 2004; Carlomagno, Anaganti et al. 2006; Chang, Adnane et al. 2007). These pro-angiogenic and tumorigenic RTKs can mediate signaling through RAF/MEK/ERK to induce proliferation and prolong the survival of vascular endothelial cells. Previous reports by others have indicated that Sorafenib induces apoptosis *in-vitro* in human leukemia, hepatocellular carcinoma, melanoma, esophageal carcinoma and a variety of other human tumors and is successfully utilized in the treatment of renal cell carcinoma (Carlomagno, Anaganti et al. 2006; Kane, Farrell et al. 2006; Chang, Adnane et al. 2007). In melanoma, single agent Sorafenib trials have had disappointing clinical outcomes and it is thus recommended in combination with other chemotherapeutic regiments that include carboplatin, paclitaxel and temozolomide (Eisen, Ahmad et al. 2006; McDermott, Sosman et al. 2008; Amaravadi, Schuchter et al. 2009; Augustine, Toshimitsu et al. ; Ott, Hamilton et al. 2010). Recently, PLX4720/PLX4032/RG7204 has been described as a specific inhibitor of *$BRAF^{V600E}$* with low affinity for other kinases and potent cytotoxicity *in-vitro* and *in-vivo* against melanoma cells bearing this particular mutation (Tsai, Lee et al. 2008; Yang, Higgins et al. 2010). A phase I clinical trial reported a response rate of 81% among patients with the *$BRAF^{V600E}$* mutation with significant shrinkage of liver, bowel and bone metastasis marked by a median progression free-survival of 7 months (Flaherty, Puzanov et al. 2010). One of the more serious side effects was the development of squamous-cell carcinoma in 32% of these patients warranting careful dermatological monitoring of patients during PLX4032 treatment (Bollag, Hirth et al. 2010; Flaherty, Puzanov et al. 2010). A phase II clinical trial showed a response rate of 52% with patients developing resistance to the drug after 2-19 months of treatment (Bollag, Hirth et al. 2010). Different paths to resistance after PLX4032 treatment has been attributed to acquisition of *N-RAS* mutations or up-regulation of PDGF-β (Nazarian, Shi et al. 2010), COT/MAP3K8 (Mitogen-activated protein kinase kinase kinase 8) expression which reactivates the MAPK pathway, (Johannessen, Boehm et al. 2010) enhanced IGF-1R (insulin like growth factor 1 receptor) signaling (Villanueva, Vultur et al. 2010) and activation of AKT (Shao and Aplin 2010). In addition to the ongoing studies with PLX4032, other BRAF inhibitors such as GDC0879 (Hoeflich, Herter et al. 2009; Wong, Belvin et al. 2009) and GSK'436 (King, Patrick et al. 2006) are currently being tested to determine their efficacy in melanoma treatment.

## 6. G-protein-coupled receptors (GPCRs)

G-protein coupled receptors (GPCRs) feature seven transmembrane spanning domains and are responsive to numerous stimuli such as odors, amino acids, peptides or large glycoproteins (Pin, Kniazeff et al. 2004). GPCRs transduce extracellular signals and mediate intracellular responses that govern cell proliferation, differentiation and apoptosis via activation of heterotrimeric G-proteins (Gutkind 1998; Rozengurt 1998; Marinissen and Gutkind 2001). Ligand binding on the receptor induces a conformation change from an inactive to an active state leading to G-protein activation (Marinissen and Gutkind 2001; Pin, Kniazeff et al. 2004). Active GPCRs stimulate GDP-GTP exchange on G-proteins inducing the dissociation of the α-GTP and βγ subunits, which regulate the activity of various effector proteins such as adenylyl cyclase, phospholipase C, ion channels, and voltage-gated calcium channels (Marinissen and Gutkind 2001; Goudet, Magnaghi et al. 2009). GPCRs have been known to have oncogenic properties since Young et al., cloned and sequenced a potential oncogene, *Mas*, harboring seven hydrophobic transmembrane domains and hydrophilic amino and carboxy terminus (Young, Waitches et al. 1986). *Mas*, was found capable of transforming murine NIH 3T3 fibroblasts with weak foci forming ability *in-vitro* and tumorigenicity in nude mice. The lack of mutations in this oncogene was the first instance documented of a normal GPCR being tumorigenic as a result of its ectopic expression. Other oncogenic GPCRs have since been recognized in gliomas, gastric carcinoma, melanoma and other human cancers (Cuttitta, Carney et al. 1985; Julius, Livelli et al. 1989; Pollock, Cohen-Solal et al. 2003; Mazzuco, Chabre et al. 2006). Melanocortin-1 receptor and metabotropic glutamate receptor 1 are some of the GPCRs implicated in melanoma development (Healy, Jordan et al. 2001; Pollock, Cohen-Solal et al. 2003).

### 6.1 Melanocortin-1 receptor (MC1R)

The melanocortin-1 receptor (*MC1R*) is expressed on epidermal melanocytes and is the receptor for α-melanocyte stimulating hormone (α-MSH). *MC1R* contributes to pigmentation by regulating the relative concentrations of eumelanin (brown/black pigment) and pheomelanin (red/yellow pigment) (Valverde, Healy et al. 1995; Barsh 1996). The binding of the ligand to the receptor stimulates cAMP production which stimulates the production of eumelanin. *MC1R* is highly polymorphic in human populations and its allelic variations are the principle determinant of pigment phenotypes and skin phototypes in humans (Valverde, Healy et al. 1995; Schioth, Phillips et al. 1999; Sturm, Duffy et al. 2003). Variants of *MC1R* have been identified in patients with sporadic melanoma due to their association with red hair, fair skin freckles and low tanning ability (Valverde, Healy et al. 1995; Smith, Healy et al. 1998; Raimondi, Sera et al. 2008; Williams, Olsen et al.). Three common variants of MC1R; R151C, R160W, and D294H contribute to the red hair phenotype and are highly associated with melanoma (Smith, Healy et al. 1998; Bastiaens, ter Huurne et al. 2001; Box, Duffy et al. 2001). The presence of these variants is thought to contribute to melanoma by impairing the ability of the epidermis to repair DNA damage after sun exposure in fair skinned and red-haired individuals (Healy, Jordan et al. 2001). This theory is however disputed as dark skinned individuals with MC1R variants also have an increased incidence of melanoma (Palmer, Duffy et al. 2000; Kennedy, ter Huurne et al. 2001). In addition, the presence of MC1R variant is thought to double the risk for melanoma in melanoma prone families with *CDKN2A* mutations (Box, Duffy et al. 2001; Chaudru, Laud et al. 2005; Fargnoli, Gandini et al. 2010). Moreover, the presence of MC1R variants in

*CDKN2A* mutation carriers is also associated with the development of multiple primary melanomas (van der Velden, Sandkuijl et al. 2001; Goldstein, Landi et al. 2005).

### 6.2 Metabotropic glutamate receptor 1 (GRM1/mGlu$_1$/mGluR1)

Excessive glutamate signaling has been shown to underlie many neurological diseases including epilepsy, spasticity, stroke, traumatic brain injury and Amyotrophic Lateral Sclerosis (ALS) (Lee, Zipfel et al. 1999; McNamara 1999). Aberrant glutamate signaling also plays roles in patho-physiological diseases such as chronic pain, depression and anxiety (Swanson, Bures et al. 2005). Recently, glutamate signaling has been shown to be involved in various neoplasms including gliomas, colon cancer, breast carcinomas and melanoma (Albasanz, Ros et al. 1997; Pollock, Cohen-Solal et al. 2003; Chang, Yoo et al. 2005). Metabotropic glutamate receptors transduce glutamate induced signaling through the activation of heterotrimeric G-proteins. These receptors are primarily localized in the central nervous system where they are involved in synaptic transmission and less prominently in somatic tissues where they regulate proliferation, migration and differentiation (Skerry and Genever 2001; Hinoi, Takarada et al. 2004; Hinoi, Takarada et al. 2004; Shin, Martino et al. 2008b). Of the 8 metabotropic glutamate receptors identified (Houamed, Kuijper et al. 1991; Masu, Tanabe et al. 1991; Conn and Pin 1997; Goudet, Magnaghi et al. 2009), metabotropic glutamate receptor 1 is the only one involved in melanoma development (Pollock, Cohen-Solal et al. 2003; Marin, Namkoong et al. 2005; Marin, Namkoong et al. 2006). This discovery was prompted by results of a transgenic mouse study utilizing a 2 KB fragment of genomic DNA (Clone B) (Chen, Tiecher et al. 1989; Colon-Teicher, Wise et al. 1993), that had been shown to commit fibroblasts to undergo adipocyte differentiation upon introduction. Of the 5 transgenic founders with the Clone B transgene and in which an expected obese phenotype was never observed, one of the founder mice (TG3) developed raised lesions on the eyes, snout, tail and peri-anal region at 8 months (Zhu, Reuhl et al. 1998). Subsequent progeny of TG3 developed similar lesions with 100% penetrance. These melanocytic lesions increased in size and number and were also invasive as illustrated by their detection in the lymph nodes, brain, muscles, lungs, choroid plexus and inner ears. These lesions were verified conclusively by histopathology as melanoma with a high degree of similarity to human melanoma. The transgene was found to be localized on a region of mouse chromosome 10 orthologous to human chromosomal band 6q23-24 (Pollock, Cohen-Solal et al. 2003). Seven to eight transgene insertions were integrated in intron 3 of the gene that encodes metabotropic glutamate receptor 1, *Grm1,* with concomitant deletion of 70 Kb of host intronic sequences. The expression of *Grm1* was confirmed in the tumors derived from the raised melanocytic lesions in the pinnae, tails and skin of TG3 mice relative to normal controls. This ectopic expression of *Grm1* in melanocytes was theorized to be the cause of the observed phenotype. Elucidation of the etiological role of aberrant *Grm1* expression in melanocytes was deduced from the targeted expression of *Grm1* in melanocytes under the regulation of melanocyte specific promoter dopachrome tautomerase (*Dct*) (Pollock, Cohen-Solal et al. 2003). Transgenic mice generated with the *Dct-Grm1* transgene, TG (*Grm1*) EPv, developed pigmented lesions on the pinnae and tail at 5-7 months which were histologically similar to those from TG3 mice and were transmitted with 100% penetrance to their offspring. This was conclusive evidence that the ectopic expression of *Grm1* in mouse melanocytes was sufficient to induce spontaneous melanoma *in-vivo.* Recently, another group generated a *Grm1* inducible model of melanoma that exhibits a similar phenotype upon expression of *Grm1* in adult mice (Ohtani, Harada et al. 2008). They showed in their model that mice with persistent *Grm1* expression in melanocytes, harbored significant tumor burden compared to those with suppressed transgene expression indicating that *Grm1* is not only necessary for the initiation of melanoma but also for their continued progression. This is also in agreement with results that show that *Grm1* is capable of transforming immortalized mouse melanocytes *in-vitro* and forming robust tumors *in-vivo* (Shin, Namkoong et al. 2008a). Further studies provide compelling evidence that *Grm1* expression can co-operate with other transformation mediators to support tumorigenicity. Akt2 has been shown to be not only a downstream target of Grm1 activation but is also involved in promoting the invasiveness exhibited by the *Grm1* transformed mouse melanocytes (Shin, Wall et al. 2010). In addition, progeny from an inducible *Grm1*-expressing transgenic mouse model crossed with a stem cell factor (*SCF*) transgenic line exhibited increased populations of melanocytes in the epidermis and shorter latency in melanoma development than in the *Grm1*-only transgenic mouse model (Abdel-Daim, Funasaka et al. 2010).

Involvement of human metabotropic glutamate receptor 1 (*GRM1*) in melanoma has also been demonstrated in melanoma biopsies and cell lines. Analyses of these samples showed that 80% of the cell lines and over 60% of the biopsy samples exhibited GRM1 expression at the level of both RNA and protein which was not detected in benign nevi (Pollock, Cohen-Solal et al. 2003; Funusaka, Harada et al. 2006; Namkoong, Shin et al. 2007). This would make GRM1 a potential therapeutic target in human melanoma. Previous reports indicated that glutamate receptor antagonists inhibit cell proliferation (Rzeski, Turski et al. 2001; Stepulak, Sifringer et al. 2005). The competitive GRM1 antagonist LY367385 or the non-competitive GRM1 antagonist Bay 36-7620 were investigated and found to suppress the growth of the GRM1 positive melanoma cells but not of GRM1 negative control cells (Namkoong, Shin et al. 2007). *GRM1* expressing human melanoma cells and *Grm1* transformed mouse melanocytes were observed to release high amounts of glutamate extracellularly which through an autocrine loop is thought to enhance cell proliferation (Namkoong, Shin et al. 2007; Shin, Namkoong et al. 2008a). Riluzole, an FDA approved drug for the treatment of ALS is an inhibitor of glutamate release (Bensimon, Lacomblez et al. 1994; Bryson, Fulton et al. 1996; Lacomblez, Bensimon et al. 2002). We demonstrated that disruption of the autocrine loop by Riluzole through the suppression of the release of glutamate inhibits GRM1 positive melanoma cell proliferation *in-vitro,* tumorigenicity *in-vivo* and induces apoptosis (Namkoong, Shin et al. 2007). In addition, Riluzole was also shown to inhibit the migration and invasion of GRM1 positive melanoma cells (Le, Chan et al. 2010). A phase 0 clinical trial of Riluzole in stage III and IV patients with resectable melanoma showed a 34% response after only 2 weeks of treatment with significant tumor shrinkage in some patients accompanied by suppression of the MAPK and PI3K/AKT pathways (Yip, Le et al. 2009). A recently completed phase II trial showed modest anti-tumor activity with 42% of the patients exhibiting stable disease (Mehnert, Wen et al. 2010). These results suggest that Riluzole might display higher efficacy in combination with other anti-melanoma therapies.

## 7. Conclusion

The future of melanoma treatment lies in the identification of drugable targets. Genetic analyses has generated copious amounts of information that illustrate the importance of "personalized medicine" matching each patient's unique genetic predisposition with the available and developing regimens. Novel finding such as the involvement of GRM1 in melanoma development might be involved in charting novel treatments for the treatment of metastatic melanoma.

## 8. References

Abdel-Daim, M., Y. Funasaka, et al. (2010). "Pharmacogenomics of metabotropic glutamate receptor subtype 1 and in vivo malignant melanoma formation." J Dermatol 37(7): 635-46.

Ackermann, J., M. Frutschi, et al. (2005). "Metastasizing melanoma formation caused by expression of activated N-RasQ61K on an INK4a-deficient background." Cancer Res 65(10): 4005-11.

Albasanz, J. L., M. Ros, et al. (1997). "Characterization of metabotropic glutamate receptors in rat C6 glioma cells." Eur J Pharmacol 326(1): 85-91.

Albino, A. P. (1992). "The role of oncogenes and growth factors in progressive melanoma-genesis." Pigment Cell Res Suppl 2: 199-218.

Albino, A. P., A. N. Houghton, et al. (1986). "Class II histocompatibility antigen expression in human melanocytes transformed by Harvey murine sarcoma virus (Ha-MSV) and Kirsten MSV retroviruses." J Exp Med 164(5): 1710-22.

Albino, A. P., D. M. Nanus, et al. (1989). "Analysis of ras oncogenes in malignant melanoma and precursor lesions: correlation of point mutations with differentiation phenotype." Oncogene 4(11): 1363-74.

Alexis, J. B., A. E. Martinez, et al. (2005). "An immunohistochemical evaluation of c-kit (CD-117) expression in malignant melanoma, and results of imatinib mesylate (Gleevec) therapy in three patients." Melanoma Res 15(4): 283-5.

Amaravadi, R. K., L. M. Schuchter, et al. (2009). "Phase II Trial of Temozolomide and Sorafenib in Advanced Melanoma Patients with or without Brain Metastases." Clin Cancer Res 15(24): 7711-7718.

American Cancer Society. (2010). Cancer facts & figures. Atlanta, American Cancer Society.

Antonescu, C. R., K. J. Busam, et al. (2007). "L576P KIT mutation in anal melanomas correlates with KIT protein expression and is sensitive to specific kinase inhibition." Int J Cancer 121(2): 257-64.

Arora, A. and E. M. Scholar (2005). "Role of tyrosine kinase inhibitors in cancer therapy." J Pharmacol Exp Ther 315(3): 971-9.

Augustine, C. K., H. Toshimitsu, et al. (2010). "Sorafenib, a multikinase inhibitor, enhances the response of melanoma to regional chemotherapy." Mol Cancer Ther 9(7): 2090-101.

Balch, C. M., A. J. Sober, et al. (2003). "The new melanoma staging system." Semin Cutan Med Surg 22(1): 42-54.

Balch, C. M., S. J. Soong, et al. (2004). "An evidence-based staging system for cutaneous melanoma." CA Cancer J Clin 54(3): 131-49; quiz 182-4.

Ballo, M. T., E. A. Strom, et al. (2002). "Adjuvant irradiation for axillary metastases from malignant melanoma." Int J Radiat Oncol Biol Phys 52(4): 964-72.

Bardeesy, N., B. C. Bastian, et al. (2001). "Dual inactivation of RB and p53 pathways in RAS-induced melanomas." Mol Cell Biol 21(6): 2144-53.

Barnhill, R. L., M. Xiao, et al. (1996). "Expression of platelet-derived growth factor (PDGF)-A, PDGF-B and the PDGF-alpha receptor, but not the PDGF-beta receptor, in human malignant melanoma in vivo." Br J Dermatol 135(6): 898-904.

Barsh, G. S. (1996). "The genetics of pigmentation: from fancy genes to complex traits." Trends Genet 12(8): 299-305.
Bastiaens, M., J. ter Huurne, et al. (2001). "The melanocortin-1-receptor gene is the major freckle gene." Hum Mol Genet 10(16): 1701-8.
Bastian, B. C., P. E. LeBoit, et al. (1998). "Chromosomal gains and losses in primary cutaneous melanomas detected by comparative genomic hybridization." Cancer Res 58(10): 2170-5.
Bastian, B. C., P. E. LeBoit, et al. (2000). "Mutations and copy number increase of HRAS in Spitz nevi with distinctive histopathological features." Am J Pathol 157(3): 967-72.
Beadling, C., E. Jacobson-Dunlop, et al. (2008). "KIT gene mutations and copy number in melanoma subtypes." Clin Cancer Res 14(21): 6821-8.
Bellacosa, A., D. de Feo, et al. (1995). "Molecular alterations of the AKT2 oncogene in ovarian and breast carcinomas." Int J Cancer 64(4): 280-5.
Bellett, R. E., M. J. Mastrangelo, et al. (1976). "Randomized prospective trial of DTIC (NSC-45388) alone versus BCNU (NSC-409962) plus vincristine (NSC-67574) in the treatment of metastatic malignant melanoma." Cancer Treat Rep 60(5): 595-600.
Bennett, D. C., P. J. Cooper, et al. (1987). "A line of non-tumorigenic mouse melanocytes, syngeneic with the B16 melanoma and requiring a tumour promoter for growth." Int J Cancer 39(3): 414-8.
Bensimon, G., L. Lacomblez, et al. (1994). "A controlled trial of riluzole in amyotrophic lateral sclerosis. ALS/Riluzole Study Group." N Engl J Med 330(9): 585-91.
Bhargava, R., W. L. Gerald, et al. (2005). "EGFR gene amplification in breast cancer: correlation with epidermal growth factor receptor mRNA and protein expression and HER-2 status and absence of EGFR-activating mutations." Mod Pathol 18(8): 1027-33.
Boguski, M. S. and F. McCormick (1993). "Proteins regulating Ras and its relatives." Nature 366(6456): 643-54.
Bollag, G., P. Hirth, et al. (2010). "Clinical efficacy of a RAF inhibitor needs broad target blockade in BRAF-mutant melanoma." Nature 467(7315): 596-9.
Bos, J. L. (1989). "ras oncogenes in human cancer: a review." Cancer Res 49(17): 4682-9.
Bottaro, D. P., J. S. Rubin, et al. (1991). "Identification of the hepatocyte growth factor receptor as the c-met proto-oncogene product." Science 251(4995): 802-4.
Boulton, T. G., S. H. Nye, et al. (1991). "ERKs: a family of protein-serine/threonine kinases that are activated and tyrosine phosphorylated in response to insulin and NGF." Cell 65(4): 663-75.
Box, N. F., D. L. Duffy, et al. (2001). "MC1R genotype modifies risk of melanoma in families segregating CDKN2A mutations." Am J Hum Genet 69(4): 765-73.
Bradl, M., A. Klein-Szanto, et al. (1991). "Malignant melanoma in transgenic mice." Proc Natl Acad Sci U S A 88(1): 164-8.
Bryson, H. M., B. Fulton, et al. (1996). "Riluzole. A review of its pharmacodynamic and pharmacokinetic properties and therapeutic potential in amyotrophic lateral sclerosis." Drugs 52(4): 549-63.
Cadena, D. L. and G. N. Gill (1992). "Receptor tyrosine kinases." Faseb J 6(6): 2332-7.
Cannon-Albright, L. A., D. E. Goldgar, et al. (1992). "Assignment of a locus for familial melanoma, MLM, to chromosome 9p13-p22." Science 258(5085): 1148-52.
Cappuzzo, F., M. Varella-Garcia, et al. (2005). "Increased HER2 gene copy number is associated with response to gefitinib therapy in epidermal growth factor receptor-positive non-small-cell lung cancer patients." J Clin Oncol 23(22): 5007-18.

Carlomagno, F., S. Anaganti, et al. (2006). "BAY 43-9006 inhibition of oncogenic RET mutants." J Natl Cancer Inst 98(5): 326-34.

Chang, A. E., L. H. Karnell, et al. (1998). "The National Cancer Data Base report on cutaneous and noncutaneous melanoma: a summary of 84,836 cases from the past decade. The American College of Surgeons Commission on Cancer and the American Cancer Society." Cancer 83(8): 1664-78.

Chang, H. J., B. C. Yoo, et al. (2005). "Metabotropic glutamate receptor 4 expression in colorectal carcinoma and its prognostic significance." Clin Cancer Res 11(9): 3288-95.

Chang, Y. S., J. Adnane, et al. (2007). "Sorafenib (BAY 43-9006) inhibits tumor growth and vascularization and induces tumor apoptosis and hypoxia in RCC xenograft models." Cancer Chemother Pharmacol 59(5): 561-74.

Chaudru, V., K. Laud, et al. (2005). "Melanocortin-1 receptor (MC1R) gene variants and dysplastic nevi modify penetrance of CDKN2A mutations in French melanoma-prone pedigrees." Cancer Epidemiol Biomarkers Prev 14(10): 2384-90.

Chedekel, M. R. and L. Zeise (1988). "Sunlight, melanogenesis and radicals in the skin." Lipids 23(6): 587-91.

Chen, L., S. Agrawal, et al. (1998). "Synergistic activation of p53 by inhibition of MDM2 expression and DNA damage." Proc Natl Acad Sci U S A 95(1): 195-200.

Chen, S., L. Tiecher, et al. (1989). "DNA commitment of mouse fibroblasts to adipocyte differentiation by DNA transfection." Science 244: 582-585.

Cheng, J. Q., A. K. Godwin, et al. (1992). "AKT2, a putative oncogene encoding a member of a subfamily of protein-serine/threonine kinases, is amplified in human ovarian carcinomas." Proc Natl Acad Sci U S A 89(19): 9267-71.

Cheng, J. Q., B. Ruggeri, et al. (1996). "Amplification of AKT2 in human pancreatic cells and inhibition of AKT2 expression and tumorigenicity by antisense RNA." Proc Natl Acad Sci U S A 93(8): 3636-41.

Cheung, M., A. Sharma, et al. (2008). "Akt3 and mutant V600E B-Raf cooperate to promote early melanoma development." Cancer Res 68(9): 3429-39.

Chin, L., J. Pomerantz, et al. (1997). "Cooperative effects of INK4a and ras in melanoma susceptibility in vivo." Genes Dev 11(21): 2822-34.

Christensen, J. G., R. Schreck, et al. (2003). "A selective small molecule inhibitor of c-Met kinase inhibits c-Met-dependent phenotypes in vitro and exhibits cytoreductive antitumor activity in vivo." Cancer Res 63(21): 7345-55.

Chudnovsky, Y., A. E. Adams, et al. (2005). "Use of human tissue to assess the oncogenic activity of melanoma-associated mutations." Nat Genet 37(7): 745-9.

Cobb, M. H., D. J. Robbins, et al. (1991). "ERKs, extracellular signal-regulated MAP-2 kinases." Curr Opin Cell Biol 3(6): 1025-32.

Cohen, Y., E. Rosenbaum, et al. (2004). "Exon 15 BRAF mutations are uncommon in melanomas arising in nonsun-exposed sites." Clin Cancer Res 10(10): 3444-7.

Colon-Teicher, L., L. S. Wise, et al. (1993). "Genomic sequences capable of committing mouse and rat fibroblasts to adipogenesis." Nucleic Acids Res. 21: 2223-2228.

Conn, P. J. and J.-P. Pin (1997). "Pharmacology and functions of metabotropic glutamate receptors." Annu. Rev. Pharmacol. Toxicol. 37: 205-237.

Curtin, J. A., K. Busam, et al. (2006). "Somatic activation of KIT in distinct subtypes of melanoma." J Clin Oncol 24(26): 4340-6.

Cuttitta, F., D. N. Carney, et al. (1985). "Bombesin-like peptides can function as autocrine growth factors in human small-cell lung cancer." Nature 316(6031): 823-6.

Dai, D. L., M. Martinka, et al. (2005). "Prognostic significance of activated Akt expression in melanoma: a clinicopathologic study of 292 cases." J Clin Oncol 23(7): 1473-82.

Dankort, D., D. P. Curley, et al. (2009). "Braf(V600E) cooperates with Pten loss to induce metastatic melanoma." Nat Genet 41(5): 544-52.

Davies, H., G. R. Bignell, et al. (2002). "Mutations of the BRAF gene in human cancer." Nature 417(6892): 949-54.

de Wit, P. E., S. Moretti, et al. (1992). "Increasing epidermal growth factor receptor expression in human melanocytic tumor progression." J Invest Dermatol 99(2): 168-73.

Dean, M., M. Park, et al. (1987). "Characterization of the rearranged tpr-met oncogene breakpoint." Mol Cell Biol 7(2): 921-4.

Demunter, A., M. R. Ahmadian, et al. (2001). "A novel N-ras mutation in malignant melanoma is associated with excellent prognosis." Cancer Res 61(12): 4916-22.

Deng, W. G., J. Kwon, et al. (2010). "IL-24 gene transfer sensitizes melanoma cells to erlotinib through modulation of the Apaf-1 and Akt signaling pathways." Melanoma Res.

DePinho, R. A. (1998). "Transcriptional repression. The cancer-chromatin connection." Nature 391(6667): 533, 535-6.

Der, C. J., T. Finkel, et al. (1986). "Biological and biochemical properties of human rasH genes mutated at codon 61." Cell 44(1): 167-76.

Dhomen, N., J. S. Reis-Filho, et al. (2009). "Oncogenic Braf induces melanocyte senescence and melanoma in mice." Cancer Cell 15(4): 294-303.

Dziadziuszko, R., S. E. Witta, et al. (2006). "Epidermal growth factor receptor messenger RNA expression, gene dosage, and gefitinib sensitivity in non-small cell lung cancer." Clin Cancer Res 12(10): 3078-84.

Earle, W. R. (1943). " Production of Malignancy in Vitro. IV. The Mouse Fibroblast Cultures and Changes Seen in the Living Cells." J. Nat. Cancer Inst.,(4): 165-212.

Eckstein, N., K. Servan, et al. (2008). "Epidermal growth factor receptor pathway analysis identifies amphiregulin as a key factor for cisplatin resistance of human breast cancer cells." J Biol Chem 283(2): 739-50.

Eddy, B. E., S. E. Stewart, et al. (1959). "Induction of tumors in rats by tissue-culture preparations of SE polyoma virus." J Natl Cancer Inst 22(1): 161-71.

Eddy, B. E., S. E. Stewart, et al. (1958). "Neoplasms in hamsters induced by mouse tumor agent passed in tissue culture." J Natl Cancer Inst 20(4): 747-61.

Eisen, T., T. Ahmad, et al. (2006). "Sorafenib in advanced melanoma: a Phase II randomised discontinuation trial analysis." Br J Cancer 95(5): 581-6.

Eisinger, J., J. Flores, et al. (1982). "Association of cytosol hemoglobin with the membrane in intact erythrocytes." Proc Natl Acad Sci U S A 79(2): 408-12.

Elenbaas, B., L. Spirio, et al. (2001). "Human breast cancer cells generated by oncogenic transformation of primary mammary epithelial cells." Genes Dev 15(1): 50-65.

Fargnoli, M. C., S. Gandini, et al. (2010). "MC1R variants increase melanoma risk in families with CDKN2A mutations: a meta-analysis." Eur J Cancer 46(8): 1413-20.

Flaherty, K. T., I. Puzanov, et al. (2010). "Inhibition of mutated, activated BRAF in metastatic melanoma." N Engl J Med 363(9): 809-19.

Flore, O., S. Rafii, et al. (1998). "Transformation of primary human endothelial cells by Kaposi's sarcoma-associated herpesvirus." Nature 394(6693): 588-92.

Fountain, J. W., M. Karayiorgou, et al. (1992). "Homozygous deletions within human chromosome band 9p21 in melanoma." Proc Natl Acad Sci U S A 89(21): 10557-61.

Funusaka, Y., T. Harada, et al. (2006). " Expression of metabotropic glutamate receptor 1 and phosphorylated extracellular signal-regulated kinase 1/2 proteins in human melanocytic lesions." Pigm. Cell Res. 19: 256.

Garnett, M. J. and R. Marais (2004). "Guilty as charged: B-RAF is a human oncogene." Cancer Cell 6(4): 313-9.

Geara, F. B. and K. K. Ang (1996). "Radiation therapy for malignant melanoma." Surg Clin North Am 76(6): 1383-98.

Gey, G. O. (1941). "Cytological and Cultural Observations on Transplantable Rat Sarcomata Produced by the Inoculation of Altered Normal Cells Maintained in Continuous Culture." Cancer Research: 787.

Goel, V. K., A. J. Lazar, et al. (2006). "Examination of mutations in BRAF, NRAS, and PTEN in primary cutaneous melanoma." J Invest Dermatol 126(1): 154-60.

Goerttler, K. and H. Loehrke (1976). "Improved tumour yields by means of a TPA-DMBA-TPA variation of the Berenrlum-Mottram experiment on the back skin of NMRI mice. The effect of stationary hyperplasia without inflammation." Exp Pathol (Jena) 12(6): 336-41.

Goerttler, K., H. Loehrke, et al. (1980). "Two-stage tumorigenesis of dermal melanocytes in the back skin of the Syrian golden hamster using systemic initiation with 7,12-dimethylbenz(a)anthracene and topical promotion with 12-O-tetradecanoylphorbol-13-acetate." Cancer Res 40(1): 155-61.

Goldstein, A. M., N. C. Dracopoli, et al. (1994). "Linkage of cutaneous malignant melanoma/dysplastic nevi to chromosome 9p, and evidence for genetic heterogeneity." Am J Hum Genet 54(3): 489-96.

Goldstein, A. M., M. T. Landi, et al. (2005). "Association of MC1R variants and risk of melanoma in melanoma-prone families with CDKN2A mutations." Cancer Epidemiol Biomarkers Prev 14(9): 2208-12.

Goudet, C., V. Magnaghi, et al. (2009). "Metabotropic receptors for glutamate and GABA in pain." Brain Res Rev 60(1): 43-56.

Greenblatt, M. S., W. P. Bennett, et al. (1994). "Mutations in the p53 tumor suppressor gene: clues to cancer etiology and molecular pathogenesis." Cancer Res 54(18): 4855-78.

Greene, M. H. F., J.F (1979). "The hereditary variant of malignant melanoma."

Gutkind, J. S. (1998). "Cell growth control by G protein-coupled receptors: from signal transduction to signal integration." Oncogene 17(11 Reviews): 1331-42.

Hahn, W. C., C. M. Counter, et al. (1999). "Creation of human tumour cells with defined genetic elements." Nature 400(6743): 464-8.

Hahn, W. C., S. A. Stewart, et al. (1999). "Inhibition of telomerase limits the growth of human cancer cells." Nat Med 5(10): 1164-70.

Hahn, W. C. and R. A. Weinberg (2002). "Modelling the molecular circuitry of cancer." Nat Rev Cancer 2(5): 331-41.

Halaban, R., J. S. Rubin, et al. (1993). "met and HGF-SF in normal melanocytes and melanoma cells." EXS 65: 329-39.

Hanahan, D. (2000). "Benefits of bad telomeres." Nature 406(6796): 573-4.

Hanahan, D. and R. A. Weinberg (2000). "The hallmarks of cancer." Cell 100(1): 57-70.

Hanahan, D. and R. A. Weinberg (2011). "Hallmarks of cancer: the next generation." Cell 144(5): 646-74.

Harris, R. J., F. C. Chesterman, et al. (1961). "Induction of tumours in newborn ferrets with Mill Hill polyoma virus." Lancet 1(7181): 788-91.

Hayflick, L. (1961). "The limited in vitro lifetime of human diploid cell strains." Exp. Cell. Res(37): 614-636.

Healy, E., S. A. Jordan, et al. (2001). "Functional variation of MC1R alleles from red-haired individuals." Hum Mol Genet 10(21): 2397-402.

Hibi, M., A. Lin, et al. (1993). "Identification of an oncoprotein- and UV-responsive protein kinase that binds and potentiates the c-Jun activation domain." Genes Dev 7(11): 2135-48.

Hinoi, E., T. Takarada, et al. (2004). "Glutamate signaling in peripheral tissues." Eur J Biochem 271(1): 1-13.

Hinoi, E., T. Takarada, et al. (2004). "Glutamate signaling system in bone." J Pharmacol Sci 94(3): 215-20.

Hirsch, F. R. and P. A. Bunn, Jr. (2005). "Epidermal growth factor receptor inhibitors in lung cancer: smaller or larger molecules, selected or unselected populations?" J Clin Oncol 23(36): 9044-7.

Hirsch, F. R., M. Varella-Garcia, et al. (2005). "Increased epidermal growth factor receptor gene copy number detected by fluorescence in situ hybridization associates with increased sensitivity to gefitinib in patients with bronchioloalveolar carcinoma subtypes: a Southwest Oncology Group Study." J Clin Oncol 23(28): 6838-45.

Hodi, F. S., P. Friedlander, et al. (2008). "Major response to imatinib mesylate in KIT-mutated melanoma." J Clin Oncol 26(12): 2046-51.

Hoeflich, K. P., S. Herter, et al. (2009). "Antitumor efficacy of the novel RAF inhibitor GDC-0879 is predicted by BRAFV600E mutational status and sustained extracellular signal-regulated kinase/mitogen-activated protein kinase pathway suppression." Cancer Res 69(7): 3042-51.

Houamed, K. M., J. L. Kuijper, et al. (1991). "Cloning, expression, and gene structure of a G protein-coupled glutamate receptor from rat brain." Science 252(5010): 1318-21.

Houben, R., J. C. Becker, et al. (2004). "Constitutive activation of the Ras-Raf signaling pathway in metastatic melanoma is associated with poor prognosis." J Carcinog 3(1): 6.

Hunter, T. (2009). "Tyrosine phosphorylation: thirty years and counting." Curr Opin Cell Biol 21(2): 140-6.

Hussussian, C. J., J. P. Struewing, et al. (1994). "Germline p16 mutations in familial melanoma." Nat Genet 8(1): 15-21.

Ikeda, T., K. Yoshinaga, et al. (2000). "Anticorresponding mutations of the KRAS and PTEN genes in human endometrial cancer." Oncol Rep 7(3): 567-70.

Ikenoue, T., Y. Hikiba, et al. (2004). "Different effects of point mutations within the B-Raf glycine-rich loop in colorectal tumors on mitogen-activated protein/extracellular signal-regulated kinase kinase/extracellular signal-regulated kinase and nuclear factor kappaB pathway and cellular transformation." Cancer Res 64(10): 3428-35.

Isabel Zhu, Y. and J. E. Fitzpatrick (2006). "Expression of c-kit (CD117) in Spitz nevus and malignant melanoma." J Cutan Pathol 33(1): 33-7.

Jafari, M., T. Papp, et al. (1995). "Analysis of ras mutations in human melanocytic lesions: activation of the ras gene seems to be associated with the nodular type of human malignant melanoma." J Cancer Res Clin Oncol 121(1): 23-30.

Jambrosic, J., M. L. Mancianti, et al. (1989). "Transformation of normal human melanocytes and non-malignant nevus cells by adenovirus 12-SV40 hybrid virus." Int J Cancer 44(6): 1117-23.

Johannessen, C. M., J. S. Boehm, et al. (2010). "COT drives resistance to RAF inhibition through MAP kinase pathway reactivation." Nature 468(7326): 968-72.

Julius, D., T. J. Livelli, et al. (1989). "Ectopic expression of the serotonin 1c receptor and the triggering of malignant transformation." Science 244(4908): 1057-62.

Kamb, A., D. Shattuck-Eidens, et al. (1994). "Analysis of the p16 gene (CDKN2) as a candidate for the chromosome 9p melanoma susceptibility locus." Nature Genet 8: 22-26.

Kamijo, T., J. D. Weber, et al. (1998). "Functional and physical interactions of the ARF tumor suppressor with p53 and Mdm2." Proc Natl Acad Sci U S A 95(14): 8292-7.

Kane, R. C., A. T. Farrell, et al. (2006). "Sorafenib for the treatment of advanced renal cell carcinoma." Clin Cancer Res 12(24): 7271-8.

Kang, K. S., W. Sun, et al. (1998). "Involvement of tyrosine phosphorylation of p185(c-erbB2/neu) in tumorigenicity induced by X-rays and the neu oncogene in human breast epithelial cells." Mol Carcinog 21(4): 225-33.

Kennedy, C., J. ter Huurne, et al. (2001). "Melanocortin 1 receptor (MC1R) gene variants are associated with an increased risk for cutaneous melanoma which is largely independent of skin type and hair color." J Invest Dermatol 117(2): 294-300.

King, A. J., D. R. Patrick, et al. (2006). "Demonstration of a genetic therapeutic index for tumors expressing oncogenic BRAF by the kinase inhibitor SB-590885." Cancer Res 66(23): 11100-5.

Kirkwood, J. M., J. G. Ibrahim, et al. (2001). "High-dose interferon alfa-2b significantly prolongs relapse-free and overall survival compared with the GM2-KLH/QS-21 vaccine in patients with resected stage IIB-III melanoma: results of intergroup trial E1694/S9512/C509801." J Clin Oncol 19(9): 2370-80.

Klein-Szanto, A., M. Bradl, et al. (1991). "Melanosis and associated tumors in transgenic mice." Proc Natl Acad Sci U S A 88(1): 169-73.

Kodaki, T., R. Woscholski, et al. (1994). "The activation of phosphatidylinositol 3-kinase by Ras." Curr Biol 4(9): 798-806.

Koprowski, H., M. Herlyn, et al. (1985). "Expression of the receptor for epidermal growth factor correlates with increased dosage of chromosome 7 in malignant melanoma." Somat Cell Mol Genet 11(3): 297-302.

Korman, A. J., K. S. Peggs, et al. (2006). "Checkpoint blockade in cancer immunotherapy." Adv Immunol 90: 297-339.

Krimpenfort, P., K. C. Quon, et al. (2001). "Loss of p16Ink4a confers susceptibility to metastatic melanoma in mice." Nature 413(6851): 83-6.

Kumar, R., S. Angelini, et al. (2003). "BRAF mutations in metastatic melanoma: a possible association with clinical outcome." Clin Cancer Res 9(9): 3362-8.

Kumar, R., J. Smeds, et al. (2001). "A single nucleotide polymorphism in the 3'untranslated region of the CDKN2A gene is common in sporadic primary melanomas but mutations in the CDKN2B, CDKN2C, CDK4 and p53 genes are rare." Int J Cancer 95(6): 388-93.

Lacomblez, L., G. Bensimon, et al. (2002). "Long-term safety of riluzole in amyotrophic lateral sclerosis." Amyotrophic Lateral Sclerosis & Other Motor Neuron Disorders 3(1): 23-9.

Land, H., L. F. Parada, et al. (1983). "Tumorigenic conversion of primary embryo fibroblasts requires at least two cooperating oncogenes." Nature 304(5927): 596-602.
Larue, L., N. Dougherty, et al. (1993). "Melanocyte culture lines from Tyr-SV40E trangenic mice: models for the molecular genetic evolution of malignant melanoma." Oncogene 8: 523-531.
Le, M. N., J. L. Chan, et al. (2010). "The glutamate release inhibitor Riluzole decreases migration, invasion, and proliferation of melanoma cells." J Invest Dermatol 130(9): 2240-9.
Lee, J. M., G. J. Zipfel, et al. (1999). "The changing landscape of ischaemic brain injury mechanisms." Nature 399(6738 Suppl): A7-14.
Lemmon, M. A. and J. Schlessinger (2010). "Cell signaling by receptor tyrosine kinases." Cell 141(7): 1117-34.
Li, L. and A. H. Ross (2007). "Why is PTEN an important tumor suppressor?" J Cell Biochem 102(6): 1368-74.
Liu, L., D. Dilworth, et al. (1999). "Mutation of the CDKN2A 5' UTR creates an aberrant initiation codon and predisposes to melanoma." Nat Genet 21(1): 128-32.
Lundberg, A. S., S. H. Randell, et al. (2002). "Immortalization and transformation of primary human airway epithelial cells by gene transfer." Oncogene 21(29): 4577-86.
Luo, R., J. Gao, et al. (2003). "Molecular identification of distinct neurogenic and melanogenic neural crest sublineages." Development 130(2): 321-30.
Lyons, J. F., S. Wilhelm, et al. (2001). "Discovery of a novel Raf kinase inhibitor." Endocr Relat Cancer 8(3): 219-25.
Ma, P. C., R. Jagadeeswaran, et al. (2005). "Functional expression and mutations of c-Met and its therapeutic inhibition with SU11274 and small interfering RNA in non-small cell lung cancer." Cancer Res 65(4): 1479-88.
Madhunapantula, S. V., A. Sharma, et al. (2007). "PRAS40 deregulates apoptosis in malignant melanoma." Cancer Res 67(8): 3626-36.
Mao, J. H., M. D. To, et al. (2004). "Mutually exclusive mutations of the Pten and ras pathways in skin tumor progression." Genes Dev 18(15): 1800-5.
Marin, Y. E., J. Namkoong, et al. (2006). "Stimulation of oncogenic metabotropic glutamate receptor 1 in melanoma cells activates ERK1/2 via PKCepsilon." Cell Signal 18(8): 1279-86.
Marin, Y. E., J. Namkoong, et al. (2005). "Grm5 expression is not required for the oncogenic role of Grm1 in melanocytes." Neuropharmacology 49 Suppl 1: 70-9.
Marinissen, M. J. and J. S. Gutkind (2001). "G-protein-coupled receptors and signaling networks: emerging paradigms." Trends Pharmacol Sci 22(7): 368-76.
Markovic, S. N., L. A. Erickson, et al. (2007). "Malignant melanoma in the 21st century, part 2: staging, prognosis, and treatment." Mayo Clin Proc 82(4): 490-513.
Masu, M., Y. Tanabe, et al. (1991). "Sequence and expression of a metabotropic glutamate receptor." Nature 349(6312): 760-5.
Mattei, S., M. P. Colombo, et al. (1994). "Expression of cytokine/growth factors and their receptors in human melanoma and melanocytes." Int J Cancer 56(6): 853-7.
Mazzuco, T. L., O. Chabre, et al. (2006). "Ectopic expression of the gastric inhibitory polypeptide receptor gene is a sufficient genetic event to induce benign adrenocortical tumor in a xenotransplantation model." Endocrinology 147(2): 782-90.

McCormick, F. (1993). "Signal transduction. How receptors turn Ras on." Nature 363(6424): 15-6.

McDermott, D. F., J. A. Sosman, et al. (2008). "Double-blind randomized phase II study of the combination of sorafenib and dacarbazine in patients with advanced melanoma: a report from the 11715 Study Group." J Clin Oncol 26(13): 2178-85.

McNamara, J. O. (1999). "Emerging insights into the genesis of epilepsy." Nature 399(6738 Suppl): A15-22.

Mehnert, J., Y. Wen, et al. (2010). "A phase II trial of riluzole, an antagonist of metabotropic glutamate receptor (GRM1) signaling, in advanced melanoma." J Clin Oncol 28:15((suppl; abstr TPS309) ).

Melber, K., G. Zhu, et al. (1989). "SV40-transfected human melanocyte sensitivity to growth inhibition by the phorbol ester 12-O-tetradecanoylphorbol-13-acetate." Cancer Res 49(13): 3650-5.

Michaloglou, C., L. C. Vredeveld, et al. (2005). "BRAFE600-associated senescence-like cell cycle arrest of human naevi." Nature 436(7051): 720-4.

Millward, M. J., C. House, et al. (2006). "The multikinase inhibitor midostaurin (PKC412A) lacks activity in metastatic melanoma: a phase IIA clinical and biologic study." Br J Cancer 95(7): 829-34.

Molven, A., M. B. Grimstvedt, et al. (2005). "A large Norwegian family with inherited malignant melanoma, multiple atypical nevi, and CDK4 mutation." Genes Chromosomes Cancer 44(1): 10-8.

Monahan, K. B., G. I. Rozenberg, et al. (2010). "Somatic p16(INK4a) loss accelerates melanomagenesis." Oncogene 29(43): 5809-17.

Montone, K. T., P. van Belle, et al. (1997). "Proto-oncogene c-kit expression in malignant melanoma: protein loss with tumor progression." Mod Pathol 10(9): 939-44.

Moyer, J. D., E. G. Barbacci, et al. (1997). "Induction of apoptosis and cell cycle arrest by CP-358,774, an inhibitor of epidermal growth factor receptor tyrosine kinase." Cancer Res 57(21): 4838-48.

Naib, Z. M., A. J. Nahmias, et al. (1969). "Genital herpetic infection. Association with cervical dysplasia and carcinoma." Cancer 23(4): 940-5.

Namkoong, J., S. S. Shin, et al. (2007). "Metabotropic glutamate receptor 1 and glutamate signaling in human melanoma." Cancer Res 67(5): 2298-305.

Natali, P. G., M. R. Nicotra, et al. (1993). "Expression of the c-Met/HGF receptor in human melanocytic neoplasms: demonstration of the relationship to malignant melanoma tumour progression." Br J Cancer 68(4): 746-50.

Nazarian, R., H. Shi, et al. (2010). "Melanomas acquire resistance to B-RAF(V600E) inhibition by RTK or N-RAS upregulation." Nature 468(7326): 973-7.

Nogueira, C., K. H. Kim, et al. (2010). "Cooperative interactions of PTEN deficiency and RAS activation in melanoma metastasis." Oncogene 29(47): 6222-32.

Noonan, F. P., J. Dudek, et al. (2003). "Animal models of melanoma: an HGF/SF transgenic mouse model may facilitate experimental access to UV initiating events." Pigment Cell Research 16(1): 16-25.

Normanno, N., C. Bianco, et al. (2003). "Target-based agents against ErbB receptors and their ligands: a novel approach to cancer treatment." Endocr Relat Cancer 10(1): 1-21.

Normanno, N., N. Kim, et al. (1995). "Expression of messenger RNA for amphiregulin, heregulin, and cripto-1, three new members of the epidermal growth factor family, in human breast carcinomas." Breast Cancer Res Treat 35(3): 293-7.

O'Brien, W., G. Stenman, et al. (1986). "Suppression of tumor growth by senescence in virally transformed human fibroblasts." Proc Natl Acad Sci U S A 83(22): 8659-63.

O'Day, S. J., O. Hamid, et al. (2007). "Targeting cytotoxic T-lymphocyte antigen-4 (CTLA-4): a novel strategy for the treatment of melanoma and other malignancies." Cancer 110(12): 2614-27.

Ohtani, Y., T. Harada, et al. (2008). "Metabotropic glutamate receptor subtype-1 is essential for in vivo growth of melanoma." Oncogene 27: 7162-7170.

Omholt, K., S. Karsberg, et al. (2002). "Screening of N-ras codon 61 mutations in paired primary and metastatic cutaneous melanomas: mutations occur early and persist throughout tumor progression." Clin Cancer Res 8(11): 3468-74.

Otsuka, T., H. Takayama, et al. (1998). "c-Met autocrine activation induces development of malignant melanoma and acquisition of the metastatic phenotype." Cancer Res 58(22): 5157-67.

Ott, P. A., A. Hamilton, et al. (2010). "A phase II trial of sorafenib in metastatic melanoma with tissue correlates." PLoS One 5(12): e15588.

Palmer, J. S., D. L. Duffy, et al. (2000). "Melanocortin-1 receptor polymorphisms and risk of melanoma: is the association explained solely by pigmentation phenotype?" Am J Hum Genet 66(1): 176-86.

Papp, T., H. Pemsel, et al. (1999). "Mutational analysis of the N-ras, p53, p16INK4a, CDK4, and MC1R genes in human congenital melanocytic naevi." J Med Genet 36(8): 610-4.

Park, M., M. Dean, et al. (1987). "Sequence of MET protooncogene cDNA has features characteristic of the tyrosine kinase family of growth-factor receptors." Proc Natl Acad Sci U S A 84(18): 6379-83.

Parmiter, A. H. and P. C. Nowell (1988). "The cytogenetics of human malignant melanoma and premalignant lesions." Cancer Treat Res 43: 47-61.

Patton, E. E., H. R. Widlund, et al. (2005). "BRAF mutations are sufficient to promote nevi formation and cooperate with p53 in the genesis of melanoma." Curr Biol 15(3): 249-54.

Pawlowski, A., H. F. Haberman, et al. (1980). "Skin melanoma induced by 7,12-dimethylbenzanthracene in albino guinea pigs and its similarities to skin melanoma of humans." Cancer Res 40(10): 3652-60.

Pearson, G., F. Robinson, et al. (2001). "Mitogen-activated protein (MAP) kinase pathways: regulation and physiological functions." Endocr Rev 22(2): 153-83.

Peggs, K. S., S. A. Quezada, et al. (2006). "Principles and use of anti-CTLA4 antibody in human cancer immunotherapy." Curr Opin Immunol 18(2): 206-13.

Pin, J. P., J. Kniazeff, et al. (2004). "The activation mechanism of class-C G-protein coupled receptors." Biol Cell 96(5): 335 42.

Pollock, P., U. Harper, et al. (2003b). "High frequency of BRAF mutations in nevi." Nature Genetics 33: 19-20.

Pollock, P. M., K. Cohen-Solal, et al. (2003). "Melanoma mouse model implicates metabotropic glutamate signaling in melanocytic neoplasia." Nat Genet 34(1): 108-12.

Pollock, P. M., G. J. Walker, et al. (2002). "PTEN inactivation is rare in melanoma tumours but occurs frequently in melanoma cell lines." Melanoma Res 12(6): 565-75.

Pomerantz, J., N. Schreiber-Agus, et al. (1998). "The Ink4a tumor suppressor gene product, p19Arf, interacts with MDM2 and neutralizes MDM2's inhibition of p53." Cell 92(6): 713-23.

Quelle, D. E., F. Zindy, et al. (1995). "Alternative reading frames of the INK4a tumor suppressor gene encode two unrelated proteins capable of inducing cell cycle arrest." Cell 83(6): 993-1000.

Raimondi, S., F. Sera, et al. (2008). "MC1R variants, melanoma and red hair color phenotype: a meta-analysis." Int J Cancer 122(12): 2753-60.

Rajagopalan, H., A. Bardelli, et al. (2002). "Tumorigenesis: RAF/RAS oncogenes and mismatch-repair status." Nature 418(6901): 934.

Rawls, W. E., W. A. Tompkins, et al. (1969). "The association of herpesvirus type 2 and carcinoma of the uterine cervix." Am J Epidemiol 89(5): 547-54.

Recio, J. A., F. P. Noonan, et al. (2002). "Ink4a/arf deficiency promotes ultraviolet radiation-induced melanomagenesis." Cancer Res 62(22): 6724-30.

Ries, L. A., P. A. Wingo, et al. (2000). "The annual report to the nation on the status of cancer, 1973-1997, with a special section on colorectal cancer." Cancer 88(10): 2398-424.

Rodriguez-Viciana, P., P. H. Warne, et al. (1994). "Phosphatidylinositol-3-OH kinase as a direct target of Ras." Nature 370(6490): 527-32.

Rouse, J., P. Cohen, et al. (1994). "A novel kinase cascade triggered by stress and heat shock that stimulates MAPKAP kinase-2 and phosphorylation of the small heat shock proteins." Cell 78(6): 1027-37.

Rozengurt, E. (1998). "Signal transduction pathways in the mitogenic response to G protein-coupled neuropeptide receptor agonists." J Cell Physiol 177(4): 507-17.

Ruley, H. E. (1983). "Adenovirus early region 1A enables viral and cellular transforming genes to transform primary cells in culture." Nature 304(5927): 602-6.

Rzeski, W., L. Turski, et al. (2001). "Glutamate antagonists limit tumor growth." Proc Natl Acad Sci U S A 98(11): 6372-7.

Salomon, D. S., R. Brandt, et al. (1995). "Epidermal growth factor-related peptides and their receptors in human malignancies." Crit Rev Oncol Hematol 19(3): 183-232.

Sato, C., S. Ito, et al. (1985). "Establishment of a mouse melanocyte clone which synthesizes both eumelanin and pheomelanin." Cell Struct Funct 10(4): 421-5.

Sattler, M., Y. B. Pride, et al. (2003). "A novel small molecule met inhibitor induces apoptosis in cells transformed by the oncogenic TPR-MET tyrosine kinase." Cancer Res 63(17): 5462-9.

Schicher, N., V. Paulitschke, et al. (2009). "Erlotinib and bevacizumab have synergistic activity against melanoma." Clin Cancer Res 15(10): 3495-502.

Schioth, H. B., S. R. Phillips, et al. (1999). "Loss of function mutations of the human melanocortin 1 receptor are common and are associated with red hair." Biochem Biophys Res Commun 260(2): 488-91.

Schmidt, L., K. Junker, et al. (1998). "Two North American families with hereditary papillary renal carcinoma and identical novel mutations in the MET proto-oncogene." Cancer Res 58(8): 1719-22.

Seger, R., U. Rodeck, et al. (2008). "Receptor tyrosine kinases: the emerging tip of systems control." IET Syst Biol 2(1): 1-4.

Serrano, M., G. J. Hannon, et al. (1993). "A new regulatory motif in cell-cycle control causing specific inhibition of cyclin D/CDK4." Nature 366(6456): 704-7.

Shao, Y. and A. E. Aplin (2010). "Akt3-mediated resistance to apoptosis in B-RAF-targeted melanoma cells." Cancer Res 70(16): 6670-81.

Sharpless, E. and L. Chin (2003). "The INK4a/ARF locus and melanoma." Oncogene 22(20): 3092-8.

Sharpless, N. E., N. Bardeesy, et al. (2001). "Loss of p16Ink4a with retention of p19Arf predisposes mice to tumorigenesis." Nature 413(6851): 86-91.

Sharpless, N. E., K. Kannan, et al. (2003). "Both products of the mouse Ink4a/Arf locus suppress melanoma formation in vivo." Oncogene 22(32): 5055-9.

Sherr, C. J. and R. A. DePinho (2000). "Cellular senescence: mitotic clock or culture shock?" Cell 102(4): 407-10.

Sherr, C. J. and J. M. Roberts (1999). "CDK inhibitors: positive and negative regulators of G1-phase progression." Genes Dev 13(12): 1501-12.

Shin, S. S., J. J. Martino, et al. (2008b). "Metabotropic glutamate receptors (mGlus) and cellular transformation." Neuropharmacology 55(4): 396-402.

Shin, S. S., J. Namkoong, et al. (2008a). "Oncogenic activities of metabotropic glutamate receptor 1 (Grm1) in melanocyte transformation." Pigment Cell Melanoma Res 21(3): 368-78.

Shin, S. S., B. A. Wall, et al. (2010). "AKT2 is a downstream target of metabotropic glutamate receptor 1 (Grm1)." Pigment Cell Melanoma Res 23(1): 103-11.

Shukla, V. K., D. C. Hughes, et al. (1989). "ras mutations in human melanotic lesions: K-ras activation is a frequent and early event in melanoma development." Oncogene Res 5(2): 121-7.

Skerry, T. M. and P. G. Genever (2001). "Glutamate signalling in non-neuronal tissues." Trends Pharmacol Sci 22(4): 174-81.

Smith, R., E. Healy, et al. (1998). "Melanocortin 1 receptor variants in an Irish population." J Invest Dermatol 111(1): 119-22.

Smolen, G. A., B. Muir, et al. (2006). "Frequent met oncogene amplification in a Brca1/Trp53 mouse model of mammary tumorigenesis." Cancer Res 66(7): 3452-5.

Sotillo, R., J. F. Garcia, et al. (2001). "Invasive melanoma in Cdk4-targeted mice." Proc Natl Acad Sci U S A 98(23): 13312-7.

Soufir, N., M. F. Avril, et al. (1998). "Prevalence of p16 and CDK4 germline mutations in 48 melanoma-prone families in France. The French Familial Melanoma Study Group." Hum Mol Genet 7(2): 209-16.

Staal, S. P. (1987). "Molecular cloning of the akt oncogene and its human homologues AKT1 and AKT2: amplification of AKT1 in a primary human gastric adenocarcinoma." Proc Natl Acad Sci U S A 84(14): 5034-7.

Stahl, J. M., A. Sharma, et al. (2004). "Deregulated Akt3 activity promotes development of malignant melanoma." Cancer Res 64(19): 7002-10.

Stambolic, V., A. Suzuki, et al. (1998). "Negative regulation of PKB/Akt-dependent cell survival by the tumor suppressor PTEN." Cell 95(1): 29-39.

Stepulak, A., M. Sifringer, et al. (2005). "NMDA antagonist inhibits the extracellular signal-regulated kinase pathway and suppresses cancer growth." Proc Natl Acad Sci U S A 102(43): 15605-10.

Stevenson, M. and D. J. Volsky (1986). "Activated v-myc and v-ras oncogenes do not transform normal human lymphocytes." Mol Cell Biol 6(10): 3410-7.

Stewart, A. L., A. M. Mhashilkar, et al. (2002). "PI3 kinase blockade by Ad-PTEN inhibits invasion and induces apoptosis in RGP and metastatic melanoma cells." Mol Med 8(8): 451-61.

Stewart, S. E., B. E. Eddy, et al. (1957). "The induction of neoplasms with a substance released from mouse tumors by tissue culture." Virology 3(2): 380-400.

Sturm, R. A., D. L. Duffy, et al. (2003). "Genetic association and cellular function of MC1R variant alleles in human pigmentation." Ann N Y Acad Sci 994: 348-58.

Sumimoto, H., F. Imabayashi, et al. (2006). "The BRAF-MAPK signaling pathway is essential for cancer-immune evasion in human melanoma cells." J Exp Med 203(7): 1651-6.

Suzuki, A., J. L. de la Pompa, et al. (1998). "High cancer susceptibility and embryonic lethality associated with mutation of the PTEN tumor suppressor gene in mice." Curr Biol 8(21): 1169-78.

Suzuki, S., Y. Dobashi, et al. (2005). "Protein overexpression and gene amplification of epidermal growth factor receptor in nonsmall cell lung carcinomas. An immunohistochemical and fluorescence in situ hybridization study." Cancer 103(6): 1265-73.

Swanson, C. J., M. Bures, et al. (2005). "Metabotropic glutamate receptors as novel targets for anxiety and stress disorders." Nat Rev Drug Discov 4(2): 131-44.

Tjin, E. P., R. W. Groen, et al. (2006). "Functional analysis of HGF/MET signaling and aberrant HGF-activator expression in diffuse large B-cell lymphoma." Blood 107(2): 760-8.

Trahey, M. and F. McCormick (1987). "A cytoplasmic protein stimulates normal N-ras p21 GTPase, but does not affect oncogenic mutants." Science 238(4826): 542-5.

Trahey, M., R. J. Milley, et al. (1987). "Biochemical and biological properties of the human N-ras p21 protein." Mol Cell Biol 7(1): 541-4.

Tran, M. A., R. Gowda, et al. (2008). "Targeting V600EB-Raf and Akt3 using nanoliposomal-small interfering RNA inhibits cutaneous melanocytic lesion development." Cancer Res 68(18): 7638-49.

Tsai, J., J. T. Lee, et al. (2008). "Discovery of a selective inhibitor of oncogenic B-Raf kinase with potent antimelanoma activity." Proc Natl Acad Sci U S A 105(8): 3041-6.

Tsao, H., X. Zhang, et al. (2000). "Relative reciprocity of NRAS and PTEN/MMAC1 alterations in cutaneous melanoma cell lines." Cancer Res 60(7): 1800-4.

Ugurel, S., R. Hildenbrand, et al. (2005). "Lack of clinical efficacy of imatinib in metastatic melanoma." Br J Cancer 92(8): 1398-405.

Ullrich, A. and J. Schlessinger (1990). "Signal transduction by receptors with tyrosine kinase activity." Cell 61(2): 203-12.

Valverde, P., E. Healy, et al. (1995). "Variants of the melanocyte-stimulating hormone receptor gene are associated with red hair and fair skin in humans." Nat Genet 11(3): 328-30.

van 't Veer, L. J., B. M. Burgering, et al. (1989). "N-ras mutations in human cutaneous melanoma from sun-exposed body sites." Mol Cell Biol 9(7): 3114-6.

van der Velden, P. A., L. A. Sandkuijl, et al. (2001). "Melanocortin-1 receptor variant R151C modifies melanoma risk in Dutch families with melanoma." Am J Hum Genet 69(4): 774-9.

van Elsas, A., S. F. Zerp, et al. (1996). "Relevance of ultraviolet-induced N-ras oncogene point mutations in development of primary human cutaneous melanoma." Am J Pathol 149(3): 883-93.

Villanueva, J., A. Vultur, et al. (2010). "Acquired resistance to BRAF inhibitors mediated by a RAF kinase switch in melanoma can be overcome by cotargeting MEK and IGF-1R/PI3K." Cancer Cell 18(6): 683-95.

Wan, P. T., M. J. Garnett, et al. (2004). "Mechanism of activation of the RAF-ERK signaling pathway by oncogenic mutations of B-RAF.[see comment]." Cell 116(6): 855-67.

Wasenius, V. M., S. Hemmer, et al. (2005). "MET receptor tyrosine kinase sequence alterations in differentiated thyroid carcinoma." Am J Surg Pathol 29(4): 544-9.

Weber, J., J. A. Thompson, et al. (2009). "A randomized, double-blind, placebo-controlled, phase II study comparing the tolerability and efficacy of ipilimumab administered with or without prophylactic budesonide in patients with unresectable stage III or IV melanoma." Clin Cancer Res 15(17): 5591-8.

Wehrle-Haller, B. (2003). "The role of Kit-ligand in melanocyte development and epidermal homeostasis." Pigment Cell Res 16(3): 287-96.

Wellbrock, C., M. Karasarides, et al. (2004). "The RAF proteins take centre stage." Nat Rev Mol Cell Biol 5(11): 875-85.

Wellbrock, C., L. Ogilvie, et al. (2004). "V599EB-RAF is an oncogene in melanocytes." Cancer Res 64(7): 2338-42.

White, R. L., Jr., D. J. Schwartzentruber, et al. (1994). "Cardiopulmonary toxicity of treatment with high dose interleukin-2 in 199 consecutive patients with metastatic melanoma or renal cell carcinoma." Cancer 74(12): 3212-22.

Wilhelm, S. M., C. Carter, et al. (2004). "BAY 43-9006 exhibits broad spectrum oral antitumor activity and targets the RAF/MEK/ERK pathway and receptor tyrosine kinases involved in tumor progression and angiogenesis." Cancer Res 64(19): 7099-109.

Williams, P. F., C. M. Olsen, et al. (2010). "Melanocortin- 1-receptor and risk of cutaneous melanoma: A meta-analysis and estimates of population burden." Int J Cancer.

Willmore-Payne, C., J. A. Holden, et al. (2005). "Human malignant melanoma: detection of BRAF- and c-kit-activating mutations by high-resolution amplicon melting analysis." Hum Pathol 36(5): 486-93.

Willmore-Payne, C., L. J. Layfield, et al. (2005). "c-KIT mutation analysis for diagnosis of gastrointestinal stromal tumors in fine needle aspiration specimens." Cancer 105(3): 165-70.

Wiltshire, R. N., P. Duray, et al. (1995). "Direct visualization of the clonal progression of primary cutaneous melanoma: application of tissue microdissection and comparative genomic hybridization." Cancer Res 55(18): 3954-7.

Wolfel, T., M. Hauer, et al. (1995). "A p16INK4a-insensitive CDK4 mutant targeted by cytolytic T lymphocytes in a human melanoma." Science 269: 1281-1284.

Wong, H., M. Belvin, et al. (2009). "Pharmacodynamics of 2-[4-[(1E)-1-(hydroxyimino)-2,3-dihydro-1H-inden-5-yl]-3-(pyridine-4-yl)-1 H-pyrazol-1-yl]ethan-1-ol (GDC-0879), a potent and selective B-Raf kinase inhibitor: understanding relationships between systemic concentrations, phosphorylated mitogen-activated protein kinase kinase 1 inhibition, and efficacy." J Pharmacol Exp Ther 329(1): 360-7.

Wu, H., V. Goel, et al. (2003). "PTEN signaling pathways in melanoma." Oncogene 22(20): 3113-22.

Wyman, K., M. B. Atkins, et al. (2006). "Multicenter Phase II trial of high-dose imatinib mesylate in metastatic melanoma: significant toxicity with no clinical efficacy." Cancer 106(9): 2005-11.

Wyman, K., Kelley, M., Puzanov, I., Sanders, K., Hubbard, F., Krozely, P., Sturgeon, D., Viar, V., and Sosman, J (2006). "Phase II study of erlotinib given daily for patients with metastatic melanoma (MM) " Clin Oncol (Meeting Abstracts) vol. 24 no. 18 suppl 18002

Yang, F. C., G. Merlino, et al. (2001). "Genetic dissection of melanoma pathways in the mouse." Semin Cancer Biol 11(3): 261-8.

Yang, H., B. Higgins, et al. (2010). "RG7204 (PLX4032), a selective BRAFV600E inhibitor, displays potent antitumor activity in preclinical melanoma models." Cancer Res 70(13): 5518-27.

Yarden, Y. (2001). "The EGFR family and its ligands in human cancer. signalling mechanisms and therapeutic opportunities." Eur J Cancer 37 Suppl 4: S3-8.

Yazdi, A. S., G. Palmedo, et al. (2003). "Mutations of the BRAF gene in benign and malignant melanocytic lesions." J Invest Dermatol 121(5): 1160-2.

Yin, Y. and W. H. Shen (2008). "PTEN: a new guardian of the genome." Oncogene 27(41): 5443-53.

Yip, D., M. N. Le, et al. (2009). "A phase 0 trial of riluzole in patients with resectable stage III and IV melanoma." Clin Cancer Res 15(11): 3896-902.

Young, D., G. Waitches, et al. (1986). "Isolation and characterization of a new cellular oncogene encoding a protein with multiple potential transmembrane domains." Cell 45(5): 711-9.

Young, J., M. A. Barker, et al. (2005). "Evidence for BRAF mutation and variable levels of microsatellite instability in a syndrome of familial colorectal cancer." Clin Gastroenterol Hepatol 3(3): 254-63.

Yuan, Z. Q., R. I. Feldman, et al. (2003). "AKT2 inhibition of cisplatin-induced JNK/p38 and Bax activation by phosphorylation of ASK1: implication of AKT2 in chemoresistance." J Biol Chem 278(26): 23432-40.

Yuen, S. T., H. Davies, et al. (2002). "Similarity of the phenotypic patterns associated with BRAF and KRAS mutations in colorectal neoplasia." Cancer Res 62(22): 6451-5.

Zepter, K., A. C. Haffner, et al. (1995). "Reduced growth factor requirements and accelerated cell-cycle kinetics in adult human melanocytes transformed with SV40 large T antigen." J Invest Dermatol 104(5): 755-62.

Zhang, Y., Y. Xiong, et al. (1998). "ARF promotes MDM2 degradation and stabilizes p53: ARF-INK4a locus deletion impairs both the Rb and p53 tumor suppression pathways." Cell 92(6): 725-34.

Zhu, H., K. Reuhl, et al. (1998). "Development of heritable melanoma in transgenic mice." J Invest Dermatol 110(3): 247-52.

Zou, H. Y., Q. Li, et al. (2007). "An orally available small-molecule inhibitor of c-Met, PF-2341066, exhibits cytoreductive antitumor efficacy through antiproliferative and antiangiogenic mechanisms." Cancer Res 67(9): 4408-17.

# Part 5

## Diagnosis

18

# Biomarkers for Melanoma Diagnosis and the Technologies Used to Identify Them

Takeshi Mori[1] and Jeong-Hun Kang[2]
[1]*Department of Applied Chemistry, Faculty of Engineering, Kyushu University, 744 Motooka, Nishi-Ku, Fukuoka 819-0395,*
[2]*Department of Biomedical Engineering, National Cerebral and Cardiovascular Center Research Institute, 5-7-1 Fujishiro-dai, Suita, Osaka 565-8565, Japan*

## 1. Introduction

Melanoma is a malignant tumor originating from melanocytes (pigment-producing cells). Although the tumor is mainly detected in skin (cutaneous melanoma), it can also be detected in the eye (uveal melanoma), gastrointestinal (GI) tract and oral mucosa and genital tract (mucosal melanoma) (Landreville et al., 2008; Akaraviputh et al., 2010; Bakalian et al., 2008; Rigel et al., 2010; Seetharamu et al., 2010). Melanoma can be classified as belonging to one of four subtypes: superficial spreading, nodular, lentigo maligna, and acral lentiginous melanoma. These subtypes are characterized based on prognosis, incidence of metastasis and the frequency of gene mutations (e.g., *BRAF* and *NRAS*) (Saldanha et al., 2006; Jaeger et al., 2007; Markovic et al., 2007; Jönsson et al., 2010). Superficial spreading melanoma is the most common form of melanoma found in Caucasian populations, while the acral lentiginous melanoma is frequently detected in Asian and African populations (Cress and Holly, 1997; Weyers et al., 1999).

Several important risk factors that have been linked to the development of melanoma have been identified. Of these risk factors, most can be considered to be either environmental factors, such as exposure to ultraviolet (UV) radiation, especially in childhood, or other host factors such as family history and melanocytic nevi (Markovic et al., 2007, Schulman and Fisher, 2009), but other cancer risk factors such as smoking (Osterlind et al., 1988), diet (Osterlind et al., 1988; Veierod et al., 1997) or hormone therapy (Naldi et al., 2005) have not been found to be associated with an increased risk of melanoma. The risk of developing melanoma is higher in Caucasian than in Asian or African populations. This is closely related to skin pigmentation as melanin has been shown to have a protective function for UV-induced melanoma and Caucasian populations show low levels of melanogenesis (Lens and Dawes, 2004; Hu et al., 2008; Jemal et al., 2010). In general, the melanocortin-1 receptor (MC1R), which is a G-protein-coupled receptor (GPCR), stimulates melanogenesis through the activation of adenylate cyclase and protein kinase A (PKA) (Jordan and Jackson, 1998; Rouzaud et al., 2003). Its genetic variants are associated with melanoma incidence and sun sensitivity (Box et al., 2001; Markovic et al., 2007). Moreover, the risk of developing melanoma is greater in males than in females over the age of 40, although the opposite effect is observed in patients under 40 years old (Lens and Dawes, 2004; Jemal et al., 2010).

The global incidence of melanoma has increased over the past decades (Markovic et al., 2007; Jemal et al., 2010, Rigel et al., 2010). The 5-year survival rate for melanoma is higher than for other prominent cancers such as tumors of the prostate, ovary, liver and bile duct, lung and bronchus, colon and rectum, and stomach. Yet, the early diagnosis and treatment of melanoma is crucial to increasing the survival rate (Jemal et al., 2010, Rigel et al., 2010).

An important early diagnostic methodology for melanoma is the ABCDE criteria, which is defined by describing changes to the appearance of the suspected lesion based on the following features: Asymmetry, Border (irregularity), Color (variegation), Diameter and Evolution (over time). Other diagnostic strategies also typically utilized include histological and/or molecular analysis (e.g., genes or proteins profiling) of biopsied material, dermoscopy (also known as dermatoscopy or epiluminescent microscopy) using a light-based magnification or digital (computer)-assisted device, ultrasound imaging and magnetic resonance imaging (Abbasi et al., 2004; Rigel et al., 2005; Markovic et al., 2007; Psaty and Halpern, 2009; Rigel et al., 2010).

Recently there has also been a move toward establishing biomarkers for malignant melanoma. These types of biological markers are not only beneficial for the diagnosis of melanoma, but also allow physicians to monitor the recurrence of melanoma after surgical resection, or to monitor the effect of radiation or anticancer drug therapies. To identify putative melanoma biomarkers in tissue samples or body fluids, a number of methodologies can be utilized, including two-dimensional gel electrophoresis (2-DE) and high throughput microarray technology.

## 2. Melanoma biomarkers

### 2.1 Cellular signals and tissue biomarkers (immunohistochemical biomarkers)

Signal transduction pathways are the mechanism through which cells respond to the extracellular signals (ligands) required to regulate or modulate downstream gene expression. These extracellular signals activate signal transduction pathways by either penetrating the cellular membrane or binding to specific receptors. The activated receptors are then able to change the quantity or intracellular distribution of the second messengers through the use of effector molecules. Second messengers also activate protein targets, which control downstream gene expression. In these cellular signal transduction pathways, phosphorylation of the target proteins (by protein kinases), or dephosphorylation or proteolytic cleavage (by proteases) play a key role in cell division and motility, apoptosis and carcinogenesis.

In melanoma cells, major signal transduction pathways are RAS/RAF/MEK/ERK and the PI3K/AKT (as known as protein kinase B)/mTOR pathway; however, other pathways such as PLC/DAG/PKC or Wnt/β-catenin pathway have also been identified (Figure 1). The interaction of a number of different ligands [e.g., fibroblast growth factor (FGF), vascular endothelial growth factor (VEGF), or epidermal growth factor (EGF)] with their respective receptors [e.g., growth factor receptors (GFRs) (tyrosine kinase receptors)] leads to the stimulation of the RAS target protein, which has three members (HRAS, KRAS, and NRAS).

Phosphorylation of RAF kinase by RAS activates downstream targets the MAPK extracellular signal-regulated kinase-1 and -2 (MEK1 and MEK2), which causes the phosphorylation of extracellular signal-regulated kinase-1 and -2 (ERK1 and ERK2). Activated ERK1 and 2 has been found to modulate the gene expression necessary for survival and proliferation of melanoma cells, and has been linked to the increase resistance of melanoma cells to apoptosis by inhibiting the activation of caspase 8 (Becker et al., 2006; Sekulic et al., 2008). The *BRAF* mutation is necessary for ERK-mediated survival and proliferation and participates in the reduction of proapoptotic proteins (e.g., Bcl-2 family), while *RAF* genes consist of *ARAF*, *BRAF*, and *CRAF* (also known as *Raf-1*) (Becker et al., 2006; Cartlidge et al., 2008; Sekulic et al., 2008). The *BRAF* mutation, predominantly V600E (substitution of glutamate to valine; previously known to V599E), frequently occurs in melanoma and is strongly related to exposure to UV radiation (Tsao et al., 2004; Wan et al., 2004; Gray-Schopfer et al., 2005; Becker et al., 2006; Sekulic et al., 2008).

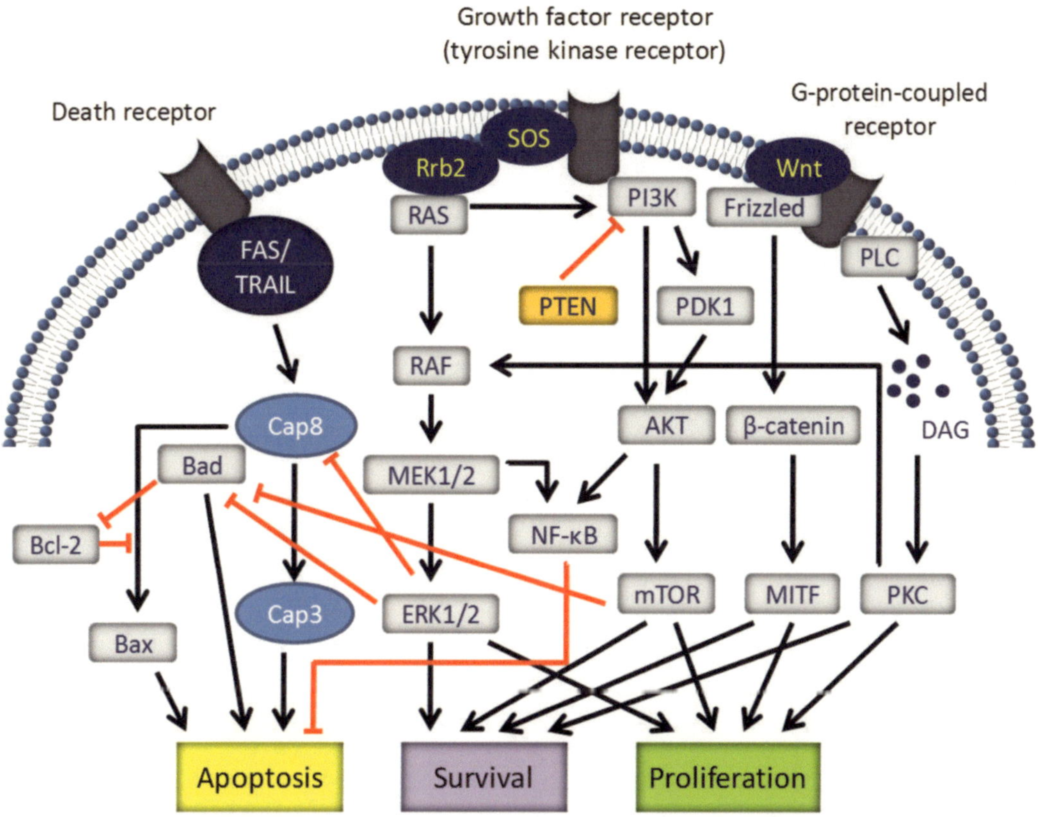


Fig. 1. Intracellular signal transduction of melanoma. RAS/RAF/MEK/ERK, PI3K/AKT/mTOR, PLC/DAG/PKC, and Wnt/β-catenin pathways are associated with survival, proliferation angiogenesis, and apoptosis of melanoma cells. Melanoma cells show an increase in the expression of survival or proliferation-associated signals and angiogenesis-associated signals, but a decrease in the expression of tumor suppressor or apoptosis-associated signals

| Biomarkers | Changes of expression | References |
|---|---|---|
| Survival or proliferation-associated molecules | | |
| GFRs (e.g., EGFR, VEGFR, FGFR, and PIGFR) 1) | Increased | Lacal et al., 2000; Ribatti et al., 2003; Odorisio et al., 2006; Diaz et al., 2007 |
| GPCRs (e.g., Wnt/fizzled receptor and chemokine receptors) 1) | Increased | Lee et al., 2008 |
| c-kit, one of GPCRs | Increased, but decreased in metastatic melanoma | Janku et al., 2005 |
| Activated PI3K | Increased | Becker et al., 2006; Sekulic et al., 2008 |
| Activated AKT | Increased | Stahl et al., 2004 |
| Activated ERK1/2 | Increased | Cohen et al., 2002 |
| Activated protein kinase C (PKC)α | Increased | Lahn and Sundell, 2004; Kang et al., 2008 |
| β-catenin 2) | Increased | Sanders et al., 1999; Widlund et al., 2002 |
| Cytokines (e.g., IL-1, IL-6, IL-8, and IL-10) | Increased | Ciotti et al., 1995 |
| Heat shock proteins (HSPs) (e.g., HSP 27 or 90) | Increased | McCarthy et al., 2008; Coupland et al., 2010 |
| Microphthalmia transcription factor (MITF) | Increased, but decreased in metastatic melanoma | Garraway et al., 2005; Fecker et al., 2006; Hoek et al., 2008 |
| Apoptosis-associated molecules | | |
| Antiapoptotic Bcl-2 family (Bcl-2, Bcl-XL, and Mcl-1) | Increased 3) | Leiter et al., 2000; Boisvert-Adamo et al., 2009 |
| Proapoptotic Bcl-2 family (multidomain proteins; Bax and Bak) | Decreased | Fecker et al., 2006; Tchernev and Orfanos, 2007 |
| Proapoptotic Bcl-2 family (BH3-only proteins; Bad, Bid, Bim, PUMA, and NOXA) | Decreased | Eisenmann et al., 2003; Karst et al., 2005; Ley et al., 2005; Qin et al., 2005; Zhang et al., 2006 |
| TRAIL-R1 (DR4) and TRAIL-R2 (DR5) | Decreased | Zhang et al., 1999; Zhuang et al., 2006 |
| Activated NF-κB | Increased | Ueda and Richmond, 2006 |
| Tumor suppressor-associated molecules | | |
| p4ARF | Decreased | Krimpenfort et al., 2001; Rizos et al., 2001 |
| p16INK4A | Decreased | Krimpenfort et al., 2001 |
| PTEN | Decreased | Stahl et al., 2003; Wu et al., 2003 |
| Inhibitor of growth family member 3 (ING3) | Decreased | Wang et al., 2007 |
| Angiogenesis-associated molecules 4) | | |
| Chemokine receptors (CXCR1 and CXCR2); one family of GPCRs | Increased | Scala et al., 2005; Varney et al., 2006; Richmond et al., 2009 |
| Matrix metalloproteinases (MMPs) | Increased | Hofmann et al., 2000 |
| Urokinase plasminogen activator receptor (uPAR) | Increased | de Vries et al., 1994; Ferrier et al., 2000 |
| Metastasis-associated proteins | | |
| Chemokine receptors (CXCR4, CCR7, and CCR10) 5) | Increased | Payne and Cornelius, 2002; Scala et al., 2005; Richmond et al., 2009 |
| Cell adhesion-associated molecules | | |
| Cytoskeleton/structure proteins (e.g., vimentin) | Increased | Coupland et al., 2010; Li et al., 2010 |

[1] These receptors also stimulate melanoma angiogenesis. [2] The β-catenin functions as a cell adhesion-associated molecule. [3] Other studies suggested a decrease in the expression of antiapoptotic Bcl-2 in metastatic melanoma (Fecker et al., 2006; Zhuang et al., 2007). [4] The angiogenesis-associated molecules take part in melanoma metastasis. [5] The chemokine receptors also play an important role in melanoma growth.

Table 1. (continues on next page) Tissue biomarkers (immunohistochemical biomarkers) for the diagnosis of melanoma and changes in their expression levels

| Biomarkers | Changes of expression | References |
|---|---|---|
| MUC18 | Increased | Lai et al., 2007 |
| Integrin αvβ3 | Increased | Hieken et al., 1995; Natali et al., 1997 |
| Integrin α6β4 | Increased | Nikolopoulos et al., 2004 |
| N-cadherin | Increased | Li et al., 2001; Qi et al., 2005 |
| P-cadherin | Decreased | Sanders et al., 1999 |
| E-cadherin 6) | Decreased | Sanders et al., 1999; Poser et al., 2001; Molina-Ortiz et al., 2009 |
| Antigens 7) | | |
| Melanocyte lineage/differentiation antigens | | |
| TRP1/gp75 | Increased | Thomson et al., 1985; Winder et al., 1994; Rad et al., 2004 |
| TRP2 | Increased | Winder et al., 1994; Rad et al., 2004 |
| Melan-A/MART-1 | Increased | Chen et al., 1998; Murer et al., 2004 |
| Tyrosinase | Increased | Sonesson et al., 1995; Stevens et al., 1996 |
| gp100/pmel-17 | Increased | Pardo et al., 2007 |
| S100 proteins (e.g., S100B) | Increased | Henze et al., 1997; Schlagenhauff et al., 2000 |
| Melanoma inhibitory activity (MIA) | Increased | Bosserhoff et al., 1999; Schmidt and Bosserhoff, 2009 |
| Cancer/testis antigens | | |
| BAGE family | Increased | Simpson et al., 2005; Barrow et al., 2006 |
| GAGE family | Increased | Simpson et al., 2005; Barrow et al., 2006 |
| MAGE family | Increased | Simpson et al., 2005; Barrow et al., 2006 |
| NY-ESO-1 | Increased | Chen et al., 1998; Simpson et al., 2005; Barrow et al., 2006 |
| Melanoma-associated antigens | | |
| A 90-kDa glycoprotein (e.g., TA-90 and periostin) | Increased | Rote et al., 1980; Kelley et al., 1998; Paulitschke et al., 2009 |
| Survivin (one of apoptosis inhibitors gene family) | Increased | Tas et al., 2004 |
| Other antigens | | |
| Cytotoxic T-lymphocyte antigen-4 (CTLA-4) (a negative regulator for T cells) | Increased | O'Day et al., 2007; Robert and Ghiringhelli, 2009 |
| Galectin-3 (a β-galactoside-binding protein) | Increased | Prieto et al., 2006; Vereecken et al., 2006 |
| Preferentially expressed antigen of melanoma (PRAME) (a repressor of retinoic acid) | Increased | Epping and Bernards, 2006 |
| Multiple myeloma 1 (MUM1) (melanoma associated antigen) | Increased | Natkunam et al., 2001 |
| Other tissue biomarkers | | |
| Nodal/Cripto-1 (nodal coreceptor) | Increased | Topczewska et al., 2006; Strizzi et al., 2009 |

6) The E-cadherin also functions as a tumor suppressor-associated molecule. 7) The antigens are found mainly in metastatic melanoma.

Table 1. (continues) Tissue biomarkers (immunohistochemical biomarkers) for the diagnosis of melanoma and changes in their expression levels

Moreover, phosphorylation of AKT kinase by phosphatidyl inositol 3-kinase (PI3K) stimulates the mammalian target of rapamycin (mTOR), which leads to the survival and proliferation of melanoma cells. The AKT/mTOR pathway suppresses apoptosis by decreasing the levels of pro-apoptotic proteins (e.g., BAD and caspase-9). Among the three AKT members (AKT1, AKT2, and AKT3), it is AKT3 that is often overexpressed in melanoma (Stahl et al., 2004) and is regulated by the phosphatase and tensin homolog (PTEN), which degrades the products of PI3K (Wu et al., 2003; Becker et al., 2006; Sekulic et al., 2008).

In addition, many antigens, which have immunostimulatory or activator roles in tumorigenesis, have been identified in metastatic melanoma. Important antigens include the melanocyte lineage/differentiation antigens [e.g., tyrosinase-related protein-1 (TRP1)/gp75, TRP2, Melan-A/MART-1] (Thomson et al., 1985; Winder et al., 1994; Murer et al., 2004; Rad et al., 2004) and cancer/testis antigens (e.g., BAGE family, GAGE family, MAGE family, and NY-ESO-1) (Chen et al., 1998; Simpson et al., 2005; Barrow et al., 2006). Melanocyte lineage/differentiation antigens are associated with the production of melanin pigments and have been identified in both normal melanocytes and melanoma (Thomson et al., 1985; Houghton et al., 1988). Cancer/testis antigens are abundant in normal tissues during development, but in mature cells, their expression is restricted to the male germ cells in the testis and to various tumors (Simpson et al., 2005).

As indicated, several gene mutations such as *NRAS* (Q61K/R), *BRAF* (V600E), *PTEN*, and *CDKN2A* mutation play an important role in the occurrence of melanoma (Tsao et al., 2004; Wan et al., 2004; Gray-Schopfer et al., 2005; Becker et al., 2006; Sekulic et al., 2008). These mutations are excellent targets for the diagnosis of melanoma. Moreover, in the context of melanoma prognosis, melanoma cells show an increase in the expression of survival or proliferation-associated molecules, angiogenesis-associated molecules, and in the expression of antigens, but a decrease in the expression of tumor suppressor-associated proteins (e.g., PTEN) or proapoptotic proteins (e.g., Bax and Bak) is observed (Table 1). Thus, these molecules, which show altered expression levels in melanoma relative to normal cells, are useful tissue biomarkers (immunohistochemical biomarkers) for melanoma diagnosis. However, in spite of these discoveries, these markers are not specific to melanoma and there are few melanoma-specific tissue biomarkers, excluding melanocyte lineage/differentiation antigens and melanoma-associated antigens (e.g., TRP1/gp75 and 2, Melan-A/MART-1, and TA-90) that are overexpressed in metastatic melanoma.

### 2.2 Serologic biomarkers for melanoma diagnosis

Many researchers have identified putative serologic biomarkers for melanoma diagnosis (Table 2), which play a key role in the growth and survival of melanoma cells. Typically, these markers activate survival and/or proliferation-associated and angiogenesis-associated signal transduction pathways after binding with their receptors. The most important receptors of this kind are GFRs (e.g., VEGFR and FGFR) and GPCRs (e.g., MC1R, Wnt/frizzled receptor, and chemokine receptor) (Halaban, 1996; Lee et al., 2008).

The primary antigens that have been observed in the serum of melanoma patients are melanocyte lineage/differentiation antigens and melanoma-associated antigens. The existence of these antigens in serum is closely associated with melanoma progression and low survival rates. Thus, these types of markers are useful as prognostic biomarkers and have potential to act as therapeutic targets.

In the absence of vascularization, the growth of melanoma is limited to 0.2 - 0.3 cm due to the limited diffusion of oxygen and nutrients into the tumor. For additional growth, angiogenesis is essential for providing adequate blood supply to the growing lesion. Angiogenesis is regulated by proangiogenic factors, such as VEGF, FGF, tumor necrosis factor (TNF), and interleukin-8 (IL-8) and by antiangiogenic factors, such as interferons (IFNs) and angiostatin. An increase in vascular density provides a greater supply of oxygen and nutrients to cells, leading to melanoma growth (Folkman, 2007; Mahabeleshwar and Byzova, 2007). High levels of proangiogenic factors in the serum of melanoma patients can be used as an indicator of melanoma at diagnosis.

Multiple cytokines (e.g., IL-1, 4, 6, 8, 10 and 14), which are correlated with melanoma growth, angiogenesis and metastasis, have been observed in the serum of melanoma patient at both the protein and/or mRNA level. Serum levels of these cytokines are increased in metastatic melanoma patients, suggesting that they can be used as an indicator of melanoma progression (Porter et al., 2001; Varney et al., 2006; Yurkovetsky et al., 2007). Moreover, the serum concentration of the soluble IL-2 receptor is elevated in patients with metastatic melanoma and elevated serum IL-2 receptor levels are associated with lowered survival rates (Boyano et al., 1997; Ottaiano et al., 2006). Interestingly, IFNs are soluble cytokines, but possess antiangiogenic and antitumor activities. An increase in the melanoma progression-associated cytokines leads to a reduction in IFNs levels, but there is a decrease in the serum levels of melanoma progression-associated cytokines in melanoma patients following immunomodulatory therapy with IFNs (mainly IFN-$\alpha$2b)(Singh and Varner, 1998; Jonasch and Haluska, 2001; Yurkovetsky et al., 2007; Dummer and Mangana, 2009; Hofmann et al., 2011). Thus, the analysis of a number of different serum cytokines may be a useful means of monitoring the efficacy of immunomodulatory therapy.

### 2.3 Urinary biomarkers for melanoma diagnosis

Urinary biomarkers for melanoma diagnosis have received much greater interest because of the relative ease of sample collection and handling compared with the analysis of blood or tissue samples, but this form of sample may lack the sensitivity required for a diagnostic biomarker. Of the urinary biomarkers of melanoma already identified (Table 3), 5SCD and 6-hydroxy-5-methoxyindole-2-carboxylic acid (6H5MI2C), are intermediate metabolites in melanin pigment formation, and have been the most extensively studied. An increase in urine levels of these markers has been associated with tumor progression and low survival rates (Kärnell et al., 1997; Bánfalvi et al., 2000; Wakamatsu et al., 2002). In healthy patients, the urinary levels of these markers are influenced by age (Meyerhöffer et al., 1998), sex (Morishima and Hanawa, 1981; Kågedal et al., 1992), skin color (Wirestrand et al., 1985) and season (Ito et al., 1987), but not by pregnancy (Carstam et al., 1985). Although both 5SCD and 6H5MI2C have been detected in the urine of melanoma patients, because of the higher levels of 5SCD, this marker is considered a more reliable urinary biomarker for melanoma than the 6H5MI2C (Kärnell et al., 1997, 2000; Wakamatsu et al., 2006). Moreover, the 90-kDa glycoprotein (TA-90)(Rote et al., 1980; Euhus et al., 1989), S100A7 (Brouard et al., 2002) and $\beta$-human chorionic gonadotropin (Carter et al., 1995) have also been identified in the urine of patients with melanoma (Table 3).

Of these urinary biomarkers, 5SCD, 6H5MI2C, and S100A7 can be considered the most melanoma-specific of the urinary biomarkers (Kärnell et al., 1997; Bánfalvi et al., 2000; Brouard et al., 2002; Wakamatsu et al., 2002).

| Biomarkers | Functions | References |
|---|---|---|
| Proangiogenic factors | | |
| VEGF 1) | VEGF receptor (VEGFR) ligand | Lacal et al., 2000 |
| FGF 1) | FGF receptor (FGFR) ligand | Ribatti et al., 2003 |
| EGF 1) | EGF receptor (EGFR) ligand | Hurks et al., 2000 |
| Placental growth factor (PIGF) 1) | Neuropilin-1 and -2 receptor ligand | Lacal et al., 2000; Odorisio et al., 2006 |
| TNF 1) | GPCR ligand | Singh and Varner 1998; Lie et al., 2005 |
| IL-8 (CXCL8) 1) | GPCR (specially, chemokine receptor CXCR1 and 2) ligand | Singh and Varner 1998; Lie et al., 2005; Varney et al., 2006 |
| Laminin-5 2) | Laminin receptor (e.g., integrin α6β4 and α7β1) ligand | Ziober et al., 1999; Nikolopoulos et al., 2004 |
| Osteopontin 2) | Integrin αvβ3 ligand | Zhou et al., 2005; Kadkol et al., 2006 |
| uPA 2) | uPAR ligand | Delbaldo et al., 1994; de Vries et al., 1994; Ferrier et al., 2000 |
| Antigens 3) | | |
| Melanocyte lineage/Differentiation antigens | | |
| Tyrosinase | Regulator enzyme in melanin synthesis; Increased in metastatic prognosis | Sonesson et al., 1995; Stevens et al., 1996 |
| gp100/pmel-17 | Melanin synthesis-associated melanosomal matrix glycoprotein; Increased in metastatic prognosis | Pardo et al., 2007 |
| S100 proteins (e.g., S100B) | Cell division and differentiation-associated acidic calcium-binding protein; Increased in metastatic prognosis | Henze et al., 1997; Schlagenhauff et al., 2000; Findeisen et al., 2009 |
| MIA | A small soluble protein; Increased in metastatic prognosis | Bosserhoff et al., 1999; Schmidt and Bosserhoff, 2009 |
| L-dopa/L-tyrosine ratio | An index of tyrosinase functional activity; Increased in metastatic prognosis | Letellier et al., 1999; Stoitchkov et al., 2002 |
| Melanoma-associated antigens | | |
| TA-90 | Potential immunostimulator or antineoplastic activator; Increased in metastatic prognosis | Rote et al., 1980; Kelley et al., 1998 |
| Survivin (one of apoptosis inhibitors gene family) | Apoptosis inhibition; Increased in metastatic prognosis | Tas et al., 2004 |
| Cytoplasmic/high-molecular-weight melanoma-associated antigen (CYT-MAA/HMW-MAA) | Unknown exactly, but may relate to melanoma progression | Vergilis et al., 2005 |

[1] These proangiogenic factors also function as an important stimulator for melanoma growth.[2] These proangiogenic factors also take part in melanoma metastasis.

Table 2. (continues on next page) Serologic biomarkers for the diagnosis of melanoma

| Biomarkers | Functions | References |
|---|---|---|
| Other antigens | | |
| Galectin-3 | A β-galactoside-binding protein; Increased in metastatic prognosis | Vereecken et al., 2006, 2009 |
| Synovial sarcoma X breakpoint-2 (SSX-2) | A family of highly homologous synovial sarcoma X (SSX) breakpoint proteins and repressive gene regulator | Kyyamova et al., 2006 |
| Gangliosides (GM2, GD2, GM3, and GD3) | Group of glycosphingolipids; Relate to interactions between melanoma cells | Ravindranath et al., 2003 |
| Cytokines and cytokine receptors 4) | | |
| IL-1 | Survival or proliferation-associated factor | Porter et al., 2001; Yurkovetsky et al., 2007 |
| IL-4 | Survival or proliferation-associated factor | Porter et al., 2001 |
| IL-6 | Survival or proliferation-associated factor | Deichmann et al., 2000; Moretti et al., 2001; Porter et al., 2001; Yurkovetsky et al., 2007 |
| IL-10 | Survival or proliferation-associated factor | Moretti et al., 2001; Porter et al., 2001 |
| IL-12 | Survival or proliferation-associated factor | Moretti et al., 2001; Yurkovetsky et al., 2007 |
| Soluble IL-2 receptor | Survival or proliferation-associated factor | Boyano et al., 1997; Ottaiano et al., 2006 |
| Other serologic biomarkers | | |
| YKL-40 | Unknown exactly, but may function as a survival or proliferation-associated factor | Johansen et al., 2006; Schmidt et al., 2006 |
| C reactive protein (CRP) | Unknown exactly, but may relate to tumor-associated inflammatory response | Deichmann et al., 2000; Findeisen et al., 2009 |
| Lactate dehydrogenase (LDH) | An indicator for liver metastasis; a prognostic indicator in metastatic melanoma | Deichmann et al., 2000; Findeisen et al., 2009; Zhuang et al., 2010 |
| Glypican-3 (GPC3) | Unknown exactly, but may function as a survival or proliferation-associated factor | Nakatsura et al., 2004; Ikuta et al., 2005 |
| PKCα | A survival or proliferation-associated protein | Kang et al., 2009 |
| 5SCD | A precursor of melanin; Increased in metastatic prognosis | Kärnell et al., 1997, 2000; Bánfalvi et al., 2000; Wakamatsu et al., 2002 |
| 6H5MI2C | A precursor of melanin; Increased in metastatic prognosis | Hara et al., 1994; Kärnell et al., 1997, 2000 |
| Serum amyloid A (SAA) | A superfamily of acute-phase proteins and proinflammatory adipokine | Findeisen et al., 2009 |
| Cystatin C | A potent inhibitor of cysteine proteases; Increased primary and metastatic melanoma | Kos et al., 1997; Ervin and Cox, 2005 |

[3] Antigens that are found in melanoma tissues become good immunohistochemical biomarkers. [4] The cytokines also take part in melanoma metastasis.

Table 2. (continues) Serologic biomarkers for the diagnosis of melanoma

| Biomarkers | References |
|---|---|
| 5SCD | Yamada et al., 1992; Kärnell et al., 1997; Bánfalvi et al., 2000; Wakamatsu et al., 2002 |
| 6H5MI2C | Yamada et al., 1992; Kärnell et al., 1997 |
| TA-90 | Rote et al., 1980; Euhus et al., 1989 |
| S100A7 | Brouard et al., 2002 |
| β-human chorionic gonadotropin | Carter et al., 1995 |

Table 3. Urinal biomarker for the diagnosis of melanoma

### 2.4 Biomarkers for early melanoma diagnosis

The early diagnosis of melanoma is closely related to an increase in survival rate. Although many prognostic biomarkers (mainly metastatic prognosis biomarkers) of melanoma have been reported, there are very few capable of allowing an early diagnosis. Glypican-3 (GPC3) is a membrane-bound heparin sulfate proteoglycan which is overexpressed in several tumors. It has been suggested that GPC3 may be a useful early stage biomarker for patients with the early stages of the disease (0 - II) (Nakatsura et al., 2004; Ikuta et al., 2005). Moreover, cyclooxygenase-2 (COX-2) (Chwirot and Kuźbicki, 2007), serum amyloid A (SAA) (Mian et al., 2005; Findeisen et al., 2009) and DNA methylation profiling (Conway et al., 2011) can be used to distinguish between early melanomas and benign nevi.

## 3. Screening techniques of melanoma biomarkers

Before the development of high throughput proteomics techniques, biomarker candidates were identified based on known melanoma molecular pathways and validated by traditional techniques such as western blotting, ELISA and immunohistochemical analysis. However, the recent development of proteomics has enabled novel biomarkers to be screened from across a much larger section of the proteome. The most widely used technique for this form of screening is one whereby the samples are first separated by 2-DE and then each protein is identified by mass spectrometry (MS). Recently, simple gel-free techniques such as shotgun proteomics (Liu et al., 2002) and surface-enhanced laser desorption/ionization time-of-flight mass spectrometry (SELDI-TOF MS)(Petricoin et al., 2002) have been developed. These techniques employ simple separation procedures such as capillary chromatography and surface chromatography prior MS analysis.

### 3.1 Screening for tumor tissues and cell lines

Biomarkers discovered from tissue samples and cultured cell lines also have utility for the development of diagnostic and prognostic assays. Tissue microarray is a high throughput technique in which many tissue samples can be screened simultaneously. This technique is suitable for the validation of candidate biomarkers, which are first obtained by other proteomics techniques. Several biomarkers of melanoma such as HSP 90 (McCarthy et al., 2008), ING3 (Wang et al., 2007), and the epidermal growth factor receptor family member HER3 (Reschke et al., 2008) were validated using this technique.

For comprehensive screening of biomarkers from lysates collected from tumor tissue and cultured cells, 2-DE combining MS is used as a standard method. The representative attempts of biomarker screening of melanoma lysates are summarized in Table 4. Since tumor tissue is heterogeneous mixture of several cell types, cultured cell lines may be preferable for the screening of biomarkers. To search for biomarkers useful for the diagnosis of metastases, primary and metastatic cell lines were compared and several candidate biomarkers were successfully discovered (Table 4) (Bernard et al., 2003; Zuidervaart et al., 2006; Al-Ghoul et al., 2008). Proteomics analysis of melanoma-associated fibroblast stromal cells revealed the aberrant expression of several proteins not detected in normal fibroblasts (Paulitschke et al., 2009). These proteins may promote tumor progression. However, the passages number of the melanoma cell lines tested was found to produce changes in the proteome, which may underscore the invasive character observed in melanoma cells line that have been passaged many times (Pardo et al., 2006).

| Screening methods | Samples | Biomarkers | Remarks | References |
|---|---|---|---|---|
| 2-DE/MALDI-TOF-MS | Primary and metastatic melanoma cell lines, and normal melanocyte lines | Hepatoma-derived growth factor (HDGF)<br>Nucleophosmin B23 | Increased in melanoma | Bernard et al., 2003 |
| 2-DE/LC-MS/MS | Uveal malignant melanoma (UM) cell lines with varying passages | MUC18<br>HMG-1 | Increased in higher passages | Pardo et al., 2006 |
| 2-DE/MALDI-TOF/TOF-MS | UM primary and metastatic cell lines | HSP 27<br>Galectin-1 | Increased in metastases | Zuidervaart et al., 2006 |
| 2-DE/MS/MS | Primary and metastatic melanoma cell lines | Cyclophilin A | Increased in metastatic melanoma | Al-Ghoul et al., 2008 |
| LC-MS/MS | Melanoma-associated fibroblasts and normal fibroblast | Periostin (a 90-kDa glycoprotein)<br>Stanniocalcin-1 (a 56-kDa glycoprotein) | Increased; melanoma-associated antigens | Paulitschke et al., 2009 |
| 2-DE/MS/MS | UM with monosomy 3 and disomy 3 | HSP 27<br>Vimentin | Increased in disomy UM | Coupland et al., 2010 |

Table 4. Biomarker screening for tumor tissues and cell lines

### 3.2 Screening biomarkers obtained from serum and secreted from cultured cell lines

Because serum samples are far less invasive to obtain than biopsied material, the discovery of serological biomarkers has received a great deal of attention. Well-defined biomarkers enable early detection, allow the appropriate classification of tumor types (which provides the clinician insight into the best choice of therapy), and enable the patient to be more thoroughly monitored for progression and regression. However, there are several difficulties with screening serological biomarkers: (1) the presence of abundant blood proteins, which may inhibit the detection of biomarkers, and (2) the low serum concentration of the biomarker after it is secreted from tumor tissue and diluted in the bloodstream (Simpson et al., 2008). Hence, processes by which the abundant blood proteins are removed from the sample or the target proteins are concentrated are essential to address these problems. As a result of these difficulties inherent in serum proteomics, the secretome has received much attention recently.

Table 5 summarizes a number of different reports in which comprehensive screening of biomarkers from serum and the secretome occurred. By comparing the secretome between melanoma and normal melanocyte, several potential biomarkers were successfully discovered (Pardo et al., 2007; Paulitschke et al., 2009). The traditional serological biomarkers of melanoma such as LDH, S100B and CRP lack sensitivity as early stage melanoma biomarkers. To search for early stage biomarkers, Findeisen et al. extensively analyzed the serum proteome of about 600 melanoma patients at each stage of the disease (stages I - IV) by SELDI-TOF-MS technique (Mian et al., 2005; Findeisen et al., 2009). This analysis led to the discovery of a new biomarker, SAA, which was found to be highly sensitive for detecting early stage melanoma.

| Screening methods | Samples | Biomarkers | Remarks | References |
|---|---|---|---|---|
| 2D-GE/LC-MS/MS | UM cell lines and normal melanocytes | gp100/pmel-17 Cathepsin D Mad-9 (syntenin 1) | Increased in melanoma | Pardo et al., 2007 |
| Multiplex immunobaed assay | Serum of melanoma patients and healthy individuals | Cytokines (e.g. IL-1, IL-6, TNF-α) | Increased in patients with longer relapse-free survival (RFS) values | Yurkovetsky et al., 2007 |
| LC-MS/MS | Malanoma cell lines and normal melanocyte | Glutathione peroxidase | Increased in malanoma | Paulitschke et al., 2009 |
| SELDI-TOF-MS | Serum of melanoma patients with different stages | SAA | Increased in early stages | Mian et al., 2005 Findeisen et al., 2009 |

Table 5. Biomarker screening for serum and secretome of cell lines

## 4. Summary and overall conclusions

Melanoma biomarkers have the capacity not only to diagnose melanoma, but also to allow patients to be monitored for recurrence after surgical resection and to allow the effect of anticancer drug treatments to be evaluated. Advanced technologies (e.g., high throughput technologies in genomics or proteomics) have contributed much to the hunt for melanoma biomarkers in tissue samples or body fluids and have typically been MS-based or array-based technologies.

Several immunohistochemical, serologic and urinary biomarkers have been reported to be very useful diagnostic and prognostic biomarkers. However, there is a paucity of data on melanoma-specific biomarkers, with the exception of the melanocyte lineage/differentiation antigens and melanoma-associated antigens, and some urinary biomarkers such as 5SCD, 6H5MI2C and S100A7.

Moreover, several melanoma biomarkers with prognostic capabilities, mainly for the detection of metastatic disease, have been applied to clinical use. However, there is s still a great need to identify melanoma early-stage melanoma biomarkers, as early detection of the disease is key to increasing the survival rate. Of several melanoma biomarkers identified, GPC3, COX-2, SAA and DNA methylation profiling may hold promise for the diagnosis of early melanoma.

## 5. References


Abbasi NR, Shaw HM, Rigel DS, Friedman RJ, McCarthy WH, Osman I, Kopf AW, Polsky D (2004). Early diagnosis of cutaneous melanoma: revisiting the ABCD criteria. *JAMA*, 292, 2771-2776.

Akaraviputh T, Arunakul S, Lohsiriwat V, Iramaneerat C, Trakarnsanga A (2010). Surgery for gastrointestinal malignant melanoma: experience from surgical training center. *World J Gastroenterol*, 16, 745-748

Al-Ghoul M, Brück TB, Lauer-Fields JL, Asirvatham VS, Zapata C, Kerr RG, Fields GB (2008). Comparative proteomic analysis of matched primary and metastatic melanoma cell lines. *J Proteome Res* 7, 4107-4118.

Bakalian S, Marshall JC, Logan P, Faingold D, Maloney S, Di Cesare S, Martins C, Fernandes BF, Burnier MN Jr (2008). Molecular pathways mediating liver metastasis in patients with uveal melanoma. *Clin Cancer Res*, 14, 951-956.

Bánfalvi T, Gilde K, Boldizsár M, Fejös Z, Horváth B, Liszkay G, Beczássy E, Kremmer T (2000). Serum concentration of 5-S-cysteinyldopa in patients with melanoma. *Eur J Clin Invest*, 30, 900-904.

Barrow C, Browning J, MacGregor D, Davis ID, Sturrock S, Jungbluth AA, Cebon J (2006). Tumor antigen expression in melanoma varies according to antigen and stage. *Clin Cancer Res*, 12, 764-771.

Becker JC, Kirkwood JM, Agarwala SS, Dummer R, Schrama D, Hauschild A (2006) Molecularly targeted therapy for melanoma. *Cancer*, 106, 2317-2327.

Bernard K, Litman E, Fitzpatrick JL, Shellman YG, Argast G, Polvinen K, Everett AD, Fukasawa K, Norris DA, Ahn NG, Resing KA (2003). Functional proteomic analysis of melanoma progression. *Cancer Res*, 63, 6716-6725.

Boisvert-Adamo K, Longmate W, Abel EV, Aplin AE (2009). Mcl-1 is required for melanoma cell resistance to anoikis. *Mol Cancer Res*, 7, 549-556.

Bosserhoff AK, Lederer M, Kaufmann M, Hein R, Stolz W, Apfel R, Bogdahn U, Buettner R (1999). MIA, a novel serum marker for progression of malignant melanoma. *Anticancer Res*, 19, 2691-2693.

Box NF, Duffy DL, Irving RE, Russell A, Chen W, Griffyths LR, Parsons PG, Green AC, Sturm RA (2001). Melanocortin-1 receptor genotype is a risk factor for basal and squamous cell carcinoma. *J Invest Dermatol*, 116, 224-229.

Boyano MD, García-Vázquez MD, Gardeazabal J, García de Galdeano A, Smith-Zubiaga I, Cañavate ML, Raton JA, Bilbao I, Díaz-Pérez JL (1997). Serum-soluble IL-2 receptor and IL-6 levels in patients with melanoma. *Oncology*, 54, 400-406.

Brouard MC, Saurat JH, Ghanem G, Siegenthaler G (2002). Urinary excretion of epidermal-type fatty acid-binding protein and S100A7 protein in patients with cutaneous melanoma. *Melanoma Res*, 12, 627-631.

Carstam R, Hansson C, Rorsman H, Rosengren E, Sjöberg NO, Wirestrand LE (1985). Urinary excretion of melanocytic metabolites in fertile women. *Acta Derm Venereol*, 65,543-545.

Carter PG, Iles RK, Neven P, Ind TE, Shepherd JH, Chard T (1995). Measurement of urinary beta core fragment of human chorionic gonadotrophin in women with vulvovaginal malignancy and its prognostic significance. *Br J Cancer*, 71, 350-353.

Cartlidge RA, Thomas GR, Cagnol S, Jong KA, Molton SA, Finch AJ, McMahon M (2008). Oncogenic BRAF(V600E) inhibits BIM expression to promote melanoma cell survival. *Pigment Cell Melanoma Res*, 21, 534-544.

Chen YT, Güre AO, Tsang S, Stockert E, Jäger E, Knuth A, Old LR (1998). Identification of multiple cancer/testis antigens by allogeneic antibody screening of a melanoma cell line library. *Proc Natl Acad Sci USA*, 95, 6919-6923.

Chwirot BW, Kuźbicki Ł (2007). Cyclooxygenase-2 (COX-2): first immunohistochemical marker distinguishing early cutaneous melanomas from benign melanocytic skin tumours. *Melanoma Res*, 17, 139-145.

Ciotti P, Rainero ML, Nicolò G, Spina B, Garrè C, Casabona F, Santi PL, Bianchi-Scarrà G (1995). Cytokine expression in human primary and metastatic melanoma cells: analysis in fresh bioptic specimens. *Melanoma Res*, 5, 41-47.

Cohen C, Zavala-pompa A, Sequeira JH, Shoji M, Sexton DG, Cotsonis G, Cerimele F, Govindarajan B, Macaron N, Arbiser JL (2002). Mitogen-actived protein kinase activation is an early event in melanoma progression. *Clin Cancer Res*, 8, 3728-3733.

Conway K, Edmiston SN, Khondker ZS, Groben PA, Zhou X, Chu H, Kuan PF, Hao H, Carson C, Berwick M, Olilla DW, Thomas NW (2011). DNA methylation profiling distinguishes malignant melanomas from benign nevi. *Pigment Cell Melanoma Res*, 24, 352-360.

Coupland SE, Vorum H, Mandal N, Kalirai H, Honoré B, Urbak SF, Lake SL, Dopierala J, Damato B (2010). Proteomics of uveal melanomas suggests HSP-27 as a possible surrogate marker of chromosome 3 loss. *Invest Ophthalmol Visual Science*, 51, 12-20.

Cress RD, Holly EA (1997). Incidence of cutaneous melanoma among non-Hispanic whites, Hispanics, Asians, and blacks: an analysis of california cancer registry data, 1988-93. *Cancer Causes Control*, 8, 246-252.

Deichmann M, Benner A, Waldmann V, Bock M, Jäckel A, Näher H (2000). Interleukin-6 and its surrogate C-reactive protein are useful serum markers for monitoring metastasized malignant melanoma. *J Exp Clin Cancer Res*, 19, 301-307.

Delbaldo C, Masouye I, Saurat JH, Vassalli JD, Sappino AR (1994). Plasminogen activation in melnocytic neoplasia. *Cancer Res*, 54, 4547-4552.

de Vries TJ, Quax PH, Denijn M, Verrijp KN, Verheijen JH, Verspaget HW, Weidle UH, Ruiter DJ, van Muijen GN (1994). Plasminogen activators, their inhibitors, and urikinase receptor emerge in late stages of melanocytic tumor progression. *Am J Pathol*, 144, 70-81.

Diaz A, Suarez E, Blanco R, Badia T, Rivero D, Lopez-Requena A, Lopez A, Montero E (2007). Functional expression of human-epidermal-growth-factor receptor in a melanoma cell line. *Biotechnol Appl Biochem*, 48, 21-27

Dummer R, Mangana J (2009). Long-term pegylated interferon-alpha and its potential in the treatment of melanoma. *Biologics*, 3, 169-182.

Eisenmann KM, VanBrocklin MW, Staffend NA, Kitchen SM, Koo HM (2003). Mitogen-activated protein kinase pathway-dependent tumor-specific survival signaling in melanoma cells through inactivation of the proapoptotic protein Bad. *Cancer Res*, 63, 8330-8337.

Epping MT, Bernards R (2006). A causal role for the human tumor antigen preferentially expressed antigen of melanoma in cancer. *Cancer Res*, 66, 10639-10642.

Ervin H, Cox JL (2005). Late stage inhibition of hematogenous melanoma metastasis by cystatin C over-expression. *Cancer Cell Int*, 5, 14.

Euhus DM, Gupta RK, Morton DL (1989). Detection of a tumor-associated glycoprotein antigen in serum and urine of melanoma patients by murine monoclonal antibody (AD1-40F4) in enzyme immunoassay. *J Clin Lab Anal*, 3, 184-190.

Fecker LF, Geilen CC, Tchernev G, Trefzer W, Assaf C, Kurbanov BM, Schwarz C, Daniel PT, Eberle J (2006). Loss of proapoptotic Bcl-2-related multidomain proteins in primary melanomas is associated with poor prognosis. *J Invest Dermatol*, 126, 1366-1371.

Ferrier CM, Suciu S, van Geloof WL, Straatman H, Eggermont AM, Koops HS, Kroon BB, Lejeune FJ, Kleeberg UR, van Muijen GN, Ruiter DJ (2000). Hign-tPA-expression in primary melanoma of the limb correlates with good prognosis. *Br J Cancer*, 83, 1351-1359.

Findeisen P, Zapatka M, Peccerella T, Matzk H, Neumaier M, Schadendorf D, Ugurel S (2009). Serum amyloid A as a prognostic marker in melanoma identified by proteomic profiling. *J Clin Oncol*, 27, 2199-2208.

Folkman, J. (2007) Angiogenesis: an organizing principle for drug discovery? *Nat. Rev. Drug Discov*, 6, 237-286.

Garraway LA, Widlund HR, Rubin MA, Getz G, Berger AJ, Ramaswamy S, Beroukhim R, Milner DA, Granter SR, Du J, Lee C, Wagner SN, Li C, Golub TR, Rimm DL, Meyerson ML, Fisher DE, Sellers WR (2005). Integrative genomic analyses identify MITF as a lineage survival oncogene amplified in malignant melanoma. *Nature*, 436, 117-122.

Gray-Schopfer VC, da Rocha Dias S, Marais R (2005). The role of B-RAF in melanoma. *Cancer Metastasis Rev*, 24, 165-183.

Halaban R (1996). Growth factors and melanomas. *Semin Oncol*, 23, 673-681.

Hara H, Walsh N, Yamada K, Jimbow K (1994). High plasma level of a eumelanin precursor, 6-hydroxy-5-methoxyindole-2-carboxylic acid as a prognostic marker for malignant melanoma. *J Invest Dermatol*, 102, 501-505.

Henze G, Dummer R, Joller-Jemelka HI, Böni R, Burg G (1997). Serum S100-a marker for disease monitoring in metastatic melanoma. *Dermatology*, 194, 208-212.

Hieken TJ, Farolan M, Ronan SG, Shilkaitis A, Wild L, Das Gupta TK (1995). $\beta_3$ integrin expression in melanoma predicts subsequent metastasis. *J Surg Res*, 63, 169-173.

Hoek KS, Eichhoff OM, Schlegel NC, Döbbeling U, Kobert N, Schaerer L, Hemmi S, Dummer R (2008). In vivo switching of human melanoma cells between proliferative and invasive states. *Cancer Res*, 68, 650-656.

Hofmann MA, Kiecker F, Küchler I, Kors C, Trefzer U (2011). Serum TNF-α, B2M and sIL-2R levels are biological correlates of outcome in adjuvant IFN-α2b treatment of patients with melanoma. *J Cancer Res Clin Oncol,* 137, 455-462.

Hofmann UB, Westphal JR, Van Muijen GN, Ruiter DJ (2000). Matrix metalloproteinases in human melanoma. *J Invest Dermatol,* 115, 337-344.

Houghton AN, Albino AP, Cordon-Cardo C, Davis LJ, Eisinger M (1988). Cell surface antigens of human melanocytes and melanoma. Expression of adenosine deaminase binding protein is extinguished with melanocyte transformation. *J Exp Med*, 167, 197-212.

Hu DN, Yu G, McCormick SA, Finger PT (2008). Population-based incidence of conjunctival melanoma in various races and ethnic groups and comparision with other melanoma. *Am J Ophthlmol*, 145, 418-423.

Hurks HM, Metzelaar-Blok JA, Barthen ER, Zwinderman AH, De Wolff-Rouendaal D, Keunen JE, Jager MJ (2000). Expression of epidermal growth factor receptor: risk factor in uveal melanoma. *Invest Ophthalmol Vis Sci*, 41, 2023-2027.

Ikuta Y, Nakatsura T, Kageshita T, Fukushima S, Ito S, Wakamatsu K, Baba H, Nishimura Y (2005). Highly sensitive detection of melanoma at an early stage based on the increased serum secreted protein acidic and rich in cysteine and glypican-3 levels. *Clin Cancer Res*, 11, 8079-8088.

Ito S, Kato T, Fujita K (1987). Seasonal variation in urinary excretion of 5-S-cysteinyldopa in healthy Japanese. *Acta Derm Venereol*, 67, 163-165.

Jaeger J, Koczan D, Thiesen HJ, Ibrahim SM, Gross G, Spang R, Kunz M (2007). Gene expression signatures for tumor progression, tumor subtype, and tumor thickness in laser-microdissected melanoma tissues. *Clin Cancer Res*, 13, 806-815.

Janku F, Novotny J, Julis I, Julisova I, Pecen L, Tomancova V, Kocmanova G, Krasna L, Krajsova I, Stork J, Petruzelka L (2005). KIT receptor is expressed in more than 50% of early-stage malignant melanoma: a retrospective study of 261 patients. *Melanoma Res*, 15, 251-256

Jemal A, Siegel R, Xu J, Ward E (2010). Cancer statistics, 2010. *CA Cancer J Clin*, 60, 277-300.

Johansen JS, Jensen BV, Roslind A, Nielsen D, Price PA (2006). Serum YKL-40, new prognostic biomarker in cancer patients? *Cancer Epidemol Biomarkers Prev*, 15, 194-202.

Jonasch E, Haluska FG (2001). Interferon in oncological practice: review of interferon biology, clinical applications, and toxicities. *Oncologist*, 6, 34-55

Jönsson G, Busch C, Knappskog S, Geisler J, Miletic H, Ringnér M, Lillehaug JR, Borg A, Lønning PE (2010). Gene expression profiling-based identification of molecular subtypes in stage melanoma with different clinical outcome. *Clin Cancer Res*, 16, 3356-3367.

Jordan SA, Jackson IJ (1998). Melanocortin receptors and antagonists regulate pigmentation and body weight. *Bioassays*, 20, 603-606.

Kadkol SS, Lin AY, Barak V, Kalickman I, Leach L, Valyi-Nagy K, Majumdar D, Setty S, Maniotis AJ, Folberg R, Pe'er J (2006). Osteopontin expression and serum levels in metastatic uveal melanoma: A pilot study. *Invest Ophthalmol Vis Sci*, 47, 802-806.

Kågedal B, Lenner L, Arstrand K, Hansson C (1992). The stability of 5-S-cysteinyldopa and 6-hydroxy-5-methoxyindole-2-carboxylic acid in human urine. *Pigment Cell Res*, 2, 304-307.

Kang JH, Asai D, Toita R, Kitazaki H, Katayama Y (2009). Plasma protein kinase C (PKC)alpha as a biomarker for the diagnosis of cancers. *Carcinogenesis*, 30, 1927-1931.

Kang JH, Asai D, Yamada S, Toita R, Oishi J, Mori T, Niidome T, Katayama Y (2008). A short peptide is a protein kinase C (PKC) $\alpha$-specific substrate. *Proteomics*, 8, 2006-2011.

Kärnell R, Kågedal B, Lindholm C, Nilsson B, Arstrand K, Ringborg U (2000). The value of cysteinyldopa in the follow-up of disseminated malignant melanoma. *Melanoma Res*, 10, 363-369.

Kärnell R, von Schoultz E, Hansson LO, Nilsson B, Arstrand K, Kågedal B (1997). S100B protein, 5-S-cysteinyldopa and 6-hydroxy-5-methoxyindole-2-carboxylic acid as biochemical markers for survival prognosis in patients with malignant melanoma. *Melanoma Res*, 7, 393-399.

Karst AM, Dai DL, Martinka M, Li G (2005). PUMA expression is significantly reduced in human cutaneous melanomas. *Oncogene*, 24, 1111-1116.

Kelley MC, Jones RC, Gupta RK, Yee R, Stern S, Wanek L, Morton DL (1998). Tumor-associated antigen TA-90 immune complex assay predicts subclinical metastasis and survival for patients with early stage melanoma. *Cancer* 83, 1355-1361.

Krimpenfort P, Quon KC, Mooi WJ, Loonstra A, Berns A (2001). Loss of $p16^{Ink4a}$ confers susceptibility to metastatic melanoma in mice. *Nature*, 413, 83-86.

Kos J, Stabuc B, Schweiger A, Krasovec M, Cimerman N, Kopitar-Jerala N, Vrhovec I (1997). Cathepsins B, H, and L and their inhibitors stefin A and cystatin C in sera of melanoma patients. *Clin Cancer Res*, 3, 1815-1822.

Kyyamova RG, Gryshkova VS, Zhyvoloup AM (2006). Expression of SSX2 tumor antigen in baculovirus expression system and its application for screening of blood serum of melanoma patients. *Exp Oncol*, 28, 110-113.

Lacal PM, Failla CM, Pagani E, Odorisio T, Schietroma C, Falcinelli S, Zambruno G, D'Atri S (2000). Human melanoma cells secrete and respond to placenta growth factor and vascular endothelial growth factor. *J Invest Dermatol*, 115, 1000-1007.

Lahn MM, Sundell KL (2004). The role of protein kinase C-alpha (PKC-$\alpha$) in melanoma. *Melanoma Res*, 14, 85-89.

Lai K, Sharma V, Jager MJ, Conway RM, Madigan MC (2007). Expression and distribution of MUC18 in human uveal melanoma. *Virchows Arch*, 451:967-976.

Landreville S, Agapova OA, Harbour JW (2008). Emerging insights into the molecular pathogenesis of uveal melanoma. *Future Oncol*, 4, 629-636.

Lee HJ, Wall B, Chen S (2008). G-protein-coupled receptors and melanoma. *Pigment Cell Melanoma Res*, 21, 415-428.

Leiter U, Schmid RM, Kaskel P, Peter RU, Krähn G (2000). Antiapoptotic bcl-2 and bcl-xL in advanced malignant melanoma. *Arch. Dermatol Res*, 292, 225-232.

Lens MB, Dawes M (2004). Global perspectives of contemporary epidemiological trends of cutaneous malignant melanoma. *Br J Dermatol*, 150, 179-185.

Letellier S, Garnier JP, Spy J, Stoitchkov K, Le Bricon T, Baccard M, Revol M, Kerneis Y, Bousquet B (1999). Development of metastases in malignant melanoma is associated with an increase in the plasma L-dopa/L-tyrosine ratio. *Melanoma Res*, 9, 389-94.

Ley R, Ewings KE, Hadfield K, Cook SJ (2005). Regulatory phosphorylation of Bim: sorting out the ERK from the JNK. *Cell Death Differ*, 12, 1008-1104.

Li G, Satyamoorthy K, Herlyn M (2001). N-cadherin-mediated intercellular interactions promote survival and migration of melanoma cells. *Cancer Res*, 61, 3819-3825.

Li M, Zhang B, Sun B, Wang X, Ban X, Sun T, Liu Z, Zhao X (2010). A novel function for vimentin: the potential biomarker for predicting melanoma hematogenous metastasis. *J Exp Clin Cancer Res*, 29, 109.

Lie G, Zhang F, Lee J, Dong Z (2005). Selective induction of interleukin-8 expression in metastatic melanoma cells by transforming growth factor-β1. *Cytokine*, 31, 241-249.

Liu H, Lin D, Yates JR 3rd (2002). Multidimensional separations for protein/peptide analysis in the post-genomic era. *Biotechniques*, 32, 898-902.

Mahabeleshwar GH, Byzova TV (2007). Angiogenesis in melanoma. *Semin Oncol*, 34, 555-565.

Markovic SN, Erickson LA, Rao RD, Weenig RH, Pockaj BA, Bardia A, Vachon CM, Schild SE, McWilliams RR. Hand JL, Laman SD, Kottschade LA, Maples WJ, Pittelkow MR, Pulido JS, Cameron JD, Creagan ET, Melanoma Study Group of the Mayo Clinic Cancer Center (2007). Malignant melanoma in the 21st century, part 1: epidemiology, risk factors, screening, prevention, and diagnosis. *Mayo Clin Proc*, 82, 364-380.

McCarthy MM, Pick E, Kluger Y, Gould-Rothberg B, Lazova R, Camp RL, Rimm DL, Kluger HM (2008). HSP90 as a marker of progression in melanoma. *Annals Oncol*, 19, 590-594.

Meyerhöffer S, Lindberg Z, Häger A, Kågedal B, Rosdahl I (1998). Urinary excretion of 5-S-cysteinyldopa and 6-hydroxy-5-methoxyindole-2-carboxylic acid in children. *Acta Derm Venereol*, 78, 31-35.

Mian S, Ugurel S, Parkinson E, Schlenzka I, Dryden I, Lancashire L, Ball G, Creaser C, Rees R, Schadendorf D (2005). Serum proteomic fingerprinting discriminates between clinicalstages and predicts disease progression in melanoma patients. *J Clin Oncol*, 23, 5088-5093.

Molina-Ortiz I, Bartolomé RA, Hernández-Varas P, Colo GP, Teixidó J (2009). Overexpression of E-cadherin on melanoma cells inhibits chemokine-promoted invasion involving p190RhoGAP/p120ctn-dependent inactivation of RhoA. *J Biol Chem*, 284, 15147-15157.

Moretti S, Chiarugi A, Semplici F, Salvi A, De Giorgi V, Fabbri P, Mazzoli S (2001). Serum imbalance of cytokines in melanoma patients. *Melanoma Res*, 11, 395-399.

Morishima T, Hanawa S (1981). Urinary excretion of 5-S-cysteinyldopa in healthy Japanese. *Acta Derm Venereol*, 61, 149-150.

Murer K, Urosevic M, Willers J, Selvam P, Laine E, Burg G, Dummer R (2004). Expression of Melan-A/MART-1 in primary melanoma cell cultures has prognostic implication in metastatic melanoma patients. *Melanoma Res*, 14, 257-262.

Nakatsura T, Kageshita T, Ito S, Wakamatsu K, Monji M, Ikuta Y, Senju S, Ono T, Nishimura Y (2004). Identification of glypican-3 as a novel tumor marker for melanoma. *Clin Cancer Res*, 10, 6612-6621.

Naldi L, Altieri A, Imberti GL, Giordano L, Gallus S, La Vecchia C, Oncology Study Group of the Italian Group for Epidemiologic Research in Dermatology (2005). Cutaneous malignant melanoma in women: phenotypic characteristics, sun exposure, and hormonal factors: a case-control study from Italy. *Ann Epidemiol*, 15, 545-550.

Natali PG, Hamby CV, Felding-Habermann B, Liang B, Nicotra MR, Di Filippo F, Giannarelli D, Temponi M, Ferrone S (1997). Clinical significance of integrin and intercellular adhesion molecule-1 expression in cutaneous malignant melanoma lesions. *Cancer Res*, 57, 1554-1560.

Natkunam Y, Warnke RA, Montgomery K, Falini B, van De Rijn M (2001). Analysis of MUM1/IRF4 protein expression using tissue microarrays and immunohistochemistry. *Mod Pathol*, 14, 686-694.

Nikolopoulos SN, Blaikie P, Yoshioka T, Guo W, Giancotti FG (2004). Integrin β4 signaling promotes tumor angiogenesis. *Cancer Cell*, 6, 471-483.

O'Day SJ, Hamid O, Urba WJ (2007). Targeting cytotoxic T-lymphocyte antigen-4 (CTLA-4): A novel strategy for the treatment of melanoma and other milignancies. *Cancer*, 110, 2614-2627.

Odorisio T, Cianfarani F, Failla CM, Zambruno G (2006). The placenta growth factor in skin angiogenesis. *J Dermatol Sci*, 41, 11-19.

Osterlind A, Tucker MA, Stone BJ, Jensen OM (1988). The Danish case-control study of cutaneous malignant melanoma, IV: no association with nutritional factors, alcohol, smoking or hair dyes. *Int J Cancer*, 42, 825-828.

Ottaiano A, Leonardi E, Simeone E, Ascierto PA, Scala S, Calemma R, Bryce J, Caracò C, Satriano RA, Gianfranco N, Franco R, Botti G, Castello G (2006). Soluble interleukin-2 receptor in stage I-III melanoma. *Cytokine*, 33, 150-155.

Pardo M, Garcia A, Antrobus R, Blanco MJ, Dwek RA, Zitzmann N (2007). Biomarker discovery from uveal melanoma secretomes: Identification of gp100 and cathepsin D in patient serum. *J Proteome Res*, 6, 2802-2811.

Pardo M, García A, Thomas B, Piñeiro A, Akoulitchev A, Dwek RA, Zitzmann N (2006). The characterization of the invasion phenotype of uveal melanoma tumour cells shows the presence of MUC18 and HMG-1 metastasis markers and leads to the identification of DJ-1 as a potential serum biomarker. *Int J Cancer*, 119, 1014-1022.

Paulitschke V, Kunstfeld R, Mohr T, Slany A, Micksche M, Drach J, Zielinski C, Pehamberger H, Gerner C (2009). Entering a new era of rational biomarker discovery for early detection of melanoma metastases: secretome analysis of associated stroma cells. *J Proteome Res*, 8, 2501-2510.

Payne AS, Cornelius LA (2002). The role of chmokines in melanoma tumor growth and metastasis. *J Invest Dermatol*, 118, 915-922.

Petricoin III EF, Ardekani AM, Hitt BA, Levine PJ, Fusaro VA, Steinberg SM, Mills GB, Simone C, Fishman DA, Kohn EC, Liotta LA (2002). Use of proteomic patterns in serum to identify ovarian cancer. *Lancet*, 359, 572-577.

Porter GA, Abdalla J, Lu M, Smith S, Montgomery D, Grimm E, Ross MI, Mansfield PF, Gershenwald JE, Lee JE (2001). Significance of plasma cytokine levels in melanoma patients with histologically negative sentinel lymph nodes. *Ann Surg Oncol*, 8, 116-122.

Poser I, Domínguez D, de Herreros AG, Varnai A, Buettner R, Bosserhoff AK (2001). Loss of E-cadherin expression in melanoma cells involves up-regulation of the transcriptional repressor Snail. *J Biol Chem*, 276, 24661-24666.

Prieto VG, Mourad-Zeidan AA, Melnikova V, Johnson MM, Lopez A, Diwan AH, Lazar AJ, Shen SS, Zhang PS, Reed JA, Gershenwald JE, Raz A, Bar-Eli M (2006). Galectin-3 expression is associated with tumor progression and pattern of sun exposure in melanoma. *Clin Cancer Res*, 12, 6709-6715.

Psaty EL, Halpern AC (2009). Current and emerging technologies in melanoma diagnosis: the state of the art. *Clin Dermatol*, 27, 35-45.

Qi J, Chen N, Wang J, Siu CH (2005) Transsendothelial migration of melanoma cells involves N-cadherin-mediated adhesion and activation of the β-catenin signaling pathway. *Mol Biol Cell*, 16, 4386-4397.

Qin JZ, Ziffra J, Stennett L, Bodner B, Bonish BK, Chaturvedi V, Bennett F, Pollock PM, Trent JM, Hendrix MJ, Rizzo P, Miele L, Nickoloff BJ (2005). Proteasome inhibitors trigger NOXA-mediated apoptosis in melanoma and myeloma cells. *Cancer Res*, 65, 6282-6293

Rad HH, Yamashita T, Jin HY, Hirosaki K, Wakamatsu K, Ito S, Jimbow K (2004). Tyrosinase-realted proteins suppress tyrosinase-mediated cell death of melanocytes and melanoma cells. *Exp Cell Res*, 298, 317-328.

Ravindranath MH, Hsueh EC, Verma M, Ye W, Morton DL (2003). Serum total ganglioside level correlates with clinical course in melanoma patients after immunotherapy with therapeutic cancer vaccine. *J Immunother*, 26, 277-285.

Reschke M, Mihic-Probst D, van der Horst EH, Knyazev P, Wild PJ, Hutterer M, Meyer S, Dummer R, Moch H, Ullrich A (2008) HER3 is a determinant for poor prognosis in melanoma. *Clin Cancer Res*, 14, 5188-5197.

Ribatti D, Vacca A, Ria R, Marzullo A, Nico B, Filotico R, Roncali L, Dammacco F (2003). Neovascularisation, expression of fibroblast growth fact-2 and mast cells with tryptase activity increase simulfaneously with pathological progression in human malignant melanoma. *Eur J Cancer*, 39, 666-674.

Richmond A, Yang J, Su Y (2009). The good and the bad of chemokines/chemokine receptors in melanoma. *Pigment Cell Melanoma Res*, 22, 175-186.

Rigel DS, Friedman RJ, Kopf AW, Polsky D (2005). ABCDE-an evolving concept in the early detection of melanoma. *Arch Dermatol*, 141, 1032-1034

Rigel DS, Russak J, Friedman R (2010). The evolution of melanoma diagnosis: 25 years beyond the ABCDs. *CA Cancer J Clin*, 60, 301-316.

Rizos H, Darmanian AP, Holland EA, Mann GJ, Kefford RF (2001). Mutations in the INK4a/ARF melanoma susceptibility locus functionally impari $p14^{ARF}$. *J Biol Chem*, 276, 41424-41434.

Robert C, Ghiringhelli F (2009). What is the role of cytotoxic T lyimphocyte-associated antigen 4 blockade in patients with metastatic melanoma? *Oncologist*, 14, 848-861.

Rote NS, Gupta RK, Morton DL (1980). Tumor-associated antigens detected by autologous sera in urine of patients with solid neoplasms. *J Surg Res*, 29, 18-22.

Rouzaud F, Annereau JP, Valencia JC, Costin GE, Hearing VJ (2003). Regulation of melanocortin 1 receptor expression at the mRNA and protein levels by its natural agonist and antagonist. *FASEB J*, 17, 2154-2156.

Saldanha G, Potter L, DaForno P, Pringle JH (2006). Cutanuous melanoma subyptes show different BRAF and NRAS mutaion frequencies. *Clin Cancer Res*, 12, 4499-4505.

Sanders DS, Blessing K, Hassan GA, Bruton R, Marsden JR, Jankowski J (1999). Alterations in cadherin and catenin expression during the biological progression of melanocytic tumours. *Mol Pathol*, 52, 151-157.

Scala S, Ottaiano A, Ascierto PA, Cavalli M, Simeone E, Giuliano P, Napolitano M, Franco R, Botti G, Castello G (2005). Expression of CXCR4 predicts poor prognosis in patients with malignant melanoma. *Clin Cancer Res*, 11, 1835-1841.

Schlagenhauff B, Schittek B, Ellwanger U, Stroebel W, Blum A, Schwarz M, Rassner G, Garbe C (2000). Significance of serum protein S100 levels in screening for melanoma metastasis: dose protein S100 early detection of melanoma recurrence? *Melanoma Res*, 10, 451-459.

Schmidt H, Johansen JS, Sjoegren P, Christensen IJ, Sorensen BS, Fode K, Larsen J, von der Maase H (2006). Serum YKL-40 predicts relapse-free and overall survival in patients with American Joint Committee on Cancer stage I and II melanoma. *J Clin Oncol*, 24, 798-804.

Schmidt J, Bosserhoff AK (2009). Processing of MIA protein during melanoma cell migration. *Int J Cancer*, 125, 1587-1594.

Schulman JM, Fisher DE (2009). Indoor ultraviolet tanning and skin cancer: health risks and opportunities. *Curr Opin Oncol*, 21, 144-149.

Seetharamu N, Ott PA, Pavlick AC (2010). Mucosal melanoma: a case-based review of the literature. *Oncologist* 15, 772-781.

Sekulic A, Haluska P Jr, Miller AJ, Genebriera De Lamo J, Ejadi S, Pulido JS, Salomao DR, Thorland EC, Vile RG, Swanson DL, Pockaj BA, Laman SD, Pittelkow MR, Markovic SN, Melanoma Study Group of Mayo Clinic Cancer Center (2008). Malignant melanoma in the 21st century: The emerging molecular landscape. *Mayo Clin Proc*, 83, 825-846.

Simpson AJ, Caballero OL, Jumngbluth A, Chen YT, Old LJ (2005). Cancer/testis antigens, gametogenesis and cancer. *Nat Rev Cancer*, 5, 615-625.

Singh RK, Varney ML (1998). Regulation of interleukin 8 expression in human malignant melanoma cells. *Cancer Res*, 58, 1523-1527.

Sonesson B, Eide S, Ringborg U, Rorsman H, Rosengren E (1995). Tyrosinase activity in the serum of patients with malignant melanoma. *Melanoma Res*, 5, 113-116.

Stahl JM, Cheung M, Sharma A, Trivedi NR, Shanmugam S, Robertson GP (2003). Loss of PTEN promotes tumor development in malignant melanoma. *Cancer Res*, 63, 2881-2890.

Stahl JM, Sharma A, Cheung M, Zimmerman M, Cheng JQ, Bosenberg MW, Kester M, Sandirasegarane L, Robertson GP (2004). Deregulated Akt3 activity promotes development of malignant melanoma. *Cancer Res*, 64, 7002-7010.

Stevens GL, Scheer WD, Levine EA (1996). Detection of tyrosinase mRNA from the blood of melanoma patients. *Cancer Epidmilo Biomarkers Prev*, 5, 293-296.

Stoitchkov K, Letellier S, Garnier JP, Bousquet B, Tsankov N, Morel P, Ghanem G, Le Bricon T (2002). Melanoma progression and serum L-dopa/L-tyrosine ratio: a comparison with S100B. *Melanoma Res*, 12, 255-262.

Strizzi L, Postovit LM, Margaryan NV, Lipavsky A, Gadiot J, Blank C, Seftor RE, Seftor EA, Hendrix MJ (2009). Nodal as a biomarker for melanoma progression and a new therapeutic target for clinical intervention. *Expert Rev Dermatol*, 4, 67-78.

Tas F, Duranyildiz D, Argon A, Oguz H, Camlica H, Yasasever V, Topuz E (2004). Serum bcl-2 and surviving levels in melanoma. *Melanoma Res*, 14, 543-536.

Tsao H, Goel V, Wu H, Yang G, Haluska FG (2004). Genetic interaction between *NRAS* and *BRAF* mutations and *PTEN/MMAC1*. *J Invest Dermatol*, 122, 337-341.

Tchernev G, Orfanos CE (2007). Downregulation of cell cycle modulators p21, p27, p53, Rb and proapoptotic Bcl-2-related proteins Bax and Bax in cutaneous melanoma is associated with worse patient prognosis: preliminary findings. *J Cutan Pathol*, 34, 247-256.

Thomson TM, Mattes MJ, Roux L, Old LJ, Lloyd KO (1985). Pigmentation-associated glycoprotein of human melanomas and melanocytes: definition with a mouse monoclonal antibody. *J Invest Dermatol*, 85, 169-174.

Topczewska JM, Postovit LM, Margaryan NV, Sam A, Hess AR, Wheaton WW, Nickoloff BJ, Topczewski J, Hendrix MJ (2006). Embryonic and tumorigenic pathways converge via Nodal signaling: role in melanoma aggressiveness. *Nat Med*, 12, 925-932.

Ueda Y, Richmond A (2006). NF-κB activation in melanoma. *Pigment Cell Res*, 19, 112-124.

Varney ML, Johansson SL, Singh RK (2006). Distinct expression of CXCL8 and its receptors CXCR1 and CXCR2 and their association with vessel density and aggressiveness in malignant melanoma. *Am J Clin Pathol*, 125, 209-216.

Veierod MB, Thelle DS, Laake P (1997). Diet and risk of cutaneous malignant melanoma: a prospective study of 50,757 Norwegian men and women. *Int J Cancer*, 71, 600-604.

Vereecken P, Awada A, Suciu S, Castro G, Morandini R, Litynska A, Lienard D, Ezzedine K, Ghanem G, Heenen M (2009). Evaluation of the prognostic significance of serum galectin-3 in American Joint Committee on Cancer stage III and stage IV melanoma patients. *Melanoma Res*, 19, 316-320.

Vereecken P, Zouaoui Boudjeltia K, Debray C, Awada A, Legssyer I, Sales F, Petein M, Vanhaeverbeek M, Ghanem G, Heenen M (2006). High serum galectin-3 in advanced melanoma: preliminary results. *Clin Exp Dermatol*, 31, 105-109.

Vergilis IJ, Szarek M, Ferrone S, Reynolds SR (2005). Presence and prognostic significance of melanoma-associated antigens CYT-MAA and HMW-MAA in serum of patients with melanoma. *J Invest Dermatol*, 125, 526–531

Wakamatsu K, Kageshita T, Furue M, Hatta N, Kiyohara Y, Nakayama J, Ono T, Saida T, Takata M, Tsuchida T, Uhara H, Yamamoto A, Yamazaki N, Naito A, Ito S (2002). Elvaluation of 5-S-cysteinyldopa as a marker of melanoma progression: 10 years' experience. *Melanoma Res*, 12, 245-253.

Wakamatsu K, Takasaki A, Kågedal B, Kageshita T, Ito S (2006). Determination of eumelanin in human urine. *Pigment Cell Res*, 19, 163-169.

Wan PT, Garnett MJ, Roe SM, Lee S, Niculescu-Duvaz D, Good VM, Jones CM, Marshall CJ, Springer CJ, Barford D, Marais R, Cancer Genome Project (2004). Mechanism of activation of the RAF-ERK signaling pathway by oncogenic mutations of B-RAF. *Cell*, 116, 855-867.

Wang Y, Dai DL, Martinka M, Li G (2007). Prognostic significance of nuclear ING3 expression in human cutaneous melanoma *Clin Cancer Res*, 13, 4111-4116.

Weyers W, Euler M, Diaz-Cascajo C, Schill WB, Bonczkowitz M (1999). Classification of cutaneous maliganat melanoma: a reassessment of histopathologic criteria for the distinction of different types. *Cancer*, 86, 288-299.

Widlund HR, Horstmann MA, Price ER, Cui J, Lessick SL, Wu M, He X, Fisher DE (2002). β-catenin-induced melanoma growth requires the downstream target *Microphthalmia*-associated transcription factor. *J Cell Biol*, 158, 1079-1087.

Winder A, Kobayashi T, Tsukamoto K, Urabe K, Aroca P, Kameyama K, Hearing VJ (1994). The tyrosinase gene family: interactions of melanogenic proteins to regulate melanogenesis. *Cell Mol Biol Res*, 40, 613-626.

Wirestrand LE, Hansson C, Rosengren E, Rorsman H (1985). Melanocyte metabolites in the urine of people of different skin colour. *Acta Derm Venereol*, 65,345-348.

Wu H, Goel W, Haluska FG (2003). PTEN signaling pathways in melanoma. *Oncogene*, 22, 3113-3122.

Yamada K, Walsh N, Hara H, Jimbow K, Chen H, Ito S (1992). Measurement of eumelanin precursor metabolites in the urine as a new marker for melanoma metastases. *Arch Dermatol*, 128, 491-494.

Yurkovetsky ZR, Kirkwood JM, Edington HD, Marrangoni AM, Velikokhatnaya L, Winans MT, Gorelik E, Lokshin AE (2007). Multiplex analysis of serum cytokines in melanoma patients treated with interferon-α2b. *Clin Cancer Res*, 13, 2422-2428.

Zhang XD, Franco A, Myers K, Gray C, Nguyen T, Hersey P (1999). Relation of TNF-related apoptosis-inducing ligand (TRAIL) receptor and FLICE-inhibitory protein expression to TRAIL-induced apoptosis of melanoma. *Cancer Res*, 59, 2747-2753.

Zhang XD, Wu JJ, Gillespie S, Borrow J, Hersey P (2006). Human melanoma cells selected for resistance to apoptosis by prolonged exposure to tumor necrosis factor-related apoptosis-inducing ligand are more vulnerable to necrotic cell death induced by cisplatin. *Clin Cancer Res*, 12, 1355-1364.

Zhou Y, Dai DL, Martinka M, Su M, Zhang Y, Campos EI, Dorocicz I, Tang L, Huntsman D, Nelson C, Ho V, Li G (2005). Osteopontin expression correlates with melanoma invasion. *J Invest Dermatol*, 124, 1044-1052.

Zhuang L, Lee CS, Scolyer RA, McCarthy SW, Zhang XD, Thompson JF, Hersey P (2007). Mcl-1, Bcl-XL and Stat3 expression are associated with progression of melanoma whereas Bcl-2, AP-2 and MITF levels decrease during progression of melanoma. *Mod Pathol*, 20, 416-426.

Zhuang L, Lee CS, Scolyer RA, McCarthy SW, Zhang XD, Thompson JF, Screaton G, Hersey P (2006). Progression in melanoma is associated with decreased expression of death receptors for tumor necrosis factor-related apoptosis-inducing ligand. *Hum Pathol*, 37, 1286-1294.

Zhuang L, Scolyer RA, Murali R, McCarthy SW, Zhang XD, Thompson JF, Hersey P (2010). Lactate dehydrogenase 5 expression in melanoma increases with disease progression and is associated with expression of Bcl-XL and Mcl-1, but not Bcl-2 protein. *Mod Pathol*, 23, 45-53.

Ziober BL, Chen YQ, Ramos DM, Waleh N, Kramer RH (1999). Expression of the laminin receptor suppresses melanoma growth and metastatic potential. *Cell Growth Different*, 10, 479-490.

Zuidervaart W, Hensbergen PJ, Wong M-C, Deelder AM, Tensen CP, Jager MJ, Gruis NA (2006). Proteomic analysis of uveal melanoma reveals novel potential markers involved in tumor progression. *Invest Ophthalmol Visual Sci*, 47, 786-793.

# Characterization of Melanoma Progression on Animal Model Using Fourier Transform Infrared Mapping

Beljebbar A.[1], Gatouillat G.[2], Morjani H.[1], Manfait M.[1] and Madoulet C.[2]
[1]*Unité MéDIAN, MEDyC CNRS UMR6237*
[2]*Laboratoire de Biochimie, IFR53 Biomolécules, UFR de Pharmacie, Université de Reims Champagne-Ardenne, 51 rue Cognacq-Jay, 51096 Reims Cedex, France*

## 1. Introduction

A majority of human cancers arise within the skin. The effective cure is surgical excision of the primary tumor (Thompson et al., 2005) when the lesions are smaller than 1 mm (James et al., 2000). Melanoma removal at early stages is almost always curative and therefore detection is essential. In fact, early detection of cancer is the most important factor in the prevention of cancer and a guarantee in most cases of an effective treatment or complete cure. Thus, the only reliable strategy to prevent death from melanoma still remains to be early diagnosis. The prognosis for a patient with stage I or II melanoma is mainly related to tumor thickness. Currently, the gold standard in most cancer diagnosis is histopathological evaluation, which involves the removal of tissue biopsies and examination by pathologists (Slater, 2000). This process includes tissue staining and morphological pattern recognition. During tissue transformation, it is expected that substantial modifications occur at molecular level before visible morphological changes become apparent. Hence, early detection is critical in melanoma treatment, and the evolution of the tumor and its penetration into the dermis are key factors to be studied in order to understand the disease (Elder, 2006). Melanoma is a tumor of melanocytes, which are a class of cells located at the epidermal-dermal junction. Observations in situ are limited, however, and tumor progression cannot be followed in humans due to ethical concerns.Therefore, appropriate animal model systems are needed. Second, the spatially distributed nature of the tumor requires the use of imaging techniques but the influence of multiple cells requires biochemical contrast especially to study subtle molecular changes in early stage disease and its progression. The first is the development of model systems to study disease and the second is the development of new imaging technologies. Similarly, there have been efforts to characterize melanoma progression in biochemical terms, (Jeffs et al., 2009) including understanding the role of cells other than melanocytes in tumor evolution (Kempen et al., 2003). While characterization of tissue and tissue models is routinely accomplished by structural imaging, a biochemical characterization typically requires destruction of the structure, thereby losing spatially specific information. A combination of biochemical and structural knowledge is often helpful and is enabled by the emerging fields of chemical imaging and microscopy.

The main objective is a detection of the source of the pathological variation at molecular level in order to further understand the molecular carcinogenic process in a range of cancers. Indeed, tumor tissues are mostly heterogeneous in nature, and this heterogeneity further depends on the stage of disease and its aggressiveness. The emergence of a novel technique, complementary to histopathology and immunohistochemistry, can thus help in the early diagnostic of tissue transformation during carcinogenesis. Fourier-transform infrared microspectroscopy (FTIRM) has emerged as a powerful tool to study molecular structure and structural interactions in biological systems. When this technique is applied to tissues, the resulting spectra is composed of characteristic absorption bands originating from all infrared-active vibrational modes of biological macromolecules present in the tissue, such as proteins, lipids, and nucleic acids (Parker, 1971). Each of these molecules provides a unique absorption spectral pattern named fingerprint through the entire infrared spectrum. This property offers a way to identify the molecule type (qualitative analysis) and the amount or quantity of this molecule in the sample (quantitative analysis) (Beljebbar et al., 2008). This method can be used as a diagnostic tool, complementary to histopathology or immunochemistry (Fernandez et al., 2005). As the image contrast is based on the intrinsic vibrational signature of the tissue components, spectral images does not require the use of added dyes or labelling methods for visualization of different chemical components in the sample (Bates, 1976). Indeed, FT-IRM imaging combined a high spatially resolved morphological and biochemical information that offer a number of advantages for ex-vivo assessment of tissue and aid the histopathologist in the identification and classification of subtle biochemical changes related to carcinogenesis (Petibois & Déléris, 2006; Cohenford & Rigas, 1998). The use of a high spectral resolution and appropriate data treatment are of fundamental importance to isolate representative spectral markers of biocomponents. Correlations of morphologic and biochemical skin tissue differences could be used to identify variations that occur between healthy and diseased tissues. The development of clinical protocols for the routine examination of tissue histology or for localized tumors using IR microspectroscopic methods has been largely used in medical diagnostics of tumors (Wong et al, 1991; Rigas et al, 1990; Krafft, 2006, 2007; Amharref et al, 2006; Beljebbar et al., 2008). Previous studies have investigated the structure of skin (Garidel, 2002, 2003), diseases (Tfayli et al., 2005, Hammody et al., 2005, 2008; Ly et al., 2008) dynamics of diffusion (Mendelsohn et al., 2003, 2006; Morganti et al., 1999; Dary et al., 2001; Tetteh et al., 2009) or use it as a model system for studies (Bhargava and Levin., 2004). In vivo Raman and IR studies have not examined skin cancers, but focus on the effect of hydration and penetration enhancers on the stratum corneum (Pirot et al, 1997; Casper et al, 2003). Ex vivo IR studies indicate differences between skin tumors and normal skin (Wong et al, 1993); however, such studies have not taken into account the effect of the heterogeneous nature of the skin.

Infrared spectra contain many overlapping bands and so data interpretation cannot be made by simple visual inspection and alternative approaches are needed. Because of the high complexity of the FTIR spectra obtained from tissues, multivariate statistical methods are required to extract biochemical information related to tissue. This would permit to objectively differentiate distinct tissue structures and for identifying origin that gave rise to the specific tissue pathology. These methods have had a major impact on the quantitative and qualitative analysis of infrared spectral data. They have been shown to improve analysis precision, accuracy, reliability, and applicability for infrared spectral analyses relative to the more conventional univariate methods of data analysis. Rather than attempting to find and use only an isolated spectral feature in the analysis of spectral data, multivariate methods derive their power from the simultaneous use of multiple intensities (i.e. multiple variables) in each spectrum (Mourant et al., 2003). During the last decade, it has been recognized that FT-IR, in combination with the appropriate multivariate analysis strategies, has considerable potential as a metabolic fingerprinting tool for the rapid detection and diagnosis of disease or dysfunction (Goodacre et al., 2004; Diem et al., 1999). Multivariate imaging techniques including Unsupervised Hierarchical Cluster Analysis (UHCA) (Jackson et al., 1998; Mohlenhoff et al., 2005), K-means clustering (Lasch et al., 2004; Zhang et al., 2003), Principal Components Analysis (PCA) (Lasch and Naumann, 1998), Linear Discriminant Analysis (LDA) (Mansfield et al, 1999), Fuzzy C-means clustering (Lasch et al., 2004; Mansfield et al., 1997) and neural networks (Lasch and Naumann, 1998) have proven to be invaluable in the identification of spectral groups or "clusters" which can be directly compared to stained tissue sections. In multivariate methods, the information of the entire spectrum can be utilized for the analysis. The high correlation of spectral clusters with anatomical and histopathological features has been conclusively demonstrated for a number of different tissue types.

Thus, the objective of this study will be to detect the source of the pathological variation at molecular level in order to further understand the molecular carcinogenic process in a range of melanoma disease, and the development of FTIRM to provide non-destructive, rapid, reproducible diagnosis, and minimize inter-observer variability. The identification and quantification of these specific molecular changes within skin can provide diagnostic information for aiding in early detection of diseases and their optimized treatment. The aim of this chapter will be the monitoring and interpretation of molecular changes associated to melanoma growth and invasion by FTIRM imaging on animal models.

## 2. FTIR characterization of normal skin tissues and melanoma progression using cluster analysis

### 2.1 Animals and cell lines

Six- to eight-week-old female B6D2F1 mice were purchased from the Charles River Laboratories (Iffa Credo, L'Arbresle, France) and housed at the animal maintenance facility of the Centre de Biotechnologies, U.F.R. Pharmacy, Reims, France. The treatments of mice protocols were according to the Institutional Animal Care and Use Committee guidelines.

B16R, a pigmented mouse melanoma cell line from C57Bl/6 (H-2b) origin resistant to 3.5 x $10^{-7}$ M doxorubicin was obtained from National Tumour Institute of Milan (Mariani et al., 1990). B16R were maintained in 5% $CO_2$ atmosphere at 37°C, in complete RPMI 1640 medium (Invitrogen, Cergy-Pontoise, France) supplemented with 10% heat-inactivated FBS (Invitrogen).

### 2.2 Tumour induction

For tumor induction, B6D2F1 mouse (five animals per group) were shaved on the right flank and subcutaneously challenged with 1 x $10^6$ viable B16R cells in NaCl 0.9%. The size of the tumors was assessed in a blinded, coded fashion twice weekly and recorded as tumor area (in square cM) by measuring the largest perpendicular diameters with callipers. The experiment was repeated twice. The melanoma tumors were obtained by the injection of melanoma cell suspension in mice skin (Odot et al., 2004; Joseph-Pietras et al., 2006, 2007). B16R melanoma cells in B6D2F1 mice after subcutaneous injection is a well-established model. This may prove to be a good model for investigation of local growth of tumor cells and their interaction with metastatic lesions. However, the histological progression from injected cells to establish local growth of melanoma has not been studied systematically. We therefore have investigated the molecular changes and growth of B16R melanoma at the injection site during eleven days post-implantation to identify spectroscopic markers associated to early detection of tissue transformation. One million B16F10 melanoma cells were injected subcutaneously in B6D2F1 mice. All animals' developed tumors with reproducible localization and size around the site of injection (Fig. 1).

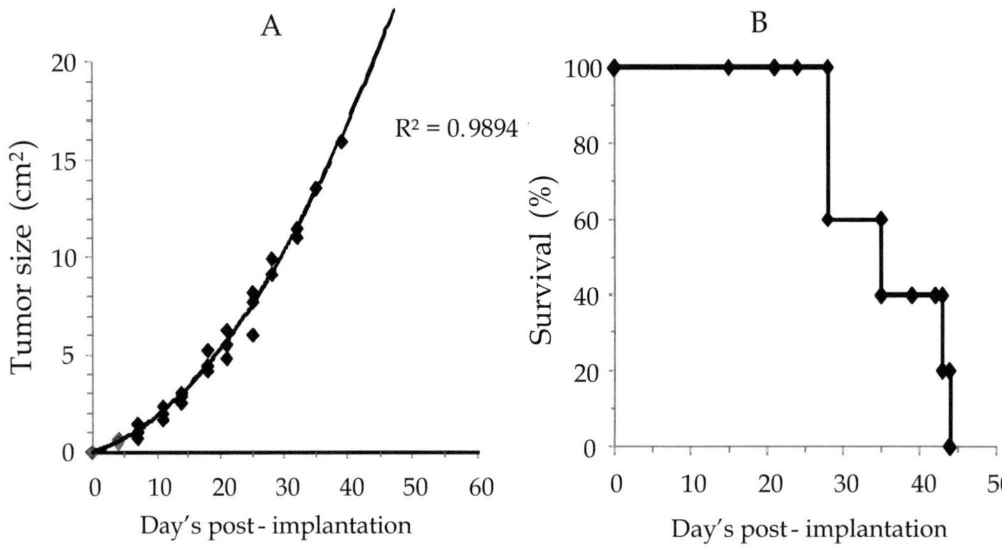


Fig. 1. Tumor development and survival of mice after subcutaneous injection of $1\times10^6$ B16R cells. Tumor size dependent on the period elapsed after injection of B16R cells. All animals with implanted B16R cells developed tumors with reproducible localization and size around the site of injection

These groups were sacrificed after 4, 7, 11 days post-implantation. After skin excision, tissue samples were snap-frozen by immersion in methyl-butane cooled down in liquid nitrogen and stored at - 80°C. Two adjacent sections were cut from each sample using a cryomicrotome. One section, 10 µm thick, was placed onto infrared transparent calcium fluoride ($CaF_2$) slides for infrared imaging. The second section, 7 µm thick, was placed on a microscope glass slide and stained with hematoxylin and eosin (H&E) for histopathological image.

### 2.3 Spectroscopic measurement

Spectra were collected using an FTIR imaging system (SPOTLIGHT, Perkin-Elmer, France) coupled to a FTIR spectrometer (Spectrum 300, Perkin-Elmer, France). This system is equipped with a liquid $N_2$ cooled Mercury-Cadmium-Telluride (MCT) line detector comprised of 16 pixel elements. The microscope was equipped with a movable, software-controlled x, y stage. In this study, FTIR images were collected from selected areas with a spatial resolution of 25 µm/pixel, in transmission mode, in the 4000–720 $cm^{-1}$ range, with a final spectral resolution of 4 $cm^{-1}$, and 16 scans per pixel. After atmospheric correction, data

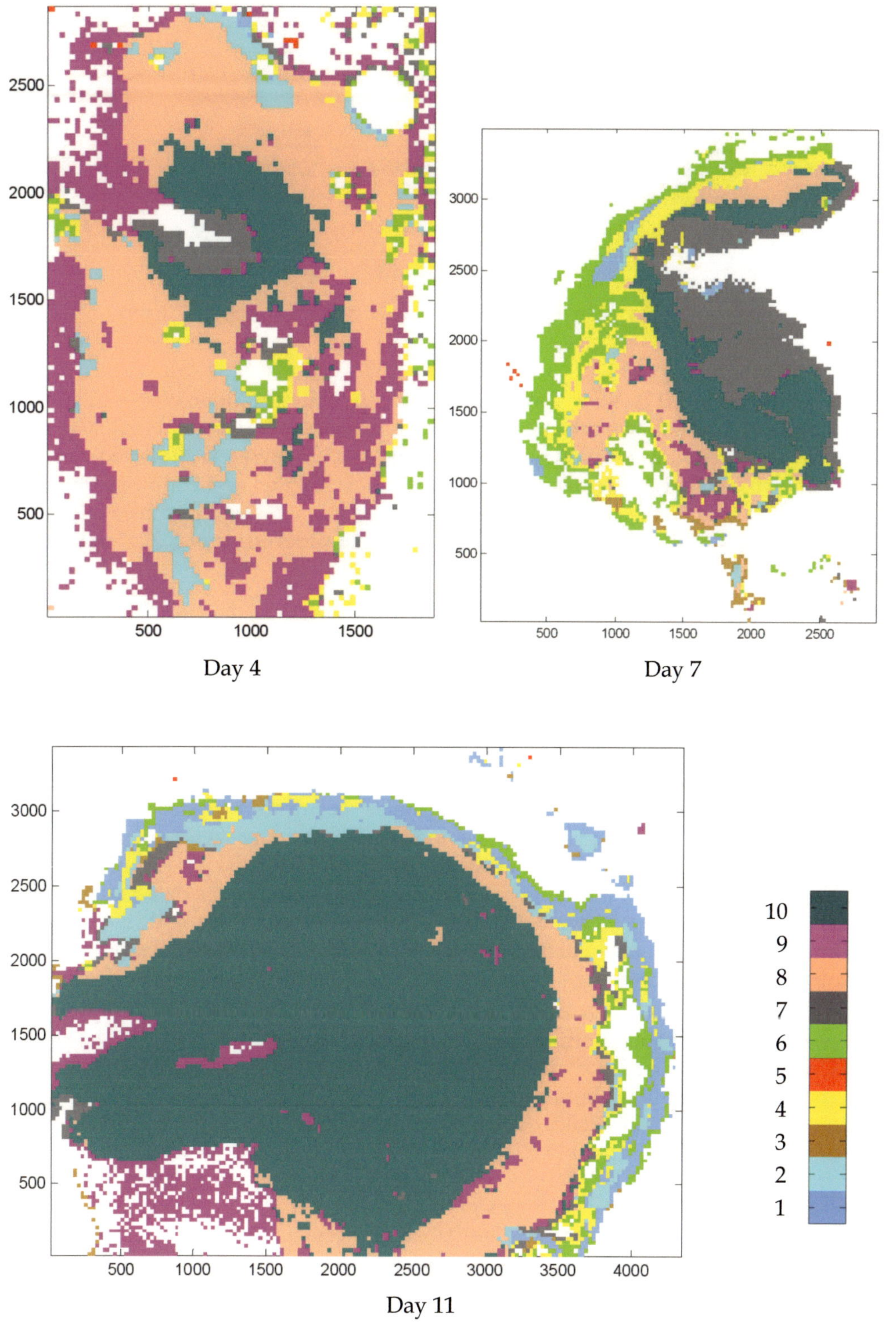
2500
2000
1500
1000
500
500 1000 1500
Day 4
3000
2500
2000
1500
1000
500
500 1000 1500 2000 2500
Day 7
3000
2500
2000
1500
1000
500
500 1000 1500 2000 2500 3000 3500 4000
Day 11
10
9
8
7
6
5
4
3
2
1

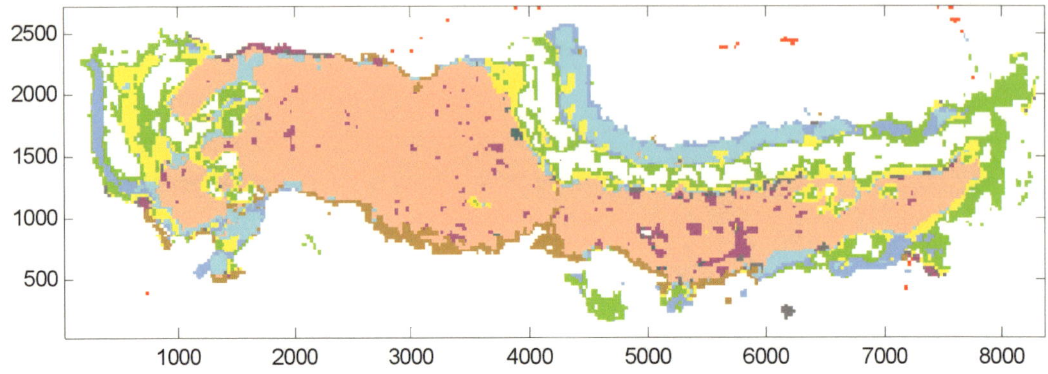


Fig. 2. All data measured on several skin tissues during tumor evolution were pooled in one dataset, processed at the same time to extract all features describing both normal and tumor tissues. Data were cut into the fingerprint region (900 to 1800 $cm^{-1}$) and cluster analysis was carried out on the first derivative spectra (to enhance the resolution of superimposed bands). K-means was calculated the cluster-membership of spectra by assigning each color to one class. Pseudo color FTIR maps on normal skin and tumor progression at 4, 7, 11 days post-implantation were constructed

were cut to fingerprint region (900 to 1800 $cm^{-1}$), converted to their first derivative, and smoothed using a seven point Savitzky-Golay algorithm in order to minimise the influence of background scatter in the spectra (Swieringa et al., 1999). The resulting spectra were then normalized using a Standard Normal Variate (SNV) procedure (Barnes and Dhanoa, 1989). A multivariate statistical analysis (Principal Component Analysis (PCA) and K-Means (KM)) was performed on this dataset. K-means clustering was performed on these principal component scores. Pseudo-color maps based on cluster analysis were then constructed by assigning a color to each spectral cluster. The cluster spectra were calculated by averaging absorbance spectra associated to each group and used for the interpretation of the chemical or biochemical differences between clusters. All data measured on normal skin and melanoma development (from 4 to 11 days growth) were pooled in one dataset, processed at the same time and the results were displayed as pseudo-color maps with the same color scale. In this way, we can easily determine all their common and discriminating features by comparing their infrared maps.

### 2.4 Discrimination between normal and melanoma progression

FTIR technique was used to identify biochemical changes associated to melanoma progression and invasion such as proteins, nucleic acid and lipids. Fig. 2 displays FTIR pseudo-color maps of skin tissues. 10 clusters describing both normal skin and cancer features were extracted and pseudo FTIR maps were constructed with the same color scale. Different clusters in the FTIR images were correlated to normal features. White color represents the area where no tissue was present. In the pseudo-color map obtained from normal skin, clusters 1 to 4 and 8 have described all normal structures. Cluster 8 encoded almost all normal skin and the other groups were associated to superficial skin layers. At day 4 post-implantation, two particular structures (clusters 7 and 10) were located in the melanoma cells injection site. These features were associated to B16 cell growth.

From day 7, the tumor is fairly large and deeply situated within the skin with massive infiltration into the tissue. Most of normal skin was destroyed by tumor tissue. Cluster 7 observed in the border of the tumor increased from 4 to 7 days post-implantation. This cluster disappeared and all tumor was described by cluster 10.

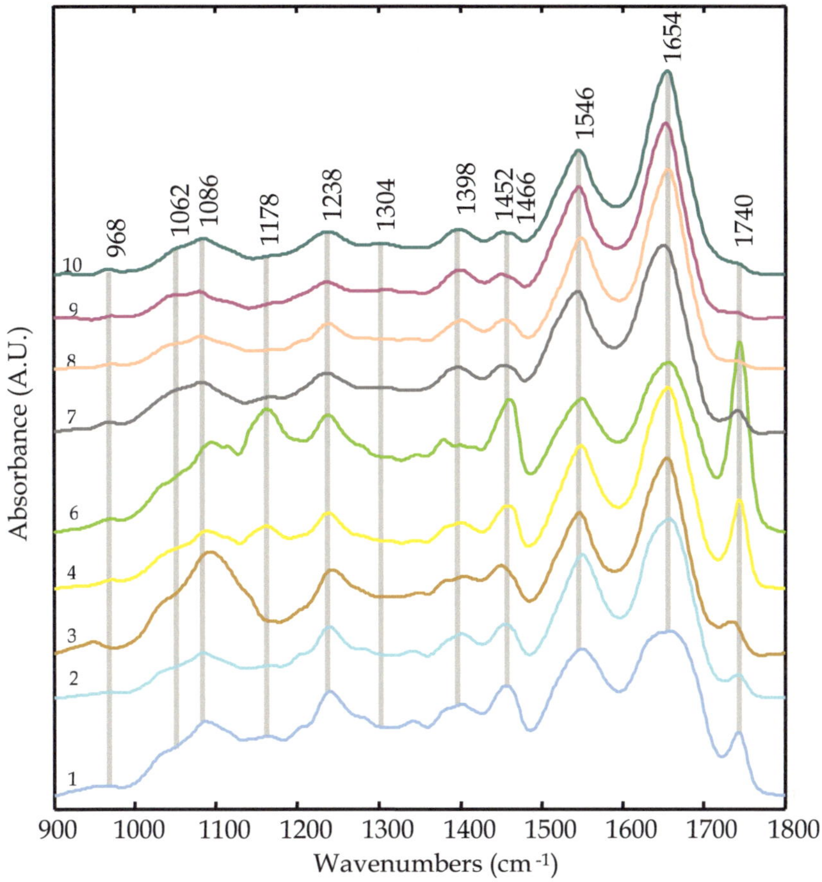


Fig. 3. Representative cluster mean FTIR spectra extracted from pseudocolor maps. Cluster averaged spectra were obtained by meaning absorbance spectra associated to each group. 10 models describing normal and melanoma skin development. Each cluster averaged spectrum assigned to one class was plotted with the same color than in pseudo-color map

Fig. 3 shows class average spectra of the normal skin and melanoma tumor tissues. These spectra are dominated by two absorbance bands at 1654 and 1546 $cm^{-1}$ known as the amide I and II, respectively. The band at 1740 $cm^{-1}$ arises from the stretching mode of C=O groups of lipids. The absorption band at 1398 is attributed to $COO^{-}$ symmetric stretching vibrations of fatty acids and amino acids. The bands at 1238 $cm^{-1}$ and 1086 $cm^{-1}$ are due to the antisymmetric and symmetric phosphate stretching mode $PO_2^{2-}$ of nucleic acids and phospholipids respectively. The relatively weak band at 1178 $cm^{-1}$, in the normal tissue is due to stretching mode of C–O groups of proteins. The band at 968 $cm^{-1}$ is attributed to the dianionic $PO_2{}^{2-}$ monoester of nucleic acids (DNA) and phospholipids. The bands at 1466

$cm^{-1}$ and 1452 $cm^{-1}$ were attributed respectively to $CH_2$ scissoring and antisymmetric deformation of $CH_3$ group. In normal skin, the intensity of antisymmetric deformation of $CH_3$ group (1452 $cm^{-1}$) is much greater than the intensity of the band at 1398 $cm^{-1}$ attributed to $COO^-$ symmetric stretching. However, in melanoma tumor, these two bands exhibit a similar intensity (clusters 7, 9, 10). Indeed, the band associated to C=O (1740 $cm^{-1}$) decreased from normal to melanoma tissues. Therefore in normal tissues, absorption from $CH_2$ groups of the lipid acyl chains dominates the band at 1466 $cm^{-1}$. In melanoma, these two bands arise predominantly from protein side chains. In a typical protein, side chains contain approximately equal proportions of $CH_2$ and $CH_3$ groups. The comparison between normal tissue and tumor counterpart shows a decreased and even disappearance of the bands at 1466 $cm^{-1}$ and 1740 $cm^{-1}$ associated to lipids and phospholipids in the melanoma tissues. Indeed, malignant tissues displayed the appearance of the band at 1062 $cm^{-1}$ attributed to the C–C stretching and a decrease in the intensity of the band at 1082 due to phospholipids diminution compared to normal tissues. The variations in the spectral characteristics between the normal and malignant tissues provided a basis for clinical application.

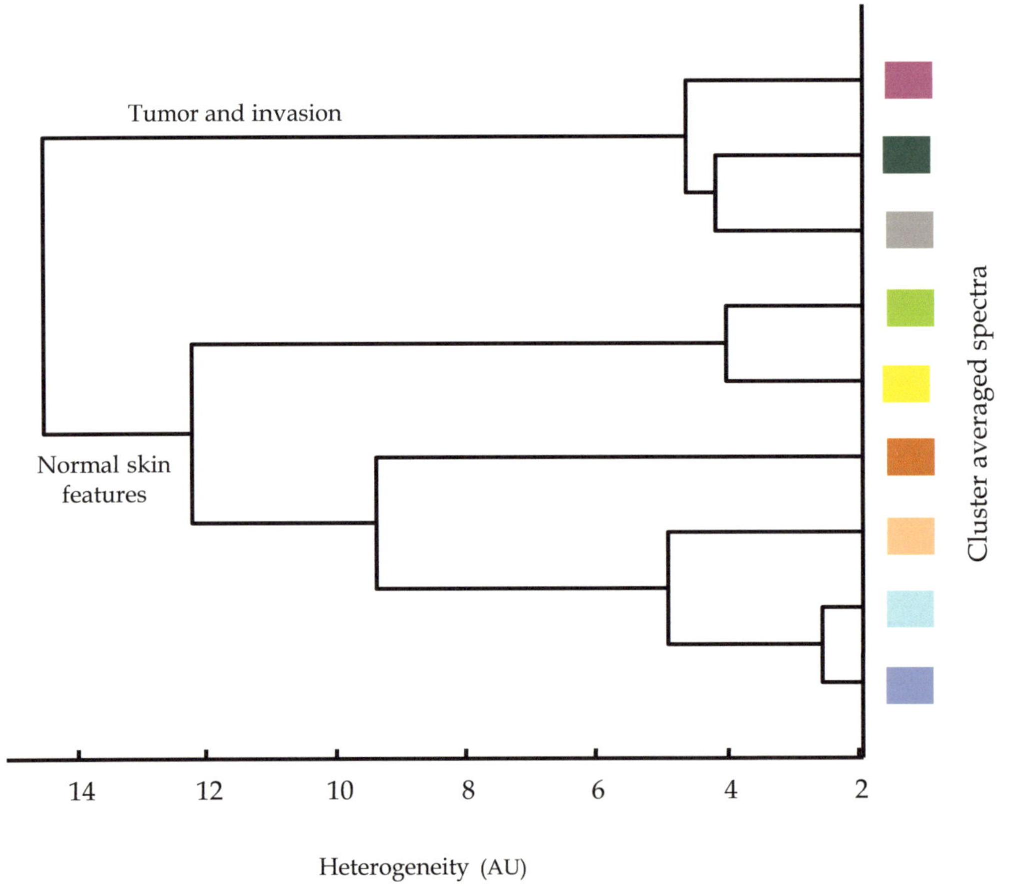


Fig. 4. Dendrogram obtained from hierarchical cluster analysis on spectral cluster averages associated to different tissue types. Heterogeneity represents the discriminating distance given by arbitrary units (AU)

We have used a cluster analysis to discriminate between normal and melanoma tissues. In fact, FTIR spectroscopy provides information on broad classes of molecules such as lipids, proteins, carbohydrates and make up the complex medium of cell and tissues. The spectrum from cells and tissues is an integration of these individual signals from all biomolecules (Diem et al., 2004). Since each molecular species is associated with specific frequencies, it may thus be possible to identify and quantify these biomolecules individually within the spectrum. Several authors have quantified individual constituents after tissue alteration. The models developed were used to explain the features present in the tissue/cellular spectra by using spectral data of pure molecules. The quantification of several biomolecules seen during tissue transformation can be used to classify disease states with high sensitivity, specificity, and accuracy. Wang et al. have investigated formalin-fixed Barrett's esophagus for predicting the underlying histopathology, the early detection and rapid staging of many diseases (Wang et al., 2007). Their model seems to be very accurate in spite of the presence of a number of common spectral features or molecular interactions and variations that can broaden individual peaks. Krafft *et al.* have developed a supervised classification model based on the LDA algorithm to IR images of three specimens from one patient (Krafft et al., 2007). There multivariate methods were used to develop a chemical/morphological model to quantify chemical composition of coronary atherosclerosis (Römer et al., 1998), breast tissue (Haka et al., 2005), porcine brain (Koljenovic et al., 2007), and molecular concentration profiles in the skin (Caspers et al., 2001).

To distinguish between normal and melanoma tissue, cluster averaged spectra obtained from pseudo-color maps were input in the hierarchical cluster analysis using Ward's clustering algorithm and the square Euclidian distance measure. Fig. 4 displayed the dendrogram associated to this classification. The result showed a clear distinction between all normal and tumor structures. Indeed, the class related to normal skin structures was divided to two sub-clusters associated to high lipid content (external layers) and low lipid constituents (internal layers).

## 3. Distribution of molecular changes in skin constituents associated to melanoma tumor

Peak ratios are commonly used to discriminate normal from tumor tissues. Krafft *et al.* have evaluated the usefulness of the lipid-to-protein ratio (2850/1655 $cm^{-1}$) as a spectroscopic marker to discriminate between normal and tumor tissue, as well as between low- and high-grade glioma tissues (krafft et al., 2007). We have investigated the spatial distribution of molecular changes between normal and melanoma. Integrated intensity bands ratio between the region 1360-1430 $cm^{-1}$ and 1430-1480 $cm^{-1}$, attributed to $COO^-$ symmetric stretching vibrations of fatty acids and amino acids and to $CH_2$ scissoring and antisymmetric deformation of $CH_3$ group respectively were calculated. Pseudo color maps scores were constructed (Fig. 5) in order to characterize the differences between healthy and pathological skin. The comparison between these pseudo color scores maps shows that high scores described the melanoma structure (colorbar). These scores decreased in the normal skin tissue. This intensity ratio was correlated to the changes in lipid content.

In our previous study, intensity ratios the 1466/1396$cm^{-1}$ (amino acid side chain from peptides and proteins at 1466 and 1396 $cm^{-1}$ were used to discriminate between normal and glioma brain tissue). Krafft et al. have demonstrated that this ratio is maximal for normal brain tissue and decreases with the progression of the disease (Krafft et al., 2007). Another study reported a significant differences between the spectra of malignant breast cancers and benign breast tissues in the relative intensity ratios of different peaks (I1640/ I1550 and I1160/I1120 for protein structures; I1640/I1460 and I1550/I1460 for relative content of protein and lipid; I1460/I1400 for lipid structures; I1310/I1240 for nucleic acid).

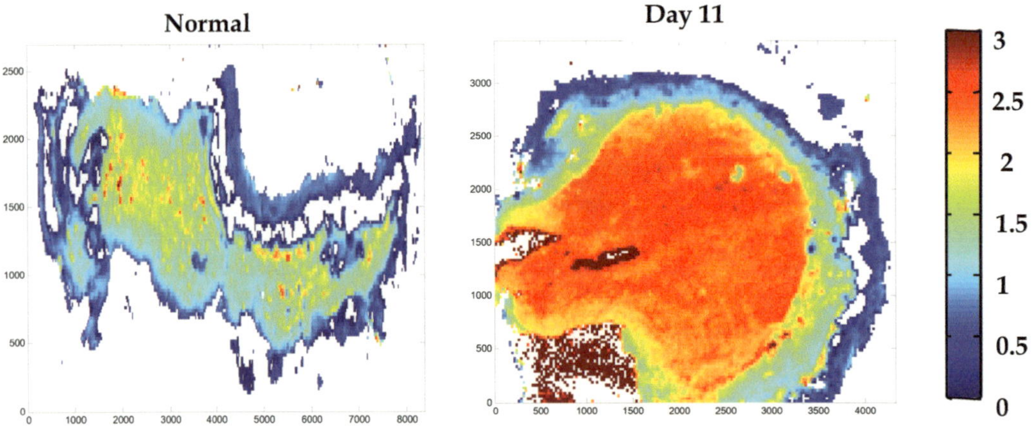


Fig. 5. Biochemical distribution of the changes in the molecular composition of tissues between normal and melanoma tumor at 11 days post-implantation. Maps of absorbance intensity ratios of bands in the region 1360-1430 and 1430-1480 were constructed and used to identify which biochemical markers could be more potential indicators of such variations between normal and melanoma tumor

## 4. Conclusion

In this study, we have demonstrated the potential of FTIR imaging combined to multivariate statistical analysis as rapid and objective tool to monitor the molecular histopathology alteration of skin tissue during melanoma growth without tissue staining. The identification and quantification of these specific molecular changes within skin can provide diagnostic information for aiding in early detection of diseases and their optimized treatment. We have monitored the molecular changes associated with melanoma growth and invasion by FTIRM imaging to better understand the tissue transformation during carcinogenesis.This study demonstrated that FT-IRM imaging, with high spatially resolved morphological and biochemical information can be used as a diagnostic tool to understand the tissue alteration. Multivariate statistical analysis such as cluster analysis allowed investigation of B16 melanoma progression (from day 4 to day 11 post implantation). Different clusters in the FTIR images were correlated to morphological and histological features. Our results showed that at 4 days after tumor implantation, FTIR investigations displayed a very small abnormal zone associated with the proliferation of B16 cells in the injection site. From this day, mice developed solid and well-circumscribed tumors. By using imaging technique, we were able to take in account the variance due to the heterogeneity of skin tissues. These constituents can be used as spectroscopic markers for early detection of tissue abnormality and discrimination among normal, invasion, and tumor.

## 5. References

Amharref, N., Beljebbar, A., Dukic, S., Venteo, L., Schneider, L., Pluot, M., Vistelle, R.. & Manfait, M. (2006). Brain tissue characterisation by infrared imaging in a rat glioma model. *Biochim. Biophys. Acta*, Vol. 1758, No. 7, (07.2006) 892-899, ISSN 00052736

Barnes, R.J., Dhanoa, M.S. & Lister, S.J. (1989). Standard normal variate transformation and de-trending of near-infrared diffuse reflectance spectra. *Appl. Spectrosc.*, Vol. 43, No. 5, (07.1989), pp. 772-777, ISSN 00037028

Bates, J.B. (1976). Fourier transform infrared spectroscopy. *Science, Vol.* 9, No. 191, 4222, (01.1976), pp. 31-37, ISSN 00368075

Beljebbar, A., Amharref, N., Lévèques, A., Dukic, S., Venteo, L., Schneider, L., Pluot, M., & Manfait, M. (2008). Modeling and quantifying biochemical changes in C6 tumor gliomas by Fourier transform infrared imaging. *Anal. Chem.*, Vol. 15, No 80, (11.2008), pp. 8406-8415, ISSN 00032700

Beljebbar, A., Amharref, N., Lévèques, A., Dukic, S., Venteo, L., Schneider, L., Pluot, M., & Manfait M. (2008). Modeling and quantifying biochemical changes in C6 tumor gliomas by Fourier transform infrared imaging. *Anal. Chem, Vol.*80, No22, (11.2008), pp. 8406-8415, ISSN 1520-6882

Bhargava, R. & Levin, I.W. (2004). Gram-Schmidt orthogonalization for rapid reconstructions of Fourier transform infrared spectroscopic imaging data. *Appl. Spectrosc.*, Vol. 58, No. 8, (08.2004), pp. 995–1000, ISSN 0003-7028

Caspers, P.J., Lucassen, G.W., & Puppels, G.J. (2003). Combined in vivo confocal Raman spectroscopy and confocal microscopy of human skin. *Biophys. J.*, Vol. 85, No. 1, (07.2003), pp.52–61, ISSN 0006-3495

Caspers, P.J., Lucassen, G.W., Carter, E.A., Bruining, H.A. & Puppels, G.J. (2001). In vivo confocal Raman microspectroscopy of the skin: noninvasive determination of molecular concentration profiles. *J. Invest. Dermatol.*, Vol. 116, No. 3, (03.2001), pp. 434-442, ISSN 0022-202X

Cohenford, M.A. & Rigas B. (1998). Cytologically normal cells from neoplastic cervical samples display extensive structural abnormalities on IR spectroscopy: implications for tumor biology. *Proc. Natl. Acad. Sci. U S A.*, Vol. 95, No. 26, (12.1998), pp. 15327–15332, ISSN 00278424

Dary, C.C., Blancato J.N. & Saleh, M.A. (2001). Chemomorphic analysis of malathion in skin layers of the rat: implications for the use of dermatopharmacokinetic tape stripping in exposure assessment to pesticides. *Regul. Toxicol. Pharmacol.*, Vol. 34, No. 3, (12.2001), pp. 234–248, ISSN 0273-2300

Diem, M., Boydston-White, S. & Chiriboga, L. (1999). Infrared spectroscopy of cells and tissues: shining light onto a novel subject. *Appl. Spectrosc.*, Vol. 53, No. 4, pp. 148-161, ISSN 00037028

Diem, M., Romeo, M., Boydston-White, S., Miljković, M. & Matthäus, C. (2004). A decade of vibrational micro-spectroscopy of human cells and tissue (1994-2004).*Analyst*, Vol. 129, No. 10, (10.2004), pp. 880–885, ISSN 0003-2654

Elder, D.E. (2006). Pathology of melanoma. *Clin. Cancer Res.*, Vol. 12, No. 7 Pt 2, (01.2006), pp. 2308s–2311s, ISSN 1078-0432

Fernandez, D.C., Bhargava, R., Hewitt, S.M.& Levin, I.W. (2005). Infrared spectroscopic imaging for histopathologic recognition. *Nature Biotechnology,* Vol. 23, No. 4, pp. 469-474, ISSN 10870156

Garidel, P. (2002). Mid-FTIR-Microspectroscopy of stratum corneum single cells and stratum corneum tissue *Phys. Chem. Chem. Phys.*, Vol. 4, No. 22, pp. 5671–5677, ISSN 1463-9076

Goodacre, R., Vaidyanathan, S., Dunn, W.B., Harrigan, G.G. & Kell, D.B. (2004). Metabolomics by numbers: Acquiring and understanding global metabolite data, *Trends Biotechnol.*, Vol. 22, No. 5, (05.2004), pp. 245–252, ISSN 01677799

Haka, A.S., Shafer-Peltier, K.E., Fitzmaurice, M., Crowe, J., Dasari, R.R. &Feld, M.S. (2005). Diagnosing breast cancer by using Raman spectroscopy. *Proc. Natl. Acad. Sci. USA*, Vol. 102, No. 35, (08.2005), pp. 12371–12376, ISSN 0027-8424

Hammody, Z., Agrov, S., Sahu, R.K., Cagnano, E., Moreh, R. & Mordechai, S. (2008). Distinction of malignant melanoma and epidermis using IR micro-spectroscopy and statistical methods. *Analyst*, Vol. 133, No. 3, (03.2008), pp. 372–378, ISSN 0003-2654

Hammody, Z., Sahu, R.K., Mordechai, S., Cagnano E. & Argov, S. (2005). Characterization of malignant melanoma using vibrational spectroscopy. *Sci. World J.*, Vol. 5, No. 5, (03.2005), pp.173–182, ISSN 1537-744X

Jackson, M., Ramjiawan, B., Hewko, M., & Mantsch, H.H.. (1998). Infrared microscopic functional group mapping and spectral clustering analysis of hypercholesteramic rabbit liver. *Cell. Mol. Biol.*, Vol. 44, No. 1, (02.1998), pp. 89–98, ISSN 01455680

James, W.D., Berger ,T.G. & D. Elston, Andrews' Diseases of the Skin, 9th ed. 2000, Philadelphia, pp. 881–889

Jeffs, A. R. , Glover, A. C., Slobbe, L. J., Wang, L. , He, S.J., Hazlett, J.A., Awasthi, A., Woolley, A.G., Marshall, E.S., Joseph W.R., Print C.G., Baguley B.C. & Eccles M.R., (2009) A gene expression signature of invasive potential in metastatic melanoma cells.PLoS One, Vol., No12, (12.2009), pp. e8461, ISSN 1932-6203

Joseph-Pietras, D., Carlier, A., Madoulet, C. & Albert, Ph. (2007). Cytostatic murine B16 cell pulsed Dendritic Cells induce effective protection against melanoma in mice. *Anticancer Res.*, Vol. 27, No. 6B, (11.2007), pp. 3863-3872, ISSN 0250-7005

Joseph-Pietras, D., Carlier, A., Madoulet, C. and Albert, Ph. (2006). Anti-tumoral activity of peripheral blood mononuclear cells against melanoma cells: discrepant *in vitro* and *in vivo* effects. *Melanoma Res.*, Vol. 16, No. 4, (08.2006), pp. 325-33, ISSN 0960-8931

Koljenovic, S. Bakker Schut, T.C.,Wolthuis, R.,Vincent, A.J., Hendriks-Hagevi, G., Santos, L., Kros, J.M.& Puppels, G.J. (2007). Raman spectroscopic characterization of porcine brain tissue using a single fiber-optic probe. *Anal. Chem.*, Vol. 79, No. 2, (01.2007), pp. 557-564, ISSN 0003-2700

Krafft, C. & Sergo V. (2006). Biomedical applications of Raman and infrared spectroscopy to diagnose tissue. *Spectrosc. Int. J.*, Vol. 20, No. 5, (01.2006), pp. 195–218, ISSN 0712-4813

Krafft, C., Neudert, L., Simat, T., & Salzer, R. (2005). Near infrared Raman spectra of human brain lipids. *Spectrochim. Acta (Part A),* Vol. 61, No. 7, (05 2005), pp. 1529-1535, ISSN 13861425

Krafft, C., Sobottka, S.B., Geiger, K.D., Schackert, G., & Salzer, R. (2007). Classification of malignant gliomas by infrared spectroscopic imaging and linear discriminant analysis. *Anal. Bioanal. Chem.*, Vol. 387, No. 5, (03 2007), pp. 1669-1677, ISSN 16182642

Krafft, C., Sobottka, S.B., Schackert, G., & Salzer R. (2006). Raman and infrared spectroscopic mapping of human primary intracranial tumors: A comparative study. *J. Raman Spectrosc.*, Vol. 37, No. 1-3, (01 2006), pp. 367-375, ISSN 03770486

Lasch, P & Naumann D. (1998). FT-IR microspectroscopic imaging of human carcinoma thin sections based on pattern recognition techniques. *Cell. Mol. Biol.*, Vol. 44, No. 1, (02.1998), pp. 189–202, ISSN 01455680

Lasch, P., Haensch, W., Naumann, D., & Diem, M. (2004). Imaging of colorectal adenocarcinoma using FT-IR microspectroscopy and cluster analysis. *Biochim Biophys Acta., Vol.* 1688, No. 2, (03.2004), pp. 176–186, ISSN 09254439

Ly, E., Piot, O., Wolthuis, R., Durlach, A., Bernard, P. & Manfait, M. (2008). Combination of FTIR spectral imaging and chemometrics for tumour detection from paraffin-embedded biopsies. *Analyst*, Vol. 133, No. 2, (02.2008), pp. 197–205, ISSN 0003-2654

Mendelsohn, R., Chen, H.C., Rerek, M.E. & Moore, D. J. (2003). Infrared microspectroscopic imaging maps the spatial distribution of exogenous molecules in skin. *J. Biomed. Opt.*, Vol. 8, No. 2, (04.2003), pp. 185–190, ISSN 1083-3668

Mendelsohn, R., Flach, C.R. & Moore, D.J. (2006). Determination of molecular conformation and permeation in skin via IR spectroscopy, microscopy, and imaging. *Biochim. Biophys. Acta, Biomembr.*, Vol. 1758, No. 7, (07.2006), pp. 923–933, ISSN 0006-3002

Mohlenhoff, B., Romeo, M., Diem, M., & Wood, B.R. (2005). Mie-type scattering and non-Beer-Lambert absorption behaviour of human cells in infrared microspectroscopy. *Biophys J., Vol.* 88, No. 5, (05.2005), pp. 3635–3640, ISSN 00063495

Morganti, F., Bramanti, E., Solaro, R., Benedetti, E., Chiellini, E., Nannipieri, E., Narducci, P., Krauser, S.F. & Samour, C.M. (1999) Thermal and spectroscopic characterization of interactions between 2-nonyl-1,3-dioxolane and stratum corneum components. *J. Bioact. Compat. Polym.*, Vol. 14, No. 2, (03.1999), pp. 162–177, ISSN 08839115

Mourant, J.R., Yamada, Y.R. Carpenter, S., Dominique, L.R. & Freyer, J.P. (2003). FTIR spectroscopy demonstrates biochemical differences in mammalian cell cultures at different growth stages. *Biophys. J.*, Vol. 85, No. 3, (09.2003) 1938–1947, ISSN 00063495

Odot, J., Albert, Ph., Carlier, A., Tarpin, M., Devy, J. & Madoulet C. (2004). *In vitro* and *in vivo* anti-tumoral effect of curcumin against melanoma cells. *Int. J. Cancer*, Vol. 111, No. 3, (09.2004), pp. 381-387, ISSN 0020-7136

Parker, F. S., (1971). *Application of infrared spectroscopy in biochemistry, biology and medicine* Plenum, New York

Petibois, C. & Déléris, G. (2006). Chemical mapping of tumor progression by FT-IR imaging: towards molecular histopathology. *Trends in Biotechnology*, Vol. 24, No. 10, (08.2006), pp. 455-462, ISSN 01677799

Pirot, F., Kalia, Y.N., Stinchcomb, A.L., Keating, G., Bunge, A. & Guy, R.H. (1997). Characterization of the permeability barrier of human skin in vivo. *Proc. Natl. Acad. Sci US, Vol.* 94, No. 4, (02.1997), pp.1562–1567, ISSN 0027-8424

Rigas, B., Morgello, S., Goldman, I., & Wong, P. (1990). Human colorectal cancers display abnormal Fourier-transform infrared spectra. *Proc. Natl. Acad. Sci. USA*, Vol. 87, No. 20, (10.1990), pp. 8140–8144, ISSN 00278424

Römer, T.J., Brennan, J.F., Fitzmaurice, M., Feldstein, M.L., Deinum, G., Myles, J.L., Kramer, J.R., Lees, R.S., Feld, M.S. (1998). Histopathology of human coronary atherosclerosis by quantifying its chemical composition with Raman spectroscopy. *Circulation*, Vol. 10, No. 9, (03.1998), pp. 878-885, ISSN 0009-7322

Savitzky, A. & Golay, M.J.E. (1964). Smoothing and differentiation of data by simplified least squares procedures. Anal. *Chem.*, Vol. 36, No. 8, (08 1964), pp. 1627-1639, ISSN 0003-2700

Slater, D.N. (2000). Doubt and uncertainty in the diagnosis of melanoma. *Histopathology*, Vol. 37, No. 5, (11.2000), pp. 469–472, ISSN 1365-2559

Swieringa, H., de Weijer A.P., van Wijk, R.J.& Buydens, L.M.C. (1999). Strategy for Constructing Robust Multivariate Calibration Models. *Chemometrics and Intelligent laboratory systems*, Vol. 49, No. 1, pp. 1-28, ISSN 0169-7439

Tetteh, J., Mader, K.T., Andanson, J.M., McAuley, W.J., Lane, M.E., Hadgraft, J., Kazarian, S.G. & Mitchell, J.C. (2009). Local examination of skin diffusion using FTIR spectroscopic imaging and multivariate target factor analysis. *Anal. Chim. Acta*, Vol. 642, No. 1-2, (05.2009), pp. 246–256, ISSN 1873-4324

Tfayli, A., Piot, O., Durlach, A., Bernard, P. & Manfait, M. (2005). Discriminating nevus and melanoma on paraffin-embedded skin biopsies using FTIR microspectroscopy. *Biochim. Biophys. Acta, Gen. Subj.*, Vol. 1724, No. 3, (08.2005), pp. 262–269, ISSN 0006-3002

Thompson, J.F., Scolyer, R.A. & Kefford, R .F. (2005). Cutaneous melanoma, *Lancet*, Vol., 365, No. 9460, (02.2005), pp. 687–701, ISSN 1474-547X

van Kempen, L.C., Ruiter, D., van Muijen, G.N. & Coussens, L.M. (2003). The tumor microenvironment: a critical determinant of neoplastic evolution. *Eur. J. Cell Biol.*, Vol. 82, No. 11, (11.2003), pp. 539–548, ISSN 0171-9335

Wang, T.D., Triadafilopoulos, G., Crawford, J.M.,, Dixon, L.R., Bhandari, T., Sahbaie, P., Friedland, S., Soetikno, R., and Contag, C.H. (2007) Detection of endogenous biomolecules in Barrett's esophagus by Fourier transform infrared spectroscopy. *Proc. Natl. Acad. Sci. USA*, Vol. 104, No. 40, (10.2007), pp. 15864–15869, ISSN 0027-8424

Wong, P.T., Wong, R.K., Caputo, T.A., Godwin, T.A. & Rigas, B. (1991). Infrared spectroscopy of exfoliated human cervical cells: Evidence of extensive structural changes during carcinogenesis. *Proc. Natl. Acad. Sci. USA*, Vol. 88, No. 24, (12.1991), pp. 10988–10992, ISSN 00278424

Wong, P.T.T., Goldstein, S.M., Grekin, R.C., Godwin, T.A., Pivik, C. & Rigas, B. (1993). Distinct infrared spectroscopic patterns of human basal cell carcinoma of the skin. Cancer Res., Vol. 53, No. 4, (02.1993), pp. 762–765, ISSN 0008-5472

Zhang, G.J., Moore, D.J., Flach, C. R. & Mendelsohn, R. (2007). Vibrational microscopy and imaging of skin: from single cells to intact tissue. *Anal. Bioanal. Chem.*, Vol. 387, No. 5, (03.2007), pp. 1591–1599, ISSN 1618-2642

Zhang, L., Small, G.W., Haka, A.S., Kidder, L.H., & Lewis, E.N. (2003). Classification of Fourier transform infrared microspectroscopic imaging data of human breast cells by cluster analysis and artificial neural networks. *Appl. Spectrosc.*, Vol. 57, No. 1, (01.2003), pp. 14–22, ISSN 00037028

Zhou, S., Xu, Z., Ling, X.F., Li, Q.B., Xu, Y.Z., Zhang, L., Zhao, H.M., Wang, L.X., Hou, K.Y., Zhou, X.S. & Wu JG. (2006). FTIR spectroscopic characterization of freshly removed breast cancer tissues. *Zhonghua Zhong Liu Za Zhi.*,Vol. 28, No. 7, (07.2006), pp. 512-514, ISSN 0253-3766

# Part 6

# Treatments and Therapies

# 20

# Ion Channels as Promising Therapeutic Targets for Melanoma

Aurélie Chantôme[1], Marie Potier-Cartereau[1], Sébastien Roger[1], Christophe Vandier[1], Olivier Soriani[2] and Virginie Joulin[3]
*[1]Inserm, U921, Tours, 37032 France; Université François Rabelais, Tours, 37032*
*[2]CNRS UMR 6543, Institut de Biologie du Développement et Cancer, 06108 Nice,*
*[3]Inserm U1009, Institut Gustave Roussy, Villejuif, 94805*
*France*

## 1. Introduction

Even cancer is far from being considered a channelopathy; the field of ion and protein channel research in cancer is highly important as an emerging and proven point of intervention in disease. Like membrane receptors, ion channels are directly connected with and sensitive to the extracellular environment. During the last decade, the number of ion-channel types expressed in various cancers, including melanoma, was rapidly increased. Moreover several ion channels are selectively expressed in aggressive cancers and seem to be implicated in metastasis development. The growing number of patents relative to cancer therapy targeting channel proteins testifies to the interest of such novel therapeutic approaches.

The physiological significance of ion channels and transporters, as illustrated by the award of four Nobel Prizes in Physiology or Medicine (1963; 1991) and Chemistry (1997, 2003), is now accepted and established. Unlike transporters and exchangers, channel proteins form a pore through membranes allowing the selective passage of one or more ions (e.g. $K^+$, $Na^+$, $Cl^-$), molecules (water) or charged atoms, through the lipid bilayer that is impermeable to these compounds. The modalities of channel opening or activation are diverse and varied: this can be performed by an external molecular stimulus (e.g. ligand), by a mechanical stimulus (e.g. cell volume, membrane tension or stretch), by electric stimuli (e.g. changes in membrane potential), by an intracellular second messenger (e.g. calcium, cAMP). Thus the classification of the channels (IUPHAR classification) is based on the channel activation mode and on the selective permeability of molecular species specific to each channel. Channel proteins are involved in the control of numerous and various physiological functions. Basically, these channels are responsible for a universal property for cellular membranes: the existence of resting membrane potential. Ion channels, mainly studied in excitable cells like muscle and neurons, are responsible for the transmission of the electric signals triggering physiological and biological phenomena such as nerve conduction or the cellular phenomenon of excitation - contraction coupling. Ion transporter ($Na^+/K^+$-ATPase or simply known as sodium pump) is the membrane pump that generates the $Na^+$ and $K^+$ gradients across the plasma membrane, driving many physiological processes. Another class of channels, water channels or aquaporins (AQP), allow water molecules to pass through the membrane much faster than by simple diffusion through the lipid bilayer, while preventing the ions to enter or exit the cell. Finally, channels participate in ionic homeostasis and in controlling the shape of the cell by regulating the water flows.

If in a physiological context, the expression of a particular channel protein is specific in one or several tissues or organs, conferring an appropriate biological function, this is not that is observed in a tumour context. As a general rule, the cancer cell hijacks a channel's normal physiological function to drive certain essential biological functions for tumour development (such as proliferation and migration/invasion). Melanoma cells are considered to be electrically non-excitable, however they express several types of voltage-activated channels (Allen et al., 1997), which is unusual in a non-excitable cell. Because melanocytes originated from neural crest-derived precursors, they have retained significant neuronal ability. It is therefore not surprising that melanocytes (and *a fortiori* melanoma cells) can express (re-express), ion channels involved in excitatory or sensory functions.

Data on the level of channel expression in melanocytes *versus* melanoma cells are highly fragmented. Few cases of aberrant expression between melanocytes *versus* melanoma cells have been described. 1) The channel is expressed only in melanoma cells but not in melanocytes and it helps in a particular biological function (*e.g.* enhanced cell migration by hijacking the $Ca^{2+}$ activated $K^{+}$ channel SK3/KCa2.3). 2) The channel is expressed by non-malignant melanocytes and is not functional in this context but acquires a function during the melanocyte-to-melanoma transition (*e.g.* anti-apoptotic activity of the P2X7 receptor). 3) Inversely, the expression of the channel belonging to transient receptor potential (TRP) cation channel subfamily M, TRPM1/Melastatin-1/MLSN-1, is decreased in melanomas according to melanoma aggressiveness and is useful as a prognostic marker for melanoma metastasis (see for review (Prevarskaya et al., 2007)). However, data and information relative to non-malignant melanocyte channel expression or function are scarce and have to be continued. Table 1 summarizes the channels expressed by and active in melanoma cells and/or melanocyte, and their assigned function.

Among channels expressed by melanoma cells, some of them contribute to cell survival, like the store-operated channel (SOC) and the P2X7R receptor, or to cell proliferation, like the SKCa channel SK2/KCa2.2 and the $Ca^{2+}$-permeable channel TRPM8. Note that the ultimate function of those $Ca^{2+}$-permeable channels is to favour $Ca^{2+}$ entry into a cell. In melanoma cells, several of channels, the voltage-dependent $Na^{+}$ channel Nav1.6, the SKCa channel SK3/KCa2.3 and the water channel AQP1, are involved in cell adherence and migration that, *in fine*, it might confer a metastatic ability.

Lastly, the significant role of channel proteins in melanomagenesis is reinforced by the systematic overexpression of the sigma 1 receptor in many types of cancer including melanoma. Even if the sigma 1 receptor is still an enigma, its most well-known action in biological systems is the regulation and modulation of many ion channels, including those known to be involved in melanoma cell biology, suggesting the existence of tumour specific channel macro-complexes. On the other hand, proliferation, apoptosis resistance and migration/adhesion of cancer cells are impaired by the modulation of sigma 1 receptor activity through mechanisms involving ion channels. By its aberrant expression in melanoma, the use of the sigma 1 receptor as a target for an imaging tracer (using a PET imaging probe) and for the specific delivery of therapeutic agents (using synthetic sigma ligands) is currently the subject of intensive investigation.

| Ion Channel Name | Ion Channel Type | Biological function in Melanoma | Expression | | References |
|---|---|---|---|---|---|
| | | | Melanocyte | Melanoma | |
| SOC | *Store Operated Channel* | Cell survival | *n.d.* | Murine (B16) melanoma cell line | (Fedida-Metula et al., 2008; Feldman et al., 2010) |
| P2X7R | *ATP-gated cation-permeable ionotropic receptor* | Cell death Cell invasiveness? | yes (not functional) | Human melanoma cell lines & MDA-MB-435S cell line | (Bringmann et al., 2001; Deli et al., 2007; Greig et al., 2003; Ohshima et al., 2010; Slater et al., 2003; Timar et al., 2006; White et al., 2005) |
| $Na^+/K^+$ pump ($\alpha$1 subunit) | *Ion transporter* | Cell survival Cell proliferation | | Human metastatic melanoma (clinical samples & cell lines) | (Mathieu et al., 2009) |
| TRPM8 | *TRPC* | Cell death | *n.d.* | Human melanoma (clinical samples & cell lines) | (Yamamura et al., 2008a) |
| SK2/KCa2.2 | *$K^+$ channel* | Cell proliferation under hypoxia | yes | Human melanoma cell lines | (Chantôme et al., 2009; Meyer et al., 1999; Tajima et al., 2006) |
| EAG | *$K^+$ channel* | Cell proliferation | *n.d.* | Melanoma cell lines | (Gavrilova-Ruch et al., 2002; Meyer et al., 1999; Pardo & Suhmer, 2008) |
| hERG | *$K^+$ channel* | Cell proliferation, migration, invasion | *n.d.* | MDA-MB-435S cell line | (Afrasiabi et al., 2010) |
| SK3/KCa2.3 | *$K^+$ channel* | Cell migration and/or invasion | no | Human melanoma cell lines | (Chantôme et al., 2009) |
| KCa3.1/IKCa | *$K^+$ channel* | Cell migration and/or invasion? | yes | Human melanoma cell lines | (Schmidt et al., 2010; Schwab et al., 1999) |
| Nav1.6 | *Voltage gated $Na^+$ channel* | Cell migration and/or invasion | *n.d.*. | Human melanoma (HTB-26) cell line | (Carrithers et al., 2009) |
| AQP1 | *Water channel* | Cell migration and/or invasion | *n.d.* | Human (WM115) & murine (B16) melanoma cell lines | (Hu & Verkman, 2006; Monzani et al., 2009; Saadoun et al., 2005) |
| Cav 1.3(a) | *Voltage gated $Ca^{2+}$ channel* | Cell migration and/or invasion | *n.d.* | Human (A375M, C8161) melanoma cell lines | (Yohem et al., 1991) |
| Sigma-1 receptor | *Chaperone protein* | Cell migration | | Human melanoma (clinical samples & cell lines) | (Friebe et al., 2001; Megalizzi et al., 2007) |
| Kv1.3 | *$K^+$ channel* | Cell adherence | *n.d.*. | Human melanoma (LOX) cell line | (Artym & Petty, 2002) |
| Pkd2 | *Non-selective cation channel* | Cell adherence | *n.d.* | Murine melanoma cell lines | (Bian et al., 2010) |

| | | | | | |
|---|---|---|---|---|---|
| TASK-3 | *Two-pore $K^+$ channel* | Unknown | yes | Human melanoma cell lines | (Pocsai et al., 2006; Rusznak et al., 2008) |
| TRPM2 | *TRPC* | Unknown | no | Melanoma cell lines | (Orfanelli et al., 2008) |
| TRPM1 | *TRPC* | Unknown | yes | No in human melanoma metastases | (Duncan et al., 1998) |
| ENaC delta | *$Na^+$ channel* | Unknown | *n.d.* | Human melanoma cell lines | (Yamamura et al., 2008b) |

(a) Expression of Cav 1.3 has been indirectly determined using Verapamil, a $Ca^{2+}$ channel blocker.
*TRPC*: Transient Receptor Potential Channel; *n.d.*: not determined

Table 1. Summary of ion channels expressed in melanoma

Our understanding of the action of channel proteins in cancer has just begun to take shape. Despite the advancements over the past two decades in defining the expression and the role of channel proteins in melanoma, many questions remain unanswered. For example, can a particular channel protein be a marker of a specific phenotype of melanoma? Is there particular intracellular signalling machinery involved for an ionic channel tumour function? As channel proteins are hijacked from their normal physiological function: Do channel proteins adopt a different folded conformation in a tumour context compared to a physiological context? Do channels form different protein complexes in a physiological context compared to tumour context? Regarding to these two last questions, do channel proteins link to a particular membrane tumour environment (*e.g.* lipid, raft)? Answering the last three questions will help design specific therapeutic approaches targeting channel proteins, that will make it possible to avoid side effects.

This review aims to identify the data of the literature that reported expression of proteins known to form ion channels and found to be expressed by cutaneous melanoma cells, and, whenever possible, to precise the biological function that has been assigned to them in this tumour context. A critical analysis on the druggable nature of these channel proteins will be presented. The cutaneous malignant melanoma being one of the cancers that has a greater metastatic potential, we shall pay a particular attention to the channels participating in the motility (migration and invasion) of the cancer cell. With the development of personalized targeted therapies, we are entitled to wonder if each channel protein, hijacked from its physiological function by the cancer cell, can indeed be considered as relevant therapeutic targets.

## 2. Ion channels and cell survival and apoptosis

### 2.1 Store-operated channels (SOCs)

Malignant melanoma is characterized by its extreme resistance to cell death-inducing factor (Becker et al., 2006; Soengas & Lowe, 2003). The molecular derangement underlying the low susceptibility of melanoma cells to apoptosis include an aberrant activation of protein kinase PKB/Akt. Indeed, high resting PKB activity in the murine metastatic melanoma clone B16BL6, promotes their serum independent growth and protects these cells from apoptosis (Assa-Kunik et al., 2003). In contrast, non-tumour cells are sensitive to cell death-inducing factors associated to a very low basal activity of PKB (Assa-Kunik et al., 2003). Elevated level of PKB activity is a common finding in lesions of advanced melanoma (Dai et al., 2005; Slipicevic et al., 2005) and inversely correlates with patient survival (Dai et al., 2005). One of the activation pathways of PKB involves the complex calcium ($Ca^{2+}$)/calmodulin associated

(Dong et al., 2007) with functional Store-Operated Channels (SOCs) (Fedida-Metula et al., 2008). In most non-excitable, cells depletion of endoplasmic reticulum (ER) stores elicits sustained $Ca^{2+}$ influx by SOCs in plasma membrane, defining the major $Ca^{2+}$ influx pathway (Putney, 1986). Following ER depletion, the ER $Ca^{2+}$ sensor Stim1 forms multimers and migrates to ER/plasma membrane junctions where they activate a non-voltage-gated channel called $Ca^{2+}$ release-activated $Ca^{2+}$ (CRAC) channel, Orai. The CRAC current is characterized by a very low single channel conductance, a high $Ca^{2+}$ selectivity, an inward rectification and a complex regulation by both intra and extracellular $Ca^{2+}$ (Parekh & Putney, 2005).

$Ca^{2+}$ storage inside the ER is an essential indicator of the cell's proliferative, metabolic and apoptotic status. The retrograde signalling process from ER $Ca^{2+}$ depletion to store-operated $Ca^{2+}$ entry (SOCE) activation has a central role for many cellular and physiological functions (Lewis, 2001). Thus, coordinated regulatory mechanisms must exist in the cell to ensure tight control of SOCs function. Among all key regulators of intracellular $Ca^{2+}$ homeostasis, trans-mitochondrial $Ca^{2+}$ transport is one of the most important, particularly in the sub-plasmalemmal and ER (Demaurex et al., 2009; Parekh, 2008) thanks to the mitochondrial uniporter (mCU) (Demaurex et al., 2009; Parekh, 2008; Rizzuto & Pozzan, 2006). In addition to regulate $Ca^{2+}$ homeostasis in these micro-domains, the ability of mitochondria to take up and release $Ca^{2+}$ impacts on SOCE process (Glitsch et al., 2002). More clearly, mitochondria have been shown to modulate SOCE by buffering incoming $Ca^{2+}$, so this dissipation of high $Ca^{2+}$ micro domains is critical for sustained $Ca^{2+}$ entry (Demaurex et al., 2009; Gilabert et al., 2001; Gilabert & Parekh, 2000; Malli et al., 2003; Parekh, 2003, 2008). In order for mitochondria to buffer efficiently $Ca^{2+}$ and to prevent the slow $Ca^{2+}$-dependant inactivation, it was proposed $Ca^{2+}$ entry attracts mitochondria to plasma membrane, close to the $Ca^{2+}$ entry channel (Quintana et al., 2006; Varadi et al., 2004).

Recent study on melanoma cells, suggests a functional relevance for $Ca^{2+}$ driven growth and survival-promoting signalling in these tumour cells due to a control of SOCE by mitochondria (Feldman et al., 2010). The authors have shown that coupling of mitochondria to SOCE sustains constitutive activation of PKB/Akt pathway leading to increase melanoma cells survival (Fig. 1). When they compared SOCE in malignant melanoma cells B16BL6-8 and in non-malignant cells Kb30 B16BL6, they described, only for malignant melanoma cells, a robust SOC function (without over-expression of Orai1 and Stim1) associated with accelerated trans-mitochondrial $Ca^{2+}$ flux (Feldman et al., 2010). Conversely, inhibition of the trans-mitochondrial $Ca^{2+}$ by the antagonist of $Na^+/Ca^{2+}$ exchanger (NCX) decreased SOCE (Feldman et al., 2010). This functional coupling allow the maintain of a strong $Ca^{2+}$ fluxes in malignant melanoma cells. $Ca^{2+}$ is, among others, an essential second messenger modulating AKT activity in many types of cells (Deb et al., 2004; Dong et al., 2007; Sandoval et al., 2007). AKT kinases, have emerged as critical mediators of signal transduction pathways downstream of activated tyrosine kinases and phosphatidylinositol 3-kinase. AKT protein is a cardinal node in diverse signalling cascades important in both normal cellular physiology and various disease states include cell proliferation and survival, intermediary metabolism, angiogenesis, and tissue invasion. Aberrant regulation of these processes result in cellular perturbations considered hallmarks of cancer, and numerous studies testify to the frequent hyperactivation of AKT signalling in many human cancers (Altomare & Testa, 2005; Bellacosa et al., 2004; Testa & Tsichlis, 2005). Recent studies have observed that $Ca^{2+}$/calmodulin may be a regulator of AKT activation and found that activity and functions of AKT are directly regulated by the $Ca^{2+}$ signal (Fig. 1). More precisely, in neutrophils, it has been described that SOCE mediates intracellular alkalinization and ERK1/2, AKT phosphorylation (pAKT) (Sandoval et al., 2007). This link was supported by the correlation between of trans-mitochondrial $Ca^{2+}$ flux triggered by SOCs and SOCE itself and levels of AKT in malignant *vs* non-tumour melanoma cells (Feldman et al., 2010). Indeed, the high basal AKT activity in malignant melanoma cells is $Ca^{2+}$ dependant and can be reversed by decreasing cytosolic $Ca^{2+}$ concentration with $Ca^{2+}$ chelator (Fedida-Metula et al., 2008) giving a special importance of SOCE in the control of intracellular $Ca^{2+}$ concentration. Thus, down-regulation of the SOCs regulator Stim1 by shRNA leading to ~ ten-fold reduction of SOCE correlated to a significantly decreased of pAKT levels compared to control transfected cells (Feldman et al., 2010). The same results have been obtained in melanoma tumour cells treated with an antagonist of $Na^+/Ca^{2+}$ exchanger: AKT inactivation and the decreased of intracellular $Ca^{2+}$ concentration coincided with an important SOCE reduction (Feldman et al., 2010). Taken together, theses studies showed a real control of AKT regulation by a positive feedback loop between trans-mitochondrial $Ca^{2+}$ transport and SOCE leading to strong cell resistance to apoptosis.

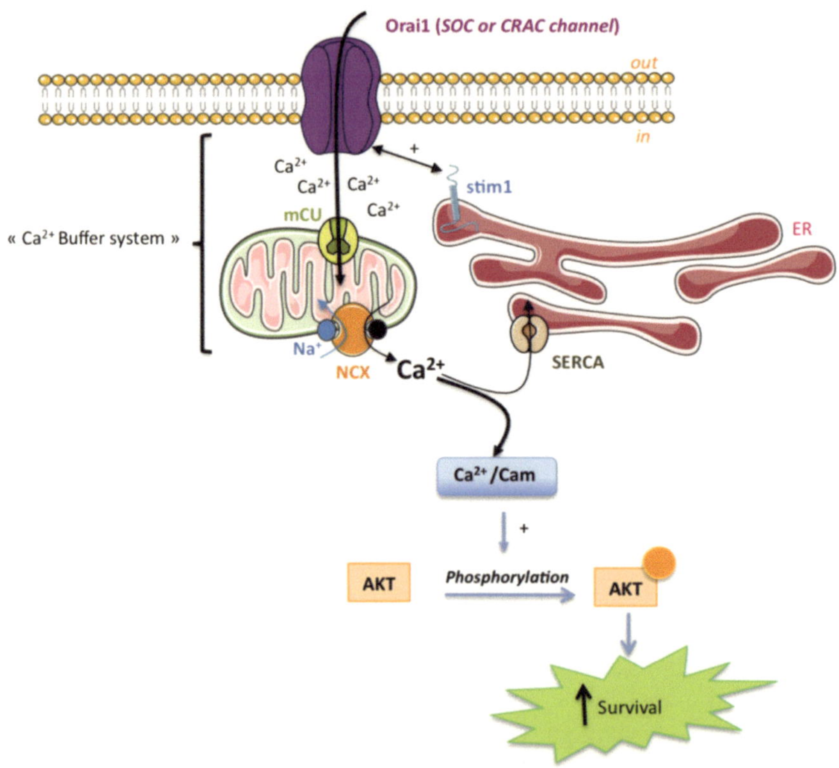


Fig. 1. AKT activation by mitochondria coupled to store-operated $Ca^{2+}$ entry. Massive $Ca^{2+}$ entry, following activation of Orai1 by Stim1, facilitates the transmitochondrial $Ca^{2+}$ flux trough the uniporter mCU and exchanger $Na^+/Ca^{2+}$ NCX. This mechanism removes high $Ca^{2+}$ level from the SOCs vinicity (as a $Ca^{2+}$ buffer) and preventing the $Ca^{2+}$ dependent slow inactivation of CRAC channel. The ability of mitochondria to buffer sub-plasmalemmal $Ca^{2+}$ sustains a robust $Ca^{2+}$ entry required for AKT activation leading to increase cell survival

The role of SOCE and trans-mitochondrial $Ca^{2+}$ transport present a real potential to develop new strategy to control AKT regulation and thus try to modulate tumour aggressiveness and death signals in cancer cells. It remains to show that these interesting and promising data, which have all been observed in murine cell lines, have a meaning in human melanomas.

### 2.2 ATP-gated ionotropic P2X7 receptor

Purine nucleotides, essential components of DNA and RNA, are key elements in replication and transcription phenomenon and therefore in cell physiology and proliferation. Among all purine nucleotides, Adenosine 5′-Triphosphate (ATP) is also recognized as being the fundamental energetic source necessary for all cellular functions. Indeed ATP is a central and a precious intracellular molecule to be kept inside the cells. After having been confronted to considerable scepticism, Geoffrey Burnstock established the existence of intercellular purines signalisations pathways allowed by the release of ATP in the extracellular compartment (Burnstock, 1972). Indeed, extracellular purines are known to modulate general cellular properties such as cell survival and proliferation, cell differentiation and motility through the activation of plasma membrane purinergic receptors. These receptors are well known in vertebrates (Burnstock, 2006) and are conserved throughout the evolution in lower organisms such as unicellular eukaryotes (Fountain et al., 2007), green algae (Fountain et al., 2008), and also in plants (Kim et al., 2006; Weerasinghe et al., 2009).

Extracellular ATP activates plasma membrane G protein-coupled P2Y receptors and/or ligand-gated cation-permeable channels ($Na^+$ / $Ca^{2+}$ / $K^+$) P2X receptors (Burnstock, 2006). Among the members of the P2X receptors family, the latest cloned P2X7 receptor (P2X7R) (Rassendren et al., 1997; Surprenant et al., 1996) is very unique in its functioning by many features, such as 1) its low sensitivity to ATP (North, 2002), 2) its increasing activity, called facilitation, under successive or sustained applications of agonist (Roger et al., 2010; Roger et al., 2008), and 3) the appearance of a large, non-selective membrane pore after sustained stimulations with ATP due to the P2X7-dependent activation of pannexin-1 (Pelegrin & Surprenant, 2006). From a physiological point of view P2X7R is expressed in cells from immune lineage and its activation by extracellular ATP at concentrations upper than 100 $\mu$M is considered as an alarming signal, and is a key step in the initiation of the inflammatory cascade through the NLP3 inflammasome (Di Virgilio, 2007; Pelegrin, 2008). Pharmacological activation of P2X7R is generally associated to membrane permeabilization and blebbing, phosphatidyl serine loss of asymmetry, cell swelling, increase of internal $Ca^{2+}$, loss of mitochondrial potential. All these phenomenon were demonstrated to be reversible under brief P2X7R activation, and called pseudoapoptosis, but were leading to cell death when prolonged stimulation (Mackenzie et al., 2005). This led to the hypothesis that P2X7R were cytolytic and that their stimulation or overexpression could be deleterious for cells (Di Virgilio et al., 1998; Mackenzie et al., 2005; Surprenant et al., 1996). Surprisingly, it was found that P2X7R was expressed at very high levels in several tumours, compared to normal tissues (Adinolfi et al., 2002; Raffaghello et al., 2006; Slater et al., 2004a; Slater et al., 2004b; Solini et al., 2008; Wang et al., 2004; Zhang et al., 2004) and was even proposed to represent an early prostate cancer marker (Slater et al., 2005), while in cervical cancer a decreased expression of P2X7R in cancer cells was reported (Li et al., 2006). Several studies indicated the overexpression of P2X7R in human (Bringmann et al., 2001; Deli et al., 2007; Slater et al.,

2003; White et al., 2005) and B16 mouse melanoma (Ohshima et al., 2010). However the role of such a receptor in melanoma cell biology remains unclear.
The most accepted view attributes pro-apoptotic effects of P2X7R stimulation in melanoma and non-melanoma skin cancers (Greig et al., 2003; White et al., 2005). This supported the use of ATP for the treatment of melanoma (White et al., 2005; White et al., 2009), as it was proposed in the 1980's for other cancers (Rapaport, 1983, 1988; Rapaport et al., 1983). Ohshima and coll. (Ohshima et al., 2010) showed that P2X7R is expressed in a B16 mouse model of melanoma and was responsible for ATP release from cancer cells induced by - irradiation. They also suggested that this release of ATP in the extracellular compartment of tumours could play as a signalling molecule between cancer cells and adjacent parenchymal cells. This should be further investigated.
In another study, P2X7R was reported to be overexpressed and functional in melanoma cells compared to normal melanocytes in which it was non-functional. In melanoma, P2X7R was associated to the overexpression of type 2 ryanodine receptor (RyR2) and contrarily to the general consensus; it displayed anti-apoptotic effects (Deli et al., 2007). The same study showed P2X7R proteins expression in melanoma cell nucleus. Therefore this raises the possibility that activation of P2X7R in melanoma could be responsible for different cell fate, depending on its subcellular localization and/or protein association. It is also possible that P2X7R proteins may be dysfunctional in some cases as it was proposed in chronic lymphocytic leukaemia with the overexpression of the loss-of-function mutant allele A1513C (Wiley et al., 2002) or in cervical cancers in which P2X7R is overexpressed under its truncated form that is inefficient to permeabilise cell membrane (Feng et al., 2006a; Feng et al., 2006b).
All these studies mainly focused on the regulation of cell proliferation / apoptosis and P2X7R participation in other parameters such as cancer cell invasiveness have not yet been assessed in melanoma. A recent study performed in MDA-MB-435s cancer cells showed the expression of the full length and fully functional P2X7R and that its activation was leading to the SK3-dependent increase in cell motility, probably through the increase of internal $Ca^{2+}$, and was dramatically increasing extracellular matrix proteolysis through the release of active cystein cathepsins (Jelassi et al., 2011). Indeed further studies will be necessary to really establish the role of such intriguing receptors in melanoma as well as in other cancer types. Depending on this, either the use of agonists, or recent antagonists, mainly developed for the treatment of inflammatory diseases (Romagnoli et al., 2008) could be considered for the treatment of melanoma.

### 2.3 Calcium channel TRPM8

The TRPM8 (express transient receptor potential melastatin subfamily member 8) channel, a cold-temperature receptor, belongs to the transient receptor potential (TRP) channel superfamily. It has been identified in sensory neuron as a $Ca^{2+}$-permeable cation channel that is stimulated by temperatures below 28°C and is modulated in a voltage channel-dependent fashion. After activation by temperature decrease or cooling compounds such as menthol or eucalyptol, TRPM8 induces membrane depolarization by $Ca^{2+}$ influx. In addition to transduction of thermal stimuli in the peripheral nervous system, TRPM8 serves other biological roles according to its expression in other tissues (*e.g.* bladder, male genital tract) (Stein et al., 2004). It is also observed that TRPM8 expression increases dramatically in many cancer types including cutaneous melanoma (Yamamura et al., 2008a). Yamamura and coll. demonstrated that TRPM8 activation by agonists suppresses human melanoma cell viability

(Yamamura et al., 2008a). Interestingly, numerous classical TRPM8 agonists are known, in addition to novel agonists (Bodding et al., 2007) that may be useful to treating most cancers in which TRPM8 channel is overexpressed in comparison to the corresponding normal tissue. Because of their inocuity, they represent a formidable pharmacological tool to evaluate this channel as target to melanoma therapy.

### 2.4 The sodium pump ($Na^+/K^+$-ATPase)

The sodium pump ($Na^+,K^+$-ATPase) is a plasma membrane binary complex with enzymatic activity that moves three $Na^+$ ions out of, and two $K^+$ ions into, the cell for each ATP that is hydrolysed. In humans, the $Na^+$ pump acts to maintain resting membrane potential, is useful as transporter, regulate intracellular ion homeostasis, and regulate cellular volume. The human sodium pump is composed of two essential protein subunits, the catalytic $\alpha$-subunit that has four isoforms ($\alpha_1$–$\alpha_4$) and the auxiliary $\beta$-subunit that has three isoforms ($\beta_1$–$\beta_3$) (Morth et al., 2011), and an optional regulatory $\gamma$-subunit with tissue-specific expression. The $\alpha_1$ and $\beta_1$ subunits of the $Na^+,K^+$-ATPase are ubiquitously expressed and form $\alpha_1\beta_1$ complex in most tissues, the other $\alpha$ and $\beta$ subunits exhibit a restricted pattern of expression specific to each subunit (Morth et al., 2011). Many cancer types over-express the different $\alpha$ sub-units, including melanoma (Boukerche et al., 2004). Interestingly, Mathieu and coll. have recently shown that more than 30% of all human melanomas, 50% of all melanoma metastases and 72% of brain melanoma metastases over-expressed sodium pump $\alpha_1$ subunit compared with only 5% of naevi. Interestingly the $\alpha_1$ subunit expression significantly correlates with tumour thickness and disease progression (Mathieu et al., 2009). Moreover, using the pharmacological drug UNBS1450 and genetic approach, the authors demonstrated that functional inhibition of $\alpha_1$ subunit in melanoma cell lines impaired cell growth, induced cell death, and improved the survival of immunodeficient mice bearing human melanoma brain metastases. Note that UNBS1450, a hemi-synthetic cardiotonic steroid, which binds to the $\alpha_1$ subunit of the sodium pump, has entered Phase I clinical trials in cancer patients.

## 3. Ion channels and melanoma cell proliferation

Information on ion channels involvement in melanoma cell proliferation is highly fragmented and unclear, although early data were published almost three decades. This research is still in its beginnings. Indeed there is good evidence that at least $K^+$ channels are involved in the cell cycle progression and proliferation in many cancer cells of different origins (Villalonga et al., 2007). Several hypotheses could explain the involvement of $K^+$ efflux in the control of the cell cycle: $Ca^{2+}$ signalling, membrane potential and cell volume (Villalonga et al., 2007). In melanoma cell lines, the inhibition of $K^+$ channel activity by unspecific $K^+$ channel blockers leads to membrane depolarization and an arrest of cell proliferation (Gavrilova-Ruch et al., 2002; Lepple-Wienhues et al., 1996; Nilius & Wohlrab, 1992). In addition, membrane depolarization of melanoma cells induced by elevated extracellular $K^+$ concentration inhibited proliferation of cycling cells (Nilius & Wohlrab, 1992). Nilius *et al.* (Nilius et al., 1993), proposed that in human melanoma cells overexpression of $K^+$ channels leads to hyperpolarisation as a result of the efflux of cations from the cell interior, which subsequently causes inward movement of $Ca^{2+}$ ions to maintain the membrane potential. The role of $Ca^{2+}$ in the transition from the G1 to the S phase during mitosis in mammalian cells is well documented and $Ca^{2+}$ acts as a pacemaker that initiates the timing of cell cycle transitions (Santella et al., 2005). Interestingly, recent evidence suggests that in addition to their $K^+$ conductance, a non-pore function of KCa3.1/SK4/IKCa and Eag1 could be observed by interacting directly with cell signalling network involved in the control of cell proliferation in non-cancer cells (Hegle et al., 2006; Millership et al., 2010). Furthermore, mutation that eliminates Eag1 ion permeation fails to completely abolish xenograft tumour formation, indicating that Eag1 contributes to tumour progression independently of its primary function as an ion channel (Downie et al., 2008).

### 3.1 Small and intermediate calcium-activated potassium channel (SKCa and IKCa)

The calcium-activated $K^+$ channel KCa family encompasses Small- (SKCa) and Intermediate- (IKCa/KCa3.1/SK4) conductance calcium activated $K^+$ channels. Functional SKCa channels result mostly in a homo or heteromeric assemblies of four subunits. There are three isoforms of SKCa subunits, named SK1/KCa2.1, SK2/KCa2.2, SK3/KCa2.3, which associate to form homo- or hetero-tetramers (Ishii et al., 1997; Monaghan et al., 2004). SK1, SK2 and SK3 proteins are principally expressed in central neurons where SKCa channels have a fundamental role in regulating neuronal excitability (Bond et al., 2005). Indeed, they hyperpolarize the plasma membrane and they contribute to the long lasting afterhyperpolarisation that follows an action potential (Bond et al., 2005). SK2 and SK3, in contrast to SK1, are not restricted to neuronal tissues and SK3 protein is expressed in vascular and visceral smooth muscle-rich tissues (Chen et al., 2004). In these muscles the activation of SK3 channel induces hyperpolarisation that respectively regulates muscle tone and cell motility (Chen et al., 2004; Herrera et al., 2003; Taylor et al., 2003). This membrane function of SK3 channel, hyperpolarisation that is dependent of $K^+$ flux, is that you except to find for $K^+$ channels in excitable cells like muscle and neuronal cells.

SKCa channel activity is independent to voltage but sensitive to elevated $Ca^{2+}$ concentrations. Involvement of theses channels have been investigated in melanoma cells because their resulting $K^+$ efflux could provide a membrane hyperpolarisation necessary to cell proliferation. In agreement with the reported restricted expression pattern of SK1 channel mainly found in neuronal tissues, transcript was no detected in melanoma cells and in normal human epidermal melanocytes NHEM (Chantôme et al., 2009; Tajima et al., 2006). In contrast, SK2 transcripts were always detected in melanocyte and melanoma cell lines but electrophysiological analyses revealed that SK2 channels were not functional in the three melanoma cell lines tested (IGR-1, SKmel-28 and 518A2) (Chantôme et al., 2009; Meyer et al., 1999; Tajima et al., 2006). Interestingly, SK2 transcripts level and KCa (SK2 et KCa3.1) currents are increase under hypoxia and only in this condition, apamin application, a non specific pore blocker of SK2, reduced cell proliferation rates in IGR-1 melanoma cells (Tajima et al., 2006). SK3 transcripts and functional SK3 channels have been found in several melanoma cells but not in untransformed melanocytes (Chantôme et al., 2009; Tajima et al., 2006). It has been clearly demonstrated that SK3-dependent efflux regulates membrane potential in 518A2 and SKmel-28 melanoma cells (Chantôme et al., 2009). However, enforced production of SK3 channels in SK3 non-expressing melanoma cells or specific SK3 channel extinction in 518A2 melanoma cells has no effect on their cell proliferation (Chantôme et al., 2009).

At last, KCa3.1/SK4 channels are widely expressed in a variety of non-excitable tissue and have been involved in cell cycle progression of different type of cancer cells such as breast, pancreatic, and endometrial cancer cells (Jager et al., 2004; Ouadid-Ahidouch et al., 2004; Wang et al., 2007). KCa3.1/SK4 transcripts are detected in NHEM and in all melanoma cell lines tested and electrophysiological analyses shown strong KCa3.1/SK4 currents (Chantôme et al., 2009; Meyer et al., 1999; Tajima et al., 2006). Application of charybdotoxin, an unspecific KCa3.1/SK4 blocker, inhibits or not cell proliferation of IGR-1 cells according to studies (Gavrilova-Ruch et al., 2002; Tajima et al., 2006). A more recent study using TRAM-34, a specific inhibitor of KCa3.1/SK4 channel (Wulff et al., 2000), demonstrated that this channel is not involved in cell proliferation of SKmel-28 melanoma cells despite actively regulated membrane polarization (Chantôme et al., 2009). Note that, TRAM-34 inhibits both $K^+$ conductance and non-pore function of KCa3.1/SK4 channels (Millership et al., 2010). In conclusion, even if membrane polarization is in part controlled by SK3 and KCa3.1/SK4 efflux in melanoma cell lines, it seems not involved or not sufficient to modulate their cell proliferation. It will be interesting to precise the mechanism through SK2 under hypoxia condition promotes cell proliferation of melanoma cells.

### 3.2 Voltage-gated potassium channels and Eag1

Voltage gated $K^+$ channels (VGKC) represent the largest ion channel family. Functional channels result from the association of alpha- (pore) and beta- (accessory) subunits (Pongs & Schwarz, 2010). Alpha subunits co-assemble in tetramers, each subunit containing a "voltage-sensor" determining the voltage threshold for channel activation. VGKC are divided up in 12 families containing up to 8 members, totalizing 40 different cloned alpha subunit isoforms (Gutman et al., 2003). Functional channels result from the association of different members inside a given family, giving rise to an extraordinary large panel of different channels with various gating kinetics and pharmacological properties. The set of alpha subunit expressed by a given cell type defines in fact its electrical signature and its function. VGKC are widely expressed in excitable and non-excitable cells and participate to the control of membrane resting potential and action potential repolarisation and firing frequency. Not surprisingly, these channels are involved in a large variety of physiological processes including neuronal excitability, hormone secretion, muscle contraction, and cardiac rhythm. Interestingly, several VGKC are abnormally expressed in cancer versus healthy tissues, including melanoma. Their initial function is then hijacked to participate to the tumour phenotype. We will more particularly focus on Eag1 and its putative role in cell proliferation, and hERG and Kv1.3 and their putative role in cell migration / invasion (see below).

Eag1 (*ether-à go-go*) channel also known as KCNH1 (gene) or Kv10.1 (protein) are a voltage-gated channel that regulates permeation of ion in response to changes in the membrane potential. Eag1 gives rise to a slowly activating and non-inactivating current in heterologous expression systems. Eag1 is mainly expressed in the brain {Martin, 2008 #283; (Martin et al., 2010). In the periphery, Eag1 expression is restricted to cell populations of the gastrointestinal tract, pancreas and male reproductive system (Hemmerlein et al., 2006; Pardo & Suhmer, 2008).

No information about its expression in melanocyte has been reported. While its function in the brain remains unknown, Eag1 has been involved in skeletal muscle development, the channel being transiently expressed in the onset of myoblasts fusion (Bijlenga et al., 1998). Remarkably, Eag1 is associated with tumours development in patients and animals. Eag1 is significantly overexpressed in up to 70% of tumour samples and cell lines (Hemmerlein et al., 2006; Pardo et al., 1999; Pardo & Suhmer, 2008), including melanoma cells (Meyer et al., 1999). The mechanisms inducing Eag1 overexpression in cancer cells is still unknown, but it has been reported that immortalization of cells by oncogenes such as papillomavirus provokes Eag1 expression (Diaz et al., 2009). The molecular and functional links between Eag1 expression and cancer development has been intensively scrutinized. Eag1 inhibition by either siRNA silencing or functional antibodies decreases cancer cell proliferation *in vitro* (Weber et al., 2006) and *in vivo* (Gomez-Varela et al., 2007). Moreover, Eag1 expression increases neovascularisation and enhances cell resistance to hypoxia by increasing Hif activity (Downie et al., 2008). Interestingly, point mutation abolishing Eag1 pore function failed to completely abolish xenograft tumour formation by transfected cells, indicating that Eag1 contributes to tumour progression independently of its primary function as an ion channel. Other study proposes that Eag-1 channels participate to cell-cycle progression in IGR-1 melanoma cells by using different unspecific blockers of $K^+$ channels (Gavrilova-Ruch et al., 2002). It will be interesting to confirm this result by using specific siRNA directed to Eag1 channels as it was already used previously in other type of cancer cell lines (Weber et al., 2006). Altogether, these data suggest that Eag1 represent a very promising target in melanoma treatment. It is noteworthy that Eag-1 is not expressed in the heart, rendering possible the use of specific Eag-1 blockers. However good selectivity *vs* the hERG cardiac channel, of the same family, (KCNH2) should be taken into account. In this perspective, functional antibodies would represented an interesting perspective to target Eag-1 in tumours, neither altering the cardiac hERG channel, nor the Eag-1 channels expressed in the CNS because of the brain blood barrier (Gomez-Varela et al., 2007).

## 4. Ion channels and melanoma cell migration / invasion / adhesion

With the occurrence of metastasis, the prognosis of melanoma is poor, with limited available treatments and an expected survival less than one year. Knowing that the metastasis occurrence involves many cellular processes including cell deformation, invasion, migration, adhesion and homing in the "metastatic" site, it is important to define the specific molecular mechanisms governing each of these various steps. This is especially important that no new treatment of metastatic melanoma has been validated for decades. Intensive research in this area has identified at least a type of ion channels involved in melanoma cell migration, the calcium-activated potassium channel SK3, and channels that contributes to melanoma cell migration / invasion / adhesion.

### 4.1 SK3 channel

Among SKCa channels, SK3 channel was found to promote breast and colon epithelial cancer cells and, melanoma cells migration by hyperpolarizing plasma cell membrane (Chantôme et al., 2009; Potier et al., 2006; Potier et al., 2010). As mentioned above, SK3 protein is produced in melanoma cells but not in untransformed melanocytes (Chantôme et al., 2009). This is not surprising if you consider that melanocytes share a neural crest origin with most SK3-expressing mature cells, *i.e.* neurons, glial cells and endocrine cells. Re-expression of embryonic genes during cancer has been widely described (Monk & Holding, 2001). It is therefore plausible that SK3 channel expression during melanoma malignancy corresponds to the re-expression of an embryonic gene expressed by a neural progenitor common to neurons and melanocytes (Klein et al., 2007; Rasheed et al., 2005).

We have reported that SK3 channel promotes melanoma cell migration by hyperpolarisating plasma membrane as observe in excitable cells (Chantôme et al., 2009). This new function of the SK3 channel in melanoma cells was revealed using pharmacological and molecular biology approaches (there is no specific inhibitor of SK3 channel); stable silencing SK3 protein inhibited melanoma cell migration, which became insensitive to apamin and inversely, a stable expression of SK3 in SK3-non expressing melanoma cells, enhanced their migration that became sensitive to apamin. If patch-clamp experiments reveal that SK3 channel hyperpolarises plasma membrane of melanoma cells, increasing external $K^+$ concentration reduced only SK3-dependant cell motility (Chantôme et al., 2009). All of these experiments demonstrate that SK3 channel promotes melanoma cell migration through its primary function as an ion channel. Since the KCa3.1 channel had no effect on melanoma cell migration despite actively regulating membrane potential we propose that the increase of melanoma cell migration by hyperpolarisation is SK3 dependent.

The mechanism by which SK3 channel regulates melanoma cell migration may involve $[Ca^{2+}]$ oscillations (frequency, amplitude) regulation (Fig. 2). Indeed, an increase of $K^+$ efflux shifts the membrane potential towards negative values (hyperpolarization) and consequently increases the $Ca^{2+}$ driving force (Potier et al., 2006; Rao et al., 2006; Rao et al., 2002). Inversely, a reduction of SK3 channel activity may depolarize the plasma membrane and reduce $Ca^{2+}$ entry. That further suggests that SK3 channel interacts in cooperation with a specific complex such as voltage-independent-calcium channel like transient-receptor - potential (TRP) that are known to be sufficient to activate $Ca^{2+}$-regulated stimulatory pathways for cell migration (Louis et al., 2008; Rao et al., 2006; Waning et al., 2007; Wondergem et al., 2008). This needs to be elucidated.

The ability of SK3 channel to promote cancer cell migration led us to create a patent that addresses the use of this protein as a tool for the *in vitro* screening of compounds that inhibits SK3-dependent cell migration and metastasis development (Potier et al., 2008).

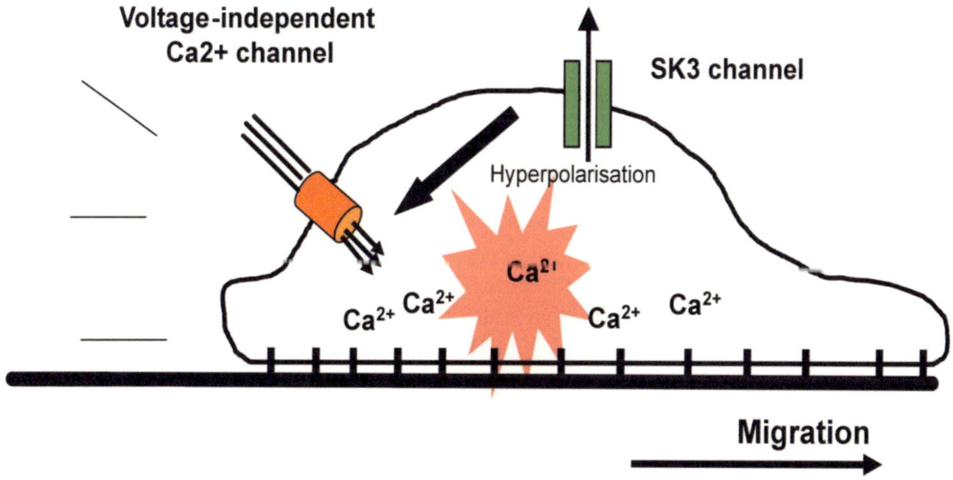


Fig. 2. Proposed model to explain how SK3 channel increase melanoma cell migration. The expression of SK3 protein lead to a functional SK3 channel that hyperpolarizes plasma membrane and increase $Ca^{2+}$ entry through voltage-independent $Ca^{2+}$ channels and intracellular $Ca^{2+}$ concentration promoting cell migration

### 4.2 IKCa/KCa3.1/SK4 channel

The KCa3.1 channel - composed of protein that is strictly expressed outside the central nervous system - is expressed in melanocytes and melanoma cell lines (Allen et al., 1997; Chantôme et al., 2009; Schmidt et al., 2010; Schwab et al., 1999; Tajima et al., 2006). This channel appears to be involved in the migration process by facilitating the retraction of the rear part of migrating cells through induction of local cell shrinkage (Schwab, 2001). Interestingly, the KCa3.1 channel was found to support melanoma inhibitory activity, a protein known to play a role in melanoma development, progression and metastasis formation (Schmidt et al., 2010). KCa3.1 channel was also found to be involved in non-cancerous cell migration o (e.g. lung mast cells or human coronary smooth muscle cells) (Cruse et al., 2006; Toyama et al., 2008). Low dose of TRAM-34 (that specifically blocks KCa3.1 channel and depolarize cell membrane) and high dose of TRAM-34 or clotrimazole (that inhibit KCa3.1 channels and other voltage dependent $K^+$ channels (Wulff et al., 2000)) did not impair melanoma cell migration (Chantôme et al., 2009). This indicates that KCa3.1 channel activity has no effect on melanoma cell migration despite its active role in regulating membrane potential.

### 4.3 Voltage-gated potassium channel hERG

The human ether-à-go-go (eag) related gene channel hERG, also known as KCNH2 (gene) and Kv11.1 (protein), is a member of the related Eag-like family of $K^+$ channel. hERG encodes a voltage-dependent $K^+$ channel that normally regulates cardiac repolarisation (Sanguinetti et al., 1995; Trudeau et al., 1995). The channel presents a unique activation kinetic: upon depolarisation, the channel opens but very rapidly inactivates, shutting down the $K^+$ efflux. During the repolarisation phase of cardiac action potential, the recovery from inactivation is faster than the deactivation, the resulting $K^+$ tail current shortening the action potential duration and decreasing the firing frequency (Schwarz & Bauer, 2004). In contrast to Eag1, hERG channel is expressed in a variety of tissue but its expression in melanocyte has not been investigated in our knowledge, but it is found in many tumour cells of different origins and exert pleiotropic effects in cancer cells (Asher et al., 2010). In a series of recent studies, the team of Arcangeli has proposed hERG as a biological marker of leukaemia and several solid tumours and leukaemia. HERG is involved in cell proliferation, apoptosis resistance and cell invasion (Bianchi et al., 1998; Lastraioli et al., 2004; Pillozzi et al., 2002). Several hERG isoforms interacting to modulate subunit trafficking and functional channel membrane expression are linked to the cell cycle and the differentiation state of myeloid and neuroblastoma cells (Crociani et al., 2003; Guasti et al., 2008). Strikingly, hERG forms membrane macromolecular complexes with β1 integrins and the growth factor receptor FLT1. Cell adhesion to extra cellular matrix components such as fibronectin activates hERG and enhances adhesion receptor signalling such as tyrosine phosphorylation of focal adhesion kinase (Cherubini et al., 2005). In AML, the hERG1b isoform is recruited by the β1 integrin to promote FLT1 signalling. In vivo, hERG positive blasts are more efficient in invading the peripheral circulation and the extramedullary sites after engraftment into immunodeficient mice (Pillozzi et al., 2007). In acute lymphoblastic leukaemia, hERG expression enhances chemotherapy-induced apoptosis and drug resistance (Pillozzi et al., 2011). In the MDA-MD-435s cell line, hERG participates to cell migration and proliferation through a MAP kinase/c-fos pathway. HERG blockers such as E-4031 or silencing by siRNA reduce both proliferation and migration, but surprisingly no current can be recorded, demonstrating that hERG is no functional as a $K^+$ pore (Afrasiabi et al., 2010). Similar to

Eag1, hERG might mediate at least in part, its effects on cell cancer behaviour through non-pore associated mechanisms. However, concerning the role of hERG in melanoma cell behaviour, data must be used cautiously since the cancer origin of MDA-MD-435s cell line is rather a basal-type breast cancer, even if MDA-MD-435s cells have a genetic basis similar to melanomas (Chambers, 2009; Rae et al., 2007; Sellappan et al., 2004).

### 4.4 Voltage-gated potassium channel Kv1.3

Kv1.3 (KCNA3) channels, another voltage-dependent $K^+$ channel, have been first isolated from Jurkat T cells (Chandy et al., 2004; DeCoursey et al., 1984). By regulating the resting membrane potential and thus the $Ca^{2+}$ driving force, this channel modulates NFAT (Nuclear Factor of Activated T cells) translocation and mitogenesis (Chandy et al., 2004). The expression level of Kv1.3 is unchanged or down regulated depending the cancer type. In breast adenocarcinoma, the promoter of the gene encoding the channel is methylated leading to a down regulation of Kv1.3 expression (Bielanska et al., 2009; Brevet et al., 2009). In the LOX melanoma cell line, Kv1.3 is associated to the β1-integrin subunit and might regulate tumour cell behaviour by influencing macro molecular complexes linked to integrins (Artym & Petty, 2002). In this way, Kv1.3 may have in melanoma cells the same function as hERG in leukaemia cells.

### 4.5 Voltage-gated sodium channel Nav1.6

Voltage-gated Na+ channels (NaV) are known to be responsible for transient inward Na+ currents in excitable cells in which they are responsible for the initial membrane depolarisation triggering and allowing the propagation of action potentials. They are blocked by the highly specific blocker tetrodotoxin (TTX) at different doses from nM to µM concentrations depending on isoforms and numerous pharmacological modulators of these channels have been developed by pharmaceutical companies for the treatment of pain or some cardiovascular diseases.

The expression and activity of pore-forming alpha subunits of NaV have been linked to cancer cell migration/invasion originating from different tissues such as prostate (Diss et al., 2001), breast (Fraser et al., 2005; Gillet et al., 2009; Roger et al., 2003), lung (Onganer & Djamgoz, 2005; Roger et al., 2007), cervix (Diaz et al., 2007), colon (House et al., 2010), ovaries (Gao et al., 2010). Depending on the tissues, pore-forming isoforms responsible for the Na+ current and for the cellular effect, i.e. the enhancement of cancer cell invasiveness are different, but appeared not to be linked to the triggering of action potentials, but rather to the cystein cathepsin-dependent extracellular matrix degradation (Gao et al., 2010). In human breast cancer cells MDA-MB-231, NaV1.5 functioning enhances the activity of the $Na^+/H^+$ exchanger type 1 (NHE-1) responsible for the perimembrane space acidification and thus promoting cystein cathepsins proteolytic activity (Brisson et al., 2011).

In melanoma there are, to our knowledge, only two studies reporting the expression of NaV. The first one was carried out in the late 1990's, on human melanoma cell lines, and had for goal to identify the electrophysiological characteristics of these cells (Allen et al., 1997). In this first article, TTX-sensitive (Kd ~ 6 nM) voltage-gated Na+ currents were recorded in about 40% of C8161 and C8146 cells tested. However, the role of these currents in melanoma biology was not identified.

Later on, a study performed by Carrithers and coll. on HTB-26 invasive human melanoma cells indicated the expression of a splice variant lacking the exon 18 of the Na+ channel SCN8A gene, encoding the NaV1.6 protein (Carrithers et al., 2009). The activity of this channel, mainly identified in intracellular vesicles, was found to be involved in melanoma invadopodia formation and cell invasiveness. This effect was proposed to depend on intracellular $Ca^{2+}$ regulation through mitochondrial $Na^+/Ca^{2+}$ exchangers and to the rapid remodelling of F-actin cytoskeleton. This regulation of intracellular $Na^+$ and $Ca^{2+}$ homeostasis could also modulate the activity of pH regulators, such as NHE-1, demonstrated to be key regulators of melanoma invasion at the front of invasive cells (Stock et al., 2007; Stock & Schwab, 2009).

## 5. Ion channel modulators as therapeutic targets

### Sigma1 receptors as ion channel regulatory partners in cancer cells

Targeting ion channels abnormally expressed in cancer cells represents an exciting new perspective for cancer treatment. Nevertheless, because these ion channels are also expressed in the heart or brain, the use of toxins is potentially hazardous and the therapeutic challenge is to specifically target ion channels in tumours. Characterizing the specific interactors of ion channels in cancer cells opens an interesting alternative strategy, providing the possibility to target ion channels through these tumour-specific partners (Arcangeli et al., 2009). The Sigma 1 receptor (Sig1R) is a 25 kDa protein anchored to the different cell membrane systems including ER, mitochondria, nucleus and plasma membranes (Tsai et al., 2009). The structure shares no homology with other mammalian proteins (Hanner et al., 1996) and includes two putative transmembrane domains (Su et al., 2010). Sig1R is distributed in the brain and peripheral tissues such as liver, kidney, ovaries or testis. Sig1R binds a large panel of exogenous drugs such as antipsychotics, opioids, antidepressants (sigma ligands) but also interacts with endogenous steroids (cholesterol and progesterone). Since the introduction of the concept thirty years ago (Martin et al., 1976) the function associated to Sig1R, mainly studied through the effects produced by sigma ligands, has been representing a challenging question. Sig1R have been involved in a huge number very different functions covering nociception, memory, drug addiction, cell electrical activity, apoptosis, cell cycle or immune response. Despite the abundant literature generated so far, the primary molecular mechanism governed by Sig1R to achieve those different functions has been missing. Recently, Su & Hayashi demonstrated in neuroblastoma cells that Sig1R physically associates to the chaperone Bip at the mitochondria-associated ER membrane (MAM) where it regulates $Ca^{2+}$ fluxes between ER and mitochondria through the stabilisation of IP3 receptors (Fig. 3) (Hayashi & Su, 2007). From these finding, the emerging concept of the Sig1R as an inter-organelle signalling modulator activated either by ligands or cell stress was proposed (Su et al., 2010). On the other hand, Sig1R interacts with various molecular families of ion channels including Kv, Cav, Nav, VRCC, NMDA or Asic channels (Herrera et al., 2008; Johannessen et al., 2009; Renaudo et al., 2007; Renaudo et al., 2004; Soriani et al., 1999a; Soriani et al., 1999b; Soriani et al., 1998). Interestingly, sigma receptors are overexpressed in many cancer cell types and the protein is now considered as a tumour biomarker (Aydar et al., 2006; Aydar et al., 2004). Many efforts have been done since the early 90's to develop specific sigma ligands for medical imagery and therapeutic applications (Collier et al., 2007). In particular, amine-amide-dithiol-[99mTc]oxotechnetium(V) complexes have been proposed as in vivo diagnostic agents for melanoma and its metastasis, with a high tumour uptake and significant tumour/non-tumour ratio (Friebe et al., 2001). Recently, sigma ligands have been used to develop nanoparticles that can systemically deliver siRNA into the cytoplasm of B16F10 murine melanoma cells, which express the sigma receptor. The targeted nanoparticles containing c-Myc siRNA sensitized B16F10 cells to paclitaxel (Taxol), inducing a strong decrease in cell growth. Treatments of c-Myc siRNA in the targeted nanoparticles also showed significant inhibition on the growth of MDA-MB-435 tumour (Chen et al., 2010). Last, the sigma1 ligand 4-IBP decreases melanoma cell migration *in vitro* (Megalizzi et al., 2007). These data raise the question of the function of sigma receptors in cancer cells. Recently, we have demonstrated that sigma ligands inhibit cell cycle by inhibiting both Kv and volume regulated chloride channels (VRCC) in leukaemia and small cell lung carcinoma cells. The alteration of these ion channels by sigma ligand provokes a reduced capacity of cell to regulate their shape and volume during at the G1/S checkpoint, leading to an accumulation of p27kip1 and the downstream reduction in cyclin A levels (Renaudo et al., 2004; Renaudo et al., 2007). Moreover, we found that the overexpression of Sig1R in cancer cells enhanced *per se* apoptosis resistance by reducing VRCC activation kinetics, this channel controlling the apoptosis volume decrease (Renaudo et al., 2007). These finding suggest that sigma1 receptors are involved in the control of cell shape through $K^+$, $Cl^-$ and water fluxes, a key factor for cancer cell division, apoptosis and migration (Habela et al., 2009; Rouzaire-Dubois et al., 2000). Interestingly, Su and coll. have shown that Sig1R regulate IP3 receptors following a cell stress (Tsai et al., 2009). It can then be suggested that the ion channel regulatory function of Sig1R is specifically potentiated in cancer cells when compared to healthy cells. However, if the effects of exogenous sigma receptor ligands on several ion channels are well described, the innate role of Sig1R regarding ion channel function or expression needs to be studied.

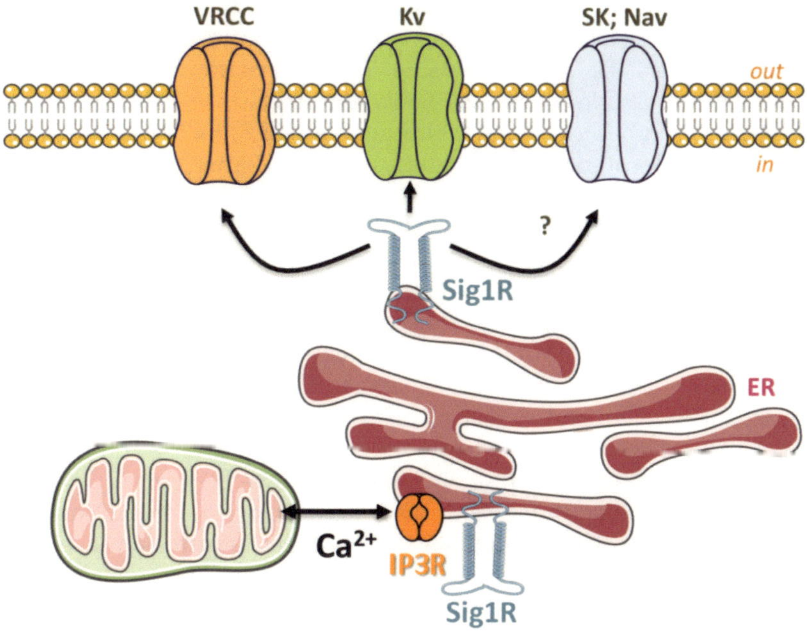


Fig. 3. Sig1R modulation on ion channels: A putative model. Under ER stress, Sig1R stabilizes IP3 receptors and regulates $Ca^{2+}$ influx from ER to mitochondria to protect cells from apoptosis (Hayashi & Su, 2007). Sig1R also modulates VRCC and Kv channels to reduce AVD, enhancing apoptosis resistance (Renaudo et al., 2004; Renaudo et al., 2007). Sig1R might target other channels such as Nav or SKCa

Altogether, these data suggest that Sig1R might be a potential therapeutic target in melanoma. While the function and mechanisms of action of Sig1R in melanoma remain to be determined, it can be speculated that the protein regulates various ion channels of interest involved in proliferation and/or invasiveness. Sigma ligands might then be used to inhibit these channels specifically in melanoma.

## 6. Channel proteins and anti-cancer therapy for melanoma

In summary, there are at least 8 channels or groups of channels that have been suggested as anticancer or antimetastatic therapeutic targets: Store-Operated Channels (SOCs) (including Stim 1 and Orai1); P2X7R; TRPM8; sodium pump ($Na^+$,$K^+$-ATPase); SK3/KCa2.3 channel; the VGKC Eag1; Nav1.6 and Sig1R. In absence of the identification of cancer-associated mutant ion channel molecules, there is no ideal and specific target in the field of ion channels, like the other potential therapeutic targets corresponding to wild-type molecules. The Sig1R does not follow this rule because it is suspected of having cancer-specific interactions with ion channels. Identification of such specific cancer associated interactions of Sig1R with channel partners would be very attractive to target tumour cells because they offer the possibility of minimizing toxic effects to non-tumour cells. As tumour eradication is obviously preferable to tumour arrest, targeting ion channels involved only in cell proliferation, which would help rather to limit tumour expansion than to eliminate it, is conceivable in combination to other therapies. However, the inhibition of melanoma SOC channels would be helpful to overcome resistance to chemotherapy-induced apoptosis, and inversely the activation of P2X7R and TRPM8 or inhibition of sodium pump might lead to cell death. Finally, since metastatic melanoma is almost incurable because of lack of effective anti-metastatic therapies, the most promising ion channel candidates for melanoma are those that would target cellular processes involved in metastasis occurrence. Fortunately at least two ion channel candidates belong to this category; SK3/KCa2.3 and Nav1.6 channels.

Due to their cellular localisation, modulation of ion channels is easy and has many advantages that make it an ideal anti-cancerous therapeutic approach (*e.g.* extracellular targeting, excepted for stim1; restricted metabolic effects). The recent robotisation of patch clamp method, the electrophysiological method that measured ion channel activity, greatly facilitates the screening of new anti-channel drugs. The exploitation of anti-channel drug as anticancer drugs is currently still underdeveloped, may be due to their unintentional side effects on non-tumour tissues. This is specifically true for channels expressed in cardiomyocyte that might cause undesirable cardiac side effects (*e.g.* hERG). Arcangeli and coll have written an excellent review that addresses the altered expression of ion channels in cancer, their pharmacological blockers potentially usable in therapy and the numerous side effects predicted or known related to their inhibition (Arcangeli et al., 2009). Thus, before developing new therapeutic approaches through new biological targets, some prerequisites must be considered to predict or avoid some side effects (expression level and biological function between tumour and non-tumour tissue). With regard to melanoma, our current knowledge are relatively fragmented and remained to be deepening, but for some channels such as SK3, TRPM8, sodium pump, Nav1.6, Sig1R, recent data are sufficient to consider them as good druggable targets. Note that for two of them, TRPM8 and sodium pump, their expression in human clinical samples has already been demonstrated. If multiple cellular targets of melanoma have been identified, pharmacological drugs remain to be developed. Note that most ion channels belong to large families of channels and that it is relatively difficult to develop specific agonists or antagonists for one particular channel. In oncology

the concept to use ion channel modulators in therapy is recent but might be compensated by the active development of these modulating agents in other medical disciplines (e. g. neurology, cardiology).
Actually, there is an increasing list of recent patents related to the use of ion channels modulators in anticancer therapy (Le Guennec et al., 2007; Villalonga et al., 2007). To date, only KCa3.1/SK4 blockers have been proposed for the treatment of prostate, pancreatic, and endometrial cancer, based on their ability to inhibit *in vitro* cell proliferation. So far only few blockers, particularly the clotrimazole analogue to TRAM-34 (Patent WO/2007/033307, 22.03.2007), emerge as promising anticancer drugs, presumably as adjuvant of cancer therapy. In this regard, SK3 channel has been proposed as a tool for the *in vitro* screening of compounds that might inhibit SK3-dependent cell migration and metastasis development (WO/2008/015267). In regards to Sig1R, the number of patents in the field of cancer is rather low, and concerns mainly imagery (PET scan) for the early detection of tumours. We believe that the identification of cancer-associated interaction between Sig1R and a specific ion channels might propose the more specific of anti-cancer therapies. Indeed if Sig1R represent a promising target for cancer therapy, physical and functional links with ion channels expressed in melanoma require to be explored, especially for the putative coupling with Nav1.6, Kv1.3, Eag1 and SK3 channels, channels that have been already link to some behaviour of melanoma cells (see above). To our knowledge, no patented molecules or drugs has been established for its ability to recognize a cancer-associated complex of Sig1R/ ion channel.

## 7. Conclusion - perspectives

In conclusion, there is now strong evidence that numerous ion channels play important roles in carcinogenesis in participating actively to determine the common features of cancer cells, such as unlimited proliferative potential, evasion of cell death, angiogenesis, reduction of adhesion, invasion and metastasis development. In melanogenesis, additional research remains to be done such, as clinical relevance related to channel type expression, prognostic information, discovery of melanoma-specific complexes, development of more potent and specific inhibitors. To expect reaching the ideal specificity of a new drug toward melanoma, effort might be done in the identification of cancer-associated mutants of ion channel molecules, in the identification of specific complexes of channels /partners or channels / subunits associated to melanoma. Nevertheless, the important work of the cell physiologists, oncologists, chemists, biologists and pharmacologists has shown the promising interest of ion channel as therapeutic targets.

## 8. Acknowledgment

Research in our groups is supported by institutional grants from INSERM and CNRS, by INCa, Canceropole Grand Ouest, Région Centre, Ligue Contre le Cancer, Ti'Toine Normandie, by Agence Nationale pour la Recherche. A.C. is the recipient of a fellowship from INCa.

## 9. References

Adinolfi, E., Melchiorri, L., Falzoni, S., Chiozzi, P., Morelli, A., Tieghi, A., Cuneo, A., Castoldi, G., Di Virgilio, F., and Baricordi, O.R. (2002). P2X7 receptor expression in evolutive and indolent forms of chronic B lymphocytic leukemia. *Blood* 99, 706-708.

Afrasiabi, E., Hietamaki, M., Viitanen, T., Sukumaran, P., Bergelin, N., and Tornquist, K. (2010). Expression and significance of HERG (KCNH2) potassium channels in the regulation of MDA-MB-435S melanoma cell proliferation and migration. *Cell Signal* 22, 57-64.

Allen, D.H., Lepple-Wienhues, A., and Cahalan, M.D. (1997). Ion channel phenotype of melanoma cell lines. *J Membr Biol* 155, 27-34.

Altomare, D.A., and Testa, J.R. (2005). Perturbations of the AKT signaling pathway in human cancer. *Oncogene* 24, 7455-7464.

Arcangeli, A., Crociani, O., Lastraioli, E., Masi, A., Pillozzi, S., and Becchetti, A. (2009). Targeting ion channels in cancer: a novel frontier in antineoplastic therapy. *Curr Med Chem* 16, 66-93.

Artym, V.V., and Petty, H.R. (2002). Molecular proximity of Kv1.3 voltage-gated potassium channels and beta(1)-integrins on the plasma membrane of melanoma cells: effects of cell adherence and channel blockers. *J Gen Physiol* 120, 29-37.

Asher, V., Sowter, H., Shaw, R., Bali, A., and Khan, R. (2010). Eag and HERG potassium channels as novel therapeutic targets in cancer. *World J Surg Oncol* 8, 113.

Assa-Kunik, E., Fishman, D., Kellman-Pressman, S., Tsory, S., Elhyany, S., Baharir, O., and Segal, S. (2003). Alterations in the expression of MHC class I glycoproteins by B16BL6 melanoma cells modulate insulin receptor-regulated signal transduction and augment [correction of augments] resistance to apoptosis. *J Immunol* 171, 2945-2952.

Aydar, E., Onganer, P., Perrett, R., Djamgoz, M.B., and Palmer, C.P. (2006). The expression and functional characterization of sigma (sigma) 1 receptors in breast cancer cell lines. *Cancer Lett* 242, 245-257.

Aydar, E., Palmer, C.P., and Djamgoz, M.B. (2004). Sigma receptors and cancer: possible involvement of ion channels. *Cancer Res* 64, 5029-5035.

Becker, J.C., Kirkwood, J.M., Agarwala, S.S., Dummer, R., Schrama, D., and Hauschild, A. (2006). Molecularly targeted therapy for melanoma: current reality and future options. *Cancer* 107, 2317-2327.

Bellacosa, A., Testa, J.R., Moore, R., and Larue, L. (2004). A portrait of AKT kinases: human cancer and animal models depict a family with strong individualities. *Cancer Biol Ther* 3, 268-275.

Bian, G.H., Cao, G., Lv, X.Y., Li, Q.W., Sun, H., Xiao, Y., Ai, J.Z., Yang, Q.T., Duan, J.J., Wang, Y.D., *et al.* (2010). Down-regulation of Pkd2 by siRNAs suppresses cell-cell adhesion in the mouse melanoma cells. *Mol Biol Rep* 37, 2387-2395.

Bianchi, L., Wible, B., Arcangeli, A., Taglialatela, M., Morra, F., Castaldo, P., Crociani, O., Rosati, B., Faravelli, L., Olivotto, M., *et al.* (1998). herg encodes a $K^+$ current highly conserved in tumours of different histogenesis: a selective advantage for cancer cells? *Cancer Res* 58, 815-822.

Bielanska, J., Hernandez-Losa, J., Perez-Verdaguer, M., Moline, T., Somoza, R., Ramon, Y.C.S., Condom, E., Ferreres, J.C., and Felipe, A. (2009). Voltage-dependent potassium channels Kv1.3 and Kv1.5 in human cancer. *Curr Cancer Drug Targets* 9, 904-914.

Bijlenga, P., Occhiodoro, T., Liu, J.H., Bader, C.R., Bernheim, L., and Fischer-Lougheed, J. (1998). An ether -a-go-go $K^+$ current, Ih-eag, contributes to the hyperpolarization of human fusion-competent myoblasts. *J Physiol* 512 ( Pt 2), 317-323.

Bodding, M., Wissenbach, U., and Flockerzi, V. (2007). Characterisation of TRPM8 as a pharmacophore receptor. *Cell Calcium* 42, 618-628.

Bond, C.T., Maylie, J., and Adelman, J.P. (2005). SK channels in excitability, pacemaking and synaptic integration. *Curr Opin Neurobiol* 15, 305-311.

Boukerche, H., Su, Z.Z., Kang, D.C., and Fisher, P.B. (2004). Identification and cloning of genes displaying elevated expression as a consequence of metastatic progression in human melanoma cells by rapid subtraction hybridization. *Gene* 343, 191-201.

Brevet, M., Haren, N., Sevestre, H., Merviel, P., and Ouadid-Ahidouch, H. (2009). DNA methylation of K(v)1.3 potassium channel gene promoter is associated with poorly differentiated breast adenocarcinoma. *Cell Physiol Biochem* 24, 25-32.

Bringmann, A., Pannicke, T., Moll, V., Milenkovic, I., Faude, F., Enzmann, V., Wolf, S., and Reichenbach, A. (2001). Upregulation of P2X(7) receptor currents in Muller glial cells during proliferative vitreoretinopathy. *Invest Ophthalmol Vis Sci* 42, 860-867.

Brisson, L., Gillet, L., Calaghan, S., Besson, P., Le Guennec, J.Y., Roger, S., and Gore, J. (2011). Na(V)1.5 enhances breast cancer cell invasiveness by increasing NHE1-dependent $H(^{+})$ efflux in caveolae. *Oncogene*. 30, 2070-2076

Burnstock, G. (1972). Purinergic nerves. *Pharmacol Rev* 24, 509-581.

Burnstock, G. (2006). Purinergic signalling. *Br J Pharmacol* 147 Suppl 1, S172-181.

Carrithers, M.D., Chatterjee, G., Carrithers, L.M., Offoha, R., Iheagwara, U., Rahner, C., Graham, M., and Waxman, S.G. (2009). Regulation of podosome formation in macrophages by a splice variant of the sodium channel SCN8A. *J Biol Chem* 284, 8114-8126.

Chambers, A.F. (2009). MDA-MB-435 and M14 Cell Lines: Identical but not M14 Melanoma? *Cancer Res* 69 5292-5293

Chandy, K.G., Wulff, H., Beeton, C., Pennington, M., Gutman, G.A., and Cahalan, M.D. (2004). $K^{+}$ channels as targets for specific immunomodulation. *Trends Pharmacol Sci* 25, 280-289.

Chantôme, A., Girault, A., Potier, M., Collin, C., Vaudin, P., Pages, J.C., Vandier, C., and Joulin, V. (2009). KCa2.3 channel-dependent hyperpolarization increases melanoma cell motility. *Exp Cell Res* 315, 3620-3630.

Chen, M.X., Gorman, S.A., Benson, B., Singh, K., Hieble, J.P., Michel, M.C., Tate, S.N., and Trezise, D.J. (2004). Small and intermediate conductance $Ca(^{2+})$-activated $K^{+}$ channels confer distinctive patterns of distribution in human tissues and differential cellular localisation in the colon and corpus cavernosum. *Naunyn Schmiedebergs Arch Pharmacol* 369, 602-615.

Chen, Y., Bathula, S.R., Yang, Q., and Huang, L. (2010). Targeted nanoparticles deliver siRNA to melanoma. *J Invest Dermatol* 130, 2790-2798.

Cherubini, A., Hofmann, G., Pillozzi, S., Guasti, L., Crociani, O., Cilia, E., Di Stefano, P., Degani, S., Balzi, M., Olivotto, M., *et al.* (2005). Human ether-a-go-go-related gene 1 channels are physically linked to beta1 integrins and modulate adhesion-dependent signaling. *Mol Biol Cell* 16, 2972-2983.

Collier, T.L., Waterhouse, R.N., and Kassiou, M. (2007). Imaging sigma receptors: applications in drug development. *Curr Pharm Des* 13, 51-72.

Crociani, O., Guasti, L., Balzi, M., Becchetti, A., Wanke, E., Olivotto, M., Wymore, R.S., and Arcangeli, A. (2003). Cell cycle-dependent expression of HERG1 and HERG1B isoforms in tumour cells. *J Biol Chem* 278, 2947-2955.

Cruse, G., Duffy, S.M., Brightling, C.E., and Bradding, P. (2006). Functional KCa3.1 $K^+$ channels are required for human lung mast cell migration. *Thorax* 61, 880-885.
Dai, D.L., Martinka, M., and Li, G. (2005). Prognostic significance of activated Akt expression in melanoma: a clinicopathologic study of 292 cases. *J Clin Oncol* 23, 1473-1482.
Deb, T.B., Coticchia, C.M., and Dickson, R.B. (2004). Calmodulin-mediated activation of Akt regulates survival of c-Myc-overexpressing mouse mammary carcinoma cells. *J Biol Chem* 279, 38903-38911.
DeCoursey, T.E., Chandy, K.G., Gupta, S., and Cahalan, M.D. (1984). Voltage-gated $K^+$ channels in human T lymphocytes: a role in mitogenesis? *Nature* 307, 465-468.
Deli, T., Varga, N., Adam, A., Kenessey, I., Raso, E., Puskas, L.G., Tovari, J., Fodor, J., Feher, M., Szigeti, G.P., *et al.* (2007). Functional genomics of calcium channels in human melanoma cells. *Int J Cancer* 121, 55-65.
Demaurex, N., Poburko, D., and Frieden, M. (2009). Regulation of plasma membrane calcium fluxes by mitochondria. *Biochim Biophys Acta* 1787, 1383-1394.
Di Virgilio, F. (2007). Liaisons dangereuses: P2X(7) and the inflammasome. *Trends Pharmacol Sci* 28, 465-472.
Di Virgilio, F., Chiozzi, P., Falzoni, S., Ferrari, D., Sanz, J.M., Venketaraman, V., and Baricordi, O.R. (1998). Cytolytic P2X purinoceptors. *Cell Death Differ* 5, 191-199.
Diaz, D., Delgadillo, D.M., Hernandez-Gallegos, E., Ramirez-Dominguez, M.E., Hinojosa, L.M., Ortiz, C.S., Berumen, J., Camacho, J., and Gomora, J.C. (2007). Functional expression of voltage-gated sodium channels in primary cultures of human cervical cancer. *J Cell Physiol* 210, 469-478.
Diaz, L., Ceja-Ochoa, I., Restrepo-Angulo, I., Larrea, F., Avila-Chavez, E., Garcia-Becerra, R., Borja-Cacho, E., Barrera, D., Ahumada, E., Gariglio, P., *et al.* (2009). Estrogens and human papilloma virus oncogenes regulate human ether-a-go-go-1 potassium channel expression. *Cancer Res* 69, 3300-3307.
Diss, J.K., Archer, S.N., Hirano, J., Fraser, S.P., and Djamgoz, M.B. (2001). Expression profiles of voltage-gated $Na(^+)$ channel alpha-subunit genes in rat and human prostate cancer cell lines. *Prostate* 48, 165-178.
Dong, B., Valencia, C.A., and Liu, R. (2007). $Ca(^{2+})$/calmodulin directly interacts with the pleckstrin homology domain of AKT1. *J Biol Chem* 282, 25131-25140.
Downie, B.R., Sanchez, A., Knotgen, H., Contreras-Jurado, C., Gymnopoulos, M., Weber, C., Stuhmer, W., and Pardo, L.A. (2008). Eag1 expression interferes with hypoxia homeostasis and induces angiogenesis in tumours. *J Biol Chem* 283, 36234-36240.
Duncan, L.M., Deeds, J., Hunter, J., Shao, J., Holmgren, L.M., Woolf, E.A., Tepper, R.I., and Shyjan, A.W. (1998). Down-regulation of the novel gene melastatin correlates with potential for melanoma metastasis. *Cancer Res* 58, 1515-1520.
Fedida-Metula, S., Elhyany, S., Tsory, S., Segal, S., Hershfinkel, M., Sekler, I., and Fishman, D. (2008). Targeting lipid rafts inhibits protein kinase B by disrupting calcium homeostasis and attenuates malignant properties of melanoma cells. *Carcinogenesis* 29, 1546-1554.
Feldman, B., Fedida-Metula, S., Nita, J., Sekler, I., and Fishman, D. (2010). Coupling of mitochondria to store-operated $Ca(^{2+})$-signaling sustains constitutive activation of protein kinase B/Akt and augments survival of malignant melanoma cells. *Cell Calcium* 47, 525-537.

Feng, Y.H., Li, X., Wang, L., Zhou, L., and Gorodeski, G.I. (2006a). A truncated P2X7 receptor variant (P2X7-j) endogenously expressed in cervical cancer cells antagonizes the full-length P2X7 receptor through hetero-oligomerization. *J Biol Chem* 281, 17228-17237.

Feng, Y.H., Li, X., Zeng, R., and Gorodeski, G.I. (2006b). Endogenously expressed truncated P2X7 receptor lacking the c-terminus is preferentially upregulated in epithelial cancer cells and fails to mediate ligand-induced pore formation and apoptosis. *Nucleosides Nucleotides Nucleic Acids* 25, 1271-1276.

Fountain, S.J., Cao, L., Young, M.T., and North, R.A. (2008). Permeation properties of a P2X receptor in the green algae Ostreococcus tauri. *J Biol Chem* 283, 15122-15126.

Fountain, S.J., Parkinson, K., Young, M.T., Cao, L., Thompson, C.R., and North, R.A. (2007). An intracellular P2X receptor required for osmoregulation in Dictyostelium discoideum. *Nature* 448, 200-203.

Fraser, S.P., Diss, J.K., Chioni, A.M., Mycielska, M.E., Pan, H., Yamaci, R.F., Pani, F., Siwy, Z., Krasowska, M., Grzywna, Z., *et al.* (2005). Voltage-gated sodium channel expression and potentiation of human breast cancer metastasis. *Clin Cancer Res* 11, 5381-5389.

Friebe, M., Mahmood, A., Bolzati, C., Drews, A., Johannsen, B., Eisenhut, M., Kraemer, D., Davison, A., and Jones, A.G. (2001). [99mTc]oxotechnetium(V) complexes amine-amide-dithiol chelates with dialkylaminoalkyl substituents as potential diagnostic probes for malignant melanoma. *J Med Chem* 44, 3132-3140.

Gao, R., Shen, Y., Cai, J., Lei, M., and Wang, Z. (2010). Expression of voltage-gated sodium channel alpha subunit in human ovarian cancer. *Oncol Rep* 23, 1293-1299.

Gavrilova-Ruch, O., Schonherr, K., Gessner, G., Schonherr, R., Klapperstuck, T., Wohlrab, W., and Heinemann, S.H. (2002). Effects of imipramine on ion channels and proliferation of IGR1 melanoma cells. *J Membr Biol* 188, 137-149.

Gilabert, J.A., Bakowski, D., and Parekh, A.B. (2001). Energized mitochondria increase the dynamic range over which inositol 1,4,5-trisphosphate activates store-operated calcium influx. *EMBO J* 20, 2672-2679.

Gilabert, J.A., and Parekh, A.B. (2000). Respiring mitochondria determine the pattern of activation and inactivation of the store-operated Ca($^{2+}$) current I(CRAC). *EMBO J* 19, 6401-6407.

Gillet, L., Roger, S., Besson, P., Lecaille, F., Gore, J., Bougnoux, P., Lalmanach, G., and Le Guennec, J.Y. (2009). Voltage-gated Sodium Channel Activity Promotes Cysteine Cathepsin-dependent Invasiveness and Colony Growth of Human Cancer Cells. *J Biol Chem* 284, 8680 8691.

Glitsch, M.D., Bakowski, D., and Parekh, A.B. (2002). Store-operated $Ca^{2+}$ entry depends on mitochondrial $Ca^{2+}$ uptake. *EMBO J* 21, 6744-6754.

Gomez-Varela, D., Zwick-Wallasch, E., Knotgen, H., Sanchez, A., Hettmann, T., Ossipov, D., Weseloh, R., Contreras-Jurado, C., Rothe, M., Stuhmer, W., *et al.* (2007). Monoclonal antibody blockade of the human Eag1 potassium channel function exerts antitumour activity. *Cancer Res* 67, 7343-7349.

Greig, A.V., Linge, C., Healy, V., Lim, P., Clayton, E., Rustin, M.H., McGrouther, D.A., and Burnstock, G. (2003). Expression of purinergic receptors in non-melanoma skin cancers and their functional roles in A431 cells. *J Invest Dermatol* 121, 315-327.

Guasti, L., Crociani, O., Redaelli, E., Pillozzi, S., Polvani, S., Masselli, M., Mello, T., Galli, A., Amedei, A., Wymore, R.S., *et al.* (2008). Identification of a posttranslational mechanism for the regulation of hERG1 $K^+$ channel expression and hERG1 current density in tumour cells. *Mol Cell Biol* 28, 5043-5060.

Gutman, G.A., Chandy, K.G., Adelman, J.P., Aiyar, J., Bayliss, D.A., Clapham, D.E., Covarriubias, M., Desir, G.V., Furuichi, K., Ganetzky, B., *et al.* (2003). International Union of Pharmacology. XLI. Compendium of voltage-gated ion channels: potassium channels. *Pharmacol Rev* 55, 583-586.

Habela, C.W., Ernest, N.J., Swindall, A.F., and Sontheimer, H. (2009). Chloride accumulation drives volume dynamics underlying cell proliferation and migration. *J Neurophysiol* 101, 750-757.

Hanner, M., Moebius, F.F., Flandorfer, A., Knaus, H.G., Striessnig, J., Kempner, E., and Glossmann, H. (1996). Purification, molecular cloning, and expression of the mammalian sigma1-binding site. *Proc Natl Acad Sci U S A* 93, 8072-8077.

Hayashi, T., and Su, T.P. (2007). Sigma-1 receptor chaperones at the ER-mitochondrion interface regulate $Ca(^{2+})$ signaling and cell survival. *Cell* 131, 596-610.

Hegle, A.P., Marble, D.D., and Wilson, G.F. (2006). A voltage-driven switch for ion-independent signaling by ether-a-go-go $K^+$ channels. *Proc Natl Acad Sci U S A* 103, 2886-2891.

Hemmerlein, B., Weseloh, R.M., Mello de Queiroz, F., Knotgen, H., Sanchez, A., Rubio, M.E., Martin, S., Schliephacke, T., Jenke, M., Heinz Joachim, R., *et al.* (2006). Overexpression of Eag1 potassium channels in clinical tumours. *Mol Cancer* 5, 41.

Herrera, G.M., Pozo, M.J., Zvara, P., Petkov, G.V., Bond, C.T., Adelman, J.P., and Nelson, M.T. (2003). Urinary bladder instability induced by selective suppression of the murine small conductance calcium-activated potassium (SK3) channel. *J Physiol* 551, 893-903.

Herrera, Y., Katnik, C., Rodriguez, J.D., Hall, A.A., Willing, A., Pennypacker, K.R., and Cuevas, J. (2008). sigma-1 receptor modulation of acid-sensing ion channel a (ASIC1a) and ASIC1a-induced $Ca^{2+}$ influx in rat cortical neurons. *J Pharmacol Exp Ther* 327, 491-502.

House, C.D., Vaske, C.J., Schwartz, A.M., Obias, V., Frank, B., Luu, T., Sarvazyan, N., Irby, R., Strausberg, R.L., Hales, T.G., *et al.* (2010). Voltage-gated $Na^+$ channel SCN5A is a key regulator of a gene transcriptional network that controls colon cancer invasion. *Cancer Res* 70, 6957-6967.

Hu, J., and Verkman, A.S. (2006). Increased migration and metastatic potential of tumour cells expressing aquaporin water channels. *FASEB J* 20, 1892-1894.

Ishii, T.M., Maylie, J., and Adelman, J.P. (1997). Determinants of apamin and d-tubocurarine block in SK potassium channels. *J Biol Chem* 272, 23195-23200.

Jager, H., Dreker, T., Buck, A., Giehl, K., Gress, T., and Grissmer, S. (2004). Blockage of intermediate-conductance $Ca^{2+}$-activated $K^+$ channels inhibit human pancreatic cancer cell growth in vitro. *Mol Pharmacol* 65, 630-638.

Jelassi, B., Chantôme, A., Alcaraz-Perez, F., Baroja-Mazo, A., Cayuela, M.L., Pelegrin, P., Surprenant, A., and Roger, S. (2011). P2X(7) receptor activation enhances SK3 channels- and cystein cathepsin-dependent cancer cells invasiveness. *Oncogene.*

Johannessen, M., Ramachandran, S., Riemer, L., Ramos-Serrano, A., Ruoho, A.E., and Jackson, M.B. (2009). Voltage-gated sodium channel modulation by sigma-receptors in cardiac myocytes and heterologous systems. *Am J Physiol Cell Physiol* 296, C1049-1057.

Kim, S.Y., Sivaguru, M., and Stacey, G. (2006). Extracellular ATP in plants. Visualization, localization, and analysis of physiological significance in growth and signaling. *Plant Physiol* 142, 984-992.

Klein, W.M., Wu, B.P., Zhao, S., Wu, H., Klein-Szanto, A.J., and Tahan, S.R. (2007). Increased expression of stem cell markers in malignant melanoma. *Mod Pathol* 20, 102-107.

Lastraioli, E., Guasti, L., Crociani, O., Polvani, S., Hofmann, G., Witchel, H., Bencini, L., Calistri, M., Messerini, L., Scatizzi, M., *et al.* (2004). herg1 gene and HERG1 protein are overexpressed in colorectal cancers and regulate cell invasion of tumour cells. *Cancer Res* 64, 606-611.

Le Guennec, J.Y., Ouadid-Ahidouch, H., Soriani, O., Besson, P., Ahidouch, A., and Vandier, C. (2007). Voltage-gated ion channels, new targets in anti-cancer research. *Recent Pat Anticancer Drug Discov* 2, 189-202.

Lepple-Wienhues, A., Berweck, S., Bohmig, M., Leo, C.P., Meyling, B., Garbe, C., and Wiederholt, M. (1996). $K^+$ channels and the intracellular calcium signal in human melanoma cell proliferation. *J Membr Biol* 151, 149-157.

Lewis, R.S. (2001). Calcium signaling mechanisms in T lymphocytes. *Annu Rev Immunol* 19, 497-521.

Li, X., Zhou, L., Feng, Y.H., Abdul-Karim, F.W., and Gorodeski, G.I. (2006). The P2X7 receptor: a novel biomarker of uterine epithelial cancers. *Cancer Epidemiol Biomarkers Prev* 15, 1906-1913.

Louis, M., Zanou, N., Van Schoor, M., and Gailly, P. (2008). TRPC1 regulates skeletal myoblast migration and differentiation. *J Cell Sci* 121, 3951-3959.

Mackenzie, A.B., Young, M.T., Adinolfi, E., and Surprenant, A. (2005). Pseudoapoptosis induced by brief activation of ATP-gated P2X7 receptors. *J Biol Chem* 280, 33968-33976.

Malli, R., Frieden, M., Osibow, K., Zoratti, C., Mayer, M., Demaurex, N., and Graier, W.F. (2003). Sustained $Ca^{2+}$ transfer across mitochondria is Essential for mitochondrial $Ca^{2+}$ buffering, sore-operated $Ca^{2+}$ entry, and $Ca^{2+}$ store refilling. *J Biol Chem* 278, 44769-44779.

Martin, S., Lino-de-Oliveira, C., Joca, S.R., Weffort de Oliveira, R., Echeverry, M.B., Da Silva, C.A., Pardo, L., Stuhmer, W., and Bel, E.D. (2010). Eag 1, Eag 2 and Kcnn3 gene brain expression of isolated reared rats. *Genes Brain Behav* 9, 918-924.

Martin, W.R., Eades, C.G., Thompson, J.A., Huppler, R.E., and Gilbert, P.E. (1976). The effects of morphine- and nalorphine- like drugs in the nondependent and morphine-dependent chronic spinal dog. *J Pharmacol Exp Ther* 197, 517-532.

Mathieu, V., Pirker, C., Martin de Lassalle, E., Vernier, M., Mijatovic, T., DeNeve, N., Gaussin, J.F., Dehoux, M., Lefranc, F., Berger, W., *et al.* (2009). The sodium pump alpha1 sub-unit: a disease progression-related target for metastatic melanoma treatment. *J Cell Mol Med* 13, 3960-3972.

Megalizzi, V., Mathieu, V., Mijatovic, T., Gailly, P., Debeir, O., De Neve, N., Van Damme, M., Bontempi, G., Haibe-Kains, B., Decaestecker, C., *et al.* (2007). 4-IBP, a sigma1 receptor agonist, decreases the migration of human cancer cells, including glioblastoma cells, in vitro and sensitizes them in vitro and in vivo to cytotoxic insults of proapoptotic and proautophagic drugs. *Neoplasia* 9, 358-369.

Meyer, R., Schonherr, R., Gavrilova-Ruch, O., Wohlrab, W., and Heinemann, S.H. (1999). Identification of ether a go-go and calcium-activated potassium channels in human melanoma cells. *J Membr Biol* 171, 107-115.

Millership, J.E., Devor, D.C., Hamilton, K.L., Balut, C.M., Bruce, J.I., and Fearon, I.M. (2010). Calcium Activated $K^+$ Channels Increase Cell Proliferation Independent of $K^+$ Conductance. *Am J Physiol Cell Physiol in press.*

Monaghan, A.S., Benton, D.C., Bahia, P.K., Hosseini, R., Shah, Y.A., Haylett, D.G., and Moss, G.W. (2004). The SK3 subunit of small conductance $Ca^{2+}$-activated $K^+$ channels interacts with both SK1 and SK2 subunits in a heterologous expression system. *J Biol Chem* 279, 1003-1009.

Monk, M., and Holding, C. (2001). Human embryonic genes re-expressed in cancer cells. *Oncogene* 20, 8085-8091.

Monzani, E., Bazzotti, R., Perego, C., and La Porta, C.A. (2009). AQP1 is not only a water channel: it contributes to cell migration through Lin7/beta-catenin. *PLoS One* 4, e6167.

Morth, J.P., Pedersen, B.P., Buch-Pedersen, M.J., Andersen, J.P., Vilsen, B., Palmgren, M.G., and Nissen, P. (2011). A structural overview of the plasma membrane $Na^+$,$K^+$-ATPase and $H^+$-ATPase ion pumps. *Nat Rev Mol Cell Biol* 12, 60-70.

Nilius, B., Schwarz, G., and Droogmans, G. (1993). Control of intracellular calcium by membrane potential in human melanoma cells. *Am J Physiol* 265, C1501-1510.

Nilius, B., and Wohlrab, W. (1992). Potassium channels and regulation of proliferation of human melanoma cells. *J Physiol* 445, 537-548.

North, R.A. (2002). Molecular physiology of P2X receptors. *Physiol Rev* 82, 1013-1067.

Ohshima, Y., Tsukimoto, M., Takenouchi, T., Harada, H., Suzuki, A., Sato, M., Kitani, H., and Kojima, S. (2010). gamma-Irradiation induces P2X(7) receptor-dependent ATP release from B16 melanoma cells. *Biochim Biophys Acta* 1800, 40-46.

Onganer, P.U., and Djamgoz, M.B. (2005). Small-cell Lung Cancer (Human): Potentiation of Endocytic Membrane Activity by Voltage-gated Na(+) Channel Expression in Vitro. *J Membr Biol* 204, 67-75.

Orfanelli, U., Wenke, A.K., Doglioni, C., Russo, V., Bosserhoff, A.K., and Lavorgna, G. (2008). Identification of novel sense and antisense transcription at the TRPM2 locus in cancer. *Cell Res* 18, 1128-1140.

Ouadid-Ahidouch, H., Roudbaraki, M., Delcourt, P., Ahidouch, A., Joury, N., and Prevarskaya, N. (2004). Functional and molecular identification of intermediate-conductance Ca(2+)-activated K(+) channels in breast cancer cells: association with cell cycle progression. *Am J Physiol Cell Physiol* 287, C125-134.

Pardo, L.A., del Camino, D., Sanchez, A., Alves, F., Bruggemann, A., Beckh, S., and Stuhmer, W. (1999). Oncogenic potential of EAG K(+) channels. *Embo J* 18, 5540-5547.

Pardo, L.A., and Suhmer, W. (2008). Eag1 as a cancer target. *Expert Opin Ther Targets* 12, 837-843.

Parekh, A.B. (2003). Store-operated $Ca^{2+}$ entry: dynamic interplay between endoplasmic reticulum, mitochondria and plasma membrane. *J Physiol* 547, 333-348.

Parekh, A.B. (2008). Mitochondrial regulation of store-operated CRAC channels. *Cell Calcium* 44, 6-13.

Parekh, A.B., and Putney, J.W., Jr. (2005). Store-operated calcium channels. *Physiol Rev* 85, 757-810.

Pelegrin, P. (2008). Targeting interleukin-1 signaling in chronic inflammation: focus on P2X(7) receptor and Pannexin-1. *Drug News Perspect* 21, 424-433.

Pelegrin, P., and Surprenant, A. (2006). Pannexin-1 mediates large pore formation and interleukin-1beta release by the ATP-gated P2X7 receptor. *Embo J* 25, 5071-5082.

Pillozzi, S., Brizzi, M.F., Balzi, M., Crociani, O., Cherubini, A., Guasti, L., Bartolozzi, B., Becchetti, A., Wanke, E., Bernabei, P.A., *et al.* (2002). HERG potassium channels are constitutively expressed in primary human acute myeloid leukemias and regulate cell proliferation of normal and leukemic hemopoietic progenitors. *Leukemia* 16, 1791-1798.

Pillozzi, S., Brizzi, M.F., Bernabei, P.A., Bartolozzi, B., Caporale, R., Basile, V., Boddi, V., Pegoraro, L., Becchetti, A., and Arcangeli, A. (2007). VEGFR-1 (FLT-1), beta1 integrin, and hERG $K^+$ channel for a macromolecular signaling complex in acute myeloid leukemia: role in cell migration and clinical outcome. *Blood* 110, 1238-1250.

Pillozzi, S., Masselli, M., De Lorenzo, E., Accordi, B., Cilia, E., Crociani, O., Amedei, A., Veltroni, M., D'Amico, M., Basso, G., *et al.* (2011). Chemotherapy resistance in acute lymphoblastic leukemia requires hERG1 channels and is overcome by hERG1 blockers. *Blood* 117, 902-914.

Pocsai, K., Kosztka, L., Bakondi, G., Gonczi, M., Fodor, J., Dienes, B., Szentesi, P., Kovacs, I., Feniger-Barish, R., Kopf, E., *et al.* (2006). Melanoma cells exhibit strong intracellular TASK-3-specific immunopositivity in both tissue sections and cell culture. *Cell Mol Life Sci* 63, 2364-2376.

Pongs, O., and Schwarz, J.R. (2010). Ancillary subunits associated with voltage-dependent $K^+$ channels. *Physiol Rev* 90, 755-796.

Potier, M., Joulin, V., Roger, S., Besson, P., Jourdan, M.L., Leguennec, J.Y., Bougnoux, P., and Vandier, C. (2006). Identification of SK3 channel as a new mediator of breast cancer cell migration. *Mol Cancer Ther* 5, 2946-2953.

Potier, M., Joulin, V., and Vandier, C. (2008). A method for the in vitro screening of anti-cancer compounds that inhibits SK3 activity, and said anti-cancer compounds. *WO2008015267*.

Potier, M., Tran, T.A., Chantôme, A., Girault, A., Joulin, V., Bougnoux, P., Vandier, C., and Pierre, F. (2010). Altered SK3/KCa2.3-mediated migration in adenomatous polyposis coli (Apc) mutated mouse colon epithelial cells. *Biochem Biophys Res Commun* 397, 42-47.

Prevarskaya, N., Zhang, L., and Barritt, G. (2007). TRP channels in cancer. *Biochim Biophys Acta* 1772, 937-946.

Putney, J.W., Jr. (1986). A model for receptor-regulated calcium entry. *Cell Calcium* 7, 1-12.

Quintana, A., Schwarz, E.C., Schwindling, C., Lipp, P., Kaestner, L., and Hoth, M. (2006). Sustained activity of calcium release-activated calcium channels requires translocation of mitochondria to the plasma membrane. *J Biol Chem* 281, 40302-40309.

Rae, J.M., Creighton, C.J., Meck, J.M., Haddad, B.R., and Johnson, M.D. (2007). MDA-MB-435 cells are derived from M14 melanoma cells--a loss for breast cancer, but a boon for melanoma research. *Breast Cancer Res Treat* 104, 13-19.

Raffaghello, L., Chiozzi, P., Falzoni, S., Di Virgilio, F., and Pistoia, V. (2006). The P2X7 receptor sustains the growth of human neuroblastoma cells through a substance P-dependent mechanism. *Cancer Res* 66, 907-914.

Rao, J.N., Platoshyn, O., Golovina, V.A., Liu, L., Zou, T., Marasa, B.S., Turner, D.J., Yuan, J.X., and Wang, J.Y. (2006). TRPC1 functions as a store-operated $Ca^{2+}$ channel in intestinal epithelial cells and regulates early mucosal restitution after wounding. *Am J Physiol Gastrointest Liver Physiol* 290, G782-792.

Rao, J.N., Platoshyn, O., Li, L., Guo, X., Golovina, V.A., Yuan, J.X., and Wang, J.Y. (2002). Activation of K(+) channels and increased migration of differentiated intestinal epithelial cells after wounding. *Am J Physiol Cell Physiol* 282, C885-898.

Rapaport, E. (1983). Treatment of human tumour cells with ADP or ATP yields arrest of growth in the S phase of the cell cycle. *J Cell Physiol* 114, 279-283.

Rapaport, E. (1988). Experimental cancer therapy in mice by adenine nucleotides. *Eur J Cancer Clin Oncol* 24, 1491-1497.

Rapaport, E., Fishman, R.F., and Gercel, C. (1983). Growth inhibition of human tumour cells in soft-agar cultures by treatment with low levels of adenosine 5'-triphosphate. *Cancer Res* 43, 4402-4406.

Rasheed, S., Mao, Z., Chan, J.M., and Chan, L.S. (2005). Is Melanoma a stem cell tumour? Identification of neurogenic proteins in trans-differentiated cells. *J Transl Med* 3, 14.

Rassendren, F., Buell, G.N., Virginio, C., Collo, G., North, R.A., and Surprenant, A. (1997). The permeabilizing ATP receptor, P2X7. Cloning and expression of a human cDNA. *J Biol Chem* 272, 5482-5486.

Renaudo, A., L'Hoste, S., Guizouarn, H., Borgese, F., and Soriani, O. (2007). Cancer cell cycle modulated by a functional coupling between sigma-1 receptors and Cl- channels. *J Biol Chem* 282, 2259-2267.

Renaudo, A., Watry, V., Chassot, A.A., Ponzio, G., Ehrenfeld, J., and Soriani, O. (2004). Inhibition of tumour cell proliferation by sigma ligands is associated with $K^+$ Channel inhibition and p27kip1 accumulation. *J Pharmacol Exp Ther* 311, 1105-1114.

Rizzuto, R., and Pozzan, T. (2006). Microdomains of intracellular $Ca^{2+}$: molecular determinants and functional consequences. *Physiol Rev* 86, 369-408.

Roger, S., Besson, P., and Le Guennec, J.Y. (2003). Involvement of a novel fast inward sodium current in the invasion capacity of a breast cancer cell line. *Biochim Biophys Acta* 1616, 107-111.

Roger, S., Gillet, L., Baroja-Mazo, A., Surprenant, A., and Pelegrin, P. (2010). C-terminal calmodulin-binding motif differentially controls human and rat P2X7 receptor current facilitation. *J Biol Chem* 285, 17514-17524.

Roger, S., Pelegrin, P., and Surprenant, A. (2008). Facilitation of P2X7 receptor currents and membrane blebbing via constitutive and dynamic calmodulin binding. *J Neurosci* 28, 6393-6401.

Roger, S., Rollin, J., Barascu, A., Besson, P., Raynal, P.I., Iochmann, S., Lei, M., Bougnoux, P., Gruel, Y., and Le Guennec, J.Y. (2007). Voltage-gated sodium channels potentiate the invasive capacities of human non-small-cell lung cancer cell lines. *Int J Biochem Cell Biol* 39, 774-786.

Romagnoli, R., Baraldi, P.G., Cruz-Lopez, O., Lopez-Cara, C., Preti, D., Borea, P.A., and Gessi, S. (2008). The P2X7 receptor as a therapeutic target. *Expert Opin Ther Targets* 12, 647-661.

Rouzaire-Dubois, B., Milandri, J.B., Bostel, S., and Dubois, J.M. (2000). Control of cell proliferation by cell volume alterations in rat C6 glioma cells. *Pflugers Arch* 440, 881-888.

Rusznak, Z., Bakondi, G., Kosztka, L., Pocsai, K., Dienes, B., Fodor, J., Telek, A., Gonczi, M., Szucs, G., and Csernoch, L. (2008). Mitochondrial expression of the two-pore domain TASK-3 channels in malignantly transformed and non-malignant human cells. *Virchows Arch* 452, 415-426.

Saadoun, S., Papadopoulos, M.C., Hara-Chikuma, M., and Verkman, A.S. (2005). Impairment of angiogenesis and cell migration by targeted aquaporin-1 gene disruption. *Nature* 434, 786-792.

Sandoval, A.J., Riquelme, J.P., Carretta, M.D., Hancke, J.L., Hidalgo, M.A., and Burgos, R.A. (2007). Store-operated calcium entry mediates intracellular alkalinization, ERK1/2, and Akt/PKB phosphorylation in bovine neutrophils. *J Leukoc Biol* 82, 1266-1277.

Sanguinetti, M.C., Jiang, C., Curran, M.E., and Keating, M.T. (1995). A mechanistic link between an inherited and an acquired cardiac arrhythmia: HERG encodes the IKr potassium channel. *Cell* 81, 299-307.

Santella, L., Ercolano, E., and Nusco, G. (2005). The cell cycle: a new entry in the field of Ca<sup>$^{2+}$</sup> signaling. In Cellular and Molecular Life Sciences (BirkhÃ€user Basel), pp. 2405-2413.

Schmidt, J., Friebel, K., Schonherr, R., Coppolino, M.G., and Bosserhoff, A.K. (2010). Migration-associated secretion of melanoma inhibitory activity at the cell rear is supported by KCa3.1 potassium channels. *Cell Res* 20, 1224-1238.

Schwab, A. (2001). Function and spatial distribution of ion channels and transporters in cell migration. *Am J Physiol Renal Physiol* 280, F739-747.

Schwab, A., Reinhardt, J., Schneider, S.W., Gassner, B., and Schuricht, B. (1999). K($^{+}$) channel-dependent migration of fibroblasts and human melanoma cells. *Cell Physiol Biochem* 9, 126-132.

Schwarz, J.R., and Bauer, C.K. (2004). Functions of erg $K^{+}$ channels in excitable cells. *J Cell Mol Med* 8, 22-30.

Sellappan, S., Grijalva, R., Zhou, X., Yang, W., Eli, M.B., Mills, G.B., and Yu, D. (2004). Lineage infidelity of MDA-MB-435 cells: expression of melanocyte proteins in a breast cancer cell line. *Cancer Res* 64, 3479-3485.

Slater, M., Danieletto, S., and Barden, J.A. (2005). Expression of the apoptotic calcium channel P2X7 in the glandular epithelium. *J Mol Histol* 36, 159-165.

Slater, M., Danieletto, S., Gidley-Baird, A., Teh, L.C., and Barden, J.A. (2004a). Early prostate cancer detected using expression of non-functional cytolytic P2X7 receptors. *Histopathology* 44, 206-215.

Slater, M., Danieletto, S., Pooley, M., Cheng Teh, L., Gidley-Baird, A., and Barden, J.A. (2004b). Differentiation between cancerous and normal hyperplastic lobules in breast lesions. *Breast Cancer Res Treat* 83, 1-10.

Slater, M., Scolyer, R.A., Gidley-Baird, A., Thompson, J.F., and Barden, J.A. (2003). Increased expression of apoptotic markers in melanoma. *Melanoma Res* 13, 137-145.

Slipicevic, A., Holm, R., Nguyen, M.T., Bohler, P.J., Davidson, B., and Florenes, V.A. (2005). Expression of activated Akt and PTEN in malignant melanomas: relationship with clinical outcome. *Am J Clin Pathol* 124, 528-536.

Soengas, M.S., and Lowe, S.W. (2003). Apoptosis and melanoma chemoresistance. *Oncogene* 22, 3138-3151.

Solini, A., Cuccato, S., Ferrari, D., Santini, E., Gulinelli, S., Callegari, M.G., Dardano, A., Faviana, P., Madec, S., Di Virgilio, F., *et al.* (2008). Increased P2X7 receptor expression and function in thyroid papillary cancer: a new potential marker of the disease? *Endocrinology* 149, 389-396.

Soriani, O., Foll, F.L., Roman, F., Monnet, F.P., Vaudry, H., and Cazin, L. (1999a). A-Current down-modulated by sigma receptor in frog pituitary melanotrope cells through a G protein-dependent pathway. *J Pharmacol Exp Ther* 289, 321-328.

Soriani, O., Le Foll, F., Galas, L., Roman, F., Vaudry, H., and Cazin, L. (1999b). The sigma-ligand (+)-pentazocine depresses M current and enhances calcium conductances in frog melanotrophs. *Am J Physiol* 277, E73-80.

Soriani, O., Vaudry, H., Mei, Y.A., Roman, F., and Cazin, L. (1998). Sigma ligands stimulate the electrical activity of frog pituitary melanotrope cells through a G-protein-dependent inhibition of potassium conductances. *J Pharmacol Exp Ther* 286, 163-171.

Stein, R.J., Santos, S., Nagatomi, J., Hayashi, Y., Minnery, B.S., Xavier, M., Patel, A.S., Nelson, J.B., Futrell, W.J., Yoshimura, N., *et al.* (2004). Cool (TRPM8) and hot (TRPV1) receptors in the bladder and male genital tract. *J Urol* 172, 1175-1178.

Stock, C., Mueller, M., Kraehling, H., Mally, S., Noel, J., Eder, C., and Schwab, A. (2007). pH nanoenvironment at the surface of single melanoma cells. *Cell Physiol Biochem* 20, 679-686.

Stock, C., and Schwab, A. (2009). Protons make tumour cells move like clockwork. *Pflugers Arch* 458, 981-992.

Su, T.P., Hayashi, T., Maurice, T., Buch, S., and Ruoho, A.E. (2010). The sigma-1 receptor chaperone as an inter-organelle signaling modulator. *Trends Pharmacol Sci* 31, 557-566.

Surprenant, A., Rassendren, F., Kawashima, E., North, R.A., and Buell, G. (1996). The cytolytic P2Z receptor for extracellular ATP identified as a P2X receptor (P2X7). *Science* 272, 735-738.

Tajima, N., Schonherr, K., Niedling, S., Kaatz, M., Kanno, H., Schonherr, R., and Heinemann, S.H. (2006). $Ca^{2+}$-activated $K^+$ channels in human melanoma cells are up-regulated by hypoxia involving hypoxia-inducible factor-1alpha and the von Hippel-Lindau protein. *J Physiol* 571, 349-359.

Taylor, M.S., Bonev, A.D., Gross, T.P., Eckman, D.M., Brayden, J.E., Bond, C.T., Adelman, J.P., and Nelson, M.T. (2003). Altered expression of small-conductance $Ca^{2+}$-activated $K^+$ (SK3) channels modulates arterial tone and blood pressure. *Circ Res* 93, 124-131.

Testa, J.R., and Tsichlis, P.N. (2005). AKT signaling in normal and malignant cells. *Oncogene* 24, 7391-7393.

Timar, J., Kasler, M., Katai, J., Soos, M., Mathiasz, D., Romany, A., Patthy, L., Kovacs, G., Jozsa, A., Szilak, L., *et al.* (2006). [Developments in cancer management by innovative genomics. 2006 report of the National Cancer Consortium]. *Magy Onkol* 50, 349-359.

Toyama, K., Wulff, H., Chandy, K.G., Azam, P., Raman, G., Saito, T., Fujiwara, Y., Mattson, D.L., Das, S., Melvin, J.E., *et al.* (2008). The intermediate-conductance calcium-activated potassium channel KCa3.1 contributes to atherogenesis in mice and humans. *J Clin Invest* 118, 3025-3037.

Trudeau, M.C., Warmke, J.W., Ganetzky, B., and Robertson, G.A. (1995). HERG, a human inward rectifier in the voltage-gated potassium channel family. *Science* 269, 92-95.

Tsai, S.Y., Hayashi, T., Mori, T., and Su, T.P. (2009). Sigma-1 receptor chaperones and diseases. *Cent Nerv Syst Agents Med Chem* 9, 184-189.

Varadi, A., Cirulli, V., and Rutter, G.A. (2004). Mitochondrial localization as a determinant of capacitative $Ca^{2+}$ entry in HeLa cells. *Cell Calcium* 36, 499-508.

Villalonga, N., Ferreres, J.C., Argiles, J.M., Condom, E., and Felipe, A. (2007). Potassium channels are a new target field in anticancer drug design. *Recent Patents Anticancer Drug Discov* 2, 212-223.

Wang, Q., Wang, L., Feng, Y.H., Li, X., Zeng, R., and Gorodeski, G.I. (2004). P2X7 receptor-mediated apoptosis of human cervical epithelial cells. *Am J Physiol Cell Physiol* 287, C1349-1358.

Wang, Z.H., Shen, B., Yao, H.L., Jia, Y.C., Ren, J., Feng, Y.J., and Wang, Y.Z. (2007). Blockage of intermediate-conductance-Ca($^{2+}$) -activated K($^{+}$) channels inhibits progression of human endometrial cancer. *Oncogene* 26, 5107-5114.

Waning, J., Vriens, J., Owsianik, G., Stuwe, L., Mally, S., Fabian, A., Frippiat, C., Nilius, B., and Schwab, A. (2007). A novel function of capsaicin-sensitive TRPV1 channels: involvement in cell migration. *Cell Calcium* 42, 17-25.

Weber, C., Mello de Queiroz, F., Downie, B.R., Suckow, A., Stuhmer, W., and Pardo, L.A. (2006). Silencing the activity and proliferative properties of the human EagI Potassium Channel by RNA Interference. *J Biol Chem* 281, 13030-13037.

Weerasinghe, R.R., Swanson, S.J., Okada, S.F., Garrett, M.B., Kim, S.Y., Stacey, G., Boucher, R.C., Gilroy, S., and Jones, A.M. (2009). Touch induces ATP release in Arabidopsis roots that is modulated by the heterotrimeric G-protein complex. *FEBS Lett* 583, 2521-2526.

White, N., Butler, P.E., and Burnstock, G. (2005). Human melanomas express functional P2 X(7) receptors. *Cell Tissue Res* 321, 411-418.

White, N., Knight, G.E., Butler, P.E., and Burnstock, G. (2009). An in vivo model of melanoma: treatment with ATP. *Purinergic Signal* 5, 327-333.

Wiley, J.S., Dao-Ung, L.P., Gu, B.J., Sluyter, R., Shemon, A.N., Li, C., Taper, J., Gallo, J., and Manoharan, A. (2002). A loss-of-function polymorphic mutation in the cytolytic P2X7 receptor gene and chronic lymphocytic leukaemia: a molecular study. *Lancet* 359, 1114-1119.

Wondergem, R., Ecay, T.W., Mahieu, F., Owsianik, G., and Nilius, B. (2008). HGF/SF and menthol increase human glioblastoma cell calcium and migration. *Biochem Biophys Res Commun* 372, 210-215.

Wulff, H., Miller, M.J., Hansel, W., Grissmer, S., Cahalan, M.D., and Chandy, K.G. (2000). Design of a potent and selective inhibitor of the intermediate-conductance $Ca^{2+}$-activated $K^{+}$ channel, IKCa1: a potential immunosuppressant. *Proc Natl Acad Sci U S A* 97, 8151-8156.

Yamamura, H., Ugawa, S., Ueda, T., Morita, A., and Shimada, S. (2008a). TRPM8 activation suppresses cellular viability in human melanoma. *Am J Physiol Cell Physiol* 295, C296-301.

Yamamura, H., Ugawa, S., Ueda, T., and Shimada, S. (2008b). Expression analysis of the epithelial $Na^{+}$ channel delta subunit in human melanoma G-361 cells. *Biochem Biophys Res Commun* 366, 489-492.

Yohem, K.H., Clothier, J.L., Montague, S.L., Geary, R.J., Winters, A.L., 3rd, Hendrix, M.J., and Welch, D.R. (1991). Inhibition of tumour cell invasion by verapamil. *Pigment Cell Res* 4, 225-233.

Zhang, X.J., Zheng, G.G., Ma, X.T., Yang, Y.H., Li, G., Rao, Q., Nie, K., and Wu, K.F. (2004). Expression of P2X7 in human hematopoietic cell lines and leukemia patients. *Leuk Res* 28, 1313-1322.

# 21

# Targeting the Proteasome in Melanoma

Rosa M. Marti et al.*
*Department of Dermatology;*
*Hospital Universitari Arnau de Vilanova. University of Lleida. IRBLLEIDA. Lleida;*
*Spain*

## 1. Introduction

Malignant melanoma, once disseminated, is a malignant neoplasm extremely resistant to conventional anticancer treatment, such as chemo or radiation therapies. Therefore, new therapeutic strategies are under investigation as, for instance, immunotherapy, gene therapy or so called targeted therapy. Proteasome appears as one of these new possible targets.

The ubiquitin proteasome pathway is a complex multicatalytic system specialized in the degradation of proteins of intracellular origin, unlike lysosomes that are specialized in the degradation of proteins of extracellular origin.

Many of the proteins degraded by the proteasome are molecules involved in cell proliferation and apoptosis, such as cyclins and cyclin dependent kinases, the proapoptotic protein p53 or the nuclear transcription factor NFkappaB. It has been demonstrated that inhibition of proteasome induces cell death, more strongly in neoplastic cells than in normal cells, and, even more, that proteasome inhibition sensitizes neoplastic cells to other proapoptotic stimulus such as chemo o radiation therapy, probably by the NFkappaB pathway. Therefore, the proteasome could be a good target for cells so resistant to apoptosis as melanoma cells are.

We and others have demonstrated that melanoma cells are sensitive *in vitro* to Bortezomib and other proteasome inhibitors, that are able to decrease melanoma cell viability, to induce a reduction in cell proliferation rate and a cell cycle arrest and to trigger apoptotic cell death through both caspase dependent and independent pathways.

Bortezomib is a commercially available proteasome inhibitor, mainly used for the treatment of multiple myeloma and other malignant hematological disorders. Although the only published phase II clinical trial using single agent Bortezomib in patients with advanced melanoma yielded disappointing results, the potential use of proteasome inhibitors for the treatment of metastatic melanoma patients is still under assessment. Based on the knowledge of the physiological role of the proteasome system and on preclinical studies, employment of proteasome inhibitors in combined therapies seems the best way to afford the use of these compounds for advanced melanoma treatment.

---

*Anabel Sorolla[1,2], Andree Yeramian[1,2], Xavier Dolcet[1,2], Leandro Abal[3], Eugenia Ortega[4], Ramon Egido[2], Xavier Matias-Guiu[2]
[1]*Laboratory of Research;* [2]*Department of Pathology and Molecular Genetics;* [3]*Department of Dermatology;* [4]*Department of Oncology; Hospital Universitari Arnau de Vilanova. University of Lleida. IRBLLEIDA. Lleida; Spain*

One of the first drugs employed to this aim was Temozolamide, a chemotherapeutic agent that has shown to exert an antitumour effect in a synergic manner when administrated with Bortezomib in melanoma animal models. A phase I clinical trial combining Bortezomib and Temozolamide that enrolled 19 patients with advanced malignant melanoma has been recently published. Although the study has been designed to define phase II dose schedule, some limited results (partial response, disease stabilization) have been observed.
Other multiple combinations containing proteasome inhibitors have been tested in both *in vitro* and *in vivo* pre-clinical studies. Some of the therapies that have been shown to synergize with proteasome inhibitors against melanoma cells are several chemotherapeutic agents, calpain inhibitors, interferon, tyrosin-kinase inhibitors, different types of cell mediated immunotherapy, etc. As proteasome inhibitors are drugs with pleiotropic effects on proliferation and suppression of apoptosis, cell invasion and angiogenesis, multiple pathways have been proposed to explain how proteasome inhibition can reduce or avoid tumor growth, but ultimate mechanisms remain unclear. In that sense, a great research effort is necessary to elucidate the molecular basis of the proteasome inhibitors action on melanoma cells in order to better design combined therapeutic strategies. We hope that in the future one or more of these or other possible combinations will reach successfully the clinical setting.
Finally, a new promise on the employment of proteasome inhibitors for the treatment of metastatic melanoma, are the second generation proteasome inhibitors. They include the peptide boronic acid analogs MLN9708 and CEP-18770, the peptide epoxyketones carfilzomib and PR-047, and the beta-lactone compound NPI-0052, all of which show a potent *in vitro* proteasome inhibitory activity. They differ in enzyme binding kinetics, which might affect their pharmacological properties, efficacy and toxicity. All these features will define their future clinical use.
In the present chapter we will review the structure and function of the proteasome, the role of proteasome inhibitors as anti-cancer agents and the current status of preclinical and clinical knowledge about the potential use of proteasome inhibitors for metastatic melanoma treatment.

## 2. The proteasome

The ubiquitin proteasome pathway is a complex multicatalytic system specialized in the degradation of proteins of intracellular origin (Voorhees 2006). Protein synthesis and protein degradation are important processes in cellular homeostasis that ensure maintenance of protein regulation (Gallastegui 2010). Nevertheless, the concept of protein turnover is quite new. At the beginning of the last century, body proteins were viewed as essentially stable constituents, and diet proteins were believed to function primarily as energy-providing products, which were independent from the structural and functional proteins of the organism. The discovery of the lysosome, as one of the compartments for cell protein processing, along with other experiments that were carried out at the same time, have strengthened the notion that cellular proteins are indeed in a constant state of synthesis and degradation (Ciechanover 2010). However, proteolysis in lysosomes is a nonspecific process. In higher eukaryotes, only membrane-associated proteins and alien proteins captured during endocytosis (viral, bacterial, etc.) are destroyed in lysosomes. Degradation of the vast majority (80-90%) of intracellular proteins is realized by the proteasome (Sorokin 2009).
The proteasome is a large cylindrical particle consisting of at least 33 subunits, with a total molecular weight of approximately 2.5 MDa. There are several variants of the proteasome

that perform slightly different functions. For example, cells of the immune system contain a particular form of the proteasome, the immunoproteasome, that produces peptides for display at the cell surface (Schrader 2009). The peptides generated by the immunoproteasome are not subjected to further degradation by cell peptidases and are used for antigen presentation (Sorokin 2009). The version of the proteasome that is found in all cells and is responsible for the specific degradation of regulatory proteins and the removal of damaged proteins is called the 26S proteasome. The 26S proteasome is composed of a 20S core particle capped by two 19S regulatory particles at both ends (Fig 1). The 20S core particle is composed by four heptameric rings, which are assembled to form a cylindrical structure. The outer two rings are made of α subunits, and the inner two rings are composed of β subunits, which contain the proteolytic active sites in a central cavity. The degradation chamber can be reached through a channel that runs along the long axis of the core particle. The entrance to the channel is narrow, such that folded proteins must be at least partially unfolded before they can be translocated into the 20S core particle and degraded. The 19S regulatory particle is composed of at least 19 subunits arranged into two subcomplexes: the lid and the base. (Schrader 2009).

Ubiquitin is a 76-amino-acid-residue protein. It is highly conservative in eukaryotes, but is absent in bacteria and archaea. In eukaryotes, several genes encode ubiquitin. Activation of ubiquitin requires processing by so called deubiquitinating enzymes (Sorokin 2009). Proteins targeted for degradation by the 26S proteasome are first "labeled" by covalent linkage of a polyubiquitin chain, via a three-step cascade mechanism utilizing the following three enzymes: E1, the ubiquitin-activating enzyme, E2, the ubiquitin-carrier protein, and E3, the ubiquitin-protein ligase. Successive conjugation of ubiquitin moieties generates a polyubiquitin chain. A polyubiquitin chain consists at minimum of four molecules. These polyubiquitinated substrates are recognized by the 26S proteasome and rapidly broken down into short peptides. One important function of the 19S regulatory particle is to recognize ubiquitinated proteins and other potential substrates of the proteasome. A second function of the 19S regulatory particle is to open an orifice in the α-ring that will allow entry of the substrate into the proteolytic chamber. Also, since a folded protein would not be able to fit through the narrow proteasomal channel, it is assumed that the 19S particle unfolds substrates and inserts them into the 20S core particle. Both the channel opening function and the unfolding of the substrate require metabolic energy, and indeed, the base of the 19S regulatory particle contains six different ATPase subunits. Following degradation of the substrate, short peptides derived from the substrate are released, as well as reusable ubiquitin (Fig. 1) (Ciechanover 2010, Kim 2011). This process has been named the "ubiquitin-dependent degradation of protein" (Sorokin 2009).

Substrates for this non lysosomal protein degradation pathway include misfolded and defective proteins, as well as others that are selectively polyubiquitin-tagged and targeted for degradation by the ubiquitin-proteasome system (Potts 2010). Proteins differ greatly from each other in lifetime, and the lifetime of protein molecules in an organism depends on their role. So, some structural proteins can remain unchanged for many years, whereas regulatory proteins are frequently required only for a few minutes to trigger a certain process and after completing their function they should be destroyed. Moreover, in the course of time, cells accumulate a large amount of aberrantly folded and oxidized protein that should be also eliminated. The proteasome is the basis of a complex multicomponent cellular machine for getting rid of these unwanted cell proteins (Sorokin 2009).

Proteasomes in eukaryotic cells are localized both in the cytoplasm and in the nucleus. Nuclear/cytoplasmic distribution of proteasomes seems to be tissue-specific. The distribution of proteasomes between the cytoplasm and the nucleus also changes remarkably during embryogenesis. In spermatozoids and ovules, proteasomes are concentrated in the cytoplasm, at early stages of subdivision they translocate to the nucleus, and by the blastocyst stage the intracellular localization of proteasomes is close to their distribution in adult somatic cells. Besides, intracellular distribution of proteasomes changes dynamically in accord with the cell cycle phase. Proteasomal degradation of cyclins in the nucleus is a necessary condition for the normal course of the cell cycle (Sorokin 2009).

During the last years, experimental data have pointed about the existence of deviations from the classical protein degradation pathway. The vast majority of examples of non-classical proteasomal degradation are associated with the ubiquitin-independent degradation of proteasome substrates. Some of the proteins that can undergo ubiquitin-independent degradation are ornithine decarboxylase, p21, p53 and oncosupressive Rb proteins (Sorokin 2009).

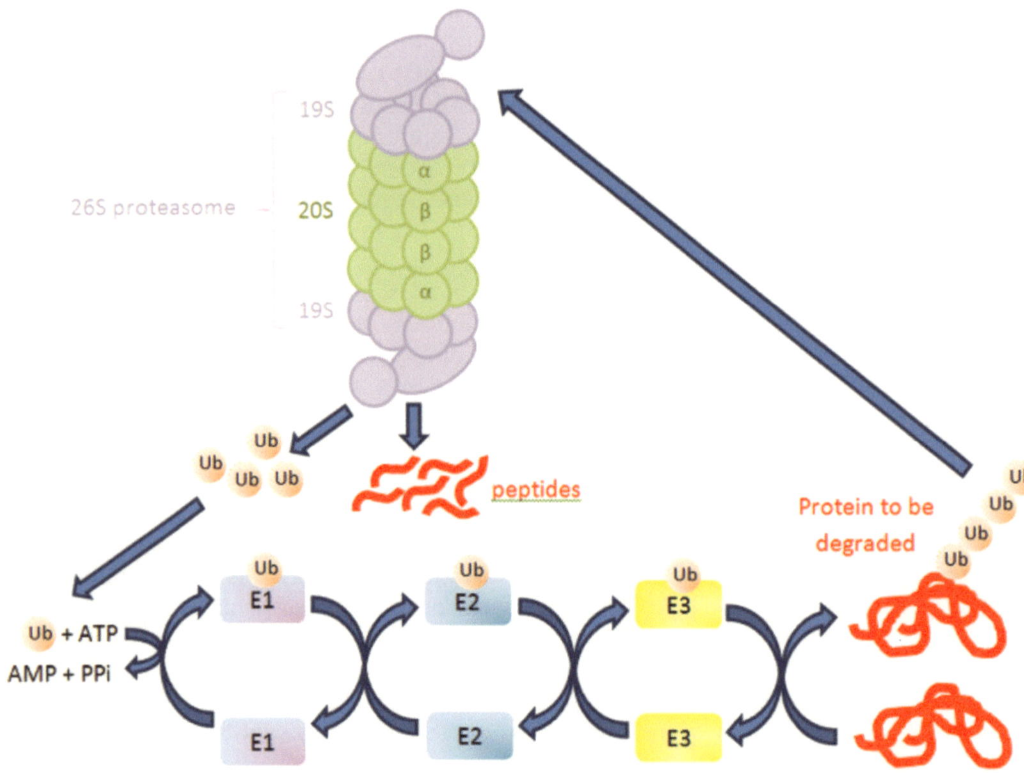


Fig. 1. The ubiquitin-proteasome pathway: The scheme shows the main steps of the ubiquitin-proteasome pathway in eukaryotic cells. First, the ATP consumption is needed for the binding of ubiquitin (Ub) with the ubiquitin activating enzyme (E1). Second, the ubiquitin-carrier protein (E2) takes the ubiquitin molecule from E1. Third, ubiquitin molecule is transferred from the E2 to the ubiquitin-protein ligase (E3). Fourth, the target proteins bind up to four molecules of ubiquitin. Fifth, the proteasome recognizes the protein and finally the protein is degraded by the catalytic core 20S, releasing free molecules of ubiquitin and digested peptides

In addition, recent emerging evidences suggest the existence of many other non-proteolytic functions of both the proteasome and ubiquitin. Non-proteolytic functions of proteasome include DNA repair, transcription initiation and transcription elongation. Ubiquitin has even more diverse non-proteolytic functions, such as membrane trafficking, protein kinase activation, DNA repair, and chromatin remodelling. The relationship of non-proteolytic functions between proteasome and ubiquitin is not clear. (Kim 2011, Kwak 2011, Livnat-Levanon 2011).

The discovery that ubiquitin modification plays a role in routing proteins to the lysosome/vacuole and that modification by specific and unique ubiquitin-like proteins controls autophagy demonstrated that the two distinct proteolytic systems, the lysosomes and the proteasome, communicate with one another (Ciechanover 2010).

With the many processes and substrates targeted by the ubiquitin pathway, it is not surprising to find that aberrations in the system underlie, directly or indirectly, the pathogenesis of many diseases (Ciechanover 2010).

## 3. Proteasome inhibitors as anticancer agents

In addition to providing a mechanism for cellular protein quality control, the ubiquitin-proteasome pathway facilitates essential cell functions ranging from antigen processing to signal transduction, cell cycle control, proliferation, differentiation, angiogenesis and apoptosis. Thus, besides involving in normal cellular functions and homeostasis, the alteration of proteasomal activity contributes to the pathological states of several clinical disorders including inflammation, neurodegeneration and cancer. These critical roles, together with the ubiquitious nature of the proteolytic 20S core particle, suggest multiple potential applications for proteasome inhibition for several pathological conditions such as inflammation / autoimmune diseases and cancer therapy (Potts 2010, Chen Current Protein 2010).

Many of the proteins degraded by the proteasome are molecules involved in cell proliferation and apoptosis, such as cyclins and cyclin dependent kinases, the proapoptotic protein p53, members of the Bcl2 family, the nuclear transcription factor NFkappaB, etc. Thus, the inhibition of proteasome activity could have important downstream consequences that can be used to advantage in tumor cells. It has been demonstrated that inhibition of the proteasome induces cell death in both normal and neoplastic cells, that cancer cells possess elevated levels of proteasome activity and are more sensitive to proteasome inhibitors than normal cells and, even more, that proteasome inhibition sensitizes neoplastic cells to other proapoptotic stimulus such as chemo o radiation therapy, probably by the NFkappaB pathway. These and other findings provided strong rationale for targeting the proteasome for the treatment of cancer (Voorhees 2006, Potts 2010, Chen 2010b).

One of the principal actions of proteasome inhibitors are the regulation of cell cycle control molecules. Ubiquitin-dependent proteolysis mediates the normal turnover of p53, the guardian of human genome. Consequently, proteasome inhibition leads to p53 accumulation and subsequently induces the transcription of cyclin-dependent kinase inhibitor p21. Proteasome inhibition also induces p53 phosphorylation. Some studies reveal that the ubiquitin-proteasome system is responsible for the degradation of p21 and p27, both of which are important cell cycle regulators whose expression are down-regulated in various malignancies. So, an important biologic effect of proteasome inhibitors is the accumulation of p27 (Voorhees 2006, Wu 2010, Chen 2010b).

Another main action of proteasome inhibitors is the regulation of pro- and anti-apoptotic proteins. The execution of apoptosis is largely governed by opposing activities of pro-(Bax, Bak, Bik,Bim, Bad, Bid, HRK, NOXA, PUMA, and BNIP3) and antiapoptotic (Bcl-2, Bcl-xL, Bcl-w, A1, and Mcl-1) members of the Bcl-2 family. Altogether, such group of proteins regulates mitochondrial membrane permeability, cytochrome C release, generation of reactive oxygen species, and caspase activation. Proteasome inhibition has been shown to favor balance to pro-apoptotic signaling. Therefore, proteasome inhibitors block the degradation and upregulate the expression of Bax, Bik, Bim, and NOXA. Proteasome inhibition also activates transcription of PUMA and promotes Mcl-1 cleavage. Moreover, proteasome inhibitors downregulate the expression of a class of proteins, known as inhibitors of apoptosis (IAPs), that suppresses the effector caspases. To this end, proteasome inhibitors reduce the expression of several IAPs, including cIAP-1, XIAP and survivins (Voorhees 2006, Wu 2010, Chen 2010b)

As above mentioned, proteasome inhibitors have been shown to synergize with several chemotherapeutic drugs inducing apoptosis of malignant cells. This action has been mainly explained by their inhibitory effect on NFκB activation. NFκB is a heterodimeric transcription factor, mostly composed of 65 and 50 kDa subunits, which is prevented from translocation into the nucleus through association with a family of inhibitory proteins called IκB. Upon stimulation through several factors (basically chemokines and cytokines, such as TNFα, free radicals, ultraviolet radiation or bacterial components) the IκB is phosphorylated, ubiquitinated and subsequently degraded in the 26S proteasome. Then, free NFκB translocates into the nucleus, where it activates transcription of genes whose products can inhibit apoptosis by mediating cellular survival responses. This signal pathway has been called "canonical" NFκB activation, in front of "non-canonical" or different mechanisms of activation of NFκB. As NFκB also regulates angiogenesis, cell cycle control, adhesion and migration, strategies employed by malignant tumors to evade antitumoral therapies include upregulation of NFkB. Thus, on the one hand, many tumor cells, in contrast to their normal counterparts, show constitutive activation of NFkB. On the other hand, treatment of malignancies with radiation therapy or some cytostatic compounds, such as anthracycline drugs, leads to induced activation of NFkB. The latter mechanism is considered a major cause for the development of inducible chemoresistance. Thus, strategies to inhibit NFkB in malignant tumors are considered a worthwhile addition to the current therapeutic options. One way to indirectly inhibit the NFκB pathway is via the inhibition of the 26S proteasome. Lack of degradation of IκB induces increased levels of the IκB inhibitory subunit that prevents NFκB from translocation into the nucleus, and subsequently activation of anti-apoptotic and survival signals. In addition, the proteasome has also shown to have a role in the "non-canonical" NFκB activation. Consequently, proteasome inhibitors are strong potential substances for NFκB blockade of and chemosenzitation of cancer cells (Voorhees 2006, Yang 2006, Testa 2009, Amschler 2010).

Thus, proteasome inhibitors induce tumoral cell-cycle arrest and apoptosis, inhibit cell-adhesion, migration and release of angiogenic factors and sensitize malignant cells to pro-apoptotic stimulus such as chemotherapeutic agents or radiation therapy (Amschler 2010, Testa 2009, Wu 2010, Chen 2010b)

Other important actions of proteasome inhibitors are the accumulation of misfolded proteins and endoplasmic reticulum stress, the induction of oxidative stress, the down regulation of the PI3K/AKT pathway, the activation of bone morphogenetic protein signaling, the repression of global protein translation, the immunosensitization of cancer cells to the cytotoxicity of lymphocytes, etc. In addition, proteasome inhibitors can induce cytoprotective responses that attenuate their antitumor efficacy, such as upregulation of heat-shock proteins, induction of macroautophagy, or activation of some other prosurvival signaling pathways, even NFκB. In summary, the specific effects and precise mechanism of action of proteasome inhibition in malignancy remain unclear and are subject to further investigation (Rajkumar 2005, Voorhees 2006, Wu 2010).

There are five main types of proteasome inhibitors that bind either reversibly or irreversibly to the active enzyme sites in the 20S proteasome, primarily the chymotrypsin-like site, thus inhibiting their proteolytic function. These types include peptide vinyl sulfones, peptide boronates, peptide epoxyketones (Epoxomycin and Eponomycin) and -lactones (Lactacystin and derivatives). Only a few compounds have progressed to clinical development, however, with others deemed unsuitable owing to metabolic instability, potency issues or lack of specificity (Dick 2010).

Bortezomib (PS-341) is the first-in-class proteasome inhibitor that reached human clinical use. Other first-in-class proteasome inhibitors, not available for clinical use in humans (such as MG-132, ALLN, Lactacystin, Epoxomicin, etc), have been extensively employed in the experimental setting in order to better understand the ubiquitin-proteasome pathway and the potential clinical use of the whole group. Bortezomib is a dipeptidyl boronic acid analog that reversibly inhibits the 26S proteasome by binding to N terminal threonine residues in the active site of the chymotrypsin-like catalytic región. It has been approved for the treatment of multiple myeloma and relapsed mantle cell lymphoma. However, it has generally been ineffective as monotherapy for the treatment of a wide variety of solid tumors. Bortezomib can overcome or reverse chemoresistance and increase sensitivity to chemotherapeutic agents, including Melphalan, Doxorubicin, Mitoxantrone, and to Dexamethasone. Such combinations have been approved for relapsed or newly diagnosed multiple myeloma. Moreover, combinations of Bortezomib and novel targeted therapies may act synergistically to increase antitumor activity and overcome specific cellular resistance and/or antiapoptotic mechanisms. Those targeted therapies include protein deacetylase inhibitors, kinase inhibitors, farnesyltransferase inhibitors, heat-shock protein 90 inhibitors, pan-Bcl-2 family inhibitors, and other classes of targeted inhibitors. Based in the results of preclinical studies, some early-phase clinical trials combining Bortezomib and other targeted therapies are ongoing, basically for the treatment of multiple myeloma patients (Voorhees 2006, Testa 2009, Orlowski 2008, Wright 2010 Eisenle 2010).

In clinical trials of multiple myeloma patients, Bortezomib adverse events have been reported in at least 10% of cases. They include anemia, anorexia, constipation, dehydration, diarrhea, dizziness, fatigue, headache, limb pain, nausea, neutropenia, peripheral neuropathy, pyrexia, rash, thrombocytopenia, vomiting, and weakness. Thrombocytopenia and neuropathy are probably the most limiting in the clinic (Orlowski 2008).

With the validation of the proteasome as a target for cancer therapy, interest has focused on the possibility that proteasome inhibitors other than Bortezomib could offer some advantages. Various second-generation agents are now in development. Among peptide boronic acid analogs, two new molecules have to be mentioned. MLN9708, which hydrolyses immediately in plasma to MLN2238, is a reversible inhibitor of the chymotrypsin-like subunit of the 20S proteasome that is distinct from Bortezomib in having a substantially shorter dissociation half-life. CEP-18770 (Cephalon) is a P2 threonine boronic acid that is another reversible inhibitor, primarily of the chymotrypsin-like activity of the proteasome. Two compounds in the peptide epoxyketone class are being developed. Carfilzomib (formerly PR-171) is an irreversible inhibitor of the chymotrypsin-like activity of the proteasome, and PR-047 is an orally bioavailable analog of Carfilzomib, again being an irreversible inhibitor of the β5 subunit. Finally, several natural compounds have been identified as inhibitors of the proteasome. Marizomib (NPI-0052, or salinosporamide A), is a β-lactone compound derived from the marine bacterium Salinospora tropica; like Carfilzomib and PR-047, it is also an irreversible inhibitor of the β5 subunit. Given their low nanomolar IC50 values for the β5 subunit, Bortezomib and the second-generation inhibitors, all represent very effective inhibitors of proteasome activity. NPI-0052 also has a low nanomolar IC50 for the trypsin-like (β2) subunit. Two second-generation agents have entered phase I trials: NPI-0052 and Carfilzomib. Both, unlike Bortezomib, bind irreversibly the proteasome, abrogating one mechanism of recovery from proteasome inhibition, such as release of the target by the drug. Preclinical studies have shown that both at least partially overcome Bortezomib resistance in vitro. Moreover, in a number of models, including multiple myeloma and chronic lymphocytic leukemia, these inhibitors have shown enhanced potency compared with Bortezomib, suggesting they may have a broader spectrum of activity. Early results from phase I studies of Carfilzomib indicate that it is well tolerated, even on a dose intense schedule, and may have less neurotoxicity than Bortezomib. Evidence of antitumor activity is being seen in multiple myeloma and Waldenstron's macroglobulinemia, including in myeloma patients with previously Bortezomib-refractory disease. In phase I clinical trials employing Marizomib for patients with leukemia, lymphoma and other solid tumors, Marizomib did not appear to induce the limiting toxicities associated with Bortezomib, such as peripheral neuropathy, neutropenia and thrombocytopenia, in spite of eliciting levels of proteasome inhibition that equal or exceed those produced by Bortezomib. Anti-tumor activity was also seen in multiple myeloma patients previously treated with Bortezomib. Marizomib phase I clinical trials combining second generation proteasome inhibitors with other targeted therapies, as for instance Marizomib plus Vorinostat (a hystone deacetilating agent), have been initiated. Second-generation proteasome inhibitors might address some of the key issues associated with Bortezomib, such as improving the efficacy of proteasome inhibition in solid tumors, and limiting therapy-associated peripheral neuropathy. Combinatory therapy employing two different proteasome inhibitors, such as Bortezomib and Marizomib has also been proposed. Extensive clinical investigation of the second-generation inhibitors will be required, however, to determine whether the pharmacologic differences between these agents and Bortezomib will result in differences in efficacy and safety in patients. (Orlowski 2008, Testa 2009, Einsele 2010, Dick 2010, Potts 2010, Bettignies 2010, Berkers 2010, Potts 2011).

Finally, another interesting concept about the use of proteasome inhibitors as anticancer agents is the role of the feedback regulation of proteasome gene expression as a possible mechanism of proteasome inhibitors resistance in solid tumors. The proteasome can be regulated at different levels. The 26S proteasome is composed of 33 distinct subunits each encoded by a different gene. Regulation of proteasome gene expression is another important mechanism that controls proteasome homeostasis. The discovery of feedback regulation of proteasome gene expression has several important implications in cancer therapy that targets the proteasome. First, it provides a clue to understand the cause of proteasome overexpression often-detected in cancers. Second, the feedback mechanism may contribute to drug resistance in cancer therapy. The feedback induction, which normally occurs only when the proteasome activity is suppressed, may become constitutively active in cancer cells. As already mentioned, Bortezomib is the only proteasome inhibitor in clinical use. Although this drug has shown promising results in the treatment of multiple myeloma and mantle cell lymphoma it has limited efficacy in other cancer types. Whereas the compromised efficacy of Bortezomib by the feedback mechanisms may still be sufficient to kill myeloma tumor cells, it may not be strong enough to be effective in other cancers, especially solid tumors. Thus, the feedback pathway presents a potential target for cancer therapy. To date, proteasome inhibitors attacking the catalytic sites of the proteasome are the only tool to reduce the proteasome activity. However, knockdown of individual proteasome genes combined with proteasome inhibitors may present a promising alternative in cancer therapy. Further investigation of these mechanisms will provide more choices for proteasome-targeting cancer therapy (Xie 2010).

## 4. Melanoma and proteasome inhibitors

Cutaneous melanoma is the most aggressive form of skin cancer. Its treatment is based on early detection and surgical excision. Once in an advanced stage, metastatic melanoma presents a very poor prognosis as it becomes resistant to conventional anticancer treatments, such as chemo or radiation therapies. At the moment, the methylating agent Dacarbazine is still the standar therapy for metastatic melanoma allowing clinical objective responses in only 10-20% of patients, with a complete response rate of less than 5%, and a short median response duration of 4-6 months. Therefore, new therapeutic strategies are under investigation as, for instance, immunotherapy or so called targeted therapy (Ibrahim 2009, Lutzky 2010).

Some of the mechanisms related to the aggressive behavior of melanoma cells are 1) constitutive activation of growth factor receptors (c-Kit, PDGFR-α, EGFR), 2) constitutive activation of the MAP-kinase pathway (RAS/RAF/MEK/ERK), 3) constitutive activation of the PI3K/AKT pathway (partially due to loss, mutation, or epigenetic silencing of PTEN tumor suppressor gene), 4) constitutive activation of transcription factor NFκB, 5) disregulation (deletions, silencing, mutations) of proteins involved in cell cycle control (CDKN2A/CDK4/CCND1), 6) impairment of transcriptional activities of proapoptotic protein p53 and 7) overexpression of antiapoptotic Bcl-2 protein family (Fecher 2007, Rother 2009, Nathanson 2010). Besides these mechanisms, directly involved in cell proliferation and survival, melanoma cells also employ other strategies that allow them to invade and migrate (p.e. aberrant expression of adhesion molecules) (Kuphal 2005, Abdullah 2010, Braeuer 2011), to grow (p.e.secretion of angiogenic factors) (Basu 2009, Ria 2010), and to escape the immune system control (Gajewski 2007). Theoretically, any molecule involved in hot points of this altered cell machinery could be a good target for melanoma treatment.

Up to now, targeted therapies that have reached the best results on the clinical setting are specific inhibitors of BRAF (PLX4032) in melanomas with the V600E BRAF mutation, c-Kit inhibitors in melanomas harboring c-Kit mutations (Davies 2010) and anti-CTLA-4 antibodies, such as Ipilimumab or Tremelimumab, that overcome the mechanisms of immunotolerance (Boasberg 2010). Although the introduction of these drugs has been a great advance for the treatment of patients with metastatic melanoma, this only represents the end of the very beginning. First, despite impressive clinical responses to PLX4032 treatment, most responsive patients ultimately relapse because of acquired resistance.

Second, melanomas with c-Kit mutations constitute only a very low percentage of the whole group of metastatic melanomas and, from what we know about other neoplasms with c-Kit mutations, relapse because of acquired resistance will also occur. Third, we continue without a good alternative for melanoma patients with tumors presenting a molecular profile different to BRAF/V600E or c-Kit mutations. And, finally, we lack biomarkers to identify subgroups of patients that will respond to anti-CTLA-4 therapy (Flaherty 2010, Shepherd 2010, Robert 2009).

For most authors, a possible therapeutic approach to avoid drug resistance developed in patients treated with single agent therapy is the use of combinatory treatments that simultaneously target different cellular pathways. In this context, proteasome inhibitors, that have pleiotropic effects on proliferation, survival, migration, invasion and angiogenesis, and that can synergize with several other drugs or therapies, appear as a good tool for metastatic melanoma treatment (Tawbi 2009).

### 4.1 Preclinical evidences of usefulness of proteasome inhibitors in melanoma

#### 4.1.1 Effect of single-agent proteasome inhibitors on melanoma cells

First observations about the *in vitro* effect of proteasome inhibitors on proliferation and survival of melanoma cells were published by our group and others during 2004-08. These studies demonstrated that several different proteasome inhibitors (Bortezomib, that was the only one used in clinical practice, and ALLN, MG-132 and Epoxomicin, that were exclusively used in experimental studies) were able to decrease the viability of melanoma cell lines by inhibiting their proliferation, causing cell cycle arrest and inducing apoptotic cell death by caspase-dependent and -independent mechanisms, AIF related (Fernandez 2005, Qin 2005, Nikiforov 2007, Sorolla 2008).

Investigation of underlying molecular mechanisms to the effect of proteasome inhibitors in melanoma cells indicated that Bortezomib-mediated release of mitochondrial death inducers is not preceded by a significant cleavage of Bid nor down-regulation of apoptotic factors frequently related with the NFκB pathway (Bcl-2, Bcl-xL, XIAP, FLIP, TRAF-2), all previously associated with melanoma chemoresistance (Fernandez 2005). Comparing benign melanocytes with melanoma cells and other neoplastic cells, these studies also showed that proteasome inhibitors have the feature of promoting a dramatic induction of the proapoptotic protein NOXA in a tumor cell-restricted manner (Fernandez 2005, Qin 2005). The induction of NOXA by proteasome inhibitors was P53 (Qin 2005), HIF-1 and E2F-1 independent but directly dependent on the oncogene c-MYC. Thus, c-MYC appeared as a direct modulator of NOXA, essential for the regulation of NOXA by the proteasome in neoplastic cells, providing a molecular explanation for the preferential selectivity of proteasome inhibitors toward tumor cells (Yerlicava 2008, Fuchs 2008). The role of NOXA in the response of melanoma cells to Bortezomib was validated in xenograft murine model systems (Fernandez 2005, Qin 2005).

A recent work presented a genome-wide siRNA screen for modulators of cell death induced by Bortezomib on colon cancer, cervical cancer and malignant melanoma cells. The authors found that a common set of 39 genes was responsible for conferring sensitivity to Bortezomib in the different tumor cell types. They causally linked Bortezomib-induced apoptosis to the accumulation of ASF1B, MYC, ODC1, NOXA, BNIP3, Gadd45α, p-SMC1A, SREBF1, and p53. These results suggested that proteasome inhibition promotes cell death primarily by dysregulating MYC and polyamines, interfering with protein translation, and disrupting essential DNA damage repair pathways; in summary, leading to the inhibition of multiple homeostatic responses that finally drive tumor cells to engage programmed cell death. They considered that such information could be useful to the design of pharmacodynamic biomarkers and the application of combination chemotherapy regimens containing Bortezomib (Chen 2010a).

Additional studies of our group and others also showed that antioxidant agents can block apoptosis triggered by proteasome inhibition in melanoma and other tumor types (Fernandez 2006, Llobet 2008). In detail, the antioxidant compound Tiron completely inhibits proteasome-induced apoptosis caused by the boronic acid-based proteasome inhibitor Bortezomib, but has no effects on the aldehyde proteasome inhibitors MG-132 and ALLN. Conversely, the antioxidant molecule, called Edaravone, blocks the MG-132 and ALLN-induced apoptosis, but does not have significant effects on apoptosis induced by Bortezomib. Vitamin C has been also shown to abrogate the ability of Bortezomib to induce apoptosis in several other cancer cell lines. (Llobet 2008, Zou 2006). These results indicated that different antioxidants are able to block different proteasome inhibitors in a specific way and may have important implications for the design of drug mixtures containing proteasome inhibitors.

Finally, Bortezomib-induced endoplasmic reticulum stress and autophagy in melanoma cells are other antineoplastic functions of proteasome inhibitors that have become a point of great interest in the last few years (Hill 2009, Armstrong 2011).

#### 4.1.2 *In vitro* and *in vivo* melanoma preclinical models about proteasome inhibitor-based combinatory therapy

As melanoma is almost universally resistant to chemotherapy and shows a constitutive activation of transcription factor NFκB, inhibition of the proteasome seemed a good option to overcome melanoma cell chemoresistance.

One of the experimental studies, that most encouraged the clinical use of combinatory therapy containing proteasome inhibitors and chemotherapeutic agents in melanoma, was published in 2004. The authors showed that Bortezomib enhanced Temozolamide induced growth inhibition of melanoma cells *in vitro* and *in vivo* in a xenograft tumor model. Tumor growth decrease was related to inhibition of nuclear translocation of NFκB, stabilization of p53 and p21 levels and, ultimately, induction of apoptosis. The combination also significantly inhibited tumoral angiogenesis when compared with the use of Temozolamide alone (Amiri 2004). Significantly enhanced killing of melanoma cells was also achieved by simultaneously triggering production of NOXA (using Bortezomib) as well as reducing Mcl-1 levels (using Fludarabine) (Qin 2006).

More recently, another study demonstrated that the proteasome inhibitor Bortezomib led to a significant synergistic enhancement of the antitumoral activity of the chemotherapeutic agent Camptothecin on melanoma cells. This effect consisted in broader induction of cell apoptosis, suppression of cell invasion, as well as inhibition of *in vivo* metastasis in a murine model. A reduced degradation of IkB and, consecutively, a reduced activity of NFκB were observed, as expected. The *in vivo* model allowed to assess the inhibition of nuclear NFkB translocation and the induction of melanoma cell apoptosis in pulmonary melanoma metastases. In addition Bortezomib exerted pleiotropic and/or off-target effects. These effects were, at least in part, independent of proteasome inhibition or independent to NFκB inhibition and differed from those induced by the selective IKKb inhibitor, KINK-1. For instance, it was found that Camptothecin-induced upregulation of the Bcl-2 family protein NOXA was markedly augmented by Bortezomib, whereas KINK-1 achieved a less

pronounced increase. Bortezomib also led to a marked increase of the Camptothecin induced release of cytochrome C (a critical step in the mitochondrial pathway of apoptosis) that was not seen after melanoma cells incubation with KINK-1 (Amschler 2010).
The second generation proteasome inhibitor Marizonib (NPI-0052 or salinosporamide A) seems also to sensitize prostate cancer and malignant melanoma cells to Cisplatinum (Potts 2011).
Other agents that showed a synergistic effect on melanoma cells when combined with proteasome inhibitors are radiation therapy (Munshi 2004), Geldanamycin and Geldanamycin analogues (that target the Hsp 90 protein chaperone) (Bonvini 2001, Mimnaugh 2004, Banerji 2009), the Hsp70 inhibitors KNK-437 and Schisandrin-B (Yerlikaya 2010), Mistletoe Lectin-I and the PPAR-A agonist Rosiglitazone (Freudlsperger 2007), Gossypol (an inhibitor of the anti-apoptotic proteins Mcl-1/Bcl-2/Bcl-xL) (Wolter 2007) and the BH3 mimetic ABT-737 (inhibitor of Bcl-2/Bcl-X(L)/Bcl-w) (Miller 2009), the cytokines Interferon-alpha (Lesinski 2008, Lesinski 2009) and IL-29 (Guenterberg 2010), Bacitracin (a protein disulfide isomerase inhibitor) (Lovat 2008), Decitabine (a demethylating agent) (Halaban 2009), Fenretinide (a synthetic retinoid inducing endoplasmic reticulum stress) (Hill 2009), Evodiamine (Wang 2010), GRP78-specific subtilase toxin (that inhibits GRP78, a vital unfolded protein response mediator) (Martin 2010) and newly developed SMAC-mimetics (Lecis 2010). A combination of the new generation proteasome inhibitor Marizomib with histone deacetylase inhibitors was also tested in preclinical melanoma models, with not yet published results (Potts 2011).
Proteasome inhibition also enhanced the effect of cell-mediated immunotherapies in melanoma animal models, such as dendritic cell-based immunization/activation (Schumacher 2006) and adoptive transfer of tumor-specific T lymphocytes (Seeger 2010, Jazirehi 2011). Nevertheless, some paradoxical responses to this type of approach have been observed (Lundqvist 2010).
Recently, our group showed that a combined exposure to the multikinase inhibitor Sunitinib and Bortezomib resulted in a synergistic decrease of cell viability and an increase in caspase activation and apoptosis in two Sunitinib sensitive melanoma cell lines (M16 and M17) (Yeramian 2011). We demonstrated that constitutive activated PDGFRα and VEGFR2, respectively, were the targets of the observed Sunitinib effect. Proteasome inhibition did not show any additive or synergistic effect on Sunitinib resistant cell lines. In Sunitinib sensitive cell lines, Sunitinib inhibited Akt phosphorylation in its two residues (Thr 308. Ser 473), suppressed the phosphorylation of ribosomal protein p70S6KSer240/244 and downregulated the levels of cyclin D1. In addition, Sunitinib partially inactivated ERK in M17 but not in M16 cell line because M16 harbored the BRAF/V600E mutation that maintains the ERK pathway active despite the complete inactivation of PDGFRα by Sunitinib. Moreover, LY294002, a PI3K inhibitor, sensitized melanoma cells to Bortezomib treatment, suggesting that down-regulation of phospho-Akt by Sunitinib mediates the synergy obtained by Bortezomib plus Sunitinib co-treatment. Altogether, our results suggest that melanoma cells harbouring an activated tyrosin-kinase receptor may be clinically responsive to pharmacologic receptor tyrosin-kinase inhibition by Sunitinib, and a strategy combining Sunitinib and Bortezomib, may provide therapeutic benefit. Moreover, our results also highlighted that subgrouping of melanomas by their molecular profile will be important in the design of personalized combined therapies containing proteasome inhibitors. Different responses to Bortezomib therapy in BRAF wild type or BRAF mutated melanoma cells have also lately described by other authors (Armstrong 2011).

### 4.2 Clinical studies employing proteasome inhibitors in patients with metastatic melanoma

Bortezomib is the proteasome inhibitor that has been preferentially clinically evaluated for the treatment of metastatic melanoma, as single agent or in combination with conventional chemotherapeutic drugs.

The first phase II clinical trial has employed Bortezomib as single agent administered twice weekly for 2 weeks, every 3 weeks at a intravenous dose of 1.5 mg/m$^2$. The study was intended to treat 45 patients, but it was closed after an interim analysis due to early evidence of insufficient clinical efficacy. Twenty-seven patients with a median age of 56 years (range, 32–77 years) were included. Objective responses were not observed. Only 6 patients (22%) achieved stable disease. Of these 6 patients, 4 were still stable after 4 cycles of treatment, but were removed from the study due to toxicity. The median time to disease progression was 1.5 months (95% confidence interval, 1.4 -1.6) and the median overall survival was 14.5 months (95% confidence interval, 9–22). No Grade 4/5 treatment-related toxicities were reported. Eleven patients (42%) had Grade 3 toxicities including sensory neuropathy, thrombocytopenia, constipation, fatigue, ileus, abdominal pain, and infection without neutropenia. After these results, the authors concluded that single-agent Bortezomib was not found to be effective in the treatment of patients with metastatic melanoma, and that exploration of combination regimens may be warranted (Markovic 2005).

Based in previous *in vitro* and *in vivo* experimental evidence of the existence of a synergic effect between Bortezomib and the chemotherapeutic agent Temozolamide on melanoma cells (Amiri 2004), a second phase I trial was designed. Objectives included defining a maximum tolerated dose for the combination, characterizing biomarker changes reflecting inhibition of both proteasome and NFκB activity in blood and tumor samples, and characterizing antitumor activity. Nineteen melanoma patients with poor prognostic factors (including 17 patients with M1c type metastasis and 10 with raised serum LDH) were enrolled onto four escalating dose levels of Temozolomide and Bortezomib. Bortezomib, 1.3 mg/m$^2$, and Temozolomide, 75 mg/m$^2$, proved to be the maximum tolerated dose. Dose-limiting toxicities were neurotoxicity, fatigue, diarrhea, and rash. Objective responses included only a partial response of 8 months of duration. Three more patients achieved stabilization. A significant reduction in proteasome-specific activity in peripheral blood mononuclear cells was observed 1 hour after infusion at Bortezomib. Nevertheless, consistent effects on NFκB activation could not be detected. Authors gave different explanations to this fact including the possibility that Bortezomib acts on melanoma cells through other mechanisms such as a c-MYC–dependent increase in NOXA. A phase II trial is already in progress (Su 2010).

Finally, a recent phase II clinical trial has been published about the effect on metastatic melanoma patients of the combination of Paclitaxel, Carboplatin, and Bortezomib. This trial was based in preclinical studies demonstrating that Bortezomib has anticancer additive/synergistic effects when combined with several chemotherapeutic agents, including Paclitaxel and Platinum, and the results of a previous phase I trial of this 3-drug combination that included patients with metastatic melanoma and other tumor types (Ma 2007). Bortezomib was administered at a dose of 1.3 mg/m$^2$ intravenously, Paclitaxel at a dose of 175 mg/m$^2$, and Carboplatin at an area under the concentration. Seventeen patients were enrolled. A median of 4 cycles were administered. Three patients discontinued treatment due to persistent grade 4 neutropenia with grade 3 leukopenia or grade 4 pulmonary embolism. Grade 3 toxicities included neutropenia, leukopenia, thrombocytopenia, and arthralgia. Two partial responses and four stabilization of disease were observed. The median progression-free survival was 3.2 months, and the median overall survival was 7.0 months. The authors concluded that the combination of Paclitaxel, Carboplatin and Bortezomib in patients with metastatic melanoma lacks sufficient clinical activity and was associated with significant toxicity to warrant further investigation (Croghan 2010).

Clinical trials of malignant melanoma patients based on combinatory treatments employing proteasome inhibitors and therapeutic strategies other than conventional chemotherapy have been not published so far.

Additional phase I clinical trials combining Bortezomib with interferon-alfa (Kendra 2008) or with Dacarbazine (Roberts 2006) have also been reported at ASCO meetings. Although the primary objective of the trials was to determine the safety, tolerability and dose limiting toxicities, the antitumoral activity of the combinations was quite limited and, to our knowledge, phase II clinical trials employing these combinatory therapies are not currently ongoing. Other two phase I clinical trials employing de second-generation proteasome inhibitor, Marizomib, have also been reported at the 2008 and 09 ASCO meetings. 23 and 30 patients with different tumor types were enrolled, including patients with myeloma, lymphomas, leukemias, and solid tumors. Stable disease was induced in one and two patients with melanoma, respectively. The toxicity profile was tolerable and dissimilar to Bortezomib in spite of reaching higher levels of proteasome inhibition (Aghajanian 2008, Townsend 2009).

## 5. Conclusion

In conclusion, biologic properties of proteasome inhibitors and preclinical studies suggested that this type of pharmacological agents could be a good therapeutic approach for the treatment of many cancer types. However, first human clinical assays employing the first commercially available proteasome inhibitor, Bortezomib, demonstrated that this drug is quite effective in some hematologic malignancies but not in solid tumors, such as malignant melanoma, nor as single agent nor in combination with conventional chemotherapeutic products. Nevertheless, multiple preclinical studies, carried out on *in vitro* or *in vivo* melanoma models, support that proteasome inhibitors could be useful in combinations with several targeted therapies or different immunotherapeutic strategies. As we currently know that melanoma is a molecular heterogeneous disease, studies designed to increase our knowledge about underlying mechanisms to the combined action of proteasome inhibitors and other treatments on the different melanoma subtypes are warranted. In this way, we could have a rational basis to select those groups of melanoma patients in which proteasome inhibitor-based therapy could be a good choice. Finally, second generation proteasome inhibitors appear as a chance for the treatment of solid tumors. Probably in the coming years we will see to what extent this can be a reality in melanoma.

## 6. Acknowledgements

This work was supported by FIS-PI060832, 2009SGR794 and RD06/0020/1034, Programa de Intensificación de la Investigación (Instituto Carlos III) and Gotta. A.Y. holds a postdoctoral fellowship from Ministerio de Educación y Ciencia (Programa Juan de la Cierva). A.S. is recipient of a predoctoral fellowship from Fundación Científica AECC, Catalunya contra el Cancer, Lleida. X.D. holds a postdoctoral fellowship from Fondo de Investigaciones Sanitarias, Ministerio de Sanidad y Consumo (CP05/00028).

## 7. References

Abdullah C, Xiaolei Wang X, Becker D. Molecular therapy for melanoma. Useful and not useful targets. *Cancer Biology & Therapy* 2010; 10: 113-118

Aghajanian CA, Hamlin P, Gordon MS, Hong DS, Naing A, Younes A, Hannah A, Palladino MA, Spear MA, Kurzrock R. Phase I study of the novel proteasome inhibitor NPI-0052 in patients with lymphoma and solid tumors [abstract]. *J Clin Oncol* 2008; 26 (suppl): 3574

Amiri KI, Horton LW, LaFleur BJ, Sosman JA, Richmond A. Augmenting chemosensitivity of malignant melanoma tumors via proteasome inhibition: implication for bortezomib (VELCADE, PS-341) as a therapeutic agent for malignant melanoma *Cancer Res* 2004; 64: 4912-4918

Amschler K, Schön MP, Pletz N, Wallbrecht K, Erpenbeck L, Schön M. NF-kappaB inhibition through proteasome inhibition or IKKbeta blockade increases the susceptibility of melanoma cells to cytostatic treatment through distinct pathways. *J Invest Dermatol* 2010; 130: 1073-1086

Armstrong JL, Corazzari M, Martin S, Pagliarini V, Falasca L, Hill DS, Ellis N, Al Sabah S, Redfern CP, Fimia GM, Piacentini M, Lovat PE. Oncogenic B-RAF Signaling in melanoma impairs the therapeutic advantage of autophagy inhibition. *Clin Cancer Res* 2011; 17: 2216-2226

Banerji U. Heat shock protein 90 as a drug target: some like it hot. *Clin Cancer Res* 2009; 15: 9-14

Basu B, Biswas S, Wrigley J, Sirohi B, Corrie P. Angiogenesis in cutaneous malignant melanoma and potential therapeutic strategies. *Expert Rev Anticancer Ther* 2009; 9: 1583-1598

Berkers CR, Ovaa H. Drug discovery and assay development in the ubiquitin-proteasome system. *Biochem Soc Trans* 2010; 38: 14-20

de Bettignies G, Coux O. Proteasome inhibitors: Dozens of molecules and still counting. *Biochimie* 2010; 92: 1530-1545

Bonvini P, An WG, Rosolen A, Nguyen P, Trepel J, Garcia de Herreros A, Dunach M, Neckers LM. Geldanamycin abrogates ErbB2 association with proteasome-resistant beta-catenin in melanoma cells, increases beta-catenin-E-cadherin association, and decreases beta-catenin-sensitive transcription. *Cancer Res* 2001; 61: 1671-1677

Braeuer RR, Zigler M, Villares GJ, Dobroff AS, Bar-Eli M. Transcriptional control of melanoma metastasis: The importance of the tumor microenvironment. *Semin Cancer Biol* 2011; 21 :83-88

Chen S, Blank JL, Peters T, Liu XJ, Rappoli DM, Pickard MD, Menon S, Yu J, Driscoll DL, Lingaraj T, Burkhardt AL, Chen W, Garcia K, Sappal DS, Gray J, Hales P, Leroy PJ, Ringeling J, Rabino C, Spelman JJ, Morgenstern JP, Lightcap ES. Genome-wide siRNA screen for modulators of cell death induced by proteasome inhibitor bortezomib. *Cancer Res* 2010; 70: 4318-4326

Chen D, Dou QP. The ubiquitin-proteasome system as a prospective molecular target for cancer treatment and prevention. *Curr Protein Pept Sci* 2010; 11: 459-470

Ciechanover A. Intracellular protein degradation: from a vague idea through the lysosome and the ubiquitin-proteasome system and onto human diseases and drug targeting. *Medicina (B Aires)* 2010; 70: 105-119

Croghan GA, Suman VJ, Maples WJ, Albertini M, Linette G, Flaherty L, Eckardt J, Ma C, Markovic SN, Erlichman C. A study of paclitaxel, carboplatin, and bortezomib in the treatment of metastatic malignant melanoma: a phase 2 consortium study. *Cancer* 2010; 116: 3463-3468

Davies MA, Samuels Y. Analysis of the genome to personalize therapy for melanoma. *Oncogene* 2010; 29: 5545–5555

Dick LR, Fleming PE. Building on bortezomib: second-generation proteasome inhibitors as anti-cancer therapy. *Drug Discov Today* 2010;15 :243-249

Einsele H. Bortezomib. *Recent Results Cancer Res* 2010; 184: 173-187

Fecher LA, Cummings SD, Keefe MJ, Alani RM. Toward a molecular classification of melanoma. *J Clin Oncol* 2007; 25: 1606-1620

Fernandez Y, Verhaegen M, Miller TP, Rush JL, Steiner P, Opipari AW, Jr., Lowe SW, Soengas MS. Differential regulation of noxa in normal melanocytes and melanoma cells by proteasome inhibition: therapeutic implications. *Cancer Res* 2005;65:6294-304

Flaherty KT, Hodi FS, Bastian BC. Mutation-driven drug development in melanoma. *Curr Opin Oncol* 2010; 22: 178–183

Freudlsperger C, Thies A, Pfuller U, Schumacher U. The proteasome inhibitor bortezomib augments anti-proliferative effects of mistletoe lectin-I and the PPAR-gamma agonist rosiglitazone in human melanoma cells. *Anticancer Res* 2007; 27: 207-13

Fuchs SY. MYC-induced sensitivity of human malignant melanoma to proteasome inhibitors - a KaMYCaze effect. *Pigment Cell Melanoma Res* 2008; 21: 9-10

Gajewski TF. Failure at the effector phase: immune barriers at the level of the melanoma tumor microenvironment. *Clin Cancer Res* 2007; 13: 5256-5261

Gallastegui N, Groll M. The 26S proteasome: assembly and function of a destructive machine. *Trends Biochem Sci* 2010; 35: 634-642

Guenterberg KD, Grignol VP, Raig ET, Zimmerer JM, Chan AN, Blaskovits FM, Young GS, Nuovo GJ, Mundy BL, Lesinski GB, Carson WE 3rd. Interleukin-29 binds to melanoma cells inducing Jak-STAT signal transduction and apoptosis. *Mol Cancer Ther* 2010; 9: 510-520

Halaban R, Krauthammer M, Pelizzola M, Cheng E, Kovacs D, Sznol M, Ariyan S, Narayan D, Bacchiocchi A, Molinaro A, Kluger Y, Deng M, Tran N, Zhang W, Picardo M, Enghild JJ. Integrative analysis of epigenetic modulation in melanoma cell response to decitabine: clinical implications. *PLoS One* 2009; 4: e4563

Hill DS, Martin S, Armstrong JL, Flockhart R, Tonison JJ, Simpson DG, Birch-Machin MA, Redfern CP, Lovat PE.Combining the endoplasmic reticulum stress-inducing agents bortezomib and fenretinide as a novel therapeutic strategy for metastatic melanoma. *Clin Cancer Res* 2009; 15: 1192-1198.

Ibrahim N, Haluska FG. Molecular pathogenesis of cutaneous melanocytic neoplasms. *Annu Rev Pathol* 2009; 4: 551-79

Jazirehi AR, Baritaki S, Koya RC, Bonavida B, Economou JS. Molecular mechanism of MART-1+/A*0201+ human melanoma resistance to specific CTL-killing despite functional tumor-CTL interaction. *Cancer Res* 2011; 71: 1406-1417

Kaehler KC, Piel S, Livingstone E, Schilling B, Hauschild A, Schadendorf D. Update on immunologic therapy with anti-CTLA-4 antibodies in melanoma: identification of clinical and biological response patterns, immune-related adverse events, and their management. *Semin Oncol* 2010; 37: 485-498

Kendra KL, Lesinski GB, Olencki TE, Carson W. A phase I study of bortezomib and interferon-alpha-2b in patients with metastatic melanoma [abstract]. *J Clin Oncol* 2008; 26 (Suppl): 20031

Kim HM, Yu Y, Cheng Y. Structure characterization of the 26S proteasome. *Biochim Biophys Acta* 2011; 1809: 67-79

Kuphal S, Bauer R, Bosserhoff A-K. Integrin signaling in malignant melanoma. *Cancer Metastasis Rev* 2005; 24: 195-222

Kwak J, Workman JL, Lee D. The proteasome and its regulatory roles in gene expression. *Biochim Biophys Acta* 2011; 1809: 88-96

Lecis D, Drago C, Manzoni L, Seneci P, Scolastico C, Mastrangelo E, Bolognesi M, Anichini A, Kashkar H, Walczak H, Delia D. Novel SMAC-mimetics synergistically stimulate melanoma cell death in combination with TRAIL and Bortezomib. *Br J Cancer* 2010; 102: 1707-1716

Lesinski GB, Raig ET, Guenterberg K, Brown L, Go MR, Shah NN, Lewis A, Quimper M, Hade E, Young G, Chaudhury AR, Ladner KJ, Guttridge DC, Bouchard P, Carson WE 3rd. IFN-alpha and bortezomib overcome Bcl-2 and Mcl-1 overexpression in melanoma cells by stimulating the extrinsic pathway of apoptosis. *Cancer Res* 2008; 68: 8351-8660

Lesinski GB, Benninger K, Kreiner M, Quimper M, Young G, Carson WE 3rd. Bortezomib pre-treatment prolongs interferon-alpha-induced STAT1 phosphorylation in melanoma cells. *Cancer Immunol Immunother* 2009; 58: 2031-2037

Livnat-Levanon N, Glickman MH. Ubiquitin-proteasome system and mitochondria - reciprocity. *Biochim Biophys Acta* 2011; 1809: 80-87

Llobet D, Eritja N, Sorolla A, Yeramian A, Schoenenberger JA, Llombart-Cussac A, Marti RM, Matias-Guiu X, Dolcet X. Antioxidants block proteasome inhibitors function in endometrial carcinoma cells. *Anti-cancer Drug* 2008; 19: 115-124

Lovat PE, Corazzari M, Armstrong JL, Martin S, Pagliarini V, Hill D, Brown AM, Piacentini M, Birch-Machin MA, Redfern CP. Increasing melanoma cell death using inhibitors of protein disulfide isomerases to abrogate survival responses to endoplasmic reticulum stress. *Cancer Res* 2008; 68: 5363-5369

Ludwig H, Khayat D, Giaccone G, Facon T. Proteasome inhibition and its clinical prospects in the treatment of hematologic and solid malignancies. *Cancer* 2005; 104: 1794-1807

Lundqvist A, Su S, Rao S, Childs R. Cutting edge: bortezomib-treated tumors sensitized to NK cell apoptosis paradoxically acquire resistance to antigen-specific T cells. *J Immunol* 2010; 184: 1139-1142

Lutzky J. New Therapeutic Options in the Medical Management of Advanced Melanoma. *Semin Cutan Med Surg* 2010; 29: 249-257

Ma C, Mandrekar SJ, Alberts SR, Croghan GA, Jatoi A, Reid JM, Hanson LJ, Bruzek L, Tan AD, Pitot HC, Erlichman C, Wright JJ, Adjei AA. A phase I and pharmacologic study of sequences of the proteasome inhibitor, bortezomib (PS-341, Velcade), in combination with paclitaxel and carboplatin in patients with advanced malignancies. *Cancer Chemother Pharmacol* 2007; 59: 207-215

Markowic SN, Geyer SM, Dawkins F, Sharfman W, Albertini M, Maples W, Fracasso PM, Fitch T, Lorusso P, Adjei AA, Erlichman C. A phase II study of bortezomib in the treatment of metastatic malignant melanoma. *Cancer* 2005; 103: 2584-2589

Martin S, Hill DS, Paton JC, Paton AW, Birch-Machin MA, Lovat PE, Redfern CP. Targeting GRP78 to enhance melanoma cell death. *Pigment Cell Melanoma* Res 2010; 23: 675-682

Miller LA, Goldstein NB, Johannes WU, Walton CH, Fujita M, Norris DA, Shellman YG. BH3 mimetic ABT-737 and a proteasome inhibitor synergistically kill melanomas through Noxa-dependent apoptosis. *J Invest Dermatol* 2009; 129: 964-971

Mlynarczuk-Bialy I, Roeckmann H, Kuckelkorn U, Schmidt B, Umbreen S, Golab J, Ludwig A, Montag C, Wiebusch L, Hagemeier C, Schadendorf D, Kloetzel PM, et al. Combined effect of proteasome and calpain inhibition on cisplatin-resistant human melanoma cells. *Cancer Res* 2006; 66: 7598-7605

Munshi A, Kurland JF, Nishikawa T et al. Inhibition of constitutively activated nuclear factor-kappaB radiosensitizes human melanoma cells. *Mol Cancer Ther* 2004; 3: 985-992

Nathanson KL. Using genetics and genomics strategies to personalize therapy for cancer: Focus on melanoma. *Biochem Pharmacol* 2010; 80:755-761

Potts BC, Lam KS. Generating a generation of proteasome inhibitors: from microbial fermentation to total synthesis of salinosporamide a (marizomib) and other salinosporamides. *Mar Drugs* 2010; 8: 835-880

Potts BC, Albitar MX, Anderson KC, Baritaki S, Berkers C, Bonavida B, Chandra J, Chauhan D, Cusack JC Jr, Fenical W, Ghobrial IM, Groll M, Jensen PR, Lam KS, Lloyd GK, McBride W, McConkey DJ, Miller CP, Neuteboom STC, Oki Y, Ovaa H, Pajonk F, Richardson PG, Roccaro AM, Sloss CM, Spear MA, Valashi E, Younes A, Palladino MA. Marizomib, a proteasome inhibitor for all seasons: preclinical profile and a framework for clinical trials. *Curr Cancer Drug Targets* 2011; 11: 254-284

Qin JZ, Ziffra J, Stennett L, Bodner B, Bonish BK, Chaturvedi V, Bennett F, Pollock PM, Trent JM, Hendrix MJ, Rizzo P, Miele L, Nickoloff BJ. Proteasome inhibitors trigger NOXA-mediated apoptosis in melanoma and myeloma cells. *Cancer Res* 2005; 65: 6282-6293

Qin JZ, Xin H, Sitailo LA, Denning MF, Nickoloff BJ. Enhanced killing of melanoma cells by simultaneously targeting Mcl-1 and NOXA. *Cancer Res* 2006; 66: 9636-9645

Rajkumar SV, Richardson PG, Hideshima T, Anderson KC. Proteasome inhibition as a novel therapeutic target in human cancer. *J Clin Oncol* 2005; 23: 630-639

Ria R, Reale A, Castrovilli A, Mangialardi G, Dammacco F, Ribatti D, Vacca A. Angiogenesis and progression in human melanoma. *Dermatol Res Pract* 2010; 2010: 185687

Robert C, Ghiringhelli F. What is the role of cytotoxic T lymphocyte-associated antigen 4 blockade in patients with metastatic melanoma? *Oncologist* 2009; 14: 848-661

Roberts JD, Ernstoff MS, Birdsell C. Phase I trial of dacarbazine and bortezomib in melanoma and soft tissue sarcoma [abstract]. *J Clin Oncol* 2006; 24 (Suppl): 18008

Rother J, Jones D. Molecular markers of tumor progression in melanoma. *Current Genomics* 2009; 10: 231-239

Schrader EK, Harstad KG, Matouschek A. Targeting proteins for degradation. *Nat Chem Biol* 2009; 5: 815-822

Schumacher LY, Vo DD, Garban HJ, Comin-Anduix B, Owens SK, Dissette VB, Glaspy JA, McBride WH, Bonavida B, Economou JS, Ribas A. Immunosensitization of tumour cells to dendritic cell-activated immune responses with the proteasome inhibitor bortezomib (PS-341, Velcade). *J Immunol* 2006; 176: 4757-4765

Seeger JM, Schmidt P, Brinkmann K, Hombach AA, Coutelle O, Zigrino P, Wagner-Stippich D, Mauch C, Abken H, Krönke M, Kashkar H. The proteasome inhibitor bortezomib sensitizes melanoma cells toward adoptive CTL attack. *Cancer Res* 2010; 70: 1825-1834

Shepherd C, Puzanov I, Sosman JA. B-RAF Inhibitors: An evolving role in the therapy of malignant melanoma. *Curr Oncol Rep* 2010; 12: 146–152

Sorokin AV, Kim ER, Ovchinnikov LP. Proteasome system of protein degradation and processing. *Biochemistry (Mosc)* 2009; 74: 1411-1142

Sorolla A, Yeramian A, Dolcet X, Perez de Santos AM, Llobet D, Schoenenberger JA, Casanova JM, Soria X, Egido R, Llombart A, Vilella R, Matias-Guiu X, et al. Effect of proteasome inhibitors on proliferation and apoptosis of human cutaneous melanoma-derived cell lines. *Br J Dermatol* 2008; 158: 496-504.

Su Y, Amiri KI, Horton LW, Yu Y, Ayers GD, Koehler E, Kelley MC, Puzanov I, Richmond A, Sosman JA. A phase I trial of bortezomib with temozolomide in patients with advanced melanoma: toxicities, antitumor effects, and modulation of therapeutic targets. *Clin Cancer Res* 2010; 16: 348-357

Tawbi H, Nimmagadda N. Targeted therapy in melanoma. *Biologics* 2009; 3: 475-484

Townsend AR, Millward M, Price T, Mainwaring P, Spencer A, Longenecker A, Palladino MA, Lloyd GK, Spear MA and Padrik P. Clinical trial of NPI-0052 in advanced malignancies including lymphoma and leukemia (advanced malignancies arm) [abstract]. *J Clin Oncol* 2009; 27 (Suppl): 3582

Voorhees PM, Orlowski RZ. The proteasome and proteasome inhibitors in cancer therapy. *Annu Rev Pharmacol Toxicol* 2006; 46:189-213

Wang C, Li S, Wang MW. Evodiamine-induced human melanoma A375-S2 cell death was mediated by PI3K/Akt/caspase and Fas-L/NF-kappaB signaling pathways and augmented by ubiquitin-proteasome inhibition. *Toxicol In Vitro* 2010; 24: 898-904

Wolter KG, Verhaegen M, Fernández Y, Nikolovska-Coleska Z, Riblett M, de la Vega CM, Wang S, Soengas MS. Therapeutic window for melanoma treatment provided by selective effects of the proteasome on Bcl-2 proteins. *Cell Death Differ* 2007; 14: 1605-1616

Xie Y. Feedback regulation of proteasome gene expression and its implications in cancer therapy. *Cancer Metastasis Rev* 2010; 29: 687-63

Yeramian A, Sorolla A, Velasco A, Santacana M, Dolcet X, Valls J, Abal L, Moreno S, Egido R, Casanova JM, Puig S, Vilella R, Llombart-Cussac A, Matias-Guiu X, Martí RM. Inhibition of activated receptor tyrosine kinases by Sunitinib induces growth arrest and sensitises melanoma cells to Bortezomib by blocking Akt pathway. *Int J Cancer* [Epub ahead of print, march 28 2011]

Yerlikaya A, Okur E, 350 Eker S, Erin N. Combined effects of the proteasome inhibitor bortezomib and Hsp70 inhibitors on the B16F10 melanoma cell line. *Mol Med Report* 2010; 3: 333-339

Zou W, Yue P, Lin N, He M, Zhou Z, Lonial S, Khuri FR, Wang B, Sun SY. Vitamin C inactivates the proteasome inhibitor PS-341 in human cancer cells. *Clin Cancer Res* 2006; 12: 3-4

# 22

# Nuclear Translocation of YB-1 Protein Induced by Ultraviolet Light and the Investigational Gallium Drug GaQ3 in Melanoma Cells

Seied Mojtaba Valiahdi[1], Michael A. Jakupec[1], Sara Daraei[2], Franz Wohlrab[3] and Bernhard K. Keppler[1]

[1]*Institute of Inorganic Chemistry, University of Vienna*
[2]*Donauspital SMZ Ost, Department of Dermatology and Venereology, Vienna*
[3]*Max F. Perutz Laboratories; Medical University of Vienna*
*Austria*

## 1. Introduction

The Y-box factors are a family of proteins that have been structurally and functionally conserved throughout evolution (Wolffe et al., 1992). They are transcription factors that are expressed in a wide range of cell types from bacteria to human cells. They are called Y-box proteins after the specificity originally shown for human YB-1 in binding the Y-box sequence CTGATTGGCCAA present in the promoter region of major histocompatibility complex class II genes (Didier et al., 1988). Y-box proteins have emerged as key players in cellular metabolism. These proteins are capable of binding one or more types of nucleic acids, single- or double-stranded DNA or RNA. The negative or positive modulation of transcription by YB-1 causes diverse biological effects on a wide array of genes, modification of chromatin (Ashizuka et al., 2002), translational masking of mRNA (Evdokimova et al., 2006), cooperation in eukaryotic redox signaling pathways (Swamynathan et al., 2002), RNA chaperoning (Matsumoto et al., 2005) and stress response regulation (Swamynathan et al, 1998). The nuclear functions of YB-1 also include a role in DNA replication (En-Nia et al., 2005) and repair (Marenstein et al., 2001) as well as mRNA transport into the cytoplasm (Soop et al., 2003) (Figure 1).

YB-1 protein is a member of the DNA-binding protein family. It binds to the Y-box, an inverted CCAAT box, in the promoter region of many oncogenes and regulates their activity, for example the human multidrug resistance 1 gene, which encodes P-glycoprotein (P-gp) (Kuwano et al., 2004; Gluz et al., 2009), the cell division cycle 6 gene, which promotes cell cycle progression (Basaki et al., 2010), and the membrane type I-matrix metalloproteinase, which facilitates tumor invasion and metastasis (Lovett et al., 2010).

P-glycoprotein was first identified by virtue of its overexpression in multidrug resistant (MDR) tumor cells, where it mediates the energy-dependent efflux of a variety of chemotherapeutic agents (Trambas et al., 1997). The human class I P-glycoprotein is known to transport phospholipids, cholesterol, calcium channel blockers, immunosuppressants, peptides, steroids and xenobiotics (Bauer et al., 2005). More recent studies suggest that

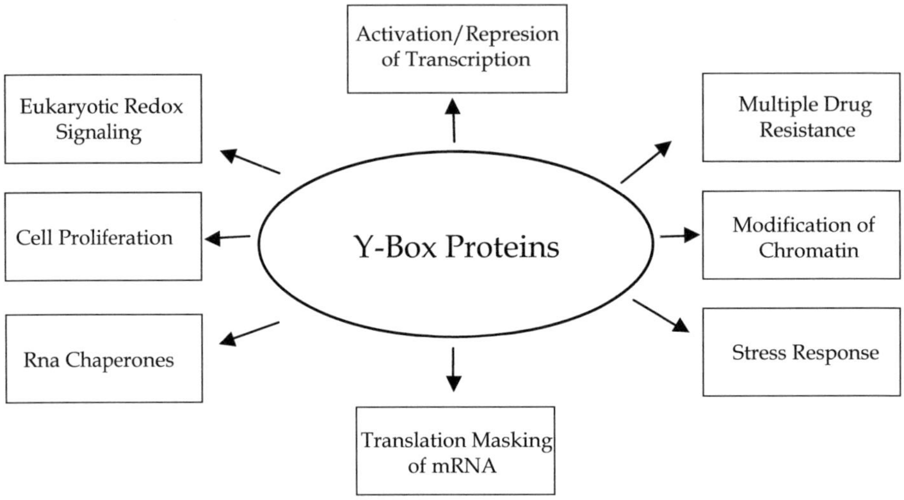


Fig. 1. Involvement of Y-box proteins in various cellular processes

upregulation of P-gp genes in tumor cells can prevent apoptosis and enhances the ability to resist chemotherapeutics (Park et al., 2006) and a wide range of apoptotic inducers, including serum starvation, fas ligand, UV irradiation, tumor necrosis factor and other stress inducer, including heat shock and chemotherapeutic agents (Hu et al., 2000). Gómez-Martínez has reported that the proximal promoter of MDR 1 contains several regulatory regions, including an inverted CCAAT box at -82 to -73 and a GC element at -56 to -42, both of which have been shown to be necessery for constitutive promoter activity in some cell types (Gómez-Martínez et al., 2007). Various environmental stimuli increase the activity of the MDR 1 promoter in response to all stimulation cascades that are dependent on the inverted CCAAT box (Kathleen & David, 1998). Interaction of the nuclear factor MDR-NF1 with this promoter region is increased when cells are exposed to UV or anticancer drugs (Ohga et al., 1996). To understand the molecular basis of MDR 1 promoter activity and the stress-dependent induction, the cDNA for MDR-NF1 has been cloned, revealing that the amino acid sequence encoded by the cloned cDNA is indentical to that of YB-1 (Ohga et al., 1996).

YB-1 was found to be expressed at much higher levels in all cisplatin-resistant cell lines than in the respective drug-sensitive parental counterparts. Two transfectants with a YB-1 antisense construct showed increased sensitivity to cisplatin, mitomycin C and UV irradiation, but not to vincristine, doxorubicin, camptothecin or etoposide, suggesting that cells with downregulated YB-1 gene expression are more sensitive to agents that induce cross-linking of DNA (Ohga et al., 1996). Nuclear localization and an upregulation of YB-1 expression are closely associated with intrinsic MDR 1 gene expression in primary human breast cancers (Bargou et al., 1997; Spitkovsky et al., 1992). YB-1 protein is localized mainly in the cytoplasm, but accumulates in the nucleus by UV exposure, hyperthermia (Stein et al., 2001), phosphorylation (Davies et al., 2011), or association with p53 (Zhang et al., 2003). This translocation may be induced by a protein kinase C-mediated signal transduction pathway, and the C-terminal region of YB-1 might be important for cytoplasmic retention of YB-1 (Koike et al., 1997). Similarly, exposure to chemotherapeutic agents stimulates accumulation in the nucleus (Valiahdi et al., 2006).

In malignant melanoma, YB-1 plays a key role for proliferation, survival and invasion and increases chemoresistance. The high expression of YB-1 in aggressive types of cancer and the evidence for a role in cell proliferation suggests a potential as a therapeutic target. YB-1 also associates with key tumor factors such as MMP-2, bcl-2, cyclinD1 and p16INK4A (Schittek et al., 2007), p53 (Okamoto et al., 2000), AP-1 (Lasham et al., 2003), Smad 3 and p300 (Higashi et al., 2003) and directly as well as indirectly regulates gene expression. An increased YB-1 expression of melanoma cells in comparison to benign melanocytes was shown in vitro and in vivo (Schittek et al., 2007). YB-1 is translocated into the nucleus in invasive and metastatic melanoma cells, and a downregulation of YB-1 by shRNA reduces the rate of proliferation and increases the rate of apoptotic cell death (Schittek et al., 2007). Translocation of the protein into the nucleus leads to its association with the family of serine/threonine kinases that inhibit apoptosis, stimulate angiogenesis, and promote tumor formation. It has also been suggested that Janus kinase and casein kinase II phosphorylate YB-1 and induce translocation of this protein into the nucleus (Sutherland et al., 2005).

Gallium has long been studied for its suitability both for imaging and therapy of malignant tumors including melanoma among others, with the most prominent effects in malignant lymphoma (Jakupec & Keppler, 2004). Through never established in clinical routine, attempts to utilize gallium-67 scintigraphy for the detection and surveillance of occult metastatic disease in melanoma patients showed that these tumors can regularly be visualized by gallium tracers, suggesting a certain affinity (Kirkwood et al., 1982). To investigate the therapeutic effect of gallium nitrate in advanced malignant melanoma, a clinical study was performed in which gallium nitrate (250-300 mg/m$^2$) was administered daily to 31 patients for 7 consecutive days. The compound was well tolerated, but only one of 31 evaluable patients experienced a partial remission (Casper et al., 1985). In a prior phase I study, 3 of 19 patients with advanced melanoma treated with gallium nitrate had experienced disease stabilization (Bedikian et al., 1978).

In order to improve the oral bioavailability and the pharmacological activity of gallium, a gallium complex has been developed by our institute (GaQ3). GaQ3 is an investigational anticancer drug in early clinical development, suitable for oral administration and well tolerable in toxicological studies (Collery et al., 1996). We demonstrated strong antiproliferative effects of GaQ3 in metastatic melanoma cell lines and in primary cultures of freshly explanted melanoma samples in comparison to established drugs (Valiahdi et al., 2009).

## 2. Experimental part

### 2.1 Drugs

Tris(8-quinolinolato)gallium (III) (GaQ3) was synthesized and isolated as a solid in high purity at the Institute of Inorganic Chemistry, University of Vienna, Austria, according to a previously established procedure (Collery et al., 1996). Gallium nitrate was purchased from Sigma-Aldrich as a hydrate of the composition $Ga(NO_3)_3 \cdot 5.8H_2O$, as determined by thermogravimetric analysis. GaQ3 was applied from fresh stock solutions in dimethylsulfoxide (DMSO) and diluted in media or buffer as appropriate to a maximum of 0.3% DMSO.

### 2.2 Cell lines and culture conditions

The human melanoma cell lines 518A2, 607B, A375, MEL-JUSO and SK-MEL-28 were kindly provided by Dr. Rodrig Marculescu (Clinical Institute of Medical and Chemical Laboratory Diagnostics, Medical University of Vienna, Austria) and chicken embryo fibroblasts (Cef32) by Prof. Dr. Wolfgang Schneider (Max F. Perutz Laboratories; Medical University of Vienna; Austria) , respectively. Cells were grown in 75 $cm^2$ culture flasks (Iwaki/Asahi Technoglass, Gyouda, Japan) as adherent monolayer cultures in complete culture medium, i.e. minimal essential medium (MEM) supplemented with 10% heat-inactivated fetal bovine serum, 1 mM sodium pyruvate, 4 mM L-glutamine and 1% non-essential amino acids (100×) (all purchased from Sigma–Aldrich, Vienna, Austria). Cultures were maintained at 37 °C in a humidified atmosphere containing 5% $CO_2$.

### 2.3 Cytotoxicity assay

Cytotoxicity was determined by a colorimetric microculture assay (MTT assay). For this purpose, 518A2, 607B, A375, MEL-JUSO and SK-MEL-28 cells were harvested from culture flasks by trypsinization and seeded into 96-well microculture plates (Iwaki/Asahi Technoglass) in densities of 1.5–3.5 × $10^4$ viable cells/well, depending on the cell line. After a 24 h preincubation, cells were exposed to dilutions of the test compounds in 200 µL/well complete culture medium for 96 h. At the end of exposure, drug solutions were replaced by 100 µL/well RPMI 1640 medium (supplemented with 10% heat-inactivated fetal bovine serum and 4 mM L-glutamine) plus 20 µL/well MTT solution (5 mg/mL) in phosphate-buffered saline (PBS) . After incubation for 4 h, medium was removed and the formazan product formed by viable cells was dissolved in DMSO (150 µL/well). Optical densities at 550 nm were measured with a microplate reader (Tecan Spectra Classic). The quantity of viable cells was expressed in terms of T/C values by comparison to untreated controls, and 50% inhibitory concentrations ($IC_{50}$) were calculated from concentration-effect curves by interpolation. Evaluation is based on means from at least three independent experiments, each comprising six replicates per concentration level.

### 2.4 Construction of plasmids expressing a GFP-YB-1 fusion protein

Because of the high levels of endogenous YB-1 in the cells, it was useful to use tagged YB-1 constructs for the study of YB-1. In this study, we developed a tagged chk-YB-1 by cloning cDNA of YB-1 into the ApaI site of the pEGFP-C1 plasmid. To investigate role of extreme C-terminus of YB-1 on translocation into nucleus, the full-length YB-1 gene was deleted at the C-terminus to create the YB-1Δ27 product (Figure 2).

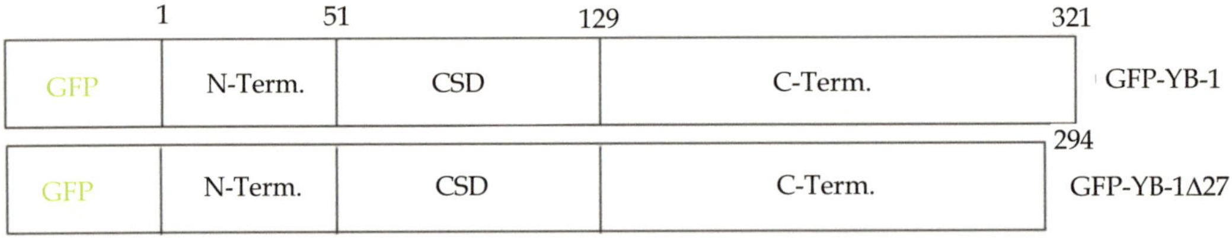


Fig. 2. Schematic representation of GFP-YB-1 and the truncated construct GFP-YB-1Δ27. The numbers represent the position of amino acids at the border between the respective domains. CSD: cold shock domain; GFP: green fluorescent protein

### 2.5 Transient transfection

Cef32 cells (chicken embryo fibroblasts) were transfected with a GFP-chk-YB-1, GFP-chk-YB-1Δ27 or GFP only construct. SK-MEL-28 cells were transfected with a pCMV-YB-1-GFP construct (kindly provided by Dr. K. Higashi, Kyoto University, Kyoto, Japan). In a six-well plate or 35-mm tissue culture plate, about 1-2 x $10^5$ cells were seeded in 2 ml of MEM supplemented with 10% fetal calf serum and grown for 24 h to a confluence of 40-60%. The cells were washed once with 2 ml of serum-free medium, and for each transfection 0.8 ml serum-free medium were added to each tube containing 200 µl jetPEI reagent-DNA complex (Qbiogene, Inc). After washing, cells were overlaid with a 1 ml mixture of jetPEI reagent-DNA complex and serum-free medium and incubated for 5-24 h at 37 °C. Then the DNA-containing medium was replaced with 2 ml of growth medium containing serum and incubated for 48-72 h. In order to assure successful transfection, the expression of the reporter gene encoding for green fluorescence protein (GFP) was visualized directly by observation of green fluorescence under the fluorescence microscope or indirectly by an anti-GFP antibody (Western blotting).

### 2.6 Nuclear and cytoplasmic cell extracts

To obtain total cell extracts, Cef32 cells were washed twice in PBS, scraped into PBS, pelleted, and resuspended in lysis buffer. Cells were washed with PBS, resuspended in 200 µl ice-cold 40% TKM buffer (50 mM Tris-HCl pH 7.4, 25 mM KCl, 5 mM $MgCl_2$, 0.2 mM EDTA) containing protease inhibitor (1 M dithiothreito (DTT), 10 mM vanadate, 1 mg/ml leupeptin, 3 mg/ml aprotinin and 100 mM phenylmethylsulfonylfluorid (PMSF)) and incubated on ice for 10 min. Then, the cells were disrupted by 25 strokes in a dounce homogenizer using a tight-fitting pestle. The homogenate was immediately diluted with the threefold volume of TKM buffer and centrifuged at 1000xg for 10 min at 4 °C. The low-speed supernatant was used as the cytoplasmic fraction. The low-speed pellet was resuspended in 400 µl TKM buffer, laid on 400 µl 60% sucrose in TKM and centrifuged at 100.000xg for 60 min at 4 °C. The sucrose was aspirated and the pellet (nuclear fraction) resuspended in 800 µl TKM buffer.

### 2.7 Western blotting

Western blots of both nuclear extracts and cytosolic fractions of untreated and UV-exposed Cef32 cells were assayed by immunoblotting using anti-chk-YB-1C (1:5000 dilution, Sigma) and primary antibodies against GFP (1:1000) (mouse IgG monoclonal antibody, clones 7.1 and 13.1, Roche). For this purpose, Cef32 cells and Cef32 cells transiently expressing EGFP-chk-YB-1 were treated with UV light (50 J/m$^2$), and whole cell lysates or fractionated cell lysates were diluted in 2x sample buffer (125 mM Tris pH 6.8, 4% sodium dodecyl sulfate (SDS), 10% glycerol, 0.006% bromophenol blue, 1.8% beta-mercaptoethanol). Denatured cellular extracts were resolved by SDS-PAGE (sodium dodecyl sulfate polyacrylamide gel electrophoresis), transferred onto nitrocellulose membranes (Amersham Hybond ECL, GE Healthcare, Little Chalfont, UK), blocked in fetal calf serum, and incubated with appropriate antibodies. Secondary anti-mouse antibody was used in dilutions of 1:10000. For visualization of the proteins, Western blotting luminal reagent (Santa Cruz Biotechnology, Santa Cruz, CA, USA) was used according to the instructions of the manufacturer, and X-ray film was exposed to the blots.

### 2.8 UV irradiation

Cef32 cells were grown in MEM medium to 80% confluence. The medium was removed and the cells were washed with PBS (37 °C). After treatment of the cells with UV light at 50 J/m$^2$

(UV Stratalinker 2400), the removed medium was added again to the cells and cells were incubated for 1 hour at 37 °C. The effect of UV irradiation was investigated either by using fluorescence microscopy or Western blotting.

## 3. Results

### Cytotoxicity in melanoma cell lines

The $IC_{50}$ values obtained with GaQ3 in five human melanoma cell lines are in a relatively narrow range of very low micromolar concentrations (0.8–2.5 µM), whereas cytotoxicity of the former investigational anticancer drug gallium nitrate is much lower, as reflected by $IC_{50}$ values between 20 and > 200 µM in the same cell lines (Table 1, Figure 3). Thus, GaQ3 shows a 23- to > 80-fold higher potency than gallium nitrate, based on the comparison of $IC_{50}$ values. The high intrinsic gallium nitrate resistance of the cell line SK-MEL-28 does not affect sensitivity to GaQ3 in equal measure.

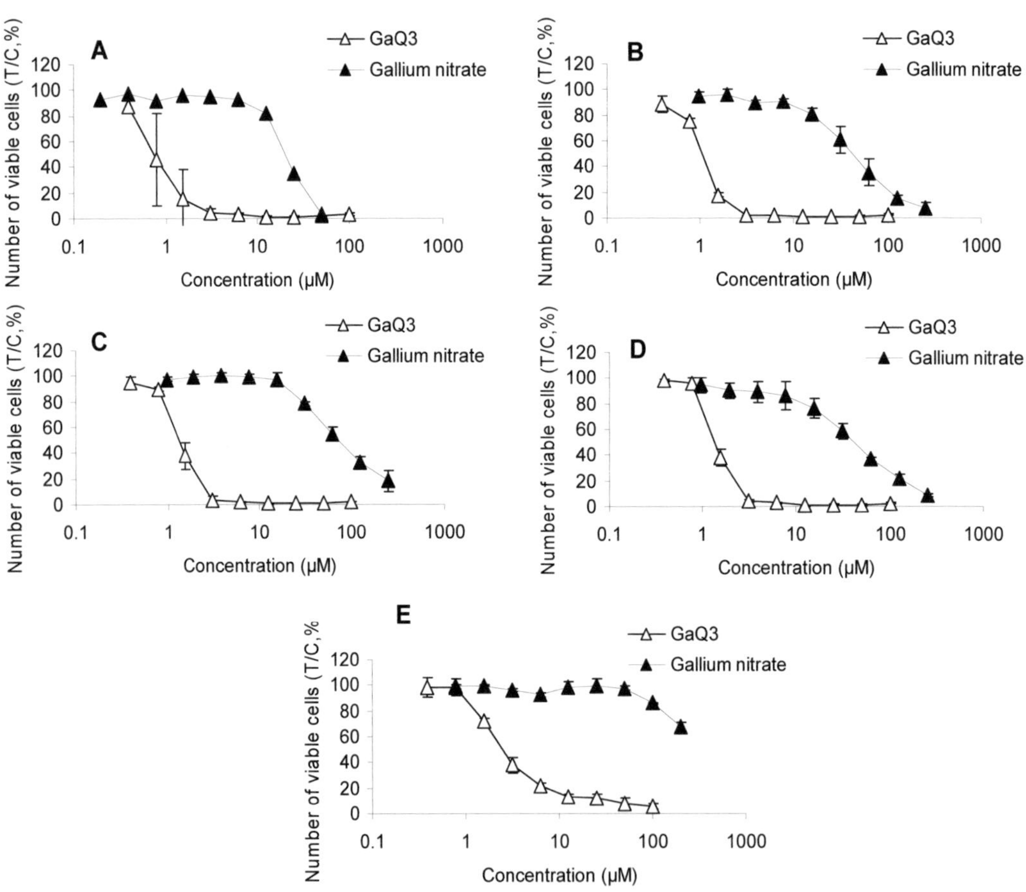


Fig. 3. Comparison of concentration-effect curves of GaQ3(-△-) and gallium nitrate (-▲-) in the human melanoma cell lines 518A2 (A), 607B (B), A375 (C), MEL-JUSO (D) and SK-MEL-28 cells (E), obtained by the MTT assay (96 h exposure)

| **Compound** | **IC$_{50}$ (μM)[a]** | | | | |
|---|---|---|---|---|---|
| | **SK-MEL-28** | **607B** | **A375** | **MEL-JUSO** | **518A2** |
| **GaQ3** | 2.45 ± 0.15 | 1.35 ± 0.09 | 1.30 ± 0.15 | 1.05 ± 0.10 | 0.855 ± 0.362 |
| **Gallium nitrate** | > 200 | 39.9 ± 4.7 | 72.4 ± 8.9 | 42.7 ± 9.1 | 20.0 ± 1.0 |

[a] 50% inhibitory concentrations in SK-MEL-28, 607B, A375, MEL-JUSO and 518A2 melanoma cells in the MTT assay, 96h exposure. Values are the mean ± standard deviation obtained from at least three independent experiments.

Table 1. Cytotoxicity of the new gallium complex (GaQ3) in comparison with gallium nitrate in five human melanoma cell lines

**Immunostaining**

Preliminary experiments showed that the chk-YB-1C antibody was unable to detect the fusion YB-1 protein, presumably due to steric hindrance. Therefore, exogenous YB-1 expression in GFP-YB-1 transfected Cef32 cells (in comparison with GFP-only-transfected cells) were indirectly detected by an anti-GFP antibody (Figure 4). The expression of the fusion protein GFP-YB-1 with a molecular weight of 77 kDa is clearly discernible in the immunoblots of total Cef32 cell extracts.

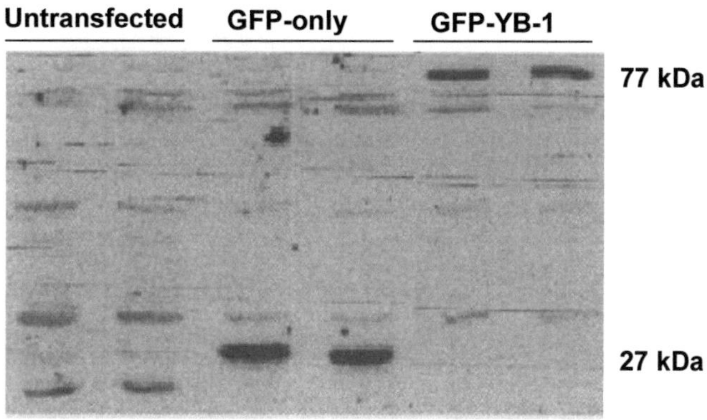


Fig. 4. Western blot of total cell extracts from Cef32 cells transiently transfected with GFP and GFP-YB-1, as well as from untransfected cells (negative control). Proteins were separated on a 10%polyacrylamide SDS gel and probed with anti-GFP antibody (1:5000 dilution)

The effect of UV irradiation on the localization of endogenous and exogenous chk-YB-1 in Cef32 cells was studied with an antibody directed against the extreme C-terminus of YB-1 (anti-chk-YB-1C), revealing that the endogenous protein in UV-exposed cells can be found in the nuclear fraction after only 1 hour incubation (Figure 5, middle blots). To indicate the exogenous YB-1 protein in Cef32 cells, we detected the presence of the GFP fusion protein in the nuclear fraction after UV irradiation by an anti-GFP polyclonal antibody, revealing the same nuclear translocation for the exogenous YB-1 protein upon UV exposure (Figure 5, upper blot).

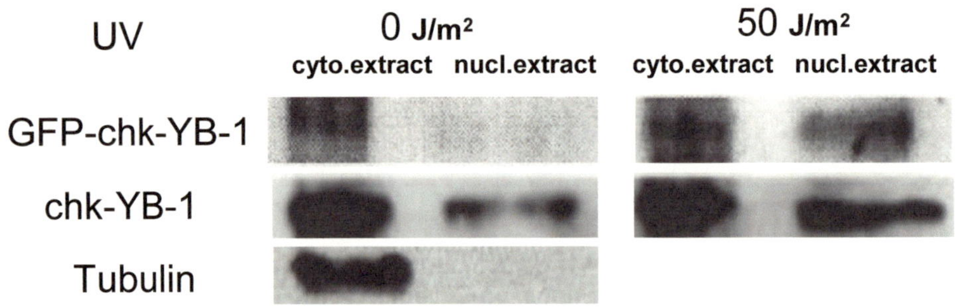


Fig. 5. Subcellular distribution of endogenous and exogenous YB-1 protein in Cef32 cells. Western blots of both nuclear extracts and cytosolic fractions of untreated and UV-exposed (50 J/m$^2$) untransfected and transfected Cef32 cells were assayed by immunoblotting using anti-GFP antibody (upper blots) and anti-chk-YB-1C antibody (middle blots). In order to exclude contamination of the nuclear fraction with cytosolic proteins, extracts were immunoblotted with anti-α-tubulin (lower blot)

**Fluorescence microscopy**

The subcellular distribution of GFP-YB-1 and the effect of UV irradition were additionally investigated by fluorescence microscopy of Cef32 cells transfected with the chk-YB-1-GFP expression construct, yielding further evidence for the nuclear accumulation of YB-1 upon UV irradiation, whereas larger amounts of YB-1 were detected in the cytosol, more at the perinuclear region than in the nucleus of untreated fibroblast cells (Figure 6).

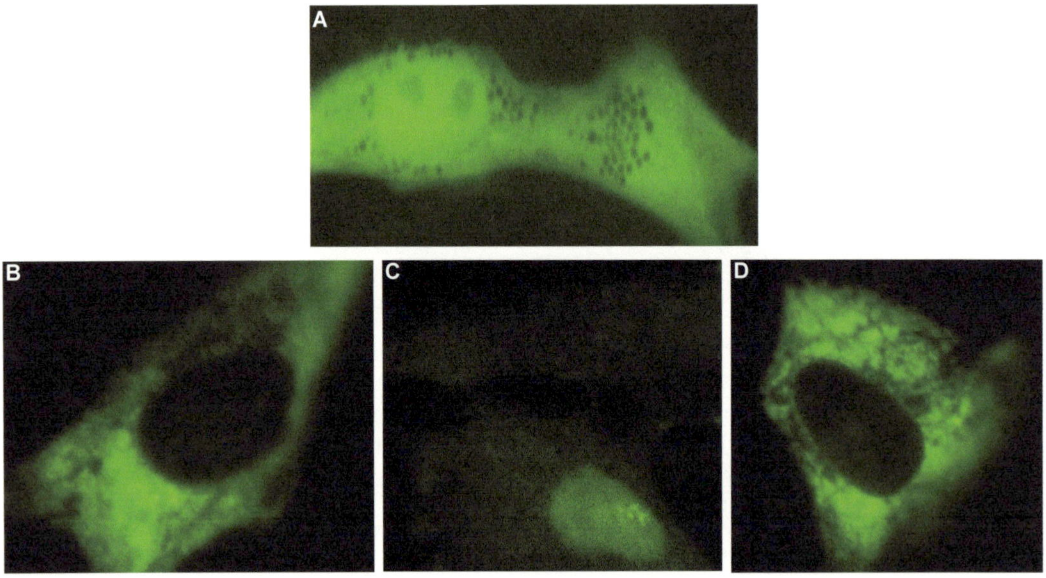


Fig. 6. Fluorescence microscopic images of Cef32 cells transfected with either pEGFP-C1 only (A) or a GFP-chk-YB-1 construct (B-D). While the fluorescence of GFP is rather evenly distributed in both cytosol and nucleus in the former cells (no difference of GFP expression in cytoplasm and nucleus) (A), untreated GFP-chk-YB-1 transfected cells show mainly cytosolic fluorescence, indicating the cytosolic expression of YB-1 (B, D). Translocation of this protein into the nucleus was observed 2 h after UV irradiation (50 J/m$^2$) (C)

To investigate the effect of the deletion of the 27 C-terminal amino acids on intracellular localization of YB-1, GFP-YB-1(27 was transfected transiently into Cef32 cells and visualized by fluorescence microscopy after 48 hours incubation at 37 °C. GFP-YB-1 and GFP-YB-1(27 lacking the C-terminus (294-321) of YB-1 were located mainly in the cytosol, but the deletion construct was located more in perinuclear regions (Figure 7 B). In contrast to cells transfected with the complete GFP-YB-1 construct, UV irradiation did not result in recognizable nuclear translocation of fluorescence in those cells transfected with the deletion construct (Figure 7C), suggesting that the C-terminal sequence is essential for translocation.

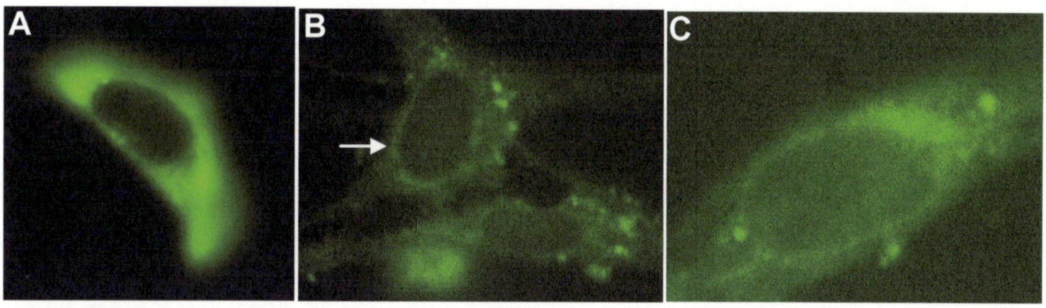


Fig. 7. Fluorescence microscopic images of Cef32 cells transiently transfected with GFP-YB-1 (A) or GFP-YB-1Δ27 (B, C). The deletion product GFP-YB-1Δ27 is mainly expressed in the cytosol, in particular in the perinuclear region, in untreated cells (B), and no pronounced translocation into the nucleus is discernible upon UV irradiation (50 J/m$^2$) (C)

Furthermore, the human melanoma cell line SK-MEL-28 was transfected with a pCMV-hYB-1-GFP plasmid (encoding for human YB-1), and the localization of YB-1 in the cell was again visualized using the fluorescence of the reporter protein GFP. The same translocation of YB-1 into the nucleus as in UV-treated Cef32 cells was observed upon GaQ3 treatment in these transiently transfected SK-MEL-28 cells (Figure 8).

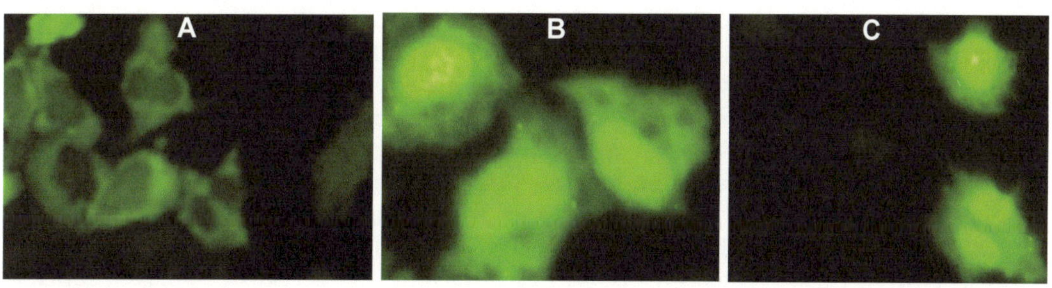


Fig. 8. Fluorescence microscopic images of SK-MEL-28 cells transiently transfected with pCMV-YB-1-GFP construct. Untreated cells show mainly a cytosolic expression of YB-1 (A), whereas translocation into the nucleus is visible after treatment with 5 μM GaQ3 for 24 h (B,C)

## 4. Discussion

The tumor-inhibiting compound GaQ3 has strong antiproliferative activity in human melanoma cells, in particular in the Human Tumor Cloning Assay (HTCA) in primary melanoma explants. The effects induced by GaQ3 in melanoma cell lines involve S phase arrest, caspase activation and poly-(ADP-ribose) polymerase cleavage, indicating induction of apoptosis, whereas no direct interactions with DNA could be observed (Valiahdi et al., 2009). The improved pharmacological properties of GaQ3 as compared to earlier gallium-based agents and in vitro data presented here warrant further studies of this compound in malignant melanoma. The mechanism of action of GaQ3 is far from understood, but seems to deviate from that of gallium nitrate and does not involve DNA interactions such as cross-linking or strand breakage (Valiahdi et al., 2009). Nevertheless, we could demonstrate that cellular responses to this investigational anticancer drug involve the Y-box protein YB-1.

Y-box proteins play multiple roles in the cell, serving as transcription factors, as a part of mRNA particles, or in cell proliferation (Matsumoto & Wolffe, 1998); however, their entire function is still unclear. The import of transcription factors into the nucleus is not a constitutive process and appears to be modulated in response to external stimuli, cell cycle and development. Regulation of the subcellular localization of proteins involves the direct phosphorylation of the transported protein, masking of the nuclear localization signals, cytoplasmic retention by binding to an anchoring protein, and the interplay among these different mechanisms (Calkhoven & Ab, 1996; Garcia-Bustos et al., 1991). It has been proposed that the YB-1 protein migrates to the nucleus in response to certain stress signals (Koike et al., 1997). However, examination of the YB-1 sequence shows no obvious nuclear localisation sequence. The question arising from this issue is: How are Y-box proteins signalized to move into the nucleus? Is phosphorylation an effective factor for nuclear translocation? To address this issue, we considered possibilities to tag the protein to study compartimental changes and to investigate what region of the protein might be responsible for this translocation. A GFP fusion protein enabled us to observe the subcellular location and intracellular movements in vitro. Observations under the fluorescence microscope showed clearly a predominant expression of GFP-YB-1 and the truncated version YB-1(27 in the cytoplasm of Cef32 cells. Kokie and colleagues have reported that the C-terminal region of YB-1 might be important for cytoplasmic retention of YB-1. In their study, they demonstrated that expression of GFP-YB-1 with the C-terminus of YB-1 was located mainly in the cytosol, but GFP-YB-1deltaC with a larger deletion at the C-terminus of YB-1 (248-317) was located in the nucleus (Kokie et al., 1997), in contrast to our observation with a different deletion at the C terminus. The C-terminal domain of YB-1 does not have a nuclear export signal such as mitogen activated protein kinase kinase (MAPKK). Since this domain has been shown to be involved in the protein-protein interaction, it was hypothesized that YB-1 could be retained in the cytoplasm by binding to an anchoring protein (Ruzanov et al., 1999), as observed for the transcription factor NF-κB interacting with I κB in the cytoplasm (Verma et al., 1995).

The recruitment of YB-1 to the nucleus after exposure to UV irradiation or cytotoxic agents suggests that YB-1 itself protects the cells against the effects of genotoxic damage (Cohen et al., 2010). The association between nuclear YB-1 and resistance against cisplatin might be a useful predictive marker for cancer multidrug resistance (Yahata et al., 2002). Recently, an association of YB-1 interacellular localization with expression levels of P-gp (P-glycoprotein, which is able to dispose drugs from the cell via the cell membrane) has been proposed (Bargou et al., 1997). This P-glycoprotein is encoded by the MDR1 gene, which responsible for drug resistance of many tumors. Bargou have reported that nuclear localization of YB-1 is closely associated with MDR1 gene expression in a human breast cancer cell line and that P-gp levels were high in untreated primary breast cancers in which YB-1 was localized in the nucleus, but were low in the breast cancers where YB-1 was localized in the cytoplasm.

These results show that in untreated primary breast cancers, nuclear localization of YB-1 protein is associated with intrinsic multidrug resistance. It was shown that YB-1 has an important role in controlling MDR 1 gene transcription, and this finding provides a basis for the analysis of molecular mechanisms responsible for intrinsic multidrug resistance in human breast cancer. However, it remains unclear whether activated YB-1 directly affects MDR1 gene expression in response to genotoxic stress. In previous studies suggests that YB-1 may itself have a key role in self-defense signaling mechanisms, being initiated in response to cellular stress. The YB-1 proteins are also integral components of a eukaryotic redox signalling pathway (Duh et al., 1995), serving as a scaffold for the assembly of other factors. All this information indicates that these Y-box proteins may be a part of mammalian stress signal transduction mechanisms.
In our studies, we investigated the dependence of intercellular localization of human-YB-1 and chk-YB-1 in metastatic melanoma cells and chicken embryo fibroblasts, respectively, by stress factors such as UV irradiation and GaQ3 treatment. Furthermore, we demonstrated that the last 27 amino acids of the C-terminus are necessary for translocation of the protein into the nucleus, since this deletion (YB-1Δ27 (294-321)) correlated with an inhibition of nuclear translocation after UV irradiation. This sequence (27 amino acids) which is rich in SH groups is a suitable substrate for posttranslational modification, in particular phosphorylation by protein kinases at serine or threonine. The frequency of these amino acids increases the negative charge of the acidic sequences and probably improves the interaction of the C-terminal domain with other proteins (carrier proteins). Protein-protein interactions may be the cause of migration of chkYB-1 into the nucleus. Molecular intervention aiming at the inhibition of nuclear translocation of YB-1 may be a strategy to improve the efficacy of anticancer drugs.
In conclusion, nuclear localization of YB-1 is a cellular response to damaging agents such as UV irradiation or the investigational anticancer drug GaQ3. YB-1 itself may be worth investigating as a potential target in cancer therapy, in particular in combination with cytotoxic drugs in malignant melanoma.

## 5. Acknowledgment

The authors are indebted to Dr. Rodrig Marculescu (Clinical Institute of Medical and Chemical Laboratory Diagnostics, Medical University of Vienna) for providing the metastases melanoma cells. We are grateful to Prof. Dr. K. Higashi (Kyoto University, Kyoto, Japan) for generous delivery of knowledge and materials for the human YB-1 construct and to Dr. Peter Unfried (Institute of Inorganic Chemistry, University of Vienna, Austria) for the synthesis of GaQ3. This work was supported by the Austrian Research Promotion Agency (FFG), the Austrian Council for Research and Technology Development and Max F. Perutz Laboratories; Medical University of Vienna; Austria.

## 6. References

Ashizuka, M., Fukuda, T., Nakamura, T., Shirasuna, K., Iwai, K., Izumi, H., Kohno, K., Kuwano, M. & Uchiumi, T. (2002). Novel translational control through an iron-responsive element by interaction of multifunctional protein YB-1 and IRP2. *Mol. Cell. Biol.* 22(18):6375-6383.

Bargou, RC., Jürchott, K., Wagener, C., Bergmann, S., Metzner, S., Bommert, K., Mapara, MY., Winzer, KJ., Dietel, M., Dörken, B. & Royer, HD. (1997). Nuclear localization and increased levels of transcription factor YB-1 in primary human breast cancers are associated with intrinsic MDR1 gene expression. *Nature Medicine.* 3, 447–450.

Bedikian, AY., Valdivieso, M., Bodey, GP., Burgess, MA., Benjamin, RS., Hall, S. & Freireich, EJ. (1978). Phase I clinical studies with gallium nitrate. *Cancer Treat. Rep.* 62: 1449–1453.

Basaki, Y., Taguchi, K., Izumi, H., Murakami, Y., Kubo, T., Hosoi, F., Watari, K., Nakano, K., Kawaguchi, H., Ohno, S., Kohno, K., Ono, M. & Kuwano, M. (2010). Y-box binding protein-1 (YB-1) promotes cell cycle progression through CDC6-dependent pathway in human cancer cells, *Eur. J. Cancer.* 46(5):954-965.

Bauer, B., Hartz, AM., Fricker, G. & Miller, DS. (2005). Modulation of p-glycoprotein transport function at the blood-brain barrier. *Exp. Biol. Med.* 230(2):118-127.

Calkhoven, CF. & Ab, G. (1996). Multiple steps in the regulation of transcription-factor level and activity. *Biochem. J.* 317 ( Pt 2): 329-342.

Casper, ES., Stanton, GF., Sordillo, PP., Parente, R., Michaelson, RA. & Vinceguerra, V. (1985). Phase II trial of gallium nitrate in patients with advanced malignant melanoma. *Cancer Treat. Rep.* 69(9): 1019-1020.

Cohen, SB., Ma, W., Valova, VA., Algie, M., Harfoot, R., Woolley, AG., Robinson, PJ. & Braithwaite, AW. (2010). Genotoxic stress-induced nuclear localization of oncoprotein YB-1 in the absence of proteolytic processing. *Oncogene.* 29(3): 403-410.

Collery, P., Domingo, JL. & Keppler, BK. (1996). Preclinical toxicity and tissue gallium distribution of a novel antitumour gallium compound: tris(8-quinolinolato)-gallium(III). *Anticancer Res.* 16: 687–692.

Davies, AH., Barrett, I., Pambid, MR., Hu, K., Stratford, AL., Freeman, S., Berquin, IM., Pelech, S., Hieter, P., Maxwell, C. & Dunn, SE. (2011). YB-1 evokes susceptibility to cancer through cytokinesis failure, mitotic dysfunction and HER2 amplification. *Oncogene.*

Didier, DK., Schiffenbauer, J., Woulfe, SL., Zacheis, M. & Schwartz, BD. (1988). Characterization of the cDNA encoding a protein binding to the major histocompatibility complex class II Y box. *Proc. Natl. Acad. Sci.* 85(19):7322-7326.

Duh, JL., Zhu, H., Shertzer, HG., Nebert, DW. & Puga, A. (1995). The Y-box motif mediates redox-dependent transcriptional activation in mouse cells. *J. Biol. Chem.* 270 : 30499-30507.

En-Nia, A., Yilmaz, E., Klinge, U., Lovett, DH., Stefanidis, I. & Mertens, PR. (2005). 1 mediates DNA polymerase alpha gene expression. *J. Biol. Chem.* 280(9): 7702-7711.

Evdokimova, V., Ruzanov, P., Anglesio, MS., Sorokin, AV., Ovchinnikov, LP., Buckley, J., Triche, TJ., Sonenberg, N. & Sorensen, PH. (2006). Akt-mediated YB-1 phosphorylation activates translation of silent mRNA species. *Mol. Cell. Biol.* 26(1):277-292.

Garcia-Bustos, J., Heitman, J. & Hall, MN. (1991). Nuclear protein localization. *Biochim Biophys Acta.* 1071(1): 83-101.

Gluz, O., Mengele, K., Schmitt, M., Kates, R., Diallo-Danebrock, R., Neff, F., Royer, HD., Eckstein, N., Mohrmann, S., Ting, E., Kiechle, M., Poremba, C., Nitz U. & Harbeck, N. (2009). Y-box-binding protein YB-1 identifies high-risk patients with primary breast cancer benefiting from rapidly cycled tandem high-dose adjuvant chemotherapy, *J. Clin. Oncol.* 27(36):6144-6151.

Gómez-Martínez A, García-Morales P, Carrato A, Castro-Galache MD, Soto JL, Carrasco-García E, García- Bautista M, Guaraz P, Ferragut JA, Saceda M. (2007). Post-transcriptional regulation of P-glycoprotein expression in cancer cell lines. *Mol. Cancer. Res.* 5(6):641-653.

Higashi, K., Inagaki, Y., Suzuki, N., Mitsui, S., Mauviel, A., Kaneko, H. & Nakatsuka, I. (2003). Y-box- binding protein YB-1 mediates transcriptional repression of human

Y-box-binding protein YB-1 mediates transcriptional repression of human alpha 2(I) collagen gene expression by interferon-gamma. *J. Biol. Chem.* 278(7): 5156-5162.

Hu, Z., Jin, S. & Scotto, KW. (2000). Transcriptional activation of the MDR1 gene by UV irradiation. Role of NF-Y and sp1. *J. Biol. Chem.* 275(4): 2979-2985.

Jakupec, MA. & Keppler, BK. (2004). Gallium in cancer treatment. *Curr. Top. Med. Chem.* 4(15): 1575-1583.

Kathleen, WS. & David, AE. (1998). Transcriptional regulation of MDR genes. *Cytotechnology.* 27: 257–269.

Kirkwood, JM., Myers, JE., Vlock, DR., Neumann, R., Ariyan, S., Gottschalk, A. & Hoffer, P. (1982). Tomographic gallium-67 citrate scanning: useful new surveillance for metastatic melanoma. *Ann Intern Med.* 97: 694-699.

Koike, K., Uchiumi, T., Ohga, T., Toh, S., Wada, M., Kohno, K. & Kuwano, M. (1997). Nuclear translocation of the Y-box binding protein by ultraviolet irradiation. *FEBS Letters.* 417(3): 390-394.

Kuwano, M., Oda, Y., Izumi, H., Yang, SJ., Uchiumi, T., Iwamoto, Y., Toi, M., Fujii, T., Yamana, H., Kinoshita, H., Kamura, T., Tsuneyoshi, M., Yasumoto, K. & Kohno, K. (2004). *The role of nuclear Y-box binding protein 1 as a global marker in drug resistance, Mol. Cancer. Ther.* 3(11):1485-1492.

Lasham, A., Moloney, S., Hale, T., Homer, C., Zhang, YF., Murison, JG., Braithwaite, AW. & Watson, J. (2003). The Y-box-binding protein, YB1, is a potential negative regulator of the p53 tumor suppressor. *J. Biol. Chem.* 278(37): 35516-35523.

Lovett, DH., Cheng, S., Cape, L., Pollock, AS. & Mertens, PR. (2010). YB-1 alters MT1-MMP trafficking and stimulates MCF-7 breast tumor invasion and metastasis, *Biochem Biophys Res Commun.* 398(3):482-488.

Marenstein, DR., Ocampo, MT., Chan, MK., Altamirano, A., Basu, AK., Boorstein, RJ., Cunningham, RP. & Teebor, GW. (2001). Stimulation of human endonuclease III by Y box-binding protein 1 (DNA- binding protein B). Interaction between a base excision repair enzyme and a transcription factor. *J. Biol. Chem.* 276(24): 21242-21249.

Matsumoto, K. & Wolffe, AP. (1998). Gene regulation by Y-box proteins: coupling control of transcription and translation. *Trends. Cell. Biol.* 8(8):318-323.

Matsumoto, K., Tanaka, KJ. & Tsujimoto, M. (2005). An acidic protein, YBAP1, mediates the release of YB-1 from mRNA and relieves the translational repression activity of YB-1. *Mol. Cell. Biol.* 25(5): 1779- 1792.

Ohga, T., Koike, K., Ono, M., Makino, Y., Itagaki, Y., Tanimoto, M., Kuwano, M. & Kohno, K. (1996). Role of the human Y box-binding protein YB-1 in cellular sensitivity to the DNA- damaging agents cisplatin, mitomycin C, and ultraviolet light. *Cancer Res.* 56(18): 4224-4228.

Okamoto,T., Izumi, H., Imamura, T., Takano, H., Ise, T., Uchiumi,T., Kuwano, M. & Kohno, K. (2000). Direct interaction of p53 with the Y-box binding protein, YB-1: a mechanism for regulation of human gene expression. *Oncogene.* 19(54): 6194-6202.

Park, SJ., Wu, CH., Choi, MR., Najafi, F., Emami, A. & Safa, AR. (2006). P-glycoprotein enhances TRAIL- triggered apoptosis in multidrug resistant cancer cells by interacting with the death receptor DR5. *Biochem Pharmacol.* 72(3):293-307.

Ruzanov, PV., Evdokimova, VM., Korneeva, NL., Hershey, JW. & Ovchinnikov, LP. (1999). Interaction of the universal mRNA-binding protein, p50, with actin: a possible link between mRNA and microfilaments. *J. Cell. Sci.* 112: 3487-3496.

Schittek, B., Psenner, K., Sauer, B., Meier, F., Iftner, T. & Garbe, C. (2007). The increased expression of Y box-binding protein 1 in melanoma stimulates proliferation and tumor invasion, antagonizes apoptosis and enhances chemoresistance. *Int. J. Cancer.* 120(10): 2110-2118.

Soop, T., Nashchekin, D., Zhao, J., Sun, X., Alzhanova-Ericsson, AT., Björkroth, B., Ovchinnikov, L. & Daneholt, B. (2003). A p50-like Y-box protein with a putative translational role becomes associated with pre-mRNA concomitant with transcription. *J. Cell Sci.* 116(Pt 8): 1493-503.

Spitkovsky, DD., Royer-Pokora, B., Delius, H., Kisseljov, F., Jenkins, NA., Gilbert, DJ., Copeland, NG. & Royer, HD. (1992). Tissue restricted expression and chromosomal localization of the YB-1 gene encoding a 42 kD nuclear CCAAT binding protein. *Nucl. Acids. Res.* 20(4):797-803.

Stein, U., Jürchott, K., Walther, W., Bergmann, S., Schlag, PM. & Royer, HD. (2001). Hyperthermia-induced nuclear translocation of transcription factor YB-1 leads to enhanced expression of multidrug resistance-related ABC transporters. *J. Biol.Chem.* 276(30): 28562-28569.

Swamynathan, SK., Varma, BR., Weber, KT. & Guntaka, RV. (2002). Targeted disruption of one allele of the Y- box protein gene, Chk-YB-1b, in DT40 cells results in major defects in cell cycle. *Biochem. Biophys. Res. Commun.* 296(2): 451-457.

Swamynathan, SK., Nambiar, A.& Guntaka, RV. (1998). Role of single-stranded DNA regions and Y-box proteins in transcriptional regulation of viral and cellular genes. *FASEB J.* 12(7):515-522.

Sutherland, BW., Kucab, J., Wu, J., Lee, C., Cheang, MC., Yorida, E., Turbin, D., Dedhar, S., Nelson, C., Pollak, M., Leighton Grimes, H., Miller, K., Badve, S., Huntsman, D., Blake-Gilks, C., Chen, M., Pallen, CJ. & Dunn, SE. (2005). Akt phosphorylates the Y-box binding protein 1 at Ser102 located in the cold shock domain and affects the anchorage-independent growth of breast cancer cells. *Oncogene.* 24(26): 4281-4292.

Trambas,CM., Muller, HK. & Woods, GM. (1997). P-glycoprotein mediated multidrug resistance and its implications for pathology. *Pathology.* 29(2):122-130.

Valiahdi, SM., Jakupec, MA., Wohlrab, F. & Keppler, BK. (2006). The intracellular localization of chk-YB-1 protein depends on a casein kinase II consensus sequence in the C-terminal part of the protein, The 5th International Annual Conference on Frontiers in Cancer Prevention Research, Boston, 2006b:94

Valiahdi, SM., Heffeter, P., Jakupec, MA., Marculescu, R., Berger, W., Rappersberger, K. & Keppler, BK. (2009). The gallium complex KP46 exerts strong activity against primary explanted melanoma cells and induces apoptosis in melanoma cell lines. *Melanoma Res.* 19(5): 283-293.

Verma, IM., Stevenson, JK., Schwarz, EM., Van Antwerp, D. & Miyamoto S. (1995). Rel/NF-kappa B/I kappa B family: intimate tales of association and dissociation. *Genes Dev.* 9 : 2723-2735.

Wolffe, AP., Tafuri, S., Ranjan, M. & Familari, M. (1992). The Y-box factors: a family of nucleic acid binding proteins conserved from Escherichia coli to man. *New Biol.* 4(4): 290-298.

Yahata, H., Kobayashi, H., Kamura, T., Amada, S., Hirakawa, T., Kohno, K., Kuwano, M. & Nakano, H. (2002). Increased nuclear localization of transcription factor YB-1 in acquired cisplatin-resistant ovarian cancer. *J. Cancer. Res. Clin. Oncol.* 128(11):621-626.

Zhang, YF., Homer, C., Edwards, SJ., Hananeia, L., Lasham, A., Royds, J., Sheard, P. & Braithwaite, AW. (2003). Nuclear localization of Y-box factor YB1 requires wild-type p53. *Oncogene.* 22(18):2782-2794.

# 23

# Novel Approach to the Characterization of Melanoma Associated-Peptide-Specific CTL Lines from Melanoma Patients

Yasuto Akiyama[1], Masaru Komiyama[1], Akira Iizuka[1],
Akifumi Yamamoto[3], Naoya Yamazaki[4] and Yoshio Kiyohara[2]
[1]*Shizuoka Cancer Center Research Institute,*
[2]*Shizuoka Cancer Center Hospital,*
[3]*Saitama Medical School,*
[4]*National Cancer Center Hospital Central*
*Japan*

## 1. Introduction

Melanoma-associated antigens are categorized as class I human leukocyte antigen (HLA)-restricted cancer/testis antigens (Renkvist et al., 2001) which are considered to be immunogenic to the immune system because they are hardly expressed in normal tissues except testis. However, melanoma is still difficult cancer to treat once it becomes advanced or metastatic. Malignant melanoma is the most well known cancer in which multiple tumor-specific antigens have been defined compared to other solid cancers, and utilized in vaccination strategies as peptide vaccines or peptide-pulsed dendritic cell (DC) vaccines (Nestle et al., 1998; Banchereau et al., 2001). Our group has been running a clinical phase I trial of peptide cocktail-pulsed DC vaccines in metastatic melanoma patients for some years. We reported that almost all cases showed more than 2 peptide-specific cytotoxic T cell (CTL) responses in blood and 2 cases had clinical responses [1 complete remission (CR), 1 partial remissions (PR)] (Akiyama et al., 2005).

We have identified some melanoma peptide-specific CTL lines and determined cDNA sequences of specific TCRs in the clinical trial. However, few studies have focused on the characterization or determination of peptide-oriented single specific CTL clones from melanoma patients treated with DC vaccines. Recently, specific CTLs or tumor-infiltrating lymphocytes (TILs) have been successfully cloned from blood or tumors of melanoma patients (Dudley et al., 2001, 2002, 2005; Yee et al., 2002). In some cases, melanoma peptide-specific CTL clones obtained from the tumor tissue were expanded, and could be utilized for adoptive immunotherapy (Dudley et al., 2002, 2005).

Interestingly, it is also reported that the same TCR repertoire specific to MART-1 peptide was recognized among blood CTLs as TIL clones isolated from tumors.

As to other types of cancers, a very small number of TILs were expanded to isolate tumor-specific clones from a bulk of TILs and utilized to search for novel tumor antigens in a tumor-derived complementary DNA library (Hoshino et al., 1997; Gohara et al., 1997). However, cloning from a bulk of CTLs is time-consuming, and usually very costly.

In the present study, we have established a novel efficient method for the expansion and separation of a very small number of melanoma peptide-specific CTLs using HLA-A2 or A24 peptide tetramer and T cell receptor (TCR)-specific monoclonal antibody (MoAb)-based cell sorting. Through the molecular cloning of melanoma peptide (MART-1, gp100 or MAGE-1)-specific TCRs, the biological characterization of each CTL line was performed in Japanese metastatic melanoma patients given DC vaccines.

## 2. Experimental design

### 2.1 Clinical trial of DC vaccines

Thirty-three cases of metastatic melanoma were enrolled into a phase I/II study of monocyte-derived DC-based immunotherapy. HLA typing showed 7 cases of HLA-A2 and 26 of A24 positive. Briefly, Enriched monocytes were obtained using OptiPrep™ from leukapheresis products, and then incubated with GM-CSF and IL-4 in a closed serum-free system. After pulsing with a cocktail of 5 melanoma-associated synthetic peptides (gp100, tyrosinase, MAGE-2, MAGE-3 and MART-1 or MAGE-1) restricted to HLA-A2 or A24 and keyhole limpet hemocyanin (KLH), cells were cryopreserved until used. Finally, thawed DCs were washed and injected subcutaneously (s.c.) into the inguinal region in a dose-escalation manner.

### 2.2 CTL induction cultures

Peripheral blood mononuclear cells (PBMCs) from 6 cases of HLA-A*0201$^+$ and 1 of HLA-A*2402$^+$ metastatic melanoma were used for *in vitro* CTL inductions (The clinical research using PBMC from melanoma patients was approved by the Institutional Review Board of Shizuoka Cancer Center, Shizuoka, Japan. All patients gave written informed consent.). All cases of metastatic melanoma were given melanoma-associated peptide-pulsed DC vaccines in clinical trial reported previously (Akiyama et al., 2005). Briefly, after non-adherent PBMCs were stimulated twice with melanoma peptide-pulsed mature DCs (most cells positively stained with CD83 MoAb), cells were boosted in RPMI1640 medium containing L-glutamine (2mM), penicillin (100U/ml), streptomycin (100U/ml) and 5% AB human serum referred to as CTL medium with 2 rounds of stimulation with peptide-pulsed T2 or T2-A24 cells. Finally, expanded peptide-specific CTLs were utilized for various experiments or cell sorting.

### 2.3 TCR repertoire profiling and function analysis

The staining profile of CTLs during the expansion procedure was monitored using a TCR Vβ repertoire kit, major populations positively stained with the specific anti-TCR antibody were determined. For function analysis, CTLs were pre-incubated with melanoma peptide-treated T2 or T2-A24 cells and stained intracellularly with anti-human IFN-γ MoAb, peptide-specific tetramer, and/or anti-specific TCR MoAb. The stained cells were analyzed on a flow cytometer.

### 2.4 CTL sorting by TCR-specific MoAb

Melanoma peptide tetramer-based or TCR MoAb-based CTL sorting was performed using the autoMACS (magnetic cell sorting) system (Miltenyi, Germany). Briefly, we used a specific PE-labeled tetramer or FITC-labeled TCR-specific MoAb as primary antibody, and anti-PE or FITC MoAb microbeads as secondary antibody. The purity of the tetramer+ or specific TCR+ CTLs was more than 98% (data not shown). Purified CTLs were sequentially used for PCR cloning of the TCR gene.

### 2.5 PCR cloning and sequencing of melanoma peptide-specific TCRBV cDNA

Total RNA of sorted CTLs was prepared with a kit, Nucleospin RNA II (Machery-Nagel, Germany), and aliquots of 2 µg were subjected to reverse transcription using oligo (dT) primer and SuperScript II (Invitrogen, CA). The first strand cDNA was amplified by PCR using KOD Polymerase (Toyobo, Japan) according to the manuacturer's instructions. Coding region-specific primers for TCRBV28 and TCRBC1 (MART-1 peptide-specific TCR), TCRBV12-4 and TCRBC2 (gp100 peptide-specific TCR) or TCRBV4 and TCRBC1 (MAGE-1 peptide specific TCR) are shown as in Table 1.

**Table 1 TCR-specific primers**

| Repertoire | Sequence |
|---|---|
| TCRBV28; | 5'-GCAGCCATGGGAATCAGGCTCCTCTGT-3' |
| TCRBV12-4; | 5'-TCTGCCATGGACTCCTGGACCCTCTGC-3' |
| TCRBV4; | 5'-GCTAGCATGGGCTGCAGGCTGCTCTGC-3' |
| TCRBC1; | 5'-TCAGAAATCCTTTCTCTTGACCATGGC-3' |
| TCRBC2; | 5'-CTAGCCTCTGGAATCCTTTCTCTTGAC-3' |

Table 1. TCR-specific primers

The PCR product was separated by electrophoresis on a 1.5% agarose gel, and the band of appropriate size (bp) was excised and extracted from the gel. The recovered DNA fragment was cloned into the plasmid pCR-Blunt (Invitrigen, CA, USA), and its sequence was determined using BigDye Terminator reagent and a 3130*xl* Genetic Analyzer (Applied Biosystems, CA).

### 2.6 TCRBV gene transduction into primary naive T cells

The plasmid vector pmax was utilized for making the construct containing GFP, cloned specific TCR genes, or vehicle. T cell transfection kit (Nucleofector™, Amaxa, Cologne, Germany) and a Nucleofector™ device (Amaxa) were used according to the manufacturer's instructions. Prior to electroporation, all lymphocytes including T cells were usually stimulated with anti-CD3 (2ug/ml) and CD28 MoAb (1ug/ml) for 5 days in GT-T503 medium and collected for the gene transduction procedure. The expression of TCR protein was analyzed on a flow cytometer using anti-TCRBV9 and BV28 (in MART-1) or anti-TCRBV12 (in gp100) MoAbs.

### 2.7 IFN-γ production by specific TCR gene-transduced naïve T cells

Two days after electroporation, naïve T cells transduced with mock, GFP, or a specific TCR gene were harvested and incubated with melanoma peptide-pulsed T2 cells or TISI cells for 24 hours. The supernatant was collected and the IFN-γ level was measured using an ELISA kit specific for human IFN-γ.

## 3. Result

### 3.1 Tetramer⁺ CTL induction and expansion

After the expansion of melanoma peptide-specific CTLs, the frequency of MART-1 tetramer$^+$ CTLs increased to 46.5 % (mean of 4 cases) compared with before stimulation (less than 1%) (Table.2). The absolute No. of MART-1 tetramer$^+$ CTLs was shown to increase 187 to 619 fold (average 415 fold) after T2 stimulations compared to prior to the stimulation. Additionally, in case 3 and 5, gp100 A2 and MAGE1 A24 tetramer$^+$ CTLs were surprisingly expanded up to 1585 and 5068 fold, respectively.

| Case No. | Peptide | Total cell No. ($x10^7$) | | | tetramer (%) | | |
|---|---|---|---|---|---|---|---|
| | | Pre | 2DC | 2DC+2T2[a] | Pre | 2DC | 2DC+2T2[a] |
| 1 | MART1 (A2) | 2.4 | 2.5 | 2.0 | 0.14 (1) | 0.89 (66) | 31.7 (186) |
| 2 | MART1 (A2) | 2.0 | 3.6 | 3.9 | 0.35 (1) | 4.64 (24) | 78.8 (396) |
| 3 | MART1 (A2) | 2.0 | 2.2 | 4.8 | 0.12 (1) | 1.73 (19) | 40.5 (619) |
| 3[b] | gp100 (A2) | 2.0 | 9.3 | - | 0.13 (1) | 44.3 (1585) | - |
| 4 | MART1 (A2) | 2.0 | 1.4 | 0.62 | 0.02 (1) | 1.32 (46) | 35.0 (458) |
| 5 | MAGE1 (A24) | 2.0 | 12.3 | 21.8 | 0.04 (1) | 3.1 (477) | 18.6 (5068) |

Pre; before starting CTL induction, 2DC; after 2 rounds of peptide-pulsed DC stimulation, 2DC+2T2; after 2 rounds of peptide-pulsed T2 stimulation in addition to 2DC, N.D.; not detected, Each value shows the mean for 2 experiments. [a] In case5, T2-A24 cells treated with MAGE1 A24 peptide were used. [b] Expansion data from gp100 A2 peptide-stimulated CTLs. Values in the parenthesis show fold increase of tetramer$^+$ CTL No. compared with pre-stimulation.

Table 2. Analysis of peptide-specific CTL production from melanoma patients

### 3.2 CTL killing activity of expanded melanoma peptide-specific CTLs

Cultured CTLs from 4 melanoma cases showed strong killing activity against MART-1 peptide-pulsed T2 cells and the C32 melanoma cell line (HLA-A*0201$^+$, MART1$^+$) (Fig. 1A). In contrast, no significant killing activity was seen in RPMI7951 (HLA-A*0201$^+$, MART1$^-$) and NCC-KT (HLA-A*0201$^-$, MART1$^+$). The killing activity was shown to be HLA-A2 and antigen (MART-1)-specific. Meanwhile, MAGE-1 A24 peptide-CTLs induced from case 5 were also demonstrated to be HLA-A24 and MAGE-1 antigen-specific in killing against TISI and cancer cell lines (Fig. 1B).

### 3.3 Intracellular IFN-γ staining of expanded tetramer⁺ CTLs from melanoma patients

The frequency of both MART-1 tetramer and IFN-γ-positive CTLs in 4 melanoma cases after peptide-pulsed T2 stimulation was 7.6%, 34.2%, 25.4%, and 9.8%, respectively. The percentage of IFN-$\gamma^+$ out of all tetramer$^+$ cells was 23.9%, 43.4%, 62.7% and 27.9%. CTLs from case 2 and 3 were more efficient in IFN-γ production than those from the other two cases (Fig. 2). In the case of MAGE-1 A24 CTLs, 49% of tetramer$^+$ cells were shown to be IFN-γ producer.

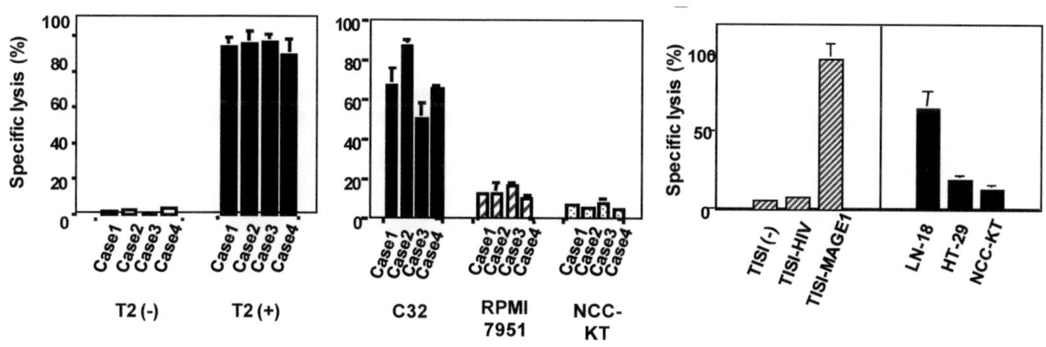


(A) (B)

Fig. 1. Cytotoxic activity of expanded melanoma peptide-specific CTL lines from melanoma patients. Target cells were labeled with fluorescence enhancing ligand and co-incubated with CTLs for 3 hrs. (A) MART1-specific CTL lines from 4 cases, T2 (-); untreated, T2 (+); treated with MART1 A2 peptide, melanoma cell lines (C32 : HLA-A*0201⁺, MART1⁺ ; RPMI7951 : HLA-A*0201⁺, MART1⁻ ; NCC-KT : HLA-A*0201⁻, MART1⁺). (B) MAGE1-specific CTL line from case 5, LN-18: HLA-A*2402⁺, MAGE1⁺ ; HT-29 : HLA-A*2402⁺, MAGE1⁻. Each column shows the mean ± S.D. for triplicate samples

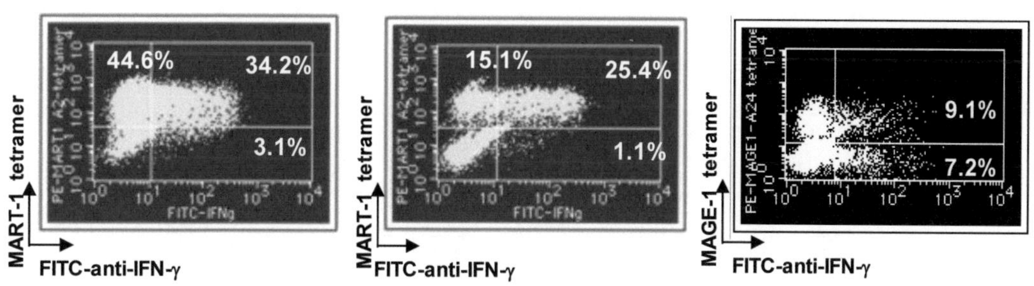


(A) (B) (C)

Fig. 2. IFN-γ production from melanoma peptide tetramer⁺ CTL lines stimulated with peptide-pulsed target cells. Each CTL line was stained first with MART-1 A2 or MAGE-1 A24 peptide tetramer and then intracellularly with anti-IFN-γ MoAb. (A) case 2, (B) case 3 and (C) case 5

### 3.4 TCR repertoire profiling in melanoma cases and its relation to cytotoxic activity

After the expansion there were 1 major and 3 minor populations with specific TCR repertoires among 78.8 % of MART-1 tetramer⁺ CTLs in case 2 (Table. 3). Case 3 had a major population in both MART-1 and gp100 A2 tetramer⁺ CTLs. In the case 5 of MAGE-1 A24 tetramer⁺ CTLs, 2 major populations were identified. Fig. 3 shows the association of IFN-γ production by peptide-stimulated CTLs (cytotoxic activity) with the specific TCR repertoire in cases 2 and 5. TCRBV9⁺ (MART1) CTL populations alone exhibited a specific killing activity in case 2 (Fig. 3A). TCRBV28⁺ (MART1) and BV12⁺ (gp100) in case 3, TCRBV4⁺ (MAGE1) in case 5 (Fig. 3B), were identified as IFN-γ producers. Those populations were specifically sorted (purity >98%) using the autoMACS system, and utilized for TCR gene cloning.

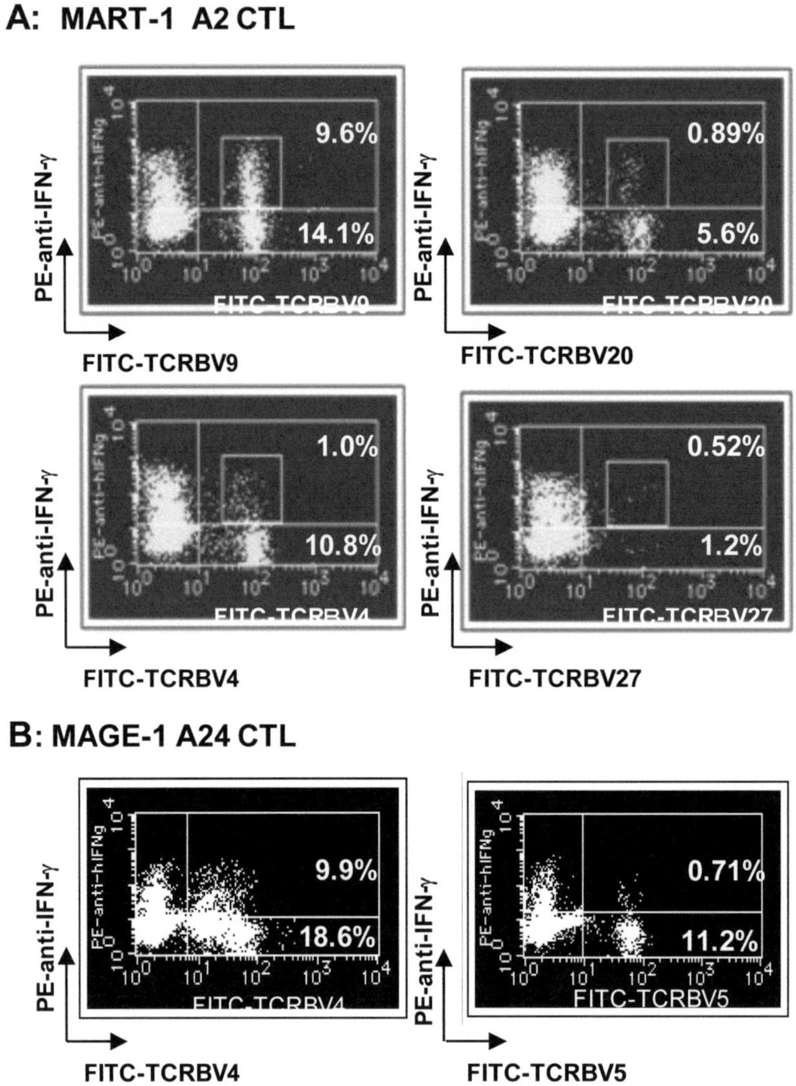


Fig. 3. IFN-γ production by CTL populations recognized by specific anti-TCR repertoire MoAb. (A) MART-1 A2 peptide-specific CTLs. MoAbs for TCRBV9, TCRBV20, TCRBV4 and TCRBV27 were used. (B) MAGE-1 A24 peptide-specific CTLs. MoAbs for TCRBV4 and TCRBV5 were used. Each CTL was stained first with anti-TCR repertoire MoAb and then intracellularly with anti-IFN-γ MoAb after target cell stimulation

### 3.5 IFN-γ production from peptide-specific CTL line sorted by TCR-specific MoAb

CTL lines sorted by FITC-labeled anti-TCRBV28, anti-TCRBV12 or anti-TCRBV4 MoAbs showed MRAT-1, gp100 and MAGE-1 peptide specific cytotoxic activity, respectively (Fig. 4). Gp100 A2-peptide specific CTL line exhibited the greater IFN-γ production than other peptide-specific lines after the various dose of peptide-pulsed target cell stimulation.

| Case No. | Peptide | Tetramer+ CTLs (%) | Repertoire | Frequency* (%) |
|---|---|---|---|---|
| 2 | MART1 | 78.8 | BV9 | 35.7 |
| | | | BV20 | 18.5 |
| | | | BV4 | 12.1 |
| | | | BV27 | 11.3 |
| 3 | MART1 | 40.5 | BV28 | 87.8 |
| 3 | gp100 | 44.3 | BV12 | 82.5 |
| 5 | MAGE1 | 18.4 | BV4 | 27.1 |
| | | | BV5 | 12.8 |

*Frequency ; percentage of tetramer+/specific TCR repertoire+ CTLs.
A TCR repertoire with a frequency of more than 10% was chosen.
Each value shows the mean for 2 experiments.

Table 3. Frequency of specific TCR repertoire+ CTLs from melanoma patients

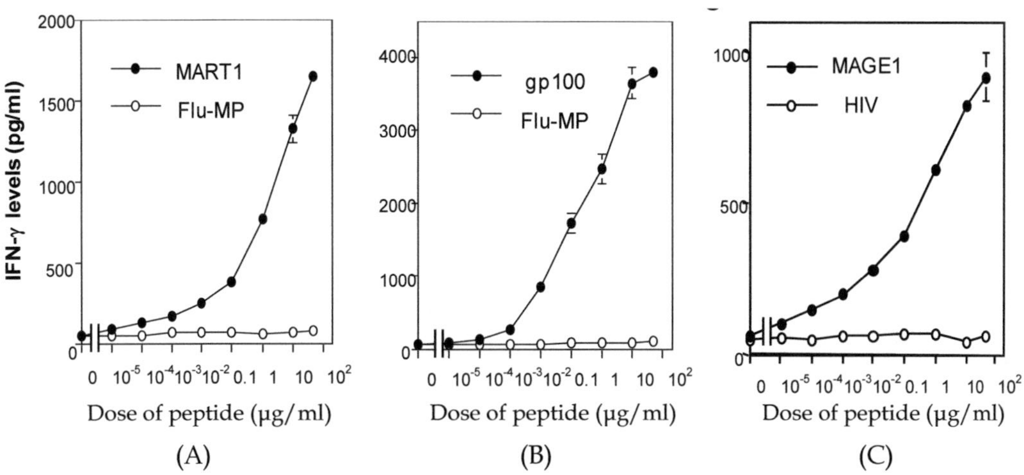


Fig. 4. Peptide dose-dependent IFN-γ productions from anti-TCR MoAb-sorted CTL lines. (A) Anti-TCRBV28 MoAb-sorted MART-1-specific CTL line, (B) anti-TCRBV12 MoAb-sorted gp100-specific CTL line, (C) anti-TCRBV4 MoAb-sorted MAGE-1-specific CTL line. These lines were stimulated with peptide-treated target cells. IFN-γ levels in the supernatant were measured using human IFN-γ-specific ELISA kit. Each point shows the mean ± S.D. of triplicate samples

### 3.6 TCR cDNA sequences in melanoma peptide-specific CTL lines

Cloned TCR cDNA sequences are shown in Fig. 5 (MART-1-specific sequence in case2, MART-1, gp100-specific sequence in case3 and MAGE1-specific sequence in case5). The TCR repertoire used was TCRBV9 in case 2, TCRBV28 and TCRBV12 in case 3, and TCRBV4 in case 5, respectively.

**Case2 MART-1 A2 CTL**

Repertoire TRBV9*01 N1 TRBD2*01 N2 P TRBJ2-7*01
Nucleotide tgtgccagcagcgtag ... gg ... gcgg ..... tc .. ag...ctcctacgagcagtacttc
Protein C A S S V G A V S S Y E Q Y F

**Case3 MART-1 A2 CTL**

Repertoire TRBV28*01 N1 TRBD1*01 N2 TRBJ1-5*01
Nucleotide tgtgccagcag....CC....cagggggc....ctgggc.....cagccccagcatttt
Protein C A S S P G G L G Q P Q H F

**Case3 gp100 A2 CTL**

Repertoire TRBV12-4*01 TRBD1*01 N2 TRBJ2-2*01
Nucleotide tgtgccagcagtttagc.....aggggg.....tt.....acaccggggagctgtttttt
Protein C A S S L A G G Y T G E L F F

**Case5 MAGE-1 A24 CTL**

Repertoire TRBV4-1*01 N1 P TRBD1*01 N2 P TRBJ1-1*01
Nucleotide tgcgccagcagccaag...tt ... cc ... gggacag....atg....a...tgaacactgaagctttcttt
Protein C A S S Q V P G Q M M N T E A F F

Fig. 5. Alignment of cloned TCR cDNA sequences from sorted CTL lines. Segments V, D, J and C were identified using a tool at the IMGT web site (JunctionAnalysis, http://imgt.cines.fr/)

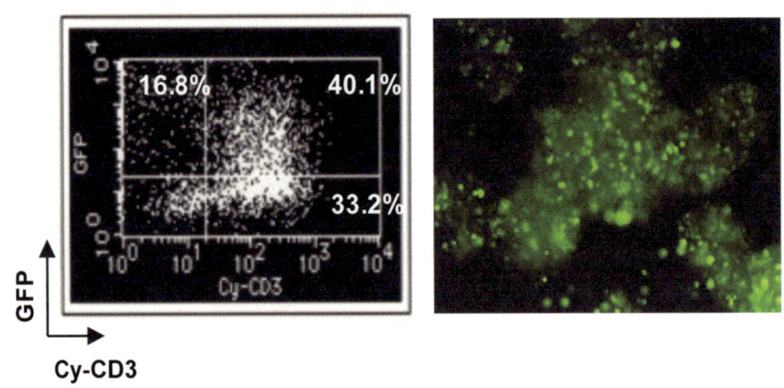


(A) (B)

Fig. 6. GFP gene transduction into melanoma patients' PBMCs using electroporation. After electroporation, cells were stained with anti-CD3 MoAb and analyzed on a flow cytometer. (A) Stimulated PBLs, (B) picture of PBLs expressing GFP. PBLs stimulated with anti-CD3 and anti-CD28 MoAb prior to electroporation

### 3.7 TCR cDNA transduction into primary naïve T cells in melanoma cases

The GFP cDNA transduction experiment after antibody-mediated T cell stimulation showed an improved transduction efficiency [unstimulated 25.9% (data not shown) vs stimulated 40.1%] (Fig. 6A). In the case of 4μg of the TCR cDNA for MART-1, gp100 and MAGE-1, the frequency of TCR-positive T Cells was 23.9% (MART-1, case2), 31.3% (MART-1, case3), 13.3% (gp100, case 3) and 32.4% (MAGE-1, case 5), respectively (data not shown).

### 3.8 IFN-γ production by TCR cDNA-transduced naïve T cells on peptide stimulation

PBMCs from melanoma patients were transduced with 4 μg of TCR cDNA (MART-1 in case2 and 3, gp100 in case3 and MAGE-1 in case 5) by electroporation and used for co-culture with peptide-pulsed target cells. PMBCs transduced with the MART-1-specific TCR cDNA (case 3) showed specific IFN-γ production against MART-1 peptide-pulsed T2 cells in a HLA and antigen-restricted manner (Fig. 7). Additionally, PBMCs transduced with another MART-1-specific (case 2), gp100-specific (case 3) and MAGE1-specific (case 5) TCR cDNAs also demonstrated moderate IFN-γ production against each of the peptide-pulsed target cells.

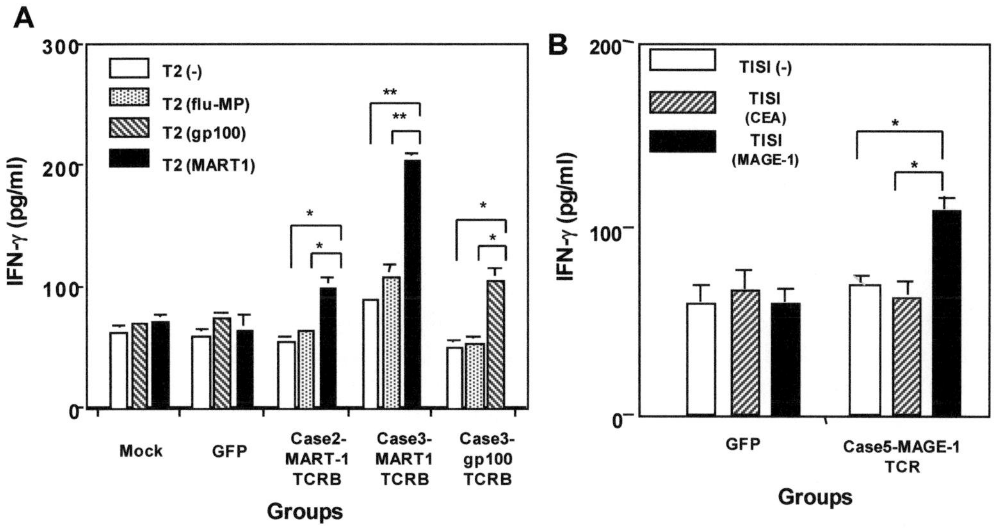


Fig. 7. IFN-γ production from specific TCR cDNA-transduced PBLs derived from a melanoma patient against target cells. Mock or TCR gene-transduced PBLs were co-incubated with peptide-treated target cells. (A) MART-1 or gp100 A2 peptide-specific CTLs from melanoma case 2 and 3. (B) MAGE-1 A24 peptide-specific CTL from melanoma case 5. The amount of IFN-γ produced in the supernatant was measured using an ELISA kit. T2 (-); untreated, T2 (peptide): treated with various peptides. Each column shows the mean ± S.D. for triplicate samples. * * ; $P< 0.01$, * ; $P<0.05$

## 4. Discussion

It is generally considered that spontaneously immunized CTL clones can be recognized at tumor sites or in peripheral blood without aggressive vaccinization, because melanomas are generally immunogenic tumors in terms of the immune response against antigens (Mandruzzato et al., 2002; Sensi et al., 1995). With regard to common melanoma antigens like MART-1, gp100, and tyrosinase and MAGEs, many heterogenous tumor-infiltrating lymphocytes (TILs) or blood CTLs specific to these peptides have been identified using clonal analysis and characterized specifically in terms of antigen avidity and cytotoxic activity against tumors (Valmori et al., 2000; Sensi et al., 1993; Yee et al., 1999; Hishii et al., 1997).

This time we characterized melanoma antigen-specific CTL lines derived from the blood of patients given DC vaccines and established an *ex vivo* expansion culture method. Finally, our group succeeded in cloning and sequencing melanoma peptide (MART-1, gp100, and MAGE-1)-specific TCR genes. Few clonal CTL analyses after the use of cancer vaccines including DCs and peptides have been performed so far (Valmori et al., 2002; Kan-Mitchell et al., 1993; Powell et al., 2006) Powell *et al.* demonstrated the efficacy of a multiple course peptide-immunization for the generation in high frequencies of tumor antigen-specific T cells, because they recognized vaccine-specific CTLs in blood even one year after the final vaccination (Powell et al., 2004). Additionally, Godelaine *et al.* reported that several potent CTL clones specific to MAGE3 A1 peptide were amplified after the use of a peptide-pulsed DC vaccine and the frequency of tetramer-positive CTLs in blood increased 20-400 fold compared with before the vaccination (Godelaine et al., 2003).

With regard to *ex vivo* CTL expansion, we established our own method to increase number of melanoma-peptide-specific blood CTLs from patients given a DC vaccine several times. Briefly, PBMCs obtained from melanoma patients were stimulated *in vitro* with patient-derived DCs pulsed with the same peptide as used in the DC vaccine, and furthermore activated with peptide-pulsed target cells like T2 and T2-A24. Finally, MART-1 and MAGE-1 tetramer-positive CTLs were able to be expanded up to 620 and 5070 fold, respectively in melanoma patients given the vaccine. In contrast, in the case of CTLs obtained from patients prior to the vaccination, the expansion was much less extensive. This observation demonstrated that utilizing PBMCs from vaccinated patients is a very efficient way of preparing numerous adoptive CTLs for clinical use. More importantly, MAGE-1 A24 peptide-specific CTL line was derived from a DC vaccinated-patient who showed a significant clinical response, and our group succeeded in cloning and sequencing of MAGE-1 A24 peptide-specific T cell receptor (TCR) cDNA for the first time.

Meanwhile, distinguishing these CTLs in terms of tumor-specific avidity and cytotoxicity is important. Generally, tetramer-positive CTLs have polyclonal effectors and the clone responsible for the genuine anti-tumor activity cannot be identified at the expansion stage. We utilized specific staining of CTLs with a combination of anti-TCR MoAb and intracellular IFN-γ staining. Using this method, the monoclonal TCR repertoire mediating the anti-tumor cytotoxicity could be elucidated. Furthermore, anti-TCR MoAb-sorted CTL clones were shown to have the very potent melanoma-peptide specific cytotoxic activity. Once the functional TCR repertoire is determined, a functional CTL clone can be purified by MoAb sorting, and finally specific DNA is cloned as we have performed. This might be a novel approach to determine the genuine clone responsible for peptide-specific cytotoxicity at the level of selection of polyclonal CTLs (Fig. 8).

Demonstrating the efficiency and capability of cancer-specific CTLs for clinical application is also important issue. Many studies of cytotoxicity or avidity for tumors comparing TILs with blood CTLs have been reported. Basically, TIL clones tend to be more cytotoxic and have greater affinity for tumor cells and a more limited TCR repertoire than blood CTLs. Cole *et al.* and others showed that the same TCR repertoire specific to MART-1 peptide was recognized among blood CTLs as TIL clones isolated from tumors, which supported the application of vaccine-boosted blood CTLs to adoptive immunotherapy (Cole et al., 1997). In the present study, TILs from melanoma tissue were not analyzed. In future, upcoming resected tumors will be used for TIL expansion according to other researchers' methods.

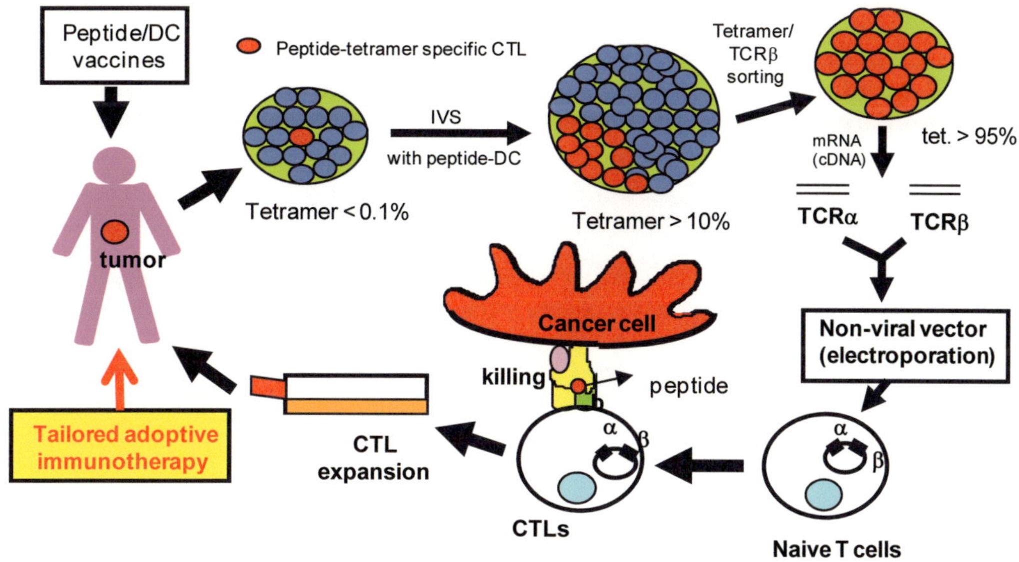


Fig. 8. Strategy for vaccinated patients-based immune-effector cell engineering for developing a novel adoptive CTL therapy

When considering the application of native adoptive CTL therapy, a great number of potent CTLs specific to cancer peptides are needed. The technology of TCR gene-engineering is possibly one efficient tool with which to expand necessary specific effector T cells. Recently, retroviral vector-mediated TCR gene transduction has been utilized in basic research and some clinical trials (Roszkowski et al., 2005; Hughes et al., 2005; Morgan et al., 2006; Tsuji et al., 2005). Recently, the use of a lentiviral vector system was shown to be the optimal way to transduce specific TCR genes into naïve T cells (Van Tendeloo et al., 2007). However, adverse effects such as leukemogenesis in stem cell-based retroriral gene transduction programs cannot be avoided completely. In the present study, a novel electroporation-based TCR gene transduction was performed and the transduction efficiency in naïve T cells derived from melanoma patients was acceptable (56% for GFP gene, 31% for MART-1 TCRBV28 gene, respectively). More importantly, anti-CD3 and anti-CD28 antibody-mediated T cell activation prior to electroporation is needed to reduce the damage to T cells and promote the transduction efficiency as previously reported (Chun et al., 2002).
DC vaccine-based efficient CTL expansion using blood CTLs from vaccinated melanoma patients, may be a good immunotherapeutic modality. This novel approach can be employed for adoptive CTL therapy followed by the use of peptide-cocktail pulsed DC vaccines and the administration of a T cell-supporting cytokine like IL-2, IL-7 or IL-15 to maintain and expand infused CTLs *in vivo*.

## 5. Conclusion

We characterized melanoma antigen-specific CTL lines derived from the blood of patients given DC vaccines and established an *ex vivo* expansion culture method. For functional analysis of CTLs, specific staining of CTLs with a combination of anti-TCR MoAb and intracellular IFN-γ staining was utilized, and monoclonal TCR repertoire mediating the anti-tumor cytotoxicity was able to be elucidated. Anti-TCR MoAb-sorted CTL clones were shown to exhibit the very potent melanoma-peptide specific cytotoxic activity. Finally, we succeeded in cloning and sequencing melanoma peptide (MART-1, gp100, and MAGE-1)-specific T cell receptor (TCR) genes. This might be a novel approach to determine the genuine clone responsible for peptide-specific cytotoxicity at the level of selection of polyclonal CTLs.

## 6. Acknowledgement

We thank Dr. Mochizuki for supplying several synthetic peptides, and Ms. Tai, Mrs. Maruyama and Kawaguchi for their excellent technical assistance. This work was supported by a grant from the cooperation of Innovative Technology and Advanced Research in Evolutional Area (CITY AREA) program from the Ministry of Education, Culture, Sports, Science and Technology.

## 7. References

Akiyama, Y.; Tanosaki, R.; Inoue, N.; Shimada, M.; Hotate, Y.; Yamamoto, A.; Yamazaki, N.; Kawashima, I.; Nukaya, I.; Takesako, K.; Maruyama, K.; Takaue, Y. & Yamaguchi, K. (2005). Clinical response in Japanese metastatic melanoma patients treated with peptide cocktail-pulsed dendritic cells. *J Transl Med* Vol.3, No.1, pp4, ISSN 1479-5876

Banchereau, J.; Palucka, AK.; Dhodapkar, M.; Burkeholder, S.; Taquet, N.; Rolland, A.; Taquet, S.; Coquery, S.; Wittkowski, KM.; Bhardwaj, N.; Pineiro, L.; Steinman, R. & Fay, J. (2001). Immune and clinical responses in patients with metastatic melanoma to $CD34^+$ progenitor-derived dendritic cell vaccine. *Cancer Res* Vol.61, No.17, pp6451-6458, ISSN 0008-5472

Chun, HJ.; Zheng, L.; Ahmad M.; Wang, J.; Speirs, CK.; Siegel, RM.; Dale, JK.; Puck, J.; Davis, J.; Hall, CG.; Skoda-Smith, S.; Atkinson, TP.; Straus, SE. & Lenardo, MJ. (2002) Pleiotropic defects in lymphocytes activation caused by caspase-8 mutations lead to human immunodeficiency. *Nature* Vol.419, No.6905, pp395-399, ISSN 0028-0836

Cole, DJ.; Wilson, MC.; Rivoltini, L.; Custer, M. & Nishimura, MI. (1997). T-cell receptor repertoire in matched MART-1 peptide-stimulated peripheral blood lymphocytes and tumor-infiltrating lymphocytes. *Cancer Res* Vol.57, No.23, pp5320-5327, ISSN 0008-5472

Dudley, ME.; Wunderlich, J.; Nishimura, MI.; Yu, D.; Yang, JC.; Topalian, SL.; Schwartzentruber, D.; Hwu, P.; Marincola, FM.; Sherry, R.; Leitman, SF. & Rosenberg, SA. (2001). Adoptive transfer of cloned melanoma-reactive T lymphocytes for the treatment of patients with metastatic melanoma. *J Immunother* Vol.24, No.4, pp363-373, ISSN 1524-9557

Dudley, ME.; Wunderlich, JR.; Robbins, PF.; Yang, JC.; Hwu, P.; Schwartzentruber, DJ.; Topalian, SL.; Sherry, R.; Restifo, NP.; Hubicki, AM.; Robinson, MR.; Raffeld, M.; Duray, P.; Seipp, CA.; Rogers-Freezer, L.; Morton, KE.; Mavroukakis, SA.; White, DE. & Rosenberg, SA. (2002). Cancer regression and autoimmunity in patients after clonal repopulation with antitumor lymphocytes. *Science* Vol.298, No.5594, pp850-854, ISSN 0036-8075

Dudley, ME.; Wunderlich, JR.; Yang, JC.; Sherry, RM.; Topalian, SL.; Restifo, NP.; Royal, RE,; Kammula, U.; White, DE.; Mavroukakis, SA.; Rogers, LJ.; Gracia, GJ.; Jones, SA.;

Jones, SA.; Mangiameli, DP.; Pelletier, MM.; Gea-Banacloche, J.; Robinson, MR.; Berman, DM.; Filie, AC.; Abati, A. & Rosenberg, SA. (2005). Adoptive cell transfer therapy following non-myeloablative but lymphodepleting chemotherapy for the treatment of patients with refractory metastatic melanoma. *J Clin Oncol* Vol.23, No.10, pp2346-2357, ISSN 0732-183X

Godelaine, D.; Carrasco, J.; Lucas, S.; Karanikas, V.; Schuler-Thurner, B.; Coulie, PG.; Schuler, G.; Boon, T. & Vanpel, A. (2003). Polyclonal CTL responses observed in melanoma patients vaccinated with dendritic cells pulsed with a MAGE-3.A1 peptide. *J Immunol* Vol.171, No.9, pp4893-4897, ISSN 0022-1767

Gohara, R.; Nakao, M.; Ogata, Y.; Isomoto, H.; Oizumi, K. and Itoh, K. (1997). Histocompatibility leukocyte antigen-A2402-restricted cytotoxic T lymphocytes recognizing adenocarcinoma in tumor-infiltrating lymphocytes of patients with colon cancer. *Jpn J Cancer Res* Vol.88, No.2, pp198-204, ISSN 0910-5050

Hishii, M.; Andrews, D.; Boyle, LA.; Wong, JT.; Pandolfi, F.; Van Den Elsen, P. & Kurnick, JT. (1997). *In vivo* accumulation of the same anti-melanoma T cell clone in two different metastatic sites. *Proc Natl Acad Sci USA* Vol.94, No.4, pp1378-1383, ISSN 0027-8424

Hoshino, T.; Seki, N.; Kikuchi, M.; Kuramoto, T.; Iwamoto, O.; Kodama, I.; Koufuji, K.; Takeda, J. & Itoh, K. (1997). HLA class-I-restricted and tumor-specific CTL in tumor-infiltrating lymphocytes of patients with gastric cancer. *Int J Cancer* Vol.70, No.6, pp631-638, ISSN 0020-7136

Hughes, MS.; Yu, YYL.; Dudley, ME.; Zheng, Z.; Robbins, PF.; Li, Y.; Wunderlich, J,; Hawley, RG.; Moayeri, M.; Rosenberg, SA. & Morgan, RA. (2005) Transfer of a TCR gene derived from a patient with a marked antitumor response conveys highly active T-cell effector functions. *Hum Gene Ther* Vol.16, No.4, pp457-472, ISSN 1043-0342

Kan-Mitchell, J.; Huang, XQ.; Steinman, L.; Oksenberg, JR.; Harel, W.; Parker, JW.; Goedegebuure, PS.; Darrow, TL. & Mitchell, MS. (1993) Clonal analysis of in vivo activated $CD8^+$ cytotoxic T lymphocytes from a melanoma patient responsive to active specific immunotherapy. *Cancer Immunol Immunother* Vol.37, No.1, pp15-25, ISSN 0340-7004

Mandruzzato, S.; Rossi, E.; Bernardi, F.; Tosello, V.; Macino, B.; Basso, G.; Chiarion-Sileni, V.; Rossi, CR.; Montesco, C. & Zanovello, P. (2002). Large and dissimilar repertoire of Melan-A/MART-1-specific CTL in metastatic lesions and blood of a melanoma patient. *J Immunol* Vol.169, No.7, pp4017-4024, ISSN 0022-1767

Morgan, RA.; Dudley, ME.; Wunderlich, JR.; Hughes, MS.; Yang, JC.; Sherry, RM.; Royal, RE.; Topalian, SL.; Kammula, US.; Restifo, NP.; Zheng, Z.; Nahvi, A.; de Vries, CR.; Roger-Freezer, LJ.; Mavroukakis, SA. & Rosenberg, SA. (2006). Cancer regression in patients after transfer of genetically engineered lymphocytes. *Science* Vol.314, No.5796, pp126-129, ISSN 0036-8075

Nestle, FO.; Alijagic, S.; Gilliet, M.; Sun, Y.; Grabbe, S.; Dummer, R.; Burg, G. & Schadendorf, D. (1998). Vaccination of melanoma patients with peptide- or tumor lysate-pulsed dendritic cells. *Nat Med* Vol.4, No.3, pp328-332, ISSN 1078-8956

Powell, Jr. DJ. & Rosenberg, SA. (2004). Phenotypic and functional maturation of tumor antigen-reactive $CD8^+$ T lymphocytes in patients undergoing multiple course peptide vaccination. *J Immunother* Vol.27, No.1, pp36-47, ISSN 1524-9557

Powell, Jr. DJ.; Dudley, ME.; Hogan, KA.; Wunderlich, JR. & Rosenberg, SA. (2006) Adoptive transfer of vaccine-induced peripheral blood mononuclear cells to patients with metastatic melanoma following lymphodepletion. *J Immunol* Vol.177, No.9, pp6527-6539, ISSN 0022-1767

Renkvist, N.; Castelli, C.; Robbins, PF. & Parmiani, G. (2001). A listing of human tumor antigens recognized by T cells. *Cancer Immunol Immunother* Vol.50, No.1, pp3-15, ISSN 0340-7004

Roszkowski, JJ.; Lyons, GE.; Kast, WM.; Yee, C.; Van Besien, K. & Nishimura, MI. (2005). Simultaneous generation of $CD8^+$ and $CD4^+$ melanoma-reactive T cells by retroviral-mediated transfer of a single T-cell receptor. *Cancer Res* Vol.65, No.4, pp1570-1576, ISSN 0008-5472

Sensi, M.; Salvi, S.; Castelli, C.; Maccalli, C.; Mazzocchi, A.; Mortarini, R.; Nicolini, G.; Herlyn, M.; Parmiani, G. & Anichini, A. (1993). T cell receptor (TCR) structure of autologous melanoma-reactive cytotoxic T lymphocyte (CTL) clone:tumor-infiltrating lymphocytes overexpress in vivo the TCR beta chain sequence used by an HLA-A2-restricted and melanocyte-lineage-specific CTL clone. *J Exp Med* Vol.178, No.4, pp1231-1246, ISSN 0022-1007

Sensi, M.; Traversari, C.; Radrizzani, M.; Salvi, S.; Maccalli, C.; Mortarini, R.; Rivoltini, L.; Farina, C.; Nicolini, G.; Wolfel, T.; Brichard, V.; Boon, T.; Bordignon, C.; Anichini, A. & Parmiani, G. (1995). Cytotoxic T-lymphocyte clones from different patients display limited T-cell-receptor variable-region gene usage in HLA-A2-restricted recognition of the melanoma antigen Melan-A/MART-1. *Proc Natl Acad Sci USA* Vol.92, No.12, pp5674-5678, ISSN 0027-8424

Tsuji, T.; Yasukawa, M.; Matsuzaki, J.; Ohkuri, T.; Chamoto, K.; Wakita, D.; Azuma, T.; Niiya, H.; Miyoshi, H.; Kuzushima, K.; Oka, Y.; Sugiyama, H.; Ikeda, H. & Nishimura, T. (2005) Generation of tumor-specific, HLA class I-restricted human Th1 and Tc1 cells by cell engineering with tumor peptide-specific T-cell receptor genes. *Blood* Vol.106, No.2, pp470-476, ISSN 0006-4971

Valmori, D.; Dutoit, V.; Lienard, D.; Lejeune, F.; Speiser, D.; Rimoldi, D.; Cerundolo, V.; Dietrich, PY.; Cerottini, JC. & Romero, P. (2000). Tetramer-guided analysis of TCR β-chain usage reveals a large repertoire of Melan-A-specific $CD8^+$ T cells in melanoma patients. *J Immunol* Vol.165, No.1, pp533-538, ISSN 0022-1767

Valmori, D.; Dutoit, V.; Schnuriger, V.; Quiquerez AL.; Pittet, MJ.; Guillaume, P.; Rubio-Godoy, V.; Walker, PR.; Rimoldi, D.; Lienard, D.; Cerottini, JC.; Romero, P. & Dietrich, PY. (2002). Vaccination with a Melan-A peptide selects an oligoclonal T cell population with increased functional avidity and tumor reactivity. *J Immunol* Vol.168, No.8, pp4231-4240, ISSN 0022-1767

Van Tendeloo, V.; Willems, R.; Ponsaerts, P.; Lenjou, M.; Nijs, G.; Vanhove, M.; Muylaert, p.; Van Cauelaert, P.; Van Broeckhoven, C.; Van Bockstaele, DR. & Berneman, ZN. (2000). High-level transgene expression in primary human T lymphocytes and adult bone marrow $CD34^+$ cells via electroporation-mediated gene delivery. *Gene Ther* Vol.7, No.16, pp1431-1437, ISSN 0969-7128

Yee, C.; Savage, PA.; Lee, PP.; Davis, MM. & Greenberg, PD. (1999). Isolation of high avidity melanoma-reactive CTL from heterogeneous populations using peptide-MHC tetramers. *J Immunol* Vol.162, No.4, pp2227-2234, ISSN 0022-1767

Yee, C.; Thompson, JA.; Byrd, D.; Riddell, SR.; Roche, P.; Celis, E. & Greenberg, PD. (2002). Adoptive T cell therapy using antigen-specific $CD8^+$ T cell clones for the treatment of patients with metastatic melanoma: in vivo persistence, migration, and antitumor effect of transferred T cells. *Proc Natl Acad Sci USA* Vol.99, No.25, pp16168-16173, ISSN 0027-8424

# 24

# Quantitative Regulation of Melanoma Growth in the Host by Tumor-Specific Serpins in Blood Serum is a Main Reason for Inefficient Tumor Treatment

Donenko F. V.[1], Kiselevskii M.V.[1] and Efferth T.[2]
[1]N. N. Blokhin Russian Cancer Research Centre, Moscow,
[2]Department of Pharmaceutical Biology, Institute of Pharmacy and Biochemistry, University of Mainz,
[1]Russia
[2]Germany

## 1. Introduction

### 1.1 Estimation of efficiency of experimental chemotherapy

The analysis of the phenomena of experimental oncology should begin with an estimation of efficiency of chemotherapy (Goldin A et.al. 1983). All criteria allow the distinction into two groups. Either or not an increase of life span (ILS) of tumor-bearing animals can be reached after treatment. Cytostatic drugs destroy a part of the tumor and, as a result these mice live longer than mice without treatment. The conclusion from this observation is that it is necessary to kill as much tumor cells as possible. Another possibility is that cytostatic drugs lead to inhibition of tumor growth, but an increase of life span does not occur. This observation shows that life span of tumor-bearing animals does not only depend on the number of killed tumor cells. To elucidate the mechanism of this unexpected phenomenon, we performed the following experiment. C57Bl mice were transplanted with $6.1 \times 10^6$ of melanoma B16 cells into the right back hip. The animals were divided into three groups. The control group was left untreated. The second group received doxorubicin i.p. (7 mg/ kg of body weight) 24 hours after melanoma cell transplantation. Another group received doxorubicin i.p. (7 mg/ kg of body weight) 9 days after transplantation. Each group contained 10 mice. In figure 1 the average life spans of animals is shown. In the control group, the average life span was 41.7 ± 1.8 days. The average life span in the second group was 67.6 ± 1.5 days ($p<0.05$ vs control). The ILS of mice after treatment by doxorubicin was 62 %. The average life span of mice in the third group was 40.8 + 2.5 days ($p>0.5$ vs control). An inhibition of a tumor growth observed between day 12 and 19 was 100% (Fig. 2). (taken from own data).
It can be concluded that the best ILS tumor-bearing mice could be reached by treatment of animals with doxorubicin injected 24 hours after tumor transplantation. This result led us to the hypothesis that tumor cells have no time to establish in the host during the first 24 hours after transplantation. At this time, dependence between the number of killed tumor cells by

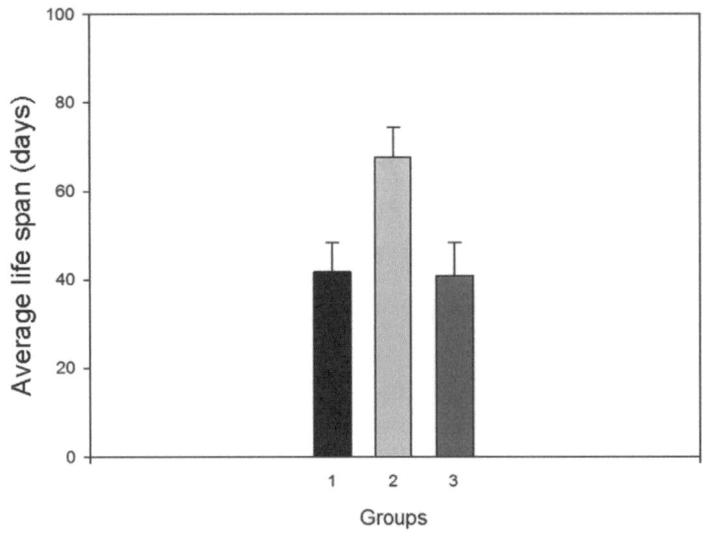


Fig. 1. Influence of the time interval between tumor transplantation and treatment with doxorubicin on average life span of B16 melanoma-bearing mice. 1. The control group was not treated with doxorubicin. 2. In the second group of animals which doxorubicin was injected 24 hours after tumor transplantation. 3. In the third group of animals, doxorubicin was injected 9 days after transplantation

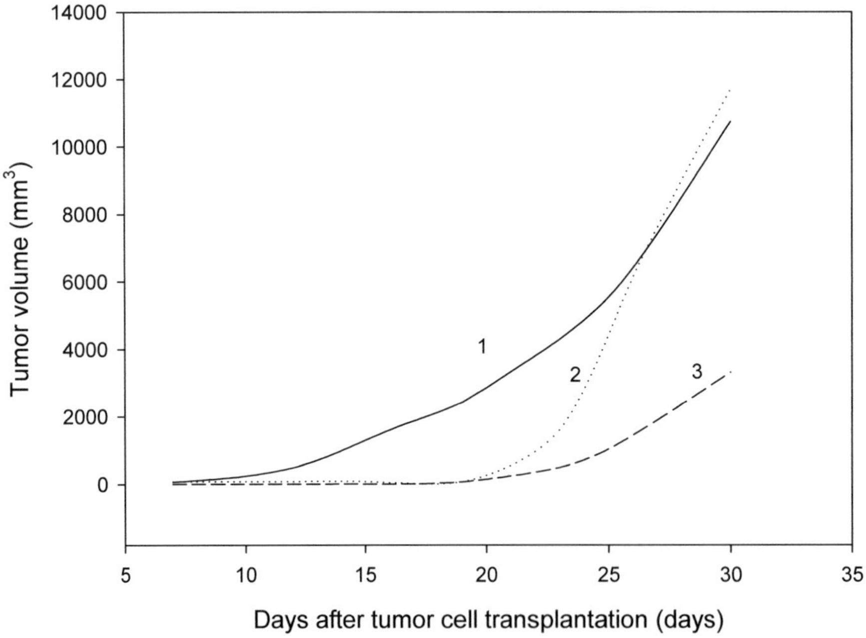


Fig. 2. Influence of the time interval between tumor transplantation and treatment by doxorubicin on tumor volume of B16 melanoma-bearing mice. Details see Figure 1. (taken from own data)

chemotherapy and ILS of animals was observed. Nine days after transplantation, tumor cells were integrated into the host. Then a molecular growth program for the tumor was set on. This program of tumor growth determines the life span of tumor-bearing animals. Therefore, a dependence between the number of killed tumor cells by chemotherapy and ILS of animals is not observed in advanced tumors.

### 1.2 Acceleration of tumor growth after removal of primary tumor

It is a well-known phenomenon that metastatic growth is boosted after removal of the primary tumor. We addressed the question, whether growth of metastases in mice with removed primary tumor really leads to a decrease of average life span. Therefore, we performed the following experiment. Mice with implanted B16 melanoma were used in the experiment. The conditions of tumor implantation are described above. All animals were divided into three groups. The first group contained control animals. In the second group, the tumor was removed 24 hours after injection of tumor cells. In the third group, the tumor was removed 9 days after implantation of the tumor. In figure 3, the results of the influence of removal of the primary tumor on average life span of mice are shown. The average life span of mice in the control group was 39.3 ± 2.4 days, in mice which received treatment 24 hours after tumor inoculation more than 70 days ($p<0.05$ vs control), and in mice where the tumors were removed 9 days later 38.3 ± 2.9 days ($p<0.5$ vs control). In the last group, in animals metastatic growth in lungs was observed. 1. After transplantation of tumor cells they were integrated into the host. 2. As a result of this integration, a program of tumor growth was activated in the host. 3. This program restored eliminated cells so that the average life span of animals did not change.

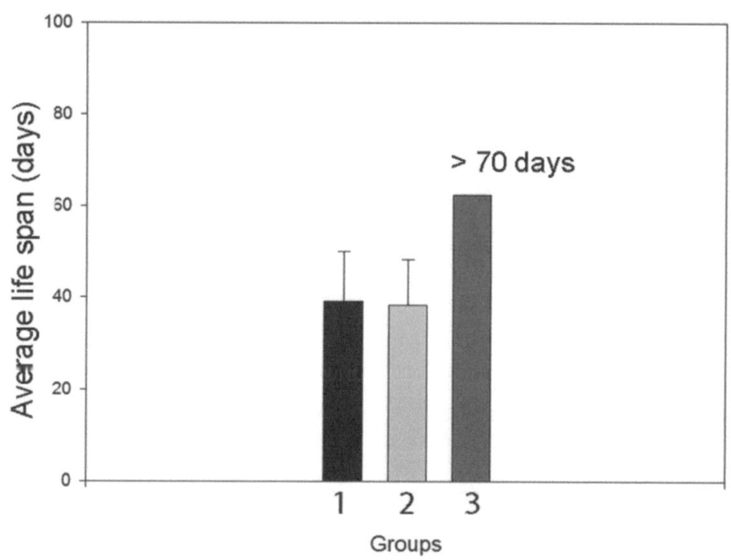


Fig. 3. Influence of the time interval passed between tumor transplantation and its removal on average life span of B16 melanoma-bearing mice. 1. Control group without tumor removal. 2. Group of animals where primary tumors were removed 9 days after transplantation of B16 melanoma cells. 3. Group of animals where primary tumors were removed 24 hours transplantation of B16 melanoma cells (taken from own data)

In the literature, this phenomenon is known as acceleration of tumor growth after removal of primary tumor. In contrast, our results did not show an acceleration of tumor growth. Animals with removed tumor died as rapid as control mice. After removal of the primary tumor the growth characteristics changed, and the tumor actively metastasized. From our point of view it is, therefore, correct to speak about a phenomenon of stability of tumor growth (Donenko et al., 1995).

### 1.3 Specific stimulation of metastatic growth

It is very easy to prove that this program of tumor growth in the host is tumor specific (Sitdikova et al., 2007). We performed the following experiment: C57Bl/6 mice or hybrids of first generation (F1) were used. B16 mouse melanoma cells were transplanted to one flank, and Ehrlich carcinoma cells were transplanted into the other side of the mice. B16 melanoma cells are black colored and it metastasizes after removal of primary tumor into the lung. Ehrlich carcinoma cells have a white color and metastasized after removal of primary tumor into the belly lymph nodes. When the melanoma was removed, melanoma-derived black metastases occured in the lung, while white metastases were not found in the belly lymph nodes. Removal of Ehrlich carcinoma was followed by the development of carcinoma-derived white metastases in the belly lymph nodes, but not of black metastases in the lung. Since melanoma and carcinoma cells were transplatend to the same mice, the constitution of growth factors, e.g. vascular endothelial growth factor (VEGF) etc. was identical. However, the response of B16 melanoma and Ehrlich carcinoma was specific. Therefore, we conclude that the mechanism which stimulated the restoration of tumor cells is specific.

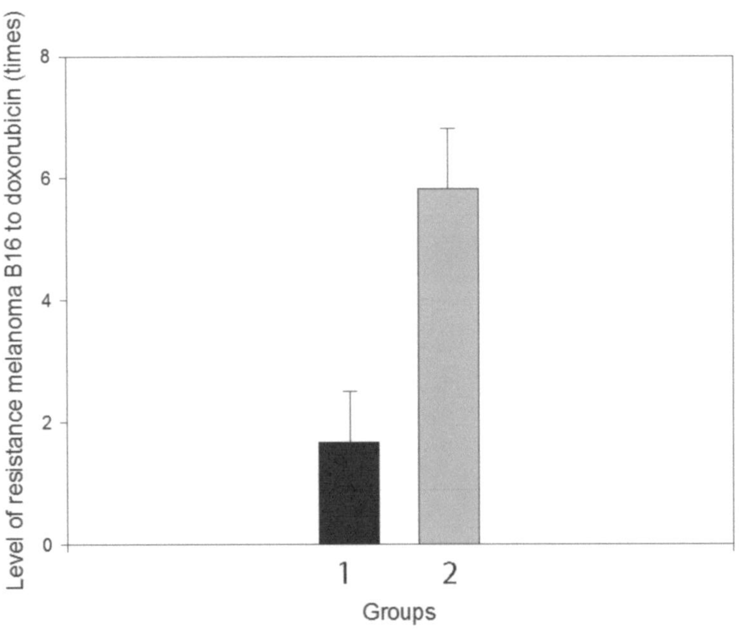


Fig. 4. Level of resistance of B16 melanoma cells towards doxorubicin after six tumor passages. 1. Doxorubicin was injected 24 hours after tumor transplantation. 2. Doxorubicin was injected 9 days after B16 melanoma transplantation to mice (taken from own data)

### 1.4 Induction of drug resistance by a tumor-specific mechanism

In another experiment, B16 melanoma-bearing C57Bl/6 mice received doxorubicin (5 mg/kg body weight). All animals were divided into two groups. In the first group, doxorubicin was injected 24 hours after tumor transplantation. After the tumors reached a volume of 1000 $mm^3$, the melanoma cells were transplanted to healthy mice. These mice received doxorubicin also 24 hours after tumor cell transplantation. Afterwards, the entire cycle was repeated. Animals of the second group were treated with doxorubicin 9 days after tumor cell inoculation. After the tumors reached a volume of 1000 $mm^3$, the melanoma cells were transplanted to healthy mice. These mice were injected with doxorubicin also 9 days after tumor transplantation. Subsequently, this cycle was repeated. The entire experiment was stopped, when the mice in the second group a reduction of tumor volume was not observed anymore after doxorubicin treatment. We concluded that resistance of melanoma cells to doxorubicin has developed (Donenko et al., 1991). The degree of resistance of B16 melanoma cells towards doxorubicin after six tumor passages was 1.7 (±0.5), if the drug was injected 24 hours after tumor transplantation. However, a significantly higher resistance (5.9 (±1.4)-fold, $p<0.05$) was observed after six passages, if doxorubicin was injected 9 days after tumor transplantation (Fig. 4).

We conclude that the mechanism restoring number of tumor cells after doxorubicin chemotherapy accelerated the selection of drug-resistant B16 melanoma cells (Sukhanov et al., 1991).

### 1.5 Influence of blood serum proteins of tumor-bearing mice on the growth rate of primary tumors

**Experiment**

Melanoma cells ($10^5$ cells) were injected into the right back leg of C57bl/6 mice. Then animals were divided into three groups. The first group of animals was the control group. The second group of animals received i.p. 0.4 ml of serum blood of healthy C57Bl/6 within one hour after tumor transplantation. The third group of animals were injected with 0.4 ml of B16 tumor-bearing of serum blood within one hour after tumor transplantation As shown in figure 5, acceleration of tumor growth was only observed in animals which received serum from tumor-bearing animals, but not in animals receiving serum of healthy animals or in control mice. Thus, we conclude that blood serum of tumor-bearing mice contains tumor-specific factors which accelerate tumor growth (Donenko et al., 1995; Donenko et al., 1997; Sitdikova et al., 2003).

### 1.6 Concomitant immunity after removal of primary tumors

This phenomenon has been described as resistance of animal to a second challenge tumor transplantation of the same tumor (Gorelik, 1983). It was found that this phenomenon is not restricted to tumors, but can also be observed with infective and parasitic diseases. This phenomenon is dependent on quantitative parameters of infections, parasitic diseases and tumor growth (Gorelik, 1983).

We performed the following experiment: Animals were divided into four groups. The first group consisted of healthy animals. Then, C57bl/6 mice were injected with three groups of B16 melanoma cells into the right back leg. Each mouse was inoculated with $10^6$ B16 melanoma cells. The second group of animals was the control group. Then, 9 days later $10^5$ melanoma cells were subcutaneously transplanted to two groups (group number 3 and 4) of

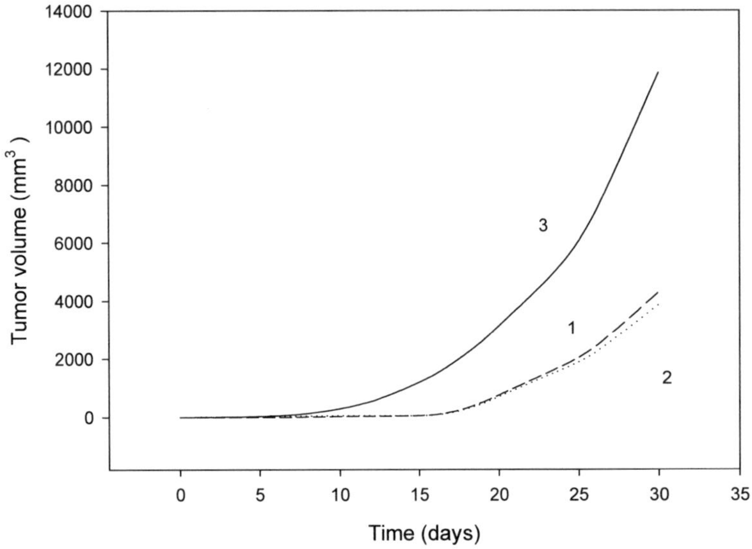


Fig. 5. Influence of serum blood proteins of tumor-bearing mice on growth of primary B16 melanoma. 1. Control group. Serum blood proteins were not injected into mice. 2. Group of mice which received serum blood proteins of healthy mice. 3. Group of mice which received serum blood proteins of B16 melanoma-bearing mice (taken from own data)

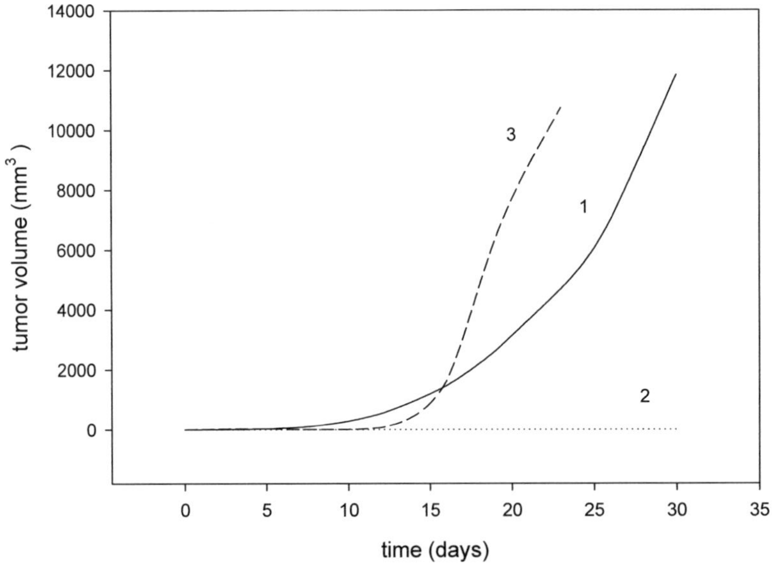


Fig. 6. Influence of concomitant immunity on growth of a second challenge with B16 melanoma transplant and subcutaneousB16 melanoma metastases after removal of the primary tumor. 1. Growth of a second challenge B16 melanoma transplant in healthy mice (group 1). 2. Growth of a second challenge in B16 melanoma-bearing mice with primary tumor or with removed primary tumor (groups 3 and 4). 3. Growth of subcutaneous metastases in mice with removed primary tumor (group 3) (taken from own data)

tumor-bearing mice and the group of healthy animals(second challenge tumor transplantat). At the same day, primary tumors were removed in mice of one of the two groups (group number 3). Figure 6 shows the results of a second challenge of tumor transplantation is shown. In the tumor-bearing animals of the third and fourth groups, the second challenges did not result in tumor growth (line 2). In the healthy animals of the first group, tumor growth was observed after a second challenge(line 1). For removal of primary tumors, the mice of the fourth group were fixed by means of clips. At the location, where the clips were fixed, we observed the growth of subcutaneous B16 melanoma metastases. Growth of these metastases is shown in line 3 of figure 6 (group 3). The growth of these metastases was faster in comparison with the growth of the second challenge. Furthermore, the growth of these metastases was associated with a damage of the hypodermic layers by the clips. It is an unexpected, but remarkable result that both the naturally occurring lung metastases and the artificial, clip-induced subcutaneous metastases were observed (group 3).
We conclude that tumor cells grow at strictly defined locations and with strictly defines speed. This phenomenon is associated with a still unknown mechanism. This mechanism determines location and growth rate of melanoma cells (Donenko et al., 1992).

## 2. Identification tumor-specific factors in blood serum

Previously, it was hypothesized that a growth-promoting factor is released by the primary tumor (Weiss, 1952). Attempts to identify this factor were unsuccessful during the past 50 years. The phenomenon of accelerated metastatic tumor growth after removal of the primary tumor represents a major reason for the relapse of the disease (Peeters et al., 2006). The mechanisms how the removal of the primary tumor influences metastatic growth are still not understood. By using six different tumor models, Fisher et al. hypothesized the existence of a growth-stimulating factor in the blood serum of animals after removal of the primary tumor ( Fisher et al., 1989).
Fisher at al. hypothesized that this growth factor is present in an inactive form and becomes active over time. An important fact for this hypothesis is that the maximal acceleration of metastatic growth was observed only within the first 24 h after removal of the primary tumor, a time period which is too short to affect neo-angiogenesis of tumors or to restore volume of the removed tumor. Rather than hypothesizing the release of a growth-promoting factor by the primary tumor as done by Fisher and co-workers, we assume that a growth-stimulating factor is constantly produced by the tumor-bearing host (see: Phenomenon of influence of proteins of serum blood of tumor-bearing mice on growth rate of primary tumor.). If this assumption is true, the removal of the primary tumor by surgery would then lead to an increase of its concentration in blood serum and to acceleration of metastatic growth. However, increasing concentrations of this factor in the serum activate a negative feedback loop resulting in a subsequent decrease of this factor in the serum and a retardation of metastatic growth. Hence, decreased proliferation of tumor cells within 24 h after removal of primary tumor might indicate the existence of a negative feedback loop. A balance between growth stimulation and retardation leads to a net increase metastatic growth (Donenko et al., 2009).
To prove our assumption, we have chosen Ehrlich ascitic carcinoma as test model And then to repeat the same effect on melanoma Cloudman S91. Ehrlich ascitic carcinoma cells have been removed together with ascitic fluid by means of a syringe. During this procedure, only the number of tumor cells in the tumor-bearing host changed. Other factors possibly influencing the biological effects of our procedure were excluded in this experimental

setting, i.e. anesthetics, surgical trauma, bleeding, change of concentration of tumor cell in the ascitic fluid, growth inhibition of the tumor by contact interaction, and the influence of tumor angiogenesis. All these factors might have stirred Fisher and co-workers investigating this phenomenon. Hence, the hypothesis is that a tumor-stimulating factor is produced by the tumor-bearing host itself. Only its continuing production by the host might accelerate the growth of the remaining tumor cells.

### 2.1 Tumor-specific factors in blood serum. How can they influence growth of a tumor?

The cell cycle analysis of ascitic fluids by flow cytometry was carried out seven days after inoculation of tumor cells. The initial percentage of proliferating cells in ascitic fluids was about 15 %. The removal of ascitic liquids caused an increase of proliferating cells to 30.8 % after 24h. This result is comparable with data of Fisher et al. After 48h, the percentage of proliferating cells decreased again to 16% and remained constant after 120h (17%) (Figure 7) (Donenko et al., 2009).

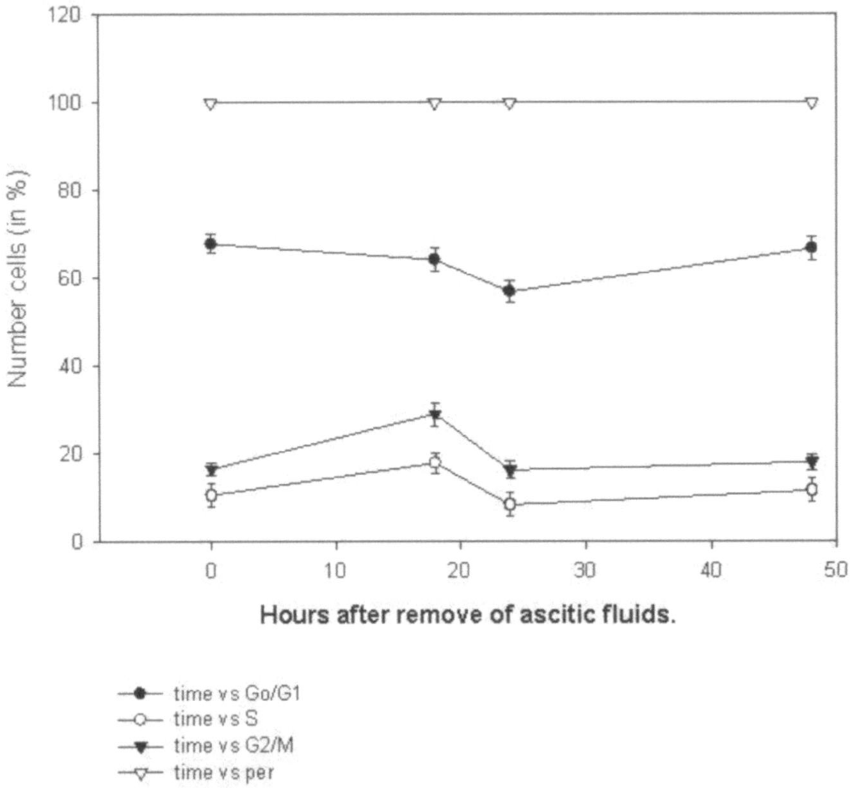


Fig. 7. Influence of removal ascitic fluids on distribution of Ehrlich carcinoma cells and peritoneal cells on cell cycle. —●— - Influence of removal ascitic fluids on distribution of Ehrlich carcinoma cells in the G0/G1 cell cycle phase. —○— - Influence of removal ascitic fluids on distribution of Ehrlich carcinoma cells in the S cell cycle phase. —▼— - Influence of ascitic fluid removal in distribution of Ehrlich carcinoma cells in the G2/M cell cycle phase. —▽— - Influence of ascitic fluid removal on distribution of peritoneal cells in G0/G1 cell cycle phase. X-axis, time (hours after remove ascitic fluids); Y-axis, number of cells (in %)

Representative histograms and gel electrophoreses of three independent experiments are shown (taken from Donenko et al., 2009 with permission).

By means of flow cytometry, it is possible to distinguish Ehrlich carcinoma cells from normal peritoneal cells. Peritoneal cells were completely in the G0/G1 phase (100%) (Figure 7). 1. Serum tumor-specific factor can increase or decrease tumor cells mitotic activity. A tumor-specific factor of the serum blood determines the mitotic index of tumor cells. It means that a serum tumor-specific factor is necessary for the entry of tumor cells into mitosis. Without such a serum tumor-specific factor the division of tumor cells is impossible. Phenomena like this have been previously described (Fisher B, et. al., 1989). For all these phenomena, an increase of life span after treatment of advanced B16 melanoma B16 was not observed. Hence, the phenomenon of stabile tumor growth can possibly explained by the regulation of mitotic tumor cell activity by a serum tumor-specific factor.

### 2.2 Negative feedback loop

It is important to note that our published experiments one the resistance of mice towards tumor transplantation have been successfully repeated by other scientists.

Decreased proliferation of tumor cells within 24h after removal of primary tumor might indicate the existence of a negative feedback loop. We hypothesized that removal of a primary tumor activates a growth-inhibitory process towards the remaining tumor cells in the tumor-bearing host. To prove this possibility, peripheral blood leukocytes (PBLC), spleen leukocytes (SLC), and PC were transferred from animals with removed ascites tumor into healthy animals together with Ehrlich tumor cells. A scheme of the experimental setting is shown in Figure 8.

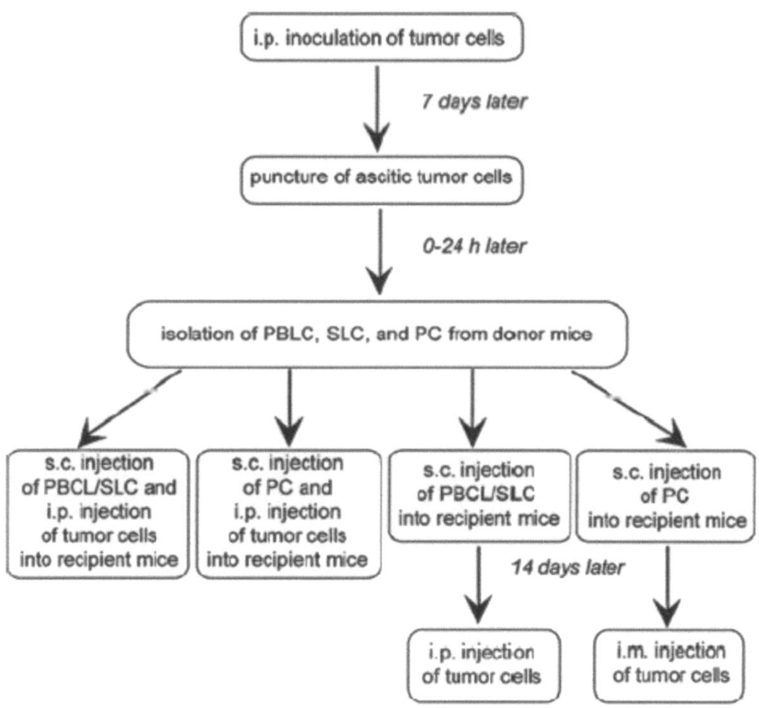


Fig. 8. Diagram of the experimental setting

| No. group | Time after tumor removal (hours) | Cell type | Resistance of mice (%) |
|---|---|---|---|
| 1. | 0 | SLC | 0 |
| 2. | 0 | PBLC | 0 |
| 3. | 0 | PC | 0 |
| 4. | 1 | SLC | 0 |
| 5. | 1 | PBLC | 0 |
| 6. | 1 | PC | 0 |
| 7. | 4 | Cells of spleen | 0 |
| 8. | 4 | SLC | 0 |
| 9. | 4 | PBLC | 0 |
| 10. | 5 | PC | 15.6 ± 2.8 |
| 11. | 5 | PBLC | 0 |
| 12. | 5 | PC | 12.5 ± 5.0 |
| 13 | 6 | SLC | 32.5 ± 5.0 |
| 14. | 6 | PBLC | 35.0 ± 5.7 |
| 15. | 6 | PC | 42.5 ± 3.1 |
| 16. | 8 | SLC | 47.5 ± 8.3 |
| 17. | 8 | PBLC | 27.5 ± 4.3 |
| 18. | 8 | PC | 28.1 ± 4.5 |
| 19. | 10 | SLC | 22.5 ± 5.0 |
| 20. | 10 | PBLC | 0 |
| 21. | 10 | PC | 0 |
| 22. | 12 | SLC | 0 |
| 23. | 12 | PBLC | 0 |
| 24. | 12 | PC | 0 |
| 25. | 24 | SLC | 0 |
| 26. | 24 | PBLC | 0 |
| 27. | 24 | PC | 0 |
| 28. | 48 | SLC | 0 |
| 29. | 48 | PBLC | 0 |
| 30. | 48 | PC | 0 |
| 31. | 120 | SLC | 0 |
| 32. | 120 | PBLC | 0 |
| 33. | 120 | PC | 0 |

Table 1. Time kinetics of donor cells to inhibit Ehrlich carcinoma cells in recipient mice after removal of Ehrlich carcinoma in donor mice. Tumor cells ($1\times10^6$ cells) were injected into mice together with peripheral blood leukocytes (PBLC), spleen leukocytes (SLC), or peritoneal cells (PC) ($3\times10^6$ cells). Ehrlich carcinoma cells were i.m. injected, if PC were co-applied. Ehrlich carcinoma cells were i.p. transplanted, if PBLC or SLC were co-applied (taken from Donenko et al., 2009 with permission)

| No. group | Time after tumor removal (hours) | Origin of cells | Resistance of mice (%) |
|---|---|---|---|
| 1. | 0 | SLC | 0 |
| 2. | 0 | PBLC | 0 |
| 3. | 0 | PC | 0 |
| 4. | 1 | SLC | 0 |
| 5. | 1 | PBLC | 0 |
| 6. | 1 | PC | 0 |
| 7. | 4 | SLC | 0 |
| 8. | 4 | PBLC | 0 |
| 9. | 4 | PC | 0 |
| 10. | 5 | SLC | 8.1 ± 4.5 |
| 11. | 5 | PBLC | 0 |
| 12. | 5 | PC | 86.7 ± 5.8 |
| 13 | 6 | SLC | 93.1 ± 5.7 |
| 14. | 6 | PBLC | 66.7 ± 5.8 |
| 15. | 6 | PC | 87.5 ± 5.0 |
| 16. | 8 | SLC | 98.5 ± 3.8 |
| 17. | 8 | PBLC | 58.0 ± 16.4 |
| 18. | 8 | PC | 82.5 ± 14.9 |
| 19. | 10 | SLC | 6.7 ± 5.8 |
| 20. | 10 | PBLC | 0 |
| 21. | 10 | PC | 0 |
| 22. | 12 | SLC | 0 |
| 23. | 12 | PBLC | 0 |
| 24. | 12 | PC | 0 |
| 25. | 24 | SLC | 0 |
| 26. | 24 | PBLC | 0 |
| 27. | 24 | PC | 0 |
| 28. | 48 | SLC | 0 |
| 29. | 48 | PBLC | 0 |
| 30. | 48 | PC | 0 |
| 31. | 120 | SLC | 0 |
| 32. | 120 | PBLC | 0 |
| 33. | 120 | PC | 0 |

Table 2. Time kinetics of donor cells to induce resistance towards Ehrlich carcinoma in untreated, healthy recipient mice after removal of Ehrlich carcinoma in donor mice. Peripheral blood leukocytes (PBLC), spleen leukocytes (SLC), or peritoneal cells (PC) ($3\times10^6$ cells) were subcutaneously injected. Ehrlich carcinoma cells were i.m. injected, if PC were co-applied. Ehrlich carcinoma cells were i.p. transplanted, if PBLC or SLC were co-applied. Then, 14 days after donor cell injection $1\times10^6$ carcinoma cells were applied (taken from Donenko et al., 2009 with permission)

PBLC, SLC, PC were taken at different time points after ascitic tumor removal (0 – 120 h). This procedure suppressed tumor growth in 20-40% of the recipient animals, if PBLC, SLC, or PC were taken only 6-8 h after tumor removal in the donor animals (Table 1). A follow-up of those mice, which showed resistance towards tumor development after injection of PBLC, SLC, or PC revealed that these mice maintained tumor resistance for at least four months, even if the number of transplanted tumor cells increased from $10^3$ to $40\times10^6$ cells. This follow-up experiment is still continuing to explore the long-term effect of this phenomenon.
To address the question, whether resistance towards tumor development is induced by the host or by the tumor cells, which where co-transplanted along with PBLC, SLC, or PC, we performed another set of experiments. PBLC, SLC, or PC were injected into mice, and Ehrlich tumor cells were inoculated 14 days later (see the scheme in Figure 8) (taken from Donenko et al., 2009 with permission).
The results in Table 2 demonstrated that tumor resistance occurred in the same time frame (6-8 h) and was more frequent than in the previous experiment (60-80% in Table 2 versus 20-40% in Table 1). This may be taken as a clue that the tumor-suppressive activity mediated by PBLC, SLC, or PC was induced by the host. Possibly, 6-8 h represents a necessary time frame for recovery of the animals from surgical interventions and also activation of defense phenomena as observed in our set of experiments.
We observed this phenomenon not only in Ehrlich carcinoma, but also in Cloudman S91 melanoma (Table 3). Recipient mice injected with PBCL, SLC, or PC from operated donor animals revealed less frequently tumors, if these cells have been taken 6-8 h after operation. The percentage of mice resistant towards tumor development could be increased, if these cells were injected repeatedly. Single injection of these cells resulted in a percentage of 20% mice with resistance towards melanoma development. Double transplantation increased the number of resistant mice up to 40-70 %, and after triple transplantation resistance was found in up to 100% of mice. These results strongly speak for tumor-suppressive effects conferred by the host organism.

### 2.3 Possible activation mechanism for the negative feedback loop

In Figure 9, the influence of removal of ascitic fluid on binding of FITC-labeled serum glycoproteins is shown in a time-dependent manner. Initially (0 h) the percentage of positive cells is zero or very low. One hour after removal of ascitic liquid the percentage of positive cells increased up to 6%, and after 7h up to 21%. A maximum of about 40% was reached 24 h after removal of the ascitic liquid. These data show that the changes in PBLC, SLC, and PC as well as in serum glycoprotein immunoreactivity occurred after 6-8 h and 18 h, respectively (Donenko et al., 2009). The chemical nature of this factor is unknown. We favor another explanation, which points to a factor initially produced by the host itself. This factor is absorbed by the tumor and is necessary for cell proliferation. After removal of the tumor, the concentration of this factor drastically increases. Then, the increased concentration of this factor in blood serum leads to a negative feedback loop resulting in a subsequent decrease of this factor in the serum. This poses the question, as to why such a hypothetical negative feedback loop is activated. A possible answer to this question is provided by our flow cytometry data. Using forward and sideward scattering, we observed a change in size of tumor cells after partial removal of the ascitic fluid. This change in tumor cell size might be associated with a change in the interaction of these cells with molecules in the ascitic fluid. This assumption is important to postulate a negative feedback loop. Ascitic fluids and blood contain many polar and hydrophobic molecules. These chemical groups are located on the surface of cells and biomacromolecules. A concentration change of these chemical groups might lead to the dissociation of these molecules from the surface or to the formation of molecule complexes. Complexes might be formed between biomacromolecules, between biomacromolecules and cells, and as conglomerates of cells. A formation of cell conglomerates may be dangerous for an organism, as it causes the development of the so-called "sludge" syndrome. For example, this syndrome occurs after dehydration of an organism or after sepsis. Dehydration causes an increase of the erythrocyte number in blood. As a result, erythrocytes form monetary column-formed structures (Hinshaw, 1996; Moore et al., 2003).

| No. group | Time after tumor removal (hours) | Cell type | Number injection of donor cells | Resistance of mice (%) |
|---|---|---|---|---|
| 1. | 6 | SLC | Single | 27.5 ± 4.9 |
| 2. | 6 | PBLC | Single | 12.5 ± 5.0 |
| 3. | 6 | PC | Single | 17.5 ± 5.0 |
| 4. | 6<br>7 | SLC + PBLC | Double | 40 ± 8.2 |
| 5. | 6<br>7 | PC + SLC | Double | 66.7 ± 5.8 |
| 6. | 6<br>7<br>8 | PBLC + PC + SLC | Triple | 86.7 ± 5.7 |
| 7. | 6 | PC | Triple | 98.5 ± 3.8 |
| 8. | 6 | PBLC | Triple | 82.5 ± 5.0 |
| 9 | 6 | SLC | Triple | 98.5 ± 3.8 |

Table 3. Influence of modes of application of donor cells on the growth of Cloudman S91 melanoma in mice. Peripheral blood leukocytes (PBLC), spleen leukocytes (SLC), or peritoneal cells (PC) ($3\times10^6$ cells) were subcutaneously injected. Single, double, or triple injections were performed. Fourteen days after donor cell injection, $1\times10^6$ Cloudman melanoma cells were subcutaneously applied (taken from Donenko et al., 2009 with permission)

Therefore, we studied the interaction of blood serum glycoproteins with peritoneal cells of mice. Our results indicate an increased binding of glycoproteins with peritoneal cells after removal of ascitic liquid. A formation of conglomerates of the remaining tumor cells in the ascitic fluid was observed after visual inspection. Hence, it is worth speculating that partial removal of ascitic fluid causes a condition in the remaining cells similar to the"sludge" syndrome. Such a condition might be dangerous to the tumor-bearing host and might possibly lead to a switch to compensatory mechanisms. As a result, the affinity of biomacromolecules to tumor and peritoneal cells might be changed. Affinity changes of proteins to cells can be measured as alterations in their glycosylation pattern. Indeed, we have shown that glycosylation of blood serum proteins changed within 6h after removal of ascitic fluid. It is reasonable to assume that lymphocytes can carry out protein glycosylation reactions by recognition and dissociation of formed complexes, which can then be released into biological fluids such as ascitic fluid (Sitdikova et al., 2005).

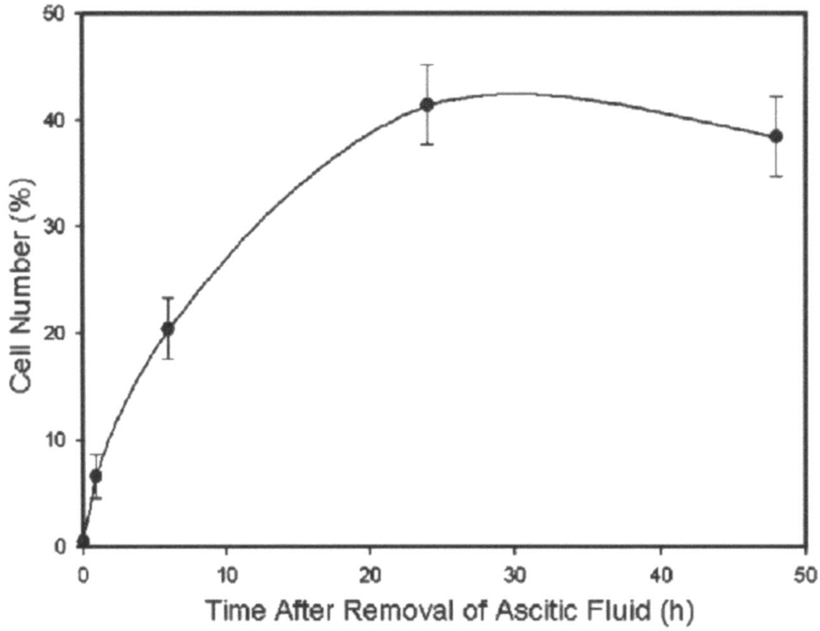


Fig. 9. Quantitative analysis of the time-dependent influence of removal of ascitic fluid on the binding of FITC-labeled serum glycoprotein's from ascitic Ehrlich carcinoma cell-bearing mice after removal of ascitic fluid injected with peritoneal cells received from i.m. transplanted Ehrlich carcinoma-bearing mice (taken from Donenko et al., 2009 with permission)

### 2.4 Identification of tumor-specific serum factors

We have received very interesting experimental model of development resistance of mice to the transplanted tumor. We have shown that increasing the levels of a hitherto uncharacterized factor induced a negative feedback mechanism, which inhibited the development of this factor by the host. This in turn led to inhibition of tumor growth as shown for Ehrlich carcinoma and Cloudman S-91 melanoma. This can be taken as a clue for the existence of an equilibrium between serum factors and target cells, which might influence each other. The infringement of such a balance resulted in the occurrence of new cellular properties, leading to resistance of mice towards tumor growth. These tumor-suppressing features became apparent upon transfer of blood serum from tumor-bearing mice to healthy mice inoculated with cancer cells. The aim of the next step of investigation was to identify tumor-specific serum factors of mice bearing Ehrlich carcinoma, which have the potential to confer resistance towards tumor development. For this purpose, we incubated isolated immune cells (peritoneal cells or spleen lymphocytes) from intact mice in vitro with blood serum or ascitic fluid from tumor-bearing mice. From our point of view during incubation immune cells from intact mice in serum of blood or in ascitic liquid of tumor-bearing animals in vitro system observes the same infringement of tumor-specific balance which is observed in vivo system in animals with the removed primary tumor. Immune cells which are received from intact mice should to react against a tumor-specific of balance of serum blood proteins or ascitic liquid. Time through which will develop this reaction it is known to us. It makes 7 hours. The experimental design is shown in Figure 10.

The results of the experiments are presented in Table 4. Mice inoculated with PC previously incubated for 7 h with ascitic fluid did not develop tumors at a frequency of 9 from 10 mice (inoculation of Ehrlich carcinoma cells after two weeks) or 100% (inoculation of Ehrlich carcinoma cells three months later). Inhibition of tumor growth was observed in mice injected both with PCs and SLCs 6 - 8 h after infringement of balance between the tumor and the tumor-bearing host. In the next step, the infringement of balance between tumor and host has been simulated in vitro by incubation of PCs and SLCs from mice without tumor with ascitic liquid or its fractions from tumor-bearing mice.

Table 4 shows the data of animals injected with PCs. However, SLCs possessed the same ability to induce resistance mice to tumor growth. Accordingly, it has previously been shown that tumor growth was not inhibited in mice which received PCs and SLCs 4 h after tumor removal. Therefore, the control group of animals received PCs 4 h after incubation with PCs and ascitic liquid or its fractions. This indicates that mice developed resistance towards tumor development. In resistant mice, after i.p. injection of $1\times10^6$ tumor cells per mice tumor growth was not detected at least for one year. By contrast, resistance towards tumor formation was not observed in the control group and life span of mice was not more than 20 days. To further analyze this phenomenon, we prepared different fractions of the ascitic fluid: fractions with proteins of >300 kDa (fraction 1), of 100-300 kDa (fraction 2), of 50-100 kDa (fraction 3), and of <50 kDa (fraction 4). Furthermore, two glycoprotein fractions were prepared, one with lower affinity than concavalin A, which were eluted by saccharose (fraction 5) and another with higher affinity than concavalin A, which was eluated by methylmannopyranoside (fraction 6). Corresponding controls were prepared for all six fractions. As shown in Table 4, fractions 1 and 2 weakly prevented tumor formation in mice. Only three out of 10 mice were resistance to tumor growth. This resistance towards tumor growth was short. At a repeated injection of ascitic cells three months later resulted in tumor growth in three hour of three all mice. The tumor growth rate in these mice was much less than in the control group. In control group, mice lived less than 20 days compared to two months in the experimental group. A strong prevention of tumor formation was obtained for fractions 3 and 5. Nine out of ten mice which received fraction 3 and seven from ten mice which received fraction 5 were resistant to tumor growth upon tumor cell inoculation two weeks after PCs. This resistance towards tumor growth was much longer. Repeated injections of ascitic cells three months later resulted in inhibited tumor growth in nine out of nine mice which received fractions 3 and six out of seven mice which received fraction 5. The best protection rate was measured using fraction 3. Resistance towards tumor formation was found in nine out of ten mice (two-week regimen) and nine out of nine mice (three-month regimen). Fractions 4 and 6 as well as all control fractions did not confer resistance on mice towards tumor development.

As a next step, we investigated the active fractions 1, 2, 3, and 5 by LC/MS, in order to identify their molecular constituents. 40 proteins were identified in the activated protein fractions from tumor-bearing mice. To determine, which of these differentially regulated serum proteins were functionally linked to resistance to tumor development, we incubated protein fraction 5 with PCs for 7 h, removed PCs by centrifugation, and subjected the fraction to LC/MS-MS. The comparison of the protein fraction before and after incubation showed that serpin ($\alpha$-1-antitrypsin) was absent from the PC-incubated fraction, indicating that this protein was bound to PCs and, thereby, purged from the protein fraction. This result obtained by LC/MS-MS was confirmed by gel electrophoresis and MALDI-TOF analyses. And at least one protein has appeared after 7 hours incubation PC-incubated fraction. As determined by mass spectrometry, this band represents cathepsin L1, with 93.9% intensity coverage (Donenko et al., 2010).

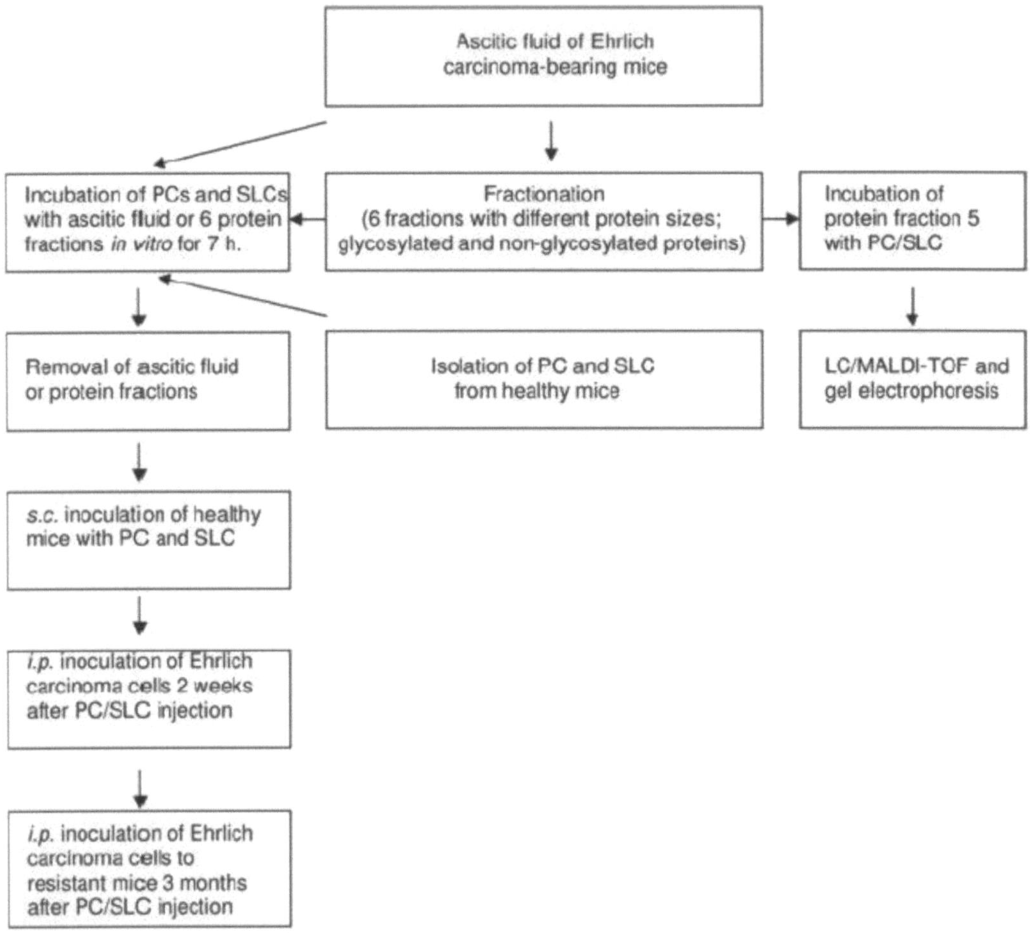


Fig. 10. Diagram of the experimental setting (taken from Donenko et al., 2010 with permission)

Peritoneal cells (PCs) ($3\times10^6$ cells) were treated in vitro with protein fractions from ascites of tumor-bearing mice and subcutaneously injected into healthy mice. Fourteen days after donor cell injection, $1\times10^6$ Ehrlich carcinoma cells were i. p. applied. Then, three months later mice which were resistant to tumor development after the first tumor cell injection (14 days) received another injection of the same type of tumor cells ($3\times10^6$ cells).

The proteomic analyses finally led to the identification of serpin ($\alpha$-1-antitrypsin) as candidate protein to explain the biological activity of fraction 5. We identified 40 different proteins, but only one protein of this fraction, serpin, disappeared in our experimental setting. Serpin is a major protein of blood serum with an amount of 200-400 mg in 100 ml blood serum. This indicates an eminent role of this protein in biological processes. The full exhaustion of serpin was accompanied by loss of tumor-specific activity of fraction 5. Absorption of serpin from fraction 5 by PC correlated with secretion of cathepsin L1.

Interestingly, it has previously been reported that squamous cell carcinoma antigen (SSCA), another serpin member inhibited cathepsin L (Takeda et al., 1995, Kato H, 1996.). It can, therefore, be speculated that the purging of serpin (α-1-antitrypsin) in our investigation might lead to a re-expression of cathepsin L1, which is otherwise repressed in the presence of serpin (α-1-antitrypsin).

| N | Fraction of ascitic fluid | Number of resistant mice compared to all mice 14 days after donor cells injection# | Number of resistant mice compared to all mice three months after donor cells injection |
|---|---|---|---|
| 1. | Ascitic fluids | 9/10 | 9/9 |
| | Control | 0/10 | 0/10 |
| 2. | Fraction 1: fraction of ascitic fluid with proteins of more than 300 kDa | 3/10 | 0/3# |
| | Control | 0/10 | 0/10 |
| 3. | Fraction 2: fraction of ascitic fluid with proteins in a range of 100 to 300 kDa | 3/10 | 0/3# |
| | Control | 0/10 | 0/10 |
| 4. | Fraction 3: fraction of ascitic fluid with proteins in a range of 50 to 100 kDa | 9/10 | 9/9 |
| | Control | 0/10 | 0/10 |
| 5. | Fraction 4: fraction of ascitic fluid with proteins of less than 50 kDa | 0/10 | |
| | Control | 0/10 | |
| 6. | Fraction 5: first fraction of ascitic fluid with glycoproteins in a range of 50 to 100 kDa | 7/10 | 6#/7 |
| | Control | 0/10 | 0/10 |
| 7. | Fraction 6: second fraction of ascitic fluid with glycoproteins in a range of 50 to 100 kDa | 0/10 | |
| | Control | 0/10 | |

Table 4. Influence of different protein fractions of ascitic fluid from tumor-bearing mice on peritoneal cells and spleen lymphocytes from healthy mice on induction of resistance towards Ehrlich carcinoma growth in healthy recipient mice. # Mice still alive after the first injection of ascitic cells were injected with tumor cells again three months later. Repeated tumor cell injection caused tumor growth. The tumors growth in early resistant mice was very slowly (about 30 – 60 days) and without development of ascitic fluid. In control groups, mice developed ascitic fluid and died within 20 days. (taken from Donenko et al., 2010 with permission).

### 2.5 (Patho)physiological processes of quantitative organ (tissue) regulation in the body

Not only tumor tissues, but all tissues of an organism may participate in the complex balance of biomacromolecules, an assumption which is supported by the literature. Removal of a kidney, a part of the liver, a salivary gland or a plaintive gland causes an increase in the proliferative activity of the remaining organ or gland ( Urie et al., 2007 ; Haxhija et al., 2007; Martin et al., 2008; Juno et al., 2002; Nelson et al., 2002; Vlastos et al., 2008; Aussilhou et al., 2008; Wilms et al., 2008). A factor appears in blood serum which enhances cell proliferation as early as 12 h after small bowel resection (Juno et al., 2003.). There are several indications in the literature that a serum factor causes an increase in vascular endothelial growth factor (VEGF) after organ resection (Parvadia et al., 2007; Schrijvers et al., 2005). This factor is not VEGF, since VEGF has no organ or tumor specificity. When mice are transplanted with two tumors of different colors, such as melanoma (black) and carcinoma (white), removal of the carcinoma is followed by the development of carcinoma-derived white metastases in the belly lymph nodes. When the melanoma is removed, melanoma derived black metastases occur in the lung. Hence, the proposed serum factor underlying this metastasis route may be revealed to have organ and tumor specificity (Sitdikova et al., 2007). The occurrence of lipomatosis after cosmetic surgery also supports our view of complex balances (Ginat et al., 2008; Puttarajappa et al., 2008; Jowett et al., 2008; Pandzic Jaksic V et al., 2008). Goshtasby et al described a case of isolated symmetrical lipomatosis of soft tissue overlying the trochanters that developed a recurrence after liposuction treatment (Goshtasby et al., 2006). Removal causes responses in the organism, such as increased cell proliferation in the remaining tissue. These data further strengthen the assumption that a balance exists between the biomacromolecules of tissues and glands from one side and the biomacromolecules of serum blood proteins from another side.

Another line of evidence comes from studies by Scheiffarth et al. (1967) and Warnatz et al. (1967). The authors showed that the spleen cells of a donor with chemically-induced hepatitis caused hepatitis in the recipient. The ability of donor lymphocytes to keep and transmit disease-mediating information about an illness is difficult to explain. However, taking our hypothesis into account, there are interesting parallels between both phenomena. Lymphocytes contribute to a healthy balance in the organism. In the above mentioned studies, lymphocytes were taken from an organism suffering from chemically-induced hepatitis. Therefore, donor lymphocytes from an unbalanced organism can transmit this information to the recipient organism, who subsequently also develops a diseased state. In the our present study, donor cells (PBLCs, SLCs or PCs) were obtained from mice with extracted tumors. We assumed that these mice had developed a condition inhibiting tumor growth, and therefore sought to identify the occurrence of a similar condition in the recipient mice. We found that the injection of PBLCs, SLCs or PCs from donor mice collected at a maximum of 6-8 h after tumor removal protected the recipient mice from tumor growth. Furthermore, this tumor-stimulating factor might be specific for each individual tumor. This specificity might be achieved by individual glycosylation patterns of blood serum.

Bearing in mind that inhibitors of proteases are frequently of low molecular weight (e.g. the pancreatic inhibitor of trypsin has a weight of only 6 kDa (Stryer L., 1981), it is noteworthy that serpin is an inhibitor of elastase in neutrophils and has a molecular weight of 45 kDa. Furthermore, serpin is a thermosensitive and glycosylated protein. It can be speculated that this protein may perform complex cellular functions, rather than non-specific enzyme inactivation. Concerning lability of protein activity, it has been reported that during isolation of serpin only 0.22% of the total serum protein fraction retained specific enzymatic activity (Mistry et al., 1991.). Serpins play a central role in the regulation of a wide variety of (patho)physiological processes, including coagulation, fibrinolysis, inflammation, development, tumor invasion, and apoptosis (Kummer et al., 2004; Law et al., 2006.).

Furthermore, serpins may protect parasites against the immune systems of the host (Yan et al., 2005). Taken together, it can be hypothesized that serpins represent a tissue- and tumor-specific anti-proteinase. The specificity of anti-proteinase activity is frequently determined by glycosylation (Lonberg-Holm et al., 1987; Silverman et al., 2004). Different glycosylation patterns of serpins might exert specific protection function in fatty tissue, muscular tissue, skin or other organs and tissues.

Thus, growth, development, and quantity of a tissue in an organism might not only be determined by growth factors, but also by a balance of protases and anti-proteases. Such proteases are produced by immune cells located in corresponding tissue or organs, while anti-proteases are produced in the liver. The fact that immune cells generate tissue-specific proteinases supports this hypothesis (Miller et al., 2002.). The phenomenon of regulation of different metabolic processes by specific proteases and antiproteases is well-known, e.g. for coagulation, fibrinolysis, kallikrein/kinin/kininogen system), but we hypothesize that this principle is even more global. The fact that serpins are ancient and well-conserved proteins throughout evolution may be taken as a clue for an ancient immune system, which controls the structure of organs and tissues. The question for the existence of such an ancient immune system arises. Previously, we have described the activity of a protease of Klebsiella pneumoniae (Trishin et al., 2004.). Surprisingly, this protease did not destroy secreted proteins from Klebsiella pneumoniae itself, whereas mammalian target proteins were effectively destroyed. This clearly indicates that microbial proteases can recognize and distinguish own and foreign proteins. This capability may be interpreted as an early step in the evolution of immunity. The quantitative regulation of a tissue in a host by serpins is determined by the suicide properties of this molecule, i.e. one molecule of serpin inactivates one molecule of proteinase in a stoichiometric manner. The production of cathepsin L1 in parallel to serpin activity allows us to assume that this proteinase may destroy other cells which are not subject to protection in this tissue or organ (homing effect and concomitant immunity phenomenon). The production of cathepsin L1 by PCs may contribute to Ehrlich carcinoma growth in mice. Possibly, cathepsins can cause protein receptors to be shed from a surface of tumor cells. As a result of removal (shedding) of these protein structures from the tumor cell, it cannot be fixed and grow in this tissue. Quantitative regulatory processes are characteristic not only for a tumor, but also for chronic infections and for parasites (Gorelik E, 1983). This explains the phenomenon of homing, where mislocated cells in a tissue or organ cannot exert their function or are destroyed. Growth factors do not possess such specificity. Examples illustrating this phenomenon are growth factors of blood vessels. Their activity increases after removal of healthy tissue, e.g. liver tissue, or a tumor. However, accelerated growth of blood vessels is observed only in the healthy removed tissue or in the removed tumor. Vessel sprouting in other tissues with other tissue-specific proteinases does not take place.

## 3. Hypothesis: Regulation of cellular physiological and patho-physiological homeostasis by proteinase-antiproteinase balance

The modern theory of immunity cannot explain many phenomena. One of the basic statements of immunity is that the immune system recognizes and distinguishes own from own antigens in another place. However, one striking example which is in contrast to this basic rule of immunity is "homing" effect, when own cells from one organ are stopped in another organ, although there are cells from the same orgamism. It is known that such «own» cells of an organism cannot further develop if thes are dislocated in the body. This phenomenon has been termed "homing" effect. The "homing" effect is the phenomenon when cells of a organism can develop only in the organ or tissue where they have been generated. We speculate that concomitant immunity is a special case of this "homing" effect. Concomitant immunity is the phenomenon, when "foreign" cells (either tumors, or microbial cells or even parasites) can develop only at that location, where they are fixed in an organism for the first time. Theviological relevance of this phenomenon is enormous. It is assumed that immunity develops by proteases-antiproteases balances at the place of penetration of fungi or other microbial parasites after 9-10 days. Then, the organism develops resistance to all subsequent attacks by these infective agents and prevent infections also at other locations of the host. A similar situation may exist in the case of tumor development. Such chronic conditions of disease (even helminthic invasion) have been described by Gorelik (1983). We point out that immunity does not necessity have to destroy all aliens in the body. If the infective agent does not lead to fatal consequences at the first attack, it may survive at the site of entry into the body. It may not distributed all over the body. This phenomenon has been termed microchimerism and describes the long-term existence of infective microorganisms in an organism (Kallenbach et al., 2011; Miech R.P., 2010). It is possible to explain this phenomenon by our hypothesis. The immune system of an organism does not try to destroy all foreign invaders (being either infective mnicroorganisms or cancer cells), but only recognize them at their site of initial location (homing effect).

The liver synthesizes different serpins with a molecular weight in the range from 45 up to 725 kDa. These serpins represent tissue-, tumor-, or microbial-specific anti-proteinases. The amount of specific serpins determines the quantity of the body`s own tissue or other foreign antigensin this organism. The amount tumor-specific serpins also determines the mitotic index and growth rate of a tumor in a host. For example, we showed that injection of hemoglobin containing complex of blood serum proteins isolated from tumor-bearing animals led to tumor regression. Some regimen of injection of these blood serum proteins decreased the growth rate of Ehrlich carcinoma for about three months. In the control group, the tumor-bearing mice did not live longer than 20 days. Slowly growing tumor cells were transplanted to healthy mice. These mice did not live longer than 20 days. Slowly growing tumor cells had mitotic indeces of 4- 5 % in comparison to 14-16 % in control mice. Blood serum proteins did not reveal cytotoxic activity in vitro. This example shows that the growth rate of a tumor was rather determined by host factors than by specific properties of tumor cells (Donenko et al., 2008).

The homing effect is provided by immune cells, which are associated with the location of infection or tumor development (organ-associated lymphocytes). As described above, these cells have a specific set proteinases in each organ (location) and synthesize specific cathepsins in response to absorption-specific serpins. All these proteinases only attack accessible surface receptors on the cell surface in this organ. Shedding of these receptors stops cellular metabolism and the mitotic cycle cannot be entered. Cells with the intact surface receptors can enter the mitotic cycle in this organ and constitute this organ.

This hypothesis postulates specific tumor-specific serum factors, which allow tumor cells to divide more quickly or more slowly. This hypothesis explains:

1. The mechanism of tumor relapse after drug treatment.
2. The phenomenon of concomitant immunity.
3. The increase of the mitotic index of tumor cells after treatment.
4. The quantitative and specific restoration of a tumor after treatment.
5. The quantitative and specific restoration of normal tissues in the host after treatment.

We envision that this hypothesis opens a new direction of treatment of oncological diseases.

## 4. Conclusion

For more than 30 years, immense efforts have been undertaken to improve cancer therapy. Still, the cure from their disease is not a common everyday reality for cancer patients. Hakomori described a unusual case of regression of a stomach cancer in a 66 years old women (Hakimori, 1986). After tumor regression, she lived further 22 years without any sign of disease. Hakomori allocated the following distinctive sign of the patient: her blood contained antibodies against all blood groups except her own. The tumor had foreign antigen determinants for the host. The patient experienced a hemotransfusion of 25 ml donor blood. The patient's reaction towards the hemotransfusion was very rough (hemolysis) (Hakomori, 1986). Researchers have established a foreign antigen on the surface of tumor cells and have generated an anticancer vaccine. However, these results could not be repeated. Subsequent vaccines on the basis of tumor-associated antigens were not that effective (Eggermont et al., 2009; Sitdikova et al., 2009).

However, this case shares many common signs with the phenomenon of cure of Ehrlich carcinoma-bearing mice described by us. Ehrlich carcinoma also has antigens foreign to the host. The treatment effect has been obtained after injection of hemolytic products into mice. On the other hand, vaccines generated on the basis of tumor-associated antigens also were not very effective. We assume that in both cases the cure effect was associated with the presence of hemolytic products and a tumor-specific infringement of balance of biomacromolecules. This infringed balance disturbed the synthesis of a tumor-specific factor of blood serum in the host. The absence such a tumor-specific serum factor in the tumor-bearing host led to full tumor regression. The experimental setting described here was repeated by other scientists. Remarkably, a similar tumor regression was also observed in their hands.

In summary, we conlude that it is necessary to block the synthesis tumor-specific factors (serpins) in the tumor-bearing host for a successful treatment of oncological diseases.

The first article about tumor-specific serum factors has been published by us only three years ago. Currently, we are generating mice resistant to the growth of B16 and Cloudman S91 melanoma by manipulating serum proteins. The potential of serpins for the improvement of cancer therapy merits further investigations in the future.

## 5. References

Goldin A, Kline I and Sofina ZP (eds.) (1980): Experimental Evaluation of Antitumor Drugs in the USA and USSR and Clinical Correlations. National Cancer Institute Monograph 55. NIH Publication no. 1933. U.S. Department of Health and Human Services. National Institutes of Health, NCI, Bethesda, Maryland.

Donenko FV, Moroz LV (1995). Phenomenon of tumor growth stability in the host's body. New approach to growth and treatment of tumors. Vestn Ross Akad Med Nauk. No. 4, pp. 14-16.

Sitdikova SM, Amandzholov BS, Kiselevskii MV, Donenko FV (2007). Specificity of relapses and metastases of experimental transplanted Ehrlich carcinoma and B16 melanoma. Bull Exp Biol Med. Vol.143, No.1, pp.80-82.

Sukhanov VA, D'iakov VL, Lalaev VV, Iakh'iaev AV, Voronkova IM, Donenko FV, Borovkova NB, Moroz LV. (1991). The expression of P-glycoprotein in leukemia P388 cells with induced doxorubicin resistance.Biull Eksp Biol Med. Vol.111, No. 3, pp.290-291.

Donenko FV, Moroz LV.(1995). Immunoglobulins from a tumor-bearing body as possible regulators of the growth rate of relapses and metastases of Ehrlich carcinoma. Biull Eksp Biol Med. Vol.119, No. 1, pp. 62-64.

Sitdikova SM, Amandzholov BS, Sel'chuk VY, Donenko FV. (2003). Tumor-specific changes in mouse serum during Ehrlich carcinoma growth.Bull Exp Biol Med. Vol.135, No. 6, pp.576-579.

Donenko FV, Sitdikova SM, Moroz LV. (1997). The role of serum humoral factors in metastasis and recurrence of Ehrlich carcinoma in mice.Biull Eksp Biol Med. Vol.124, No. 10, pp.443-445.

Donenko FV, Efferth T, Mattern J, Moroz LV, Volm M. (1991). Resistance to doxorubicin in tumor cells in vitro and in vivo after pretreatment with verapamil. Chemotherapy. Vol. 37, No. 1, pp. 57-61.

Gorelik E (1983). Concomitant tumor immunity and the resistance to a second tumor challenge. Adv Cancer Res Vol. 39, pp. 71-120.

Donenko FV, Sitdikova SM, Kabieva AO, Moroz LV. (1992). The characteristics of Ehrlich carcinoma recurrence and metastasis. Biull Eksp Biol Med. Vol.114, No. 12, pp. 652-654.

Weiss P (1952). Self-regulation of organ growth by its own products. Science Vol.114, p. 487.

Peeters CF, de Waal RM, Wobbes T, Westphal JR and Ruers TJ. (2006). Outgrowth of human liver metastases after resection of the primary colorectal tumor: a shift in the balance between apoptosis and proliferation Int J Cancer Vol. 119, pp. 1249-1253.

Fisher B, Gunduz N, Coyle J, Rudock C and Saffer E. Presence of a growth-stimulating factor in serum following primary tumor removal in mice. Cancer Res Vol. 49, pp. 1996-2001.

Donenko FV, Sitdikova SM, Syrtsev AV, Gradyushko AT, Kiselevsky MV, Serebryakova MV, and Efferth T. (2008).

Hemoglobin-associated proteins isolated from blood serum of Ehrlich carcinoma-bearing mice. Int J Oncol,Vol. 32, pp. 885-893.

Donenko FV, Ziganshin RK, Sitdikova SM, Amandzholov BS, Kiselevskii MV and Efferth T. (2009). Induction of resistance towards murine tumor development is associated with alterations in glycosylation of blood serum proteins. Mol. Med. Reports Vol. 2, pp. 487- 495.

Sitdikova SM, Amandzholov BS, Kiselevskii MV, Donenko FV. (2005). Lectin binding to mouse blood lymphocytes during tumor growth. Bull Exp Biol Med. Vol.140, No. 4, pp.445-448.

Donenko FV, Ziganshin RK, Anisimova N. Yu., Voyushin K.E., Sitdikova SM, Amandzholov BS, Kiselevskii MV and Efferth T. (2010). Identification of serpins ($\alpha$-1-antitrypsin) as serum growth inhibitory factor in murine Ehrlich carcinoma by proteomics. Cancer Genomics and Proteomics, Vol. 7, pp.147-156.

Hinshaw L.B. (1996). Sepsis/septic shock: participation of the microcirculation: an abbreviated review. Crit Care Med Vol. 24, pp.1072-1078.

Moore K, Thompson C and Trainer P. (2003). Disorders of water balance. Clin Med Vol. 3, pp. 28-33.

Takeda A, Yamamoto T, Nakamura Y, Takahashi T and Hibino T. (1995). Squamous cell carcinoma antigen is a potent inhibitor of cysteine proteinase cathepsin L. FEBS Lett Vol. 359, pp. 78-80.

Kato H. (1996). Expression and function of squamous cell carcinoma antigen. Anticancer Res Vol.16, pp. 2149-2153.

Urie BK, Tillson DM, Smith CM, Brawner WR, Almond GT, Beard DM, Lenz SD and Lothrop CD Jr. (2007). Evaluation of clinical status, renal function, and hematopoietic variables after unilateral nephrectomy in canine kidney donors. J Am Vet Med Assoc Vol. 230, pp. 1653-1656.

Haxhija EQ, Yang H, Spencer AU, Sun X and Teitelbaum DH (2007). Intestinal epithelial cell proliferation is dependent on the site of massive small bowel resection. Pediatr Surg Int Vol. 23, pp. 379-390.

Martin CA, Bernabe KQ, Taylor JA, Nair R, Paul RJ, Guo J, Erwin CR and Warner BW. (2008). Resection-induced intestinal adaptation and the role of enteric smooth muscle. J Pediatr Surg Vol. 43, pp. 1011-1017.

Juno RJ, Williams JL, Knott AW, Erwin CR, O'Brien DP and Warner BW. (2002). A serum factor after intestinal resection stimulates epidermal growth factor receptor signaling and proliferation in intestinal epithelial cells. Surgery Vol. 132, pp. 377-383.

Nelson LA, O'Brien DP, Kemp CJ, Williams JL, Dunke-Jacobs E, Erwin CR and Warner BW. (2002). Intestinal and hepatic response to combined partial hepatectomy and small bowel resection in mice. Am J Surg Vol. 183, pp. 435-440.

Vlastos IM, Parpounas K, Economides J, Helmis G, Koudoumnakis E and Houlakis M. (2008). Tonsillectomy versus tonsillotomy performed with scissors in children with tonsillar hypertrophy. Int J Pediatr Otorhinolaryngol Vol. 72, pp. 857-863.

Aussilhou B, Lesurtel M, Sauvanet A, Farges O, Dokmak S, Goasguen N, Sibert A, Vilgrain V and Belghiti J. (2008). Right portal vein ligation is as efficient as portal vein embolization to induce hypertrophy of the left liver remnant. J Gastrointest Surg Vol. 12, pp. 297-303.

Wilms C, Mueller L, Lenk C, Wittkugel O, Helmke K, Krupski-Berdien G, Rogiers X and Broering DC. (2008). Comparative study of portal vein embolization versus portal vein ligation for induction of hypertrophy of the future liver remnant using a mini-pig model. Ann Surg Vol. 247, pp. 825-834.

Juno RJ, Knott AW, Erwin CR and Warner BW. (2003). A serum factor(s) after small bowel resection induces intestinal epithelial cell proliferation: effects of timing, site, and extent of resection. J Pediatr Surg Vol. 38, pp. 868-874.

Ginat DT, Bhatt S and Dogra VS. (2008). Replacement lipomatosis of the kidney: sonographic features. J Ultrasound Med Vol. 27, pp.1393-1395.

Puttarajappa C and Dhoble A. (2008). Mediastinal lipomatosis as a cause of low voltage complexes on electrocardiogram and widened mediastinum: A case report. Cases J 1, p. 171.

Jowett C, Mitra P, O'Donnell P and Singh DS. (2008). Synovial lipomatosis of hindfoot tendon sheaths: case reports and literature review. Foot Ankle Int Vol. 29, pp. 752-755.

Pandzic Jaksic V and Bozkov V. (2008). From ancient enigmas to novel paradigms: a depiction of multiple symmetric lipomatosis. Coll Antropol Vol. 32, pp. 637-640.

Goshtasby P, Brooks G and Fielding LP. (2006). Lipomatous disorder of the peri-trochanteric soft tissue: case report and review. Curr Surg Vol. 63, pp. 338-344.

Scheiffarth F, Warnatz H and Mayer K. (1967). Studies concerning the importance of mononuclear cells in development of experimental hepatitis. J Immunol Vol. 98, pp. 396 - 401.

Warnatz et al (Warnatz H, Scheiffarth F, Wolf F and Schmidt HJ. (1967). Autoradiographic experiments concerning the importance of mononuclear cells in development of experimental hepatitis. J Immunol Vol. 98, pp. 402-405.

Stryer L. (1981). Biochemistry, Stanford University, Second Edition W.H. Freeman and Company, San Francisco.

Mistry R, Snashall PD, Totty N, Guz A and Tetley TD. (1991). Isolation and characterization of sheep α-proteinase inhibitor. Biochem J Vol. 273, pp. 685-690.

Kummer JA, Strik MCM, Bladergroen BA and Hack CE. (2004). Production, characterization, and use of serpin antibodies. Methods Vol. 32, pp. 141-149.

Law RHP, Zhang Q, McGowan S, Buckle AM, Silverman GA, Wong W, Rosado CJ, Langendorf CG, Pike RN, Bird PI and Whisstock JC. (2006). An overview of the serpin superfamily. Genome Biology Vol. 7, pp. 1-11.

Yan Y, Liu S, Song G, Xu Y and Dissous C. (2005). Charaterization of novel vaccine candidate and serine proteinase inhibitor from Schistosoma japonicum (Sj serpin). Vet Parasitol Vol. 131, pp. 53-60.

Lonberg-Holm K, Reed DL, Roberts RC, Hebert RR, Hillman MC and Kutney RM. (1987). Three high molecular weight protease inhibitors of rat plasma. J Biol Chem Vol. 262, pp. 438-445.

Silverman GA and Lomas DA. (2004). Serpin identification, production, and characterization. Methods Vol. 32, pp. 71-72.

Miller HRP and Pemberton AD. (2002). Tissue-specific expression of mast cell granule serine proteinases and their role in inflammation in the lung and gut. Immunology Vol. 105, pp. 375-390.

Trishin AV, Zhdanovich MIu, Savvateeva LV, Toptygin AIu, Donenko FV, Kiselevskiĭ MV, Kurbatova EA, Gruber IM, Elkina SI and Kalina NG. (2004). Protease activity of Klebsiella pneumoniae of different virulence. Zh Mikrobiol Epidemiol Immunobiol Vol. 4, pp. 7-11.

Kallenbach LR, Johnson KL, Bianchi DW. (2011). Fetal cell microchimerism and cancer: a nexus of reproduction, immunology, and tumor biology Cancer Res. Vol. 71, No. 1, pp. 8-12.

Miech RP. The role of fetal microchimerism in autoimmune disease. (2010). Int J Clin Exp Med. Vol. 3, No. 2, pp. 164-168.

Hakomori S.(1986). Glycosphingolipids. Scientific American, Vol. 254, No. 5, pp.44 -53.

Eggermont A.M.M. (2009).Therapeutic vaccines in solid tumours: Can they be harmful? Eur. J.of Cancer. Vol. 45, p.2087 - 2090.

Sitdikova SM, Kiselevskii MV, Sel'chuk VY, Amandzholov BS, Kurbatova EA, Donenko FV. (2009). Evaluation of immunotherapy efficiency in mouse CaO-1 ovarian carcinoma treated by vaccines based on dendritic cells. Bull Exp Biol Med. Vol.147, No. 2, pp. 226-228.

# 25

# Molecular Profiling of A375 Human Malignant Melanoma Cells Treated with Kojic Acid and Arbutin

Jung-Feng Hsieh[1], Shui-Tein Chen[2] and Sun-Long Cheng[3]
[1]*Department of Food Science, Fu Jen Catholic University*
[2]*Institute of Biological Chemistry and Genomics Research Center, Academia Sinica*
[3]*Department of Plastic Surgery, Chung Shan Medical University, Chung Shan Medical University Hospital*
*Taiwan*

## 1. Introduction

Malignant melanoma is a serious type of skin cancer that begins in the pigmentation system of the skin. Malignant melanomas, characterized by their high capacity for invasion and metastasis, are one of the most frequent forms of skin cancer. Primary cutaneous melanomas have been divided into four groups based on histopathology: superficial spreading melanoma, nodular melanoma, lentigo maligna melanoma and acral lentiginious melanoma[1]. Superficial spreading melanoma is the most common type of melanoma and grows outwards at first to form an irregular pattern on the skin with an uneven color. It usually starts by spreading out across the surface of the skin in what is known as the radial growth phase. Nodular melanoma occurs most often on the chest or back. It tends to grow deeper into the skin and grows quite deeply if not removed. This type of melanoma is often raised above the rest of the skin surface and feels like a bump. It may be very dark brown-black or black. Lentigo maligna melanoma is most commonly found on the face of elderly people. It grows slowly and may take several years to develop. Acral lentiginious melanoma is usually found on the palms of the hands, soles of the feet or around the toenails. Although melanoma is almost always curable in its early stage, it may be too late if the melanomas spread to other parts of the body. Early diagnosis of melanoma is therefore very important, and it is necessary to develop additional methods of melanoma therapy[2].

Malignant melanoma usually develops from the transformation and proliferation of melanocytes that normally reside in the basal cell layer of the epidermis. It also develops when the melanocytes no longer respond to normal control mechanisms of cellular growth. The melanocytes may then invade nearby structures or spread to other organs in the body (metastasis), where again they invade and compromise the function of that organ. To better understand the molecular and cellular mechanisms involved in the progression of cutaneous melanoma, human malignant melanoma cells have been widely used as a melanoma skin model for *in vitro* testing. This is because it is highly reproducible, quantifiable and easily handled in culture. Not only is it a structural cell model that closely parallels the progression of melanoma *in vivo*, it is also a cost-effective alternative to animal and clinical testing. The antiapoptotic mechanisms regulating cell death have been implicated in conferring drug resistance in tumor cells[3]. Therefore, further knowledge on the nature of this resistance and a better understanding of the signal transduction pathways leading to tumor cell death could allow the identification of new target molecules to overcome drug resistance and improve melanoma therapy. In recent years, toxicogenomics has represented the merging of toxicology with genomics and bioinformatics. There have been significant practical challenges in pharmacology to develop both predictive and mechanism-based toxicology in an effort to identify candidate drugs and toxic agents more quickly and economically[4].

Kojic acid (5-hydroxy-2-hydroxymethyl-1,4-pyrone) is a secondary metabolic product widely used as a food additive for preventing enzymatic browning of raw crabs and shrimps and as a skin lightening or bleaching agent in cosmetic preparations[5,6]. Kojic acid is also used as an important material in antibiotic and pesticide productions and has been shown to act as a competitive and reversible inhibitor of animal and plant polyphenol oxidases, xanthine oxidase, and D- and some L-amino acid oxidases[7,8]. Acute or subchronic toxicity resulting from an oral dose of kojic acid has never been reported, but convulsions may occur if kojic acid is injected. Continuous administration of high doses of kojic acid in mice resulted in thyroid adenomas in both sexes[9]. Moreover, some reports have evaluated the tumorigenic potential of kojic acid, and the genotoxic risk for humans using kojic acid as a skin-lightening agent has also been studied[10]. However, kojic acid at high doses has certain side effects. For example, it affects thyroid function when given at a massive dose or in a long administration period by inhibiting iodine organification in the thyroid, decreasing triiodothyronine (T3) and thyroxine (T4) levels and increasing thyroid-stimulating hormone (TSH)[11]. Recently, kojic acid was found to be a tumor promoter and an enhancer of hepatocarcinogenesis in rats and in mice[12]. However, the topical use of kojic acid as a skin-lightening agent results in minimal exposure that poses a negligible or no risk of genotoxicity or toxicity to the consumer.

Arbutin, a natural compound of hydroquinone beta-D-glucopyranoside, is widely used as an ingredient in skin care products[13]. It is effective in the treatment of various cutaneous hyperpigmentations and inhibits melanogenesis in melanoma cells[14]. However, recent findings have raised serious concerns regarding both the safety and side effects of arbutin. Although the mechanisms of some inhibitory effects of arbutin on melanogenesis in melanoma cells have been elucidated, the comprehensive study of its biological effects on the regulation of malignant melanogenesis through the functional effect on carcinogenesis is not clear and rarely reported on a human genomics level. The general risk factors for melanoma include sun exposure, fair skin that burns easily, blistering sunburn, previous melanoma, previous nonmelanoma skin cancer, family history of melanoma, large numbers of moles and abnormal moles. During the progression of melanoma, different proteolytic enzyme systems, including the plasminogen-activator system and matrix metalloproteinases, play an important role in the degradation and remodeling of the extracellular matrix and basement membranes[15]. Tyrosinase is the main enzyme regulating melanogenesis, and it catalyzes three distinct reactions in the melanogenic pathway: hydroxylation of monophenol (L-tyrosine), dehydrogenation of catechol (L-DOPA) and dehydrogenation of dihydroxyindole. By contrast, catalase is the proteolytic enzyme that regulates the removal of $H_2O_2$, which is a potent inhibitor of tyrosinase. Peroxidase also serves to increase eumelanin polymer formation from monomers in the presence of $H_2O_2$ and metal ions, especially copper, which enhance the conversion of monomers to polymers[16]. Thus, changes in enzyme levels, including modifications in protein- and gene-expression levels, influence melanogenesis in melanomas. The complex regulatory control of the biosynthesis machinery involved in melanogenesis also includes receptor-mediated pathways activated by hormones, neurotransmitters, cytokines, growth factors and eicosanoids. Additionally, receptor-independent mechanisms are activated or modified by nutrients, micromolecules, microelements, pH, cation and anion concentrations, and the oxidoreductive potential in the physicochemical milieu. Soluble factors can reach target melanocytes by circulation, by release from nerve endings or by local production to act as positive or negative regulators of melanogenesis.

Toxicogenomic applications are increasingly used to evaluate preclinical drug safety and to explain toxicity associated with compounds at the mechanistic level. Recently, a high-throughput DNA microarray technique gained an important role in genomic research by allowing the simultaneous study of the function of thousands of genes showing differential gene expression profiles. This opened the door to the discovery of biomarkers or special gene markers intended for pharmaceutical applications and disease therapy[17]. High-throughput DNA microarray technology is a powerful tool for genomic research because it allows the study of the function of thousands of genes simultaneously, reveals different gene expression profiles and elucidates the exact mechanisms and defects in genetic aberrations. Recently, microarrays have been used to analyze gene expression profiles of human melanomas. However, only a few such analyses have been reported in A375 melanoma cells. For example, the metastasis of A375 melanoma cells has been studied in nude mice by microarray analysis[18].

Proteomics is the study of the proteome, the protein complement of the genome. The terms "proteomics" and "proteome" were coined by Marc Wilkins and colleagues in the early 1990s and mirror the terms "genomics" and "genome," which describe the entire collection of genes in an organism[19]. In fact, the proteomic approach is a powerful tool for the simultaneous determination of the protein composition of complex samples. Proteomics consists of several tools, including two-dimensional polyacrylamide gel electrophoresis (2-D PAGE) and mass spectrometry[20]. 2-D PAGE takes advantage of two unique biochemical characteristics of proteins, combining isoelectric focusing (IEF), which separates proteins according to their isoelectric point, with SDS-PAGE, which further separates them according to their molecular mass. 2-D PAGE allows simultaneous detection and quantification of up to thousands of protein spots on the same gel[21]. Mass spectrometry has been in use for many years, but it could not be applied to macromolecules such as proteins and nucleic acids. The m/z measurements are taken on molecules in the gas phase, and the heating or other treatment needed to convert a macromolecule to the gas phase usually caused its rapid decomposition. In 1988, two different techniques were developed to overcome this problem. In one of the techniques, proteins are placed in a light-absorbing matrix. With a short pulse of laser light, the proteins are ionized and then desorbed from the matrix into the vacuum system. This process, known as matrix-assisted laser desorption/ionization mass spectrometry (MALDI MS), has been successfully used to measure the mass of a wide range of macromolecules[22]. MALDI time of flight (TOF) MS is advantageous due to the rapid and direct analysis of complex mixtures and its tolerance to buffer salts or detergents in the samples.

Although the tumorigenic potential and some genotoxic effects of kojic acid and arbutin on human skin cell lines have been widely studied, the effect of these compounds on gene and protein expression levels that may be involved in many biological functions in human skin has never been reported. In this study, we used DNA microarrays and 2-D PAGE to investigate the biological effects of kojic acid and arbutin on gene and protein expression profiles of A375 human malignant melanoma cells and on melanocytic tumorigenesis and other related side effects of cancer therapy. These candidate genes and proteins may consequently aid in the development of early diagnostic and therapeutic applications.

## 2. Toxicogenomic analysis of kojic acid-treated A375 melanoma cells

### 2.1 Inhibitory effect of kojic acid on A375 melanoma cells

Previous examination showed that cell growth of A375 melanoma cells was directly inhibited by increasing kojic acid concentrations[18]. After treatment with kojic acid for 72 h, the highest concentration of kojic acid (1000 μg/ml) inhibited A375 melanoma cell growth less than 40%, whereas the lower concentrations of 0.32, 1.6, 8 and 40 μg/ml kojic acid inhibited A375 melanoma cell growth less than 20% (Fig. 1).

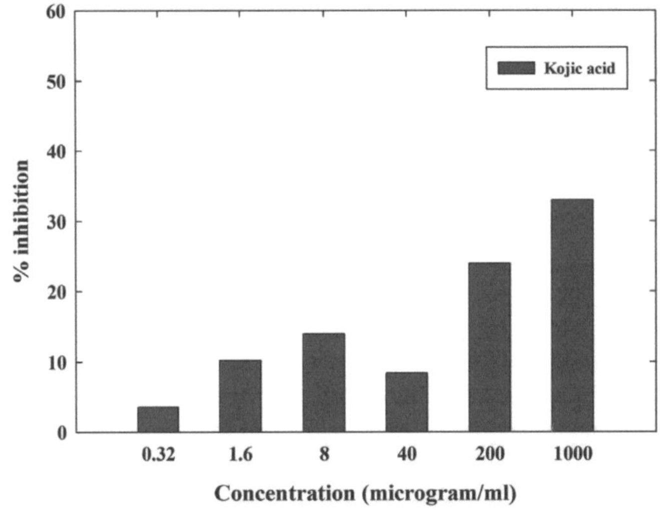


Fig. 1. Effect of different kojic acid concentrations on the growth inhibition of A375 cells at 72 h

These results indicate that the inhibition of A375 melanoma cell growth was not strongly affected by all concentrations of kojic acid. In addition, there was no morphological change of A375 melanoma cells over 24 h in the presence of 8 μg/ml kojic acid, which is a mild concentration and the recommended dosage of kojic acid for human skin safety[24]. To study the early-stage gene expression profile of A375 melanoma cells following stimulation by kojic acid, comparable to conditions used in human skin therapy, we chose the 24 h time point for the following microarray analysis.

### 2.2 Microarray analysis of kojic acid-treated A375 melanoma cells

Messenger RNA from control and kojic acid-treated A375 melanoma cells was labeled with Cy3- or Cy5-dCTP, respectively, using a single round of reverse transcription and hybridization with the oligonucleotide microarray chip. The microarray results showed different fluorescence intensities of Cy3 and Cy5 depending on the gene expression level[18].

| Gene name | Accession No. | Ratio | Description |
|---|---|---|---|
| PSCDBP | NM_004288 | 15.34 | Pleckstrin homology, Sec7 and coiled-coil domains |
| TM4SF3 | NM_004616 | 10.99 | Transmembrane 4 superfamily member 3 (TM4SF3), mRNA |
| KRT7 | NM_005556 | 10.71 | Keratin 7 (KRT7), mRNA |
| KLHL13 | NM_033495 | 10.13 | Kelch-like 13 (Drosophila) (KLHL13), mRNA |
| WBSCR19 | NM_175064 | 9.58 | Williams Beuren syndrome chromosome region 19 (WBSCR19) |
| BC031966 | BC031966 | 8.53 | cDNA clone MGC:43036 IMAGE:4839025, complete cds. |
| CRSP2 | NM_004229 | 6.23 | Cofactor required for Sp1 transcriptional activation, subunit 2 (CRSP2) |
| FGF12 | NM_004113 | 5.95 | Fibroblast growth factor 12 (FGF12), transcript variant 2, mRNA |
| FLJ46156 | NM_198499 | 5.78 | FLJ46156 protein (FLJ46156), mRNA |
| ENST00000316004 | ENST00000316004 | 5.75 | Olfactory receptor 4H12 (Fragment). |
| SPP1 | NM_000582 | 5.38 | Secreted phosphoprotein 1 (SPP1), mRNA |
| PLAGL1 | NM_002656 | 5.14 | Pleiomorphic adenoma gene-like 1 (PLAGL1) |
| MGC35118 | NM_152453 | 5.07 | Hypothetical protein MGC35118 (MGC35118), mRNA |
| TTC9 | D86980 | 4.83 | mRNA for KIAA0227 gene, partial cds. |
| AQP1 | NM_000385 | 4.50 | Aquaporin 1 (channel-forming integral protein, 28 kDa) (AQP1) |
| PHCA | NM_018367 | 4.47 | Phytoceramidase, alkaline (PHCA), mRNA |
| FBXO16 | NM_172366 | 4.21 | F-box only protein 16 (FBXO16), mRNA |
| PARG | NM_003631 | 4.05 | Poly (ADP-ribose) glycohydrolase (PARG), mRNA |
| SOAT2 | NM_003578 | 4.02 | Sterol O-acyltransferase 2 (SOAT2), mRNA |
| THC1991976 | THC1991976 | 3.67 | AF244540 immunodominant membrane protein precursor |
| PSCD3 | NM_004227 | 3.49 | Pleckstrin homology, Sec7 and coiled-coil domains 3 (PSCD3), mRNA |
| HIST1H2AC | NM_003512 | 3.34 | Histone 1, H2ac (HIST1H2AC), mRNA |
| FLJ23018 | NM_024810 | 3.32 | Hypothetical protein FLJ23018 (FLJ23018), mRNA |
| PPP4R1 | NM_005134 | 3.01 | Protein phosphatase 4, regulatory subunit 1 (PPP4R1), mRNA |
| CPE | NM_001873 | 2.98 | Carboxypeptidase E (CPE), mRNA |
| C6orf128 | NM_145316 | 2.97 | Chromosome 6 open reading frame 128 (C6orf128), mRNA |
| CCAR1 | NM_018237 | 2.91 | Cell division cycle and apoptosis regulator 1 (CCAR1), mRNA |
| FBN2 | NM_001999 | 2.86 | Fibrillin 2 (congenital contractural arachnodactyly) (FBN2), mRNA |
| IL22RA1 | NM_021258 | 2.85 | Interleukin 22 receptor, alpha 1 (IL22RA1), mRNA |
| F10 | NM_000504 | 2.80 | Coagulation factor X (F10), mRNA |
| GPR32 | NM_001506 | 2.79 | G protein-coupled receptor 32 (GPR32), mRNA |
| PDCD1LG1 | NM_014143 | 2.65 | Programmed cell death 1 ligand 1 (PDCD1LG1), mRNA |
| HIP1 | NM_005338 | 2.64 | Huntingtin interacting protein 1 (HIP1), mRNA |
| JMJD2D | NM_018039 | 2.61 | Jumonji domain containing 2D (JMJD2D), mRNA |
| ARMC4 | AK001238 | 2.57 | cDNA FLJ10376 fis, clone NT2RM2001982 |
| CAB39L | NM_030925 | 2.54 | Calcium binding protein 39-like (CAB39L), mRNA |
| FLJ13089 | NM_024953 | 2.54 | Hypothetical protein FLJ13089 (FLJ13089), mRNA |
| OTX1 | NM_014562 | 2.51 | Orthodenticle homolog 1 (Drosophila) (OTX1), mRNA |
| COLQ | NM_080542 | 2.49 | Collagen-like tail subunit of asymmetric acetylcholinesterase |
| PDCL | NM_005388 | 2.44 | Phosducin-like (PDCL), mRNA |
| ENST00000307033 | ENST00000307033 | 2.42 | Olfactory receptor 4D5. |
| FLJ23311 | NM_024680 | 2.41 | FLJ23311 protein (FLJ23311), mRNA |
| RASSF3 | AK129920 | 2.39 | cDNA FLJ26410 fis, clone HRT09622 |
| LOC220929 | NM_182755 | 2.34 | Hypothetical protein LOC220929 (LOC220929), mRNA |
| EPHA4 | NM_004438 | 2.26 | EphA4 (EPHA4), mRNA |
| HH114 | NM_032499 | 2.23 | Hypothetical protein HH114 (HH114), mRNA |
| DOCK4 | AB018259 | 2.14 | mRNA for KIAA0716 protein, partial cds. |
| CPNE5 | NM_020939 | 2.11 | Copine V (CPNE5), mRNA |

Table 1. Up-regulated genes (48 genes, ratio > 2.0) in kojic acid-stimulated A375 cells

Analysis of gene expression changes at the RNA level using a human 1A oligonucleotide microarray complementary to 20,173 60-mer oligonucleotide probes showed a total number of 83 differentially expressed genes in kojic acid-stimulated A375 melanoma cells, including 48 up-regulated genes (Table 1, ratio > 2.0) and 35 down-regulated genes (Table 2, ratio < 0.3). We suggest that all of the differentially expressed genes may be regulated by various gene networks in the regulation of malignant tumorigenesis.

### 2.3 RT-qPCR validation of microarray results

Genes with a significant change in expression in the array analysis, determined by a mean degree of regulation with $p<0.01$, were chosen for RT-qPCR examination. Differentially expressed genes were grouped by biological function correlated with carcinogenesis and the significantly changed genes were selected according to the order of P values. The selected genes were validated by RT-qPCR analysis to confirm the microarray data.

RT-qPCR results showed the gene expression levels of seven expressed genes in kojic acid-stimulated A375 melanoma cells agreed with the DNA microarray expression data[18]. One gene chosen for RT-qPCR examination was the apolipoprotein B RNA editing deaminase (APOBEC1) gene[25]. The comparison of the gene expression level of sAPOBEC1 by microarray and RT-qPCR is shown in Table 3. This gene was downregulated in kojic acid-stimulated A375 melanoma cells and functions as a tumor suppressor in the regulation of carcinogenesis.

## 3. Toxicogenomic analysis of arbutin-treated A375 melanoma cells

### 3.1 Inhibitory effect of arbutin on A375 melanoma cells

A375 melanoma cell growth was directly inhibited by increasing arbutin concentrations[26]. After 72 h, the highest concentration of arbutin (1000 µg/ml) inhibited A375 cell growth up to 40%, while the lower concentrations of 0.32, 1.6, 8 and 40 µg/ml arbutin inhibited cell growth by less than 20% (Fig. 2).

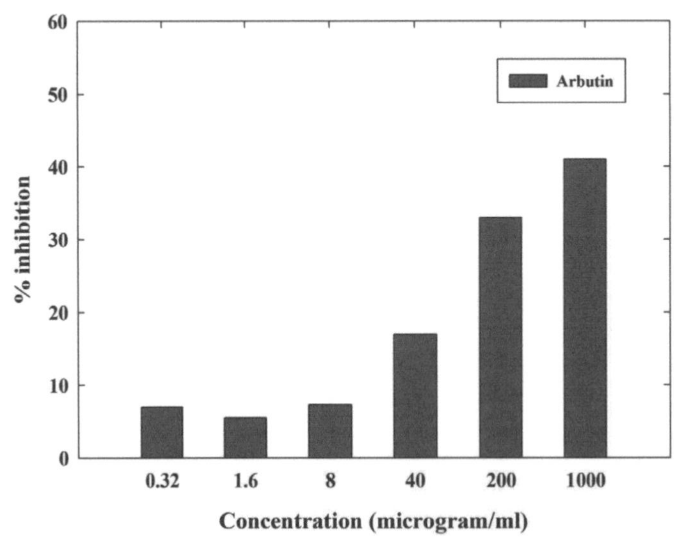


Fig. 2. Effect of arbutin concentrations on the growth inhibition of A375 cells at 72 h

| Gene name | Accession | Ratio | Description |
|---|---|---|---|
| DMXL1 | NM_005509 | 0.16 | Dmx-like 1 (DMXL1), mRNA |
| NUDT10 | NM_153183 | 0.16 | Nudix (nucleoside diphosphate linked moiety X)-type motif 10 (NUDT10) |
| SAA4 | NM_006512 | 0.17 | Serum amyloid A4, constitutive (SAA4), mRNA |
| DSPP | NM_014208 | 0.17 | Dentin sialophosphoprotein (DSPP), mRNA |
| IL6ST | NM_002184 | 0.18 | Interleukin 6 signal transducer (gp130, oncostatin M receptor) (IL6ST) |
| PEX5L | NM_016559 | 0.18 | Pex5p-related protein (PEX5R), mRNA |
| BC032472 | BC032472 | 0.18 | Similar to caspase 4, apoptosis-related cysteine protease |
| AK096677 | AK096677 | 0.19 | cDNA FLJ39358 fis, clone PEBLM2004015 |
| FLJ14297 | NM_024903 | 0.20 | Hypothetical protein FLJ14297 (FLJ14297), mRNA |
| THRB | NM_000461 | 0.20 | Thyroid hormone receptor, beta (THRB), mRNA |
| HLF | NM_002126 | 0.21 | Hepatic leukemia factor (HLF), mRNA |
| APOBEC1 | NM_001644 | 0.22 | Apolipoprotein B mRNA editing enzyme, catalytic polypeptide 1 |
| FGF5 | NM_004464 | 0.22 | Fibroblast growth factor 5 (FGF5), transcript variant 1, mRNA |
| ACMSD | NM_138326 | 0.22 | Aminocarboxymuconate semialdehyde decarboxylase (ACMSD), mRNA |
| SIN3B | AB014600 | 0.23 | mRNA for KIAA0700 protein, partial cds. |
| KIAA0565 | AB011137 | 0.24 | mRNA for KIAA0565 protein, partial cds. |
| MGC34837 | NM_152377 | 0.25 | Hypothetical protein MGC34837 (MGC34837), mRNA |
| TAL1 | NM_003189 | 0.25 | T-cell acute lymphocytic leukemia 1 (TAL1), mRNA |
| SLC17A2 | NM_005835 | 0.25 | Solute carrier family 17 (sodium phosphate), member 2 (SLC17A2) |
| CPB1 | NM_001871 | 0.25 | Carboxypeptidase B1 (tissue) (CPB1), mRNA |
| USP44 | NM_032147 | 0.26 | Ubiquitin specific protease 44 (USP44), mRNA |
| ZNF192 | NM_006298 | 0.26 | Zinc finger protein 192 (ZNF192), mRNA |
| PAH | NM_000277 | 0.27 | Phenylalanine hydroxylase (PAH), mRNA |
| FLJ14503 | NM_152780 | 0.28 | Hypothetical protein FLJ14503 (FLJ14503), mRNA |
| ZP2 | NM_003460 | 0.29 | Zona pellucida glycoprotein 2 (sperm receptor) (ZP2), mRNA |
| ST18 | NM_014682 | 0.29 | Suppression of tumorigenicity 18 (ST18), mRNA |
| PDZK10 | AB002314 | 0.29 | mRNA for KIAA0316 protein, partial cds. |
| TCN1 | NM_001062 | 0.29 | Transcobalamin I (vitamin B12 binding protein, R binder family) (TCN1) |
| ABCA13 | NM_152701 | 0.29 | ATP binding cassette gene, sub-family A (ABC1), member 13 (ABCA13) |
| ABCC13 | NM_138726 | 0.29 | ATP-binding cassette, sub-family C (CFTR/MRP), member 13 (ABCC13) |
| ADAM20 | NM_003814 | 0.29 | A disintegrin and metalloproteinase domain 20 (ADAM20), mRNA |
| AF090929 | AF090929 | 0.29 | Clone HQ0477 PRO0477p mRNA, complete cds. |
| D82326 | D82326 | 0.29 | mRNA for $Na^{+}$-independent neutral and basic amino acid transporter |
| LILRB5 | NM_006840 | 0.29 | Leukocyte immunoglobulin-like receptor, subfamily B, mRNA |
| MFAP4 | NM_002404 | 0.29 | Microfibrillar-associated protein 4 (MFAP4), mRNA |

Table 2. Down-regulated genes (35 genes, ratio < 0.3) in kojic acid-stimulated A375 cells

A375 cell growth was not strongly affected by all arbutin concentrations. In addition, there were no morphological changes in cells treated with 0.32-40 µg/ml arbutin. According to the safety recommendations for a 1% prescription drug in human skin care products, the concentration of 8 µg/ml arbutin is safe and within the recommended concentration[27]. Also, there was no morphological change in the cells within 24 h in the presence of 8 µg/ml arbutin, and the inhibition of cell growth was less than 10%. However, the biological effect of arbutin on the gene expression profile in A375 melanoma cells and other genotoxic side effects have never been reported. Therefore, a purpose of this study was to investigate the genotoxic effect of arbutin on human skin and on tumorigenesis.

| Gene name | P value | Microarray | RT-qPCR | (primer sequence) |
|---|---|---|---|---|
| APOBEC1 | < 0.0001 | 0.22 | 0.12 | Forward 5'-TGGATGATGTTGTACGCACTGG-3' |
| | | | | Reverse 5'-TGGCGGAATCGTTTGGTAATGG-3' |

Table 3. Comparison of gene expression levels of the APOBEC1 gene in kojic acid-treated A375 cells by microarray and RT-qPCR analysis

### 3.2 Microarray analysis of arbutin-treated A375 melanoma cells

The microarray results show different fluorescence intensities of Cy3 (control) and Cy5 (arbutin-treated A375 melanoma cells), corresponding to the expression level of thousands of genes. The differences in Cy3 and Cy5 signal intensities with a p-value of less than 0.01 ($p$<0.01) were considered to be significantly different[26].

| Gene name | Accession | Ratio | Description |
|---|---|---|---|
| KLHL13 | NM_033495 | 9.31 | Kelch-like 13 (Drosophila) (KLHL13) |
| EPX | NM_000502 | 8.42 | Eosinophil peroxidase (EPX) |
| TSC1 | NM_000368 | 8.31 | Tuberous sclerosis 1 (TSC1) |
| SCN1B | NM_001037 | 6.32 | Sodium channel, voltage-gated, type I, beta (SCN1B) |
| GAGED3 | NM_130777 | 4.54 | G antigen, family D, 3 (GAGED3) |
| IL3RA | NM_002183 | 4.50 | Interleukin 3 receptor, alpha (low affinity) (IL3RA) |
| FBXO16 | NM_172366 | 4.22 | F-box only protein 16 (FBXO16) |
| VPS39 | NM_015289 | 4.10 | Vacuolar protein sorting 39 (VPS39) |
| PARG | NM_003631 | 4.05 | Poly (ADP-ribose) glycohydrolase (PARG) |
| NRP2 | NM_201266 | 3.94 | Neuropilin 2 (NRP2), transcript variant 1, mRNA |
| ANKRD23 | NM_144994 | 3.65 | Ankyrin repeat domain 23 (ANKRD23) |
| FLJ13611 | NM_024941 | 3.61 | Hypothetical protein FLJ13611 (FLJ13611) |
| THC1991976 | THC1991976 | 3.55 | AF244540 immunodominant membrane protein precursor |
| AEBP2 | NM_153207 | 3.54 | AE binding protein 2 (AEBP2) |
| ZBTB20 | NM_015642 | 3.36 | Zinc finger protein 288 (ZNF288) |
| NR2F1 | NM_005654 | 3.27 | Nuclear receptor subfamily 2, group F, member 1 (NR2F1) |
| KLRC4 | NM_013431 | 3.24 | Killer cell lectin-like receptor subfamily C, member 4 (KLRC4) |
| CAPNS2 | NM_032330 | 3.17 | Calpain small subunit 2 (CAPNS2) |
| APOM | NM_019101 | 3.12 | Apolipoprotein M (APOM) |
| SLC23A3 | NM_144712 | 2.65 | Solute carrier family 23, member 3 (SLC23A3) |
| C18orf11 | NM_022751 | 2.62 | Chromosome 18 open reading frame 11 (C18orf11) |
| DDEF1 | NM_018482 | 2.58 | Development and differentiation enhancing factor 1 (DDEF1) |
| HIST1H2AC | NM_003512 | 2.55 | Histone 1, H2ac (HIST1H2AC) |
| HH114 | NM_032499 | 2.49 | Hypothetical protein HH114 (HH114) |
| CPE | NM_001873 | 2.35 | Carboxypeptidase E (CPE) |
| TARDBP | NM_007375 | 2.28 | TAR DNA binding protein (TARDBP) |
| ADAM7 | NM_003817 | 2.20 | A disintegrin and metalloproteinase domain 7 (ADAM7) |
| KIAA1706 | NM_030636 | 2.16 | KIAA1706 protein (KIAA1706) |
| CCAR1 | NM_018237 | 2.11 | Cell division cycle and apoptosis regulator 1 (CCAR1) |
| CPNE5 | NM_020939 | 2.10 | Copine V (CPNE5) |
| GPR32 | NM_001506 | 2.04 | G protein-coupled receptor 32 (GPR32) |
| HAND1 | NM_004821 | 2.02 | Heart and neural crest derivatives expressed 1 (HAND1) |

Table 4. Up-regulated genes (32 genes, ratio > 2.0) in arbutin-stimulated A375 cells

Analysis of changes in gene expression using the human oligonucleotide array revealed a total of 73 differentially expressed genes, including 32 up-regulated genes (Table 4, ratio > 2.0) and 41 down-regulated genes (Table 5, ratio < 0.3). Therefore, these genes may be useful candidate markers for early diagnostic and therapeutic applications of melanoma carcinogenesis.

| Gene name | Accession | Ratio | Description |
|---|---|---|---|
| ZNF41 | NM_153380 | 0.13 | Zinc finger protein 41 (ZNF41) |
| F13B | NM_001994 | 0.16 | Coagulation factor XIII, B polypeptide (F13B) |
| THC1910111 | THC1910111 | 0.17 | BC022679 D13Ertd275e protein |
| HSD3B1 | NM_000862 | 0.17 | Hydroxy-delta-5-steroid dehydrogenase, 3 beta-and steroid delta-isomerase |
| PF4 | NM_002619 | 0.18 | Platelet factor 4 (chemokine (C-X-C motif) ligand 4) (PF4) |
| IL6ST | NM_002184 | 0.18 | Interleukin 6 signal transducer (IL6ST) |
| LOC162967 | NM_207333 | 0.19 | Hypothetical protein LOC162967 (LOC162967) |
| RFPL3 | NM_006604 | 0.20 | Ret finger protein-like 3 (RFPL3) |
| NTF5 | NM_006179 | 0.20 | Neurotrophin 5 (neurotrophin 4/5) (NTF5) |
| GPR155 | NM_152529 | 0.20 | G protein-coupled receptor 155 (GPR155) |
| CASP8 | NM_033357 | 0.20 | Caspase 8, apoptosis-related cysteine protease (CASP8) |
| C20orf17 | NM_173485 | 0.20 | Chromosome 20 open reading frame 17 (C20orf17) |
| AK025116 | AK025116 | 0.20 | cDNA: FLJ21463 fis, clone COL04765 |
| MYO3B | NM_138995 | 0.21 | Myosin IIIB (MYO3B) |
| ZNF167 | NM_018651 | 0.22 | Zinc finger protein 167 (ZNF167) |
| RFPL2 | NM_006605 | 0.22 | Ret finger protein-like 2 (RFPL2) |
| PDZK1 | NM_002614 | 0.22 | PDZ domain containing 1 (PDZK1) |
| NEGR1 | NM_173808 | 0.22 | Neuronal growth regulator 1 (NEGR1) |
| GPC3 | NM_004484 | 0.22 | Glypican 3 (GPC3) |
| DMXL1 | NM_005509 | 0.22 | Dmx-like 1 (DMXL1) |
| ZNF141 | NM_003441 | 0.23 | Zinc finger protein 141 (clone pHZ-44) (ZNF141) |
| SLC7A3 | NM_032803 | 0.23 | Solute carrier family 7, member 3 (SLC7A3) |
| SEMG1 | NM_003007 | 0.23 | Semenogelin I (SEMG1) |
| L17325 | L17325 | 0.23 | Pre-T/NK cell associated protein (1D12A2) |
| FMNL3 | NM_175736 | 0.23 | Formin-like 3 (FMNL3) |
| CPB1 | NM_001871 | 0.23 | Carboxypeptidase B1 (tissue) (CPB1) |
| ADAMTS9 | NM_020249 | 0.23 | A disintegrin-like and metalloprotease with thrombospondin type 1 motif |
| FGF5 | NM_004464 | 0.24 | Fibroblast growth factor 5 (FGF5) |
| C14orf148 | NM_138791 | 0.24 | Hypothetical protein FLJ32809 (LOC122945) |
| BMPR1B | NM_001203 | 0.24 | Bone morphogenetic protein receptor, type IB (BMPR1B) |
| ABCA10 | NM_080282 | 0.24 | ATP-binding cassette, sub-family A (ABC1), member 10 (ABCA10) |
| PKHD1 | NM_138694 | 0.25 | Polycystic kidney and hepatic disease 1 (PKHD1) |
| NM_152768 | NM_152768 | 0.25 | Hypothetical protein FLJ25378 (FLJ25378) |
| ABCC13 | NM_138726 | 0.25 | ATP-binding cassette, sub-family C (CFTR/MRP), member 13 (ABCC13) |
| SLC15A3 | NM_016582 | 0.27 | Solute carrier family 15, member 3 (SLC15A3) |
| LGALS14 | NM_020129 | 0.27 | Placental protein 13-like protein (PPL13) |
| C6orf97 | NM_025059 | 0.27 | Chromosome 6 open reading frame 97 (C6orf97) |
| AX721299 | AX721299 | 0.27 | Sequence 259 from Patent WO0220754 |
| C15orf26 | NM_173528 | 0.28 | Hypothetical protein FLJ38615 (FLJ38615) |
| ADAM20 | NM_003814 | 0.29 | A disintegrin and metalloproteinase domain 20 (ADAM20) |
| ACMSD | NM_138326 | 0.29 | Aminocarboxymuconate semialdehyde decarboxylase (ACMSD) |

Table 5. Down-regulated genes (41 genes, ratio < 0.3) in arbutin-stimulated A375 cells

## 4. Proteomic analysis of kojic acid-treated A375 melanoma cells

### 4.1 2-D PAGE of A375 melanoma cells following kojic acid treatment

To investigate the anticancer effect of kojic acid on the protein expression pattern of A375 melanoma cells, cells were treated with kojic acid for 24, 48 and 72 h and analyzed by 2-D PAGE[28]. The 2-D gel images of the untreated control and kojic acid-treated A375 melanoma cells are shown in Fig. 3.

Most of the proteins have p*I* ranges of 3.5-5.0 or 6.5-8.5 with molecular weights of more than 25 kDa. Using PDQuest image analysis software, approximately 540 spots were detected in control and treatment groups with no significant difference of the mean numbers among groups. Most of the differentially expressed protein spots have a high molecular weight of 45-100 kDa, especially at acidic pH.

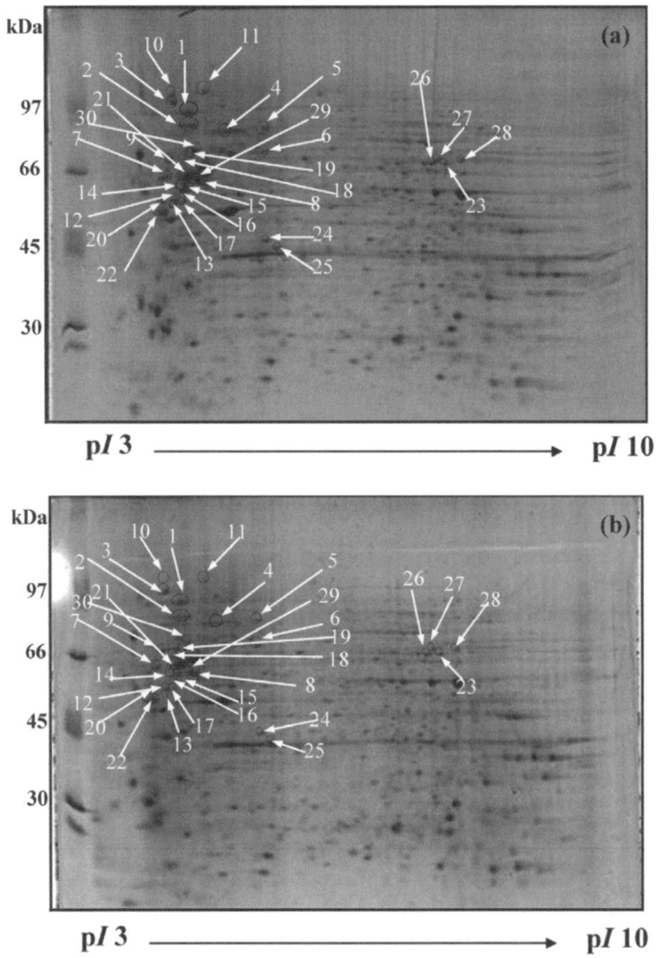


Fig. 3. 2-D PAGE images of A375 human malignant melanoma cells after control (a) and 72 h treatment (b) with arbutin. The images in the panels are the regions showing differentially expressed spots for protein identification. The pointed arrows indicate the protein spots identified in this study

To study the biological effect of kojic acid on late-stage protein expression in A375 melanoma cells, the time point of 72 h was chosen to quantify protein expression changes between the control and treatment groups, and the differentially expressed protein spots were used to further identify the proteins. There were 30 differentially expressed protein spots, including 2 up-regulated protein spots, for which the threshold of change in expression level was 1.5-fold, and 28 down-regulated protein spots, for which the threshold of change in expression level was 0.9-fold. Seven interesting proteins that have biological functions associated with the p53 tumor suppressor protein or are involved in tumor biology were then selected for validation by Western blot or RT-PCR.

### 4.2 Protein identification of differentially expressed proteins

With the use of MASCOT protein identification search software for identifying both peptide mass fingerprinting (PMF) and MS/MS ion mass data, 30 differentially expressed protein spots were successfully identified[28]. A list of identified proteins, the apparent and theoretical MW, p*I* and fold change in expression level (up- or down-regulation) are shown in Table 6. Most of identified proteins were downregulated in kojic acid-treated A375 melanoma cells when compared to the control group. There were multiple isoforms of 5 heat shock proteins, 2 endoplasmin precursors, 2 protein disulfide isomerases, 6 vimentins and 2 aldehyde dehydrogenases, which comprised about 56.7% of the identified proteins, which might be due to post-translational modifications. In addition, the prediction of protein interaction partners is shown in Table 6. The identified proteins were found at different locations within the cell. The proteins have diverse functions, especially in protein binding, and play key roles in virtually all biological processes, including apoptosis, mammalian cell-cycle progression, regulation of angiogenesis, regulation of cell proliferation, regulation of cell differentiation and the immune response. Interestingly, 11 identified proteins (36.7% of total proteins), including heat shock proteins (HS90B, GRP75, GRP78, ENPL (x2), HSP7C), T-complex protein 1 subunit epsilon (TCPE), protein disulfide isomerases (PDIA6, PDIA1), nucleolin (NUCL) and annexin A11 (ANX11), are chaperone proteins, which were found in melanosomes from stage I to stage IV with different functions.

### 4.3 Validation by Western blotting and RT-PCR

Of the identified proteins, GRP75, heat shock protein HS90B, ENPL and pyruvate kinase isozyme M1/M2 (KPYM) were validated by RT-PCR, while GRP75, VIME and serine/threonine-protein phosphatase 2A (2AAA) were validated by Western blotting (Fig. 4).

Protein and gene expression levels of 7 differentially expressed proteins were in agreement with the 2-D PAGE expression data[28]. The proteins GRP75, VIME, HS90B and ENPL were downregulated in kojic acid-treated A375 melanoma cells, while the proteins 2AAA and KPYM were upregulated.

## 5. Proteomic analysis of arbutin-treated A375 melanoma cells

### 5.1 2-D PAGE of A375 melanoma cells following arbutin treatment

The 2-D PAGE images of A375 melanoma cells without treatment (control) and with arbutin treatment at 24, 48 and 72 h are shown in Fig. 5.

| Sopt No. | Protein Name | Accession no. | Mr (Exp) | p*I* (Exp) | Mr (Cal) | p*I* (Cal) | Fold-change | Predicted protein interaction partners |
|---|---|---|---|---|---|---|---|---|
| 1 | Heat shock protein HSP 90-beta | P08238 | 97.00 | 4.20 | 83.2 | 4.97 | -2.50 | •TP53/p53 |
| 2 | Heat shock 70 kDa protein | P11021 | 91.80 | 4.20 | 72.3 | 5.07 | -2.50 | •ENPL •PDIA6 •GRP75 •p53 |
| 3 | Endoplasmin precursor (ENPL) | P14625 | 100.00 | 4.00 | 92.4 | 4.76 | -1.51 | •GRP75 •GRP78 •PDIA4 receptor •Tyrosinase-protein kinase erbB-2 |
| 4 | Heat shock cognate 71 kDa (HSP7C) | P11142 | 86.64 | 4.67 | 70.85 | 5.37 | -2.00 | •Bcl-2 binding athanogene-1, -3 •HSP86 •HSP60 |
| 5 | Stress-70 protein, mitochondrial precursor (GRP75) | P38646 | 89.22 | 5.10 | 73.64 | 5.87 | -2.21 | •p53 •DnaJ homologue subfamily A and B members •HSP90B1 |
| 6 | T-complex protein 1 subunit epsilon (TCPE) | P48643 | 76.32 | 5.10 | 59.63 | 5.45 | -2.20 | •T-complex protein 1 different subunits |
| 7 | Endoplasmin precursor (ENPL) | P14625 | 68.00 | 3.95 | 92.41 | 4.76 | -1.10 | •GRP75 •GRP78 •PDIA4 receptor •Tyrosinase-protein kinase erbB-2 |
| 8 | Protein disulfide-isomerase A6 precursor (PDIA6) | Q15084 | 63.00 | 4.60 | 48.09 | 4.95 | -2.00 | •Beta-Actin •ERp31 • GRP78 |
| 9 | Protein disulfide-isomerase precursor (PDIA1) | P07237 | 71.20 | 4.00 | 57.08 | 4.76 | -2.10 | •ERp31 •GRP78 |
| 10 | Nucleolin (NUCL) | P19338 | 102.00 | 4.00 | 76.57 | 4.60 | -2.20 | •DNA topoisomerase •p53 •Proliferation-associated protein 2G4 |
| 11 | Vimentin (VIME) | P08670 | 103.00 | 4.40 | 53.62 | 5.06 | -2.25 | •RAF-1 •Proteosome subunit alpha type1 •Protein kinase N1 |
| 12 | Vimentin (VIME) | P08670 | 58.50 | 4.25 | 53.62 | 5.06 | -2.15 | •RAF-1 •Proteosome subunit alpha type1 •Protein kinase N1 |
| 13 | Vimentin (VIME) | P08670 | 57.00 | 4.22 | 53.62 | 5.06 | -2.10 | •RAF-1 •Proteosome subunit alpha type1 •Protein kinase N1 |
| 14 | Vimentin (VIME) | P08670 | 63.00 | 4.34 | 53.62 | 5.06 | -2.10 | •RAF-1 •Proteosome subunit alpha type1 •Protein kinase N1 |
| 15 | Vimentin (VIME) | P08670 | 62.50 | 4.40 | 53.62 | 5.06 | -2.00 | •RAF-1 •Proteosome subunit alpha type1 •protein kinase N1 |
| 16 | Vimentin (VIME) | P08670 | 61.30 | 4.30 | 53.62 | 5.06 | -2.15 | •RAF-1 •Proteosome subunit alpha type1 •Protein kinase N1 |
| 17 | Gamma-enolase (EC 4.2.1. 11) | P09104 | 58.00 | 4.17 | 47.24 | 4.91 | -2.00 | •Pyruvate kinase isoenzyme M1/M2 •Enzymes in glycolytic pathway |
| 18 | Pyruvate kinase isozymes M1/M2 (KPYM) | P14618 | 71.16 | 4.40 | 57.90 | 7.96 | +2.15 | •Alpha enolase •Beta enolase •Pyruvate dehydrogenase E1 subunits |
| 19 | Serine/threonine-protein phosphatase 2A 65 kDa regulatory subunit A alpha isoform (2AAA, PP2A) | P30153 | 76.30 | 4.25 | 65.18 | 4.96 | +1.52 | •RAF proto-oncogene serine/threonine kinase •Serine/threonine protein phosphatase isoforms •Protein KIAA0889 |
| 20 | Ribonuclease inhibitor (RINI) | P13489 | 58.50 | 3.90 | 49.94 | 4.71 | -2.18 | •TNF-α •TNF-R1 •NF-kappa-B-essential modulator |
| 21 | Tubulin beta chain (TBB5) | P07437 | 65.00 | 4.40 | 49.64 | 4.78 | -0.99 | •Kinesin-like protein (KIF1A) •Mitogen-activated protein kinase 10 •Dual specificity protein kinase TTK |
| 22 | Melanoma-associated antigen 4 (MAGA-4) | P43358 | 55.00 | 3.90 | 34.91 | 4.68 | -2.30 | •26S proteosome regulatory subunit p28 •B melanoma antigen 3 precursor •Cancer/testis antigen 2 |
| 23 | Annexin A11 (Calcyclin-associated annexin 50) (ANX11) | P50995 | 71.20 | 6.18 | 54.36 | 7.53 | -1.55 | •Programmed cell death protein 6 •40S ribosomal protein 24 •Calcyclin •DNA-directed RNA polymerase III |
| 24 | Eukaryotic translation initiation factor 3 subunit 2 | Q13347 | 48.00 | 5.10 | 36.48 | 5.38 | -1.00 | •Eukaryotic translation initiation factor subunits |
| 25 | 60S acidic ribosomal protein P0 (RLAO) | P05388 | 45.50 | 5.15 | 34.25 | 5.71 | -0.95 | •Ribosomal proteins •Elongation factor 1-gamma |
| 26 | Inosine-5'monophosphate dehydrogenase 2 (EC 1.1.1.205) (IMDH2) | P12268 | 71.16 | 6.00 | 55.77 | 6.44 | -2.00 | •Inosine-5'monophosphate dehydrogenase 1 •GMP synthase •GMP reductase 1 and 2 •AMP deaminase 1 and 3 |
| 27 | Aldehyde dehydrogenase 1A3 (EC 1.2.1.5) (AL1A3) | P47895 | 72.00 | 6.25 | 56.07 | 6.99 | -1.02 | •3-Hydroxyisobutyrate dehydrogenase •Acetyl-coenzyme A synthetase 2-like |
| 28 | Aldehyde dehydrogenase 1A3 (EC 1.2.1.5) (AL1A3) | P47895 | 72.00 | 6.35 | 56.07 | 6.99 | -0.99 | •3-Hydroxyisobutyrate dehydrogenase •Acetyl-coenzyme A synthetase 2-like |
| 29 | ATP synthase subunit beta, mitochondrial precursor (EC 3.6.3.14) | P06576 | 64.00 | 4.50 | 56.52 | 5.26 | -1.00 | •ATP synthase isoforms •NADH-ubiquinone oxidoreductase |
| 30 | Rab GDP dissociation inhibitor alpha (Rab GDI alpha) | P31150 | 76.32 | 4.30 | 50.55 | 5.00 | -0.97 | •RAB4A •RAB5A •RAB2 •RAB11A •RAB9A |

Table 6. Protein identification of differentially expressed proteins in kojic acid-treated A375 cells and the prediction of protein interaction partners

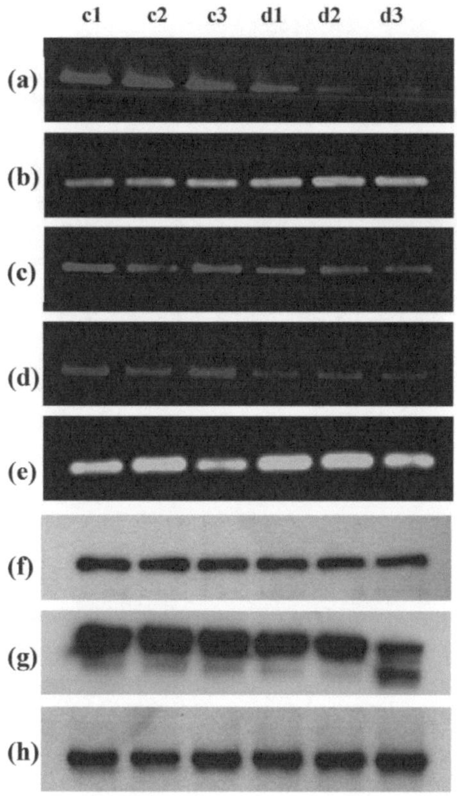


Fig. 4. Validation of differentially expressed proteins by Western blot and RT-PCR analyses. RT-PCR of (a) GRP75, (b) 2AAA, (c) HS90B (d) ENPL and (e) KPYM. Western blot of (f) GRP75, (g) VIME, and (h) 2AAA. c1, c2 and c3 indicate the control groups at 24, 48 and 72 h, respectively. d1, d2 and d3 indicate the treatment groups at 24, 48 and 72 h, respectively

The molecular weights of the proteins were distributed within the range of 25 to 97 kDa, and the differentially expressed protein spots had isoelectric points distributed between acidic and basic pH[29]. Using PDQuest image analysis software, approximately 540 spots were found in the control and treatment groups with no significant difference between the groups. There were 40 differentially expressed protein spots, including 10 up-regulated protein spots with a threshold of change in expression level of 1.0-fold, and 40 down-regulated protein spots with a threshold of change in expression level of 0.9-fold.

### 5.2 Identification of differentially expressed proteins

Using the MASCOT protein identification search software for identifying both PMF and MS/MS ion mass data, 26 differentially expressed proteins were successfully identified[29]. Among these proteins, there were five up-regulated and 15 down-regulated proteins (including their isoforms). Most of the identified proteins were downregulated in arbutin-treated A375 melanoma cells, and 13 isoforms of six identical proteins were observed. There were two vimentins, two heterogeneous nuclear ribonucleoproteins A2/B1, two heterogeneous nuclear ribonucleoproteins A1, two peroxiredoxin-1 proteins, three glyceraldehyde-3-phosphate dehydrogenases and two alpha-enolases, accounting for about

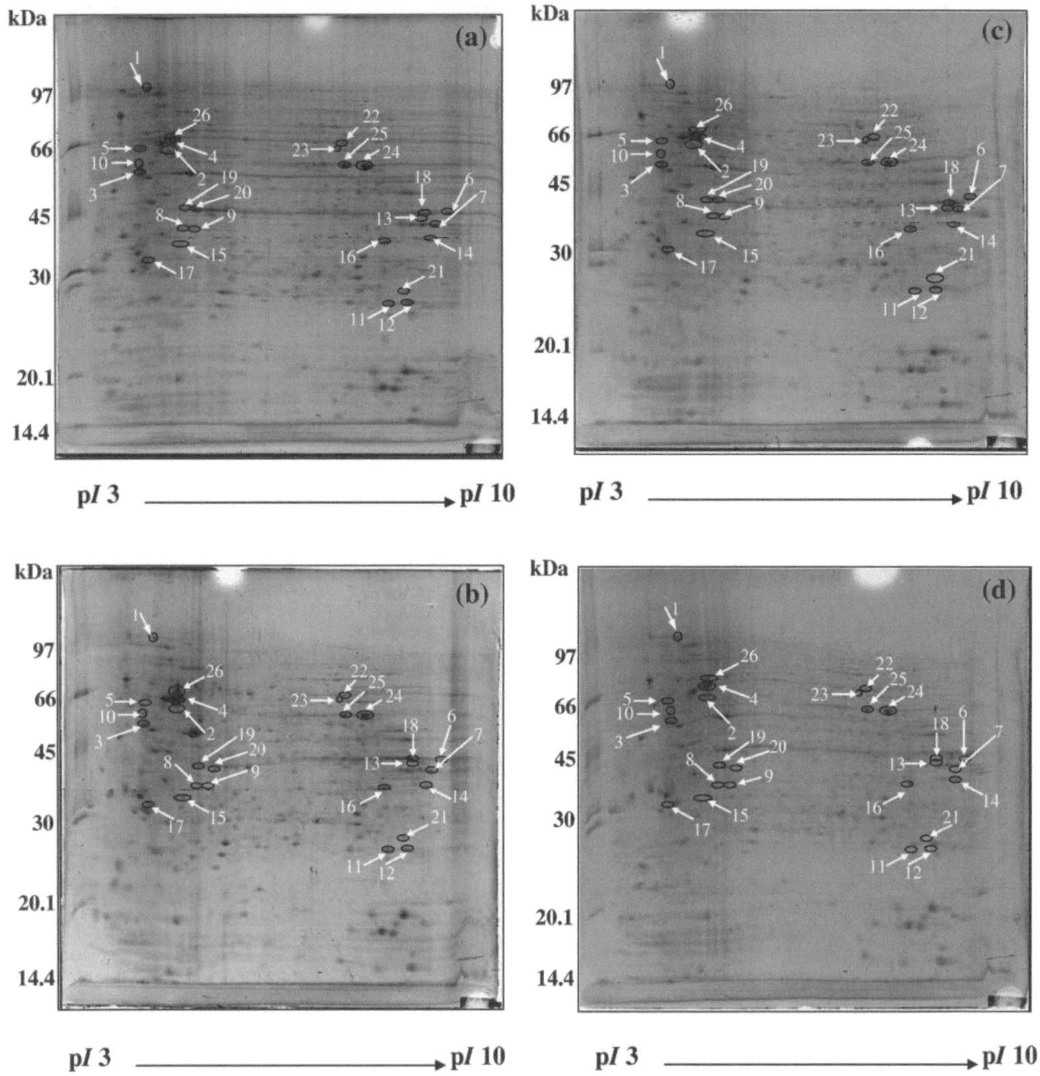


Fig. 5. 2-D PAGE images from A375 human malignant melanoma cells under the following conditions: (a) control, (b) 24-h arbutin treatment, (c) 48-h arbutin treatment and (d) 72-h arbutin treatment. The samples were separated on a homogeneous 12.5% SDS-PAGE gel using a pH 3–10 NL IPG strip. The pointed arrows indicate the protein spots identified in this study

50% of all identified proteins possibly due to post-translational modifications. The protein interaction partners are also predicted. The identified proteins are distributed to many locations within the cell, have diverse functions and play important roles in many biological processes, especially in cancer biology, such as apoptosis, angiogenesis, cell proliferation, cell differentiation and the immune response. Interestingly, five identified proteins, heat shock protein 90 kDa beta member 1 (ENPL), voltage-dependent anion-selective channel protein 1 (VDAC-1), chloride intracellular channel protein 1 (CLIC1), guanine nucleotide-binding protein subunit beta (GBLP) and 14-3-3 protein gamma (14-3-3G) (19% of total proteins), were found to play important roles in apoptosis and signal transduction. Additionally, six identified proteins (nine spots including their isoforms, 34.6% of total proteins), nuclear ribonucleoprotein H (HNRH1), ribonucleoproteins A2/B1 (ROA2), ribonucleoprotein A1 (ROA1), ribonuclease inhibitor (RINI), 14-3-3G and alpha-enolase (ENOA), function in nucleic acid processing or transcriptional regulation. Moreover, four identified proteins (seven spots including their isoforms, 27% of total proteins), malate dehydrogenase (MDHM), glyceraldehyde-3-phosphate dehydrogenase (G3P), glucose-6-phosphate 1-dehydrogenase (G6PD) and ENOA are involved in carbohydrate metabolism pathways and have additional functions in the regulation of cell growth and maintenance of cellular functions.

### 5.3 Validation by Western blot or RT-PCR

Of the identified proteins, vimentin (VIME), 14-3-3G, peroxiredoxin-1 (PRDX1), ENPL, inosine-5′-monophosphate dehydrogenase 2 (IMDH2), ENOA, VDAC-1 and p53 were validated by RT-PCR (Fig. 6). The protein and gene expression levels of eight differentially expressed proteins were in agreement with the 2-D PAGE expression data[29]. 14-3-3G, VDAC-1 and p53 were upregulated in the arbutin-treated A375 melanoma cells, whereas VIME, PRDX1, ENPL, IMDH2 and ENOA were downregulated in the arbutin-treated A375 melanoma cells.

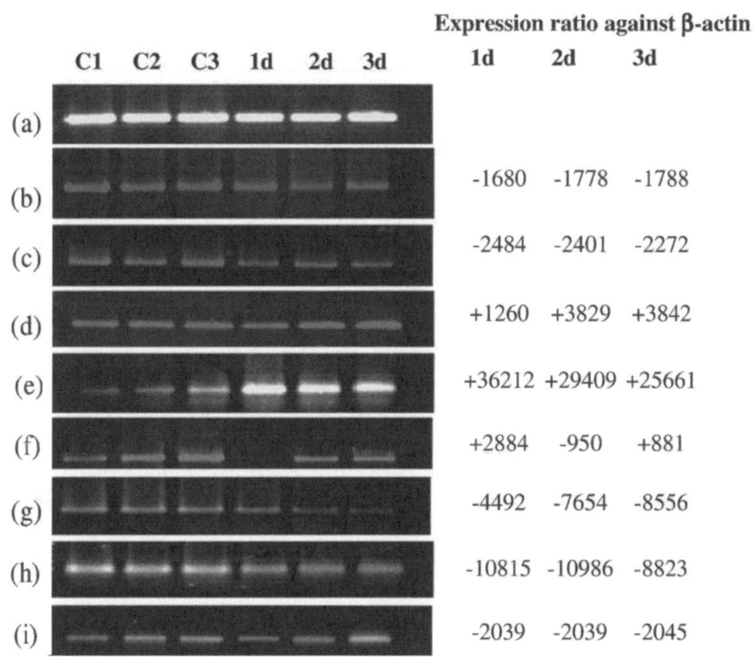


Fig. 6. Validation of differentially expressed proteins by RT-PCR analyses. (a) β-actin, (b) VIME, (c) ENPL, (d) 14-3-3G, (e) VDAC-1, (f) ENOA, (g) PROX1, (h) IMDH2 and (i) p53. C1, C2 and C3 indicate the control group at 24, 48 and 72 h, respectively. 1d, 2d and 3d indicate the treatment groups at 24, 48 and 72 h, respectively

## 6. Discussion

Although some of the biological applications and potential effects of kojic acid have been partially elucidated[30], the effects of kojic acid on a human genomics level, including gene regulatory mechanisms, are not clear and has rarely been reported. In this study, we used A375 human skin malignant melanoma cells to examine the genotoxicity of kojic acid in carcinoma therapy, not including its skin-whitening effect. To examine the genotoxicity effect of kojic acid on the gene expression profile of A375 melanoma cells, microarray technology providing a high-throughput method for easily screening the number of differentially expressed genes was used. It has been used for analysis of gene expression in dermatological studies, including studies of human melanomas[31]. However, the study of gene expression in kojic acid-stimulated A375 melanoma cells by DNA microarray has never been reported. It is challenging to use the high-throughput technology of DNA microarray for studying the effect of kojic acid on the large numbers of differentially expressed genes in A375 melanoma cells and its anti-tumorigenic function to regulate the malignancy of melanoma. We used the human 1A oligonucleotide microarray to analyze gene expression of human skin A375 melanoma cells for the following reasons: (i) the human 1A oligonucleotide microarray is comprised of 20,173 oligonucleotide probes that span conserved exons across transcripts of 18,716 human genes, is compatible with human skin A375 melanoma cells and could screen large numbers of differentially expressed human genes at a single time. (ii) The human 1A oligonucleotide microarray uses a convenient two-color labeling procedure that reduces experimental variability by allowing biological samples to be directly compared with each other on the same microarray after undergoing the same hybridization incubation. This microarray platform allowed the analysis of kojic acid-responding genes in A375 melanoma cells that may be used as gene markers of malignant melanoma for diagnostic and therapeutic applications in human skin. We examined the effect of various concentrations (0.32, 1.6, 8, 40, 200 and 1000 μg/ml) of kojic acid on growth inhibition of A375 melanoma cells. Not all kojic acid concentrations strongly inhibited the cell growth of A375 melanoma cells, even at the longer incubation time of 72 h. When using microarray technology to study the overall effects of kojic acid on gene expression of A375 melanoma cells, we used 8 μg/ml (0.8%) kojic acid because this is the mildest concentration that could inhibit A375 melanoma cells less than 20% while avoiding potential differences in gene expression data resulting from the cell death response due to cytotoxicity from higher concentrations of kojic acid. The safe level of kojic acid in human skin care products for general use is up to 1% without a prescription[24]. Therefore, 8 μg/ml kojic acid (0.8%) is safe for human skin and can be used to study the gene expression profile of A375 melanoma cells and identify the regulatory functions of these genes in carcinogenesis therapy. After microarray data were collected, we used bioinformatic tools to identify the differentially expressed genes and searched Gene Ontology for useful information. The information obtained can be used to further study regulatory mechanisms and gene markers for applications in early cancer diagnosis and therapy. For a number of differentially expressed genes, we selected significant genes involved in carcinogenesis and compared microarray analysis data with RT-qPCR data to validate changes in gene expression. RT-qPCR offered confirmatory quantitative results under stringent conditions. We show the quantification of kojic acid-responding genes from RT-qPCR is in agreement with the DNA microarray expression data. This indicates that the validation of genes in the robust biomarkers lists was done using precise data. These validated genes may become useful biomarkers to understand the biochemistry of a drug/small molecule response in future clinical studies. Interestingly, we have found seven significant kojic acid-responsive genes downregulated in kojic acid-stimulated A375 melanoma cells. Most of the genes are related to the regulation of carcinogenesis. Apolipoprotein B mRNA editing enzyme, catalytic polypeptide 1 (APOBEC1), is the central component of an RNA editosome, whose physiological role is the deamination of apoB mRNA cytidine-6666 to uracil in gastrointestinal tissues, thereby creating a premature stop codon[32]. Uncontrolled cytidine deamination could generate inappropriately folded polypeptides, dominant-negative proteins, or mutations in tumor suppressor genes and thus contribute to tumor formation[33] . Overexpression of APOBEC1 has led to the development of a number of different cancers, such as gastrointestinal cancer, colon cancer and heptocellular cancer, in a variety of tissues. This implies that inappropriate expression of a member of the DNA deaminase family could have potential oncogenic activity[34]. Furthermore, most human carcinomas are caused by APOBEC1-mediated mRNA editing[35]. Thus, down-regulated APOBEC1 may potentially deactivate the tumor progression of A375 melanoma cells.

In conclusion, we used high-throughput DNA microarray and RT-qPCR techniques for the global analysis of differentially expressed genes responding to kojic acid in A375 human melanoma cells. The differentially expressed genes were classified depending on cellular localization, molecular function and biological process, and they led to an exploration of the more valuable data on the regulation of melanoma carcinogenesis against kojic acid. In addition, seven of the down-regulated genes that showed significantly different expression in A375 melanoma cells after kojic acid treatment function as tumor suppressors and may disrupt the regulation of melanoma tumorigenesis in human malignant melanoma cells. These genes may be useful markers in further diagnostic and therapeutic applications. Moreover, our findings show the probable side effects and disadvantages of kojic acid due to its effect on the immune system, bone development and maintenance. However, we will further study the effects of kojic acid on biological and molecular mechanisms in human melanoma skin cells, including in other parts of the body, and also examine other biological functions of kojic acid in its cosmetic and/or therapeutic applications. We also examined the effect of different arbutin concentrations on the growth inhibition of A375 melanoma cells and found that the concentrations used did not strongly inhibit cell growth, even though the incubation time was up to 72 h. We used 8 μg/ml (0.8% w/v) arbutin because (i) this was the same concentration of kojic acid used[18], because this concentration was lower than the safety recommendation of 1% in prescription human skin care products[36]; (ii) this concentration inhibited cell growth less than 10% with no morphological change of cells; and (iii) it avoids changes in gene expression data resulting from the cell death response due to cytotoxicity from a high concentration of arbutin. Therefore, 8 μg/ml arbutin, which is safe for use on human skin, was used to study the genotoxic effect on the gene expression profile of A375 melanoma cells and for examining the differential gene expression and other side effects of altered signaling pathways for cancer therapy. To study the effect of arbutin on the gene expression level of A375 melanoma cells, RNA was isolated from cells 24 h after arbutin treatment to study gene expression levels with microarray analysis.

We also used high-throughput DNA microarray and bioinformatic tools in a global analysis of differentially expressed genes in arbutin-treated A375 malignant melanoma cells. These genes were classified by Gene Ontology and led to an exploration of more valuable data on the regulation of melanoma carcinogenesis. In addition, four down-regulated genes are candidate tumor suppressor genes in A375 melanoma cells following arbutin treatment.

They may disrupt the regulation of malignant tumorigenesis in human malignant melanoma cells and may be useful markers for further diagnostic and therapeutic applications. Moreover, the genotoxic effect of arbutin on the gene expression profile of A375 melanoma cells was similar to kojic acid, which indicates a similar regulation of malignant tumorigenesis by these drugs. However, we will conduct further studies on the effects of arbutin on biological and molecular mechanisms in human skin cells. We will also examine other biological characteristics of arbutin for therapeutic applications. According to our study investigating the toxicogenomic effects of kojic acid on the gene expression profile of A375 melanoma cells using microarray analysis, the cell growth inhibition was not strongly affected by all concentrations of kojic acid at a longer treatment time of 72 h[18]. There was no morphological change of A375 melanoma cells over the 72 h exposure to 8 μg/ml kojic acid, which is a mild concentration and the recommended safe dose of kojic acid for human skin. The early stage of the kojic acid stimulatory effect on the gene expression profile of A375 melanoma cells also uncovered some tumor suppressor genes. Although one gene makes one protein, protein modifications leading to changes in biological and physiological functions may not be caused by gene modifications. To examine the effects of kojic acid on protein expression levels in A375 melanoma cells, the same concentration of kojic acid (8 μg/ml) as in the microarray study, which is compliant with the safety recommendation in human skin care products, and various treatment times (24, 48 and 72 h) were used in this study. 2-D PAGE identified 30 differentially expressed proteins that showed a significant change in expression levels following 72 h of drug treatment. We used combined databases to propose a protein interaction network in which 16 differentially expressed proteins are involved in the regulation of apoptosis via major signaling proteins, such as p53, Ras, MEK/ERK, RAF-1 and Bcl-2. Interestingly, 11 chaperone proteins were downregulated in kojic acid-treated A375 melanoma cells and were found to interact with each other. It is well known that heat shock proteins are required for cell survival during stress and also have key functions in controlling cellular metabolism[37]. In cancer biology, heat shock proteins are expressed at high levels during facilitated tumor cell growth and survival[38]. In addition, GRP75, GRP78 and HSP90 interact with the p53 tumor suppressor[39]. HSP90B has a principal role in the regulation of mitogenesis and cell cycle progression and could interact with HSP70 or GRP75 to participate in the protein degradation process and protection from programmed cell death. HSP7C interacts with the Bcl-2 binding proteins athanogene-1 and athanogene-3 and other chaperone proteins, including HS90B and ENPL.
According to our results of down-regulated heat shock proteins in kojic acid-treated A375 melanoma cells, cellular stress in malignant melanoma cells was observed following kojic acid treatment. Kojic acid could suppress the expression of heat shock proteins, which support tumor growth and may lead to an antiapoptosis effect. Alternatively, because a primary mechanism for the regulation of heat shock proteins in normal cells involves the tumor repressor p53 and the related protein p63, the downregulation of heat shock proteins may be involved in the suppression of p53 expression. It has also been reported that p53 and p63 proteins suppress the transcription of heat shock protein-encoding genes via their promoter binding sites for the transcription factor NF-Y[40]. The suppression of heat shock protein expression by kojic acid may play an important role in its antitumor activity. The 70-kDa heat shock cognate protein (HSP7C) is a member of the HSP70 heat shock protein family. HSC/HSP70 function is regulated by the chaperone Bcl-2-associated gene product-1 (BAG-1), which acts as a coupling factor between HSC/HSP70 and a proteasome component[41]. BAG-family proteins also contain the BAG-domain, which mediates a direct

interaction with HSP70, the ATPase domain and a number of client proteins, including the protein kinase Raf-1[42]. Raf-1 is an important signaling molecule that functions in the Ras pathway to transmit mitogenic, differentiative and oncogenic signals to the downstream kinases MEK and ERK[43]. According to the BioCarta pathway of melanogenesis, Raf-1, Ras, MEK and ERK are important regulatory proteins in melanocytes. HSP70 also has an important role in the cotranslational maturation pathway of the human type I membrane glycoprotein tyrosinase, which interacts with calreticulin and BiP/Grp78 during its ER transit[44]. Thus, the HSP7C associated with heat shock proteins can interact with regulatory molecules in the melanogenesis pathway, in which these proteins are upstream regulators of other melanogenic enzymes, including tyrosinase and tyrosinase related protein-1.

The protein phosphatase 2AAA (or PP2A) was found to interact with hyperphosphorylated/desensitized Raf-1[45]. 2AAA is required for recycling of Raf-1 to an activation-competent state and for melanosome aggregation, and it interacts with p53, Raf-1 and Bcl-2. 2AAA is also a major Ser/Thr phosphatase implicated in the regulation of many cellular processes, including many signal transduction pathways and cell-cycle progression[46]. In cancer cells, 2AAA has been proposed to negatively regulate cellular growth and might function as a tumor suppressor[47]. Confirmation by Western blot analysis showed 2AAA is upregulated in kojic acid-treated A375 melanoma cells at 48 and 72 h. It has been suggested that kojic acid may stimulate the expression of 2AAA, leading to suppression of signaling molecules in melanogenesis. According to 2-D gel analysis, 6 isoforms of vimentin were downregulated in kojic acid-treated A375 melanoma cells. It is well known that vimentin regulates cell migration, membrane trafficking, granular secretion, protein kinase activation and regulation of stress response proteins[48]. The modification of vimentin isoforms might be caused by phosphorylation, which has a central role in regulating the dynamics of vimentin assembly into polymers as well as in regulating the connections between intermediate filament (IF) and IF-associated proteins[49]. There are many phosphorylation events affecting vimentin. For example, phosphorylation by Raf-1-associated vimentin kinase results in the proper structure of vimentin filaments[50] and phosphorylation by protein kinase C (PKC) creates isoforms that participate in the regulation of organelle movement in melanophores and many signal transduction pathways involving tyrosine kinase, nucleotide exchange factor, serine/threonine kinase, Raf-1, PKC, cytoskeletal protein actin, proteosome component and HSC70[51]. In addition to phosphorylation, the different spots of vimentin seen on the 2-D gel may be due to association with other molecules, such as protein kinase C, integrin or other associated proteins in signal transduction pathways. Changes in vimentin expression levels are also generated by stress, such as heat shock and oxidative stress[52]. Cleavage of vimentin precedes the recognition of cytoskeletal filaments in apoptosis and programmed cell death mechanisms. Downregulation of vimentin expression inhibits migration and invasion of colon and breast cancer cell lines[53]. According to our Western blot analysis, down-regulated vimentin may suppress tumorigenesis and regulate apoptosis in kojic acid-treated A375 melanoma cells. Moreover, the presence of more than one protein band recognized by the monoclonal antibody of vimentin may be caused by post-translational modifications. Another protein that leads to tumor suppression is pyruvate kinase isoenzyme (KPYM). It is a key sensor for energy consumption and regulation of the glycolytic pathway, in which KPYM links energy-rich metabolites from the flow of glucose carbons to nucleic acid[54]. In yeast cells, overexpression of pyruvate kinases leads to an inhibition of cell proliferation by depletion of glycolytic phosphometabolites. Likewise, pyruvate kinases in eukaryotic cells are involved in such fundamental processes as cell proliferation, tumor formation and apoptosis[55]. Energy used by cancer cells is preferentially produced from glycolysis, in which p53 was found to modulate the balance between the utilization of the respiratory and glycolytic pathways[56]. According to our results from 2-D PAGE and Western blot data, KPYM upregulated in kojic acid-treated A375 melanoma cells may play an important role in the suppression of tumor growth and metastasis. In summary, we identified a number of differentially expressed proteins in kojic acid-treated A375 melanoma cells. Most of these proteins were key factors involved in a wide variety of cellular processes, including cell proliferation, regulation of gene expression, signaling, and chromatin and cytoskeleton organization. Interestingly, our proposed interaction network reveals proteins associated with the regulation of apoptosis, which may lead to suppression of the melanogenesis and tumorigenesis of cancer cells. Moreover, these proteins may be useful biomarkers for use in diagnostic and therapeutic applications of skin cancer. Further functional studies of these proteins may lead to better understanding of the pathogenic mechanisms and cellular response to kojic acid treatment.

According to our investigation of the toxicogenomic effects of arbutin on the gene expression profile of A375 melanoma cells using microarray[26], there was no growth inhibition or morphological change of A375 melanoma cells after 72 h in the presence of 8 μg/ml arbutin, which is a mild arbutin concentration and safe for human skin. The gene expression data showed some tumor suppressor genes as biomarkers in A375 melanoma cells. Although one gene makes one protein, post-translational modifications of proteins can lead to changes in biological and physiological functions that may not result from gene modification. To examine the effects of arbutin on protein expression levels in A375 melanoma cells, the same concentration of arbutin (8 μg/ml) at different treatment times of 24, 48 and 72 h was used. Among the differentially expressed proteins validated by RT-qPCR, VIME, 14-3-3G and VDAC-1 were found to interact with Raf-1. VIME, an IF protein, is the major cytoskeleton component of developing cancer cells. VIME is phosphorylated by Raf-1-associated vimentin kinase, resulting in the regulation of the vimentin filament structure[57]. VIME is also a target for phosphorylation by PKC, which is involved in many signal transduction pathways including the regulation of organelle movement in melanophores[58], cytoskeletal function and programmed cell death (apoptosis)[59]. In carcinoma cell lines, downregulation of VIME expression resulted in impaired migration and adhesion[60]. Likewise, our RT-qPCR results show that VIME is downregulated in arbutin-treated A375 melanoma cells, suggesting an effect on the IF network that ultimately leads to impaired migration and adhesion of A375 melanoma cells. Because VIME is involved in the regulation of stress response proteins[61], the heat shock protein ENPL, also found to be downregulated in A375 melanoma cells in this study, may be involved in VIME regulation. ENPL is a member of the heat shock protein HSP90 complex found in the melanosome. It is well known that heat shock proteins are overexpressed in a wide range of human cancers and are implicated in tumor cell proliferation, differentiation and recognition by the immune system[62]. Therefore, the ENPL downregulated in arbutin-treated A375 melanoma cells may suppress tumor progression and metastasis and cause the decreased immune response.

ENPL was also found to be associated with other types of heat shock proteins and interacts with p53 and 14-3-3 proteins, both of which play important roles in apoptosis. 14-3-3 proteins act as control points for many cellular processes and therefore play significant roles in cell-fate determination and in several apoptotic pathways in animals[63]. 14-3-3 proteins have been reported to have important interactions with other regulatory proteins. They display important anti-apoptotic characteristics by inhibiting the pro-apoptotic Bcl-2-antagonist of cell death (BAD) and the transcription factor FKHRL-1. Major roles ascribed to the mammalian 14-3-3 proteins include activation of tyrosine and tryptophan hydroxylases, regulation of PKC, exocytosis, especially in mediating interactions between protein kinases, and other signal transduction proteins[64]. 14-3-3 was found to activate the Ras-Raf mitogenic pathway and can elicit a physiologically significant activation of Raf-1 in mammalian cells[65]. Because 14-3-3 proteins are involved in a great number of interactions, the effects of knocking out or overexpressing specific 14-3-3 genes or 14-3-3 target genes will likely have effects on other 14-3-3-regulated cellular processes. Studies have found that 14-3-3 proteins activate p53 function *in vivo*; thus, the up-regulation of 14-3-3G protein expression in arbutin-treated A375 melanoma cells implies that arbutin can stimulate changes in signal transduction pathways by stabilizing or increasing the expression of 14-3-3[66]. The increase in protein expression might involve a critical response of cell proliferation, differentiation and apoptosis of arbutin-treated A375 melanoma cells. The change in the expression of 14-3-3 might alter the biological activities of p53, RAF-1, CLIC1, ENPL, Bcl2 and kinesin-like proteins. Interestingly, the partial functions of ENPL and VDAC-1 on ion channel activity and ion sequestering ability are involved in energy metabolism, which is important for survival. The cellular location of these proteins at the cell membrane and mitochondria implies that the effect of arbutin on membrane and mitochondria may cause changes in cellular physiology and metabolic events. VDAC-1, a major mitochondrial outer membrane transporter, is a component of the permeability transition (PT) and plays an important role in apoptosis by participating in the release of intermembrane space proteins, including cytochrome c, and by its involvement in $Ca^{2+}$ signaling[67]. VDAC-1 has also been found to be associated with the Bax/Bak and Bcl-2 families of proteins, which are essential regulators of cell death and exert their primary pro- or anti-apoptotic roles at the mitochondrial outer membrane. Therefore, the upregulation of VDAC-1 expression in arbutin-treated A375 melanoma cells may play a crucial role in mitochondria-mediated apoptosis, mitochondrial membrane permeability transition and intracellular $Ca^{2+}$ transport. Alternatively, p53 tumor suppressor proteins have been reported to have additional roles in the regulation of glycolysis.

In this study, four proteins identified as glycolytic enzymes, G3P, ENOA, G6PD and MDHM, were found to be involved in glucose metabolism, but only ENOA was validated by RT-PCR. The low expression of ENOA in arbutin-treated A375 melanoma cells may be implicated in metastasis and may also change the associated signaling pathways that modulate cellular metabolism. In addition to regulating glycolysis in cancer cells, p53 also helps to regulate both apoptosis and intracellular reactive oxygen species (ROS) levels. Additionally, peroxiredoxin-1 (PROX1) is one of the antioxidant enzymes and is involved in cellular proliferation and differentiation. The ability of PROX1 to enhance cell survival is traditionally attributed to its capacity to remove ROS[68]. Indeed, lower PROX1 activity increased levels of ROS and induced p53 expression. Therefore, the level of p53 is a major determinant of the effect of decreased PROX1 expression on tumor growth and the response of cells to treatment. This agrees with our results showing up-regulated p53 and down-regulated PROX1 in arbutin-treated A375 melanoma cells. In addition to energy metabolism, arbutin may also affect nucleotide metabolism because ribonucleoproteins (HNRH1, ROA2, ROA1), ribonuclease inhibitor (RINI) and inosine-5′-monophosphate dehydrogenase (IMDH2) were affected by arbutin treatment. IMDH2 is a regulatory enzyme of guanine nucleotide biosynthesis and is also strategically positioned in the metabolic pathway of thiopurines. Increased mRNA expression levels and enzymatic activity of IMPDH2 have been observed in rapidly proliferating tumor cells. IMDH2 has been established as an anticancer target. Therefore, downregulation of IMDH2 may suppress nucleotide biosynthesis, cell proliferation and malignancy of A375 melanoma cells. According to our proteomic results, many identified proteins, including heat shock proteins, glucose-regulated proteins and other proteins, were found to be associated with p53, which is a major tumor-suppressor protein and plays significant roles in many biological processes in cancer development. Moreover, p53 has biological roles in pigmentation. Tumor suppressor p53 could down- and upregulate tissue-specific expression of the tyrosinase gene in human melanoma cell lines. Therefore, arbutin has potent effects on both protein and gene expression and leads to the suppression of melanogenesis and tumorigenesis of A375 melanoma cells. However, the correlation of protein and gene expression with biological function will be further studied to better understand the effect of arbutin on the biology of A375 malignant melanoma cancer cells. In summary, we identified differentially expressed proteins in arbutin-treated A375 melanoma cells. Most of these proteins were key players in a wide variety of cellular processes, including cell proliferation, regulation of protein expression and signaling pathways.

## 7. References

[1] Braud, F.; Khayat, D.; Kroon, B. B. R.; Valdagni, R.; Bruzzi, P. & Cascinelli, N. (2003). Malignant melanoma. *Critical Reviews in Oncology/Hematology*, 47(1), 35-63.

[2] Cheng, S. L.; Huang-Liu, R.; Sheu, J. N.; Chen, S. T.; Sinchaikul, S. & Tsay G. J. (2007). Toxicogenomics of A375 human malignant melanoma cells. *Pharmacogenomics,* 8 (8), 1017-1036.

[3] Soengas, M. S.; Capodieci, P.; Polsky, D.; Mora, J.; Esteller, M.; Opitz-Araya, X.; McCombie, R.; Herman, J. G.; Gerald, W. L.; Lazebnik, Y. A.; Cordón-Cardó, C. & Lowe, S. W. (2001). Inactivation of the apoptosis effector *Apaf-1* in malignant melanoma. *Nature*, 409, 207-211.

[4] Pennie, W. D.; Tugwood, J. D.; Oliver, G. J. A. & Kimber, I. (2000). The principles and practical of toxicogenomics: applications and opportunity. *Toxicol. Sci.*, 54 (2), 277-283.

[5] Kwak, M. Y. & Rhee, J. S. (1992). Cultivation characteristics of immobilized *Aspergillus oryzae* for kojic acid production. *Biotechnol Bioeng*, 39 (9), 903-906.

[6] Masse, M. O.; Duvallet, V.; Borremans, M. & Goeyens, L. (2001). Identification and quantitative analysis of kojic acid and arbutin in skin-whitening cosmetics. *International Journal of Cosmetic Science*, 23(4), 219-232.

[7] Beard, R. L. & Walton, G. S. (1969). Kojic acid as an insecticidal mycotoxin. *Journal of Insect Physiology*, 14(1), 53-59.

[8] Higa, Y.; Ohkubo, A.; Kitajima, S.; Moriyasu, M. & Kariya K. (2002). Effects of kojic acid on thyroidal functions in rats by single-dose administration and in cultured rat thyroid cells (frtl-5 cells). *The Journal of Toxicological Sciences*, 27, 423-431.

[9] Lee, H. F.; Boltjes, B. & Eisenman, W. (1950). Kojic acid as an inhibitor of tubercle bacilli. *Am. Rev. Tuberculosis*, 61(5), 738-741.

[10] Nohynek, G. J.; Kirkland, D.; Marzin, D.; Toutain, H.; Leclerc-Ribaud, C. & Jinnai, H. (2004). An assessment of the genotoxicity and human health risk of topical use of

kojic acid [5-hydroxy-2-(hydroxymethyl)-4H-pyran-4-one]. *Food and Chemical Toxicology*, 42(1), 93-105.

[11] Hirose, M.; Nishikawa, A.; Shibutani, M. & Mitsumori K. (2001). Environmental agents, endocrine disrupting chemicals and rat thyroid carcinogenesis. *Joural of Toxicologic Pathology*, 14, 71-77.

[12] Takizawa, T.; Imai, T.; Onose, J. I.; Ueda, M.; Tamura, T.; Mitsumori, K.; Izumi, K. & Hirose M. (2004). Enhancement of hepatocarcinogenesis by kojic acid in rat two-stage models after initiation with *N*-bis(2-hydroxypropyl)nitrosamine or *N*-diethylnitrosamine. *Toxicology Sciences*, 81, 43-49 (2004).

[13] Tomita, K.; Fukuda, M. & Kawasaki, K. (1990). Mechanism of arbutin inhibitory effect on melanogenesis and effect on the human skin with cosmetic use. *Fragrance J.* 6, 72-77.

[14] Sugimoto, K.; Nishimura, T.; Nomura, K.; Sugimoto, K. & Kuriki, T. (2004). Inhibitory effects of α-arbutin on melanin synthesis in cultured human melanoma cells and a threedimensional human skin model. *Biol. Pharm. Bull.*, 27(4), 510-514.

[15] Slominski, A.; Tobin, D. J.; Shibahara, S. & Wortsman, J. (2004). Melanin pigmentation in mammalian skin and its hormonal regulation. *Physiol. Rev.*, 84, 1155-1228.

[16] Shibata, T.; Prota, G. & Mishima, Y. (1993). Non-melanosomal regulatory factors in melanogenesis. *J. Invest. Dermatol.*, 100, S274-S280.

[17] Mantripragada, K. K.; Buckley, P. G.; Stahl, T. D. & Dumanski J. P. (2004). Genomic microarrays in the spotlight. *Trends in Genetics*, 20(2), 87-94.

[18] Cheng, S. L.; Liu, H. R.; Sheu, J. N.; Chen, S. T.; Sinchaikul, S. & Tsay, G. J. (2006). Toxicogenomics of kojic acid on gene expression profiling of A375 human malignant melanoma cells. *Biol. Pharm. Bull.*, 29, 655-669.

[19] O'Donnell, R.; Holland, J. W.; Deeth, H. C. & Alewood, P. (2004). Milk proteomics. *Int. Dairy J.*, 14, 1013-1023.

[20] Larsen, L. B.; Wedholm, A.; Møller, H. S.; Andrén, A. & Lindmark-Månsson, H. (2007). Proteomic study of regressions between milk yield and whey protein composition. *J. Anim. Feed Sci.*, 16, 200-206.

[21] Chevalier, F. & Kelly, A. L. (2010). Proteomic quantification of disulfide-linked polymers in raw and heated bovine milk. *J. Agric. Food Chem.*, 58(12), 7437-7444.

[22] Nelson, D. L. & Cox, M. M. (2005). Amino acids, Peptides, and Proteins. New York: W. H. Freeman and Company. pp. 79-95.

[23] Miralles, B.; Leaver, J.; Ramos, M. & Amigo, L. (2003). Mass mapping analysis as a tool for the identification of genetic variants of bovine β-casein. *Journal of Chromatography A*, 1007(1-2), 47-53.

[24] Burdock, G. A.; Soni, M. G. & Carabin, I. G. (2001). Evaluation of health aspects of kojic acid in food. *Toxicol. Pharmacol.*, 33, 80-101.

[25] Fujino, T.; Navaratnam, N. & Scott, J. (1998). Human apolipoprotein B RNA editing deaminase gene (APOBEC1). *Genomics*, 47, 266-275.

[26] Cheng, S. L.; Liu, R. H.; Sheu, J. N.; Chen, S. T.; Sinchaikul, S. & Tsay, G. J. (2007). Toxicogenomics of A375 human malignant melanoma cells treated with arbutin. *J. Biomed. Sci.*, 14, 87-105.

[27] Tiedtke, J.; Morel, J. & Marks, O. (2004). Depigmentation factor bioflavonoids-a safe and effective skin lightener based on encapsulated citrus bioflavonoids. *Cosmetochem* 2, 12-17.

[28] Nawarak, J.; Huang-Liu, R.; Kao, S. H.; Liao, H. H.; Sinchaikul, S.; Chen, S. T. & Cheng, S. L. (2008). Proteomics analysis of kojic acid treated A375 human malignant melanoma cells. *J Proteome Res.*, 7: 3737-3746.

[29] Nawarak, J.; Huang-Liu, R.; Kao, S. H.; Liao, H. H.; Sinchaikul, S.; Chen, S. T. & Cheng, S. L. (2009). Proteomics analysis of A375 human malignant melanoma cells in response to arbutin treatment. *Biochim Biophys Acta.*, 1794: 159-167.

[30] Wiechers, J. W.; Rawlings, A. V.; Garcial, C.; Chesne, C.; Balaguer, P.; Nicolas, J. C.; Corre, S. & Galibert, M. D. (2005). A new mechanism of action for skin whitening agents: binding to the peroxisome proliferator-activated receptor. *Int. J. Cosmetic Sci.*, 27(2), 123-132.

[31] Kunz, M.; Ibrahim, S. M.; Koczan, D.; Scheid, S.; Thiesen, H. J. & Gross, G. (2004). DNA microarray technology and its applications in dermatology. *Exp. Dermatol.*, 13(10), 593-606.

[32] Petersen-Mahrt, S. K. & Neuberger, M. S. (2003). *In vitro* deamination of cytosine to uracil in single-stranded DNA by apolipoprotein B editing complex catalytic subunit 1 (APOBEC1). *J. Biol. Chem.*, 278, 19583-19586.

[33] Morgan, H. D.; Dean, W.; Coker, H. A.; Reik, W. & Petersen-Mahrt, S. K. (2004). Activation-induced cytidine deaminase deaminates 5-methylcytosine in DNA and is expressed in pluripotent tissues. *J. Biol. Chem.*, 279, 52353-52360.

[34] Beale, R. C. L.; Petersen-Mahrt, S. K.; Wat, I. N.; Harris, R. S.; Rada, C. & Neuberger, M. S. (2004). Comparison of the differential context-dependence of DNA deamination by APOBEC enzymes: correlation with mutation spectra *in vivo*. *J. Mol. Biol.*, 337(3), 585-596.

[35] Chester, A.; Scott, J.; Anant, S. & Navaratnam, N. (2000). RNA editing: cytidine to uridine conversion in apolipoprotein B mRNA. *Biochim. Biophys. Acta*, 1494(1-2), 1-13.

[36] Tiedtke, J.; Morel, J. & Marks, O. (2004). Depigmentation factor bioflavonoids-a safe and effective skin lightener based on encapsulated citrus bioflavonoids. *Cosmetochem*, 2, 12-17.

[37] Beere, H. M. (2004). The stress of dying: the role of heat shock proteins in the regulation of apoptosis. *J. Cell Sci.*, 117, 2641-2651.

[38] Ciocca, D. R. & Calderwood, S. K. (2005). Heat shock proteins in cancer: diagnostic, prognostic, predictive, and treatment implications. *Cell Stress Chaperones*, 10, 86-103.

[39] Muller, L.; Schaupp, A.; Walerych, D.; Wegele, H. & Buchner, J. (2004). Hsp90 regulates the activity of wild type p53 under physiological and elevated temperatures. *J. Biol. Chem.* 279, 48846-48854.

[40] Wu, G.; Osada, M.; Guo, Z.; Fomenkov, A.; Begum, S.; Zhao, M.; Upadhyay, S.; Xing, M.; Wu, F.; Moon, C.; Westra, W. H.; Koch, W. M.; Mantovani, R.; Califano, J. A.; Ratovitski, E.; Sidransky, D. & Trink, B. (2005). ΔNp63alpha up-regulates the *Hsp70* gene in human cancer. *Cancer Research*, 65, 758-766.

[41] Luders, J.; Demand, J. & Hohfeld, J. (2000). The ubiquitin-regulated BAG-$_1$ provides a link between the molecular chaperones Hsc$_{70}$/Hsp$_{70}$ and the proteosome. *J. Biol. Chem.* 275, 4613-4617.

[42] Takayama, S.; Bimston, D. N.; Matsuzawa, S.; Freeman, B. C.; Aime-Sempe, C.; Xie, Z.; Morimoto, R. I. & Reed, J. C. (1997). BAG-1 modulates the chaperone activity of Hsp70/Hsc70. *EMBO J.*, 16, 4887-4896.

[43] Wang, N.; Daniels, R. & Hebert, D. N. (2005). The cotranslational maturation of the type I membrane glycoprotein tyrosinase: The heat shock protein 70 system hands off to the lectin-based chaperone system. *Mol. Biol. Cell* 16, 3740-3752.

[44] Popescu, C. I.; Paduraru, C.; Dwek, R. A. & Petrescu, S. M. (2005). Soluble tyrosinase is an endoplasmic reticulum (ER)-associated degradation substrate retained in the ER by calreticulin and BiP/GRP$_{78}$ and not calnexin. *J. Biol. Chem.*, 280, 13833-13840.

[45] Dougherty, M. K.; Muller, J.; Ritt, D. A.; Zhou, M.; Zhou, X. Z.; Copeland, T. D.; Conrads, T. P.; Veenstra, T. D.; Lu, K. P. & Morrison, D. K. (2005). Regulation of Raf-1 by direct feedback phosphorylation. *Mol. Cell*, 17(2), 215-224.

[46] Janssens, V. & Goris, J. (2001). Protein phosphatase 2A: a highly regulated family of serine/threonine phosphatases implicated in cell growth and signalling. *Biochem. J.*, 353, 417-439.

[47] Schonthal, A. H. (2001). Role of serine/threonine protein phosphatase 2A in cancer. *Cancer Letter*, 170, 1-13.

[48] Wang, N. & Stamenovic, D. (2002). Mechanics of vimentin intermediate filaments. J. Muscle Res. *Cell Motil.*, 23, 535-540.

[49] Ku, N. O.; Liao, J. & Omary, M. B. (1998). Phosphorylation of human keratin 18 serine 33 regulates binding to 14-3-3 proteins. *EMBO J.*, 17, 1892-1906.

[50] Janosch, P.; Kieser, A.; Eulitz, M.; Lovric, J.; Sauer, G.; Reichert, M.; Gounari, F.; Büscher, D.; Baccarini, M.; Mischak, H. & Kolch, W. (2000). The Raf-$_1$ kinase associates with vimentin kinases and regulates the structure of vimentin filaments. *FASEB J.*, 14, 2008-2021.

[51] Ivaska, J.; Vuoriluoto, K.; Huovinen, T.; Izawa, I.; Inagaki, M. & Parker, P. J. (2005). PKC$\varepsilon$-mediated phosphorylation of vimentin controls integrin recycling and motility. *EMBO J.*, 24, 3834-3845.

[52] Paron, I.; D'Elia, A.; D'Ambrosio, C.; Scaloni, A.; D'Aurizio, F.; Prescott, A.; Damante, G. & Tell, G. (2004). A proteomic approach to identify early molecular targets of oxidative stress in human epithelial lens cells. *Biochem. J.*, 378, 929-937.

[53] Sheikh, M. S. & Fornace Jr, A. J. (2000). Death and decoy receptors and p53-mediated apoptosis. *Leukemia* ,14, 1509-1513.

[54] Ginisty, H.; Sicard, H.; Roger, B. & Bouvet, P. (1999). Structure and functions of nucleolin. *J. Cell Sci.*, 112, 761-772.

[55] Daniely, Y.; Dimitrova, D. D. & Borowiec, J. A. (2002). Stress-dependent nucleolin mobilization mediated by p53-nucleolin complex formation. *Mol. Cell. Biol.*, 22, 6014-6022.

[56] Brazill, D. T.; Thormer, J. & Martin, S. (1997). Mck1, a member of the glycogen synthase kinase 3 family of protein kinase, is a negative regulator of pyruvate kinase in the yeast Saccharomyces cerevisiae. *J. Bacteriol.*, 179, 4415-4418.

[57] Janosch, P.; Kieser, A.; Eulitz, M.; Lovric, J.; Sauer, G.; Reichert, M.; Gounari, F.; Büscher, D.; Baccarini, M.; Mischak, H. & Kolch, W. (2000).The Raf-$_1$ kinase associates with vimentin kinases and regulates the structure of vimentin filaments. *FASEB J.*, 14, 2008-2021.

[58] Ivaska, J.; Vuoriluoto, K.; Huovinen, T.; Izawa, I.; Inagaki, M. & Parker, P. J. (2005). PKC$\varepsilon$-mediated phosphorylation of vimentin controls integrin recycling and motility. *EMBO J.*, 24, 3834-3845.

[59] Yang, X.; Wang, J.; Liu, C.; Grizzle, W. E.; Yu, S.; Zhang, S.; Barnes, S.; Koopman, W. J.; Mountz, J. D.; Kimberly, R. P. & Zhang, H. G. (2005). Cleavage of p53–vimentin complex enhances tumor necrosis factor-related apoptosis-inducing ligand-mediated apoptosis of rheumatoid arthritis synovial fibroblasts. *Am. J. Pathol.*, 167(3), 705-719.

[60] McInroy, L. & Maatta, A. (2007). Down-regulation of vimentin expression inhibits carcinoma cell migration and adhesion. *Biochem. Biophys. Res. Comm.*, 360, 109-114.

[61] Benitez-King, G. (2000). PKC activation by melatonin modulates vimentin intermediate filament organization in N1E-115 cells. *J. Pineal. Res.*, 29(1), 8-14.

[62] Ciocca, D. R. & Calderwood, S. K. (2005). Heat shock proteins in cancer: diagnostic, prognostic, predictive, and treatment implications. *Cell Stress Chaperones*, 10(2), 86-103.

[63] Tzivion, G. & Avruch, J. (2002). 14-3-3 proteins: active cofactors in cellular regulation by serine/threonine phosphorylation. *J. Biol. Chem.*, 277, 3061-3064.

[64] Aitken, A. (1996). 14-3-3 and its possible role in coordinating multiple signaling pathways. *Trends Cell Biol.*, 6(9), 341-347.

[65] Li, S.; Janosch, P.; Tanji, M.; Rosenfeld, G. C.; Waymire, J. C.; Mischak, H.; Kolch, W. & Sedivy, J. M. (1995). Regulation of Raf-1 kinase activity by the 14-3-3 family of proteins. *EMBO J.*, 14(4), 685-696.

[66] Waterman, J. L.; Shenk, J. L. & Halozonetis, T. D. (1995).The dihedral symmetry of the p53 tetramerization domain mandates a conformational switch upon DNA binding. *EMBO J.* 14(3), 512-519.

[67] Shoshan-Barmatz, V. & Gincel, D. (2003). The voltage-dependent anion channel: characterization, modulation, and role in mitochondrial function in cell life and death. *Cell Biochem. Biophys.*, 39, 279-292.

[68] Kim, Y. J.; Ahn, J. Y.; Liang, P.; Ip, C.; Zhang, Y. & Park, Y. M. (2007). Human *prx1* gene is a target of Nrf2 and is up-regulated by hypoxia/reoxygenation: implication to tumor biology. *Cancer Res.*, 67, 546-554.

# 26

# Anticancer Effects of a Micronutrient Mixture on Melanoma – Modulation of Metastasis and Other Critical Parameters

M.W. Roomi, T. Kalinovsky, A. Niedzwiecki and M. Rath
*Dr. Rath Research Institute, USA*

## 1. Introduction

Melanoma causes the most skin cancer-related deaths, due to metastasis to other areas of the body, such as lymph nodes, lungs, liver, brain or bone. Though often curable in its early stages, metastatic malignant melanoma is an extremely aggressive cancer with no current viable treatment. Thus, any successful treatment for melanoma has to target metastasis. Invasion of host tissues by cancer cells requires alteration of cancer cell adhesion, cell migration and proteolytic degradation of the extracellular matrix (ECM) (Fidler, 1990). Dr. Rath proposed that optimizing the stability and structure of the ECM and controlling its proteolytic degradation would be the most effective and universal approach to controlling cancer invasiveness and tumor growth (Rath & Pauling, 1992). Degradation of the extracellular matrix (ECM) by matrix metalloproteinases (MMPs) plays a critical role in the formation of tumors and metastasis and has been found to correlate with the aggressiveness of tumor growth and invasiveness of the cancer (Fidler, 1990; Duffy, 1992; Stetler-Stevenson, 2001). Since this process is involved not only in metastasis, but also in angiogenesis and tumor growth, control of proteolytic activity of ECM provides an opportunity to modulate key common aspects of malignancy.

Rath and Pauling suggested the use of nutritional components, such as vitamin C and lysine and lysine analogues to target plasmin-mediated connective tissue degradation as a universal approach to controlling common pathomechanisms of cancer (Rath & Pauling, 1992). Lysine interferes with the activation of plasminogen into plasmin by tissue plasminogen activator (tPA) by binding to plasminogen active sites, thereby affecting the plasmin-induced MMP activation cascade (Rath & Pauling, 1992). Our subsequent studies confirmed this approach and resulted in identifying a novel formulation composed of lysine, ascorbic acid, proline and green tea extract and other micronutrients (NM) which has shown significant anticancer activity against a large number (~40) of cancer cell lines, blocking cancer growth, tissue invasion and MMP expression both *in vitro* and *in vivo* (Roomi et al., 2010). Furthermore, NM demonstrated significant antiangiogenic activity utilizing the chorioallantoic membrane (CAM) assay in chick embryos and bFGF-induced vessel growth in C57BL/6J female mice in the mouse Matrigel plug assay (Roomi et al, 2005). In addition, *in vitro*, NM decreased the expression of pro-angiogenic factors of VEGF, angiopoietin-2, bFGF, PDGD and TDGβ-1 by U2OS cells (Roomi et al., 2005).

## 2. Selecting active compounds for the micronutrient mixture

Individual components of the NM were chosen for their potent activity on critical physiological targets in cancer progression and metastasis, such as optimization of collagen structure and stability, inhibition of MMPs, cellular migration and invasion, and induction of apoptosis . The anticancer effects of these individual constituents of the NM have been reported in both clinical and experimental studies. Optimal ECM formation and structure requires adequate supplies of ascorbic acid and the amino acids lysine and proline, since these nutrients enable proper synthesis and hydroxylation of collagen fibers. Manganese and copper are also essential for collagen formation. Lysine also acts as a natural inhibitor of plasmin-induced proteolysis to contribute to ECM stability (Rath & Pauling, 1992; Sun et al., 2002). Green tea extract has been shown to control cancer cell growth, metastasis, angiogenesis, and other aspects of cancer progression (Kemberling et al., 2003; Sato & Matsushima, 2003; Valcic et al., 1996; Muhktar & Ahmed, 2000; Yang et al., 1998; Taniguchi et al, 1992; Hara, 2001). N-acetyl cysteine and selenium have been reported to inhibit tumor cell invasion and expression of MMP-9, as well as migration of endothelial cells through ECM (Kawakami et al., 2001; Morini et al., 1999; Yoon et al., 2001). Ascorbic acid has been reported to exert cytotoxic and antimetastatic actions on malignant cell lines (Maramag et al., 1997; Koh et al., 1998; Chen et al., 2005; Kurbacher et al, 1996); in addition, low levels of ascorbic acid have been reported in cancer patients (Nunez et al, 1995; Anthony & Schorah, 1982 ). Arginine is a precursor of nitric oxide (NO); any deficiency of arginine can limit the production of NO, which has been shown to predominantly act as an inducer of apoptosis (Cooke & Dzau, 1997). Combining these micronutrients expands metabolic targets maximizing the biological impact with lower doses of components by nutrient synergy. Furthermore, effective lower doses of components using nutrient synergy also assure overcoming absorption barriers characteristic for high vitamin doses.

## 3. Nutrient synergy controls metastasis

Treatment failure of patients with melanoma is mainly due to tumor metastasis to such sites in the body as lymph nodes, lungs, liver, brain or bones. Therefore, we investigated the effectiveness of the micronutrient mixture in controlling metastasis utilizing melanoma B16FO cells *in vivo.*

### 3.1 Pulmonary metastasis

We investigated pulmonary metastasis in 6-7 week-old female C57BL/6 mice, which were divided into 6 groups of 6 mice each (Roomi et al, 2006a). B16FO melanoma cells (5 X $10^4$/mouse), were injected via tail vein into mice in Groups 1-4 and group 5 animals were injected in the tail vein with the same number of B16FO melanoma cells pretreated with NM (500 µg/mL for 18 hours). Group 6 (untreated control) was injected with the vehicle saline. Subsequently the mice were placed on the following dietary regimens and administration routes for NM: Groups 1 and 5 were fed Purina mouse chow, the control diet; group 2 mice were given NM intraperitoneally (IP) (4 mg/mouse, 3 x/week x 2 weeks) and fed the control diet; group 4 was give NM intravenously (IV) (4 mg/mouse, 3 x/week x 2 weeks and fed the control diet. Group 6 mice were fed the control diet. Two weeks later the mice were sacrificed, and their lungs were excised, weighed, and processed for histopathologic examination. The weights of the lungs were obtained and the number of metastases and number of cells in each metastatic lesion were counted.

Lungs isolated from mice injected with 5 X $10^4$ B16FO cells and fed the NM 0.5% diet (group 2) demonstrated a significant reduction in metastatic colonies (by 63%, $p<0.0001$) compared to the lungs of mice fed the control diet (group 1), as shown in Figure 1. Pulmonary colonization was inhibited by 86% ($p<0.0001$) in mice receiving NM by IP and IV injections (groups 3 and 4). The lungs from mice injected with viable melanoma cells pretreated with NM (group 5) were free from any metastasis. Thus, exposing melanoma cells to NM inhibited their ability to metastasize without the need for diet supplementation, suggesting profound changes on a cellular level. Our *in vitro* studies on B16FO cells suggest that pretreatment with 500 µg/mL NM prior to injection of the cells affected cell viability of melanoma by inhibiting cell proliferation (by 44%) and inducing profound apoptosis (over 90% of cells in apoptosis). Those in vitro results are discussed in sections 5.2 and 5.3.

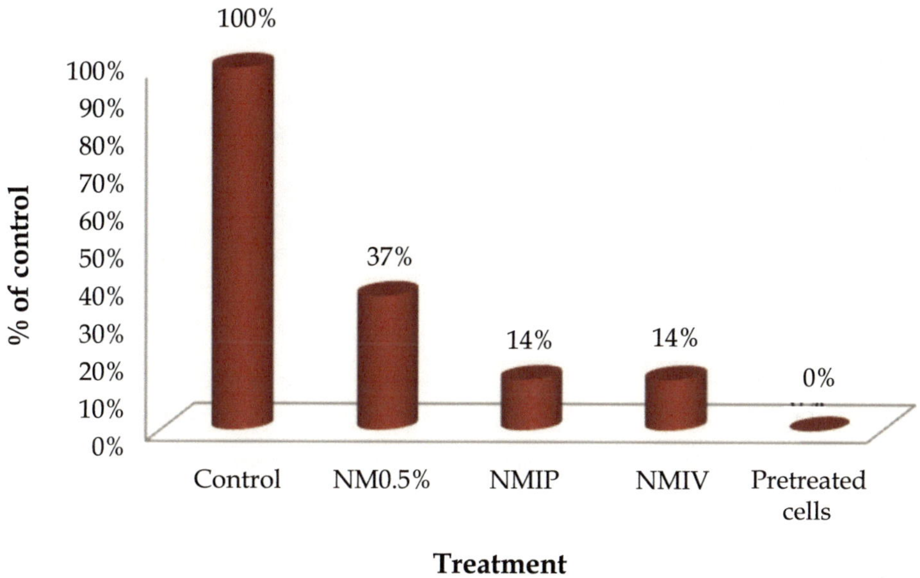


Fig. 1. Effect of NM on pulmonary colonization of B16FO cells (5x$10^4$) injected into C57BL/6 mice. Legend: NM 0.5% (NM 0.5% dietary supplementation); NM IP and NM IV (NM 4 mg/mouse, 3 x/week x 2 weeks, either IP or IV, as indicated and fed the control diet); pretreated cells (injected B16FO melanoma cells pretreated with NM 500 µg/mL for 18 hours)

### 3.2 Hepatic metastasis

In order to obtain a more clinically relevant model, we employed an orthotropic model of evaluating the effects of NM on hepatic metastasis. Orthotopic models have been suggested as the growth environment influences cancer behavior and thus animal models selected should recreate disease at the specific organs of interest.

In this study, athymic nude mice, 10-12 weeks old, received $10^6$ B16FO melanoma cells by injection into the spleen and divided into two treatment groups (Roomi et al., 2009). The control group of mice received Purina mouse chow and the NM group received the regular diet supplemented with NM 0.5%. After two weeks, animals were sacrificed and spleens, livers, kidneys and lungs were excised from all animals, examined, weighed and processed for histology.

Mice in the control group developed large black spleens and livers indicating growth in the spleen and metastasis to the liver. However, the mice supplemented with NM not only showed less tumor growth in the spleen as the control mice, but also drastically
reduced metastasis to the liver (Figures 2A-B). Intrasplenic tumor growth (mean spleen weight) was reduced significantly (by 64%, p=0.001) in the NM-supplemented group compared to the control group. Hepatic metastasis in NM-supplemented mice was reduced by 55% (p=0.006) compared to the control group, based on mean liver weights of the groups. In all groups, no metastasis to the kidneys and lungs was evident, Multiple, nodular, metastatic lesions replaced most of the examined liver sections of control mice. In contrast, only two to five small metastases were noted in the liver sections of NM-supplemented mice.

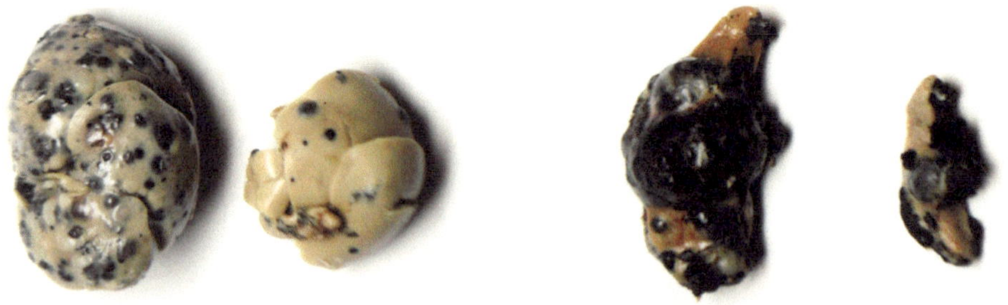

Conrol NM 0.5% Control Nm 0.5%

(A) (B)

Fig. 2. Representative livers (A) and spleens (B) from the Control and NM-supplemented athymic mice that received intrasplenic injections of $10^6$ B16FO melanoma cells

We also studied the effect of NM dietary treatment on the survival time of C57BL/6 mice after receiving an injection of $10^6$ B16FO cells IP (Roomi et al., 2008). Group 1 (n=6) received no B16FO cells and regular Purina mouse chow, group 2 (n=6), $10^6$ B16FO cells IP and regular Purina mouse chow, group 3, $10^6$ B16FO cells IP and 0.5% NM-supplemented Purina mouse chow, and group 4, $10^6$ B16FO cells IP, regular Purina mouse chow and 2 mg NM injected 3 x/week. The number of animals surviving was counted daily. The NM dietary treatment group (3) demonstrated increased mean survival time (16.7 days) over the Control diet group (2) mice with a mean survival time of 15.2 days. The longest survival time (22 days) for groups was reached by a mouse in Group 3. Group 4 mice had a mean survival time of 15.2 days.

## 4. Micronutrient synergy modulates invasive parameters of melanoma

Since proteases, especially MMP-2 and MMP-9, play key roles in tumor cell invasion and metastasis, we also investigated the effects of NM *in vitro* on melanoma A2058 and B16FO MMP-2 and MMP-9 secretion (by gelatinase zymography), migration by scratch test and invasion through Matrigel. Interestingly, B16FO melanoma cells neither expressed any MMPs nor exhibit invasion through Matrigel.

### 4.1 MMP-2 and MMP-9 secretion

Human melanoma cells A2058 grown to confluence were treated with NM dissolved in media and tested at 0, 10, 100, 500, and 1000 μg/mL in triplicate at each dose. Parallel sets of cultures were treated with phorbol 12-myristate 13-acetate (PMA) 100 ng/mL. Conditioned media were collected, centrifuged at 3000 rpm and the supernatant was collected and used for gelatinase zymography. Gelatinase zymography was performed in 10% Novex Pre-Cast SDS Polyacrylamide Gel (Invitrogen Corporation) as suggested by the manufacturer (Novex). Samples were not boiled before electrophoresis. Following electrophoresis the gels were washed twice in 2.5% Triton X-100 for 30 minutes at room temperature to remove SDS. The gels were then incubated at 37⁰C overnight in substrate buffer containing 50mM Tris-HCl and 10mM $CaCl_2$ at pH 8.0 and stained with 0.5% Coomassie Blue R250 in 50% methanol and 10% glacial acetic acid for 30 minutes and destained. Upon renaturation of the enzyme, the gelatinases digested the gelatin in the gel, producing clear bands against an intensely stained background. Protein standards were run concurrently and approximate molecular weights were determined by plotting the relative mobilities of known proteins. Gelatinase zymograms were scanned using CanoScan 9950F scanner at 300 dpi.

Zymography detected MMP-2 in untreated melanoma A2058 cells and induction of MMP-9 by PMA (100 ng/mL). MMP-2 and MMP-9 expression was inhibited by NM in a dose-dependent fashion with virtual complete blockage of MMP-9 at 100 µg/ml and MMP-2 at 500 µg/mL, as shown in figures 3A-D (Roomi et al., 2010).

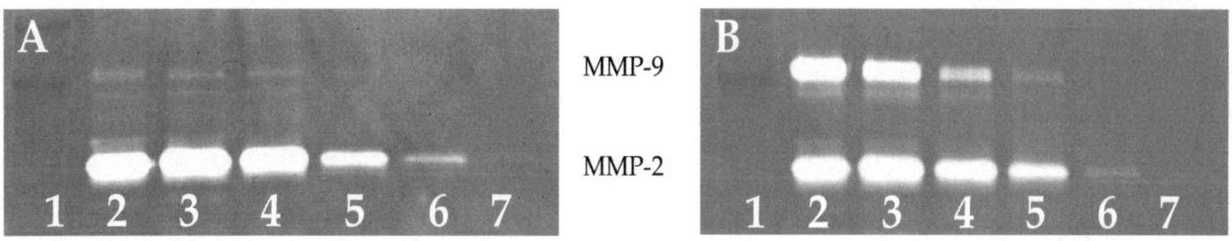


1-Marker, 2-Control,
3-7: 10, 50, 100, 500, 1000 µg/mL NM

1-Marker, 2-Control, 3-7: 100ng/mL PMA
and 10, 50, 100, 500, 1000 µg/mL NM

Fig. 3. Effect of NM on MMP-2 and -9 expression by normal (A) and PMA 100 ng/mL-treated melanoma A2058 cells: gelatinase zymography (B)

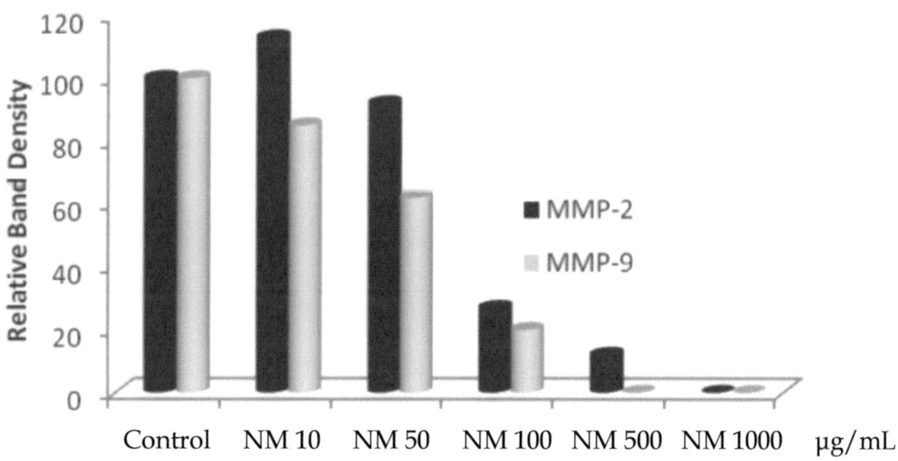


Fig. 3. (C) Effect of NM on normal melanoma A2058 MMP-2 and MMP-9 expression: densitometric analysis

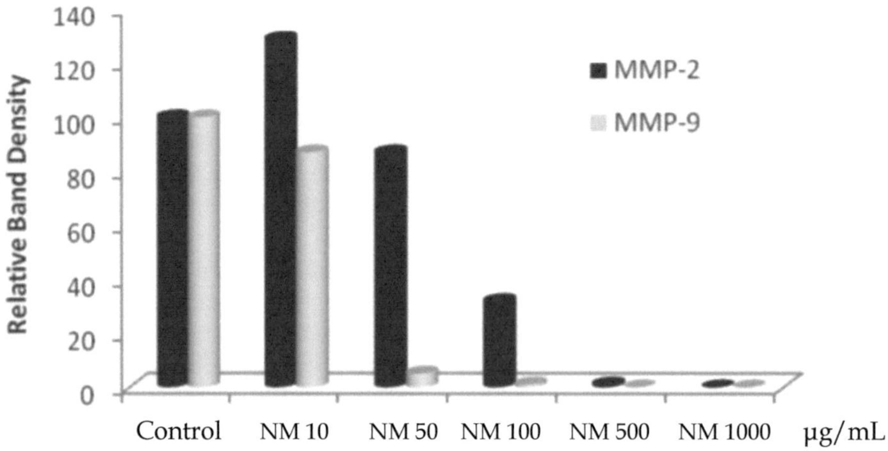


Fig. 3. (D) Effect of NM on PMA (100 ng/mL)-treated melanoma A2058 MMP-2 and MMP-9 expression: densitometric analysis

### 4.2 Matrigel invasion

Invasion studies were conducted using Matrigel (Becton Dickinson) inserts in 24-well plates. Suspended in medium, melanoma A2058 cancer cells were supplemented with nutrients, as specified in the design of the experiments and seeded on the insert in the well. Thus both the medium on the insert and in the well contained the same supplements. The plates with the inserts were then incubated in a culture incubator equilibrated with 95% air and 5% $CO_2$ for 24 hours. After incubation, the media from the wells were withdrawn. The cells on the upper surface of the inserts were gently scrubbed away with cotton swabs. The cells that had penetrated the Matrigel membrane and migrated onto the lower surface of the Matrigel were stained with hematoxylin and eosin and visually counted under the microscope.

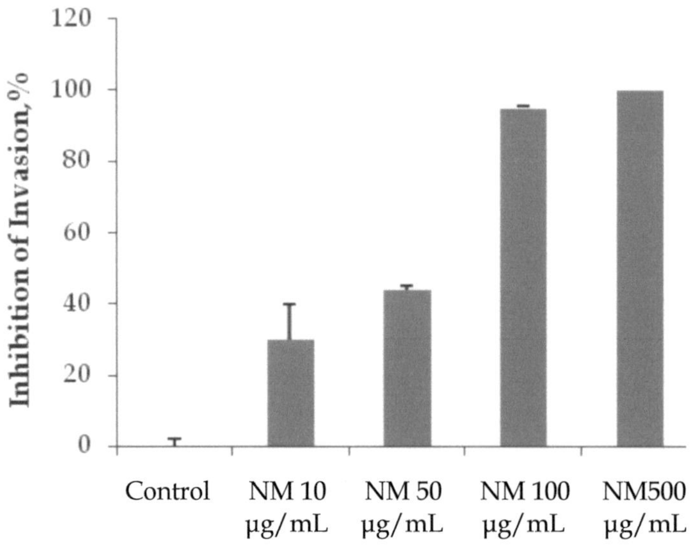


Fig. 4. Effect of NM on invasion of melanoma A2058 cells through Matrigel

Invasion of melanoma A2058 cells through Matrigel was inhibited by 30%, 44%, 95% and 100% by 10, 50,100, and 500 µg/mL of NM, respectively ($p<0.0001$), as shown in Figure 4 (Roomi et al., 2006b).

### 4.3 Cell migration: Scratch test

To study cell migration, a 2-mm wide single uninterrupted scratch was made from the top to bottom of culture plates of melanoma A2058 and B16FO cells grown to confluence. Culture plates were washed with PBS and incubated with NM in medium and tested at 0, 50, 100, 250 and 500 µg/mL, in triplicate at each dose for 24h. Cells were washed with PBS, fixed and stained with H&E and photomicrographs were taken. NM reduced cell migration in a dose-dependent manner in both cell lines, with complete block of A2058 at 500 µg/ml and B16FO at 250 µg/ml. Photomicrographs of the results for the scratch tests for melanoma A2058 (Figure 5) and B16FO (Figure 6) are shown below.

## 5. Micronutrient synergy inhibits cancer cell growth and apoptosis

ECM degradation is a prerequisite for cancer metastasis, but also it is essential to tumor growth and expansion and angiogenesis. Therefore, we investigated the effects of nutrient synergy on these important aspects of malignancy

### 5.1 Inhibition of tumor growth (xenografts)

The effect of dietary NM 0.5% on tumor growth was studied in athymic male nude mice using the model of melanoma A2058 and B16FO xenografts (Roomi et al., 2006b). Male athymic mice six weeks of age (n=12) were inoculated subcutaneously with 3 $x10^6$ A2058 cells in 0.2 mL PBS and 0.1 mL Matrigel. After injection, the mice were randomly divided into two groups; group A mice were fed regular Purina mouse chow and group B the regular diet supplemented with 0.5% NM (w/w). After four weeks, the mice were sacrificed and their tumors were excised and processed for histology. Dimensions (length and width) of tumors were measured using a digital caliper, and the tumor burden was calculated using the following formula: 0.5 x length x width. Mean weight of mice at initiation of study and termination of study did not differ significantly between the groups. NM supplementation demonstrated significant reduction in tumor weight (by 57%, $p<0.0001$ over control) and tumor burden by 31%, as well as decrease in vascularity.
Tissue samples were fixed in 10% buffered formalin, embedded in paraffin and cut at 4-5 microns for histological evaluation. After deparaffinization and appropriate epitope retrieval, the sections were incubated with primary antibody. Detection was by biotinylated goat anti-mouse antibodies followed by streptavidin conjugated to horseradish peroxidase with the use of diaminobenzidine as the chromogen. Polyclonal rabbit anti-human antibodies were used for MMP-9, MMP-2, VEGF, fibronectin and ki-67. Histological evaluation noted inhibition of MMP-9 and VEGF (an indicator of angiogenesis) secretion and mitotic index (ki-67) in mice fed the NM diet, as shown in Figure 7. There is a strong positive correlation between high ki-67 index and high-grade histopathology of neoplasms.
The effect of dietary NM 0.5% on tumor growth in athymic male nude mice was also studied using melanoma B16FO xenografts (Roomi et al, 2008). The nutrient-supplemented mice developed significantly smaller tumors (reduction in weight by 47%, $p=0.0002$). Reduction of tumor weight in melanoma A2058 and B16FO cell xenografts in nude mice is presented in Figure 8.

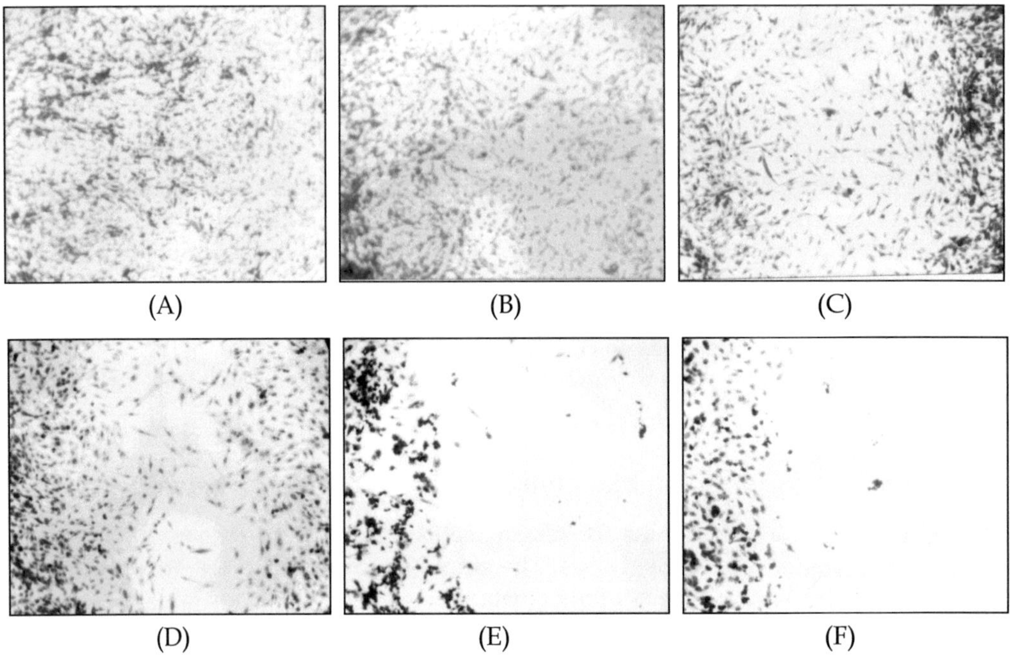


Fig. 5. Effect of NM on melanoma A2058 cell migration: scratch test: A – pre-scratch, B – control, C – NM 50 µg/mL, D – NM 100 µg/mL, E – NM 250 µg/mL, F- NM 500 µg/mL

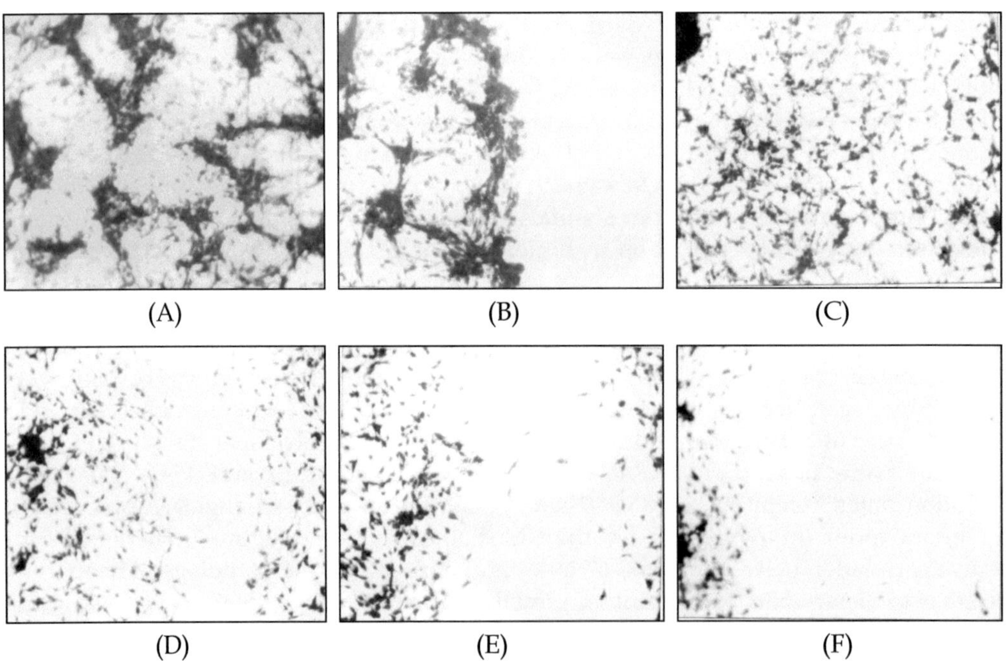


Fig. 6. Effect of NM on melanoma B16FO cell migration: scratch test: A – pre-scratch, B-scratch, C– control, D – NM 50 µg/mL, E – NM 100 µg/mL, F – NM 250 µg/mL

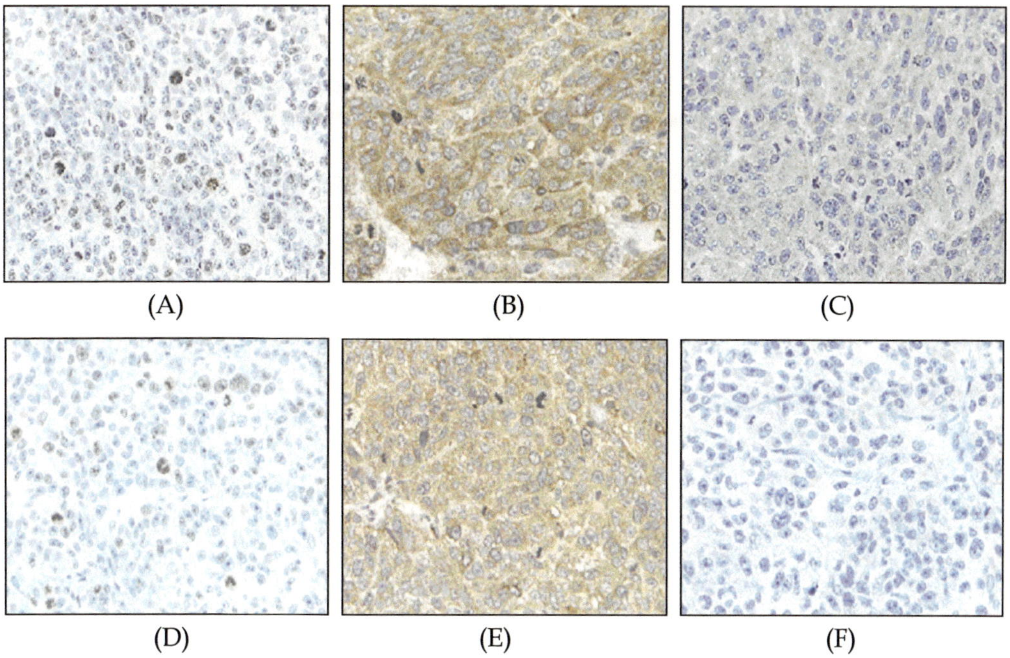


Fig. 7. Effect of NM on MMP-9, VEGF and ki-67 in A2058 xenograft tumors: A - Control Ki-67, B - Control MMP-9, C – Control VEGF, D – NM Ki-67, E – NM MMP-9, F – NM VEGF

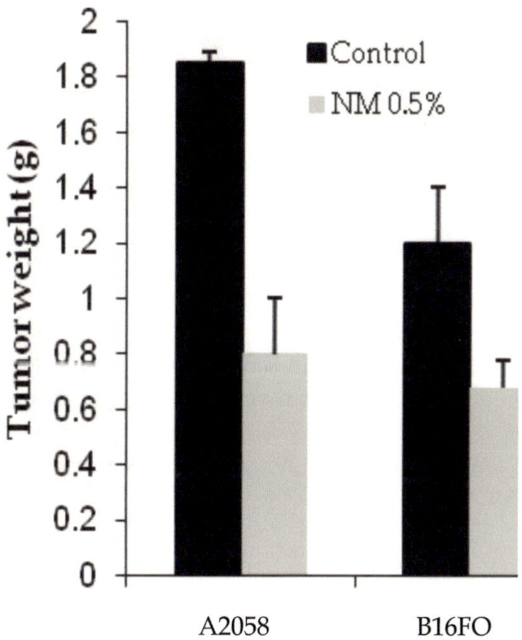


Fig. 8. Effect of supplementation with 0.5% NM on mean tumor weight of melanoma A2058 and B16FO xenografts in nude mice

### 5.2 Decreased cancer cell proliferation in the presence of nutrient synergy

We evaluated the effect of various concentrations of NM on the viability of melanoma A2058 and B16FO cells utilizing the MTT assay, a colorimetric assay based on the ability of viable cells to reduce a soluble yellow tetrazolium salt [3-(4,5-dimethylthiazol-2-yl) 2,5-diphenyl tetrazolium bromide] (MTT) to a blue formazan crystal by mitochondrial succinate dehydrogenase activity of viable cells. This test is a good index of mitochondrial activity and thus of cell viability. NM had minimal (10%) antiproliferative effects on A2058 cells at 100 µg/mL, but at 500 µg/mL, inhibited cell viability by 64% ($p<0.0001$) (Roomi et al., 2006b). Melanoma B16FO cell proliferation was not inhibited up to 100 µg/ml, but at 500 and 1000 µg/ml, inhibited cell viability by 44% ($p=0.001$) (Roomi et al., 2006b). See Figure 9 for graphic representation of NM effect on melanoma B16 and A2058 cell proliferation.

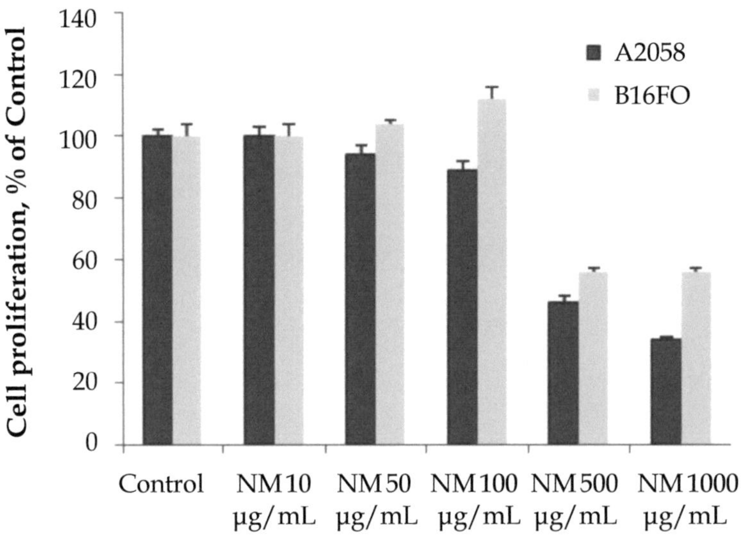


Fig. 9. Effect of NM on melanoma A2058 and B16FO cell proliferation

### 5.3 Induction of cancer cell apoptosis NM

We investigated pro-apoptotic effects of NM in both melanoma B16FO and A2058 cell lines utilizing the live-green caspases kit. To study the effect of NM on apoptosis of cancer cells, cells were grown to confluence, challenged with NM dissolved in media at 0, 100, 500, and 1000 µg/mL and incubated for 24 h. The cell culture was washed with PBS and treated with the caspase reagent as specified in the manufacturer's protocol (Molecular Probes Image-IT™ Live Green Poly Caspases Detection Kit 135104, Invitrogen). The cells were photographed under a fluorescence microscope and counted. Green-colored cells represent viable cells, while yellow orange represents early apoptosis and red, late apoptosis.

Dose-dependent induction of apoptosis in melanoma A2058 and B16FO cell lines was confirmed with NM challenge. Treatment of A2058 cells with NM demonstrated: 95.5% of cells were viable and 4.5% in apoptosis at 0 µg/mL NM; 0.7% were viable, 35.5% in early apoptosis and 63.8% in late apoptosis at 100 µg/mL NM; and 1.3% of cells were viable, 10.3% in early apoptosis, and 88.4% in late apoptosis at 500 µg/mLNM. Virtually all cells exposed to 1000 µg/mL NM were in late apoptosis. Photomicrographs of apoptotic cells and quantitative analysis of live, early and late A2058 apoptotic cells are shown in Figures 10 and 11.

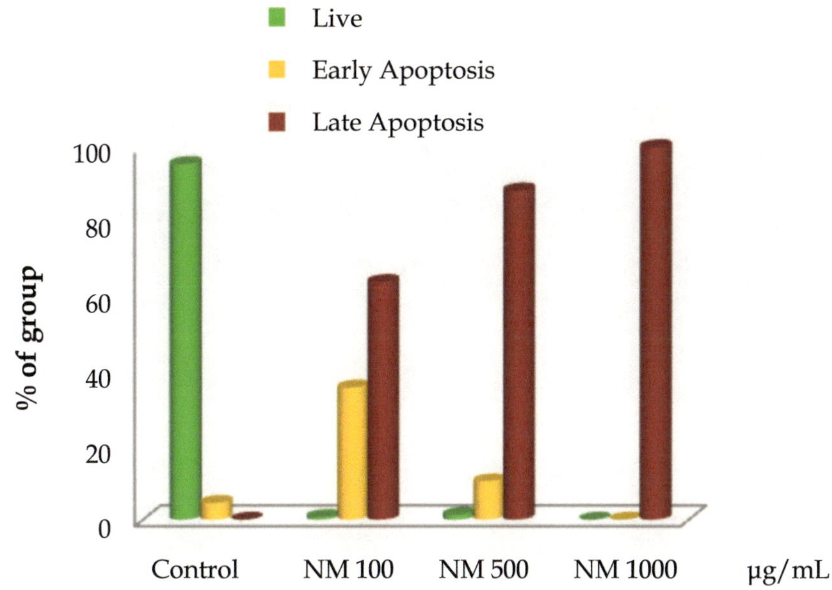


Fig. 10. Effect of NM on induction of melanoma A2058 apoptosis: quantitative analysis

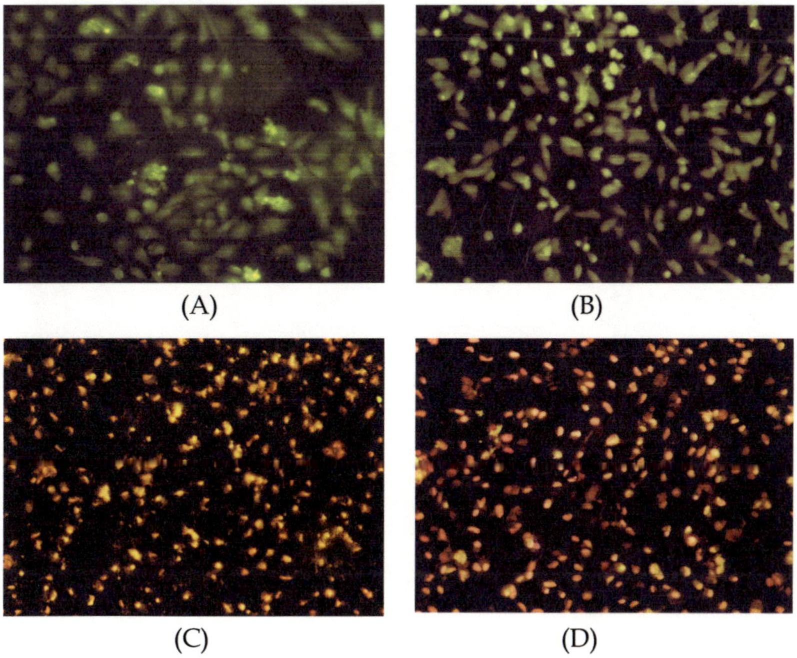


Fig. 11. Effect of NM on induction of melanoma A2058 apoptosis: photomicrographs
A - Control, B - NM 100 μg/mL, C - NM 500 μg/mL, D - NM 1000 μg/mL

B16FO cells treated with NM also shown dose-dependent apoptosis with slight induction of apoptosis ( 46% live, 33.3% early apoptosis and 20.6% late apoptosis) at 100 μg/mL NM, moderate (15%live, 4.3% early apoptosis and 82.2% late apoptosis) at 500 μg/mL NM, and extensive apoptosis (9.6% live, 0.2% early apoptosis and 86.2% late apoptosis) at 1000 μg/mL NM, as shown in Figures 12 and 13 (Roomi et al., 2008).

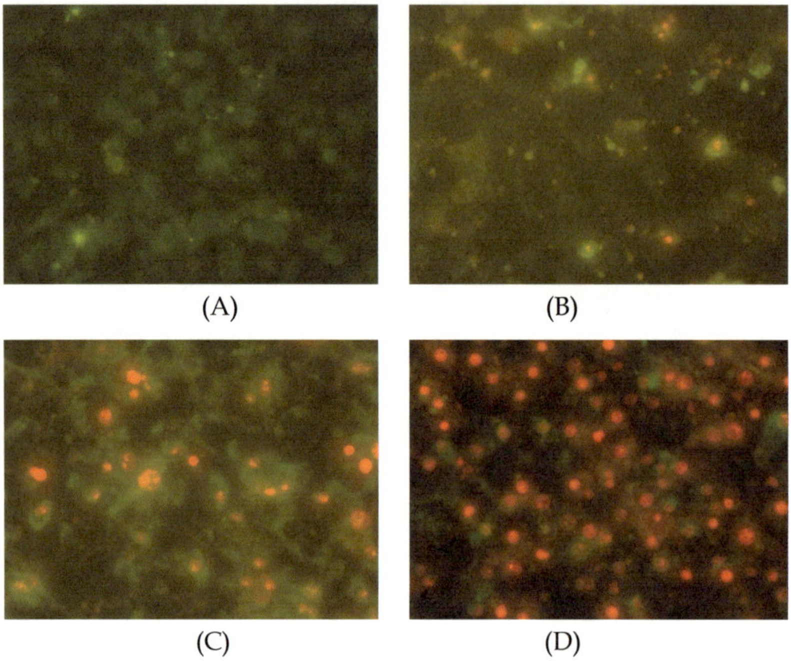


Fig. 12. Effect of NM on induction of melanoma B16FO apoptosis: photomicrographs: A - Control, B - NM 100 μg/mL, C - NM 500 μg/mL, D - NM 1000 μg/mL

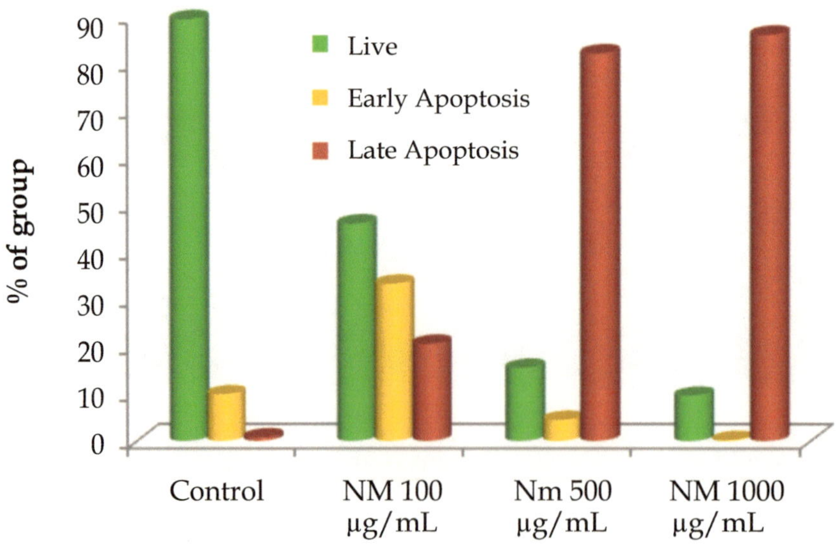


Fig. 13. Effect of NM on induction of melanoma B16FO cell apoptosis: quantitative analysis

### 5.4 Nutrient synergy modulates cancer cell cycle

We also studied the effect of NM on cell cycle in melanoma cells since deregulation of the cell cycle components may lead to tumor formation. Melanoma cells A-2058 were cultured in a 6-well plate at a concentration of 0.5 X $10^6$ cells per well. The cells were incubated with NM at 0, 10, 100 and 1000 µg/mL for 24 hours and harvested. The cells were washed once with PBS and fixed in 70% ethanol. Cell pellets were suspended in 2 µL of 10 µg/ml RNase containing 0.5% Triton and the same volume of 20 µg/mL propidium iodide, followed by incubation in the dark at room temperature for 30 minutes. Cell fluorescence was measured in the Coulter EPIC Flow Cytometer.

Melanoma A-2058 cells exposed to NM showed dose-dependent increase of % of cells in the G-1 phase and decrease in G-2 and G-3 phases, indicating decrease in cells ready to undergo mitosis. See Figure 14.

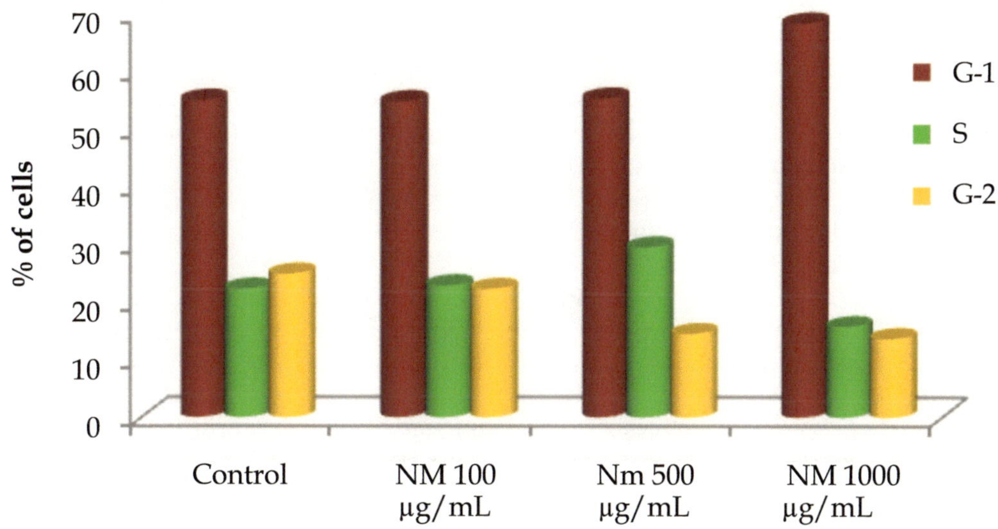


Fig. 14. Effect of NM on cell cycle of melanoma A-2058 cells

## 6. Conclusion

In conclusion, the results from these studies clearly indicate the strong anticancer potential of the micronutrient mixture based on its effective inhibition of melanoma B16FO and A2058 cells in vivo and in vitro. The NM showed profound inhibitory effects on melanoma B16FO pulmonary metastasis and hepatic metastasis and intrasplenic growth in C57BL/6 mice. Furthermore, tumor growth of melanoma A2058 and B16FO xenografts were significantly inhibited by dietary supplementation with NM. The in vitro studies supported these findings as they demonstrated inhibition of MMP-2 and MMP-9 secretion, cell migration, Matrigel invasion and cell proliferation, and induction of apoptosis. Furthermore, use of the nutrient mixture would not pose any toxic effect clinically, especially in the relevant doses, as in vivo safety studies demonstrate. During an in vivo study on possible toxicity from NM, we found that NM had neither adverse effect on vital organs (heart, liver, and kidney), nor on the associated functional serum enzymes (Roomi et al., 2003).

## 7. References

Anthony, H.M. & Schorah, C.J. (1982). Severe hypovitaminosis C in lung-cancer patients: The utilization of vitamin C in surgical repair and lymphocyte-related host resistance. *Br J Cancer*, Vol 46, pp. 354-367.

Chen, Q., Espey, M.G., Krishna, M.C., Mitchell, J.B., Corpe, C.P., Buettner, G.R., Shacter, E., Levine, M. (2005). Pharmacologic ascorbic acid concentrations selectively kill cancer cells: Action as a pro-drug to deliver hydrogen peroxide to tissues. *PNAS*, Vol 102, No 38, pp 13604-13609.

Cooke, J.P & Dzau, V.J. (1997). Nitric oxide synthase: Role in the genesis of vascular disease. *Annu Rev Med,* Vol 48, pp 489-509.

Duffy, M. J. (1992). The role of proteolytic enzymes in cancer invasion and metastasis. *Clin Exp Metastasis,* Vol 10, pp 145-155.

Fidler I.J. (1990). Critical factors in the biology of human cancer metastasis: twenty-eighth G.H.A. Clowers Memorial Award Lecture. *Cancer Res,* Vol 50, pp 6130-6138.

Hara, Y. (2001) *Green tea: Health Benefits and Applications*, Marcel Dekker, New York, Basel.

Kawakami, S., Kageyama, Y., Fujii, Y., Kihara, K. & Oshima, H. (2001). Inhibitory effects of N-acetyl cysteine on invasion and MMP 9 production of T24 human bladder cancer cells. *Anticancer Res,*Vol 21, pp 213-219.

Kemberling, J.K., Hampton, J.A., Keck, R.W., Gomez, M.A.& Selman, S.H. (2003). Inhibition of bladder tumor growth by the green tea derivative epigallocatechin-3-gallate. *J Urol,* Vol 170, No 3, pp 773-6.

Koh, W.S., Lee, S.J., Lee, H., Park, C., Park, M.H., Kim, W.S., Yoon, S.S., Park, K., Hong, S.I., Chung, M.H.& Park, C.H. (1998). Differential effects and transport kinetics of ascorbate derivatives in leukemic cell lines. *Anticancer Res*, Vol 8, pp 2487-2493.

Kurbacher, C.M., Wagner, U., Kolster, B., Andreotti, P.E., Krebs, D.& Bruckner, H.W. (1996). Ascorbic acid (vitamin C) improves the antineoplastic activity doxorubicin, cisplatin and paclitaxel in human breast carcinoma cells in vitro. *Cancer Lett*ers, Vol 103, No 2, pp 183-189.

Maramag, C., Menon, M., Balaji, K.C., Reddy, P.G. & Laxmanan, S. (1997). Effect of vitamin C on prostate cancer cells in vitro: effect on cell number, viability and DNA synthesis. *Prostate,* Vol 32, pp 188-95.

Morini, M., Cai, T., Aluigi, M.G., Noonan, D.M., Masiello, L., De Floro, S., D'Agostinin, F., Albini, A. & Fassima, G. (1999). The role of the thiol N-acetyl cysteine in the prevention of tumor invasion and angiogenesis. *Int J Biol Markers,* Vol 14, pp 268-271.

Mukhtar, H. & Ahmed, N. (2000). Tea polyphenols: prevention of cancer and optimizing health. *Am J Clin Nutr*, Vol 71, pp 1698s-1702s.

Naidu, K.A., Karl, R.C. & Coppola, D. (2003). Antiproliferative and proapoptotic effect of ascorbyl stearate in human pancreatic cancer cells: association with decreased expression of insulin-like growth factor 1 receptor. *Dig Dis Sci*, Vol 48, No 1, pp 230-7.

Niedzwiecki, A., Roomi, M.W., Kalinovsky, T. & Rath M. (2010). Micronutrient synergy – a new tool in effective control of metastasis and other key mechanisms of cancer. *Cancer Metastasis Rev,* Vol 29, No3, pp 529-543.

Nunez, C., Ortiz de Apodaca, Y.& Ruiz, A. (1995). Ascorbic acid in the plasma and blood cells of women with breast cancer. The effect of consumption of food with an elevated content of this vitamin. *Nutr Hosp,* Vol 10, pp 68-372.

Rath, M. & Pauling, L. (1992). Plasmin-induced proteolysis and the role of apoprotein(a), lysine and synthetic analogs. *Orthomolecular Medicine,* Vol 7, pp 17-23.

Roomi, M.W., Ivanov, V., Netke, S.P., Niedzwiecki, A. & Rath, M. (2003) Serum markers of the liver, heart, and kidney and lipid profile and histopathology in ODS rats treated with nutrient synergy. *J AM Coll Nutr,* Vol 22, pp 77, Abstract 86.

Roomi, M.W., Roomi, N., Ivanov, V., Kalinovsky, T., Niedzwiecki, A. & Rath, M. (2005). Inhibitory effect of a mixture containing ascorbic acid, lysine, proline, and green tea extract on critical parameters in angiogenesis. *Oncol Rep,* Vol 14, No 4, pp 807-815.

Roomi, M.W., Ivanov, V., Kalinovsky, T., Niedzwiecki, A. & Rath, M. (2006a). Inhibition of pulmonary metastasis of melanoma B16FO cells in C57BL/6 mice by a nutrient mixture consisting of ascorbic acid, lysine, proline, arginine, and green tea extract. *Exp Lung Res,* Vol 32, No 10, pp 517-30.

Roomi, M.W., Ivanonv, V., Netke, S., Kalinovsky, T., Niedzwiecki, A., Rath, M. (2006b). In vivo and in vitro antitumor effect of ascorbic acid, lysine, proline and green tea extract on human melanoma cell line A2058. *In Vivo,* Vol 20, pp 25-32.

Roomi, M.W., Kalinovsky, T., Roomi, N.W., Monterrey, J., Rath, M. & Niedzwiecki, A. (2008). Suppression of growth and hepatic metastasis of murine B16FO melanoma cells by a novel nutrient mixture. *Onc Rep,* Vol 20, pp 809-817.

Roomi, M.W., Kalinovsky, T., Roomi, N.W., Monterrey, J., Rath, M. & Niedzwiecki, A. (2009). A nutrient mixture suppresses hepatic metastasis in athymic nude mice injected with murine B16FO melanoma cells. *BioFactors,* Vol 33, pp 181-189.

Roomi, M.W., Monterrey,J.C., Kalinovsky, T., Rath, M. & Niedzwiecki, A. (2010) Inhibition of invasion and MMPs by a nutrient mixture in human cancer cell lines: a correlation study. *Exp Oncol,* Vol 32, pp 243-248.

Sato, D. & Matsushima, M. (2003). Preventive effects of urinary bladder tumors induced by N-butyl-N-(4-hydroxybutyl)-nitrosamine in rat by green tea leaves. *Int J Urol,* Vol 10, No3, pp 160-6.

Stetler-Stevenson, W.G. (2001). The role of matrix metalloproteinases in tumor invasion, metastasis and angiogenesis. *Surg Oncol Clin N Am,* Vol 10, pp 383-392.

Sun, Z., Chen, Y.H., Wang, P., Zhang, J., Gurewich, V., Zhang, P. & Liu, J.N. (2002). The blockage of high-affinity lysine binding sites of plasminogen by EACA significantly inhibits prourokinase-induced plasminogen activation. *Biochem Biophys Acta,* Vol 1596, pp182-192.

Taniguchi, S., Fujiki, H., Kobayashi, H., Go, H., Miyado, K., Sadano, H. & Shimikawa, R. (1992). Effect of (-) epigallocatechin gallate, the main constituent of green tea, on lung metastasis with mouse B16 melanoma cell lines. *Cancer Lett,* Vol 65, pp 51-54.

Valcic, S., Timmermann, B.N., Alberts, D.S., Wachter, G.A., Krutzsch, M., Wymer, J. & Guillen, J.M. (1996). Inhibitory effect of six green tea catechins and caffeine on the growth of four selected human tumor cell lines. *Anticancer Drugs,* Vol 7, pp 461-8.

Yang, G.Y., Liao, J., Kim, K., Yurtow, E.J. & Yang, C.S. (1998). Inhibition of growth and induction of apoptosis in human cancer cell lines by tea polyphenols. *Carcinogenesis*, Vol 19, pp 611-616.

Yoon, S.O., Kim, M.M., & Chung, A.S. (2001). Inhibitory effects of selenite on invasion of HT 1080 tumor cells. *J Biol Chem*, Vol 276, pp 20085-20092.

# 27

# RANK/RANKL Axis in Melanoma

Kanji Mori[1], Kosei Ando[1],
Frédéric Lézot[2] and Dominique Heymann[2]
[1]*Shiga University of Medical Science;*
[2]*Nantes University,*
[1]*Japan*
[2]*France*

## 1. Introduction

The TNF receptor superfamily member 11A known as receptor activator of nuclear factor κB (RANK/TNFRSF11A), its ligand RANKL (TNFSF11) and the decoy receptor for RANKL called osteoprotegerin (OPG/TNFRSF11B) have been shown to be key regulators of bone remodeling (Simonet et al., 1997; Lacey et al., 1998; Theoleyre et al., 2004). Indeed, RANKL mediates osteoclastogenesis and activates mature osteoclasts, whereas OPG negatively regulates RANKL binding to RANK, reduces the half-life of membranous RANKL and finally inhibits bone resorption by osteoclasts (Tat et al., 2006). Together with such part in bone, the RANK/RANKL axis is also involved in a variety of physiologic functions. Certainly, the RANK/RANKL axis controls the lymph-node organogenesis, the thymic medullary epithelial cells differentiation, the central thermoregulation, the formation of lactating mammary gland during pregnancy and the proliferation of epithelial cells of the epidermo-pilosebaceous unit (Dougall et al., 1999; Kong et al., 1999; Fata et al., 2000; Rossi et al., 2007; Hanada et al., 2009; Duheron et al., 2011).

In parallel to its physiologic functions, the RANK/RANKL axis has been also implicated in several pathologies, in particular in tumors with bone connections as bone primitive tumors and bone metastasis forming tumors. Thus, functional RANK expression has been reported in cells of different tumors, such as prostate and breast cancers, osteosarcoma and melanoma (Jones et al., 2006; Wittrant et al., 2006; Mori et al. 2007a, b, c). Moreover, RANKL was shown to trigger the migration of these RANK-expressing cells (Jones et al., 2006; Mori et al., 2007a). According to these observations, the RANK/RANKL axis might have a great impact on melanoma development. The aim of the present chapter is to discuss, based on the actual knowledge, the feasibility of targeting RANK/RANKL axis for the treatment of melanoma.

## 2. RANK/RANKL axis interest for melanoma treatment

### 2.1 RANK/RANKL, skin-appendages and skin

The RANK/RANKL axis has emerged as an important physiologic player in epithelial cell growth and differentiation. First evidences came from expression patterns of both RANK and RANKL during the development of skin-appendages as hairs, teeth and mammary glands (Ohazama et al., 2004; Mikkola, 2008; Tanos & Brisken, 2008; Duheron et al., 2011). Regarding mammary glands, RANK and its ligand are both expressed in epithelial cells and control the development of a lactating mammary gland during pregnancy. In absence of RANK/RANKL signaling, the formation of lobulo-alveolar structures, necessary to a functional lactating mammary gland, is severely impaired leading to milk secretion defect.

Concerning hairs, RANK is expressed by the hair follicle germ, bulge stem cells and epidermal basal cells. Interestingly, these cell-types are implicated in the renewal of the epidermo-pilosebaceous unit. Its ligand (RANKL) is actively transcribed by the hair follicle at initiation of its growth phase, providing a mechanism for RANK-expressing stem cell engagement and hair-cycle entry. Mice deficient in RANKL are unable to initiate a new growth phase of the hair cycle and display arrested epidermal homeostasis. Furthermore, transgenic mice overexpressing RANK in the hair follicle or administration of recombinant RANKL both activate the hair cycle and epidermal growth. Finally, RANK signaling is dispensable for the formation of the stem cell compartment and the induction of hair follicle mesenchyme, but RANK-RANKL axis regulates hair renewal and epidermal homeostasis and provides a link between these two activities.

The RANK/RANKL axis also plays essential roles on immune system including participation in T-cell/dendritic cell communications (Leibbrandt & Penninger, 2010). Interestingly, RANKL over-expression in keratinocytes results in functional alterations of epidermal dendritic cells and systemic increases of regulatory CD4(+)CD25(+) T cells. Consequently, epidermal RANKL expression can modify dendritic cell functions to maintain the number of peripheral CD4(+)CD25(+) regulatory T cells. Finally, environmental stimuli at the skin level can rewire the local and systemic immune system by means of RANKL.

### 2.2 RANK/RANKL and bone-associated cancers

Since the late nineteenth century, it has been thought that the microenvironment of the local host tissue actively participates in the tendency of some cancers to metastasize to specific organs (Paget, 1889). However, the specific factors involved are still unknown.

Bones are continuously remodeled throughout life by two complementary processes: bone matrix formation (apposition) regulated by osteoblasts and bone resorption managed by osteoclasts. The precise inter-relation between osteoblasts and osteoclasts leading to osteoclastogenesis is only partly deciphered. The discovery of certain key factors involved in the control of osteoclastogenesis has moved bone research into a new era. Current findings have revealed that the RANKL/RANK/OPG molecular triad constitutes a key regulator for both normal and pathological bone metabolism (Brown et al., 2001; Goltzman, 2001; Chen, et al. 2006). The prevention of different tumors metastases inheritance in bone by RANKL inhibitors [*i.e.*, OPG or soluble RANK (sRANK) or RANK blocking antibodies (RANK-Fc)] in established animal models of bone metastases, highlights the critical role of this triad in cancer-induced bone manifestations (Zhang et al., 2001, 2003; Corey et al., 2005; Whang et al., 2005; Mountzios et al., 2007; Canon et al, 2008). Interestingly, such anti-tumor effects appear to be restricted to bone models. Indeed, such effects have not been observed in any other models, including classical subcutaneous models (Zhang et al., 2001, 2003). Thus, it was first believed that anti-tumor effects induced by RANKL/RANK interaction blockage were the result of an indirect effect *via* osteoclasts.

In turn, functional RANK expression was recently reported in bone-associated tumors, more precisely in cells of breast cancer, prostate cancer, osteosarcoma and malignant melanoma (Jones et al., 2006; Wittrant et al., 2006; Mori et al., 2007a, b, c; Armstrong et al., 2008). According to the fact that RANK-expressing tumor cells migration was induced by RANKL stimulation (Armstrong et al., 2008; Jones et al., 2006; Mori et al., 2007a), the direct effect of RANKL on RANK-expressing tumor cells was in fine disclosed. Consequently, RANKL works, in bone, as one of the "soil" factors of Paget's theory (Fig. 1).

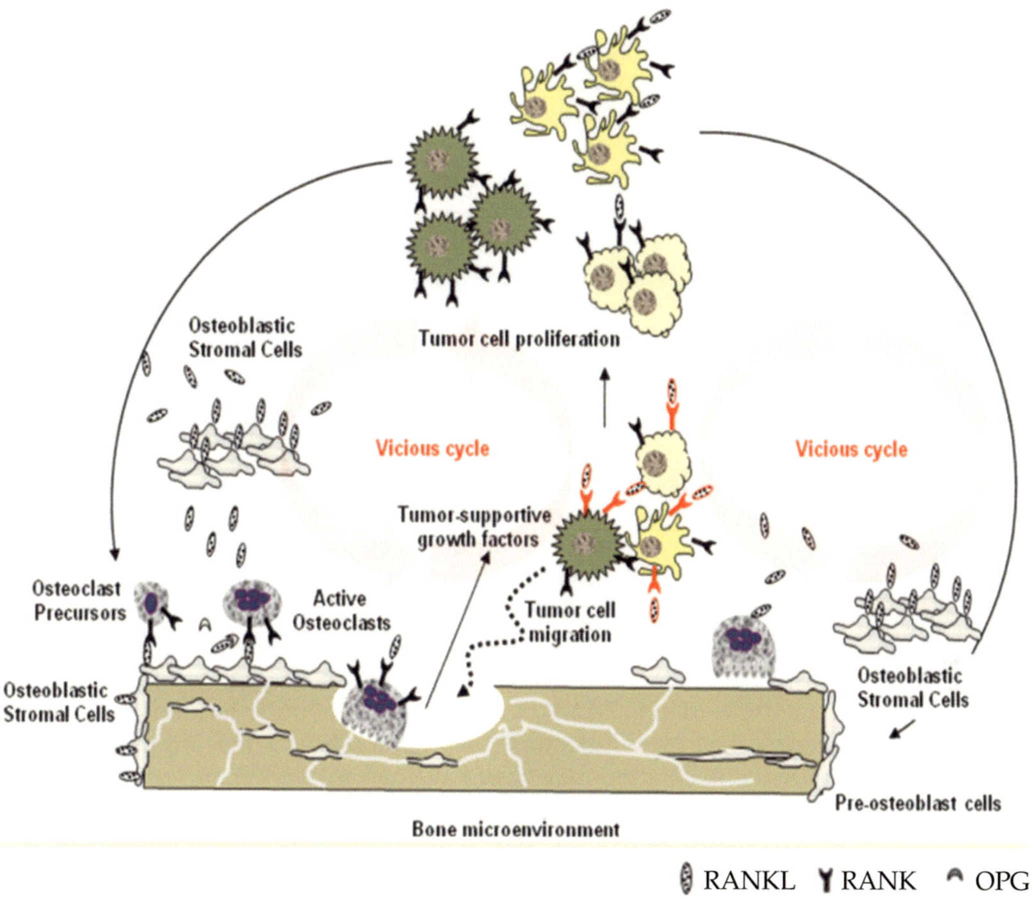


Fig. 1. Schematic representation of the putative interactions between RANK-expressing tumor cells (*i.e.,* prostate cancer, breast cancer and malignant melanoma) and bone cells (osteoblasts and osteoclasts) in the tumoral bone microenvironment

In fact, RANK-expressing tumor cells would preferentially targeted bone microenvironment where RANKL concentration is elevated. In the bone tumoral environment, RANKL produced by osteoblasts and bone stromal cells has two potential targets: on the one hand the osteoclast precursor and the osteoclast, and on the other hand the RANK-expressing tumor cell. So RANKL acts as a "soil" factor that facilitates cancer metastasis settlement in bone by activating both kinds of RANK-expressing cells.

### 2.3 Melanomas: skin tumors with bone metastasis

Melanoma belongs to the large family of skin tumors (see WHO classification of skin tumors: In Pathology and Genetics of Skin Tumors edited by P.E. LeBoit, G. Burg, D. Weedon and A. Sarasin, IARC Press, Lyon, 2006). From a clinical and public health point of view, malignant melanomas are the most important group of skin tumors. Although less common than basal and squamous cell tumors of the skin, they are much more often fatal, due to their intrinsic propensity to metastasis. The major environmental risk factor for melanoma is recurrent expositions to high-doses of UV radiations. Endogenous factors are often combined as genetic susceptibility. Bone metastasis is a poor prognostic for patient and corresponds to the ultimate stage of the pathology. The precise implication of RANK/RANKL axis in the bone metastatic process has been controversial but nowadays it seems clear that this signalization plays successive parts in this complex process. Indeed, RANK/RANKL axis is implicated in tumor cell migration (as previously described) and later in tumor cell settlement in the bone microenvironment and induction of osteolysis (Mundy, 2002; Jones et al., 2006). Consequently, targeting RANK/RANKL signalization might be a promising strategy to prevent melanoma bone metastasis and subsequent damages.

### 2.4 Targeting RANK/RANKL axis for melanoma treatment: benefit/risk

According to the disastrous consequences of melanoma metastasis in term of patient survival, any treatments that enable confinement of tumor cells to their initial site has to be considered as therapeutically beneficial. RANK/RANKL inhibitors, due to the implication of RANK/RANKL axis in metastatic process, are so potentially highly relevant therapeutic agents for melanoma. They may reduce the incidence of metastasis and synergized with anti-tumoral drugs. Indeed, several studies has been reported such beneficial effect of OPG (Lamoureux et al., 2007), OPG peptide (Heymann et al., 2005), RANK-Fc (Lamoureux et al., 2008) and Denosumab (fully human anti-RANKL antibody) (Abrahamsen et al., 2005) as RANK/RANKL inhibitors for the treatment of bone-associated cancers.

However, as presented above, the RANK/RANKL signalization is implicated in various physiological processes during development and takes part to the immune response. So targeting this pathway in children may have developmental consequences that need to be evaluated. Moreover, whatever the age of the patient, the potential impact of such inhibitor on the immune response as to be taken into account and may in fine limited their use.

## 3. Conclusion

The use of drugs targeting the RANK/RANKL axis in melanoma appears to be a promising strategy to reduce the mortality of this skin cancer. Such drugs should reduce the metastatic process and enforce the action of classical anti-tumoral treatment. However, further studies will be necessary to evaluate the impact of these drugs on RANK/RANKL signaling physiological functions, more specifically during growth, and to deal with these drugs potential wrong impact on immune system.

## 4. Acknowledgment

This work was supported by INSERM and by the French Ministry of Research.

## 5. References

Abrahamsen, B. & Teng, A.Y. (2005). Technology evaluation: denosumab, Amgen. *Curr Opin Mol Ther* Vol.7, No.6, (December), pp. 604-610, ISSN 1464-8431

Armstrong, A.P.; Miller, R.E.; Jones, J.C.; Zhang, J.; Keller, E.T. & Dougall, W.C. (2008). RANKL acts directly on RANK-expressing prostate tumor cells and mediates migration and expression of tumor metastasis genes. *Prostate* Vol.68, No.1, (January), pp. 92-104, ISSN 0270-4137

Brown, J.M.; Corey, E.; Lee, Z.D.; True, L.D.; Yun, T.J.; Tondravi, M. & Vessella, R.L. (2001). Osteoprotegerin and rank ligand expression in prostate cancer. *Urology* Vol.57, No.4, (April), pp. 611-616, ISSN 0090-4295

Canon, J.R.; Roudier, M. & Bryant, R. (2008). Inhibition of RANKL blocks skeletal tumor progression and improves survival in a mouse model of breast cancer bone metastasis. *Clin Exp Metastasis* Vol.25, No.2, pp. 119-129.

Chen, G.; Sircar, K.; Aprikian, A.; Potti, A.; Goltzman, D. & Rabbani, S.A. (2006). Expression of RANKL/RANK/OPG in primary and metastatic human prostate cancer as markers of disease stage and functional regulation. *Cancer* Vol.107, No.2, (July), pp. 289-298, ISSN 0008-543X

Corey, E.; Brown, L.G.; Kiefer, J.A.; Quinn, J.E.; Pitts, T.E.; Blair, J.M. & Vessella, R.L. (2005). Osteoprotegerin in prostate cancer bone metastasis. *Cancer Res* Vol.65, No.5, (March), pp. 1710-1718, ISSN 0008-5472

Dougall, W.C.; Glaccum, M.; Charrier, K.; Rohrbach, K.; Brasel, K.; De Smedt, T.; Daro, E.; Smith, J.; Tometsko, M.E.; Maliszewski, C.R.; Armstrong, A.; Shen, V.; Bain, S.; Cosman, D.; Anderson, D.; Morrissey, P.J.; Peschon, J.J. & Schuh, J. (1999). RANK is essential for osteoclast and lymph node development. *Genes Dev* Vol.13, No.18, (September), pp2412–2424, ISSN 0890-9369

Duheron, V.; Hess, E.; Duval, M.; Decossas, M.; Castaneda, B.; Klöpper, J.E.; Amoasii, L.; Barbaroux, J.B.; Williams, I.R.; Yagita, H.; Penninger, J.; Choi, Y.; Lézot, F.; Groves, R.; Paus, R. & Mueller, C.G. (2011). Receptor activator of NF-{kappa}B (RANK) stimulates the proliferation of epithelial cells of the epidermo-pilosebaceous unit. *Proc Natl Acad Sci U S A*. Vol.108, No.13, (March), pp. 5342-5347, ISSN 0027-8424

Fata, J.E.; Kong, Y.Y.; Li, J.; Sasaki, T.; Irie-Sasaki, J.; Moorehead, R.A.; Elliott, R.; Scully, S.; Voura, E.B.; Lacey, D.L.; Boyle, W.J.; Khokha, R. & Penninger, J.M. (2000). The osteoclast differentiation factor osteoprotegerin-ligand is essential for mammary gland development. *Cell* Vol.103, No.1, (September), pp. 41–50, ISSN 0092-8674

Goltzman, D. (2001). Osteolysis and cancer. *J Clin Invest* Vol.107, No.10, (May), pp. 1219-1220, ISSN 0021-9738

Hanada, R.; Leibbrandt, A.; Hanada, T.; Kitaoka, S.; Furuyashiki, T.; Fujihara, H.; Trichereau, J.; Paolino, M.; Qadri, F.; Plehm, R.; Klaere, S.; Komnenovic, V.; Mimata, H.; Yoshimatsu, H.; Takahashi, N.; von Haeseler, A.; Bader, M.; Kilic, S.S.; Ueta, Y.; Pifl, C.; Narumiya, S. & Penninger, J.M. (2009). Central control of fever and female body temperature by RANKL/RANK. *Nature* Vol.462, No.7272, (November), pp. 505–509, ISSN 0028-0836

Heymann, D.; Fortun, Y.; Rédini, F. & Padrines, M. (2005). Osteolytic bone diseases: physiological analogues of bone resorption effectors as alternative therapeutic tools. *Drug Discov Today* Vol.10, No.4, (February), pp. 242-247, ISSN 1359-6446

Jones, D.H.; Nakashima, T.; Sanchez, O.H.; Kozieradzki, I.; Komarova, S.V.; Sarosi, I.; Morony, S.; Rubin, E.; Sarao, R.; Hojilla, C.V.; Komnenovic, V.; Kong, Y.Y.; Schreiber, M.; Dixon, S.J.; Sims, S.M.; Khokha, R.; Wada, T. & Penninger, J.M. Regulation of cancer cell migration and bone metastasis by RANKL. (2006) *Nature* Vo.440, No.7084, (March), pp. 692-696, ISSN 0028-0836

Kong, Y.Y.; Yoshida, H.; Sarosi, I.; Tan, H.L.; Timms, E.; Capparelli, C.; Morony, S.; Oliveira-dos-Santos, A.J.; Van, G.; Itie, A.; Khoo, W.; Wakeham, A.; Dunstan, C.R.; Lacey, D.L.; Mak, T.W.; Boyle, W.J. & Penninger, J.M. (1999). OPGL is a key regulator of osteoclastogenesis, lymphocyte development and lymph-node organogenesis. *Nature* Vol.397, No.6717, (January), pp. 315–323, ISSN 0028-0836

Lacey, D.L.; Timms, E.; Tan, H.L.; Kelley, M.J.; Dunstan, C.R.; Burgess, T.; Elliott, R.; Colombero, A.;, Elliott, G.; Scully, S.; Hsu, H.; Sullivan, J.; Hawkins, N.; Davy, E.; Capparelli, C.; Eli, A.; Qian, Y.X.; Kaufman, S.; Sarosi, I.; Shalhoub, V.; Senaldi, G.; Guo, J.; Delaney, J. & Boyle, W.J. (1998). Osteoprotegerin ligand is a cytokine that regulates osteoclast differentiation and activation. *Cell* Vol.93, No.2, (April), pp. 165-176, ISSN 0092-8674

Lamoureux, F.; Richard, P.; Wittrant, Y.; Battaglia, S.; Pilet, P.; Trichet, V.; Blanchard, F.; Gouin, F.; Pitard, B.; Heymann, D. & Redini, F. (2007). Therapeutic relevance of osteoprotegerin gene therapy in osteosarcoma: blockade of the vicious cycle between tumor cell proliferation and bone resorption. *Cancer Res* Vol.67, No.15, (August), pp. 7308-7318, ISSN 0008-5472

Lamoureux, F.; Picarda, G.; Rousseau, J.; Gourden, C.; Battaglia, S.; Charrier, C.; Pitard, B.; Heymann, D. & Rédini, F. (2008). Therapeutic efficacy of soluble receptor activator of nuclear factor-kappa B-Fc delivered by nonviral gene transfer in a mouse model of osteolytic osteosarcoma. *Mol Cancer Ther* Vol.7, No.10, (October), pp. 3389-3398, ISSN 1535-7163

Leibbrandt, A. & Penninger, J.M. (2010). Novel Functions of RANK(L) Signaling in the Immune System. *Adv Exp Med Biol* Vol.658, pp. 77-94, ISSN 0065-2598

Mikkola, M.L. (2008). TNF superfamily in skin appendage development. *Cytokine Growth Factor Rev* Vol.19, No.3-4, (June-August), pp. 219-230, ISSN 1359-6101

Mori, K.; Le Goff, B.; Charrier, C.; Battaglia, S.; Heymann, D. & Rédini, F. (2007a). DU145 human prostate cancer cells express functional receptor activator of NFkappaB: new insights in the prostate cancer bone metastasis process. *Bone* Vol.40, No.4, (April), pp. 981-90, ISSN 8756-3282

Mori, K.; Le Goff, B.; Berreur, M.; Riet, A.; Moreau, A.; Blanchard, F.; Chevalier, C.; Guisle-Marsollier, I.; Léger, J.; Guicheux, J.; Masson, M.; Gouin, F.; Rédini, F. & Heymann, D. (2007b). Human osteosarcoma cells express functional receptor activator of nuclear factor-kappa B. *J Pathol* Vol.211, No.5, (April), pp. 555-562, ISSN 0022-3417

Mori, K.; Berreur, M.; Blanchard, F.; Chevalier, C.; Guisle-Marsollier, I.; Masson, M.; Rédini, F. & Heymann, D. (2007c) Receptor activator of nuclear factor-kappaB ligand (RANKL) directly modulates the gene expression profile of RANK-positive Saos-2 human osteosarcoma cells. *Oncol Rep* Vol.18, No.6, (December), pp.1365-1371, ISSN1021-335X

Mountzios, G.; Dimopoulos, M.A.; Bamias, A.; Papadopoulos, G.; Kastritis, E.; Syrigos, K.; Pavlakis, G. & Terpos, E. (2007). Abnormal bone remodeling process is due to an imbalance in the receptor activator of nuclear factor-kappaB ligand (RANKL)/osteoprotegerin (OPG) axis in patients with solid tumors metastatic to the skeleton. *Acta Oncol* Vol.46, No.2, pp. 221-229, ISSN 0284-186X

Ohazama, A.; Courtney, J.M. & Sharpe, P.T. (2004). Opg, Rank, and Rankl in tooth development: co-ordination of odontogenesis and osteogenesis. *J Dent Res* Vol.83, No.3, (March), pp. 241-244, ISSN 0022-0345

Paget, S. (1889). The distrubution of secondary growths in cancer of the breast. Lancet Vol.1, pp. 571-572, ISSN 0140-6736

Rossi, S.W.; Kim, M.Y.; Leibbrandt, A.; Parnell, S.M.; Jenkinson, W.E.; Glanville, S.H.; McConnell, F.M.; Scott, H.S.; Penninger, J.M.; Jenkinson, E.J.; Lane, P.J. & Anderson, G. (2007). RANK signals from CD4(+)3(-) inducer cells regulate development of Aire-expressing epithelial cells in the thymic medulla. *J Exp Med* Vol.204, No.6, (June), pp. 1267–1272, ISSN 0022-1007

Simonet, W.S.; Lacey, D.L.; Dunstan, C.R.; Kelley, M.; Chang, M.S.; Lüthy, R.; Nguyen, H.Q.; Wooden, S.; Bennett, L.; Boone, T.; Shimamoto, G.; DeRose, M.; Elliott, R.; Colombero, A.; Tan, H.L.; Trail, G.; Sullivan, J.; Davy, E.; Bucay, N.; Renshaw-Gegg, L.; Hughes, T.M.; Hill, D.; Pattison, W.; Campbell, P.; Sander, S.; Van, G.; Tarpley, J.; Derby, P.; Lee, R. & Boyle, W.J. (1997). Osteoprotegerin: a novel secreted protein involved in the regulation of bone density. *Cell* Vol.89, No.2, (April) pp. 309-319, ISSN 0092-8674

Tanos, T. & Brisken, C. (2008). What signals operate in the mammary niche? *Breast Dis* Vol.29, pp.69-82,

Tat, S.K.; Padrines, M.; Theoleyre, S.; Couillaud-Battaglia, S.; Heymann, D.; Redini, F. & Fortun, Y. (2006). OPG/membranous -RANKL complex is internalized via the clathrin pathway before a lysosomal and a proteasomal degradation. *Bone* Vol.39, No.4, (October) pp. 706-715, ISSN 8756-3282

Theoleyre, S.; Wittrant, Y.; Tat, S.K.; Fortun, Y.; Redini, F. & Heymann, D. (2004). The molecular triad OPG/RANK/RANKL: involvement in the orchestration of pathophysiological bone remodeling. *Cytokine Growth Factor Rev* Vol.15, No.6, (December), pp. 457-475, ISSN 1359-6101

Whang, P.G.; Schwarz, E.M.; Gamradt, S.C.; Dougall, W.C. & Lieberman, J.R. (2005) The effects of RANK blockade and osteoclast depletion in a model of pure osteoblastic prostate cancer metastasis in bone. *J Orthop Res* Vol.23, No.6, (November), pp. 1475-1483, ISSN 0736-0266

Wittrant, Y.; Lamoureux, F.; Mori, K.; Riet, A.; Kamijo, A.; Heymann, D. & Redini, F. (2006) RANKL directly induces bone morphogenetic protein-2 expression in RANK-expressing POS-1 osteosarcoma cells. *Int J Oncol* Vol.28, No.1, (January), pp. 261-269, ISSN 1019-6439

Zhang, J.; Dai, J.; Qi, Y.; Lin, D.L.; Smith, P.; Strayhorn, C.; Mizokami, A.; Fu, Z.; Westman, J. & Keller, E.T. (2001). Osteoprotegerin inhibits prostate cancer-induced osteoclastogenesis and prevents prostate tumor growth in the bone. *J Clin Invest* Vol.107, No.10, (May), pp. 1235-1244, ISSN 0021-9738

Zhang, J.; Dai, J.; Yao, Z.; Lu, Y.; Dougall, W. & Keller, E.T. (2003) Soluble receptor activator of nuclear factor kappaB Fc diminishes prostate cancer progression in bone. *Cancer Res* Vol.63, No.22, (November), pp. 7883-7890. ISSN 0008-5472

# 28

# Isolation of Cellular Clones of Murine Melanoma Resistants to the Photodynamic Therapy and Characterization of Some Mechanisms Involved in the Radioresistance

Ramón-Gallegos E.[1], Rosas-Flores L.[1], Barrera-Mendoza C.C.[1], Herrera-Carrillo Z.[1], González-Agüero G.[1], Estrada-Manrique G.[1] and Cruz-Orea A.[2]
[1]*Lab. de Citopatología Ambiental, Escuela Nacional de Ciencias Biológicas, Instituto Politécnico Nacional, Campus Zacatenco, Unidad Profesional "Adolfo López Mateos" Calle Wilfrido Massieu esquina Cda. Manuel Stampa Zacatenco, Del. Gustavo A. Madero, C.P. 07738,*
[2]*Departamento de Física, Centro de Investigación y Estudios Avanzados-IPN, México*

## 1. Introduction

In the world, the skin cancer is by far the most common of all cancers. Melanoma accounts for less than 5% of skin cancer cases but causes 75% of skin cancer deaths (ACS, 2011). 132,000 melanoma skin cancers occur globally each year (WHO, 2011). In Mexico there is an evident increase of this neoplasia, with a growth of almost 500% in the last few years (Hernandez, 2005). The malignant melanoma is the most lethal of all skin cancers, due to its great capacity to produce metastasis and its chemotherapy-resistant properties that stand as challenging barriers to successful treatment (Kim, et al., 2010). For melanoma there is not an effective treatment, in the 95% of cases surgery is the choice therapy. Other alternatives included chemotherapy, immunotherapy, radiotherapy and a combination of these. Another strategy being explored is photodynamic therapy (PDT), a non-invasive selective therapy that opens new perspectives on the treatment of cancer. PDT emerges like a hopeful treatment for cancer and other diseases (Paras, 2003), is a low invasive treatment based on photosensitizer drugs that are administrated to the patients and can be retained on a selective mode for the ill tissue more than the normal tissue (Mang, 2004). This therapeutic procedure has been applied in the treatment of many hyper proliferative diseases of keratinocytes (Bugaj et al., 2004).

The action of photodynamic therapy is based on the use of visible light or near infrared, a photosensitizer and the presence of molecular oxygen ($O_2$) on transformed cells (like tumor cells); light is absorbed for the photosensitizer and this action is used to activate the oxygen (Bonnett, 2000) present into cancerous cells and to generate reactive oxygen species (mainly singlet oxygen), that are potentially cytotoxic causing lethal damage to the cell and/or inhibits angiogenesis (Bugaj et al., 2004). Various photosensitizing drugs have been developed, such as 5-aminolevulinic acid (ALA) that unlike other PDT drugs is not a photosensitizer. When taken up by cancerous cells it is converted by a naturally occurring biosynthetic process into the photosensitizer protoporphyrin IX (PpIX). It is known that PpIX is present at low concentrations in normal cells and high concentration in tumor cells, the enzyme ferrochelatase, which converts protopophyrin IX to heme, has been found to be reduced, whereas the opposite situation has been found for porphobilinogen deaminase (Van-Hillegerberg et al., 1994). ALA can be applied topically, and was approved by the FDA in 1999 for the treatment of actinic keratosis (Zhu & Finlay, 2008). In dermatology the use of ALA has had good results on superficial tumors, however, this treatment is not recommended for pigmented tumors, like melanoma (Juzenas et al., 2002). There are many hypotheses where this problem has been discussed; maybe the presence of melanin on tumoral cells absorbs the light use on PDT on the tumor (Sheleg et al., 2004) in addition it has been considered an interaction between melanin and porphyrins, this can reduce the absorbance and generate non fluorescent compounds. However, there is little information available about PDT efficiency using ALA and derivates on the treatment of melanoma (Juzenas et al., 2002).

The aim of the present study was to obtain resistant clones of murine melanome by several photodynamic treatments and to study some factors that could be involved in the PDT-resistant such as: biosynthesis capacity of PpIX stimulated by ALA, concentration melanin and mitochondrial activity.

## 2. Material and methods

### 2.1 Cell lines and culture conditions

Murine melanoma cells B16F0 (metastatic melanoma, number CRL-6322, ATCC) and B16F10 (number CRL-6475, ATCC) both isolated from the primary tumor C57BL/6J were cultured in DMEM-F12 medium supplemented with 10% fetal bovine serum (FBS) and 100 U/mL of penicillin and 100 U/mL of streptomycin. Cells were cultured at 37 °C in 5% $CO_2$.

### 2.2 Determination of intra and extra-cellular PpIX induced by ALA

Cells were plated into 6-well plates at a cell density of $8x10^5$ per well in 2 mL of DMEM supplemented with 10% FBS. After 24 h the medium was removed and cells were exposed to 0, 25, 50, 75, 100 and 150 μg of ALA/mL of serum-free medium for 4 h in darkness at 37ºC. Afterward, the medium was removed and collected in centrifuge tubes that contained 200 μL of celita in 5% saline to its subsequent analysis. The cells were washed with saline phosphate buffer (PBS, pH 7.4) and detached with 500 μL trypsin/EDTA. Following cells were spun at 200xg, supernatant was removed and cells were rinsed once in PBS, then collected by centrifugation and lysed in 0.2 mL of 5% celite. To quantify the intra and extra-cellular PpIX it was used the Piomelli spectrofluorometry assay for free erythrocyte porphyrins (Piomelli, 1973) as adapted for cultured cells was used to quantify PpIX (Ramón et al., 1999). PpIX levels were read directly as μg/cells using a Perkin Elmer LS-2B spectrofluorometer calibrated with coproporphyrin I (0.05 μg/mL; Sigma) stock solution (excitation wavelength 408 nm, emission 608 nm). All assays were performed in triplicate. A blank was prepared in parallel by replacing the cellular suspension with 40 μL of saline solution.

### 2.3 Photodynamic treatment

30,000 cells/well were seeded in 96 well plates and these were exposed to 0, 25, 50, 75, 100, 125, 150 µg of ALA/mL of culture medium serum free for 4h. This proceeding was applied to the parental lines, B16F0 and B16F10, and irradiated with an argon laser with 70 mW of power and with a light dose of 64.3 J/cm$^2$. The used groups were: negative control (cells without ALA and irradiation), irradiation control (irradiated cells only), and treated cells group (cells with ALA and irradiation). In all the experiments the B16F0 and B16F10 cells were conserved in darkness before and after irradiation.

### 2.4 Cell survival rate by red neutral-red assay

After exposing cells to the different conditions mentioned above cell viability was measured by neutral-red spectrophotometric assay (Borenfreud and Shopis, 1985). The medium containing ALA was removed from the wells and replaced with 100 µL of fresh medium per well containing 100 µL of neutral red. The plates were then returned to the incubator for 3 h. Medium was subsequently removed, and the cultures were washed rapidly with a mixture of 40% formaldehyde and 10% $CaCl_2$ V/V (4:1). A mixture of 1% V/V acetic acid and 50% V/V ethanol (1:1) was then added to extract the neutral red. The plate was shaken for 60 s and left to stand at room temperature for 15 min. The absorbance of the solubilized dye was subsequently read at 540 nm. Quantification of the extracted dye was correlated with the live cell number. Control wells were prepared in parallel, and these cells were exposed to neutral red, but not to ALA. The percentage of viable cells in the cell population at each concentration of the test agent was calculated by means of the equation 1.

$$\% \text{ viability} = \frac{\text{Mean absorbance of treated cells}}{\text{Mean absorbance of control cells}} \times 100 \quad (1)$$

### 2.5 Obtainment PDT-resistant clones (PDTR)

B16F0 and B16F10 cells were seeded into each well of a 96-well plate before treatment. Cells were incubated for 24 h following administration of ALA at a concentration of 125 and 150 µg/mL respectively, in serum-free medium. After, they were exposed to PDT with a light dose of 64.3 J/cm$^2$ in one exposition. 24h after irradiation, cells were harvested with EDTA-trypsin and centrifuged for 2 min at 224xg. The supernatant was discarded and cells were resuspended in 1.0 mL of medium supplemented with FBS and plated in a culture bottle. In parallel one experiment was realized with the same conditions utilizing a light dose of 64.3 J/cm$^2$. In both cases the viability was measured with neutral red method.

### 2.6 Melanin determination

This quantification was performed for all cell lines. Cells were exposed to their respectively ALA concentration and incubated for 4 h. Medium was recovered for measure extracellular melanin and cells were washed with PBS and detached with trypsin-EDTA, this solution was quenched after 15-20 min with 1 mL of DMEM supplemented with 10% FBS. Cells were centrifuged at 224xg and washed with 1 mL PBS, resuspended in 1 mL NaOH 1M in DMSO 10% and incubated at 80°C for 2h. It was centrifuged at 224xg and supernatant was recovered to measure intracellular melanin. A blank of 1M NaOH in DMSO 10% was prepared in parallel. Absorbance was measured at 420 nm, the amount of melanin was expressed in absorbance units (a.u.) per cell number, according to the methodology described by Rad (Rad, et al., 2004).

### 2.7 Assessment of mitochondrial activity by MTT assay

The mitochondrial activity was determined by the 3-(4,5-dimethylthiazol-2-yl)-2,5-diphenyltetrazolium bromide (MTT) assay (Mossman, 1983). The cell lines B16F0, B16F10 and cellular clones PDT-resistant were exposed to 0, 25, 50, 75, 100, 125, 150 μg of ALA/mL for 4 h. Then, the medium containing ALA was removed from the wells and replaced with 100 μL of MTT reagent diluted in DMEM medium serum-free (25 μg/mL) at 37ºC. After 4h, the obtained formazan products were reconstituted in 0.04 N HCl in isopropyl alcohol. The reduction of MTT by the viable cells was measured by an absorbance maximum at 540 nm.

### 2.8 Determination of mitochondrial abundance by MitoTracker Green FM®

In order to evaluate the mitochondrial abundance were used the MitoTracker Green FM® selective probes (Invitrogen). It was used according to manufacturer´s conditions. Fluorescence was observed in a Nikon EFD-3.

### 2.9 Statistical analysis

Two-way analysis of variance (ANOVA) was performed for all the assessments made. In the case of the determination of mitochondrial abundance the Mann-Whitney rank-sum test was performed. The level of significance was set at $P < 0.05$. The tests were performed with SigmaStat version 3.1 for Windows (Jandel Scientific).

## 3. Results

### 3.1 Obtainment of PDT-resistant clones (PDTR)

Before of obtaining PDT-resistant melanoma clones from parental melanoma cells it was necessary to know the ALA concentration that induces the maximum intracellular accumulation of PpIX and afterwards to find this information in the PDT-resistant melanoma clones.

### 3.2 Intra and extracellular PpIX accumulation induced by ALA for 24 hours in B16F0 and B16F10 with their clones PDT-resistant

It was found that all ALA concentrations tested (25, 50, 75, 100, 125 and 150 μg of ALA/mL) induced significatively the intracellular accumulation of PpIX in comparison to the basal level (0 mg of ALA/mL) (Table 1). B16F10 accumulates 43.0 times more PpIX than basal level of B16F0, in basal conditions, did not accumulate PpIX but its concentration reached up to 2 μg of PpIX/8x$10^5$ cells and when it is compared with their intracellular PpIX concentration (1.64 μg/8x$10^5$ cells) at lest ALA concentration is possible to found that B16F0 accumulates 1.4 times. From this results it was selected the ALA concentration for PDT application; for the B16F0 was 125 μg/mL and for B16F10 was 150 μg/mL. The low level of extracellular PpIX (Table 1) shows that the majority of PpIX is keept into the cells, this is important because the PpIX acts intracellularly as a response to PDT. The B16F0 cells accumulate from 2 to 9 times more PpIX than B16F10 at ≤125 μg/mL of ALA (Figure 1A).

After obtaining cellular PDT-resistant clones the parental cells were irradiated at 64.3 J/cm$^2$ with a concentration of ALA of 125 μg/mL for B16F0 and 150 μg/mL for B16F10. Resistant cells are the ones that survive to this irradiation conditions. To determinate if PpIX accumulation were accumulated in PDT-resistant clones a similar experiment was performed (Table 2). B16F0-PDTR cells in basal condition accumulated PpIX (Tables 1 and 2) and when these cells were exposed to ALA at minimal concentration tested (25 μg/mL) accumulated 11 times more PpIX in comparison to basal level and 30 times at 125 μg/mL of ALA. B16F10-PDTR has a similar response; in basal conditions has 3 times more PpIX than B16F10, but when this is compared with ALA at 125 and 150 μg/mL intracellular PpIX concentration increases 44 and 16 times more, in comparison with the basal level. Therefore, in the PDT-resistant clones obtained (B16F0-PDTR and B16F10-PDTR) it can be seen that these when exposed to ALA accumulated the highest concentration of PpIX in comparison to parental melanoma cells, in the other hand using low ALA concentration is possible to obtain high levels of intracellular PpIX. The B16F0-PDTR cells accumulated from 2 to 8 times more PpIX than B16F10-PDTR at ≤150 μg/mL of ALA (Figure 1B).

| ALA (μg/mL) | PpIX in B16F0 | | PpIX in B16F10 | |
|---|---|---|---|---|
| | Intracellular (μg/8x10$^5$ cells) | Extracellular (μg/mL of culture medium) | Intracellular (μg/8x10$^5$ cells) | Extracellular (μg/mL of culture medium) |
| 0 | 0.00± 0.001 | 0.011 ± 0.001 | 0.06 ± 0.02 | 0.011 ± 0.000 |
| 25 | 1.64 ± 0.11 | 0.038 ± 0.001 | 0.18 ± 0.02 | 0.041 ± 0.004 |
| 50 | 1.89 ± 0.10 | 0.051 ± 0.001 | 0.35 ± 0.02 | 0.037 ± 0.001 |
| 75 | 2.24 ± 0.07 | 0.058 ± 0.004 | 0.53 ± 0.00 | 0.045 ± 0.001 |
| 100 | 2.04 ± 0.06 | 0.058 ± 0.003 | 0.99 ± 0.07 | 0.057 ± 0.003 |
| 125 | 2.21 ± 0.04 | 0.062 ± 0.001 | 1.46 ± 0.13 | 0.057 ± 0.002 |
| 150 | 2.00 ± 0.19 | 0.071 ± 0.000 | 2.45 ± 0.02 | 0.062 ± 0.004 |

Table 1. Intra and extracellular PpIX in B16F0 and B16F10 cells exposed to different ALA concentration for 24h

| ALA (μg/mL) | PpIX in B16F0-PDTR | | PpIX in B16F10-PDTR | |
|---|---|---|---|---|
| | Intracellular (μg/8x10$^5$cells) | Extracellular (μg/mL of culture medium) | Intracellular (μg/8x10$^5$cells) | Extracellular (μg/mL of culture medium) |
| 0 | 0.20 ± 0.00 | 0.017 ± 0.001 | 0.19 ± 0.00 | 0.022 ± 0.00 |
| 25 | 2.21 ± 0.02 | 0.046 ± 0.002 | 0.28 ± 0.00 | 0.051 ± 0.004 |
| 50 | 4.42 ± 0.17 | 0.054 ± 0.004 | 2.41 ± 0.1 | 0.073 ± 0.002 |
| 75 | 5.46 ± 0.35 | 0.054 ± 0.000 | 4.88 ± 0.19 | 0.074 ± 0.004 |
| 100 | 5.44 ± 0.47 | 0.059 ± 0.002 | 5.51 ± 0.47 | 0.086 ± 0.004 |
| 125 | 5.98 ± 0.09 | 0.057 ± 0.001 | 8.39 ± 0.09 | 0.081 ± 0.001 |
| 150 | 6.12 ± 0.22 | 0.060 ± 0.004 | 3.11 ± 0.09 | 0.084 ± 0.001 |

Table 2. PpIX accumulation in B16F0-PDTR and B16F10-PDTR clones exposed to different ALA concentration for 24h

The ALA dose that induced the highest accumulation of intracellular PpIX in the cell line B16F0-PDTR was of 150 μg/mL (6.12 ± 0.22μg / 8x10$^5$ cells). Two-way ANOVA statistical analysis showed a significant difference in PpIX content between the lines B16F10 and B16F10-PDTR ($p<0.05$) starting from 25 μg/mL of ALA (Fig. 1-A). With regard to B16F10-PDTR PpIX levels obtained were higher compared with the B16F10 (Fig. 1-B) and also with those obtained in B16F0 or B16F0 PDTR. The highest level of accumulation of PpIX in B16F10-PDTR was 8.39±0.09 with 125 μg/mL of ALA, this level is four times higher than that obtained with 150 μg/mL in B16F10.

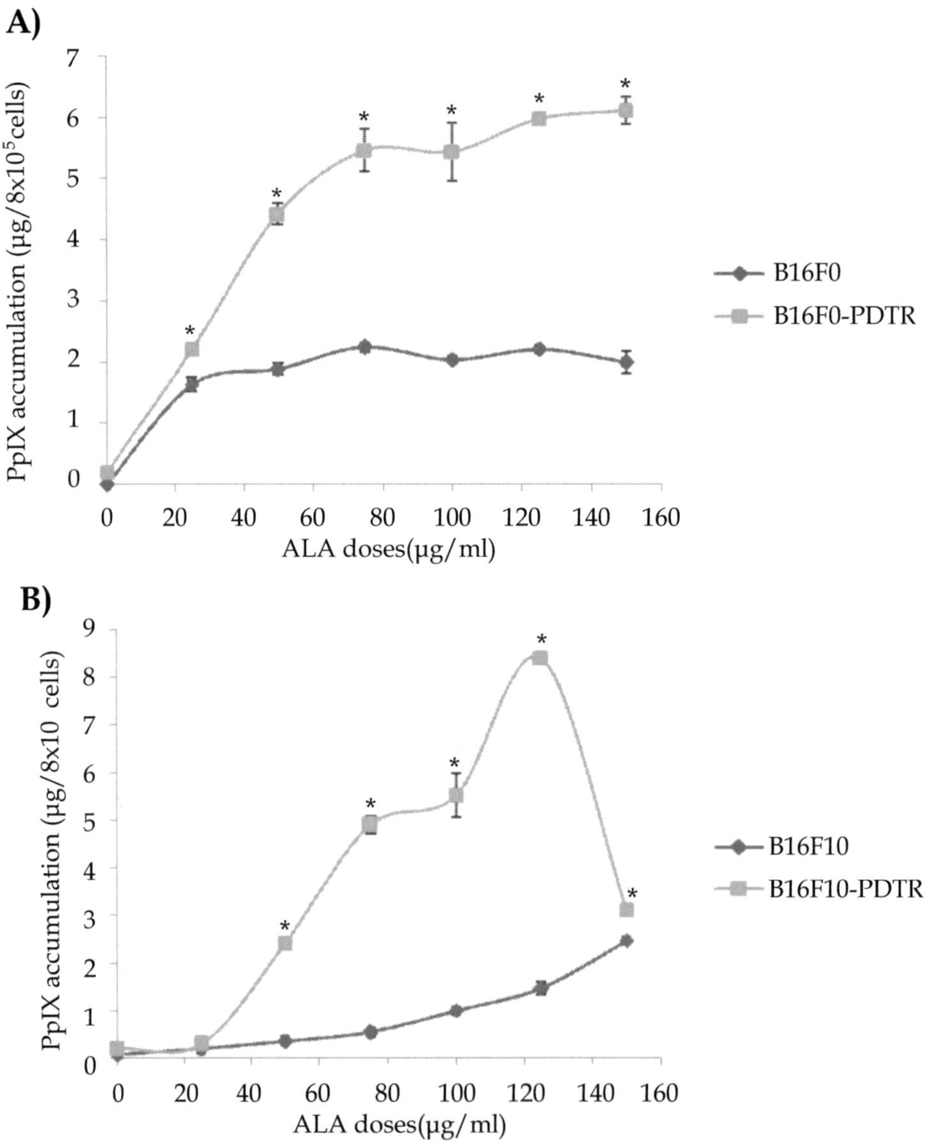


Fig. 1. Comparison of the accumulation of PpIX between B16F0 and B16F0-PDTR (A) and between B16F10 and B16F10-PDTR (B), * $p < 0.05$

### 3.3 PDT effect on cell mortality in different cell lines

The evaluation of cytotoxicity of PDT in the four cell lines was evaluated by neutral red technique. The results are expressed as percentage of mortality at different doses of ALA (125 and 150 µg/mL) exposed to a light doses of 64.3 J/cm² of irradiation. For B16F0 and B16F0-PDTR clone the mortality values ranged from 95-97%. B16F0-PDTR had a higher sensitivity to PDT in comparison with B16F0 ($p<0.05$). With regards to B16F10 and B16F10-PDTR the mortality index, as well as the previous cell lines, was higher (96±0.3% to 100%) in B16F10-PDTR. The PDT had a higher phototoxic effect when it was compared with B16F10, B16F0 and B16F0-PDTR (Fig. 2).

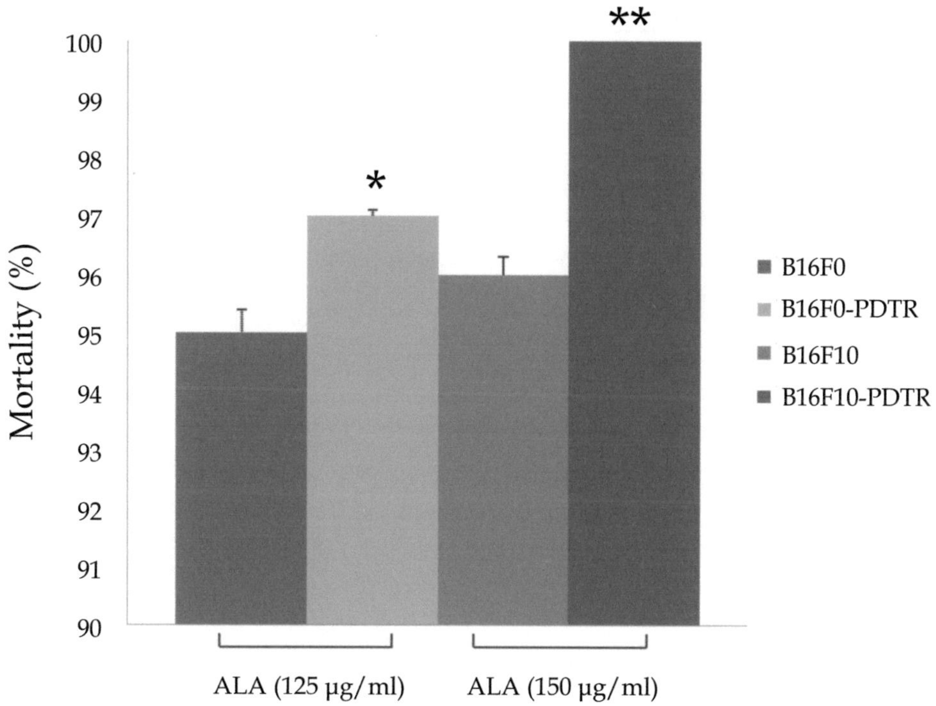


Fig. 2. Mortality percentage in the four cell lines exposed to a light doses of 64.3 J/cm². The four cell lines were treated with ALA at different doses; afterwards they were irradiated with 64.3 J/cm², *($p<0.05$) when comparing B16F0-PDTR with B16F0 and B16F10-PDTR with B16F10

| ALA (µg / mL) | Mortality (%) | | | | | | | |
|---|---|---|---|---|---|---|---|---|
| | 15 J/cm² | | | | 64.3 J / cm² | | | |
| | B16F0 | B16F0-PDTR | B16F10 | B16F10-PDTR | B16F0 | B16F0-PDTR | B16F10 | B16F10-PDTR |
| 0 | 0 | 0 | 0 | 0 | 0 | 0 | 0 | 0 |
| 125 | 44.39±3.6 | 85.31±0.43 | _ | _ | 95.0±0.4 | 97±0.1 | _ | _ |
| 150 | _ | _ | 91.00±0.51 | 96.82±0.24 | _ | _ | 96±0.3 | 100 |

Table 3. Percentage of mortality in the four cell lines with a light dose of 15 and 64.3 J/cm²

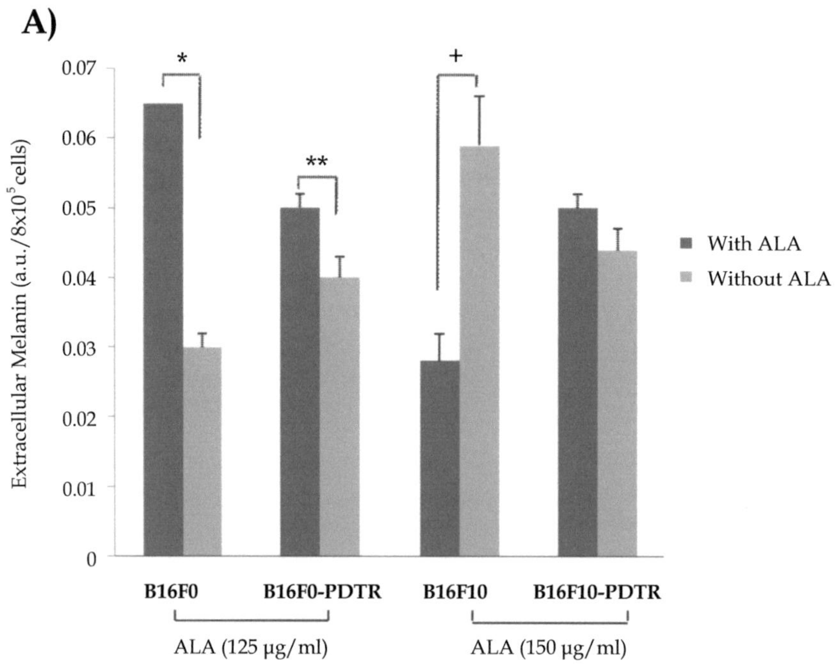


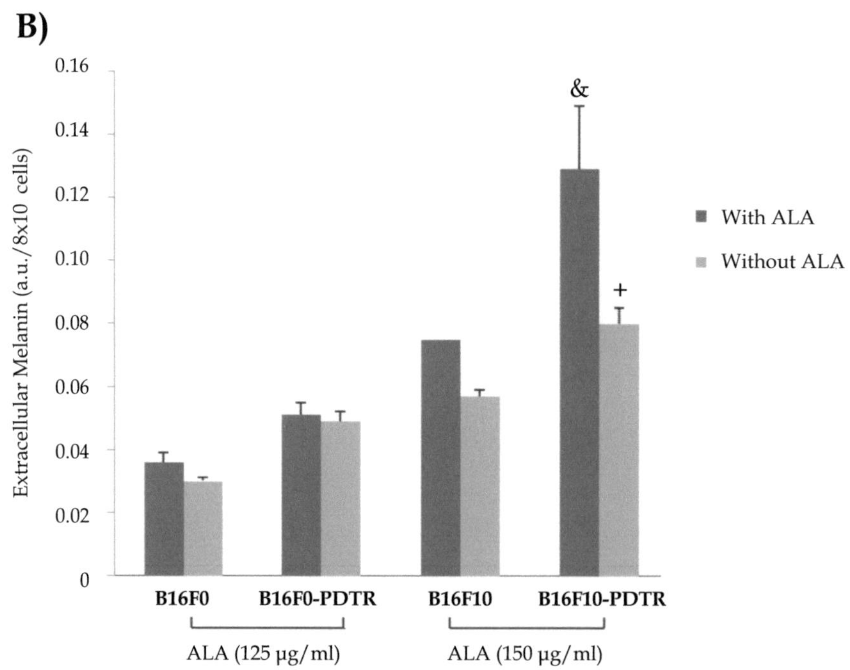


Fig. 5. Melanin concentration in four cell lines with and without ALA. A) Extracellular, B) Intracellular *($p<0.05$) when comparing B16F0 without ALA, ** ($p<0.05$) when comparing B16F0-PDTR with B16F10-PDTR without ALA, +($p<0.05$) with B16F10 with ALA, &($p<0.05$) with B16F0, B16F0-PDTR and B16F10

The effectiveness of PDT on *in vitro* murine melanoma lines have been previously reported with a light dose of 15 J/cm$^2$ or minor (Vena, et al, 2004), thus in this work it was decided to find if the four lines used suffer changes in its sensitivity to PDT using a ALA dose of 125 and 150 µg/mL with a irradiation of 15 J/cm$^2$ (Table 3).
The data observed in table 3 are similar to the ones obtained with an irradiation of 64.3 J/cm$^2$. B16F10-PDTR was the most sensitive cell line with a mortality rate of 96.82± 0.24 and B16F0 had the highest survival capacity (55.61%).

### 3.4 Concentration of extra and intracellular melanin

One of the possible mechanisms involved in the resistance to PDT is the melanin content in the cells, therefore a comparative analysis was performed between original lines and resistant clones at two levels (intracellular and extracellular). Results showed significant differences in melanin content (Fig. 5). It was observed a major concentration of intracellular melanin. The extracellular melanin content showed that B16F0 accumulates higher concentration in comparison with B16F0-PDTR (0.065 and 0.050±0.002 a.u./8x10$^5$ cells), in addition B16F10-PDTR accumulates a higher concentration of melanin than its parental line (0.050±002 and 0.028±0.004 a.u./8x10$^5$ cells) (Fig. 5-A). Resistant cell lines accumulate a higher intracellular concentration than their parental cell line. B16F10-PDTR was the cell line that accumulates the highest intracellular melanin concentration (Fig. 5-B). The presence of ALA does not interfere with the intracellular melanin contain.

### 3.5 Determination of mitochondrial activity by MTT assay

Another variable to be analyzed was the determination of mitochondrial activity in order to study functional changes in the mitochondria caused by ALA through MTT assay. The

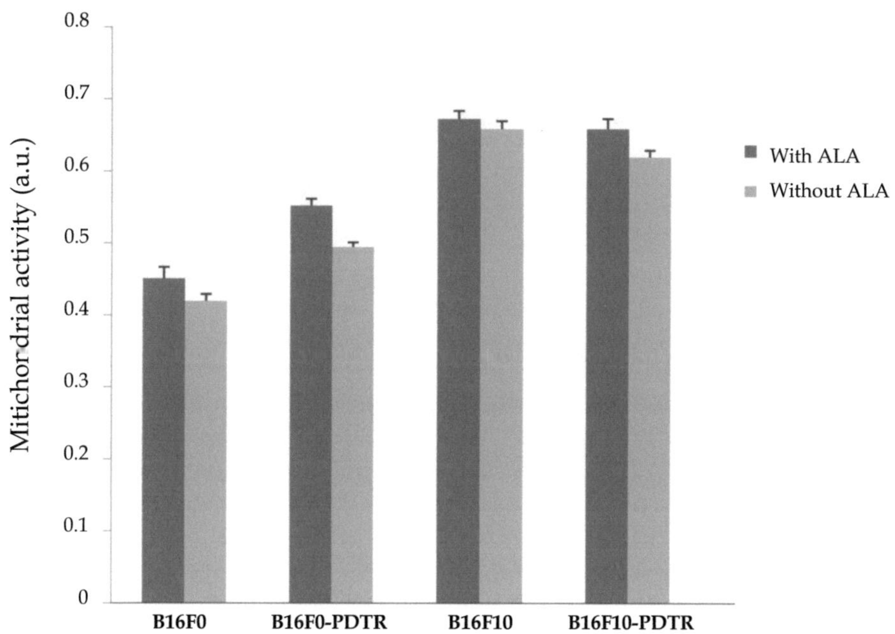


Fig. 6. Mitochondrial activity evaluated by MTT assay for B16F0, B16F0-PDTR, B16F10 and B16F10-PDTR

mitochondrial activity was evaluated in the four cell lines. The results showed an increment in the level of mitochondrial activity in the four lines when exposed to ALA, being more evident for B16F10 and its clone in comparison with B16F0 or B16F0-RPDT (Fig. 6).
The statistical analysis of mitochondrial activity between B16F0 and B16F0-RPDT showed significant differences ($p<0.05$). B16F0-PDTR showed a higher mitochondrial activity than B16F0 with or without ALA treatment. With regard to B16F10 and B16F10-RPDT lines, statistical analysis by two-way ANOVA only showed a significant difference between them without ALA ($p<0.05$), in addition B16F10-RPDT had a higher mitochondrial activity than B16F10, however they did not show significant differences in the treatment with ALA.

### 3.6 Mitochondrial abundance determination using fluorescent probes

As can be observed in table 4 B16F0 showed a higher mitochondrial light intensity (47.14±1.40) than the other three cell lines follower by B16F10-PDTR (45.01±1.04), B16F10 (34.75±0.71) and finally B16F0-PDTR (31.23±0.77) (Table 4).

| Fluorescent probe | Light Intensity (%) | | | |
|---|---|---|---|---|
| | Cell line | | | |
| | B16F0 | B16F0-PDTR | B16F10 | B16F10-PDTR |
| MitotrackerGreen FM | [a]47.14±1.40 | [a] 31.23±0.77 | [b]34.75±0.71 | [b] 45.01±1.04 |

Table 4. Mitochondrial abundance in cell lines measured by fluorescent probes. [a]26 fields, [b]30 fields

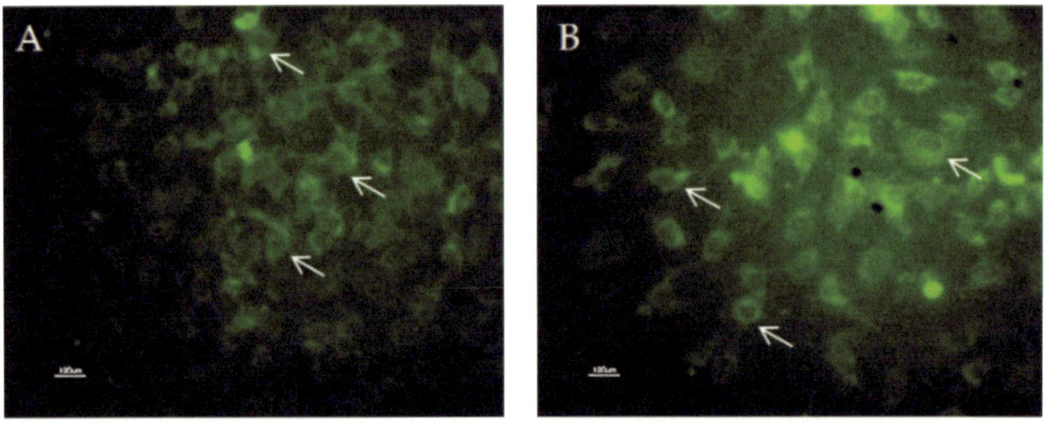


Fig. 7. Shows a representative image of the mitochondrial abundance in B16F10 (A) and B16F10-PDTR (B). The resistant cells B16F10-PDTR show a high light intensity compared with original cells, this suggests that there are a great number of mitochondria in these cells that could be involved in the process of resistance to PDT. Arrows indicate cells with fluoresce

### 3.7 Global analysis between the Photodynamic effect on parental melanoma cells and their resistant clones and the PpIX, melanin concentration, mitochondrial activity and mitochondrial concentration

A global analysis of the results is shown in table 5. The photodynamic effect can be observed by means of cellular death using two light doses (16 and 64.3 $J/cm^2$) and by observing that the cells that survive the first irradiation (B16F0-PDTR and B16F10-PDTR) when are irradiated for the second time become more sensitive; probably this effect is not clearly seen when it is used the wave length of 64.3 J/cm$^2$, but when it is used a wave length of 16 J/cm$^2$ the mortality in the resistant cells of the line B16F0 exposed to µg ALA/mL doubles in the resistant line, it as from 44.39 % of mortality to 85.31 %, this correlates with the concentration of extracellular melanin, it increases significantly when cells are exposed to ALA. Since it is so high the mortality in the line B16F10 this only increases 2 % and the extracellular melanin has no change. The mitochondrial activity increased significantly in the resistant clona B16F0-PDTR, whereas in the other lines though there is an increase from 10 to 20 % this one is not significant. In addition it can be observed that the concentration of PpIX increased in resistant cells.

| Cell line | ALA (µg ALA/mL) | Intracell PpIX µg/8x10$^5$ cel | PpIX ratio | Photodynamic effect (% Mortality) | | Melanin concentration (a.u./8x10$^5$ cells) | | Mito-chondrial activity | Mito-chondrial abundance |
|---|---|---|---|---|---|---|---|---|---|
| | | | | 16 J/cm$^2$ | 64.3 J/cm$^2$ | Intra-cellular | Extra-cellular | | |
| B16F0 | 0 | 0 [d] | - | 0 | 0 | 0.03 | 0.03 [a] | 0.43 | 47 |
| | 125 | 2.21 [d] | 1.2 | 44.39 | 95 | 0.039 | 0.07 [a] | 0.45 | - |
| B16F0-PDTR | 0 | 0.20 [e] | - | 0 | 0 | 0.048 | 0.04 [b] | 0.48 [c] | 31.23 |
| | 125 | 5.98 [e] | 30 | 85.31 | 97 | 0.05 | 0.06 [b] | 0.65 [c] | - |
| B16F10 | 0 | 0.06 [f] | - | 0 | 0 | 0.06 | 0.06 | 0.65 | 34.75 |
| | 150 | 2.45 [f] | 40 | 95 | 96 | 0.65 | 0.03 | 0.68 | - |
| B16F10-PDTR | 0 | 0.19 [g] | - | 0 | 0 | 0.08 | 0.045 | 0.63 | 45 |
| | 150 | 3.11 [g] | 16 | 97 | 100 | 0.12 | 0.05 | 0.65 | - |

PpIX ratio=[PpIX at 125 or 150 µg ALA/mL]/[PpIX at 0 µg ALA/mL]. [a,b,c,d,e,f,g] $p<0.01$

Table 5. Global analysis between the Photodynamic effect on parental melanoma cells and their resistant clones

## 4. Discussion

Malignant melanoma is one of the most aggressive cancer, in addition is resistant to the ordinary therapies (chemotherapy, immunotherapy and radiotherapy) (Gray et al., 2007), thus is necessary to look for new treatments; photodynamic therapy is a hopeful therapy that presents some advantajes over surgery and radiotherapy, however clinical results have been variable. The aim of this work was to evaluate the possibles mechanism involved in resistance to PDT of two differents resistant melanoma cell lines (B16F0-PDTR, B16F10-PDTR) derived from a invasive weakly and strong metastatic melanoma cell lines (B16F0 and B16F10).

In this work were obtained clonas of murine melanoma resistant to PDT as well as previous studies have obtained resistant clonas of colon adenocarcinome HT29-P14 to PDT (Hanlon et al., 2001) and mouse fibrosarcome Rif-8A (Di Prospero et al., 1997).

One of the mechanisms evaluated in this project was the concentration of intracellular PpIX because the amount of photosentizer induces the generation of reactive oxygen species (ROS) that leads to the increment cellular death. The results obtained showed that the PpIX is concentrated intracellularly and not extracellularly, also it was observed an accumulation of PpIX highly significant ($p<0.05$) in B16F0-PDTR compared with B16F0 in all ALA doses evaluated. A similar behavior was observed in B16F10-PDTR from 50 μg/mL. The higher concentration of PpIX of isolated cells with regard to parental lines could be due to different factors such as the difference in the expression of enzymes involved in the hemo biosynthesis (Ruiz et al., 2007), which showed differences between retinoblastoma cell lines Y-79 and WERI-Rb-1, mediated RT-PCR found that protoporphyrinogen oxidase, uroporphyrinogen synthase, and 5-aminolevulinate synthase were over expressed, these enzymes favored the synthesis of PpIX. On the other hand, it has been reported that ferrochelatase enzyme is decreased in its activity in cancer cells; therefore this contributes to the intracellular accumulation of PpIX (Li et al., 2001). Another factor that allows the biosynthesis of PpIX is the assimilation of ALA like as it was observed in murine fibrosarcoma cells MethA (Ohgari et al., 2005). Acording with the results obtainned in this work the chossen concentration of ALA was 125 μg/mL to B16F0 and 150 μg/mL to B16F10. Another important factor that is involved in PDT is the light intensity, previous studies evaluated PDT with murine melanoma using 15 J/cm$^2$ or low doses (Inuma et al., 1994; Vena et al.2004), in this work it was compared the efficency of PDT using 15 J/cm$^2$ and 64.3 J/cm$^2$, our results showed that the use of a higher light dose increases cells mortality in the 4 cell lines tested, but the higher mortality was observed in isolated clones.

In this study was eliminated between 95-100% of melanoma cells and its clones, the most susceptible cells were the B16F10-PDTR, highly metastatic melanoma cells resisted the first application of the PDT, but were totally sensitively to the second irradiation.

Other parameter analyzed in the resistant to PDT was the melanin content. The results showed a higher intracellular accumulation of melanin. In relation with this its has been reported that PpIX can induced melanogenesis since PpIX is one activator of melanin synthesis through guanilate ciclase activation (Soo-Kyeong et al., 2005). Previous studies showed that pigmented melanoma does not has a good efficiency using PDT because the melanin interfere with the light absorption, as melanin absorbs and disperse light and decrees the production of ROS (Dea-Seon et al., 2004). Nevertheless the melanin that seems to be involved in the resistance in the melanoma cells studied in this work is extracellular, nevertheless the melanin that seems to be involved in the resistance of the melanoma cells studied in this work is the extracellular, probably this effect is not clear when it was used the density of energy of 64.3 J/cm$^2$, but when it was used a density of 16 J/cm$^2$ the cellular death in the resistant cells of the line B16F0 exposed to 125 μg ALA/mL doubles in the resistant line, goes from 44.39 to 85.31% of mortality.

With regard to the analysis of the concentration and mitochondrial activity, only the latter appears to be involved, for example in the table 5 it can be observed that this activity only increases significantly in the resistant clone B16F0-PDTR, while in other lines though there is an increase from 10 to 20% it is not significant ($p>0.05$). Consequently, it could be carefully inferred that the increase in mitochondrial activity makes the cells susceptible to PDT only if there are significant amounts of PpIX and extracellular melanin.

## 5. Conclusion

The resistant clones (B16F0-PDTR, B16F10-PDTR) accumulate more PpIX than the parental lines (B16F0 and B16F10).

The factors involved in the resistance of melanoma cells are extracellular melanin (the higher the concentration of melanin the bigger the resistant to PDT), mitochondrial activity (the decrease of mitochondrial activity promotes resistance) and the concentration of PpIX (the smaller PpIX there is less cell death). It seems that the irradiation stimulates changes in cellular metabolism related with the mitochondria that diminishes the resistance of melanoma cells, thus it would be recommendable irradiate the cells several times and at densities of 64.3 J/cm$^2$ or more. With the implementation of a laser of argon and irradiating to 64.3 J/cm$^2$ it was achieved a mortality between 95-100% of PDTR B16F0, B16F10-PDTR, B16F0 and B16F10 cells.

## 6. Acknowledgment

The Authors are grateful to Anayansi Molina and F. Arena-Huertero, PhD, Departamento de Neurociencias, Instituto de Fisiología Celular-Universidad Nacional Autónoma de México for kindly providing us with the fluorescence microscopy. ER-G received EDI, COFAA, and SNI fellowships. Financing for this study was provided by the Secretaria de Investigación y Posgrado (SIP) of Instituto Politécnico Nacional through project 20090324 and CONACyT through project 57326.

## 7. References

ACS, 2011. American Cancer Institute. Date of access: March 24, 2011, Available from: <http://www.cancer.org/Cancer/SkinCancer-Melanoma/DetailedGuide/melanoma-skin-cancer-key-statistics>

Bonnett, R. (2000). Chemical Aspects of Photodynamic Therapy. Singapore: Gordon and Breach Science Publishers.

Borenfreud, E. S. (1985). Toxicity monitored with a correlated set of cell-cultured assays. *Xenobiotica, 85*, 705.

Bugaj, A., Morliére, P., Haigle, J., & Stanislaw, D. (2004). Photototicity of Protoporphyrin IX, Diarginine Diprotoporphyrinate and N,N-Dyphenylalanyl Protopprphytin Toward Human Fibroblast and Keratinocytes In Vitro: Effect of 5-Methoxypsoralen. Photochemestry and Photobiology, 80_468-491.

Dea-Seon, L., Hwan, S., & Won-Yo, L. (2004). Silkworm-pheophorbide a mediated photodinamic against B16F0 pigmented melanoma. Journal of photochemistry and photobiology B: Biology, 74: 1-6.

Di Prospero, L., Singh, G., Wilson, B., & Rainbow, A. (1997). Cross-resistance to photofrin-mediated photodynamic therapy and UV light and recovery form photodynamic therapy damage in Rif-8A mouse fibrosarcoma cells measured using viral capacity. Journal of Photochemestry and Photobiology, 38:143-151.

Gray, S., Willbrock, C., & R, M. (2007). Melanoma biology and new target theraphy. 44: 851-857.

Hanlon, J., Adams, K., Rainbow, A., Gupta, R., & Singh, G. (2001). Induction of Hsp60 by photofrin-mediated photodynamic therapy. Journal of Photochemestry and photobiology, 56:55-61.

Inuma, S., Farshi, S., B, O., & Hasan, D. (1994). A mechanistic study of cellular photodestruction with 5-aminolevulinic acid- induced porphyrin. British Journal of cancer, 70: 21-28.

Juzenas, P., Juzeien, A., Stakland, S., Iani, V., & Moan, J. (2002). Photosensitizing effecf of protoporphyrin IX in pigmented melanoma mice. Biochemical and Biophysical Research Comunications, 297:468-472.

Kim, M., Koh, Y. J., Kim, K. E., Koh, B. I., Nam, D.-H., Alitalo, K., Kim, I., Koh, G. Y. CXCR4 Signaling Regulates Metastasis of Chemoresistant Melanoma Cells by a Lymphatic Metastatic. Cancer Res; 70(24); 10411–21.2010.

Li, W., Shang, W., Ohnishi, K., Yamada, I., Ohno, R., & Hashimoto, K. (2001). 5-aminolevulinic acid- mediated photodynamic therapy in multidrug resistant leukemia cells. Journal of photochemistry and photobiology B:Biology, 60: 79-86.

Mang, T. (2004). Lasers and Light sources for PDT: past, present and future. Photodiagnosis and Photodynamic Therapy, 1:43-48.

Martínez SH. El primer Consenso Nacional de Expertos en Melanoma. Gac Mex Oncol 2005;4(2):11-13.

Mossman, T. (1983). Rapid colorimetric assay for cellular growth and survival application to proliferation and citotoxicity assays. *Journal of Immunological Methods*, 65, 55.

Mossman, T. (1983). Rapid colorimetric assay for cellular growth and survival application to proliferation and citotoxicity assays. Journal of Immunological Methods, 65, 55.

Ohgari, Y., Nakayasu, Y., Kitajima, S., Sawamoto, M., Mori, H., Shimokawa, O. M., y otros. (2005). Mechanisms involved in 5-aminolevulinic acid (ALA)- induced photosensitivity of tumor cells: Relation of ferrochelatase and uptake of ALA to the accumulation of protoporphyrin. Biochemical Pharmacology, 71:42-49.

Paras, P. (2003). Introduction to Biophotonics. New Jersey, USA. John Wyley and Sons; 433-445.

Piomelli, S. A. (1973). Micromethod for free erythrocyte porphyrins: The FEP test. J. Lab. Clin. Med., 932-940.

Rad, H. H., Yamashita, T., Y., J. H., Hirosaki, K., Wakamatsu, K., Ito, S. (2004). Tyrosinase-related proteins suppress tyrosinase-mediated cell death of melanocytes and melanoma cells. Exp Cell Res, 298, 317.

Ramón, G. E., DeLeón, R. I., Martínez, G. L., & Pérez, Z. A. (1999). In vitro study of biosynthesis of protoporphyrin IX induced by d-aminolevulinic acid in normal and cancerous cells of the human cervix. 30, 163-170.

Ruiz, G., Arenas, H., & Ramon, G. (2007). Expression of genes involved in hemo biosynthesis in the human retinoblastoma cell lines WERI-Rb-1 and Y-79: implications for photodynamic therapy. J. Exp. Clin. Cancer Research, 195-200

Sheleg, S., Zhavrid, E., Khodina, T., Kochubeev, G., Istomin, Y., Chalov, V., y otros. (2004). Photodynamic therapy with chorine e6 for skin metastases of melanoma. Photodermatology Photoinmunology and Photomedicine, 20:21-26.

Van-Hillegerberg VR, Kort WJ., Wilson JH., Current status of photodynamic therapy in oncology. Drug 1994;48:510.

Vena, F., Turchiello, R., Laville, I., Pigaglio, S., Blais, J., & Tudesco, A. (Lasers in medical Science). 5-aminolevulinic acid ester- induced protoporphyrin IX in a murine melanoma cell line. 2004, 19: 119-126.

WHO, 2011. World Health Organization. Date of access: March 24, 2011, Available from: <http://www.who.int/uv/faq/skincancer /en/index1.html>

Zhu, T., & Finlay, J. (2008). The role of photodynamic therapy (PDT) physics. Am. Assoc. Phys. Med, 3127-3136.

# 29

# Non-Thermal Effects of Near-Infrared Irradiation on Melanoma

Yohei Tanaka and Kiyoshi Matsuo
*Department of Plastic and Reconstructive Surgery, Shinshu University School of Medicine*
*Japan*

## 1. Introduction

Malignant melanoma is considered to be the most aggressive form of skin neoplasms. Over the past few decades, the incidence rate of melanoma has steadily risen throughout the world.

The risks of developing melanoma consist of intrinsic and environmental factors. Intrinsic factors generally include a family history and an inherited genotype, while the most relevant environmental factor is sun exposure. Exposure to ultraviolet (UV) radiation is the most important environmental carcinogen (Travers et al., 2008) and plays a significant role in the development of melanoma (Wolf et al., 1994). Sunscreens reduce the effects of UV radiation on human skin (Ananthaswamy et al., 1997). Nevertheless, sunscreens have failed to protect against an increase in UV radiation-induced melanomas (Wolf et al., 1994).

Various kinds of UV blocking materials, such as sunblocks, films, paints, and fibers are often used to prevent skin damage from UV exposure. Although individuals all over the world use various kinds of sunscreens, unwanted biological influences such as rosasea, erythema ab igne, long-term vasodilation, muscle thinning, and sagging still occur (Tanaka et al., 2010c).

Most sunscreens can only block UV and not visible light or near-infrared (NIR) radiation. Sunlight that reaches the human skin contains solar energy composed of 6.8% UV light, 38.9% visible light, and 54.3% infrared (IR) radiation (Kochevar et al., 1999). In addition to natural NIR, human skin is increasingly exposed to artificial NIR from medical devices and from electrical appliances (Schieke et al., 2003; Schroeder et al., 2008). Thus, we are exposed to tremendous amounts of NIR.

Both UV and visible light radiation are attenuated by melanin (Anderson & Parrish, 1981), whereas NIR can penetrate deep into human tissue where it can cause photochemical changes (Karu, 1999). We previously reported that NIR penetrates the skin and is absorbed by sweat on the skin surface, water in the dermis (Tanaka et al. 2009a, 2009b), hemoglobin in dilated vessels (Tanaka et al., 2009b, 2011c), myoglobin in the superficial muscle (Tanaka et al., 2010c), bone cortical mass, and is scattered by adipose cells (Tanaka et al., 2011b). NIR irradiation induces strand breaks and cell death by apoptosis (Tirlapur & König, 2001) as well as the cell death of cancer cells and bone marrow cells (Tanaka et al., 2010b, 2011b). In addition, NIR irradiation is used as a therapeutic option for the treatment of wound healing disorders (Danno et al., 2001; Horwitz et al., 1999; Schramm et al., 2003) and malignant tumors (Bäumler et al., 1999; Kelleher et al., 1999; Dees et al., 2002; Orenstein et al., 1999).

Despite the widespread therapeutic potential of NIR, the mechanisms responsible for the therapeutic actions of photobiomodulation with NIR have not been elucidated in detail. However, we found that NIR induced muscle thinning (Tanaka et al., 2010c, 2011a), bone marrow damage (Tanaka et al., 2011b), and had a cytocidal effect on cancer cells, which is likely due to apoptosis (Tanaka et al., 2010b).

NIR is easily absorbed by water, since water molecules are resonated by NIR due to the O-H intramolecular hydrogen bonds and electrical dipole moment (Tsai et al., 2001). NIR increases the amount of water retained in the dermis by inducing vasodilation and the expression of collagen, elastin, and water-binding proteins (Tanaka et al., 2009b). The NIR spectrum of biological materials results from the overtones and combination of O-H, C-H, and N-H groups' bond stretching vibrations (Weyer, 1985). Both collagen and elastin possess helical structures and hydrogen bonds. Elastin has higher absorption properties than water (Tsai et al., 2001). These findings suggest that we have acquired biological defense mechanisms in which induced helical structures and hydrogen bonds are resonated by NIR and absorb NIR to protect the subcutaneous tissues from this type of radiation.

NIR is also absorbed by choromophores, such as hemoglobin, or myoglobin, which have many alpha helices (Ferrari et al., 2004; Nancini et al., 1994). Alpha helices are thought to be resonated by NIR and have strong amide bands in the infrared spectra, which have characteristic frequencies and intensities (Nevskaya & Chirgadze, 1976). This implies that NIR induces the resonance of alpha helices in the oxygen-carrying proteins as well as the degeneration of proteins containing alpha helices, which results in damage to the storage and transport of oxygen, and therefore may be one of the mechanisms of apoptosis.

Nuclear lamins also have a central alpha helical structure (Prokocimer et al., 2009). Alpha helical structures of nuclear lamins are surmised to absorb NIR and protect the nucleus and DNA from NIR. NIR exposure appears to damage nuclear lamins and induce DNA damage. Nuclear lamina is transiently disassembled during mitosis (Gerace & Blobel, 1980; Nigg, 1992; Yang et al., 1997). In addition, actively proliferating cells show increased sensitivity to NIR (Karu et al., 1994; Tafur & Milles, 2008), and IR irradiation induces DNA strand breaks and apoptosis (Tirlapur & König, 2001). Therefore, these findings suggest that lamins may absorb NIR to protect the nucleus. Moreover, NIR may damage DNA of cells in the mitotic phase due to the absence of nuclear lamin protection, resulting in apoptotic cell death.

Thus, NIR irradiation has a potential application for transient mass reduction of proliferative malignant cancer, such as breast cancer and melanoma before surgery (Tanaka et al., 2010b), or for the treatment for terminal patients.

Continuous NIR exposure may damage lamins and induce mutations in the nuclear lamina genes. Alterations of nuclear lamins could also be involved in common disease processess, such as cancer (Foster et al., 2010), and may differentiate cancer cells from normal cells (Prokocimer et al., 2009). Skin tumors in mice appeared faster after irradiation with a full lamp spectrum containing UV, visible, and NIR compared to irradiation with UV alone (Bain et al., 1943). NIR irradiation may also induce carcinogenesis (Schieke et al., 2003) and enrich CD34-positive stem cells (Tanaka et al., 2011b). In this study, the mechanism of tumor cell death induced by NIR appeared to differ from a standard apoptosis mechanism, because high levels of activated caspase-3 expression and single-stranded DNA (ssDNA)-positive cells appeared gradually after NIR irradiation. However, tumor shrinkage occurred rapidly. Therefore, NIR may induce apoptosis of highly proliferative melanoma cells, stimulate stem cells, and then induce apoptosis of the cells which are unnecessary to promote the development of melanoma. This appears to be a part of the mechanism for the effects of NIR.

The necessity to protect cells from NIR in order to prevent tissue damage has not been well investigated. Many studies have proven the effects of sun and UV exposure on melanoma, but have not investigated the long-term effects of NIR exposure on human skin and skin cancers.

Persons with fair skin, multiple atypical nevi or dysplastic nevi, or born with giant congenital melanocytic nevi are at increased risk of melanoma (Bliss et al., 1995). Fair skin with sparse melanin and a thin dermis might allow NIR radiation to penetrate deeper into human tissue than dark skin, which has dense melanin and a thick dermis (Tanaka et al., 2010c). Thus, sunscreens should also protect against NIR (Pujol & Lecha, 1993; Schieke et al., 2003; Tanaka & Matsuo, 2008; Tanaka et al., 2010c, 2011b, 2011c). Our preliminary studies suggest that we should consider the effect of not only UV, but also NIR on melanoma. In this study, we present an overview of our current understanding of the biological effects of NIR radiation on melanoma through experimental studies.

## 2. Experimental part

### 2.1 NIR irradiation

#### 2.1.1 NIR device and wavelength

NIR irradiation was performed with a broadband infrared source (Titan; Cutera, Brisbane, CA, USA). The NIR device emits an NIR spectrum between 1100 to 1800 nm, with water filtering to remove wavelengths between 1400 and 1500 nm (Figure. 1), and simulates solar NIR radiation that reaches the skin of humans on the Earth's surface. This device delivers NIR without the wavelengths that are strongly absorbed by water and haemoglobin, which allow for the safe delivery of NIR energy deeper into tissue. The horizontal spot size of the irradiation was 10 × 30 mm.

To avoid thermal effects, the sapphire contact cooling tip was set to a fixed temperature of 20 °C to provide contact cooling. The sapphire block was cooled with fluids using thermoelectric coolers. Cooling fluids were circulated by a pump and a cooling system. Pre- and parallel-irradiational cooling of the superficial layers was accomplished using this temperature-controlled sapphire window, which further prevented excessive superficial heating.

These specific wavelengths and the cooling system enabled the delivery of NIR to deeper tissues without pain or epidermal burns.

#### 2.1.2 NIR irradiation and output

We previously reported that 3 rounds of NIR irradiation consisting of 2 passes at 20 J/cm$^2$ was sufficient to induce histological changes in the epidermis of rats, but that higher energies had a greater response and were preferable to see effects in deeper tissues.

The correlation with efficacy seemed to be highest with total delivered energy, not per pulse fluence, since multiple irradiations with a lower output appeared as equally effective as higher fluence irradiations.

Therefore, we performed NIR irradiation at 40 J/cm2 for the *in vivo* study.

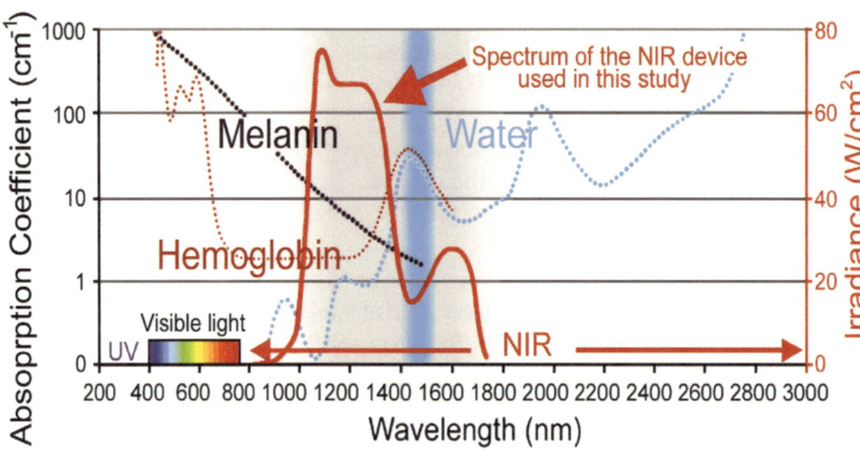


Fig. 1. The absorption coefficients and wavelength of the NIR device. This graph shows the absorption coefficients of melanin (brown), hemoglobin (red), and water (blue). The NIR device used in our study emits a spectrum of NIR from 1100 to 1800 nm (bold red), with filtering of wavelengths between 1400 and 1500 nm (blue belt) that are strongly absorbed by water and hemoglobin. These specific wavelengths and the cooling system enabled the delivery of NIR to deeper tissues without pain or epidermal burns. Cited and revised from Fig. 2. Tanaka et al. (2010). Long-lasting muscle thinning induced by infrared irradiation specialized with wavelength and contact cooling: A preliminary report. *ePlasty*. 10:e40

### 2.2 *In vitro* tumorigenicity and treatment

#### 2.2.1 Cell culture

Testing was conducted on cultures of 2 melanoma cell lines: B16F0 melanoma cells and MDA-MB435 melanoma cells. B16F0 and MDA-MB435 melanoma cell lines were obtained from the American Type Culture Collection (ATCC, Manassas, VA, USA). B16F0 and MDA-MB435 cells were maintained in DMEM (Invitrogen, Carlsbad, CA, USA) medium supplemented with 10% fetal bovine serum and antibiotics. Cells were seeded in 96-well microtitre plates at a concentration of 5 x $10^3$ cells per well in 100 µL of medium. All cells were grown at 37°C in a humidified incubator with 5% $CO_2$. A total of 768 wells of cancer cell lines were prepared for this study.

#### 2.2.2 Cell culture and NIR irradiation

Cancer cells from the 2 melanoma cultures were divided based on the number of individual NIR exposures in a single session and the total irradiation received. The numbers of exposures performed per round were 3, 10, and 20 exposures using two separate fluence settings per exposure of 20 J/$cm^2$ and 40 J/$cm^2$, because our preliminary results indicated that 3 shots at 10 J/$cm^2$ on cultured cancer cells (B16F0 cells) were not effective. This resulted in 7 different groups (including the control group) for each of the 2 cancer cell lines. The irradiated groups were exposed to a single round of irradiation. The MTS assay was performed after a 3-day incubation period following the exposure session.

#### 2.2.3 Cell proliferation assay

We performed an MTS cell proliferation assay to evaluate the effects of NIR irradiation. Cell proliferation was analyzed using a CellTiter 96 Aqueous Cell Proliferation Assay kit (Promega,

Madison, WI, USA). Aliquots of 20 µL of MTS reagent were added to the wells and incubated at 37°C in a humidified incubator for 2 hours. Absorbance at 490 nm ($OD_{490}$) was monitored with a Powerscan HT microplate reader (Dainippon Pharmaceutical, Osaka, Japan).

### 2.3 *In vivo* tumorigenicity and treatment

Animals were housed in a temperature-controlled environment under a 12-h light-dark cycle with free access to water and standard mouse chow. Body weight and tumor size were measured every other day. Tumor volumes were defined as 4/3 x π x (longest diameter)/2 x (shortest diameter)/2 x (shortest diameter)/2. This study was approved by the Shinshu University Institutional Review Board for Animal Study. In addition, national and international principles of laboratory animal care were followed throughout the study.
Forty female nude mice (Crlj:CD1-Foxn1nu) were obtained from Charles River Laboratories (Yokohama, JAPAN). MDA-MB435 cells (5.0 x $10^6$ cell/100µL/mouse) were implanted subcutaneously in the right flank of 6-week-old mice. Twenty-eight mice were divided into two groups when the tumor volume expanded to approximately 100 $mm^3$. The mice were divided into groups 19 days after tumor transplantation, which was defined as day 1 for testing. Groups consisted of two equal groups ($n$ = 14 for each group): one group (control group) was untreated, whereas the other group was treated with NIR irradiation. NIR irradiation was started on days 1 and 31. Treatments were performed once daily for 13 days. All treatments consisted of 10 exposures of IR irradiation at 40 J/$cm^2$. Animals were euthanized at 99 days after tumor transplantation (day 80).

#### 2.3.1 Histological investigation

MDA-MB435 tumors were taken from nude mice on days 3 ($n$ = 4), 9 ($n$ = 4), 45 ($n$ = 4), and 80 ($n$ = 16) for histological examination. Specimens were fixed in 20% neutral buffered formalin and processed for paraffin embedding. MDA-MB435 tumors were serially sectioned in the vertical plane (3–4 $\mu$m thickness). Specimens were evaluated by hematoxylin and eosin (H&E) staining, transferase-mediated dUTP nick-end labeling (TUNEL) technique, and immunohistological staining using an anti-Ki67 antibody, caspase-3, and single-stranded DNA as readouts. The sections were photographed under an Olympus BX51 microscope (Olympus, Tokyo, Japan) equipped with a digital camera system (DP50; Olympus). The digital photographs were processed using Adobe Photoshop (Adobe, San Jose, CA, USA).

### 2.4 *In vivo* bone marrow assessment

Thirty-five male Wistar rats (*Rattus norvegicus albinus*) weighing 360 - 440 g were used. Thirty-five rats were either irradiated ($n$ = 25) or not irradiated (control; $n$ = 10). The centre of the dorsal portion of the irradiated rats was subjected to 3 rounds of irradiation at 40 J/$cm^2$ on days 0, 7, and 14 without application of topical anesthesia. One round of treatment consisted of two passes of NIR irradiation.

#### 2.4.1 Histological investigation

Specimens, which included the spinous process of the sixth lumbar vertebra and the overlying subcutaneous tissues, were isolated from the experimental group (5 rats per time point) at 7, 30, 60, 90, and 180 d after the final -dose of irradiation (d7, d30, d60, d90, and d180, respectively). Control samples were only isolated at day 0 and day 180 (5 rats per time point).

The specimens were fixed in 20% neutral buffered formalin, paraffin embedded, and serially sectioned along the sagittal plane (3 - 4 μm thickness). Tissue sections were stained with H&E as well as with an anti-CD34 antibody for immunohistochemical analysis to detect CD34-positive hematopoietic stem cells in the bone marrow.
The percentage of the area occupied by bone marrow adipocytes, the number of hematopoietic bone marrow cells, and the number of CD34-positive stem cells were calculated in a superficial area 1.5 mm deep in the spinous process.
Images were scanned and quantified in 5 representative fields per section and subsequently averaged to obtain a final score. The sections were photographed under an Olympus BX51 microscope (Olympus, Tokyo, Japan) equipped with a digital camera system (DP50; Olympus). The digital photographs were processed using Adobe Photoshop (Adobe, San Jose, CA, USA).

### 2.5 Statistical analysis

The differences between groups at each time point were examined for statistical significance with a Student *t*-test for the melanoma studies and the Mann-Whitney U -test for the stem cell studies. $P < 0.05$ was considered to be statistically significanct.

## 3. Results

### 3.1 Cell viability measured by the MTS assay

The $OD_{490}$ values of irradiated cell cultures decreased significantly compared to controls in both B16F0 and MDA-MB435 cell lines, except at the lowest dose of irradiation with three, 20 J/cm$^2$ exposures (group 20 J x 3) ($P < 0.001$) (Fig. 2).

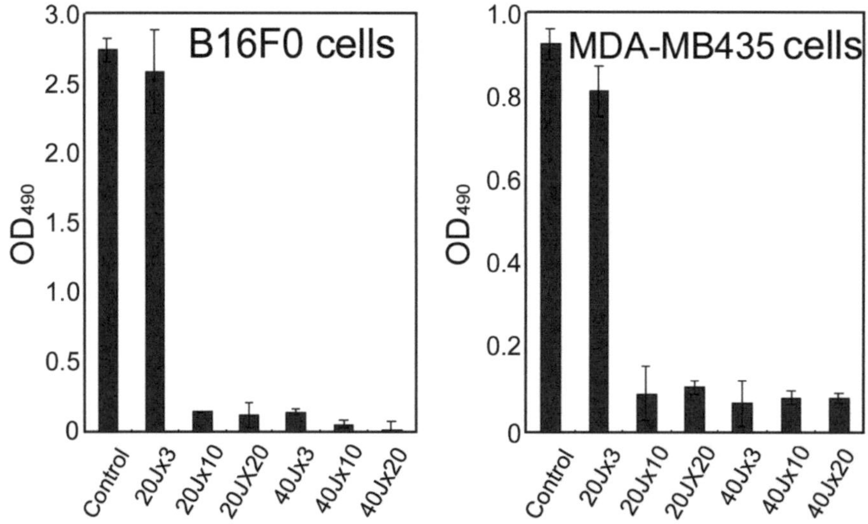


Fig. 2. The values of $OD_{490}$ in B16F0 melanoma cells (left) and MDA-MB435 melanoma cells (right). The $OD_{490}$ values of irradiated cell cultures, with the exception of the lowest NIR irradiation group of 3 exposures at 20 J/cm$^2$, decreased significantly ($P < 0.001$, compared to controls) in all cultures. Cited and revised from Fig. 2. Tanaka et al. (2010). Non-thermal cytocidal effect of infrared irradiation on cultured cancer cells using specialized device. *Cancer Science.* 101:1396-402

Group 20 J x 3 showed the smallest decrease in cell viability in MDA-MB435 cells that was still significant ($P$ = 0.034), but only modest reductions were observed in B16F0 cells. No statistically significant intra-group differences were observed between the 20 and 40 J/cm$^2$ treatment groups (excluding group 20 J x 3). This was consistently observed for both cancer cell lines.

Ten exposures at 20 J/cm$^2$ achieved a comparable significant reduction in cell count as that of 3 exposures at 40 J/cm$^2$. Three exposures at 20 J/cm$^2$ appeared close to a threshold energy dosage.

### 3.2 *In vivo* tumor volume

Significant differences were observed in tumor volume between the control group and NIR irradiated group from day 5 up to day 77 (Fig. 3).

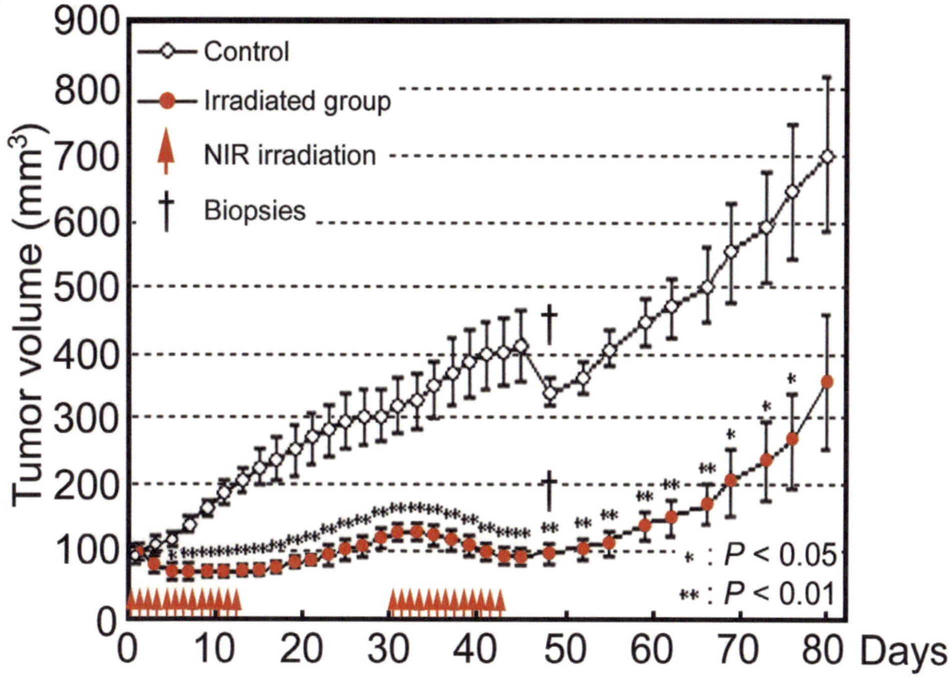


Fig. 3. Relative tumor volume of MDA-MB435. Significant differences were observed in tumor volume between the control group and NIR irradiated group from day 5 up to day 77. NIR irradiation was started on day 1 when the tumor volume expanded to approximately 100 mm$^3$, and then restarted on day 31. Treatments were performed once daily and all treatments consisted of 10 exposures of NIR irradiation at 40 J/cm$^2$. Significant differences were observed in MDA-MB435 tumor volume between the control group and NIR irradiated group from day 5 up to day 77. Significant differences are indicated (*: $P < 0.05$, **: $P < 0.01$). The cross sign indicates when two animals of each group were euthanized for histological investigation (day 45). Cited from Fig. 4. Tanaka et al. (2010). Non-thermal cytocidal effect of infrared irradiation on cultured cancer cells using specialized device. *Cancer Science.* 101:1396-402

The mean tumor volume of MDA-MB435 cells in the control group was 99.0 ± 26.85 $mm^3$ on day 1 of the treatment and increased continuously to 700.5 ± 333.8 $mm^3$ on day 80. The mean tumor volume for the irradiated MDA-MB435 group was 100.0 ± 26.06 $mm^3$ on day 1 of the treatment. Tumor volume decreased after the 1st round of IR irradiation and continued to reduce through day 5 to a minimum volume of 67.0 ± 15.75 $mm^3$. After day 5, the mean tumor volume gradually increased in the irradiated group through day 15, resulting in a tumor volume of 129.0 ± 44.05 $mm^3$ on day 31 when the second treatment started. Following the second round of irradiation, the mean tumor volume again decreased, reducing the tumor volume to 94.0 ± 41.22 $mm^3$ by day 45. Subsequently, the mean tumor volume began to increase gradually and reached 357.3 ± 297.2 $mm^3$ by day 80.

### 3.2.1 Histology of transplanted melanoma

The histology of the irradiated groups showed tumor shrinkage in MDA-MB435 cells (Figures 4-6). Injured cells were observed in the vertical histological section of NIR irradiated MDA-MB435 melanoma tumors on day 45 (Figure 4).

Significant differences between the control and irradiated groups were observed in the frequencies of Ki67-positive and TUNEL-positive on day 9 as well as caspase-3-positive and ssDNA-positive cells on day 45 ($P < 0.05$) (Figure. 8). The frequencies of Ki67-positive cells in the control group and irradiated group on day 9 were 13.82 ± 6.53% and 0.76 ± 0.12%, respectively. The frequencies of Ki67-positive cells in the control group and irradiated group on day 45 were 35.22 ± 16.10% and 31.78 ± 3.48%, respectively.

The frequencies of TUNEL-positive cells in the control group and irradiated group on day 9 were 0.84 ± 0.47% and 3.71 ± 2.22%, respectively. The frequencies of TUNEL-positive cells in the control group and irradiated group on day 45 were 1.09 ± 0.44% and 18.58 ± 21.48%, respectively. The frequencies of caspase-3-positive cells in the control group and irradiated group on day 9 were 0.36 ± 0.22% and 1.60 ± 0.86%, respectively. The frequencies of caspase-3-positive cells in the control group and irradiated group on day 45 were 0.89 ± 0.53% and 23.06 ± 7.32%, respectively. The frequencies of ssDNA-positive cells in the control group and irradiated group on day 9 were 0.13 ± 0.01 % and 0.31 ± 0.12 %, respectively. Finally, the frequencies of ssDNA-positive cells in the control group and irradiated group on day 45 were 0.18 ± 0.03% and 4.42 ± 2.95%, respectively.

### 3.2.2 *In vivo* NIR irradiation

NIR irradiation did not induce pain and the mice did not withdraw despite a lack of anesthesia during the NIR irradiation procedure. No side effects, such as epidermal burns, were observed during the study.

### 3.2.3 Histology of bone marrow

Hematopoietic bone marrow cell counts in the irradiated groups decreased significantly at day 7 and then increased gradually from day 30 to day 180 (Figures. 9-10). Significant decreases were observed between samples at days 7, 30, 90, and 180 as well as the non-irradiated controls at days 0 and 180 ($P < 0.05$).

The percentage of the area occupied by bone marrow adipocytes also increased dramatically at day 7, but gradually decreased thereafter. Significant increases were observed at days 7, 30, 90, and 180 compared to the non-irradiated controls at days 0 and 180 ($P < 0.05$).

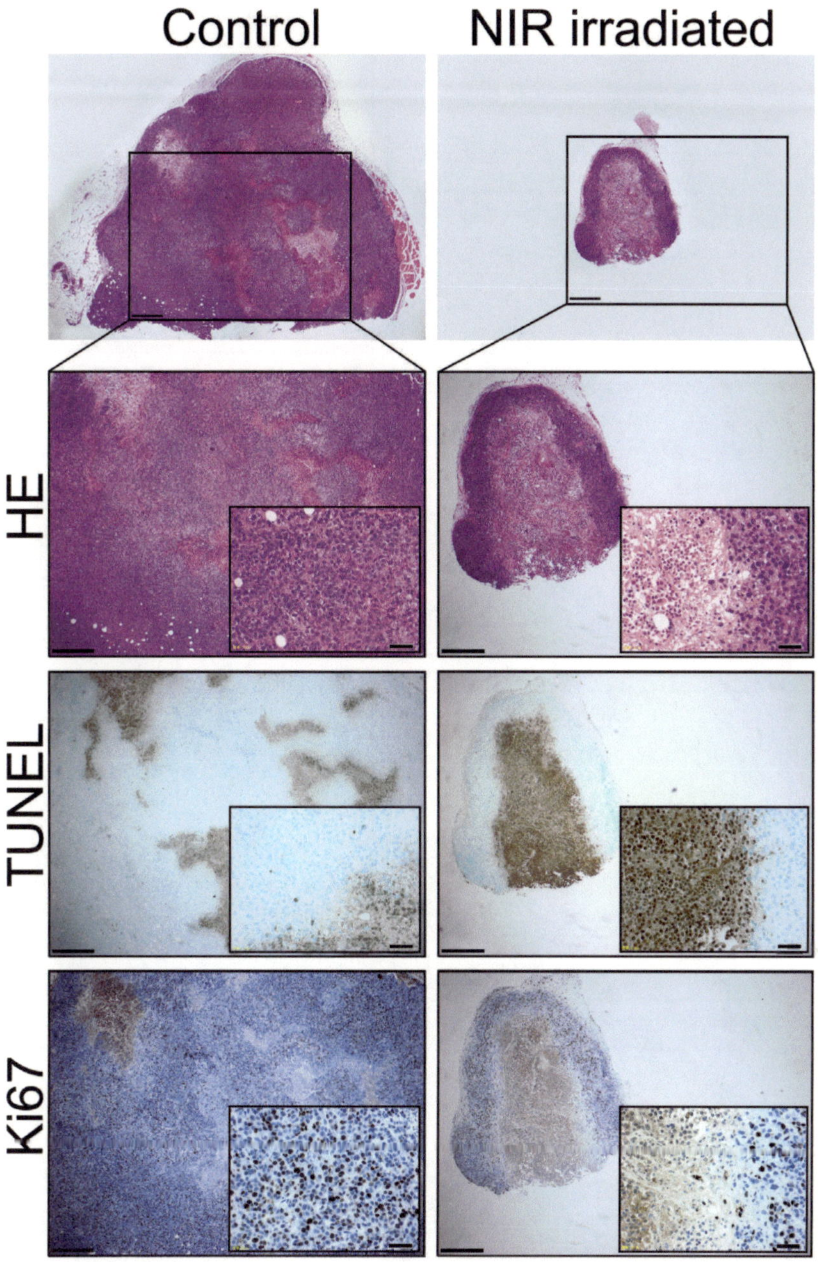


Fig. 4. Vertical histological sections of control and NIR irradiated MDA-MB435 melanoma tumors on day 45. The left column shows control tissues and the right column shows NIR irradiated tissues. Images from top to bottom show H&E staining, TUNEL staining, and immunohistological staining using an anti-Ki67 antibody. Scale bars = 400 $\mu$m (×40 magnification); insets: Scale bars = 40 $\mu$m (×400 magnification). Cited from Fig. 6(b). Tanaka et al. (2010). Non-thermal cytocidal effect of infrared irradiation on cultured cancer cells using specialized device. *Cancer Science.* 101:1396-402

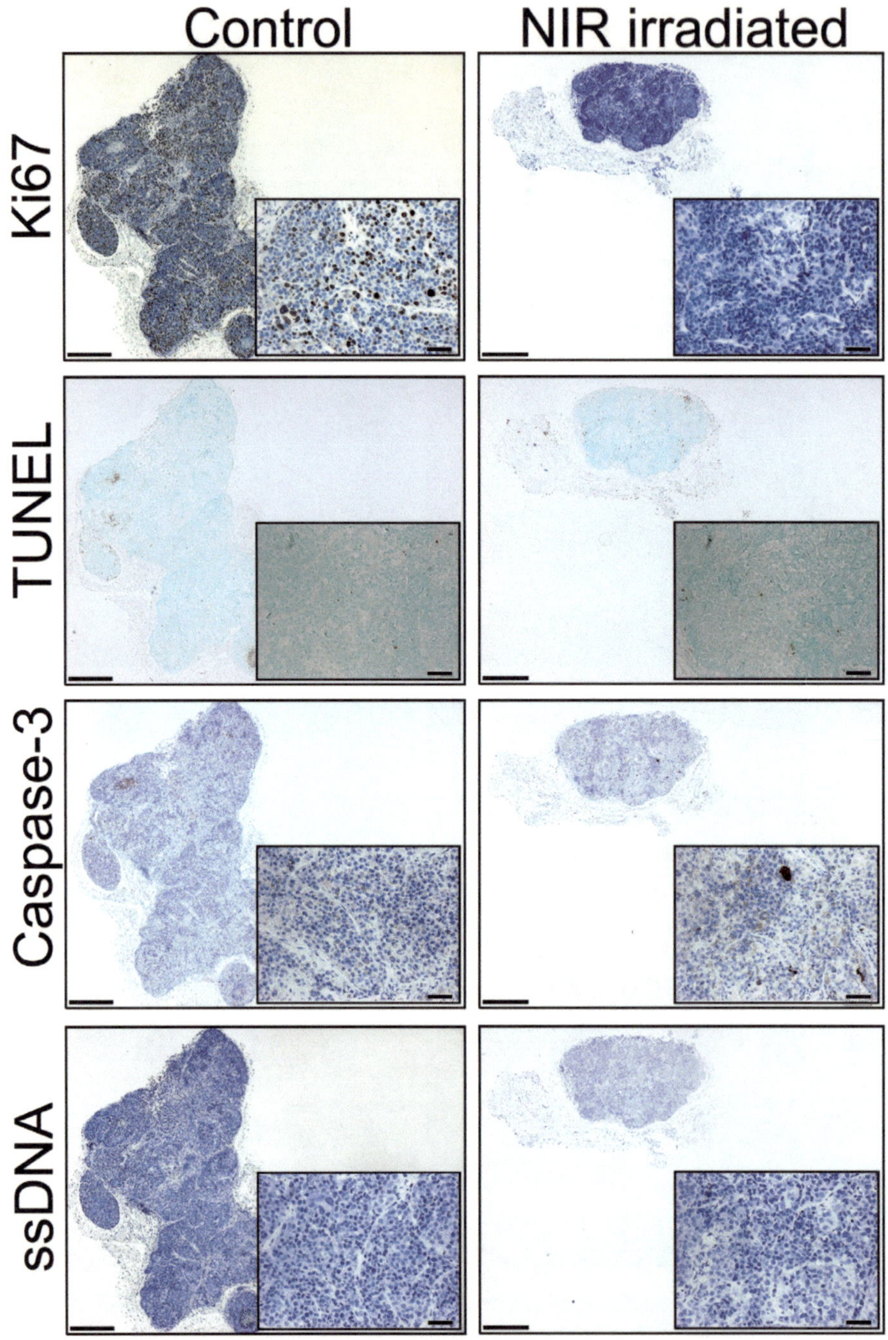


Fig. 5. Horizontal histological sections of control and NIR irradiated MDA-MB435 melanoma tumors on day 9. The left column shows control tissues and the right column shows NIR irradiated tissues. Images from top to bottom show immunohistological staining using an anti-Ki67 antibody, caspase-3, and single-stranded DNA. Scale bars = 400 $\mu$m (×40 magnification); insets: Scale bars = 40 $\mu$m (×400 magnification)

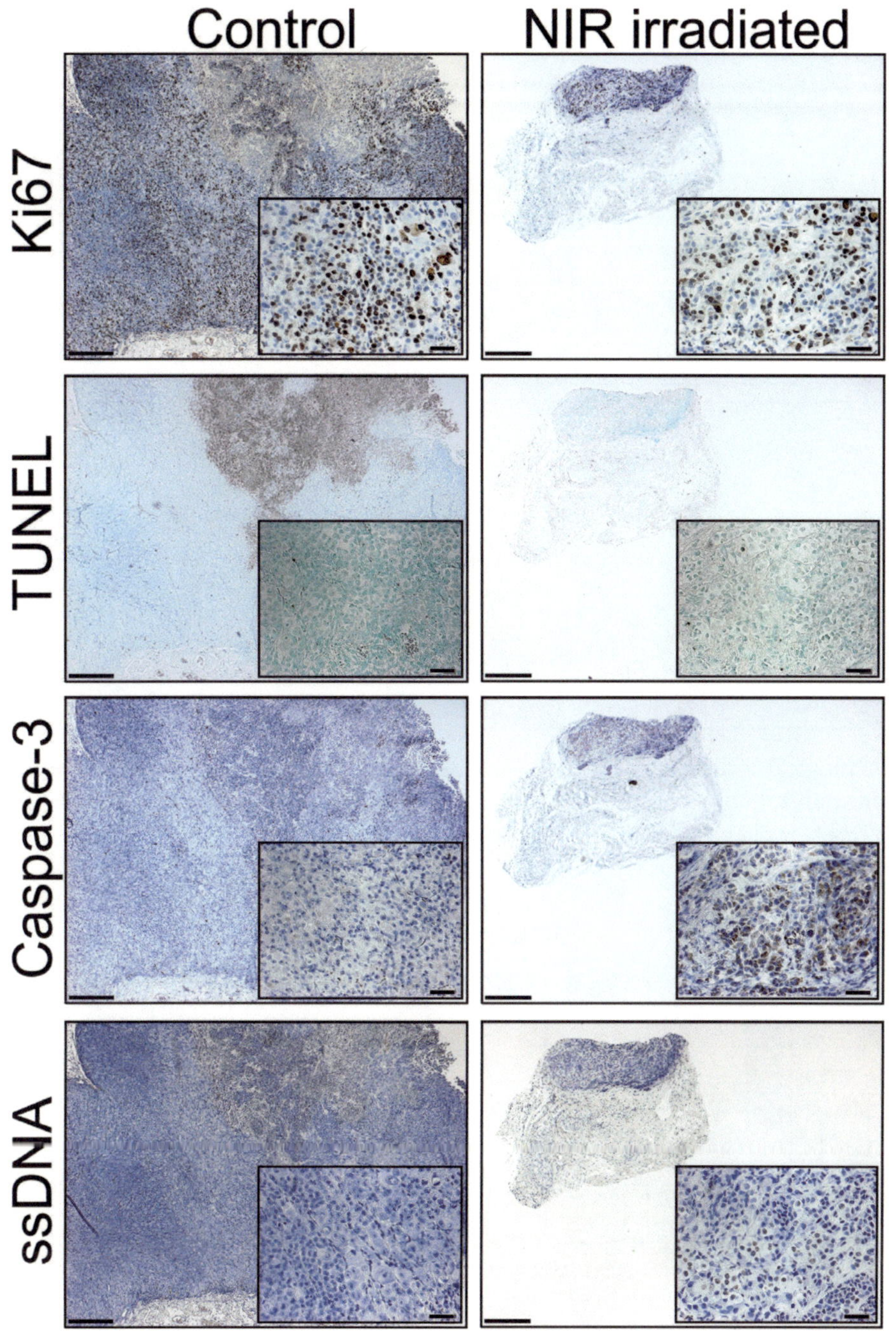


Fig. 6. Horizontal histological sections of control and NIR irradiated MDA-MB435 melanoma tumors on day 45. The left column shows control tissues and the right column shows NIR irradiated tissues. Images from top to bottom show immunohistological staining using an anti-Ki67 antibody, caspase-3, and single-stranded DNA. Scale bars = 400 $\mu$m (×40 magnification); insets: Scale bars = 40 $\mu$m (×400 magnification)

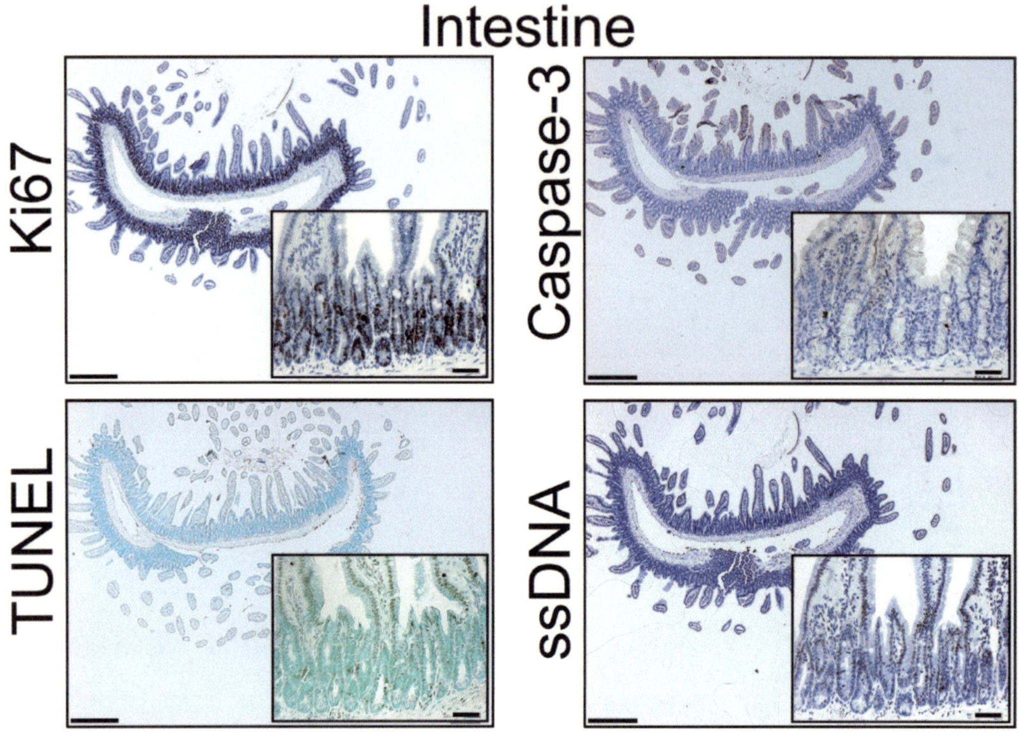


Fig. 7. Histological sections of intestine as a staining control. Images from top to bottom show immunohistological staining using an anti-Ki67 antibody, caspase-3, and single-stranded DNA. Scale bars = 400 $\mu$m; insets: Scale bars = 40 $\mu$m

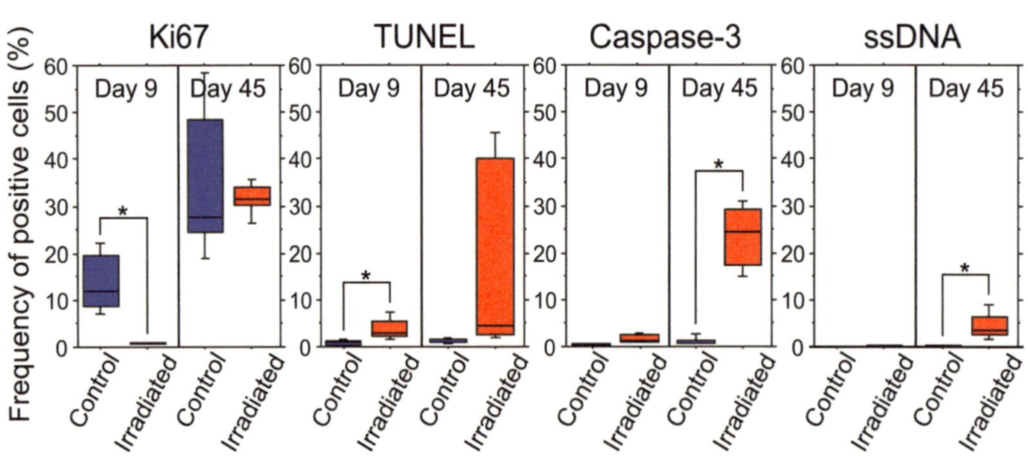


Fig. 8. Mean scores of frequencies of Ki67-, TUNEL-, caspase-3-, and ssDNA-positive cells. Significant differences (*: $P < .05$) between control and irradiated groups were observed in frequencies of Ki67-positive cells on day 9, TUNEL-positive cells, caspase-3-positive cells, and ssDNA-positive cells on day 45

The number of CD34-positive stem cells in the bone marrow dramatically increased at day 7, which persisted until day 180. Significant increases in cell number were observed on days 7, 30, 90, and 180 compared to the non-irradiated controls at days 0 and 180 ($P < 0.05$). Moreover, a majority of the CD34-positive stem cells in bone marrow were observed at the inner surface of the bone cortex.

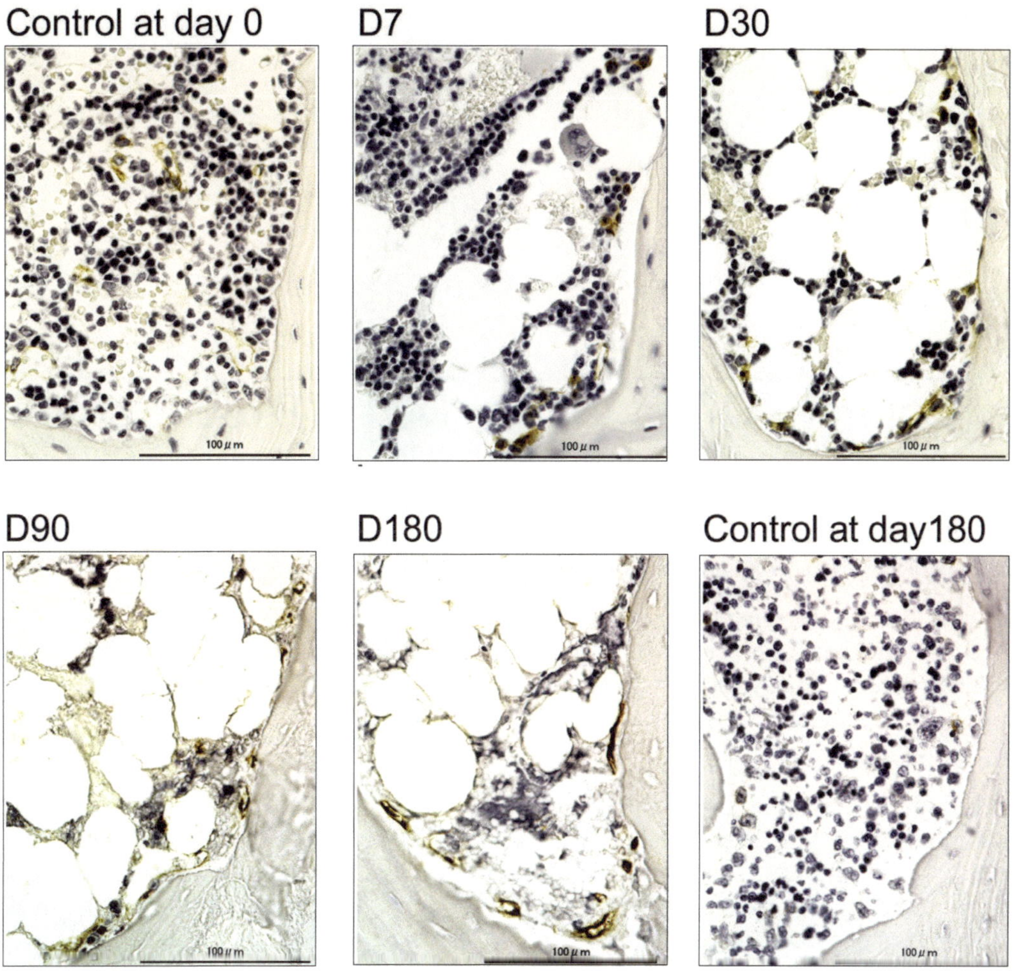


Fig. 9. Immunohistochemical staining of the spinous process with an anti-CD34 antibody

CD34-positive cells (stained brown) in the control at day 0 and 180 as well as the experimental samples at day 7, 30, 90, and 180 are shown. Scale bars = 100 $\mu$m.

Cited and revised from Fig. 2. Tanaka et al. (2011). Near-Infrared Irradiation Non-thermally affects Subcutaneous Adipocytes and Bone. *ePlasty*. 11:e12.

Hematopoietic bone marrow cell counts in the irradiated groups decreased significantly at day 7 and then increased gradually from day 30 to day 180. The percentage of the area occupied by bone marrow adipocytes also increased dramatically at day 7, but gradually decreased thereafter. The number of CD34-positive stem cells in the bone marrow dramatically increased at day 7, which persisted until day 180.

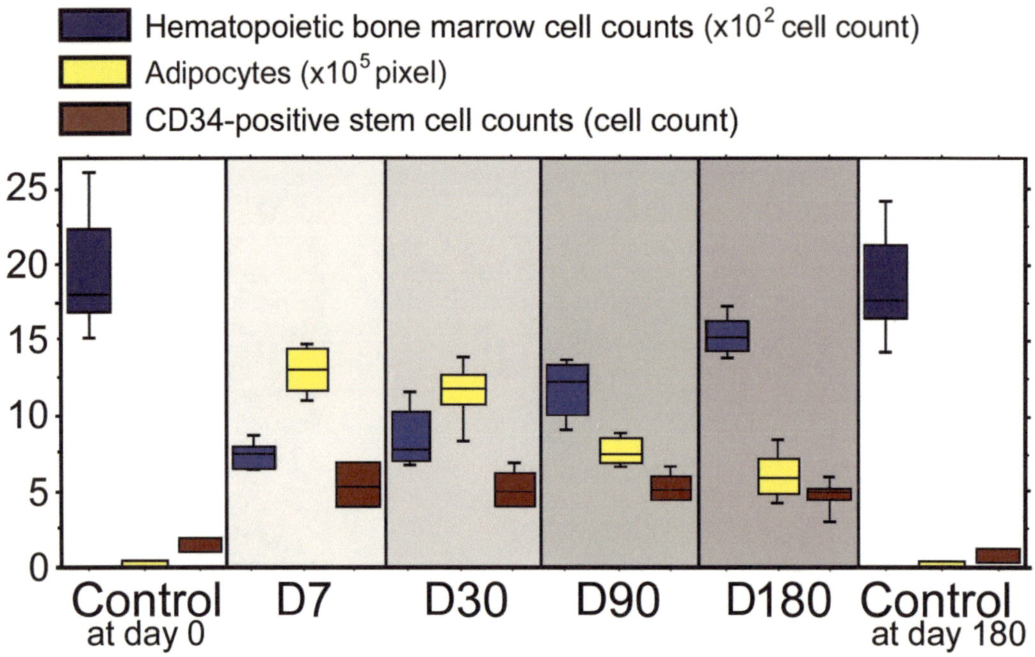


Fig. 10. Chronological changes in the hematopoietic bone marrow cell counts are indicated in blue, the percentage of the area occupied by bone marrow adipocytes in yellow, and the CD34-positive stem cell counts in brown

All were located in an area of superficial depth (1.5 mm) in the spinous process.
Cited and revised from Fig. 3 (b). Tanaka et al. (2011). Near-Infrared Irradiation Non-thermally affects Subcutaneous Adipocytes and Bone. *ePlasty*. 11:e12.

## 4. Discussion

### 4.1 UV and NIR in the natural sunlight

Individuals enjoy spending time under the sun, and UV blockers are often used to prevent skin damage by UV exposure. Exposure to UV radiation is the most important environmental carcinogen (Travers et al., 2008) and plays a significant role in the development of melanoma (Wolf et al., 1994).

Sunscreens reduce the effects of UV radiation on human skin (Ananthaswamy et al., 1997). Nevertheless, sunscreens have failed to protect against the increase in UV radiation-induced melanomas (Wolf et al.,1994). Various kinds of UV blocking materials, such as sunblocks, films, paints, and fibers are often used to prevent skin damage from UV exposure. Although individuals all over the world use various types of sunscreens, unwanted biological influences, such as rosasea, erythema ab igne, long-term vasodilation (Tanaka et al., 2011c), muscle thinning, and sagging still occur (Tanaka et al., 2010c). Most sunscreens can only block UV, but not visible light and IR (Tanaka & Matsuo, 2008).

In natural sunlight, however, humans are also continually exposed to IR. Solar IR that reaches the Earth's surface is predominantly infrared. In actuality, 54.3% of incident solar energy is composed of infrared, whereas the energy contributions of UV and visible light radiation are 6.8 and 38.9%, respectively (Kochevar, 1999). IR radiation ranging from 760 nm to 1 mm is non-ionizing radiation located 'below the red', i.e. adjacent to the red part of the visible radiation range and extending up to the microwave range. The IR spectral region is arbitrarily divided according to wavelength into sub-regions of NIR (760-3000 nm), middle IR (3000–30 000nm), and far IR (30 000 nm–1 mm). NIR radiation from the sun is selectively filtered by atmospheric water (Anderson & Parrish, 1981; Gates, 1966); thus, most NIR radiation that reaches the Earth's surface readily penetrates the superficial layers of the skin. In addition to natural NIR, human skin is increasingly exposed to artificial NIR from medical devices and electrical appliances (Schieke et al., 2003; Schroeder et al., 2008). Therefore, we are exposed to tremendous amounts of NIR every day (Tanaka & Matsuo, 2008).

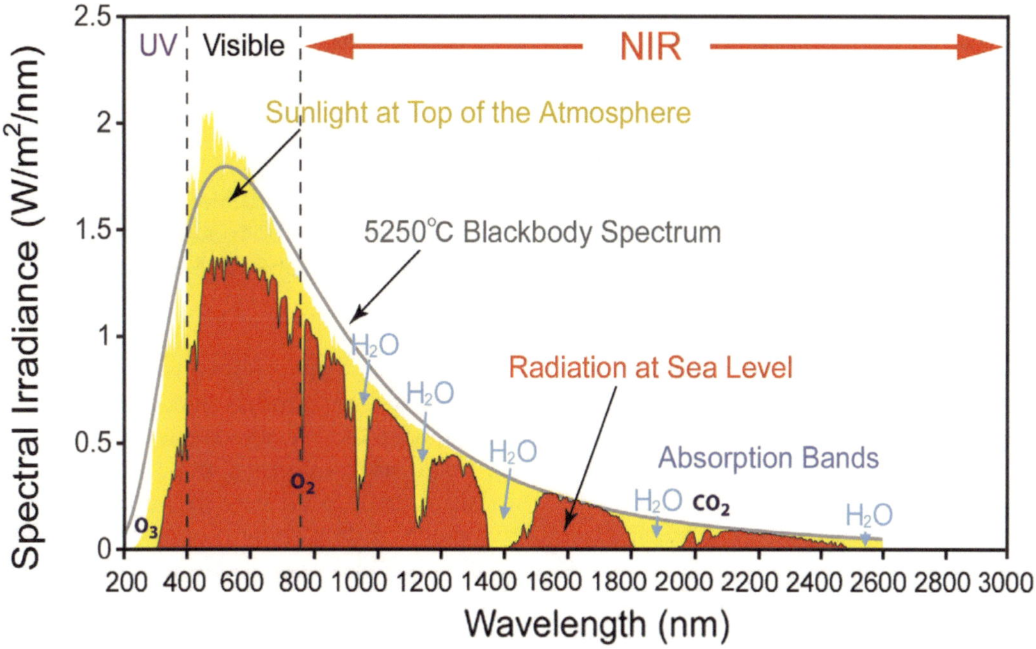


Fig. 11. Solar radiation. This graph shows the radiation spectrum for direct light both at the top of the Earth's atmosphere (yellow) and at sea level (red). The sun produces light with a distribution similar to that expected from a 5250°C blackbody (gray), which is approximately the temperature of the Sun's surface. As light passes through the atmosphere, some is absorbed by gases with specific absorption bands (blue). These curves are based on the American Society for Testing and Materials Terrestrial Reference Spectra, which are standards adopted by the photovoltaic industry to ensure consistent test conditions and are similar to the light levels expected in North America. Regions for UV, visible, and NIR are indicated

Cited and revised from Fig. 2. Tanaka et al. (2010). Long-lasting muscle thinning induced by infrared irradiation specialized with wavelength and contact cooling: A preliminary report. *ePlasty*. 10:e40.

Mr. Robert Rohde (GlobalWarmingArt.com) generously gave us precise data and the file for this figure.

### 4.2 Properties of NIR

NIR is an electromagnetic wave that simultaneously exhibits both wave and particle properties and is strongly absorbed by water, hemoglobin, and myoglobin (Tanaka et al., 2011c). As a consequence, NIR irradiation can penetrate the skin and affect the subcutaneous tissues, including muscles and bone marrow, with both its wave as well as its particle properties.

NIR irradiation was shown to induce the expression of collagen (Tanaka et al., 2009a), elastin, and water-binding proteins (Tanaka et al., 2009a, 2009b) without scar formation (Tanaka et al., 2010a). Further, near-infrared irradiation non-thermally induced long-lasting muscle thinning (Tanaka et al., 2010c), muscle relaxation (Tanaka et al., 2011a), bone marrow damage (Tanaka et al., 2011b), a cytocidal effect on cancer cells (Tanaka et al., 2010b), and stimulation of stem cells (Tanaka et al., 2011b).

The penetrating 600-1300 nm wavelength region causes photochemical changes and affects a large volume and depth of tissue (Anderson & Parrish, 1981). Actively proliferating cells show increased sensitivity to red and NIR (Karu et al.,1994; Tafur & Mills, 2008). NIR irradiation induces strand breaks and apoptosis (Tirlapur & König, 2001) as well as cell death of cancer cells and bone marrow cells (Tanaka et al., 2010b, 2011b). NIR irradiation is used as a therapeutic option in the treatment of wound healing disorders (Danno et al., 2001; Horwitz et al., 1999; Schramm et al., 2003) and malignant tumors (Bäumler et al., 1999; Dees et al., 2002; Kelleher et al., 1999; Orenstein et al., 1999). While NIR irradiation appears to damage tumor tissue, it has also been shown to reduce cellular protein damage produced by biological oxidants in normal cells (Kujawa et al., 2004).

### 4.3 The effects of NIR on human skin

Both UV and visible light radiation are attenuated by melanin (Anderson & Parrish, 1981), whereas NIR is strongly absorbed by hemoglobin and fluids. We previously reported that NIR is absorbed by sweat on the skin surface, water in the dermis, and hemoglobin in dilated vessels (Tanaka et al., 2009b, 2011c). The dermis tends to increase the amount of fluid by inducing an increase in collagen, elastin, and water-binding protein in order to protect subcutaneous tissues from NIR (Tanaka et al. 2009a, 2009b). Pre-exposure of NIR prevents UV-induced toxicity (Danno K et al., 1992; Frank et al., 2004; Menezes et al., 1998), and this effect is independent of heat shock protein induction and cell division (Menezes et al., 1998). These findings suggest that NIR irradiation prepares skin to better resist the subsequent damage of UV or NIR.

Similar to UV, NIR seems to exert biologic effects on human skin (Schieke et al., 2003). NIR irradiation was shown to cause skin changes similar to those observed in solar elastosis, and enhanced UV-induced dermal damage (Kligman, 1982). NIR irradiation is able to activate mitogen-activated protein kinases and induce gene transcription and is likely to increase collagen degradation (Kim et al., 2006; Schieke et al., 2003; Schroeder et al., 2008). NIR radiation elicits a retrograde signaling response, which subsequently induces an increase in dermal MMP-1 expression that is a key symptom of photoaging. Epidemiological data and clinical reports points to the ability of NIR to cause and enhance actinic skin damage, implying that NIR is not innocuous to human skin (Kligman LH & Kligman AM, 1984; Dover et al., 1989; Schieke et al., 2003).

Both thermal and non-thermal damage to tissue can occur when skin is exposed to NIR radiation.

The mean facial surface area that is covered with wrinkles is significantly smaller in African Americans than in Caucasians, and characteristics of age-related periorbital changes seem to occur at a more accelerated rate in Caucasians (Odunze et al., 2008). In addition, fair skin is more sensitive to skin aging (Guinot et al., 2002; Nagashima et al., 1999). These findings support the observation that fair skin tends to wrinkle and sag earlier in life (Rawlings, 2006; Tsukahara et al., 2004), because fair skin is thinner and is more susceptible to NIR damage to the underlying frontalis, orbicularis oculi, and platysma muscles than dark skin (Tanaka & Matsuo, 2008). NIR is attenuated by thick water-containing dermis. Thus, skin with sparse melanin and a thin dermis might allow NIR radiation to penetrate deeper into human tissue than skin with dense melanin and a thick dermis.

Repeated exposure to sources of heat and NIR, such as fires and stoves, results in a skin lesion described as erythema ab igne (Findlayson et al., 1996), which is clinically characterized by a reticular hyperpigmentation and teleangiectasia accompanied histologically by epidermal atrophy, vasodilation, and dermal melanin and hemosiderin deposits. After many years, these lesions may develop thermal keratoses, such as hyperkeratosis, keratinocyte dysplasia, and dermal elastosis which are similar to the changes that occur in actinically damaged skin (Arrington & Lockman, 1979). Similar to actinic keratoses, thermal keratoses are precancerous lesions that exhibit epidermal dysplasia, which may develop into invasive squamous cell carcinoma. There are several reports of carcinomas arising from heat induced erythema ab igne (Kligman LH & Kligman AM, 1984; Hewitt et al., 1993; Jones et al., 1988). NIR radiation, similar to UV radiation, induces photoaging and potentially photocarcinogenesis (Schieke et al., 2003). In addition, skin tumors in mice appeared faster after irradiation with the full lamp spectrum containing UV, visible, and NIR compared to irradiation with UV alone (Bain et al., 1943).

### 4.4 The effect of NIR on human subcutaneous tissues

Although there have been many studies regarding the superficial effects of NIR irradiation, the damage of deeper tissues has not been well investigated. Since the permeability of NIR is extremely high, the influence on deeper tissues should be considered.

NIR is an electromagnetic wave that simultaneously exhibits both wave and particle properties and is strongly absorbed by water, hemoglobin, and myoglobin (Tanaka et al., 2011c). As a consequence, NIR irradiation can penetrate the skin and affect the subcutaneous tissues (Tanaka et al., 2009a, 2009b), including muscle and bone marrow (Tanaka et al., 2010c, 2011a, 2011b).

NIR radiation induces vasodilation, collagen, and elastin, and increases the number of superficial granular adipocytes to protect the deeper tissues against NIR (Tanaka et al., 2011b). Continual long-term exposure to incident solar NIR radiation causes long-lasting thinning of the superficial facial muscles and the muscle extensions to the dermis, which ultimately leads to facial skin ptosis. Additional factors that are thought to contribute to brow ptosis include the gradual loss of forehead skin elasticity and a reduction in the tone of the frontalis muscles (Knize, 1996; Niechajev, 2004). The use of NIR irradiation for smoothing forehead wrinkles also caused brow ptosis. These results may have major implications in superficial tissue aging.

The widespread use of sunscreens has helped to reduce some of the deleterious effects of UV radiation on human skin (Ananthaswamy et al., 1997), however sunscreens that protect from NIR radiation should also be used to prevent damage to deeper tissues (Tanaka & Matsuo, 2008; Tanaka et al., 2010c, 2011b, 2011c).

### 4.5 NIR device

NIR irradiation is known to induce dermal heating, which results in skin laxity tightening. Many studies have shown the influence of superficial tissues. For example, wavelength selection directly influences target selection and penetration depth (Figure 1.).

NIR devices without a water filter or contact cooling have been used in previous studies to evaluate photobiological effects on the human body. However, with these treatments, a substantial amount of energy is absorbed in the superficial layers of skin and only limited NIR energy can be delivered to deeper tissues. Wavelengths below 1100 nm are preferentially absorbed by melanin in the superficial layers of the skin. Wavelengths between 1400 and 1500 nm and those above 1850 nm are absorbed heavily by water in the superficial layers of the skin, which results in heating and can lead to painful sensations and burns (Kelleher et al., 1999). NIR radiation from the sun is selectively filtered by atmospheric water (Anderson & Parrish, 1981; Gates, 1966); thus, most NIR radiation that reaches the Earth's surface readily penetrates the superficial layers of the skin.

In this study, we used an NIR device that emitted a spectrum of NIR irradiation from 1100 to 1800 nm with a water-filter that excluded wavelengths between 1400 and 1500 nm, which are strongly absorbed by water and hemoglobin (Figure. 1). Filtering out the wavelengths below 1100 nm, around 1450 nm, and above 1850 nm enabled for the delivery of NIR irradiation to deeper tissues (Davenport et al., 2006) and also simulated solar NIR radiation that reaches the skin of humans on the Earth's surface. Therefore, an NIR device with a water-filter mimics the natural situation and allows for the evaluation of solar NIR radiation that reaches the skin. However, in reality, both solar NIR radiation with an atmospheric water filter and the NIR device with a water filter increase the skin surface temperature and induce perspiration and blood vessel dilation that mediate the absorption of NIR radiation by water and hemoglobin, respectively. To counter this effect, in this study, we used contact cooling through a temperature-controlled sapphire window to reduce the skin surface temperature and thereby reduce perspiration and blood vessel dilation.

These specific wavelengths and the cooling system enabled NIR irradiation to penetrate the skin surface without pain or epidermal burns (Davenport et al., 2006; Goldberg, et al., 2007), which was evidenced by the ability to treat animals and humans without anesthesia and without contact burns or other adverse events.

### 4.6 The effects of NIR on cancer cells

#### 4.6.1 Wavelength of NIR anticancer therapy

Photodynamic therapy (PDT) is the most common antitumor therapy using IR for select forms of cancer (Dougherty et al., 1998). Photodynamic therapy is based on the accumulation of a photosensitizing agent in tumors and uses wavelengths near 800 nm as a photoactivating wavelength to achieve maximum penetration depth (Bäumler et al., 1999; Lobel et al., 2001; Orenstein et al., 1999). This wavelength, however, also has high melanin absorption, which limits the ability to deliver light to highly pigmented tumors (Busetti et al., 1998).

Although wavelengths near 800 nm are the standard activators for PDT, other wavelengths have also shown treatment promise. Santana et al. reported that NIR at 904 nm may have antitumor activity, as shown by an increase in cytomorphological changes as well as apoptosis in neoplastic cells (Santana-Blank et al., 2002). In a study using NIR irradiation at 904 nm, irradiation was shown to increase cytomorphologic changes with programmed cellular death in neoplastic cells; however, no apparent changes were observed in non-neoplastic cells (Santana-Blank et al., 2002). Unlike wavelengths beyond 1100 nm, where melanin absorption is negligible (Anderson & Parrish, 1981), absorption at 904 nm was significant. This may limit the possible uses of the 904 nm wavelength for certain body areas in races with skin that is rich in melanin.

Actively proliferating cells show increased sensitivity to red and IR irradiation (Karu et al., 1994; Tafur & Mills, 2008). IR irradiation alone appears to induce DNA strand breaks and apoptosis (Tirlapur & König, 2001), which elicits photodisruptive destruction of tumor tissue (Dees et al., 2002). While IR irradiation appears to damage tumor tissue, it has also been shown to reduce cellular protein damage produced by biological oxidants in normal cells (Kujawa et al., 2004).

Various types of IR devices and lasers are used in antitumor therapies, such as PDT and hyperthermia, and typically utilize wavelengths between 750 to 3000 nm. Wavelength selection directly influences target selection and penetration depth, and wavelengths below 1100 nm are absorbed preferentially by melanin in the superficial layers of skin (Figure. 1). Wavelengths between 1400 to 1500 nm and above 1850 nm are absorbed heavily by water, which results in the heating of the superficial layers of the skin. The delivery of NIR energy safely to deeper tissues without significant superficial heating requires wavelengths between 1100 nm and 1850 nm, excluding the range from 1400–1500 nm (Davenport et al., 2006).

Although many studies have shown the thermal effects of NIR irradiation on cancer cells in the field of hyperthermia, non-thermal effects of NIR irradiation were not investigated in detail. We first reported on the non-thermal effects of NIR irradiation using a specialized broad spectrum light source emitting light between 1100–1800 nm (with a filter to exclude wavelengths between 1400 and 1500 nm) on cancer cells and suggested the possibility of beneficial uses for cancer treatment (Tanaka et al., 2010b).

### 4.6.2 The effects of NIR on *in vitro* cancer studies

In our *in vitro* studies, proliferation of MDA-MB435 and B16F0 melanoma cells was significantly suppressed by NIR irradiation. Total NIR output appeared to correlate with cell survival. NIR irradiated cell cultures showed significant decreases in cell counts in all cultures, except at the lowest dose of irradiation in group 20 J x 3. A correlation with efficacy seemed to be highest with total delivered energy, and not per pulse fluence, since multiple irradiations with a lower output appeared equally effective as higher fluence irradiations. Ten exposures at 20 J/cm$^2$ achieved a comparable significant reduction in cell count as that of 3 exposures at 40 J/cm$^2$. In addition, three exposures at 20 J/cm$^2$ appeared close to a threshold energy dosage. Further studies are required to determine the accurate correlations between irradiation dose and cell survival as well as the different effects on each cancer cell line.

In our previous studies, increased temperature appeared not to play a role in the cell culture survival rate. Results in the 20 J/cm$^2$ group (excluding group 20 J x 3) were statistically equivalent to the 40 J/cm$^2$ group, and the maximum temperature rise during exposure in the 20 J/cm$^2$ group was only 3.76°C (temperature = 40.76°C). This is roughly equivalent to a illness-induced fever. In addition, elevated temperatures only remained above 40°C for 3.6

seconds, which was far short of the damages observed during prolonged high-grade fevers. The rationale of hyperthermia is based on a direct cytocidal effect at temperatures above 41-42°C (Dewey, 1994). With whole-body hyperthermia, tumor growth suppression requires temperatures of approximately 42°C and an exposure of at least 60 minutes (Wust et al., 2002). Although the extent and duration of temperature elevation were not significant in relation to the cases of hyperthermia, irradiated cell cultures showed significant decreases in cell counts in our studies. This level of temperature rise was not associated with tumor growth suppression, indicating a factor other than hyperthermia is responsible for growth suppression of these cancer cell lines. NIR is known to induce molecular vibrations (Pujol & Lecha, 1993; Schieke et al., 2003). The molecular vibrations of water and the resonance of alpha helices in proteins appeared to be related to the cytocidal effect of NIR on cancer cells.

### 4.6.3 The effects of NIR on *in vivo* cancer studies

In our *in vivo* studies, NIR irradiation significantly inhibited the tumor growth of MDA-MB435 melanoma cells transplanted in nude mice *in vivo*. Significant differences between the control and irradiated groups were observed for tumor volume and frequencies of Ki67-positive, TUNEL-positive (Tanaka et al., 2010b), activated caspase-3, and single-stranded DNA-positive cells.

The histological findings showed tumor shrinkage and dying cells in the center of the tumor mass, which supports the hypothesis that NIR electromagnetic properties induce these biological effects non-thermally.

NIR penetrates the skin and reaches the subcutaneous tissues without a significant increase in skin temperature (Schieke et al., 2003). The effects of NIR are independent of the generation of heat (Danno et al., 2001). If the cytocidal effect of NIR was induced thermally, the histology would show a gradient cytocidal effect from the superficial layer to the center of the tumor, and thermal effect would be reduced by the contact cooling (20 °C) of the NIR device. Due to surface cooling, NIR can penetrate deeper tissue and induce a drastic non-thermal cytocidal effect in the center of the tumor mass.

NIR treatment with very low output and fewer exposures (10 exposures of NIR at 20 and 40 $J/cm^2$) also inhibited tumor growth. This output was so low that on human skin, the sensation of heat would not be felt due to contact cooling. This NIR irradiation induced no pain, and the mice did not withdraw from the treatment even though NIR treatment was performed without anesthesia. In addition, side effects, such as epidermal burns, were not observed, and the mice looked healthy throughout the study. Further studies are necessary to determine if more output, increased frequency of treatments, and/or longer periods of irradiation may be even more effective in suppressing tumor growth.

It is still unknown why NIR induces a cytocidal effect in cancer cells. However, we found that NIR induced muscle thinning (Tanaka et al., 2010c, 2011a), bone marrow damage (Tanaka et al., 2011b), and a cytocidal effect in cancer cells (Tanaka et al., 2010b), which was most likely due to a different type of apoptosis. A significant reduction in tumor volume and a high level of TUNEL-positive cells in the irradiated group indicated that NIR irradiation induces apoptosis in cancer cells. The frequency of Ki67-positive cells on day 9 in the irradiated group were significantly lower than the control group, which supports the hypothesis that NIR irradiation can suppress the proliferation of cancer cells. However, the mechanism of NIR-mediated tumor cell death appeared to be different than standard apoptosis because high levels of activated caspase-3 expression and ssDNA-positive cells appeared gradually after NIR irradiation, although tumor shrinkage happened rapidly.

On the other hand, NIR irradiation induced the stimulation of CD34-positive bone marrow stem cells in our previous study (Tanaka et al., 2011b), and the frequency of Ki67-positive cells on day 45 was significantly higher than the irradiated group on day 9. These results suggest that NIR irradiation may stimulate stem cells.

The immunohistological staining results suggested that NIR may induce cell death of highly proliferative tumor cells, stimulate stem cells, and then induce apoptosis of the cells which are unnecessary to promote the development of melanoma. These steps appeared to be a part of the mechanism driving the effects of NIR on cancer cells.

The advantages of this NIR irradiation schedule include reducing discomfort, limiting side effects, and the low cost. Taken together, these characteristics were facilitated by repeated irradiations, which if proven beneficial for cancer cell reduction in humans, may provide an alternative or adjunct treatment for a transient mass reduction before surgery, offer improved results, and/ or improve patient quality-of-life. NIR irradiation is frequently administered at a level of 40 $J/cm^2$ for other indications, with a very high safety record and no significant complications (Goldberg et al, 2007).

#### 4.6.4 The effect of NIR on molecular structure: is it mainly alpha helices?

NIR is absorbed by water, hemoglobin, and myoglobin. The NIR spectrum of biological materials is a result of the overtones and combination of O-H, C-H, and N-H groups' bond stretching vibrations (Weyer, 1985). Water is a polar molecule with an electrical dipole moment and possesses hydrogen bonds. A water molecule will be resonated by NIR and absorb NIR due to the O-H intramolecular hydrogen bonds and electrical dipole moment (Tsai et al., 2001). Since T2 weighted MRI enhances water as well as active proliferating cancer cells, active proliferating cells may have a rich water content, which strongly absorbs NIR.

Hemoglobin has four heme-binding subunits, each largely made of alpha helices, and myoglobin consists of eight alpha helices that are connected through turns with an oxygen binding site. The similarity between hemoglobin and myoglobin resides in the heme binding sites and alpha helices. Heme is a prosthetic group that consists of an iron atom located in the center of a large heterocyclic organic ring called porphyrin. Our results of long-lasting muscle thinning and vasodilation induced by NIR suggest that NIR might resonate and damage heme. However, our collagen, elastin, and cancer studies suggest that NIR may mainly resonate helical structures, alpha helices, and DNA. Alpha helices are thought to be resonated by NIR and have strong amide bands in the IR spectra, which have characteristic frequencies and intensities (Nevskaya & Chirgadze, 1976). Both hemoglobin and myoglobin are the oxygen-carrying proteins and have many alpha helices. It is possible that NIR induces resonance of alpha helices in the oxygen-carrying proteins and degenerates proteins containing alpha helices, which results in damage to the storage and transport of oxygen. This could be one of the mechanisms of apoptosis. In our previous study, we evaluated the effect of NIR on myoglobin; however, similar effects may also be found for hemoglobin (Tanaka et al., 2011c).

NIR increases the amount of water retained in the dermis by inducing vasodilation and the expression of collagen and elastin (Tanaka et al., 2009b). Both collagen and elastin possess helical structures and hydrogen bonds. Elastin has higher absorption properties than that of water (Tsai et al., 2001). These findings suggest that we have acquired biological defense mechanisms in which induced helical structures and hydrogen bonds are resonated by NIR and absorb NIR to protect the subcutaneous tissues against NIR.

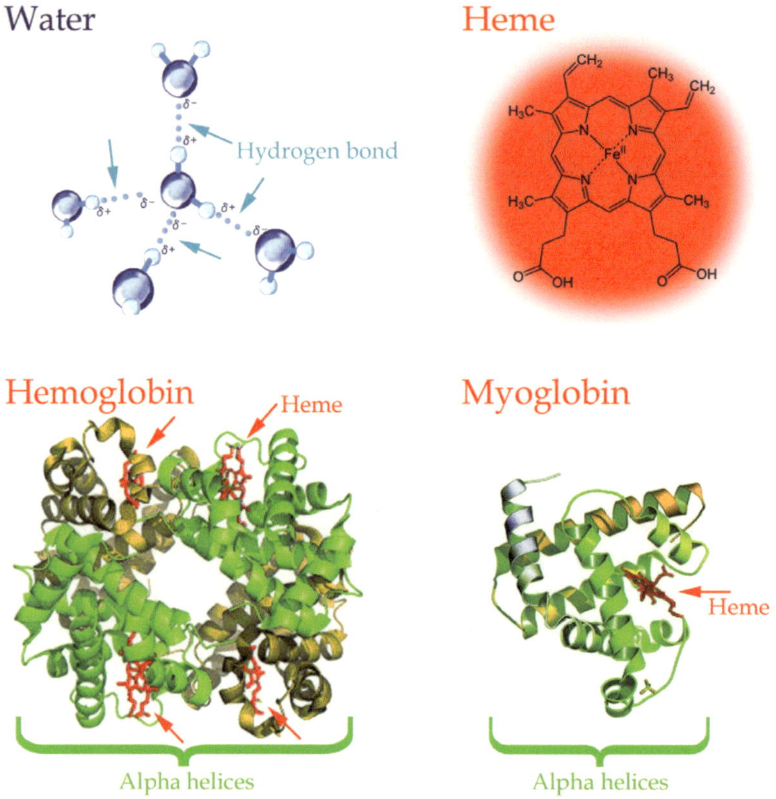


Fig. 12. The structure of water, heme, hemoglobin, and myoglobin. Water is a polar molecule with an electrical dipole moment and possesses hydrogen bonds (*light blue dots*). Heme is a prosthetic group that consists of an iron atom located in the center of a large heterocyclic organic ring called porphyrin. The hemoglobin molecule has four heme-binding subunits, each largely made of alpha helices (*green*). Myoglobin consists of eight alpha helicies (*green*) and possesses heme as an oxygen binding site. The red arrow indicates heme. Cited and revised from Wikipedia

Similarly, DNA consists of two long strands in the shape of a double helix, which is stabilized by two forces: hydrogen bonds between nucleotides, and base-stacking interactions among the aromatic bases. Many studies regarding DNA and cancer imaging have been performed using an NIR spectroscopy, since biological molecules such as proteins, lipids, and nucleic acids provide a unique absorption spectral pattern, and NIR induces the vibration of DNA. IR irradiation alone appears to induce DNA strand breaks and apoptosis (Tirlapur & König, 2001). DNA will be also resonated and absorb NIR, which is most likely due to its helical structures.

#### 4.6.5 The effects of NIR on lamin

The nuclear lamina is a proteinaceous structure located underneath the inner nuclear membrane that forms a stress-resistant elastic network where it associates with the peripheral chromatin (Prokocimer et al., 2009). It contains lamins and lamin-associated proteins, including many integral proteins of the inner nuclear membrane, chromatin modifying proteins, transcriptional repressors, and structural proteins (Hutchison & Worman, 2004; Mounkes & Stewart, 2004; Smith et al., 2005; Broers et al., 2006).

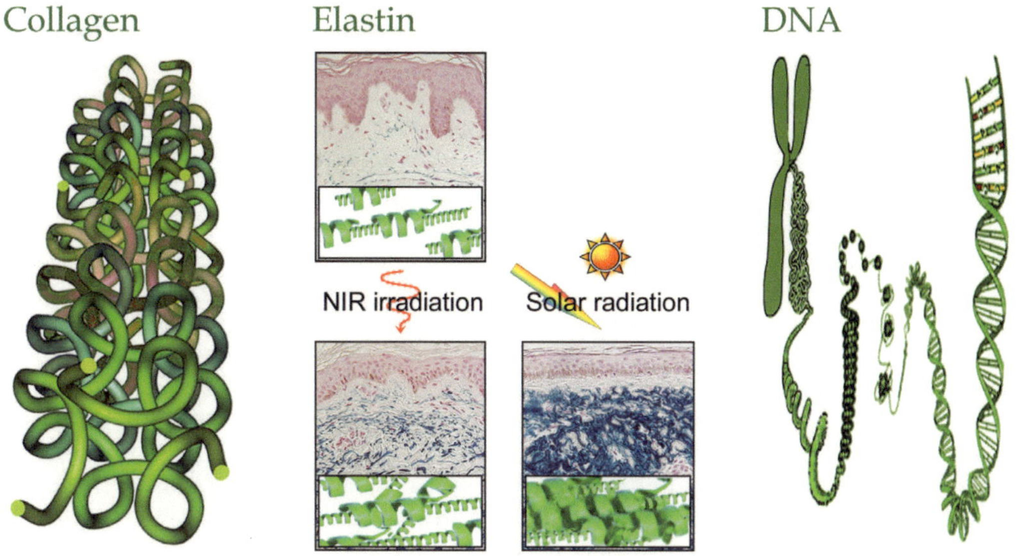


Fig. 13. The structure of collagen, elastin, and DNA. Collagen (left), elastin (center), and DNA (right) possess many alpha helices. Representative histologies of sun-protected skin (center, left) and sun-exposed skin (center, right) stained with Victoria Blue stain. Sun-protected skin taken from the thigh of a 33-year-old Japanese man. Control skin (center, above). Thirty days after NIR irradiation at 36 J/cm$^2$ (center, below). Sun-exposed skin taken from the cheek of a 72-year-old Japanese female (center, right). Solar elastosis stained blue are observed in the dermis.A schema of elastic fibers (green) is enclosed in the smaller box below each picture. Cited and revised from Wikipedia for collagen and DNA structures

Lamins are type-V intermediate filament proteins located in the nucleus, primarily in the periphery, and underlie the nuclear envelope (Mounkes & Stewart, 2004). Lamins have a conserved alpha helical central rod domain and variable head and tail domains (Prokocimer et al., 2009; Stuurman et al., 1998; Zaremba-Czogalla et al., 2011) (Fig. 14). Alpha helical structures are surmised to absorb NIR and protect the nucleus and DNA from NIR. The nuclear lamina was thought to provide structural support to the nucleus and protect the peripheral chromatin; however, it is now known that the nuclear lamina is involved in a number of fundamental molecular processes ranging from DNA replication and RNA transcription (Spann et al., 2002) to genome silencing and DNA repair (Reddy et al., 2008). The lamins and their associated proteins are required for most nuclear activities, including mitosis, and for linking the nucleoplasm to all major cytoskeletal networks in the cytoplasm. The lamin A gene has been linked to longevity and was proposed to be a guardian of somatic cells during their lifetime (Hutchison & Worman, 2004). Mutations in the lamin A gene cause a spectrum of 20 age-related human disorders, termed laminopathies, which affect the maintenance of one or more tissues of mesenchymal origin. Remarkably, many tissues affected by mutations in the lamin A gene are also affected in many degenerative conditions common to old age. The compromised tissue functions in laminopathy diseases are proposed to be a consequence of decreased cellular proliferation (Pekovic et al., 2007), a failure to maintain a differentiated state, and/or a loss of tissue repair during regeneration (Mounkes & Stewart, 2004; Bakay et al., 2006). Lamin A knock-out mouse models as well as mutated lamin A knock-in or transgenic mice manifesting either muscular dystrophy (Sullivan et al., 1999; Arimura et al., 2005) or premature ageing (Mounkes et al., 2003; Yang et al., 2005; Varga et al., 2006) have shortened lifespans and die prematurely. Moreover, mouse models null for the pre-lamin A gene also have shortened lifespans and show progeria-like pathologies of bone and muscle (Bergo et al., 2002; Pendas et al., 2002).

Lamins play important roles in DNA replication, chromatin organization, adult stem cell differentiation, aging, and tumorigenesis. In addition, mutations in lamin lead to laminopathic diseases (Prokocimer et al., 2009).

Nuclei assembled in vitro in the absence of lamins are more prone to breakage than nuclei assembled in the presence of a full complement of lamins (Sullivan et al., 1999; Newport et al., 1990). Disruption of the lamins results in abnormal mitosis, chromosomal segregation, and cell death (Liu et al., 2003).

During mitosis, lamin molecules are transiently disassembled into monomers (Gerace & Blobel, 1980; Yang et al., 1997) through phosphorylation (Peter et al., 1990) by the protein kinase p34cdc2 (Nigg, 1992). In addition, actively proliferating cells show increased sensitivity to NIR (Karu et al., 1994; Tafur & Milles, 2008), and IR irradiation induces DNA strand breaks and apoptosis (Tirlapur & König, 2001). Therefore, these findings suggest that NIR exposure appears to damage nuclear lamins and DNA in the mitotic phase due to absence of nuclear lamins protection, which results in apoptotic cell death.

Thus, NIR irradiation has a potential application for transient mass reduction of proliferative malignant cancer, such as breast cancer and melanoma before surgery (Tanaka et al., 2010b), or for the treatment for terminal patients.

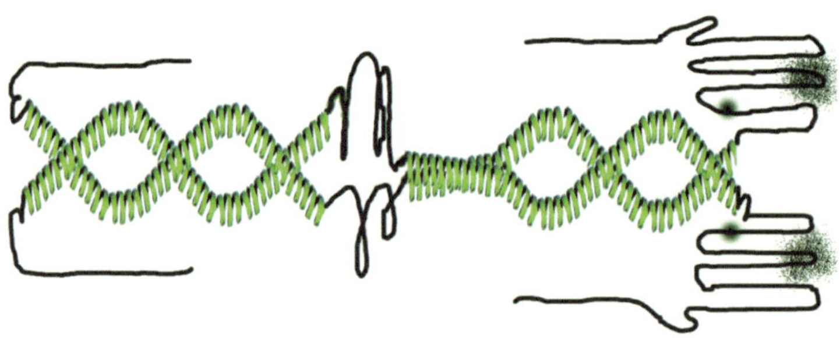

Fig. 14. The structure of lamin dimers. A pair of alpha helical central rods forms the lamin dimer. Cited and revised from Prokocimer, et al (2009). Fig. 1. Nuclear lamins: key regulators of nuclear structure and activities. *J Cell Mol Med.* 13(6):1059-85

#### 4.6.6 Lamin and cancer

Malignant transformation is a multi-step process of sequential alterations that occur in the critical genes involved in cancer regulating pathways as well as various mediators, which mediate the "cross-talk" between them. These molecular events are accompanied by nuclear structural alterations, which are involved in common diseases, particularly cancer (Foster et al., 2010), and differentiate cancer cells from normal cells (Prokocimer et al., 2009). Nuclear lamins are responsible for the distortion of the nuclear envelope, and nuclear margin

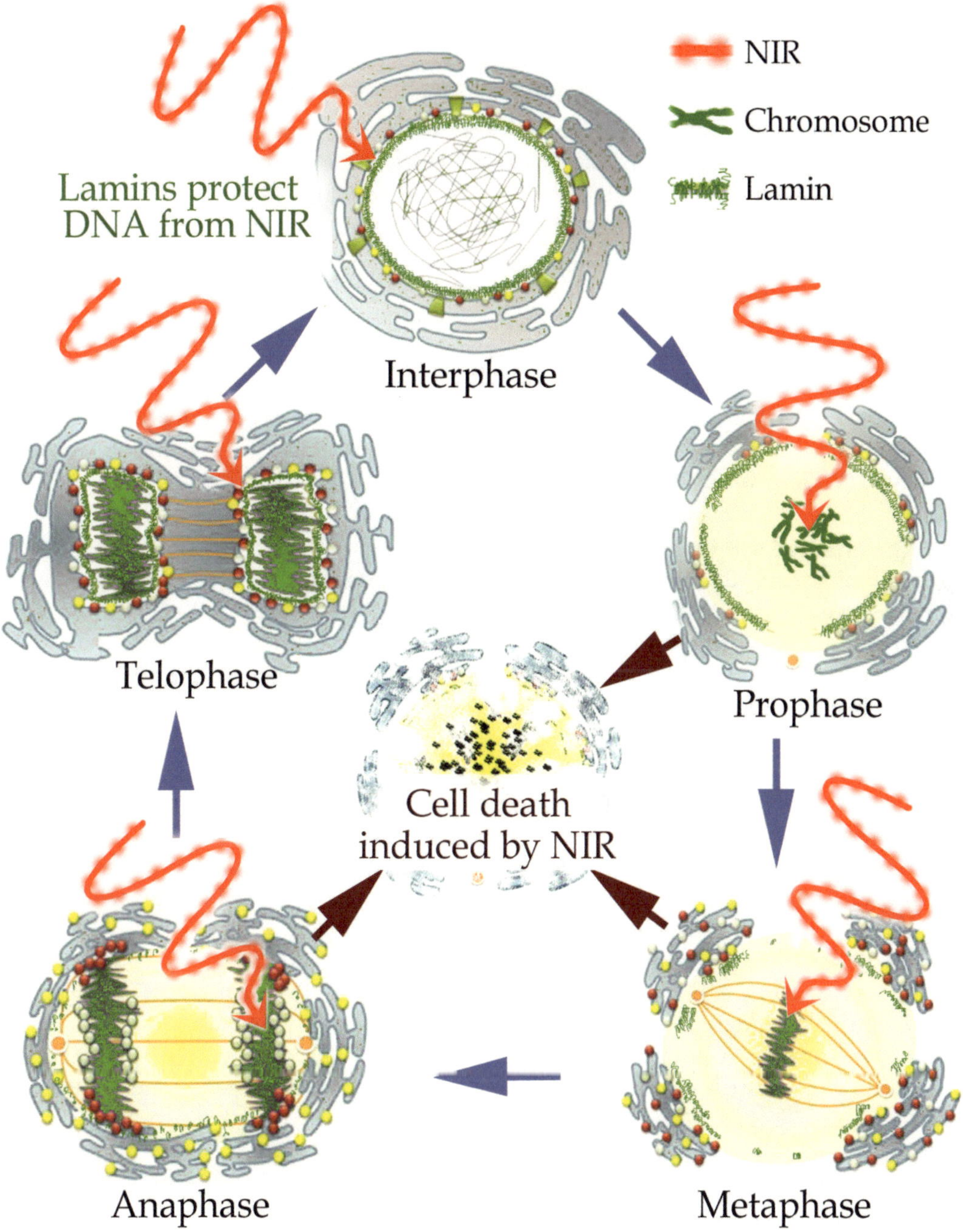


Fig. 15. A schematic of the cell cycle and effects of NIR. NIR cannot penetrate the nuclear envelope due to the protection of nuclear lamins in interphase and telophase. NIR may damage the chromosomes of mitotic cells in prophase, metaphase, and anaphase due to the absence of nuclear lamin protection, which results in apoptotic cell death. Cited and revised from Wikipedia

irregularity is an important diagnostic feature of malignant cells (Dey, 2009). Lamin expression in tumor cells may potentially serve as a cancer-related biomarker for diagnosis, prognosis, and surveillance. Alterations of the nuclear lamina are being recognized as an additional event involved in malignant transformation (Prokocimer et al., 2009). Altered lamin expression in cancer cells contributes to the characteristic changes in nuclear architecture, including alterations of nuclear structure and chromatin texture, which occurs in all cancer subtypes (Zink D et al., 2004).

Nuclear lamins also have a crucial role in maintaining chromosomal stability for the prevention of cancer progression, and are also involved in tumor suppressive pathways that trigger apoptosis or senescence (Prokocimer et al., 2009). Thus, alterations in lamins allow cancer cells to escape the normal control of cell proliferation and cell death, which yields a pro-cancerous effect (Vogelstein & Kinzler, 2004). Lamin A is absent in hyperproliferative basal cell skin carcinomas, and its presence or absence may directly influence the proliferative status of the tumor (Venables et al., 2001). Moreover, the poor outcome associated with lamin A/C-positive tumors may be reflective of a more stem-cell-like phenotype (Willis et al., 2008).

#### 4.6.7 The effect of NIR on stem cells

NIR irradiation abruptly induced subcutaneous adipocytes on the panniculus carnosus and CD34-positive cells around the subcutaneous adipocytes (Tanaka et al., 2011b). Adipose-derived stem cells express CD34 in higher percentages than bone marrow-derived mesenchymal stem cells (Yoshimura et al., 2009). CD34-positive human adipose-derived stem cells have a greater replicative capacity compared to CD34-negative cells (Suga et al., 2009). These results suggest that NIR irradiation may enrich and stimulate CD34-positive adipose-derived stem cells to increase subcutaneous adipocytes on the panniculus carnosus. Optically, fatty tissue can scatter NIR (Srinivasan et al., 2003), and fatty acids are the major NIR absorbing materials in soft tissues (Tsai et al., 2001). The oil in the liquid phase is transparent, whereas the oil in the solid phase is highly scattering to NIR (Van et al., 2005). The long-lasting induction of subcutaneous adipocytes may protect the underlying tissues, including the panniculus carnosus, against NIR damage.

NIR irradiation that simulated solar radiation non-thermally affected the subcutaneous tissues, cortical bone, and bone marrow (Tanaka et al., 2011b). The apoptotic damage to bone marrow cells might be minimized by a biological defense against NIR irradiation by means of an increase in subcutaneous and bone marrow adipocytes as well as cortical bone mass through the enrichment of CD34-positive stem cells at the inner surface of the bone cortex.

Lamin A and pre-lamin A regulate stem cell maintenance and differentiation by influencing key signaling pathways in stem cells (Prokocimer et al., 2009). Lamin A/C expression seems to be reduced or absent in undifferentiated or proliferative cells, but is observed in differentiated or non-proliferative cells, such as quiescent adult stem cells (Pekovic, 2008). Lamin A regulates stem cell maintenance through a range of regenerative signaling pathways, which suggests that the regulation of adult stem cell ageing may occur at a number of different pathway steps that intersect with lamin A, including adult stem cells, their progenitors, and/or stem cell niches (Pekovic, 2008). These results suggest that NIR radiation may stimulate stem cells, including cancer stem cells.

## 5. Conclusion

This simple technique of NIR irradiation might have a potential application for the transient mass reduction of melanoma before surgery, since the schedule reduces discomfort and side effects, reaches the deep subcutaneous tissues, and facilitates repeated irradiations.

In contrast, solar NIR radiation may also cause unexpected muscle thinning and stimulation of stem cells, including cancer stem cells, in areas of the body that are exposed to the sun. Therefore, exposed skin should be protected with sunscreens that block not only UV, but also NIR radiation, in order to prevent overlying skin ptosis, ageing, and oncogenicity. Additional non-thermal studies are required to decipher the effects on melanoma induced by both UV and NIR in humans.

## 6. Acknowledgements

We thank Ikuo Matsuyama for histological staining.

## 7. References

Ananthaswamy HN, Loughlin SM, Cox P, Evans RL, Ullrich SE, Kripke ML. (1997). Sunlight and skin cancer: Inhibition of p53 mutations in UV-irradiated mouse skin by sunscreens. *Nature Med.*3, 510-4.

Anderson RR, Parrish JA. (1981). The optics of human skin. *J Invest Dermatol* 77: 13-9.

Arimura T, Helbling-Leclerc A, Massart C, et al. (2005) Mouse model carrying H222P-Lmna mutation develops muscular dystrophy and dilated cardiomyopathy similar to human striated muscle laminopathies. *Hum Mol Genet.* 14, 155–69.

Arrington JH III, Lockman DS. (1979). Thermal keratoses and squamous cell carcinoma in situ associated with erythema ab igne. *Arch Dermatol.* 115: 1226–8.

Bain JA, Rusch HP, Kline BE. (1943). The effect of temperature upon ultraviolet carcinogenesis with wavelength 2,800–3,400A°. *Cancer Res.* 3: 610–12.

Bakay M, Wang Z, Melcon G, et al. (2006) Nuclear envelope dystrophies show a transcriptional fingerprint suggesting disruption of Rb-MyoD pathways in muscle regeneration. *Brain.* 129, 996–1013.

Bäumler W, Abels C, Karrer S, Weiss T, Messmann H, Landthaler M, Szeimies RM. (1999). Photo-oxidative killing of human colonic cancer cells using indocyanine green and infrared light. *Br J Cancer.* 80(3-4):360-3.

Bergo MO, Gavino B, Ross J, Schmidt WK, Hong C, Kendall LV, Mohr A, Meta M, Genant H, Jiang Y, Wisner ER, Van Bruggen N, Carano RA, Michaelis S, Griffey SM, Young SG. (2002). Zmpste24 deficiency in mice causes spontaneous bone fractures, muscle weakness, and a prelamin A processing defect. *Proc Natl Acad Sci USA.* 99:13049–54.

Bliss J, Ford D, Swerdlow A, Armstrong B, Cristofolini M, Elwood J, Green A, Holly E, Mack T, MacKie R. (1995). Risk of cutaneous melanoma associated with pigmentation characteristics and freckling: systematic overview of 10 case-control studies. The International Melanoma Analysis Group (IMAGE). *Int J Cancer.* 62 (4): 367–76.

Broers JL, Ramaekers FC, Bonne G, Yaou RB, Hutchison CJ. (2006). Nuclear lamins: laminopathies and their role in premature ageing. *Physiol Rev.* 86(3):967-1008.

Busetti A, Soncin M, Jori G, Kenney ME, Rodgers MA. (1998). Treatment of malignant melanoma by high-peak-power 1064 nm irradiation followed by photodynamic therapy. *Photochem Photobiol.* 68: 377–81.

Danno K, Horio T, Imamura S. (1992). Infrared radiation suppresses ultraviolet B-induced sunburn-cell formation. *Arch Dermatol Res.* 284: 92–94.

Danno K, Mori N,Toda K, Kobayashi T, Utani A. (2001). Near-infrared irradiation stimulates cutaneous wound repair: laboratory experiments on possible mechanisms. *Photodermatol Photoimmunol Photomed.*17:261-5.

Davenport SA, Gollnick DA, Levernier M, Spooner GJR. (2006). Method and system for treatment of post-partum abdominal skin redundancy or laxity. United States Patent 20060052847. Available at: http://www.freepatentsonline.com/y2006/0052847.html

Dees C, Harkins J, Petersen MG, Fisher WG, Wachter EA. (2002) Treatment of murine cutaneous melanoma with near infrared light. *Photochem Photobiol.* 75: 296-301.

Dewey WC. (1994). Arrhenius relationships from the molecule and cell to clinic. *Int J Hyperthermia.* 10: 457–83.

Dey P. (2009). Nuclear margin irregularity and cancer: a review. *Anal Quant Cytol Histol.* 31(5):345-52.

Dougherty TJ, Gomer CJ, Henderson BW, Jori G, Kessel D, Korbelik M, Moan J, Peng Q. (1998). Photodynamic therapy. *J Natl Cancer Inst.* 90: 889–905.

Dover, J.S., Phillips, T.J. & Arndt, K.A. (1989). Cutaneous effects and therapeutic uses of heat with emphasis on infrared radiation. *J. Am. Acad. Dermatol.* 20, 278-86.

Ferrari M, Mottola L, Quaresima V. (2004). Principles, techniques, and limitation of near infrared spectroscopy. *Can J Appl Physiol.* 29(4):463-87.

Findlayson GR, Sams WM Jr, Smith JG. (1966). Erythema ab igne. A histopathological study. *J Invest Dermatol.* 46:104–7.

Foster CR, Przyborski SA, Wilson RG, Hutchison CJ. (2010). Lamins as cancer biomarkers. *Biochem Soc Trans.* 38:297-300.

Frank S, Oliver L, Lebreton-De Coster C, Moreau C, Lecabellec MT, Michel L, Vallette FM, Dubertret L, Coulomb B. (2004). Infrared radiation affects the mitochondrial pathway of apoptosis in human fibroblasts. *J. Invest. Dermatol.* 123:823-31.

Gates DM. (1966). Spectral distribution of solar radiation at the earth's surface. *Science.* 151:523-9.

Gerace L, Blobel G. (1980). The nuclear envelope lamina is reversibly depolymerised during mitosis. *Cell.* 19:277-87.

Goldberg DJ, Hussain M, Fazeli A, Berlin AL. (2007). Treatment of skin laxity of the lower face and neck in older individuals with a broad spectrum infrared light device. *J Cosmet Laser Ther.* 9:35-40.

Guinot C, Malvy DJ, Ambroisine L, Latreille J, Mauger E, Tenenhaus M, Morizot F, Lopez S, Le Fur I, Tschachler E. (2002). Relative contribution of intrinsic vs. extrinsic factors to skin aging as determined by a validated skin age score. *Arch Dermatol.* 138:1454-60.

Hewitt JB, Sherif A, Kerr KM, Stankler L. (1993). Merkel cell and squamous-cell carcinomas arising in erythema ab igne. *Br J Dermatol.* 128: 591–2.

Horwitz LR, Burke TJ, Carnegie D. (1999). Augmentation of wound healing using monochromatic infrared energy. Exploration of a new technology for wound management. *Adv Wound Care.* 12(1):35-40.

Hutchison CJ, Worman HJ. (2004). A-type lamins: guardians of the soma? *Nat Cell Biol* 6, 1062–7.

Jones CS, Tyring SK, Lee PC, Fine JD. (1988). Development of neuroendocrine (Merkel cell) carcinoma mixed with squamous-cell carcinoma in erythema ab igne. *Arch Dermatol.* 124: 110–3.

Karu T, Pyatibrat L, Kalendo G. (1994). Irradiation with He-Ne laser can influence the cytotoxic response of HeLa cells to ionizing radiation. *Int J Radiat Biol* 65: 691-7.

Karu T. (1999) Invited Review. Primary and secondary mechanisms of action of visible to near-IR radiation on cells. *J Photochem Photobiol B: Biol* 49: 1-17.

Kelleher DK, Thews O, Rzeznik J, Scherz A, Salomon Y, Vaupel P. (1999). Hot topic. Water-filtered infrared-A radiation: a novel technique for localized hyperthermia in combination with bacteriochlorophyll-based photodynamic therapy. *Int J Hyperthermia.* 15:467-74.

Kim MS, Kim YK, Cho KH, Chung JH. (2006). Infrared exposure induces an angiogenic switch in human skin that is partially mediated by heat. *Br J Dermatol.*155, 1131-8.

Kligman LH. (1982). Intensification of ultraviolet-induced dermal damage by infrared radiation. *Arch. Dermatol. Res.* 272, 229-38.

Kligman LH & Kligman AM. (1984). Reflections on heat. *Br. J. Dermatol.*110, 369-75.

Knize DM. (1996). An anatomically based study of the mechanism of the eyebrow ptosis. *Plast Reconstr Surg.* 97:1321-33.

Kochevar IE, Pathak MA, Parrish JA. (1999). Photophysics, photochemistry and photobiology. In: Freedberg IM, Eisen AZ, Wolff K, et al, eds. *Fitzpatrick's Dermatology in General Medicine.* New York: McGraw-Hill:220-9.Gates DM. (1966). Spectral distribution of solar radiation at the earth's surface. *Science.*151:523-9.

Kujawa J, Zavodnik IB, Lapshina A, Labieniec M, Bryszewska M. (2004). Cell survival, DNA, and protein damage in B14 cells under low-intensity near-infrared (810nm) laser irradiation. *Photomed Laser Surg.* 22: 504-8.

Liu J, Lee KK, Segura-Totten M, Neufeld E, Wilson KL, Gruenbaum Y. (2003). MAN1 and emerin have overlapping function(s) essential for chromosome segregation and cell division in Caenorhabditis elegans. *Proc Natl Acad Sci USA.* 15;100(8):4598-603.

Lobel J, MacDonald IJ, Ciesielski MJ, Barone T, Potter WR, Pollina J, Plunkett RJ, Fenstermaker RA, Dougherty TJ. (2001). 2-(1-hexyloxyethyl)-2-devinylpyropheophorbide-a (HPPH) in a nude rat glioma model: implications for photodynamic therapy. *Lasers Surg Med.* 29: 397–405.

Menezes S, Coulomb B, Lebreton C, Dubertret L. (1998). Non-coherent near infrared radiation protects normal human dermal fibroblasts from solar ultraviolet toxicity. *J. Invest. Dermatol.* 111;629-633.

Mounkes LC, Kozlov S, Hernandez L, Sullivan T, Stewart CL. (2003). A progeroid syndrome in mice is caused by defects in A-type lamins. *Nature.* 423, 298–301.

Mounkes LC, Stewart CL. (2004). Aging and nuclear organization: lamins and progeria. *Curr Opin Cell Biol* 16, 322–27.

Nagashima H, Hanada K, Hashimoto I. (1999). Correlation of skin phototype with facial wrinkle formation. *Photo Photodermatol Photoimmunol Photomed.* 15:2-6.

Nancini DM, Bolinger L, Li H, Kendrick K, Chance B, Wilson JR. (1994). Validation of near-infrared spectroscopy in humans. *J Appl Physiol.* 77:2740-7.

Nevskaya NA, Chirgadze YN. (1976). Infrared spectra and resonance interactions of amide-I and II vibrations of alpha-helix. *Biopolymers.* 15(4):637-48.

Newport JW, Wilson KL, Dunphy WG. (1990). A lamin-independent pathway for nuclear envelope assembly. *J Cell Biol.* 111(6):2247-59.

Niechajev I. (2004). Transpalpebral browpexy. *Plast Reconstr Surg*. 113:2172-80.

Nigg EA. (1992). Assembly and cell cycle dynamics of the nuclear lamina. *Semin Cell Biol.* 3(4):245-53. Odunze M, Rosenberg DS, Few JW. (2008). Periorbital aging and ethnic considerations: A focus on leteral canthal complex. *Plast Reconstr Surg*.121:1002-8.

Orenstein A, Kostenich G, Kopolovic Y, Babushkina T, Malik Z. (1999). Enhancement of ALA-PDT damage by IR-induced hyperthermia on a colon carcinoma model. *Photochem Photobiol.* 69(6):703-7.

Pekovic V, Harborth J, Broers JL, et al. (2007). Nucleoplasmic LAP2alpha-lamin A complexes are required to maintain a proliferative state in human fibroblasts. *J Cell Biol.* 176, 163–72.

Pendas AM, Zhou Z, Cadiñanos J, Freije JM, Wang J, Hultenby K, Astudillo A, Wernerson A, Rodríguez F, Tryggvason K, López-Otín C. (2002). Defective prelamin A processing and muscular and adipocyte alterations in Zmpste24 metalloproteinase-deficient mice. *Nat Genet.* 31:94–9.

Peter M, Nakagawa J, Dorée M, Labbé JC, Nigg EA. (1990). In vitro disassembly of the nuclear lamina and M phase-specific phosphorylation of lamins by cdc2 kinase. *Cell.* 61(4):591-602.

Prokocimer M, Davidovich M, Nissim-Rafinia M, Wiesel-Motiuk N, Bar DZ, Barkan R, Meshorer E, Gruenbaum Y. (2009). Nuclear lamins: key regulators of nuclear structure and activities. *J Cell Mol Med.* 13(6):1059-85.

Przyborski SA, Wilson RG and Hutchison CJ. Lamins as cancer biomarkers. (2010). *Biochem. Soc. Trans.* 38:297-300.

Pujol JA, Lecha M. (1993). Photoprotection in the infrared radiation range. *Photodermatol Photoimmunol Photomed.* 9:275-278.

Rawlings AV. (2006) Ethnic skin types: are there differences in skin structure and function? Review article. *Int J Cosmet Sci.* 28:79-93.

Reddy KL, Zullo JM, Bertolino E, Singh H. (2008). Transcriptional repression mediated by repositioning of genes to the nuclear lamina. *Nature.* 13;452(7184):243-7.

Santana-Blank LA, Rodriguez-Santana E, Vargas F, Reyes H, Fernández-Andrade P, Rukos S, Santana-Rodríguez KE. (2002). Phase I trial of an infrared pulsed laser device in patients with advanced neoplasias. *Clin Cancer Res.* 8: 3082–91.

Schieke SM, Schroeder P, Krutmann J. (2003). Review article. Cutaneous effects of infrared radiation: from clinical observations to molecular response mechanisms. *Photodermatol Photoimmunol Photomed.* 19: 228-234.

Schramm JM, Warner D, Hardesty RA, Oberg KC. (2003). A unique combination of infrared and microwave radiation accelerates wound healing. *Plast Reconstr Surg.* 111(1):258-66.

Schroeder P, Lademann J, Darvin ME, Stege H, Marks C, Bruhnke S, Krutmann J. (2008). Infared radiation-induced matrix metalloproteinase in human skin: Implications for protection. *J Invest Dermatol.* 128:2491-7.

Smith ED, Kudlow BA, Frock RL, Kennedy BK. (2005).A-type nuclear lamins, progerias and other degenerative disorders. *Mech Ageing Dev.* 126(4):447-60.

Spann TP, Goldman AE, Wang C, Huang S, Goldman RD. (2002). Alteration of nuclear lamin organization inhibits RNA polymerase II-dependent transcription. *J Cell Biol.* 18;156(4):603-8.

Srinivasan S, Pogue BW, Jiang S, Dehghani H, Kogel C, Soho S, Gibson JJ, Tosteson TD, Poplack SP, Paulsen DK. (2003). Interpreting hemoglobin and water concentration, oxygen saturation, and scattering measured *in vivo* by near-infrared breast tomography. *Proc Natl Acad Sci U S A*. 100: 12349–54.

Stuurman N, Heins S, Aebi U. (1998). Nuclear lamins: their structure, assembly, and interactions. *J Struct Biol*. 122(1-2):42-66.

Suga H, Matsumoto D, Eto H, Inoue K, Aoi N, Kato H, Araki J, Yoshimura K. (2009). Functional implications of CD34 expression in human adipose derived stem/progenitor cells. *Stem Cells Dev*. 18:1201-9.

Sullivan T, Escalante-Alcalde D, Bhatt H, Anver M, Bhat N, Nagashima K, Stewart CL, Burke B. (1999). Loss of A-type lamin expression compromises nuclear envelope integrity leading to muscular dystrophy. *J Cell Biol*. 147(5):913-20.

Tafur J, Mills PJ. (2008). Low-intensity light therapy: exploring the role of redox mechanisms. *Photomed Laser Surg*. 26: 321-326.

Tanaka Y, Matsuo K. (2008). Protective agent against damage of biological tissue caused by near-infrared ray and product comprising the same. PCT/JP2008/063558, US2010/0129426 A1.

Tanaka Y, Matsuo K, Yuzuriha S, Shinohara H. (2009a). Differential long-term stimulation of type I versus type III collagen after infrared irradiation. *Dermatol Surg*. 35:1099-104.

Tanaka Y, Matsuo K, Yuzuriha S. (2009b). Long-term evaluation of collagen and elastin following infrared (1100 to 1800 nm) irradiation. *J Drugs Dermatol*. 8:708-12.

Tanaka Y, Matsuo K, Yuzuriha S. (2010a) Long-Term Histological Comparison between Near-Infrared Irradiated Skin and Scar Tissues. *J Clin Cosmet Invest Dermatol*. 3:143-49.

Tanaka Y, Matsuo K, Yuzuriha S, Yan H, Nakayama J. (2010b). Non-thermal cytocidal effect of infrared irradiation on cultured cancer cells using specialized device. *Cancer Science*. 101:1396-402.

Tanaka Y, Matsuo K, Yuzuriha S. (2010c). Long-lasting muscle thinning induced by infrared irradiation specialized with wavelength and contact cooling: A preliminary report. *ePlasty*. 10:e40.

Tanaka Y, Matsuo K, Yuzuriha S. (2011a).Long-lasting relaxation of corrugator supercilii muscle contraction induced by near infrared irradiation. *ePlasty*. 11:e6.

Tanaka Y, Matsuo K, Yuzuriha S. (2011b). Near-Infrared Irradiation Non-thermally affects Subcutaneous Adipocytes and Bone. *ePlasty*. 11:e12.

Tanaka Y, Matsuo K, Yuzuriha S. (2011c). Near-Infrared Irradiation Non-thermally Induces Long-lasting Vasodilation by Causing Apoptosis of Vascular Smooth Muscle Cells. *ePlasty*. 11:e22.

Tirlapur UK, König K. (2001). Femtosecond near-infrared laser pulse induced strand breaks in mammalian cells. *Cell Mol Biol*. 47: 131-4.

Travers JB, Edenberg HJ, Zhang Q, Al-Hassani M, Yi Q, Baskaran S, Konger RL. (2008). Augmentation of UVB radiation-mediated early gene expression by the epidermal platelet-activating factor receptor. *J. Invest. Dermatol*. 1284:55-60.

Tsai CH, Chen JC, Wang WJ. (2001). Near-infrared absorption property of biological soft tissue constituents. *J Med Biol Eng*. 21:7-14.

Tsukahara T, Fujimura T, Yoshida Y, Kitahara T, Hotta M, Moriwaki S, Witt PS, Simion FA, Takema Y. (2004). Comparison of age-related changes in wrinkling and sagging of the skin in Caucasian females and in Japanese females. *J Cosmet Sci*. 55:373-85.

Varga R, Eriksson M, Erdos MR, Olive M, Harten I, Kolodgie F, Capell BC, Cheng J, Faddah D, Perkins S, Avallone H, San H, Qu X, Ganesh S, Gordon LB, Virmani R, Wight

TN, Nabel EG, Collins FS. (2006). Progressive vascular smooth muscle cell defects in a mouse model of Hutchinson-Gilford progeria syndrome. *Proc Natl Acad Sci USA*. 103:3250–5.

Van Veen RL, Sterenborg HJ, Pifferi A, Torricelli A, Chikoidze E, Cubeddu R. (2005). Determination of visible near-IR absorption coefficients of mammalian fat using time- and spatially resolved diffuse reflectance and transmission spectroscopy. *J Biomed Opt*. 10:054004.

Venables RS, McLean S, Luny D, Moteleb E, Morley S, Quinlan RA, Lane EB, Hutchison CJ. (2001). Expression of individual lamins in basal cell carcinomas of the skin. *Br J Cancer*. 84(4):512-9.

Vogelstein B, Kinzler KW. (2004). Cancer genes and the pathways they control. *Nat Med*. 10:789-99.

Weyer LG. (1985). Near-infrared spectroscopy of organic substances. *Appl Spectrosc Rev*. 21:1-43.

Willis ND, Wilson RG, Hutchison CJ. (2008). Lamin A: a putative colonic epithelial stem cell biomarker which identifies colorectal tumours with a more aggressive phenotype. *Biochem Soc Trans*. 36:1350-3.

Wolf P, Donawho CK, Kripke ML. (1994). Effect of Sunscreens on UV radiation-induced enhancements of melanoma in mice. *J. Nat. Cancer. Inst.* 86 (2): 99–105.

Wust P, Hildebrandt B, Sreenivasa G, Rau B, Gellermann J, Riess H, Felix R, Schlag PM. (2002). Review article. Hyperthermia in combined treatment of cancer. *Lancet Oncol*. 3: 487–97.

Yang L, Guan T, Gerace L. (1997). Integral membrane proteins of the nuclear envelope are dispersed throughout the endoplasmic reticulum during mitosis. *J Cell Biol*. 137(6):1199-210.

Yang SH, Bergo MO, Toth JI, Qiao X, Hu Y, Sandoval S, Meta M, Bendale P, Gelb MH, Young SG, Fong LG. (2005). Blocking protein fornesyltransferase improves nuclear blebbing in mouse fibroblasts with a targeted Hutchinson-Gilford progeria syndrome mutation. *Proc Natl Acad Sci USA*. 102:10291–6.

Yoshimura K, Suga H, Eto H. (2009). Adipose derived stem/progenitor cells; roles in adipose tissue remodeling and potential use for soft tissue augumentation. *Regen Med*. 4:265-73.

Zaremba-Czogalla M, Dubińska-Magiera M, Rzepecki R. (2011). Laminopathies: the molecular background of the disease and the prospects for its treatment. Cell Mol Biol Lett. 16(1):114-48.

Zink D, Fisher AH, Nickerson JA. (2004). Nuclear structure in cancer cells. *Nat Rev Cancer*. 4:677-87.